The Process of
Human Development

The Process of Human Development
A Holistic Life-Span Approach

SECOND EDITION

Clara Shaw Schuster, Ph.D, R.N.
Assistant Professor of Nursing
Otterbein College
Westerville, Ohio;
Instructor of Nursing
Kent State University
Kent, Ohio;
Child and Family Development Specialist;
Developmental/Educational Consultant

Shirley Smith Ashburn, M.S., R.N.
Professor of Nursing
Cypress College
Cypress, California

Little, Brown and Company/Boston/Toronto

Library of Congress Cataloging-in-Publication Data

Schuster, Clara Shaw.
   The process of human development.

   Includes index.
   1. Developmental psychology.   2. Life cycle, Human.
3. Developmental biology.   I. Ashburn, Shirley Smith.
II. Title.
BF713.S36   1986   155   85–19811
ISBN 0–316–77536–3

Library of Congress Catalog Card No. 85–19811

ISBN 0-673-39404-2

5678910–WKK–949392919089

Printed in the United States of America

Photo Credits

Cover (clockwise from top): Hazel Hankin/Stock, Boston; Ed Slaman; Nancy Bates/The Picture Cube; Ed Slaman; Ken Buck.

*Figures 1–2, 8–3, 8–8, 10–1C, 11–9, 12–2, 12–4, 14–10,
14–11, 15–6, 15–8, 15–9, 17–2B, 17–3, 18–2, 18–3, 18–8,
19–6, 19–7, 19–8, 19–10, 19–15, 22–10, 23–2, 23–3, 23–4,
23–7, 24–3, 24–7 (left), 25–8, 26–1, 26–2, 26–4, 26–6, 26–7,
26–9, 27–1, 27–3, 27–5, 27–6, 27–7, 27–8, 27–9 (left), 28–1,
28–2, 28–3, 28–5, 29–2, 29–3 (right), 33–3, 33–4, 33–7, 33–8,
33–9, 35–4, 36–2, 36–3, 36–4, 37–1, 37–2, 37–3, 37–5, 37–6,
37–7, 38–2, 39–1, 39–2, 39–3, 39–5, 39–6, 39–9, 40–2, 40–5,
41–1, 41–2, 41–3, 41–5, 41–6, 41–7, 41–8, 42–1, 42–2, 42–4,
42–6:* Mt. Vernon News.

(continued on page 919)

Our thanks and praise to the Lord for providing
   resources,
   wisdom,
   strength,
   beyond our natural endowments

For their inspiration,
   patience,
   love,
   support,
in thanks we dedicate this book to:
   our mentors,
   our students, and
   our family members:
   Richard,
   Elizabeth,
   Jodi

Contents

Contributing Authors

James R. Abel, M.D.
Chapter 22

Coordinator, Pediatric Department/Senior Staff Physician, University Health Services, University of Massachusetts, Amherst, Massachusetts

Shirley Smith Ashburn, M.S., R.N.
Chapters 7, 8, 9, 10, 11, 12, 13, 24, 27, 36, and Appendix B

Professor of Nursing, Cypress College, Cypress, California

Robert Bornstein, Ph.D.
Chapters 37, 40

Associate Professor of Psychology, Miami University, Oxford, Ohio

Thomas Clifford, Ph.D.
Chapter 23

Psychologist, Southwest Forensic Center, Columbus, Ohio

Douglas W. Degelman
Chapter 24

Associate Professor, Psychology, Eastern Nazarene College, Quincy, Massachusetts

M. Patricia Donahue, Ph.D., R.N.
Chapter 21

Associate Professor, College of Nursing, The University of Iowa, Iowa City, Iowa

Johanna E. Flynn, M.A., R.N.C.
Chapter 39

Associate Professor, Nell Hodgson Woodruff School of Nursing, Emory University, Atlanta, Georgia

Sheila M. Goff, Ph.D.
Chapter 13

Associate Professor, Emeritus, Department of Communication, The Ohio State University, Columbus, Ohio

William A. Grimm, Ph.D.
Chapter 13

Chief, Communicative and Sensory Disorders Unit, Ohio Department of Health, Columbus, Ohio

Elizabeth R. Mabry, Ed.D., R.N.C.
Chapter 39

Professor of Nursing, Nell Hodgson Woodruff School of Nursing, Emory University, Atlanta, Georgia

Darlene E. McCown, Ph.D., R.N.
Chapter 21

Associate Professor, Azusa Pacific College, Azusa, California

Leona A. Mourad, M.S.N., R.N.
Chapter 36

Associate Professor, Emeritus, College of Nursing, The Ohio State University, Columbus, Ohio

Cecil R. Paul, Ph.D.
Chapter 28

Professor of Psychology and Director of Graduate Studies, Eastern Nazarene College, Quincy, Massachusetts

Joseph A. Rapalje, Ed.D.
Chapter 24

Associate Professor, Psychology, Eastern Nazarene College, Quincy, Massachusetts

Judith L. Robinson, M.A.
Chapter 41

Doctoral Candidate, Department of Psychology, Miami University, Oxford, Ohio

Clara Shaw Schuster, Ph.D., R.N.
Chapters 1, 2, 3, 4, 5, 6, 8, 9, 11, 13, 14, 15, 16, 17, 19, 20, 22, 25, 29, 30, 31, 32, 33, 35, 42, Epilogue, and Appendix C, E

Assistant Professor of Nursing, Otterbein College, Westerville, Ohio; Instructor of Nursing, Kent State University, Kent, Ohio; Child and Family Development Specialist; Developmental/Educational Consultant

Helen J. Smith, M.S.W., A.C.S.W.
Chapter 29

Principal Social Worker, Child Protection Services, Hennepin County Bureau of Social Services, Minneapolis, Minnesota

Jayne A. Tapia, M.S.N., R.N.
Chapter 34

Executive Director, Visiting Nurse and Community Health, Inc., Arlington, Massachusetts

Nancy M. Whitacre, M.A., R.N.
Chapter 38

Adjunct Professor, Division of Humanities, Franklin University, Columbus, Ohio

Gerald A. Winer, Ph.D.
Chapter 26

Associate Professor of Psychology, The Ohio State University, Columbus, Ohio

F. Franklyn Wise, Ph.D.
Chapter 18

Professor Emeritus of Christian Education and Psychology, Olivet Nazarene College, Kankakee, Illinois

Preface

Let each become all that he was created, capable of
being: expand, if possible, to his full growth, and
show himself at length in his own shape and
stature, be these what they may.

—Thomas Carlyle

The process of human development is at once both
simple and complex: simple when we can observe the
uncomplicated evolution of an individual as described by the theoretical frameworks of Erikson,
Havighurst, or Piaget; complicated when we consider
all the variations in human development created by
the interaction of the developing individual with the
environment.

Each of us is unique—we, the authors, and you, the
readers. The variations in the inherited potentials, interests, and background experiences of individuals
can both enrich and frustrate relationships. When our
interests and experiences are similar to those of
another person, we are more likely to feel comfortable with that person and to seek more frequent contact. When our experiences are widely divergent from
those of another person, we may find that person hard
to understand. We may have a tendency to dislike or
even to avoid persons who are different from ourselves. We do not understand such persons, and consequently we are uncomfortable when forced into
closer contact with them as co-workers or in a
practitioner-client relationship.

The Process of Human Development is designed to
explore comprehensively (holistically) the experience
of being human in western cultures. Since each of us
is human, it is the study of our own development and

potential futures. Information is considered relevant when it facilitates the answering of questions and offers opportunity for better understanding of both ourselves and others. This understanding can lead to the ability to accept and to work with other people more objectively, less judgmentally, with more compassion, and with greater effectiveness.

This text focuses on the development of healthy individuals—persons functioning at their highest potentials in spite of limitations, not just individuals free of illness. The four major domains (biophysical, cognitive, affective, and social) of normal human development are discussed from a pragmatic perspective in an attempt to meet the overlapping needs of students who are preparing for people-oriented professions. An attempt is made to identify the major factors that affect the development of these domains, which inspire the beauty and diversity of humanity. Also discussed are conceptual, situational, or developmental crises and the common variations in development that may be exceptional but are not considered pathological.

To facilitate study, the authors present the four domains separately and chronologically from conception through old age. The authors emphasize, however, that **each individual must be approached as a unique entity, not as a stereotyped representative of a particular age group or social environment.** The multidisciplinary approach offers a foundation for the holistic assessment of individuals and families.

Throughout the book, readers are encouraged to analyze the empirical data and theories independently and to synthesize this with their previous and current experiences. The underlying goal is to facilitate the reader's ability to create and to evaluate intervention strategies designed to maximize the potentials of each individual in all four domains. This book is dedicated to opening the mind of the reader rather than merely filling it.

A frost pattern on a winter window beautifully captures the authors' view of human development. Each pattern, like each one of us, is unique. The potential for growth is always present. The form, direction, and expressions of both are influenced by environmental conditions. Although each entity is unique in itself, there are commonalities and explanations for the patterns and behaviors displayed (even though we may not be able to identify them). The beauty of both is in the eye of the beholder; none is inherently good, bad, or deformed. Each time we look, we see a new feature or develop a renewed appreciation for the uniqueness and value of the patterns and the person.

With these thoughts in mind, we challenge you to a richer, more meaningful relationship with yourself and others as you begin a multidisciplinary and holistic study of the process of human development through the life cycle.

C.S.S.
S.S.A.

Acknowledgments

There are many persons over the course of the years who have contributed directly or indirectly to the content, the scope, and the approach of this book. Only a few can be formally recognized, but without their expertise and advice, the quality of the text would have been greatly diluted. We particularly express our thanks to the following persons for reviewing parts of the manuscript in process; their input has contributed to a more comprehensive and comprehensible text:

Jack Archer, D.D.
Robert C. Atchley, Ph.D.
Gwen Carr, M.A.
G. Maureen Chaisson-Stewart, Ph.D., R.N.
Marilyn Coleman, Ed.D.
Sarah Cook, M.Ed., R.N.
Catherine Cox, M.Div., R.N.
Gregory Cramm, D.D.S.
Marsha Driscoll, Ph.D.
Rose Ann Florentine, M.S.N., R.N.
James L. Gilmore, Ph.D.
Patricia L. Gump
Raymond Hatton, M.D.
Ronald Haxton, M.D.
Muriel Jacoby, M.S., R.N.
Susan Lech, M.D.
Jim Lynch, M.R.E.

Sandra Mott, M.S., R.N.
Joan Mulligan, Ph.D., R.N.
Jean O'Neil, Ed.D., R.N.
Loraine Parry, M.A.
William Parmenter, M.S.W.
Jack Pulec, M.D.
Jan Ream, M.S.
Anne C. Richards, Ph.D.
Mildred M. Seltzer, Ph.D.
Mark Tuel, B.A.
Janet Winckler, M.N., C.C.R.N.

The authors are most appreciative of the artwork by Elizabeth L. Haley.

Thanks are also extended to the following persons for their assistance in obtaining pictures and x-rays:

Sharon Claggett, R.T.
Robert Ronk, D.D.S.

Douglas McLeod, D.D.S.
Glenn Jackson, Ph.D.

We especially wish to thank Hal Clawson, Editor of the *Mount Vernon News*, Mount Vernon, Ohio, who opened his picture file to us. He and his staff try to report on the broad spectrum of life, and not just the tragic or exhilerating extremes. Their sensitivity to the richness of everyday scenarios is reflected in the quality of the pictures they so willingly shared.

For her dedicated, accurate typing, we extend our thanks to Pat Bosch.

For his unfailing support and patience, his assistance in verifying bibliographies and his assiduous typing and collating of the manuscript, we are especially grateful to Richard Schuster.

Last, but not least, we wish to thank Ann West of Little, Brown and Company, for her encouragement and support of our efforts to produce a viable, vibrant second edition.

Introduction for the Professor

If you really understand an important and interesting subject [sic], . . . it is a genuine happiness to explain them to others, to feel your mind grappling with their difficulties, to welcome every new book on them, and to learn as you teach.

—Gilbert Highet, *The Art of Teaching*

Several years ago we were asked to design and implement a one-year course on human growth and development for students of nursing at a major university. By pooling our personal and professional experiences, we identified the areas of information about normal human development and its variations that appeared to be most salient in guiding interpersonal relationships and that served as a foundation for a holistic approach to client evaluation and intervention.

We found that before we could treat or teach a person as a patient, we had to meet and to reach the patient as a person. This meant understanding and accepting the patient's actions, reactions, and interactions on the basis of developmental levels and perceived needs. (For example, a knowledge of both intellectual and emotional development was essential in order to gain the cooperation of a 3-year-old for an injection; an appreciation of emotional and social development was essential when an elderly person verbalized that he wished he would "hurry up and die.") We found that the clients' priorities were not always the same as the practitioners' priorities. In each case, the client's perceived needs had to be met before he or she was able to attend to what the practitioner identified as more critical matters. Often the client's perceived needs fell outside the traditional focus of the profession.

Our observations indicated that it was essential to have a comprehensive knowledge of normal development and its variations to be able to understand and to meet the needs of those with whom we worked. We also found that we needed to know ourselves better—what and why we were thinking and feeling the way we were in a given situation before we could plan or intervene objectively and appropriately. A broad data base was also fundamental for us to be able to communicate information that would help an individual to feel comfortable with his or her differences. For example, a husband may develop headaches or nausea during his wife's pregnancy, a newborn may develop jaundice, or a 15-year-old girl may not yet be menstruating. Are these signs of pathology or merely variations of the normal?

We also became acutely aware that development does not end at 18 or 20 years of age. The 24-year-old client is very different from the 54-year-old or the 84-year-old individual; each one has his or her own goals, interests, and roles in life. These differences had to be taken into account as we established and maintained effective communication with these individuals and tried to help them maximize their potentials.

We quickly became aware that much of the knowledge we sought and utilized was not unique to, nor circumscribed by, the profession of nursing. All these situations and many more made us aware that the professional person's knowledge about human growth and development must go beyond the confines of a professional data base and encompass information from many disciplines in order to obtain a truly holistic view.

After compiling and organizing our ideas, we searched for a text that would facilitate the presentation of our concept of a holistic, practical, life-span approach to human development. We found none. Our students had to purchase seven different textbooks in order to locate the information we felt was essential.

Although our course was developed for nursing students, word soon spread around campus that the course content was both interesting and valuable. Students from many other disciplines requested permission to take the course. Those who did felt that the content was just as applicable to their professions as it was to nursing.

This text has been developed to be used for an introductory undergraduate course in human growth and development. It has also been suggested that the text might be used with senior undergraduate students in an integrative course to help them apply information studied in isolated courses. A number of doctoral programs have used the first edition as a foundation for a holistic approach to further professional development.

The text is not geared toward any one discipline; the material in this book has been developed to meet the needs of practitioners who serve individuals in almost any capacity. Therefore, practitioners already in the field, such as social workers, counselors, teachers, nurses, rehabilitation therapists, physicians, lawyers, and ministers, have also found this book to be a valuable reference. As a text, it is intended to lay a broad foundation for understanding the ontogenetic process of human development, to clarify the misconceptions acquired during earlier years, and to raise some questions for further personal and professional development. The book may be used as a text for students who do not plan to take additional courses in human development, but it is the intent of the authors that the student will acquire more depth of knowledge in those areas that are germane to his or her chosen profession.

This volume combines the knowledge and skills of a number of contributing authors from diverse disciplines. The authors are of the opinion that no single authority or discipline could adequately cover an area as complex or multidisciplinary as normal human development. Since the text attempts a broad coverage of data with which persons in any profession should be acquainted, the professor may wish to identify those areas that the students of a particular discipline should be encouraged to explore in greater depth.

Finding a balance between covering too much and covering too little has been difficult at times. The approach we use offers opportunity for expansion of data in the classroom or through special assignments. Some topics have been covered in more depth because of the relative scarcity of data or the difficulty in collecting pertinent resources. This book is not intended to replace a text in general psychology, sociology, or physiology. Students who have had courses in general biology and general psychology prior to using this text may find some areas easier to understand, but the authors have endeavored to present enough information to facilitate comprehension by even the most naive student. It should be noted that the text is geared toward students who are preparing for professions in applied settings. Thus, empirical data are the base for the text, but clinical applicability is the focus.

The text is organized into 13 units, which are developmentally sequenced. Unit I may be considered the introduction to the text and Unit XIII the conclusion. Insofar as possible, the first two or three chapters of most units cover the normal development of the individual. Unit VI covers critical concepts and maturational or situational crises that may transcend more than one phase of the life cycle. Since the text is designed for a one-year course, the units and chapters are arranged to accommodate easily to either a quarter or a semester system.

It is suggested that the chapters be read in sequence. However, unique situations and professorial preferences may call for longitudinal study of one domain. The reader should keep in mind that a holistic approach necessitates integration of domains; therefore, the chapters dealing with critical concepts and maturational crises may touch on several domains. At the same time, a single experience or construct may be approached from different aspects in as many chapters.

Unit X presents the family—its formation, development, maintenance, and problems. The family is the unit through which society transmits its values to an individual. In our culture, the family provides the major environment that influences the individual's development. Events that affect the family will also affect the development of the individual and vice versa.

To help you get the most out of this text, an **Instructor's Manual** and **Test Bank** have been developed by Kathleen B. Ammon, B.S.N., M.N.Ed., Ph.D., Associate Professor of Nursing, Carlow College, Pittsburgh, PA. Included in the Instructor's Manual are Objectives, Terminology, Teaching-learning activities, and Discussion Questions, all geared to each chapter of the text. The Instructor's Manual also includes transparency masters from which a set of transparencies can be made. The Test Bank provides objective-type test questions for each chapter of the text. Both ancillaries are available through your Little, Brown College Division Sales Representative or may be requested on school letterhead directly from Little, Brown and Company, Inc.

We hope that this book will facilitate your teaching of human growth and development. We also hope that you will feel comfortable recommending the book to practitioners already in the field to refresh their knowledge of human development and to serve as a reference on normal development. We would appreciate your comments on content.

Introduction for the Student

Determination to be wise is the first step toward becoming wise! And with your wisdom, develop common sense and good judgment.

—Solomon, Proverbs 4:7, *TLB*

It has been suggested that the real title of this book should be *What You Always Wanted to Know About What Makes People Tick But Didn't Know Where to Go or Who to Ask.* Even with such an impressive title, however, the book is not an encyclopedia of human behavior; rather, it is an **overview** of human development from conception to old age. We have attempted to focus on the priorities of data from many disciplines and to offer explanations of how and why people function as they do. You may not always agree with each view offered, but our professional experience has proved to us that knowledge of many views is essential in assessing and planning intervention strategies. This is considered an eclectic approach.

Sometimes you will recognize yourself or someone you know in the descriptions of development. You may laugh; you may even cry. At other times you may become angry or even argue with the data presented, wondering how any rational person could ever propose such a theory or think and behave in such a manner. People are different—that is what makes them so interesting to study and to know, and at times, it is also what makes them so frustrating. Throughout this book, you will consciously and unconsciously begin to develop your own theories (a process we hope you will continue throughout your life-span).

As you study how you have developed and will continue to develop and learn how others have developed through life experiences quite different from your own, it is hoped that you will discover many of your stereotypes beginning to mellow and your appreciation for others increasing. The study of individuals who possess common traits (e.g., age, gender, disability, living circumstances) is helpful in understanding trends, but **each individual must be viewed in light of his or her unique combination of traits.**

Since professional persons need to be aware of what data are available to the lay public through literature and the mass media, you are encouraged to review and to read articles written in the lay literature. Many of these articles are authoritative and well written. Such sources often generate many questions or requests for help from your clients. At times you may find it helpful to refer clients to a particular article during professional contacts with them.

We hope that you will enjoy this book. We have included what we wished we had known or understood earlier in our own professional and personal lives. We have attempted to present you with comprehensible material that is relatively free of professional jargon, yet comprehensive in scope. Most important, we hope this text will help you to obtain a solid foundation on which you can and will build in the years ahead of you as a professional person.

The Process of
Human Development

I
Prologue

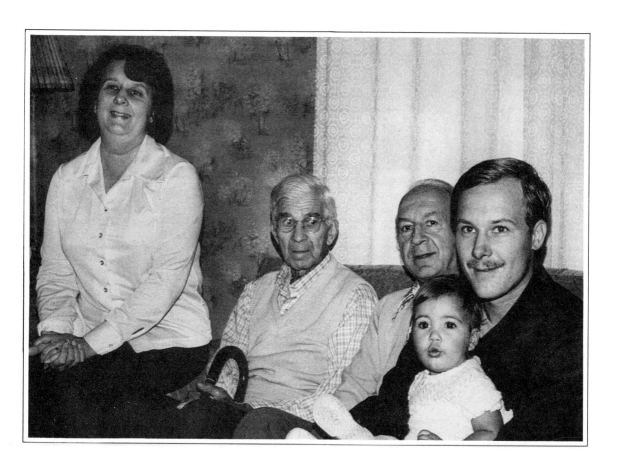

1
Study of the Human Life Span

Clara S. Schuster

> It takes a lot of knowledge to know how little
> we know.
>
> —Dagobert D. Runes

The process of human development is strongly influenced by two interacting forces: biophysical endowment and psychosocial environment. Both factors begin to influence our lives before we are ever born. The genetic potential for the development of each person is contained within the fertilized ovum. Each individual has a unique genetic makeup determined at the moment of conception that sets a ceiling on ultimate levels of personal achievement.

Our psycho-sociocultural heritage is just as powerful an influence as our biological heritage. Realization of genetic potential, or self-fulfillment, depends on the nurturing available and on the opportunities for expressing one's potentials as allowed or encouraged by the individual's environment. Variables such as the neighborhood where our family lives (urban or rural), economic level, basic attitude of our parents toward us (i.e., whether we were wanted and loved), religious orientation, educational opportunities, size of our family, and availability of medical care all influence the formation of our attitudes toward life. Each person is a unique expression of the total combination of hereditary and environmental factors touching his or her life—not the sum of each, but the result of their interactions.

Our own history influences our response to another's life-style, and vice versa. A better understanding of human development can contribute in a very practical way to the improvement of the quality of life. As you proceed in the formal study of the process of human development, you cannot ignore your own life experiences. Identifying and segregating some of the factors influencing development can help you work toward maximizing the expression of your own potentials and those of the people with whom you will eventually be working.

The process of human development has almost as many interpretations and theories as there are people to give their views. We are like the proverb about the five blind men who each gave a different description of the elephant they examined by touch (one felt the tail, one an ear, another the trunk, a fourth felt a leg, and the last the side). Each of us tends to explain human nature, the sequences of development, and cause-effect relationships on the basis of our own experiences, observations, or experiments, and the opinions and experiences of others we consider knowledgeable. Each discipline, likewise, tends to investigate selectively and to organize those attributes of the individual that are considered relevant to the particular field. These different orientations frequently appear to offer incompatible or conflicting concepts. As in the example of the five blind men, however, when humans are viewed from a more holistic perspective, these varying concepts are shown to be highly interrelated. One begins to realize that it becomes inappropriate to discuss the "rightness" or "wrongness" of a theory. The significant point is the usefulness of the theory in explaining the behaviors under scrutiny at the moment.

This book attempts to draw some of these findings and views together. We have attempted to pull the most significant observations and theories from multiple disciplines and our own experience and present them in one book. The information chosen for inclusion is not meant to be final or complete; it represents an attempt to introduce some order and integration into the increasing bulk of available knowledge. The one overriding criterion for inclusion was relevance to life in technologically oriented societies. We have avoided focusing on developmental research per se in favor of a practical approach to understanding human behaviors in today's world as explained by research, concepts, and theories. This book reflects the conceptualizations of various disciplines; therefore, it offers an interdisciplinary approach to development through the life span. Developmental changes that are significant to professionals in all areas are highlighted.

The rapidity of change is a significant factor in deciding the amount of space allotted to each developmental level. During the first days of life, hours are significant; during the first weeks of life, days are significant; during the first months of life, weeks are significant; during the first years of life, months are significant. Gradually, years become adequate guides for study, and during the adult years, phases are appropriate parameters.

The concept of qualitative differences in functioning based on age or developmental levels is relatively recent. The following review of history, research methodology, and theories of human nature will offer a foundation for the remainder of the text.

HISTORICAL PERSPECTIVE

Everyday life is influenced by the history of the human race. Advances in technology and medical care, increased affluence, and more effective contraceptive practices have influenced not only the quality of life, but also cultural standards, family identity, and the value of children. Other eras and other cultures have not and do not always recognize distinct developmental phases in the life cycle. Remnants of earlier attitudes toward children can still be found in individual families and in many American subcultures today.

Ancient Eras

"The history of childhood is a nightmare from which we have only recently begun to awaken. The further back in history one goes, the lower the level of child care, and the more likely children are to be killed, abandoned, beaten, terrorized and sexually abused"[11]. Prior to the Middle Ages, life was so uncertain that adults lived mainly for immediate gratification. Only males of the upper classes were viewed as fully human. Consequently, females and slaves were considered subhuman, with the same status as pets or working animals. As such, severe corporeal punishment or even death penalties for infractions of the "master's" desires were justified. Many felt that infanticide, especially for females, was essential for economic, familial, and societal survival. The male-female ratio is estimated to have been as high as 4:1 [11]. Even though laws against infanticide emerged as early as 374 A.D., many persons felt that infanticide was defensible since infants were not seen as fully human and therefore would not be counted as sinners if they died [11]. Those who were allowed to live were so tightly swaddled that movement was impossible and circulation was frequently impaired. The arms were bound as long as four months, and the legs for up to nine months. Motor development was markedly delayed compared to today's expectations. Many babies were underfed and became withdrawn and passive.

Harsh discipline was used to extract the evil from the child. Beatings, mutilation, and whippings were standard procedure. Jewish and Christian priests, playing an advocacy role, had some influence in reducing physical punishment, but many parents merely switched to locking the children in closets or drawers for hours or even days [11].

The parents, concerned with their own pleasures, obtained wet nurses to care for the infants so that the woman would be freely available for sexual relationships, and her body would not be disfigured by nursing. Many doctors, recognizing the adverse effect on the infants, enticed mothers to nurse their own babies because it would give the mother "a thousand delights" by cooing, smiling, and fondling her; that is, the baby would meet the **mother's** sensual needs, would parent **her.** "The child's facility in mothering adults was often its salvation"[11]. A reversal of roles was common. Many parents even dressed the child in costumes of the style worn by their own biological mother (even boys), and literally as well as symbolically made a parent out of their own child. Many parents did love their children and expressed tender feeling toward them at times, but love was conditional and given to meet the parents' projected needs rather than those of the child. The parents lacked the emotional maturity essential to see the child as a separate individual.

Middle Ages

For the average person, life was very difficult during the Middle Ages. Causes of disease were not understood, and hygiene measures were unknown. The family existed in reality but not in concept. "The density of society left no room for the family"[3]. Living quarters were small and crowded, and communal family living was common. The family consisted of anyone living under the same roof, including servants and friends [13]. Social demands were stronger than the individual need for privacy, which was uncommon—even on the wedding night. The life span was short, pleasures were few, and death was certain. Although infanticide was now rare, infant and child mortality rates were high, which discouraged emotional, social, and educational investment by the parents in their offspring. Children were rarely coddled and were often ignored [3].

The philosophy of the day appears to have been "Eat, drink, and be merry, for tomorrow you die." There was no time or place for childhood; one had to live life before it ended. The advent of pregnancy and birth were necessary evils. Child care was considered a bother and not one of the joys of life. Once the infant began to walk and to use language, the youngster was on his own—often competing with adults to meet the basic necessities of life.

Little time was devoted to, or available for, forming warm family relationships. Children were encouraged to make a very rapid transition from the nursing infant to the weaned adult. Only two phases of life were recognized—infancy and adulthood. The concept of childhood was unknown in this society. As soon as the child was weaned and able to separate from his mother, he entered the world of adulthood.

By 3 or 4 years of age, the child had already joined in adult leisure and recreational activities and had participated actively in the rowdiness and sexual play of that era. If a male child survived to age 7, he was sent to live with a craftsman as an apprentice. The 7-year-old was not seen as qualitatively different from adults—only quantitatively. Children were viewed as miniature adults. If one looks at medieval works of art, the children are portrayed with adult faces and bodies even shortly after birth. Clothing is a miniature version of adult attire. At the age of 7 and in some cases sooner, the child entered the adult work force, assuming responsibilities alongside grown men and women.

Society felt that children under 7 were in a transitional period between eternity and life. It was believed that young children had no mental activities, so their death was no real loss. Childhood death was frequently seen as a necessary waste, and the child was buried as we bury a pet today [3]. Very few records were kept of childhood mortality, since childhood was viewed as such an insignificant phase of life. One expected to have many children in order to keep a few. This attitude is consistent with the technology existing at that time; without methods for improving the quality of life, the quantity of life (number of children) became important and valued by the culture and its institutions.

Sixteenth and Seventeenth Centuries

The idea that children had special and unique needs evolved very gradually. Much of this new sensitivity appears to be related to the influence of a fifteenth century religious teacher by the name of Gerson [3]. Gerson was appalled by the amount of open talk, coarse jokes and gestures, and sexual exposure that was considered normal and acceptable in front of children. Since children were thought to be unaware of or indifferent to sex prior to the age of puberty, playing with a child's genitalia and sharing the same bed were common practice. Gerson, through the church, preached that masturbation and causing erections in children represented "pollution and sodomy"—that is, premature sexuality [3].

Under Gerson's teaching, Western European society of the era of enlightenment and romanticism began to protect children. At the end of the sixteenth century, sexual references began to be removed from books used for educating children. During the seventeenth century, society began to accept the idea of the innocence of childhood. The pendulum of sexual expression in public began to swing in the opposite direction. Modesty became the rule; bodies were to be scrupulously concealed even from family members and persons of the same gender.

The emergence of a new, commercial middle class in the latter part of the seventeenth century also had great impact on the value and roles of children through changes in both social and family structures. Although the lower classes continued to prefer the extended family—the communal family or collective society of the Middle Ages—the middle class began to separate

itself in disgust from the lower classes and in contempt from the upper classes of society. These smaller middle class family units began to realize that children were not ready to face the rigors of adult life. Children were seen as weak and innocent and therefore as being in need of education and discipline. As trades and craftsmanship assumed more importance, the economic demands of trade-bargaining and the need for high levels of skill, combined with Gerson's teachings, impressed the middle class family that it was responsible for the academic and moral training of children as well as for the transmission of name and inheritance.

Portraits painted during the sixteenth and seventeenth centuries indicate that the childhood phase of life began to have more value. Separation of adulthood and childhood was indicated by differences in costuming. Children began to wear clothing reminiscent of styles worn 100 years earlier. Although males profited first from the emergence of the concept of childhood innocence and need for education, females also began to receive more equal treatment by the end of the seventeenth century in some circles [3]. The poor continued to make little change or distinction based on age or gender.

At the end of the seventeenth century, John Locke, an English philosopher, advocated the theory that the child's mind was a blank slate or **tabula rasa** and that therefore parents must educate children from "their very cradles" [26]. The significance attached to environmental influences put much responsibility on the home and family. In the American colonies, religion invaded every aspect of life. An "other-world" attitude was consciously fostered in children as the rigid Puritan sought early spiritual conversion as preparation for untimely death.

Eighteenth Century

In the eighteenth century, marked differences were observed in the status and value of children depending on the socioeconomic level and religious orientation of the family. The Industrial Revolution in Europe created significant changes in social structure. The geographic movement of family units from rural to urban areas changed social status and increased the individual's sense of isolation. (Although the population density was increased, psychological isolation intensified.) Individual and family rights became stronger with this increased isolation. Status began to be based on economics. In Europe, poor children were forced to work long, hard hours in mills and coal mines under conditions that today would be considered inhumane. As more families entered the middle class, more time was

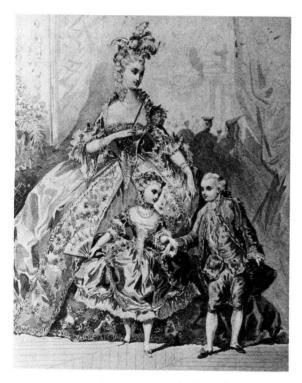

Figure 1–1. Persons from previous centuries viewed children as miniature adults. Children were quantitatively but not qualitatively different.

available for leisure, and money was available to support children for a longer period of time before they had to work to assist in meeting the financial obligations of the family. Increases in technology emphasized the need for more education. Age-graded schools emerged under the influence and direction of the church. Society encouraged the refinement of manners for the upper class and the values of responsibility and hard work for the lower class.

In Europe, the attitude toward older people began to change as a result of industrialization and the limited contact with an extended family: The elderly were no longer considered useful and worthy of respect in urban areas. Consequently, the concept of four phases of life emerged during the eighteenth century: (1) infancy (birth through age 5); (2) childhood (ages 6 through 14); (3) adulthood (postpuberty); and (4) old age.

In America, a man's home became his castle. Privacy was valued. Roles became age-graded and gender-related; males were trained for superordinate positions and females for subordinate positions. Children continued to be subjected to rigid rules to "make them pure" and "keep them in their place." Often they were fed separately, and frequently they were not allowed to enjoy adult luxuries, such as spiced foods or adequate bedcovers for warmth. Children in this "theological age" were to be seen and not heard. Time and talents were to be focused toward an eternal end. Fear and repression were predominant [24]. Hard work was emphasized; this era was the first to be influenced by the Protestant work ethic (i.e., evil can be overcome by hard work). The following excerpt illustrates the attitude of the Puritans toward children:

> Those that survived infancy, tho' probably as dearly loved as are children today, were denied all the normal sources of joy and happiness. Childish manners were formal and meek. A pert child was generally thought to be delirious or bewitched. Of course, to the stern Puritan, inexorably utilitarian, what afforded amusement seemed sinful. Child nature being depraved and wicked must be dampened. Play instincts were inexcusable [6].

Only gradually did the philosophy that children were naturally evil change to the philosophy that they were naturally good. This change in outlook was fostered by the French philosopher, Jean-Jacques Rousseau, who felt that children would instinctively know right from wrong (the idea of the "noble savage") if they were allowed to develop with less parental interference [40]. As happiness gradually became more significant than the issue of sin, theological dogma was exchanged for rules of good conduct (e.g., honesty, industry, sobriety)

as the basis for child guidance in the home. Improved knowledge of the transmission of disease increased concerns about hygiene. Increased affluence allowed more time for both education and leisure during childhood. The availability of primitive birth control methods allowed the married couple more control over family size.

The American Revolution also appears to have been a turning point for improving the quality of life for children. It marked not only the beginning of freedom for the American people but also the emancipation of the child [24]. Parents became more concerned with child welfare and disease prevention through improved hygiene, diet, clothing, and education. Juvenile literature began to change from theological philosophies to more instructive and humorous material. Printer John Newbery began to print books especially for children in 1744 [24], a welcome relief from the former stark readers. Many of our classic poems (Mother Goose) and fairy tales (Cinderella, Sleeping Beauty, Puss-in-Boots, Red Riding Hood) originated in the latter half of the eighteenth century.

Nineteenth Century

In the nineteenth century the status of the child continued to advance with democracy. From the American Revolution to the 1830s, more stress was placed on industry and knowledge. This period has been labeled the "utilitarian age." Unfortunately, many families were still so busy clearing and settling the land that there was little time for education. Nevertheless, respect for childhood had been established. Children became precious possessions, to be coddled, guided, and cherished. Children were valued for their economic contribution and enjoyed for their social contribution. Children were seen as the hope for the future. A couple without children was to be pitied.

The spirit of humanitarianism encouraged improvement in social conditions. The newly industrialized society recognized that lives could be improved through education. Public schools and compulsory education laws were adopted in almost every state. Equality before the law included the right to education [39]. Massachusetts led the way with the first free public nonsectarian high school in 1821 and the first compulsory school attendance law in 1852.

In the post-Victorian era, society began to denounce the artificial standards fostered by the Puritanical heritage. Restrictions on child behavior were released. Parents encouraged individuality, self-control, and initiative in their children. Society became truly child-centered. Adult classes were offered in child care [24], and attempts were made to understand the child better. Parents no longer attributed childhood accidents to the "will of God" as punishments for their own sins. They took an active part in accident prevention [11] and began to purchase life insurance for children [43].

It was during this period that Freud developed his theory on the nature of man, and educators began to take sides on the nature-nurture issue. Environmentalists used Locke's philosophy that the child is passively molded by the environment. Hereditarians found support in Rousseau's view that children actively fit themselves to the world through problem solving. Baby diaries or biographies began to appear; in fact, Charles Darwin was one of the first to use this method of gathering data. Although these diaries added little in the way of concrete data, they did focus attention on the qualitative differences between children and adults. Writers like Mark Twain helped people to see childhood pranks as funny and natural, rather than sinful. Parents began to encourage play activities both for merriment and to facilitate the use of the body.

During this era, there was a narrowing of the generation gap. Parents began to make friends with their children, and older people were once again respected and appreciated for their social contribution to the family.

Twentieth Century

Technology and industrialization have advanced very rapidly during the twentieth century. Advances in medical sciences have improved both the quality and length of life. Child mortality rates have been reduced so dramatically that by 1970 many death insurance policies were rewritten as education insurance policies [43]. Mobility has increased as a result of the availability of employment opportunities and improved means of transportation. The financial status of many families allows them to spend more money on leisure activities and luxuries; no longer must every penny be allocated toward pure survival. Contraceptive methods have become so effective that couples can plan both family size and spacing.

As higher levels of education became more essential for employment, the length of time the child remained within the home increased. Childhood was recognized as having two distinct phases—the school age years and the adolescent years. The period of infancy was also subdivided into a true infancy as it is known today, and early childhood. During the early 1900s, then, six developmental phases were recognized: infancy, early childhood, school age, adolescence, adulthood, and old age.

Table 1–1. Phases of the Life Cycle

Phase	Ages	
Fetus	Conception to birth	
Neonate	0 to 28 days	
Infant	0 to 15 months	
Toddler	16 to 30 months	
Preschooler	2½ to 5 years	
School-ager	6 to 10 years	
Pubescent	10 to 12 years ⎱	(varies
Adolescent	13 to 18 years ⎰	widely)
Youth	18 years to ?	
Young adult	18 to 35 years	
Middlescent	35 to 65 years	
Senescent	65 years to ?	

As society, educators, and psychologists became increasingly sensitive to the qualitative differences in individuals, the period of early childhood was further subdivided into **toddlers** and **preschoolers.** In the 1960s the preadolescent phase **pubescence** was qualitatively differentiated by Fritz Redl, and **youth** as a postadolescent but preadult phase was described by Kenneth Keniston. In the early 1970s, the **neonate** (first 28 days of life) became differentiated as a subphase of infancy. During the middle and late 1970s, the adult years began to attract more attention as having distinct and qualitatively different developmental characteristics. The concept of **middlescence** has emerged as a phase of life separating young adulthood from **senescence,** or older adulthood.

The authors recognize 12 phases of the human life cycle, as described in Table 1–1. Specific ages are attached to the phases, not to indicate discrete stages, but to give the reader the **approximate ages** of individuals in each phase. These age ranges are of particular importance in the biophysical domain; much greater variance will be seen in the other domains. **Developmental phases should be recognized as part of a continuous process and not as a set of discrete stages.**

RESEARCH IN HUMAN DEVELOPMENT

As society began to appreciate and value children more highly during the nineteenth century, it began to realize that there was a need to understand children if society and families were to help them maximize their potentials. Teachers, psychologists, and scientists became aware that a better understanding of childhood would (1) contribute in a practical way to improving the quality of life and (2) have implications for the development of theories of human behavior that could be used both to interpret and to predict behaviors [4]. The earliest research efforts were directed toward describing and differentiating age-related behaviors in order to develop theories and establish norms. **Norms** are the social behaviors, the biophysical skills, and the physiological parameters (boundaries) and responses considered to be descriptive or normal for a defined age group based on observations or assessments of large populations. The information can serve as a guideline for assessing developmental progress and identifying variations and deviations. Norms can be helpful as guides for anticipating and facilitating the emergence of skills and behaviors.

There is a wide range of variability among individuals that can be considered normal behavior. What is considered normal is often qualified by the individual's reference group (e.g., family, peers, ethnic group, racial inheritance); what is considered normal behavior in one group may be unacceptable in another. Few people are "normal" in every area. The unique combination of individual variations establishes our individuality. Parents are sometimes guilty of thinking that norms in one area of development or domain will predict norms in others. Although highly interrelated, each domain evolves at its own pace. The infant who walks at 7 months, therefore, is not automatically assured the position of valedictorian of the high school class.

Psychologists and parents soon realized that norms did not explain why variations and deviations occurred. Consequently, researchers began to look for antecedent-consequence relationships. Could theories predict as well as describe? A good theory should have both explanatory and heuristic power. During the 1940s and the 1950s, psychologists began to test the theories developed from descriptions of norms. The approaches to toilet training and weaning, maternal employment, and other specific factors were evaluated for their potential effects on child and adult personality. Although some correlations were identified, there were too many other variables involved to predict adult behaviors accurately from a single childhood experience. To say that one event **caused** a later event was impossible.

Today, research in human development has become even more specific and more refined. The neonate is attracting much attention; research is being directed toward identifying neonatal competencies as potential predictors of future competencies. The early mother-infant contact, the socialization process, cognitive development, and language development have also become foci for contemporary research. The other end of the life cycle is also attracting attention. What factors contribute to satisfaction with life for the elderly? How can functioning be maximized?

The state of the art is still more descriptive than predictive. However, as more refined measurement techniques and analysis procedures become available, more strongly correlated relationships between antecedents and consequences are being identified that have implications both for theory building and for clinical application.

Sources of Knowledge

Each individual develops hypotheses about human behavior. The major source of knowledge is **experience.** Because people have observed or participated in an event personally, they hold tenaciously to their own views. Unfortunately, this source of knowledge is severely limited. What the person fails to consider is that every other person who observes or participates in the same or similar event will also formulate a hypothesis and will be equally convinced of its truth. Such views are selective and biased. Because events are uncontrolled, they may bear little, if any, resemblance to the truth. The contribution of experience should not be underestimated, but knowledge gained through experience must be validated before it can be accepted without question.

A more reliable source of knowledge is the opinion or the experience of an **expert** in the field. Identifying with the name or the theory of a respected researcher offers more credence to personal observations or theories. However, even the most astute authority is not infallible.

A third source of insight is through the **a priori** or intellectual approach: A theory is developed through reasoning. One proceeds logically from a known fact to an assumed effect. A theory or an hypothesis may be developed through **deductive reasoning,** in which a specific idea is extracted from a general concept or theory through logical reasoning. In **inductive reasoning,** specific observations are logically combined to develop a more general theory or viewpoint. A good theoretical-empirical relationship involves both deductive and inductive reasoning. This method is very useful but is not always reliable. Two qualified people may come to equally supportable but opposite viewpoints. The history of science indicates that the understanding of phenomena has frequently been impeded by the acceptance of "obvious" assumptions that are not true.

The most valid and reliable knowledge is obtained

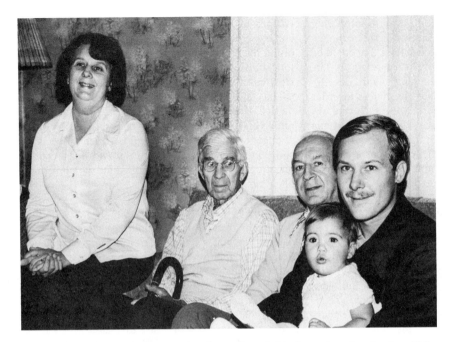

Figure 1–2. The life experiences of each member of this five-generation family will be significantly different because of world events, technological advances, and educational opportunities. Nevertheless, parents transmit a part of their philosophic and ethical values to offspring that provide some cultural continuity.

through the use of a **scientific approach** to explaining phenomena, described here in four steps. First, as an individual interacts with the environment, he or she becomes aware of a problem. Over a period of time, the problem becomes more clearly identified and delineated. Parameters are established and variables (critical factors) are identified. Second, through an a priori approach to knowledge, the individual formulates these factors into a theory—a statement that will explain and predict. Theories are developed to cover the greatest number of empirical facts as simply as possible. Third, further observations or experiments are performed in order to test hypotheses or substatements that are derived from the theory. Fourth, the data are evaluated for the degree to which the research supports each hypothesis. If the data collected do not support the hypothesis, then the theory must be reevaluated. The scientific approach is a continuous process with self-corrective mechanisms when used properly.

Descriptive Research

Critical to the effective use of a scientific approach is adequate identification of problems, parameters, and variables. Descriptive research usually focuses on the first two stages of the scientific approach.

OBSERVATIONS

The baby biographies of the late eighteenth and nineteenth centuries are examples of **natural observations.** In 1877 Charles Darwin, in his efforts to identify the place of humans in the evolutionary chain, observed and described his son's development in a natural setting. His interest in childhood spurred further interest and research in the area. However, he was never able to prove that humans are a direct descendant of animals (the **phylogenetic** approach to the study of humanity). Other investigators since Darwin have identified many characteristics that humans share with animals; however, at this time there is still no concrete evidence that humans are a higher link in the phylogenetic evolutionary chain [39]. This book is restricted to the study of developmental events occurring in the human species (the **ontogenetic** approach).

The person who is planning to observe children or adults in a natural setting needs to approach the assignment thoughtfully and thoroughly. Nancy Carbonara [7] offers the following suggestions for naturalistic observation:

1. The observer is a passive member of the environment. He should not disrupt normal activities and interactions.

2. The process of observation requires extreme concentration, empathy, and sensitivity to clues. All antecedent and sequential behaviors must be noted. The observer must also be aware of his own biases.
3. Observations should be very thorough and specific.
   a. Observe the entire setting, people and objects present, time of day, overview of activities, "tempo" of the group, and any significant antecedent events.
   b. Draw a sketch of the environment.
   c. Focus attention on one activity or one individual for 10 to 15 minutes.
   d. Record all objective and subjective observations— behaviors, verbal and nonverbal communication efforts, responses to others, and so forth.
   e. Be succinct but specific, using key words and abbreviations.
4. The observer should write a rough draft of his observations as soon as possible after notetaking, or minor details will be forgotten.
5. The observer should be objective and descriptive, using adjectives and adverbs freely in order to capture the client's individuality.
6. The summary should include the observer's interpretation of the behaviors.

Contrived observations can be made by placing and observing individuals in restricted environments or by posing problems in order to elicit response. Piaget used this method to evaluate cognitive processes in young children.

SURVEYS

In 1891 G. Stanley Hall pioneered the technique of systematic study of large groups of children with the use of a questionnaire. This method was an example of a **cross-sectional** research design (many individuals of the same age, gender, cultural background, and so forth are evaluated for the identification of norms). In a **longitudinal** design, the same individuals are evaluated for changes that occur over time—a technique used successfully by Piaget.

EX POST FACTO STUDIES

Many problems in education, medicine, and human development do not lend themselves to experimental research. Consequently, relationships between variables must be identified through careful history taking. Case studies fall into this category. Because the researcher has no control over the variables, no correlation between factors can be offered as absolute proof of any relationships observed.

CORRELATIONAL RESEARCH

When a large number of variables have been identified as being potentially related to a problem, a researcher, through detailed study and high-level statistical evaluation, may attempt to identify the degree to which two or more factors are related to each other. Like the ex post facto design, this method offers no proof of cause-effect relationships—only strength of relatedness. Both factors may actually be under the influence of an as yet unknown third variable.

Experimental Research

The four research designs just discussed can identify significant relationships that the researcher may weave into a theory. Experimental designs test the ability of a theory to generate hypotheses that can predict a result. As such, they can assess the possible existence of a causal relationship.

The true experimental design is identified by two criteria: first, by randomization in (1) selection of subjects (for external validity), (2) assignment of the subjects to groups (for internal validity), and (3) assignment of treatment to the group; second, by control of variables that are significant to the research. Environmental consistency is essential for the interpretation of results. The identification of causal relationships will inevitably lead to further questions.

Ethics in Research

Much human research remains in the descriptive category because of the technical and humane problems inherent in experimenting with humans. One cannot deliberately subject a pregnant woman to severe stress to see if it will cause birth defects in the offspring; neither does one deliberately avoid all talking to infants in order to discover "natural" language (an experiment that was performed in the 1200s (see p. 171). Some experiments could cause severe or permanent psychological or physical damage. Such problems require that the researcher locate a population of subjects who experience an alteration in a significant variable because of naturally occurring events. Although this method means more detective work for the researcher and fewer conclusive results, the rights of clients to full participation in life are protected.

The right to privacy has become a critical issue. Researchers are required by research standards to keep subjects informed of the purpose, nature, and potential side effects of research projects, and to obtain signed consent from participants. In the case of children, parents or legal guardians must give permission, but the child must also be informed as much as possible about the research design.

Many hypotheses that cannot be adequately tested in humans because of ethical and financial problems or the constraints of time in research design can be successfully tested in animals. Animal research has had immeasurable impact on theories of learning, biophysical growth, and socialization.

THEORIES OF HUMAN DEVELOPMENT

No one theory has yet been created that encompasses all aspects of human development. At best, we have partial theories that are age-specific or domain-specific. The "truth" is very elusive in the study of humans; therefore, we work with what we know until new theories are developed that are able to account for more of the behavioral variability we observe. People tend to lean toward a particular theory because it helps them to understand their own past experience or blends with their philosophy of life. **Theories reflect the culture and the life experiences of those who develop them.**

The most common and traditional approach to describing and classifying human behavior is according to chronological age. However, the chronological age approach to development does not account for the normal variations that exist among individuals and offers no explanations of cultural and biological factors that influence behaviors. (It is interesting to note that American society very much adheres to this age-dependent concept of development by using age as the criterion for school entrance, marriage without parental permission, and mandatory retirement.)

Theorists go one step beyond description of behavior according to chronological age by attempting to identify meaningful relationships in these behaviors. Complex behaviors are reduced to simple frames by the identification of core problems, tasks, or accomplishments for each phase of life.

One of the tasks of science is to transform observable data into theoretical constructs that facilitate understanding, prediction, and control of phenomena. Because of the difficulty in identifying, measuring, or manipulating variables with humans, many theories are developed through inductive reasoning. These theories or concepts are often so broad and abstract (e.g., self-esteem, inferiority, love) that measurement by empirical research methods is very difficult, and, according to some, impossible. When these broad concepts are broken down into smaller, researchable hypotheses, they become too narrow, artificial, or sterile to have broad practical application. The models de-

veloped from these narrower perspectives do not lend themselves to a life-span developmental theory. Consequently, many theories of development still have a poor empirical foundation. Despite this state of the art, theories are as important as facts in the study of human development. A theoretical framework interprets and orders facts so that an integrated view will emerge. Theory imparts meaning to facts, providing a frame of reference in which to consider and apply information [20]. Developmental theories attempt to explain both change and consistency over time.

The theorists of human development differ in two major ways. They first differ in their presupposition (initial assumption) about the origin of behavior; thus Rousseau's and Locke's views on hereditary versus environmental influences still provoke controversy in theory development and child rearing practices today. Is the child a passive or an active learner? Should nature be allowed to take its course, or should adults actively shape a child's development? The second major area of controversy concerns how the theorists explain the nature of developmental changes over time. Although all developmental theories recognize orderly, sequential changes from simple to more complex behaviors, some theories characterize these changes as smooth, and continuous, whereas other theories emphasize abrupt changes in behavior patterns.

Continuity concepts of development focus on quantitative changes in behavior that occur continuously and gradually over time until the target behavior is achieved (successive approximations). In other words, earlier skills are strengthened and lead to the development of later skills.

The stage or **discontinuity** theories emphasize that the organization of behavior is qualitatively different from one period of the life cycle to the next. Many behaviors may change simultaneously, heralding the entrance to a new level of functioning. Each new stage integrates past and present experiences into new, more complex response patterns. The behavior patterns for each stage can be described and interrelated around a core problem, a task, or an ability for that stage. The core problem or the task must be partially or completely resolved before the next stage is entered. During transition periods, an individual may exhibit behaviors of two successive stages. The stages are sequentially arranged so that the order cannot be changed, nor can a stage be skipped if the final goal is to be reached. However, it is acknowledged that the speed of passing through various stages may be accelerated or delayed as a result of genetic or environmental factors.

A holistic approach to development acknowledges both types of change: continuous and discontinuous. Motor, social, and cognitive behaviors gradually become more complex through five processes [15]:

1. Addition. New skills are gradually added to already existing skills. (The infant learns to grasp and later learns to release.)
2. Substitution. An old skill is completely replaced by a new skill. (The child begins to hold a pencil with the fingers and the thumb instead of the palm.)
3. Modification. A new skill resembles but extends or differentiates an earlier skill. (The finger-thumb grasp used for holding a writing instrument is extended to holding silverware for eating or vice versa.)
4. Inclusion. An earlier skill becomes an integral part of a more complicated task. (The child begins to use the plural forms of nouns and the past tense forms of verbs.)
5. Mediation. A skill becomes an essential link or stepping stone for a later skill. (Crawling is discarded as a form of mobility once the child can walk.)

Psychodynamic View

The psychodynamic view of human development emerged during the late nineteenth century. Artificial social standards and puritanical prudery prevailed in the late Victorian upper- and middle-class European circles. It was in this context that Sigmund Freud, a medical doctor, began to encourage his clients to reiterate their childhood experiences (ex post facto) in search of antecedents to current "phobias" and "hysterias." He felt that all behavior was meaningful and was determined by earlier events. Freud combined the data gathered from these interviews with his own life experiences and intuitive inductive reasoning to develop the first major theory on personality development. Many other theorists have used his theory as a point of departure for developing their own.

Psychodynamic theories view people as being basically affective (emotional) and irrational. The energy to act and react originates in genetically or biologically determined passions and impulses (instincts). Even the infant's growth is motivated by unconscious, irrational pleasure-seeking urges. Only gradually, under the influence of societal restrictions, does the child begin to control these impulses and passions rationally. These theories portray people as being in a constant state of conflict between natural instinctual impulses and unnatural societal mores. Psychodynamic theories also put very heavy emphasis on the importance of the mother-infant relationship for adequate resolution of conflicts.

According to the psychodynamic views of human development, we are neither active nor passive in shaping our personalities; we merely attempt to balance the internal and external forces in such a way that we can live adaptively with them. This dynamic process of balancing or maintaining homeostasis continues throughout life. Growth occurs because of the "succession of interactional imbalances (crises) within the child's personality structures and between the child and his milieu" [25]. The adjustment process helps to change personality structures so that the child interacts differently with the environment in the future. The sense of having coped successfully "strengthens the child's capacity and willingness to meet new challenges" [25]. Through this constant process of disequilibrium and homeostasis, identity is formed. Pathologies of the adult years are believed to be remnants of a poor mother-infant relationship.

THEORY OF FREUD

Sigmund Freud postulated that as the child matures, his or her instinctual sexual/sensual energy (libido) is sequentially invested in biologically predetermined areas of the body. In each stage, one body organ dominates the mode of interaction with other people. First the mouth, then the anus, and finally the genital organs become the primary focus (investment) for stimulation, input, output, and control. Each investment was seen by Freud as a separate stage of development. If the conflict was not adequately resolved (because of overindulgence or underindulgence), the child would "fixate" at that stage; evidences of fixation would then become manifest during the adult years. According to Freud, oral fixations (infancy) are characterized by obsessive eating, talking, or smoking; alcoholism; and unrealistic self-confidence or depression. Anal fixations (toddler) are exhibited through obstinacy, compulsiveness, autocratic dogmatism, extravagance, passive resistance, and aggression. Phallic fixations (preschooler) are characterized during the adult years by homosexuality, narcissism, arrogance, flamboyance, and chauvinism.

According to Freud, the major tasks of personality development were completed by about age 6 with the resolution of the oedipal complex (see Chap. 16). The school years were labeled **latency,** since he felt that all sexual curiosity and activity were submerged during that period. During adolescence (genital stage), the conflicts of early childhood were revived. If these conflicts had been handled well in earlier stages, the in-

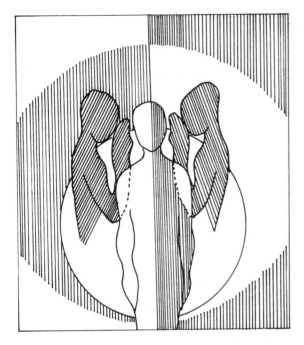

Figure 1-3. According to psychodynamic theory, the self or ego must balance the impulses of the id with the constraints of the superego to meet the realities of everyday life.

dividual would be able to resolve the conflicts and to enter into normal heterosexual relationships during the adult years. From Freud, then, came the belief that personality development is complete by the end of adolescence.

THEORY OF ERIKSON

Erik Erikson translated Freud's theory into a more relevant format to meet the needs of American culture of the mid-twentieth century. He stressed the need for social integration in place of Freud's infantile sexuality. Whereas Freud looked for the origin of pathology, Erikson looked for components that were conducive to growth. Erikson recognized eight stages of development, which continued into the adult years [12]. Partial resolution of each psychosocial crisis was essential to entering the next stage. He proposed a core crisis or task for each phase, a basic virtue that developed with successful resolution, and the affective-social counterpart of unsuccessful resolution.

According to Erikson, the infant is faced with the task of learning to **trust** life, and from this basic trust springs hope. Lack of resolution can lead to mistrust

of others, of the environment, even of self. The toddler strives for **autonomy** and expression of will: "Me do." Too many restrictions on this new-found independence lead the toddler to feelings of shame and doubt about his or her own skills. The preschooler begins to take **initiative** and to show directed purpose in activities. If these traits are not accepted, guilt results. The school-age child develops competence through **industry** or attention focused toward task accomplishment. If the child cannot achieve, feelings of inferiority arise.

The central task of adolescence is to find one's unique **identity,** which is based on previously recognized competencies and fidelity or friendships. Role confusion results when inadequate support systems are available. Once an identity has been firmly established, the young adult can share values, views, dreams, and fears without fear of ridicule from others. Even if others disagree, self-identity is stable enough not to shatter under criticism. The **intimate** person learns to share love in its many forms—parent love, spouse love, child love, friend love, spiritual love. Those who are unable to express themselves openly—as intimate people—become socially and emotionally isolated. They block and hide from other people who they really are. These people play an accepted role, but they do not truly express themselves in life.

During the middle years people who have learned to accept themselves can accept others and extend themselves to help others begin to enjoy a fuller life. Erikson calls this **generativity**—the creation of others. This activity is not accomplished through the biological bearing of children but through the psychological giving of self, through parenting, teaching, artistic endeavors, and so forth. People who are unable to find creative outlets begin to stagnate. In the last phase, **ego integrity,** the individual looks back on life realistically and says, "It's been good." Although errors are recognized, individuals can live with the idea that they did their best. A new wisdom emerges. As the infant learned to trust life, now the older adult learns to trust death. Those who cannot trust the idea of death will experience despair, feeling that life was not worth it. They are afraid of the next step.

THEORY OF ADLER

Alfred Adler spent 9 years studying with Freud but finally left him because he was unable to accept the concept of infantile sexuality. Adler believed that the desire for power offers impetus for growth; likewise, feelings of inferiority offer the impetus to strive to improve one's skills and behaviors. Although one is engaged in continuous, interpersonal competition throughout life, the basic foundations of personality structure are formed by age 6. Adler believed that feelings of inferiority may originate from real or perceived (1) organic deficiencies (malformation or immaturity), (2) spoiling (overprotectiveness that prevents growth), or (3) neglect (a child is forced to be responsible for himself before prerequisite skills are developed) [2].

THEORY OF SULLIVAN

Harry Stack Sullivan, a neo-Freudian, retained Freud's idea of developmental levels and the significance of the maternal relationship in personality development. He felt that security, rather than Adler's need for superiority, is a major goal in life. Security is achieved through satisfying social relationships. The anxiety that arises from perceived or real distance in relationships serves to motivate the individual to new, growth-producing, adaptive behaviors.

Behaviorist View

The theories of the behaviorists were developed in direct rebellion against the global, intangible theories presented by the psychodynamic theorists. Mental activity and unconscious motivations are dismissed as being outside the scientific realm. How can one observe, measure, and validate trust, inferiority, anxiety, or other mental processes and instincts? The behaviorist works on the assumption that all mental behaviors must be translated into physical behaviors before they can be observed and measured (provided they can be identified and adequate measurement tools are available).

The behaviorists, adopting Locke's "passive man," tabula rasa philosophy, assert that the infant starts life with a "blank slate" and innate tendencies that are shaped, strengthened, and modified by experiences offered by the environment. Human behavior is seen as the direct result of these experiences. The basic theory is quite simple: All behavior is under the control of environmental responses or contingencies. The primary determinants of behavior are the antecedent stimuli or needs that elicit responses. In other words, these stimuli set the occasion for the response or behavior. Secondary determinants of behavior are the consequences (contingencies) supplied by the environment when the behavior is emitted.

A basic presupposition of behaviorist theory is that people are pleasure-seeking creatures and will behave in ways that result in pleasant consequences. The forces maintaining behaviors, then, are the secondary determinants of behavior. The key is for the individual—consciously or unconsciously—to identify the

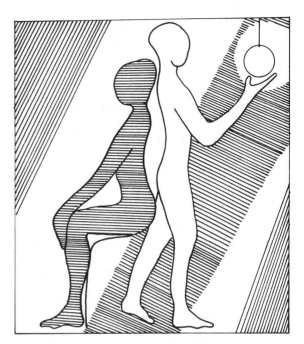

Figure 1–4. According to behaviorist theory, a person emits a certain behavior because of the reinforcement received after performing the behavior.

consequences of a behavior. If the consequence is seen as desirable, then the environment is reinforcing the behavior, and the behavior is more likely to be increased in frequency or intensity. If the environment does not respond or if the behavior results in unpleasant consequences, then the behavior gradually decreases in frequency or intensity until it becomes extinguished. The cognitive behaviorists attempt to identify the mechanisms of acquisition (learning) and those of encoding, accumulation, and retrieval (memory) as they affect behavior. Knowledge of individuals' responses in past situations can be used to predict their responses in the future.

The behaviorist offers no comprehensive framework of human development. Heredity and physical maturation are underemphasized, primarily because they are uncontrollable. The behaviorists are more concerned with systematic research than with a comprehensive theoretical position. Through systematic experimentation and observation, they attempt to identify long-term as well as short-term antecedent-behavior correlations. They use carefully designed research methodology to avoid subjective evaluation of events and to enable them to identify causal relationships. The behaviorist position has proved to be extremely valuable in developing scientific, effective teaching strategies.

It is assumed by the behaviorists that a developmental theory will eventually evolve from the synthesis of analyzed data [25]. The mind is seen as a "quantitative accumulation and association of elements supplied by the environment" [25]. (Note that mental activity thus defined is not directly observable.) Limited response elements are gradually organized by association into larger, more complex response patterns that can be transferred or generalized to new situations. The theoretical aim of behaviorists concerned with developmental profiles is to "formulate the long-term efficient causality of the child's behavior, that is, how earlier events in life are remembered and may influence responses to stimulation later in life" [25]. As a result of "progressive association between the stimuli of the external world" [25] and subjective responses, the infant's and young child's responses gradually become unified, organized behavior patterns and habits. Behavior continues to change during the entire life cycle as a result of adding new behaviors, modifying old behaviors, and losing other behaviors. "Social conditions dictate the existence of developmental phases" [28] by differentially responding to age-dependent skills, roles, and responsibilities. The environmental reinforcement of successive approximations to the final desired behaviors is responsible for much of the shaping or the modification that occurs in behavior over time. This view obviously assumes that all behavior has an antecedent and leaves little room for spontaneous actions or the will on the part of the individual. Individual differences are seen to be the result of differences in experiences or genetic influences. The mature individual has internalized the antecedents and consequences of behavior to become self-regulating and less dependent on concrete environmental events [25]. In other words, the individual internally reinforces his or her behavior.

THEORY OF THORNDIKE
The precursor of the behaviorist view was formulated by E. L. Thorndike around the turn of this century [8]. His theory of "connectionism" sought to identify stimulus-response (S-R) relationships. The "law of effect" was used to explain changes in behavior or learning. Thorndike's work provided the stimulus and prototype for experimentation in child development and learning theories.

THEORY OF PAVLOV
A contemporary of Thorndike, Ivan Pavlov, noted that dogs salivated (unconditioned response) to a visual or an auditory stimulus (conditioned stimulus) if the stimulus was regularly paired with food (unconditioned stimulus). Pavlov developed the theory of conditioned learning (respondent paradigm) based on his experiments [34] and is considered the father of modern learning theory [10].

THEORY OF WATSON
J. B. Watson is considered the "father of American behaviorism" because of his clarification and formalization of philosophy around 1915 [27]. He completely rejected the concepts of mind and consciousness, since neither was objectively observable, and demonstrated that both emotions and motor responses could be "taught" through environmental experiences [8]. When he paired furry animals with a loud noise in the presence of infants, the infants soon exhibited fear when they saw the furry animal. Watson also felt that language development was the product of conditioning. He developed the theory of operant learning: Behaviors are shaped by their consequences.

THEORY OF SKINNER
B. F. Skinner is probably the most famous name in behaviorism because of his formalization and use of behaviorist learning principles in the mid-twentieth century to systematically change behavior. Critics feel that the data from his animal experiments should not be applied to human learning. Advocates of Skinner's research indicate that elementary learning is the same regardless of the animal species. Because it is easier to control the variables with animals, generalization to human learning is by implication. It must be noted that every behaviorist principle has been demonstrated at each level of phylogeny—fish, rats, pigeons, apes, and humans.

THEORY OF BANDURA
In the 1960s Albert Bandura observed that all learning did not occur in isolation or through trial and error while the individual struggled to learn the significant relationships and consequences. He proposed that much learning occurred through observation of other individuals with replication of the model's behaviors [5]. Bandura recognized the joint influence of social modeling and cognitive processing on behavior patterns. An internal representation is used to guide behaviors. He acknowledged that all internalized behaviors were not necessarily reproduced. Expectations of the desirability of the consequence serve as a self-restraint or a motivator. Bandura's social learning theory has marked implications for the effects of family life and television on the development of aggression and affection, prosocial and antisocial behaviors, sex roles, and self-discipline.

Organic Maturation View

The maturationalist postulates that there is an auto-genetic, species-typical path (creod or canalization), which all members of a species follow given a normal, expected environment. Individuals have strong self-righting tendencies if the environment is atypical [32]. Biological maturation serves as the impetus for the emergence of social and cognitive skills. Psychological functioning grows out of biological functioning and is considered its highest form [25]. Generally, organic maturation theories are narrower in scope than the other views.

The individual actively guides his or her own development through (1) possession of genetically endowed sensitivities or skills for initial interactions with the environment, (2) organizing one's inner world in order to interact meaningfully with the outer world, (3) determining one's own orientation to both self and the world and thereby constructing one's own experiences, and (4) actively seeking experiences to actualize genetic potentials [25]. Individuals (consciously and unconsciously) internally organize, integrate, and transform themselves in order to maintain meaningful, adaptive interaction with the environment. Mastery of skills is seen as being self-generative toward higher levels of achievement.

Although discontinuous developmental stages are identified, personal continuity is maintained as each new stage emerges. "The thesis is that evolution is a synthetic process that interweaves two antithetical organismic tendencies: to maintain continuity in order to conserve one's integrity (survival and organizational coherence) and to elaborate discontinuity in order to develop" [25]. One subview of this theory, orthogenesis, sees development as progressive hierarchical integration or "nesting" of skills and associations, with the result that all mental operations gradually merge to a holistic organization in which more highly developed systems regulate less highly developed skills. A second subview, equilibration, postulates that periods of disequilibrium are experienced by an individual as new skills are being mastered. The temporary instability accompanying the transition period is healthy, since it represents and facilitates progress toward stability [25]. Periods of disequilibrium occur less frequently as the individual matures physically, socially, cognitively, and emotionally.

THEORY OF PIAGET

Jean Piaget's theory of cognitive development has probably generated more discussion on child development and more research with educational practices than any other single theory. Piaget feels that an in-

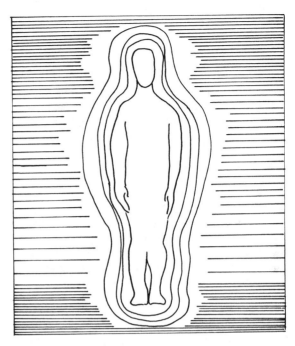

Figure 1-5. According to the organic maturation view, individuals proceed through a series of increasingly complex skills as body systems mature and the opportunity is available to practice these skills.

dividual's basic goal is to learn to master the environment (both external and internal) [14]. The pleasure received from mastery spurs curiosity, problem solving, imitation, practice, and play activities [38]. His assumption is that human nature is essentially rational.

In Piaget's theory, cognitive development is divided into four developmental periods, each of which is characterized by specific interaction patterns with the environment [35]. During the **sensorimotor** period (birth to age 2), development proceeds from the reflexive activities of the neonate to sensorimotor solutions to problems. The child of the **preoperational** period (2–7 years) solves simple motor problems internally through the use of symbols and language. The **concrete operational** child (7–11 years) is able to provide logical solutions to specific, practical problems. Abstract thought processes are not achieved until the **formal operations** period (11–15 years). Mature thought processes are developed that enable the individual to think scientifically. After this phase, quantitative but not qualitative changes in intellectual functioning occur [36].

Piaget suggests that there are four major cognitive processes: (1) a schema, which is a unit or category of thought, a classification for an object or an action (see

Chap. 8); (2) assimilation, the process whereby stimuli are recognized, absorbed or integrated, and fitted into an already existing schema; (3) accommodation, the creation of a new schema or the modification of an old one, which allows for newly recognized differences in a behavior or stimuli; and (4) equilibration, the balance a person attempts to maintain between assimilation and accommodation. The last process is the one used for coping with discrepancies at a comfortable pace.

THEORY OF HAVIGHURST

Robert Havighurst, an educator, proposed that at each life phase the individual has a set of core tasks that must be mastered. These tasks are both organically and socially determined [19]. Accomplishment of lower-level tasks prepares one for higher-level skills. Havighurst's tasks can be quite helpful in developing an individualized educational program (see Appendix C).

THEORY OF GESELL

Arnold Gesell made very detailed longitudinal observations of infant and child development. From these observations he proposed that maturation of the neuromuscular system allows for progressive organization of behaviors. He was impressed by the emergence of behavior patterns that he felt offered descriptive norms of specific age levels. Although his research was limited to a relatively small number of upper-middle-class children, he felt that his description of the cyclic emergence of periods of equilibrium and disequilibrium was useful in predicting intrapersonal and interpersonal relationships [20, 21].

Like the other two organic maturationists discussed here, Gesell felt that the environment influences many of an individual's modes of expression, but that the emergence of behavior patterns is basically determined from within [21]. The evolution of every type of behavior (physical, social, cognitive, and emotional) exhibits remarkably predictable stages. From Gesell comes the concept that "the child is just going through a stage: he'll outgrow it." Gesell recognized the influence of individual temperament as a critical variable in the amount of fluctuation observed between periods of equilibrium versus those of disequilibrium. He also proposed that the cycle begins at birth and continues during the adult years (this concept is discussed further in Chap. 2).

Humanistic View

The humanistic view of development (the "Third Force") emerged during and mid-twentieth century as a reaction against both the psychodynamic and behaviorist models. Humanistically-oriented psychologists could not accept the theory that people were in constant conflict between societal mores and inner impulses, nor could they accept the view that individuals responded mechanically to environmental forces. Earlier theorists, such as Freud, developed their theories of human development from interviews or observations of individuals who exhibited pathological behavior in adaptation to life; consequently, their idea of "constant conflict" was quite valid on the basis of the populations studied—mentally disturbed people.

The humanists accepted Rousseau's philosophy that humans are basically good and need only a supportive environment in order to express and maximize their innate potentials. Consequently, they looked for normal, healthy subjects to interview and analyze before developing their theory of the healthy, self-actualizing individual who is constantly growing toward successively higher levels of personal integration. They contend that the "will to health" or the incentive toward growth is innate. The basic drive is to grow, to find meaning in life, unity in experiences, and to actualize one's innate potentials. Humanistic theories attempt to explain how the world looks to the individual. Behavior is ambiguous or confusing unless its meaning and intent are understood from the point of view of the particular individual. For example, one person may cry as an expression of intense joy; another, as an expression of pity or relief.

Humanistically-oriented psychologists emphasize the distinctively human characteristics of choice, will, creativity, values, and self-realization. The uniqueness of each individual, rather than norms, is a primary focus. Each individual is endowed with "value" and "dignity." From the humanistic viewpoint, each individual, regardless of the degree of innate potential, has the right to develop his or her potentials maximally [1]. Human development is never complete, and growth experiences may be painful. Humans are constantly assimilating and organizing experiences to construct their own growth. Happiness does not become a goal in life but is a by-product of proactive, self-actualizing activity [1]. One can enjoy or appreciate his or her current self while at the same time evolving or becoming a more authentic self. It should be noted that, at this point, humanistic theories have little predictive value. These theories offer an interesting and valuable synthesis of observations and thoughts but are difficult to subject to empirical verification.

In contrast to the maturationists' concept of canalization, humanistic psychologists generally believe that "our inner nature is not strong, like instincts in animals, rather it is subtle, delicate, and in many ways

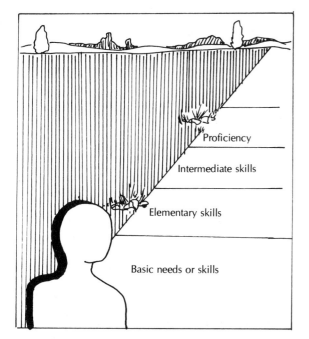

Figure 1–6. According to the humanist view, potentials for growth are always present and need only a nurturing environment to develop.

weak. It is easily drowned out by learning, by cultural expectations, by fear, by disapproval, etc." [31]. Maslow is the only representative of the humanistic position who has identified sequential developmental changes. Other humanistic psychologists present a core unifying goal, which guides interactions with the environment.

THEORY OF ALLPORT
Gordon Allport was one of the first to develop a theory of "becoming"—the conscious striving toward adaptive realization of self within the culture. He felt that one could intentionally create one's own life-style. He stressed the development of proactive coping behaviors, in contrast to Freud's reactive defense mechanisms. In other words, the boulder blocking the pathway becomes a stepping-stone to further growth with Allport's coping, but a stumbling block if one accepts Freud's defense mechanisms. (These concepts are discussed in more depth in Chap. 42.)

THEORY OF MASLOW
Abraham Maslow is generally acknowledged as the founder of the "third force." After the birth of his first child, he could no longer accept the behaviorist view of development. He stressed the need to provide chil-

dren with physical comfort and nurturing, protection, love, acceptance, a feeling of belonging, and a sense of personal value or esteem. Maslow felt that children should be allowed and encouraged to make choices in a supportive environment. In this framework, children are allowed to grow, to become individuals, and to maximize potentials.

Maslow offers a five-level hierarchy of needs that serve as motivators for behavior (see Chap. 42 and Appendixes B and C). As the needs of each level are met, the individual is able to advance to the next level. Lower-level needs are always present, but they require minimal attention once they are adequately met. Maslow recognizes that the environment can stifle the full expression of an individual's potentials. One may return to focusing on lower-level needs given certain changes in the environment. Once a person stops looking to the future and consciously planning or anticipating events, stagnation occurs. Maslow estimates that only about 1 percent of those in the Western culture ever reach complete self-actualization or full maximization of potentials [31].

THEORY OF WHITE
Robert White postulates that the individual's quest for competence is the major organizer of energy throughout life [42]. This view stresses constructive interaction with the environment. On the surface, White's theory may appear similar to Adler's, but White's concept of motivation, which emphasizes personal assessment and goal setting, has no place for Adler's interpersonal competition view that emphasizes peer influence.

THEORY OF COMBS
Arthur Combs (originally in association with Donald Snygg) proposes that behavior is a symptom, an external representation of inner life [9]. As a consequence, he believes that attempts to describe and analyze behavior apart from feelings, beliefs, values, thoughts, and aspirations, artificially bisect the individual, and insult the integrity of the person as a holistic unit. Because behavior is controlled by the individual's perception of his or her environment, behavior can only be understood and predicted by understanding its meaning to the individual (perceptual psychology). In this view, the same stimulus may have a different meaning to two individuals.

Perception is defined as the quantitative and qualitative differentiations an individual uses to interpret, store, and retrieve environmental information. Perception is the individual's interpretation and definition of reality as well as a guide to action. Combs' theory can be loosely construed as developmental because directional changes occur as the individual strives to meet the basic need that Combs identifies as efforts to maintain and enhance the production of a more adequate self. The more adequate the self, the broader the field of awareness (the perceptual field), and the wider the range of available responses. When Combs' theory is studied in depth, it becomes apparent that it embodies almost every other theory, including general systems theory (see Chap. 2). Perceptual psychology offers a holistic theory for studying individuals holistically. The basic goal of this view is to uphold the dignity and the uniqueness of the human being.

SUMMARY

The concept that qualitative differences in cognitive, biological, and psychological functioning accompany various stages of the life cycle is a relatively recent discovery. This recognition has been facilitated by advances in technology and medicine that have resulted in reduced attention to survival needs and greater attention to needs for security, self-esteem, and self-actualization. However, many adults in today's Western society still view children in ways that are reminiscent of earlier eras. These attitudes must be identified and acknowledged if the professional hopes to maximize potentials within the family unit.

In ancient eras, children were barely recognized and seldom treated as fully human. During the Middle Ages, children were viewed as little adults—there were no qualitative differences between children and adults; children merely needed time to get stronger. During the sixteenth and seventeenth centuries qualitative differences began to be recognized. However, many adults felt that children were ignorant, and therefore detested them for their stupidity instead of consciously and systematically attempting to help them to learn. In the eighteenth century children were seen as being in need of guidance but were disparaged as subordinate persons of little value. By the nineteenth century children became precious possessions to be protected and coddled. Attitudes of the twentieth century toward children vary widely, reflecting both the historical views and the views of contemporary theorists. Western culture, under the humanistic view, is beginning to appreciate the individuality of each person and to stress the need for the approaches by both family and society that maximize the individual's potentials without violating the rights of others.

Research with human subjects is very difficult because of the researchers' inability to identify and control all the critical variables as well as the potential for violation of human or individual rights. Although not all theories and views can be supported by empirical studies, they do offer frameworks for understanding, explaining, or predicting human behavior.

Four different views of development have been presented. No one theory has a corner on the truth. The authors find that knowledge of each view is essential in order to obtain a holistic view of human nature. At this point we echo Piaget, who says, "clearly, though the modest facts assembled in this work may have permitted us to answer a few minor outstanding questions, they continue to pose a host of problems. This may well perturb even the most patient of readers, but does not daunt the research worker to whom new problems are often more important than the accepted solutions" [38]. We must work with what we know—or think we know—until research or another great theoretician can explain development better. Although there are many contradictory points among the four views, they can be used in tandem to explain behavior or to plan individualized approaches.

This chapter has covered three major areas very rapidly. Further information can be obtained by consulting some of the references at the end of the chapter. Courses in sociology, anthropology, research design, general psychology, and theories of personality will give the student greater depth in those areas of interest. Appendix B gives a brief history and expands on some of the psychological theories of personality development; Appendix C provides a quick reference to the basic theoretical frameworks of theorists, offering a sequential stage approach to development.

REFERENCES

1. Allport, G. W. *Becoming.* New Haven: Yale University Press, 1955.
2. Ansbacher, H. L., and Ansbacher, R. R. (Eds.). *Individual Psychology of Alfred Adler; A Systematic Presentation in Selections from His Writings.* New York: Harper & Row, 1956.
3. Ariès, P. *Centuries of Childhood: A Social History of Family Life.* Translated by R. Baldick. London: Jonathan Cape, 1973.
4. Baldwin, A. L. The Study of Child Behavior and Development. In P. H. Mussen (Ed.), *Handbook of Research Methods in Child Development.* New York: Wiley, 1960.
5. Bandura, A. *Social Learning Theory.* Englewood Cliffs, N.J.: Prentice-Hall, 1977.
6. Calhoun, A. W. *A Social History of the American Family from Colonial Times to the Present.* New York: Arno Press, 1973.
7. Carbonara, N. T. *Techniques for Observing Normal Child*

Behavior. Pittsburgh, Pa.: University of Pittsburgh Press, 1961.

8. Charles, D. C. Historical Antecedents of Life-Span Developmental Psychology. In L. R. Goulet and P. B. Baltes (Eds.), *Life-Span Developmental Psychology.* New York: Academic, 1970.

9. Combs, A. W., Richards, A. C., and Richards, F. *Perceptual Psychology: A Humanistic Approach to the Study of Persons.* New York: Harper & Row, 1976.

10. Crain, W. C. *Theories of Development: Concepts and Applications.* Englewood Cliffs, N.J.: Prentice-Hall, 1980.

11. deMause, L. (Ed.). *The History of Childhood.* New York: Psychohistory Press, 1974.

12. Erikson, E. H. *Childhood and Society* (2nd ed.). New York: Norton, 1963.

13. Flandrin, J. L. *Families in Former Times: Kinship, Household and Sexuality.* Translated by R. Southern. Cambridge: Cambridge University Press, 1979.

14. Flavell, J. H. *The Developmental Psychology of Jean Piaget.* New York: Van Nostrand, 1968.

15. Flavell, J. H. An analysis of cognitive developmental sequences. *Genet. Psychol. Monogr.* 86:279, 1972.

16. Freud, S. *A General Introduction to Psycho-analysis.* Authorized English translation of the revised edition by J. Riviere. New York: Liveright, 1935.

17. Hall, C. S., and Lindzey, G. *Theories of Personality* (3rd ed.). New York: Wiley, 1978.

18. Hall, G. S. The contents of children's minds on entering school. *Pedagogical Seminary* 1:139, 1891.

19. Havighurst, R. J. *Developmental Tasks and Education* (3rd ed.). New York: McKay, 1972.

20. Horrocks, J. E. *The Psychology of Adolescence* (4th ed.). Boston: Houghton Mifflin, 1976.

21. Ilg, F. L., Ames, L. B., and Baker, S. M. *Child Behavior.* New York: Barnes and Noble, 1982.

22. Jones, E. *The Life and Work of Sigmund Freud,* Vol. 1. New York: Basic Books, 1953.

23. Kerlinger, F. N. *Foundations of Behavioral Research* (2nd ed.). New York: Holt, Rinehart & Winston, 1973.

24. Kiefer, M. M. *American Children Through Their Books, 1700–1835.* Philadelphia: University of Pennsylvania Press, 1948.

25. Langer, J. *Theories of Development.* New York: Holt, Rinehart & Winston, 1969.

26. Locke, J. *Some Thoughts Concerning Education* (abridged in P. Gay [Ed.], John Locke on Education). New York: Bureau of Publications, Teachers College, Columbia University, 1964.

27. Mahoney, M. J. *Cognition and Behavior Modification.* Cambridge, Mass.: Ballinger, 1974.

28. Maier, H. W. *Three Theories of Child Development* (3rd ed.). New York: Harper & Row, 1978.

29. Maslow, A. H. A theory of human motivation. *Psychol. Rev.* 50:370, 1943.

30. Maslow, A. H. Some theoretical consequences of basic need-gratification. *J. Pers.* 16:402, 1948.

31. Maslow, A. H. *Toward a Psychology of Being* (2nd ed.). New York: Van Nostrand, 1968.

32. McCall, R. B. Nature-nurture and the two realms of development: A proposed integration with respect to mental development. *Child. Dev.* 52:1–12, 1981.

33. Munn, N. L. *The Evolution of the Human Mind.* Boston: Houghton Mifflin, 1971.

34. Pavlov, I. P. *Lectures on Conditional Reflexes,* Vol. 1. Translated by W. H. Gantt. New York: International Publishers, 1928.

35. Piaget, J. *Play, Dreams, and Imitation in Childhood.* Translated by C. Gattengo and F. M. Hodgson. New York: Norton, 1962.

36. Piaget, J. *The Psychology of Intelligence.* Translated by M. Piercy and D. E. Berlyne. Totowa, N.J.: Littlefield, Adams, 1966.

37. Piaget, J. Piaget's Theory. In P. H. Mussen (Ed.), *Carmichael's Manual of Child Psychology* (3rd ed.), Vol. 1. New York: Wiley, 1970.

38. Piaget, J. *Success and Understanding.* Translated by A. J. Pomerans. Cambridge, Mass.: Harvard University Press, 1978.

39. Power, E. J. *Main Currents in the History of Education* (2nd ed.). New York: McGraw-Hill, 1970.

40. Rousseau, J. J. *Émile.* Translated by W. Boyd, 1962. In W. Boyd (Ed.), *The Émile of Jean Jacques Rousseau.* New York: Bureau of Publications, Teachers College, Columbia University, 1962.

41. Whaley, D. L., and Malott, R. W. *Elementary Principles of Behavior.* Englewood Cliffs, N. J.: Prentice-Hall, 1971.

42. White, R. W. Motivation reconsidered: the concept of competence. *Psychol. Rev.* 66:297–333, 1959.

43. Zeilzer, V. A. The price and value of children: The case of children's insurance. *Am. J. Sociol.* 86:1036–1056, 1981.

2
The Holistic Approach

Clara S. Schuster

Creating a new theory is not like destroying an old barn and erecting a skyscraper in its place. It is rather like climbing a mountain, gaining new and wider views, discovering unexpected connections . . . but the point from which we started out still exists although it appears smaller and forms a tiny part of our broad view.

—Albert Einstein

Every individual is a unique entity, functioning as a total unit. At any given moment, our behavior is influenced by the cumulative repertoire of skills and experiences, current physiological state, goals, values, and the cultural milieu as well as our perception of the immediate environment. Yet in order to understand how people function, each discipline examines a separate aspect of development. The educator looks at cognitive development; the medical practitioner, at biophysical development; the social worker, at social development; the psychologist, at affective and cognitive development; and the clergyman, at spiritual development. These focused approaches are essential in the identification of cause-effect relationships. However, there is an inherent danger to this segmentation: the focus of a discipline can become so narrow that the individual is seen as an interesting entity rather than as a total person.

When a person exhibits a **variation** (alternative, predictable behavior) or **deviation** (unpredictable or pathological behavior) from the norm, the **practitioner** (professionally trained person) of a specific discipline frequently concentrates so heavily on that one aspect of the life of the **client** (person needing assistance) that the other, more normal aspects may be ignored. In other words, the practitioner fails to recognize the client's strengths while trying to remedy his weaknesses. In extreme cases, several practitioners may be concurrently working with a client, and using opposing therapies because they have failed to capitalize on the client's strengths, to see him as a total person, or to communicate with other practitioners. The client, as a total person, may actually "get lost in the shuffle."

The holistic view emerged to prevent compartmentalized study and treatment of clients [32]. The individual is viewed as an indivisible totality, a **unitas multiplex,** who must be seen in the context of the **umwelt** (total internal and external environment) in which he or she is embedded [41]. **Holism,** a term coined in 1926 [35], is a philosophy that supports the need to be concerned with all aspects of a client's life and uses a team approach to develop **intervention** (supportive or therapeutic) strategies. The **holistic** approach recognizes the individual as a total entity and considers the interdependent functioning of the affective, biophysical, cognitive, and social domains. The individual's family, history, environment, goals, and roles are all considered significant. This holistic or integrated organismic approach to understanding the individual is most heavily supported by the humanistic view because this view addresses concepts, such as self, value, meaning, purpose, and intention [14, 32].

The holistic approach to the study of human development acknowledges interindividual differences and similarities. Each one of us is like all other people in some aspects, like some other people in other aspects, and like no other person in still others. Only through a holistic approach can these similarities and differences be identified and their uniqueness respected. The holistic approach also recognizes that most people experience intraindividual discrepancies; that is, we approach normalcy in some aspects of our lives but exhibit variations and deviations in other aspects.

A **concept** is an idea, based on knowledge and experience, which a person has about a particular phenomenon. As such, a concept is an individualized view that is not necessarily independent of the views held by others. One's concepts may change with exposure to new knowledge and experiences. From a holistic viewpoint, the practitioner must take into account the client's concepts when developing intervention strategies.

This chapter will identify some major approaches to facilitate the viewing of individuals holistically. The remainder of the text is segmented to help the reader more easily study specific behaviors. It will be up to the reader to place each aspect back into a holistic perspective.

THE FOUR DOMAINS

In the preface, the idea of four basic aspects or domains of human behavior was introduced: biophysical, cognitive, affective, and social. In focusing attention on these four major domains, we do not rule out the potential for the existence of other domains, major or minor (e.g., the spiritual or transcendental domains). However, the study of these four domains appears to organize and capture what is currently known about how human beings function. The practitioner must be cognizant of the developmental changes expected in each of these areas if a truly holistic approach is to be assumed in meeting client needs and helping clients to maximize potentials. This multidomain approach to working with clients enables the practitioner to appreciate and work with the intraindividual differences exhibited by clients. We present here an overview of each domain and some basic principles of development (Table 2–1).

Definitions

The term **growth** refers to the addition of new components or skills. In the biophysical domain, growth means increase in body size by the addition of new cells (hyperplastic growth). **Development,** on the other hand, refers to the refinement, the improvement, or the expansion of a component or a skill. Development involves evolutionary change from an undifferentiated or simple state to a complex but highly organized state. Development also implies "a long series of interactions between physiologic maturing and environmental accommodation" [2]. There is progressive change in adaptive functioning. In the biophysical domain, development means increase in body size by enlarge-

Table 2–1. The Four Domains (Overview)

Domain	Dimensions
Biophysical	Genetics, physiological processes, biological functioning, health maintenance, safety
Cognitive	Perception, memory, learning, thinking, organizing, creativity, language, problem solving
Affective	Internal responses to events, emotions, values, motivations, self-concept, self-discipline
Social	External responses to events, relationships with others, enculturation, affiliations

ment of cells already present (hypertrophic growth). **Maturation,** a concept similar to development, is the process of achieving full or optimal development of a component or a skill. In the biophysical domain, maturation means the final differentiation or refinement in the functioning of cells, tissues, and organs, and the establishment of cooperation among the components of the body so that minimal energy is expended in maintaining optimal functioning.

Throughout the text, there is reference to the term **maximization of potentials.** This concept does not imply that one must function at maximum capacity in all domains at all times—the organism would soon "burn out." The top athlete can run 1 mile in less than 4 minutes, but the same pace cannot be maintained in a 20-mile marathon. Maximization of potentials refers to optimal utilization of one's powers or assets in order to keep energy expenditures at a minimum while focusing toward the achievement of a goal.

Maximization of potentials implies the concept of **high level wellness.** If viewed from an interindividual perspective, high level wellness refers to a person's ability to function (in one or more domains) at or above the expected norms. On an intraindividual level, however, high level wellness refers to the ability of the individual to utilize potentials optimally in order to meet the exigencies of everyday living. This view accepts the presence of disability or even acute and chronic disease. However, it is a proactive definition; one that implies optimal utilization of current potentials. This perspective recognizes the uniqueness of each person and allows different levels of performance to be considered high level wellness.

High level wellness is the optimal level of functioning of which a person (or a family) is capable when total loads (deficits) and powers (assets) are considered. This holistic definition considers developmental level, past experiences, present situation, disabilities, and the environment. This approach to high level wellness and maximization of potentials requires that the practitioner have a wide background of both knowledge and experience, and that he or she works **with** the client in the assessment of loads and powers and in the establishment of goals and intervention strategies.

Biophysical Domain

The biophysical domain encompasses all the tangible aspects of self—the body. It includes every aspect of genetic, chemical, and physical self, from conception until death; from the fertilized egg through fetal de-velopment, infancy, childhood, adulthood, and the aging processes. It covers how we inherit characteristics from our parents, and how these characteristics in turn are transmitted to our offspring. Study of the biophysical domain is concerned not only with what happens, but why and how an event affects the functioning of the individual, and how to use this knowledge to maintain high level wellness.

From a philosophical viewpoint, one can say that our body is merely a tool for the expression of our spirit. From this perspective, the chapters in this book that cover the biophysical aspects of development will explore the efficiency or competencies of this tool at various points in the life cycle.

PATTERNS OF GROWTH

Physical growth appears to be governed by genetically determined, harmoniously channeled time schedules. Although the sequence of growth and development appears to be the same for all persons, the rate of development and the end product are very individual. The stage of physical growth and the development achieved is known as the **biological age,** which is not always identical with the **chronological age** (time since birth). Knowledge of the expected sequences can help the parent or the clinician to support optimal physical development by the establishment of realistic goals based on these developmental sequences and by the provision of appropriate experiences to encourage the emergence of skills.

Just as a plant needs adequate water, food, and sunshine to develop, so the individual requires adequate nutrition, exercise, and stimuli to develop and maintain optimal biophysical functioning. A holistic view recognizes that the other domains do not develop in isolation from the biophysical domain. Intact sensory modalities (visual, auditory, haptic, gustatory, and olfactory) are prerequisites for perception of the environment and subsequent cognitive organization of the information. The inadequately nourished child frequently has inadequate energy to attend to stimuli, and thus perception or organization of information by the cognitive domain may be altered. Inadequate stimuli may alter the motivation to interact with the environment (see Chaps. 14 and 39).

Some practitioners indicate that if appropriate stimuli are not given at the time the individual is biophysically programmed or ready to receive and utilize particular types of stimuli for the development of a specific psychomotor skill, the skill will be more difficult to learn later in the developmental sequence (critical period theory). Examples might include language acquisition, learning to eat solids, to run, to use scissors, or to ride a bicycle. However, since the learning of each of these skills is also heavily influenced by sociocultural factors, it is difficult to negate psychological factors, which may also inhibit the acquisition of the skill (a more holistic view).

The acquisition of skills, especially for young children, is heavily determined by neurological development. Since the nervous system develops from the brain toward the feet (cephalocaudal), children raise their heads before they can sit, and they must sit before they can crawl or walk. The nervous system also develops from the spinal cord toward the extremities (proximodistal). Consequently, **gross motor** (large muscle) activities precede **fine motor** (small muscle) activities. Children will grasp an object with the palm (palmar grasp) before they will grasp it with the finger and the thumb (pincer grip); they will catch a ball with their arms before they can catch it with their hands.

The early growth of the individual, especially during the fetal period and early infancy, is primarily through **hyperplasia** (increase in the number of cells). Gradually, hyperplastic growth is replaced by **hypertrophic** growth (increase in the size of cells). After the adolescent years, increase in body size is a result of hypertrophic growth only. Each body organ has its own optimal periods of growth. These growth periods will be discussed throughout the text; it is sufficient to indicate here that body tissues are most sensitive to permanent damage during periods of the most rapid hyperplastic growth [34]. Differences in the developmental maturity of various organ systems can lead to intraindividual differences. At times these differences can create temporary functional imbalances, such as the hormonal imbalances frequently experienced during the pubertal years or the "growing pains" of the school-age years, which are related to differences in the growth rate of the bones and muscles (see Chap. 20).

The aging process actually begins with the formation of each new cell. However, the cumulative effects of aging do not usually become readily apparent until the middlescent years when the individual may begin to recognize changes in energy level, appearance, and functioning. The longer one lives, the greater is the chance of living beyond the average life expectancy. For persons living in the United States in 1980, the years of life expected at birth for males was 70.7 years, for females 77.7 years [43]. However, a 70-year-old man can expect to live 11.1 more years, and a woman at 70 can expect 14.7 more years of life (Table 2–2). Good

Table 2–2. Expected Remaining Years of Life for Given Ages in the United States in 1978

Age (years)	Expected Remaining Years	
	Male	Female
Birth	69.5	77.2
5	65.8	73.3
10	60.9	68.4
20	51.4	58.7
40	33.2	39.5
60	17.1	22.1
70	11.1	14.7
80	6.9	8.9
85	5.5	6.9

Source: Figures obtained from *Demographic Yearbook 1980*, 32nd issue. New York: The United Nations, 1980.

health care and the avoidance of illness and accidents can increase the life span, but these measures cannot postpone death indefinitely. With increased longevity, the maintenance of high level wellness becomes a challenge; the key frequently is maintaining an interest in one's environment and continuing to actively participate in the activities of daily living.

PHYSIOLOGICAL PARAMETERS

Some physiological parameters (measurements), such as the concentration of oxygen in the blood, remain fairly stable throughout the life cycle. Other parameters, such as the body temperature, undergo minor changes depending on age, gender, hormonal balance, and time of day. Some parameters change markedly during the life cycle. For instance, changes in pulse rate and fluid intake are related to changes in body surface area and organ size or maturity. The varying metabolic (growth, maintenance, and repair) needs of each growth period also determine the caloric and protein requirements of each developmental stage. These parameters are given in Appendix E; the reader is advised to consult them as necessary throughout the text.

The patterns for physical growth and development, especially in the areas of height and weight, can be predicted both for the "average" person and for individual children (see Appendixes D and E). Height and weight charts are helpful primarily for quick reference and identification of gross abnormalities. "Normal" ranges are wide; therefore, the practitioner should focus on the child, not on the norms. Particularly in the areas of height and weight, a child must serve as his own guide to normalcy. Hereditary factors set a pattern that can be readily distinguished by 3 years of age.

By plotting changes on a height-weight grid, the practitioner can identify otherwise nonapparent, deviant (pathological) changes in a child's growth pattern. Any child who falls below the tenth percentile should receive additional attention to potential growth-inhibiting factors.

BIOLOGICAL RHYTHMS

The rising and the setting of the sun, work schedules, the seasons, and other periodically recurring events help to establish a rhythm to physiological functioning. Blood pressure, temperature, electrolyte excretion, blood values, pulse rate, and even sensory activity have all demonstrated patterned fluctuations during a 24-hour day [38]. Therefore, the "normal" parameters must provide enough leeway to accept these variations. Although it is not known whether biological rhythms are endogenous (internally mediated) or exogenous (externally imposed), it is obvious that an internal, or "living," clock somehow signals the time for the onset of physiological activities. The most commonly studied rhythm is the 24-hour day, the circadian rhythm (**circa,** about; **dies,** day). This internal clock signals when it is time to eat, to rest, and to sleep; it may even tell a person when to wake up. Regular sleep-wake cycles begin to emerge around 3 weeks of age. By the eighteenth week, a 24-hour periodicity is well established, and adult-like fluctuations in body functions are achieved by the ninth month [13, 30].

Studies indicate a positive correlation between body temperature and variations in mood or performance. For instance, the body temperature of "larks" (morning people) rises and declines earlier in the day than that of "owls" (night people). One's best performance also correlates with the peak of temperature. For most people, this occurs in the middle of the waking period. The body excretes more epinephrine during these periods of high alertness [24], which is one explanation that is offered to account for the morning versus the evening person (although correlations are not necessarily causes).

Biological rhythms can affect the ability to adapt to the environment. "Failure to realize our natural cycles can lead to unnecessary trauma, whereas understanding them may lead to elimination of useless worry and dependency on prescribed medicines" [29]. These rhythms are easily disrupted. Those who have experienced jet lag are acutely aware of the dissynchrony between the internal clock and the external stimuli. When the clocks are set forward or back 1 hour in the spring and fall, it takes 2 days for the blood pressure to make the shift and 5 days for the body temperature

to reestablish its rhythm [37]. People who work rotating shifts also experience symptoms of dissynchrony (fatigue, anorexia, nervousness, hunger and sleepiness at inappropriate times, tension, decreased mental alertness, and delayed reaction time). Because these symptoms can reduce work efficiency, employers should consider the implications of mandatory shift work versus monetary incentives for regular employment at the less desirable hours.

Some biological rhythms repeat themselves at periods greater than 24 hours. The menstrual cycle repeats itself about every 4 weeks; some energy cycles repeat themselves on a weekly basis or every 3 to 4 days. The reader may wish to keep a record to discover his or her own high and low energy cycle. People are most efficient when they can work with, rather than in spite of, their cycles.

Many people experience energy dips at midmorning, after lunch, and in the early evening. These decreases in energy are not due to food consumption or to temperature decrease, but often appear to be part of a basic rest-activity cycle [24]. These cycles of approximately 90 minutes appear even during sleep periods after the eighth month of fetal life [3]. Human growth hormone secretion in infants is highest during rapid eye movement (REM) sleep and depends on rhythmic recurrences of sleep [31]. Fifty percent of infant sleep and 20 percent of adult sleep is spent in active REM sleep. During waking times, a person should work with these natural rest-activity rhythms in order to enhance productivity. A good example is a 10- to 15-minute break from one's studies every 1½ to 2 hours. One should not study for 4 hours straight; nor should one study for 15-minute periods, because these short intervals do not allow sufficient time for integration and continuity. Matching cognitive and social activities to one's internal clock can promote optimal adaptive behaviors. The assessment of a client's circadian rhythms can help the client to identify and utilize points of high energy to increase activity and independence [19].

Cognitive Domain

The cognitive domain encompasses all those aspects involved in perceiving, interpreting, organizing, storing, retrieving, coordinating, and using stimuli received from the internal and external environments. It also includes problem solving and the creative activities involved in forming new combinations of information to adapt to the unique needs of a new situation. In short, the cognitive domain is concerned with our processes of thinking and memory—our intellectual processes.

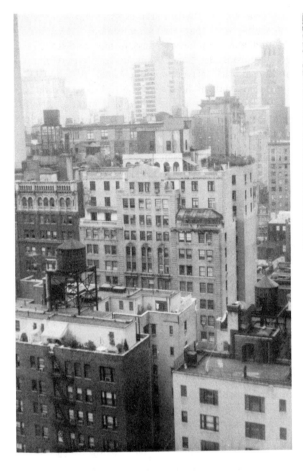

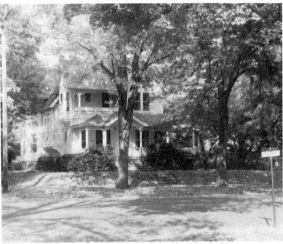

Figure 2–1. Different people may find their natural pace or temperament more suited to one environment than another. The environment has definite effects on development of all four domains. Attitudes and life-style are greatly affected by the community in which the individual lives.

PATTERNS OF GROWTH

The growth in the cognitive domain appears to be heavily dependent on the development of the central nervous system as well as on individual experiences. As in the biophysical domain, growth appears to be governed by a genetically determined time schedule. The sequence of growth and development appears to be the same for all persons, but the rate of development and the end product are very individual. Current views hold that the highest point of cognitive potential is genetically determined, but the level that one achieves is environmentally mediated. One cannot progress beyond the biologically determined levels, but the individual can function maximally within those levels if the environment is optimally supportive.

The growth in both the cognitive and the biophysical domains proceeds from the simple to the complex. Simple skills are gradually incorporated into more complex skills. To the behaviorist, these earlier skills are known as prerequisite skills, because the end skill cannot be achieved unless the earlier skills have been mastered. For example, teachers find that a child must be able to match (recognition skill) similar stimuli before the child can differentiate (receptive knowledge) a target stimulus from a group of stimuli upon request. This skill precedes the ability to name or replicate (expressive knowledge) a stimulus without the presence of the model. The child cannot understand the concept of subtracting 3 from 5 until he or she can first understand the meaning of 5, count 5 objects, add numbers to 5, subtract 1 from 5, and subtract 2 from 5. The process of advancement from lower-level to higher-level skills is known as **successive approximations**—each skill takes the individual one step closer to the end goal. This concept can be very helpful to the parent or the teacher. By breaking a goal down into smaller steps (task analysis), both the child and the adult can experience more frequent successes, and progress toward the goal becomes more obvious. The same principle holds true for any teaching-learning situation whether it is directed by a social worker, a dietician, a nurse, a physical therapist, or another practitioner.

Cognitive development also proceeds from concrete experiences to abstract thought processes. Piaget's framework for cognitive development currently offers the best explanation of this process. Benjamin Bloom maintains that cognitive behaviors progress through six major hierarchically ordered classes: knowledge, comprehension, application, analysis, synthesis, and evaluation [7].

FACTORS AFFECTING GROWTH
Changes in the environment have the greatest effect on the individual during periods of rapid change [8]. Thus the experiences with the environment during the early months and years are critical to the development of the individual. Throughout life, change must be frequent enough to draw interest and provide challenge, but not so rapid as to prevent comprehension of events. Ideally, novel experiences must be paced to the individual's needs.

Interactions between the environment and the individual are measurable and observable. However, the individual's mental organization and representation of the environment can only be inferred from observable behaviors. A person's internal representations and thought processes change consciously or unconsciously only when he or she recognizes that a discrepancy exists between current knowledge and environmental input. Learning does not consist merely of a successive accumulation of bits of knowledge, and cognitive processes cannot be accelerated merely by enriching the environment. What is learned and how it is learned depend both on the environment and on the cognitive processes available to the individual. Studies indicate that "both affective and organizational (intellectual) disequilibrium are necessary conditions for the child's engagement in the adaptive, constructive mental activities that constitute the sources of cognitive change and development" [28]. Studies repeatedly indicate that an individual cannot incorporate the reasoning involved in stages that are beyond the person's current level of cognitive development.

The teacher or the parent can facilitate the child's concept formation by (1) assisting the child to gain experiences and knowledge, and (2) helping the child to assess the validity of a concept in relation to personal experiences and knowledge. In short, the child needs to be taught **how**, not **what**, to think. "Once the basic

capacities for complex thinking have emerged, training may considerably enhance the child's ability and readiness to use complex cognitive processes efficiently and effectively" [28]. As the child becomes aware of discrepancies in his thought processes, the child will strive to reorganize and reintegrate current structures or to create new ones that will assure greater equilibrium.

Chronological age and cognitive age are not always synonymous. This discrepancy is the basis of intelligence testing. Intraindividual discrepancies can be readily observable in the infant or the young child who experiences advanced cognitive age but normal biological age. The child knows what needs to be done to achieve a goal but cannot manipulate the body adequately to perform the required psychomotor task. For example, an infant may pick up two pop beads, yet not be able to snap them together. The toddler will attempt unsuccessfully to tie shoes, and the preschooler will create a lopsided drawing. Each knows what is wrong but cannot adequately command the body to perform as desired. The resulting frustration of unachieved goals may precipitate anger or passivity, depending on other environmental factors. It is important for the adult to help the child to achieve success through appropriate supportive activities (see Chap. 14).

Adequate nutrition and exercise in the form of appropriate stimuli and challenges are as essential to cognitive growth as they are to biophysical growth. During the early years, a child needs adequate opportunities to explore objects, the environment, and new-found skills in order to test reality and to develop sufficient concrete experiences and images, which lay a foundation for the internal manipulation of objects and for later abstract thought processes. Children (and adults) must have the emotional security that will allow them the freedom to explore novel experiences and a sufficient number of these experiences to allow them to accurately predict an outcome. Exploration and prediction are basic to a constructive interaction with the environment.

Affective Domain
The affective domain encompasses all the emotional aspects of self—feelings, longings, values, motivations, aspirations, commitments, frustrations, restraints, and identifications. In short, the affective domain is concerned with internal responses to external events, other people, and self—one's basic attitude toward life.

Regardless of a person's genetic potentials for development in the biophysical and cognitive domains, most individuals should be able to achieve very high level wellness in the affective domain. There are no limits to a person's ability to achieve happiness through loving, sharing, and achieving, except those imposed by an inadequately supportive environment. Nevertheless, in spite of the fact that there are few known genetically imposed limitations on emotional growth, personality theorists, mental health clinics, formal research, and personal observations all indicate that a large percentage of people function at much lower levels of affective development than chronological age or potentials in other domains would predict.

THE MIND-BODY CONTINUUM

Although we have separated the human organism into four major divisions for study purposes, it would be both foolish and detrimental to continue this approach in working with clients. The body and the mind cannot be so readily separated in our everyday interactions. When talking with a friend, one responds to the total being, not just the mind. "Failure to appreciate the integrity of the human being commonly leads the therapeutic specialist to believe that the aspect of human functioning he is qualified to treat is all-important"[32].

Much evidence has been accumulated that indicates that the health of one domain affects the health of other domains. Body configuration often affects how an individual feels about the self as a person; this phenomenon is mediated by sociocultural factors or values placed on particular characteristics (see Chap. 19). When a person is physically ill, it is common also to become discouraged, even depressed. Energies are invested back into the self; perceptions and cognitive thought processes may be altered and attention span shortened.

When a person is severely depressed or upset emotionally, this state of mind can affect cognitive processes. For example, it is difficult to take an examination the day of a major confrontation with a roommate, or after breaking up with one's fiancé. Likewise, more household and automobile accidents occur following confrontations. Concentration on maintaining the internal integrity appears to limit attention to external events and to delay cognitive processing.

If the level of emotional depression or tension is high enough, the functioning of the biophysical domain can also be affected (see Chap. 42). Many people have changes in appetite (desire to overeat or anorexia) when they are upset. Studies on infants who fail to thrive indicate that severe depression can interfere with biological growth (see Chap. 9).

Is hunger or thirst merely a biophysical state? Mas-

low says no: The total person—the integrated, organized whole—is hungry or thirsty. All energies will be focused on satisfying these needs. The mind and body function as a unit to maintain the integrity of the organism in illness and in health. Maslow feels that higher-level needs (e.g., belonging) also reflect the integrated functioning of a person and that "motives are states of the whole person and can be understood only in those terms" [32].

PATTERNS OF GROWTH

Although the growth of the affective domain has received attention by both philosophers and psychologists for centuries, normalcy and the factors that affect healthy development are still very poorly understood. This lack of understanding is due to three factors:

1. Affective development is a very personal matter. It is not observable and, consequently, cannot be directly measured.
2. Development, or the internal responses, must be inferred from external behaviors, many of which are culturally influenced and therefore may not give a true picture of a person's internal state. Moreover, the same external behaviors may be mediated by entirely different internal forces [14, 23]; thus obedience to a parent's command may be motivated by either love or fear.
3. Each person is heavily biased or influenced by subjective emotional states, and this influences the interpretation of one's observations. Very few people can adequately extricate themselves from their own biases to interpret events with complete objectivity.

This last point is particularly true if the individual under study is functioning at a higher level of emotional development than that of the observer. Just as Piaget indicates that a person cannot completely understand or appreciate reasoning processes beyond the current level of functioning, theorists such as Maslow, Kohlberg, and Erikson indicate that a person cannot truly understand or appreciate the motivations or affective processes involved in stages beyond a current level of affective development.

The major theory of affective development presented in this text is that of Erik Erikson. Erikson offers a proactive, universal approach to affective development. His frame of reference has been found to be extremely useful and flexible both in assessing clients and in establishing a supportive milieu. Observations would indicate that inadequately supportive environments impede progress or complete resolution of the earlier stages; consequently, many individuals continue to struggle with Erikson's levels 5 and 6 during most of their adult years (see Chap. 28).

Researchers at the Gesell Institute observed that children exhibit cycles of behavior that are reflective of the internal state of adaptation of self to the environment. In a way, these cycles are similar to the biological rhythms discussed earlier. Each cycle, however, becomes progressively longer as the individual matures. This cyclical development may continue into the adult years (e.g., midlife crisis, retirement); however, no one has, to our knowledge, continued this investigation beyond age 16. The cycle consists of six phases. The child begins the cycle in **good equilibrium**; behavior is smooth and consolidated. This is followed by a period of **marked disequilibrium** between the self and the environment. A period of **relative equilibrium** is then followed by **pronounced withdrawal** or inward introspection; this period is characterized by marked touchiness and sensitivity to events, emotional lability, and pessimism—a phase that is followed by periods of **extreme expansiveness,** even to the point of endangering one's life. The child then goes through another period of **neurotic disequilibrium** before returning to good equilibrium [21] (Table 2-3).

"Failure to achieve growth in the affective domain may be the most serious failure of all" [25], because growth in this domain mediates not only the energies available for cognitive processes but also the tone of social relationships. Inadequate growth can leave one full of tensions and disquietude; adequate growth can lead to true joy in living as well as emotional "highs" and clarity of thought unobtainable by any other means.

Social Domain

The social domain encompasses those aspects that identify a person's "niche" or relationship with society or the culture—roles, affiliations, communication styles, adaptive behaviors, expressions of internal response, and interactional patterns. In short, the social domain is concerned with the individual's external response to external events, other people, and self—one's interpersonal relationships.

It is almost impossible to separate the social domain from the affective domain. In fact, to do so is purely academic, since external responses or behaviors are mediated by cognitive processing and affective interpretation of stimuli or events. The individual's ability to respond appropriately or according to socially sanctioned behaviors is dependent on the level of affective development and the state of tension at the time. For example, a person's ability to assume responsibility depends on previous experiences with the prerequisite cognitive skills and the resolution of Erikson's fourth crisis (industry). A person who has not learned to receive satisfaction from a job well done will make a poor employee.

A person's ability to communicate with others also depends on the security of his or her own identity (Erikson's fifth crisis). During earlier levels of development, the child finds identity through identification with a strong, significant person. However, with normal development, the child begins to differentiate and appreciate a separate identity. The insecure person (functioning at a lower level) will exhibit the need to quote other people frequently or to express only those opinions that are accepted by a current peer group. The person who is secure in self-identity is not afraid to express and support opinions even though others may disagree violently. This individual is able to maintain personal integrity by consciously separating personal (spiritual or affective) self from cognitive or philosophical self. The person who has a secure self-identity is able to respect the uniqueness of other people and to appreciate or to value the dignity of other individuals as well as the self (see Chap. 28). The level of development in the social domain, then, closely reflects the intrapersonal relationships of the affective

Table 2-3. Cycles of Behavior

4 weeks	4 months	10 months	2 yrs	5 yrs	10 yrs	Good equilibrium
5 weeks	5 months	11 months	2½ yrs	5½–6 yrs	11 yrs	Marked disequilibrium
6 weeks	6 months	12 months	3 yrs	6½ yrs	12 yrs	Relative equilibrium
8 weeks	7 months	15 months	3½ yrs	7 yrs	13 yrs	Pronounced withdrawal
10 weeks	8 months	18 months	4 yrs	8 yrs	14 yrs	Extreme expansiveness
12 weeks	9 months	21 months	4½ yrs	9 yrs	15 yrs	Neurotic disequilibrium

Source: Based on systematic research by the Gesell Institute. (Extracted from F. L. Ilg and L. B. Ames, *Child Behavior.* New York: Dell, 1955.)

domain. Erikson's theory reflects this duality. This text will combine discussion of these two domains under the term **psychosocial development.**

PATTERNS OF GROWTH

Growth in the social domain also develops from simple to complex and from proximal to distal relationships. The young infant's world is autistic (totally self-centered). The infant attends only to the self and to those external events that directly impinge upon the senses or meet needs. Gradually the infant begins to realize that external events are controlled by a separate entity—the mother (or mother substitute). A very intense symbiotic relationship then develops between them [26]. This simple, one-to-one relationship gradually extends to other members of the family during the toddler and preschool years. During the school-age years, relationships are extended to peers in the school and neighborhood settings. The ability to travel independently and the diversification of skills and interests lead the adolescent into the larger community to seek satisfying relationships and experiences. During the adult years, the individual is obviously free to leave home and community and to extend relationships or social horizons around the world if finances and interests permit. The individual learns to separate from the family of origin by experiencing brief separations that begin during infancy. Staying with a babysitter and attending Sunday school prepare the younger child for school experiences. Overnight stays (e.g., summer camp experiences) gradually prepare the older child for college and a separate apartment.

Early experiences can significantly affect later development. A person's reciprocal experiences with the external world can significantly affect self-concept and thus establish a framework for social interaction. "Launched on the right trajectory, the person is likely to accumulate successes that strengthen the effectiveness of his orientation to the world, while at the same time he acquires the knowledge and skills that make further success more probable" [12]. Figure 2–3 illustrates the concept of cycles of competence and incompetence ("benign" and "vicious" cycles). These conceptual frameworks also embody the **epigenetic** concept that one's past experiences or levels of development heavily influence the anticipation of future events and goals and thus modify current perceptions and behaviors.

Such frameworks are helpful to keep in mind for consideration of the enculturation process. Parents frequently attempt to transmit intact to their children their roles, values, customs, skills, and goals. In his book, *Future Shock,* Alvin Toffler indicates that relationships and responsibilities are changing so rapidly in our technological society that the roles and values of the parents may be grossly inadequate to meet the relationships and responsibilities faced by the children [36]. In order to cope with a rapidly changing world, chil-

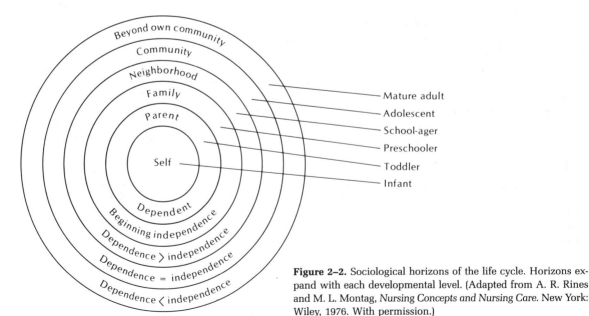

Figure 2–2. Sociological horizons of the life cycle. Horizons expand with each developmental level. (Adapted from A. R. Rines and M. L. Montag, *Nursing Concepts and Nursing Care.* New York: Wiley, 1976. With permission.)

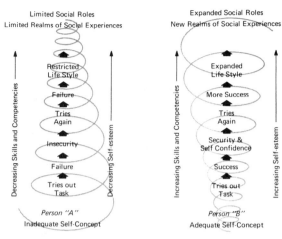

Figure 2–3. "Vicious" and "benign" cycles involved in the development of competent and incompetent people. (From J. O. Lugo and G. L. Hershey, *Human Development: A Psychological, Biological, and Sociological Approach to the Life Span* [2nd ed.]. New York: Macmillan, 1979. With permission.)

dren need experiences that are developmentally sequenced to support (1) the formation of a positive self-identity, (2) the establishment of meaningful relationships, (3) the development of sensitivity to the needs of others, (4) the ability to solve novel problems creatively, and (5) the learning of social competencies that enable them to retain their personal identity while fostering the capacity for growth. These competencies are most effectively learned within a warm, supportive, respecting family system that provides both strong role models and consistent, loving guidance.

THE INTERDEPENDENCE CONTINUUM

The developing individual progresses through various levels of dependence and independence while approaching maturity. However, no one is ever completely dependent on other people except during a critical illness, and few if any people are completely independent in all domains. Dependence-independence is a relative concept embodied within the framework of the interdependence continuum. The term **interdependence** describes the reciprocity of interaction between two or more persons. Since it is recognized that both partners in this relationship may not assume the same degree of responsibility or need for maintaining the relationship, the polar ends of the continuum are designated as **dependence** and **independence.**

Not even the neonate is completely dependent on

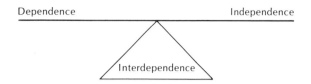

Figure 2–4. Each person must balance the quest for independence against the need for dependence.

others. The neonate's ability to capture attention through crying, eye contact, mouthing behaviors, suckling, and vocalizations make the infant an active participant in the social interaction. In fact, evidence is accumulating to indicate that a mother may lose interest in a baby who is unable to give her adequate feedback for her caretaking efforts (see Chap. 14).

Not even the millionaire is completely independent, depending on other people to help manage financial affairs, maintain a home, cook meals, or type letters. Even if he or she can handle these affairs alone, the banker must handle the money, the farmer must produce the food, and the service station attendant sells the gasoline to run the car. Every interaction requires some dependency. Perhaps the person who comes closest to complete independence is the hermit who lives alone in the desert or forest; yet even the hermit is dependent on local and federal security personnel to keep a domain free from intrusion by land theft or war. The real value of the concept of interdependence is revealed in the following section on systems.

GENERAL SYSTEMS THEORY

A **system** is an identifiable complex of two or more interacting components functioning independently and in interaction as a single unit to meet previously specified objectives. It is more than the simple sum of its parts. A holistic approach to the study of human development requires an understanding of general systems theory, since one cannot obtain a realistic perspective of human functioning by examining only one component. If one part of the body is ill, the functioning of other aspects is affected. A headache will decrease the appetite and the desire for body movement, socialization, or study. If one approaches the study of human development from a family context, then each family member both affects and is affected by the behaviors of the others, and all members are critical to the functioning of the total family as a separate system within society.

Characteristics of an Open System

General systems theory (GST) is not a separate discipline but rather a way of thinking about, organizing, or approaching complex organizations. The historical roots of GST lie in cybernetics, the theory of information-feedback systems. Ludwig von Bertalanffy first introduced GST in 1937 as a theoretical, conceptual approach to analyzing organized entities and to facilitate communication and cooperation among practitioners of the applied sciences [6]. He observed that scientific disciplines had been dissecting nonlinear, multilevel, complex entities in order to analyze them—to find the minute, significant elements of these entities. He did not deny the importance of this process but felt that the clinical sciences must think in terms of the total entity (systems in mutual interaction) if they were to be effective in understanding and helping the system to maximize its potentials [5]. He felt that the structural relationships among system components were frequently more important in determining system behavior than the individual components themselves.

An understanding of a system does not confer control over it, but it may reveal why changes occur. GST offers a framework to disciplines on which to build theories, to hang their knowledge [9]. GST makes possible " . . . a more value-free exploration of the relational determinants of behavior through its focus on a synchronic analysis of interacting systems" [22].

Von Bertalanffy identified two types of systems. The **closed system** is an entity or complex of components that is isolated from its environment. Once the components are in the system, no new components are added from the environment. A chemical experiment performed within a test tube is a good example; the final product depends on the initial composition. The composition of elements within the system tends to become equally distributed over time (homogeneous mixture).

All living organisms, such as humans or social systems, are classified as **open systems** because they are characterized by the ability to exchange energy, matter, and information with the environment in order to evolve into higher levels of heterogeneity, organization, and order (negentropy). The environment will influence, but will not determine, the final state. The final products tend to resemble each other (equifinality) even though they began with different initial components, because of this dynamic interaction of the system with the environment and the ability for self-direction and monitoring.

The components of an open system are hierarchically arranged into **subsystems.** The environment, or **suprasystem,** consists of those people, things, resources, and systems outside of the target system that affect the system and are in turn affected by it [18]. Hierarchically arranged examples of physical environments that provide constraints within which the human organism as a system must operate are as follows: (1) immediate environment (air); (2) shelter (home or work); (3) topography (mountain, ocean); (4) continent; (5) zones, hemisphere; (6) world. The designations of subsystem and suprasystem are at times arbitrary; thus it is important to identify clearly the **parameters** (boundaries) of the system under discussion. A specific component may be the subsystem of one target system but the suprasystem for another. Therefore, one must identify the level of analysis and the component parts in order to discuss meaningfully and clearly the relationships between the components. Higher levels of organization become increasingly complex because they incorporate all systems below them (Table 2–4).

The subsystems of a target system are constantly in a state of interdependence, and communication is maintained between them. The degree of dependence or independence varies with the subsystem delineated, the time of the evaluation, and the effects of the suprasystem on the system. Although the specific activities vary with the ultimate goals and the specific nature of a system, four main functions of open systems are identifiable [10]:

1. Containing. The boundaries of the system must be well established and selectively permeable in order to maintain its separate identity and prevent entrance of undesirable or extraneous matter, energy, or information from the environment.
2. Obtaining. The system must have a means for securing the matter, the energy, or the information essential for growth, development, and maintenance of its life.
3. Maintaining. The system must be able to retain and process what it needs to sustain life.
4. Disposing: A mechanism must be established for relinquishing a product and harmful or excess matter, energy, and information.

Each subsystem is assigned specific tasks, which are critical to the maintenance of the total organism. The role of the subsystems gradually become better defined and more complex as the system evolves. The subsystem is responsible for carrying out its task independently, yet in concert with the functioning of the other subsystems. Because of the close interdependence, a

Table 2–4. Examples of Levels of System Analysis

Physical Realm	Social Realm
Cell	—
Tissue	—
Organ	—
Physiological system	—
Human being as an organism	Human being as an organism
Family	Family
Clan	Community
Race	Culture
Humanity	Nation
Humanity	World

Each level can be divided into subsystems drawn from the components of the next lowest level. The next higher level constitutes the system's immediate environment or suprasystem.

change in one component affects other components and thus the functioning of the total system. The efficiency of total system performance frequently depends on the degree of communication the subsystems maintain with each other. The job of delegating tasks or decision making is usually relegated to one "master" subsystem in order to facilitate system functioning by minimizing energy expenditure for goal achievement [17].

Open systems have semipermeable boundaries that allow for dynamic, selective exchange with the environment. When matter, energy, or information is brought into the system (**input**), it must be processed (**throughout**) by the components in order to create a product (**output**) that is consistent with the goals of the system. A sensitive feedback mechanism allows the system to monitor the exchanges in order to maintain a fairly steady state by preventing overload or underload to the system. Open systems are characterized by importing more energy, information, or matter than is essential to maintain the status quo. This type of system allows for evolutionary, self-directed growth, and for storage of energy for emergency use [11].

The purpose or goal of a system determines its work and, therefore, its stability or ability to adapt to the environment (suprasystem) [33]. An open system attempts to maintain a steady state or equilibrium, which enables the system to maximize its potentials into productive work. This steady state can be achieved only when management is clearly delineated and when (1) the system remains oriented and focused toward the same goal regardless of changes in the environment; (2) progress is maintained toward the goal; (3) the ca-

pacities of the system are matched with the demands of the environment; (4) the system is able to regulate itself to maintain its focus on goal achievement; and (5) the subsystems are committed to the goals of the system, yet maintain sufficient autonomy to function independently [16].

Heinz Werner, a psychologist who studied the developmental aspects of systems, used the **orthogenetic principle** to explain the evolution of any level of system from an initial state of "relative globality and lack of differentiation to a state of increasing differentiation, articulation, and hierarchical integration" [40]. The orthogenetic principle may be easily applied to biological development by following the development of the fetus, but it may also be applied to the development of social relationships (e.g., Mahler's theory), cognitive development (e.g., Piaget's theory), or even perceptual or language development (if one chooses to conceptualize perception or language as a separate system).

Werner identified six aspects, or continuums, along which developmental levels can be objectively evaluated.

1. Undifferentiated-differentiated. As the system matures, subsystems become more clearly identified and independent in their functioning.
2. Interfused-subordinated. As the system matures, the components assume hierarchical relationships designed to maximize efficiency while reducing duplication of activity and unnecessary energy expenditure.
3. Diffuse-articulated. As the system matures, the organizational patterns for communication and cooperation increase between the subsystems.
4. Syncretic-discrete. As the system matures, external and internal input stimuli are more clearly differentiated and separately processed, and output behaviors become more specifically focused toward goal achievement.
5. Rigid-flexible. As the system matures, it is able to use alternative routes for goal achievement (the means become secondary to the end rather than vice versa).
6. Labile-stable. As the system matures, it becomes more independent of the suprasystem in goal setting and focuses energies toward goal achievement (increased resistance to distractors).

The state of health of a system can be identified by determining (1) how well it adapts to the constraints of the environment, (2) how closely its output meets the goals of the system, (3) how efficient it is in using internal and external resources for meeting goals, and (4) the degree of differentiation among component parts and their ability to function cooperatively to meet system goals.

When the system finds that its usual adaptation mechanisms or responses fail, then it can (1) alter itself, (2) alter the environment, (3) withdraw from the environment, or (4) alter its purpose, goal, or concept of desirable state [39]. It is in these areas that the practitioner, by using a systems perspective, can offer assistance. Since the systems approach is concerned with relationships as well as components, the practitioner can draw on a wide variety of theoretical frameworks as a basis for clinical assessment and intervention. This synthesizing approach allows the practitioner to keep the total human being as the central focus of intervention. Since growth is recognized as the central goal of living systems, GST offers a very positive view of human development and recognizes the value of alternative intervention strategies for achieving system goals [33]. Since the system creates its own meanings from input, the response to the environment is unique to the needs and the interpretation of the system. Combs' concept of perceptual psychology is based on this same premise. A system thus can be highly adaptive, and success can be built on failures [11].

The Systems Approach to Human Development

One cannot understand a system without evaluating all the forces that influence it. Therefore, in order to understand a system, the practitioner needs to specify:

1. The components of the system and the specific boundaries
2. The suprasystem, environment, resources, and constraints of the system
3. The relationship between the components and the efficiency of the communication system
4. The objectives or goals of the total system
5. The roles or responsibilities of the component subsystems and the efficiency with which the subsystems carry out their responsibilities
6. The management component of the system
7. The feedback or regulating mechanism for the system
8. The history or time perspective of the system

After these aspects have been identified, the practitioner can, with the system, identify ways to improve: (1) the efficiency of a subsystem(s), (2) the degree of differentiation among subsystems, (3) interaction or communication between subsystems, (4) utilization of environmental resources, or (5) sensitivity to the feedback mechanism. Intervention then may occur on one or more levels and may not even include the offending subsystem.

THE INDIVIDUAL

"A general systems perspective presents a humanistic view of man as a holistic, goal-directed, self-maintaining, self-creating individual of intrinsic worth, capable of self-reflection upon his own uniqueness" [33]. Using the systems approach, the practitioner must first identify the components of the system. For this text, the first subsystem would be the four domains. If one wishes to restrict the focus to only one domain, then the subcomponents of that domain must also be identified. The identification of the relevant subsystem will change with the suprasystem of influence at the moment.

A systems approach recognizes that disequilibrium occurs when the demands of the suprasystem are not synchronized with the needs or skills of the system or do not allow the system time to enhance, elaborate, or reorganize its subsystems in order to achieve a new steady state. Disequilibrium, in reasonable amounts, can challenge the system to become more than it is [1]; this process provides for growth and development as well as restoration.

We assume that a human being, as a system, has a limited range for absorption, processing, and retention of stimuli. A systems overload in the form of cognitive overstimulation leads to an increased need for decision making. Distortion of stimuli (assimilation) is an adaptive response of the system to facilitate processing even though the resulting output may appear to be maladaptive. A systems underload, or deprivation, is also detrimental to efficient functioning because a person cannot draw upon reserves forever. Either extreme can lead to a breakdown of the system, or low level wellness. A gross overload (flooding) can lead to the inability to process the stimuli with resultant blockage (refusal to acknowledge or accept input) or gross disorganization of behavioral output. A gross underload may lead to self-stimulatory behaviors designed to create controlled diversionary input for the individual.

In humans, the major physiological tasks of the system are carried out by the body systems, which are well-differentiated and well-organized. The integumentary system provides the physiological boundaries, allowing access only in limited ways. The gastrointestinal system is organized both to receive in-

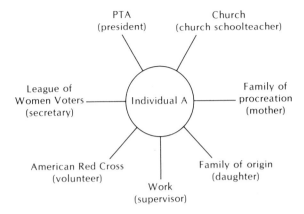

PTA
(president)

Church
(church schoolteacher)

League of
Women Voters
(secretary)

Individual A

Family of
procreation
(mother)

American Red Cross
(volunteer)

Work
(supervisor)

Family of origin
(daughter)

Figure 2–5. Individuals experience role changes according to the system of affiliation. Consequently, one person may participate in various levels of leadership and responsibility.

put (nourishment) and to excrete output (feces). The neurological system also is organized to receive input (stimuli and information) and to discharge a product (language, movement). Each body system can be analyzed in terms of its contribution to the total functioning of the body.

Allport indicates that the affective domain of the human system has a limited range of abilities, attitudes, and motives that can be evoked by differing environments. He suggests that a person's culture, class, family, and traditions must be observed to determine why an individual has accepted or rejected the suprasystem. To view personality purely in terms of role interaction and culture will depreciate the intrinsic concept of personality [1]. In other words, one must look at the input and the throughput before evaluating the output. Behavior cannot be evaluated in isolation from the *umwelt* [42], or meaning [14].

Chapter 19 presents many examples of alternative approaches to high level wellness for the total system when one or more parts of the physical domain fail to function appropriately; readers can formulate many examples of their own. The significant point is that once the goals of the system are identified, one can usually identify several options or alternative methods for achieving these goals (e.g., through increasing the input of matter, energy, or information or through reorganization of responsibilities). These options allow the system to maintain adequate functioning even when one subsystem fails to perform its assigned task. This view has multiple implications for, and challenges to, the creativity of the individual and the practitioner.

A word of caution is in order: It is very difficult to be objective when studying human functioning and personality because one's own experiences predispose to subjective biases [1]. Any practitioner becomes a part of the client's suprasystem and will be affected by, as well as affect, the client. The practitioner must be careful, therefore, to become a resource and a power for the client rather than a stressor or a load. This position requires a broad data base and a sensitivity to the feedback from the client; it also requires that the practitioner attempt to view the environment or suprasystem from the client's perspective in order to help the client to reestablish equilibrium with it. The practitioner must share the client's goals and identify resources or alternative routes to achievement. This approach often requires attention to the client's immediate suprasystem—the family.

THE FAMILY
The general systems approach broadens the practitioner's definition of client and provides a rationale for interest in, and utilization of, the environmental resources or suprasystem to meet the needs of the client [36]. Since the family generally provides the supportive, protective milieu for its members, a healthy family can help its members to achieve maximal health.

The family is a special kind of social system, comprised of two or more interdependent persons, that remains united over time and serves as a mediator between the needs of its members and the forces, the demands, and the obligations of society [20]. This definition goes beyond the traditional or the legal definition of family (marriage, blood, or adoption) and includes how people view themselves as a family. Family-type relationships may also be achieved through economic obligations, a code of rights and responsibilities (roles), religious values, sexual mores, or any other commitment based on dynamic social interactions. This definition is not meant to be loose or all-inclusive but is meant to alert the practitioner to the fact that in today's world, a client's family bonds may not be those traditionally recognized by society. The client should be allowed and encouraged to identify his or her own family and support systems; thus a client's roommate or lover of several years may be of more support during an illness or crisis than a sibling or parent.

When a person is ill or in crisis, the practitioner must approach the person as a part of a family and intervene at one or several points of the system. Frequently, especially for social or affective dysfunction, the intervention may not include the person at all but may be

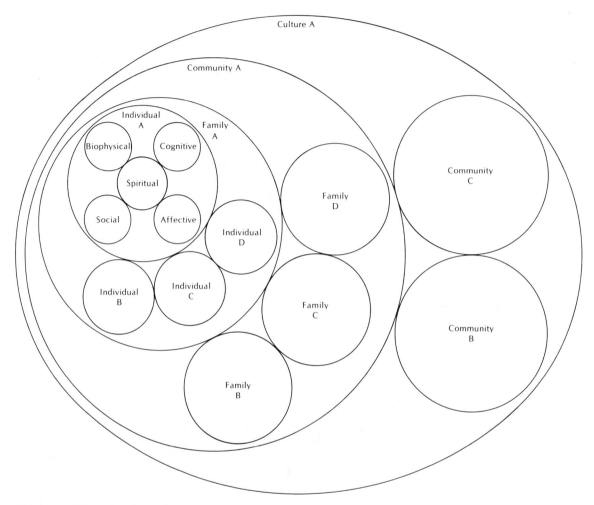

Figure 2–6. Hierarchy of social systems. When working with an individual, the practitioner must clearly identify the significant suprasystems and subsystems affecting the behavior of the system.

geared toward strengthening the entire system. Too narrow an intervention can actually fractionalize the system, "creating damage in the name of protection" [27]; this occurs frequently in cases of child abuse. The child may arbitrarily be removed from the family setting, but unless the total system is strengthened and supported, the events frequently recur.

Families have many different ways of organizing time, space, roles, and values. Many of these combinations are compatible with the healthy development of its members, but some are more appealing or more adaptive to the suprasystem (culture) than others [27]. When one thinks of the subsystems of a family, one usually identifies the number of persons in the family and designates each as a separate subsystem. However, subsystems can also be composed of interactional

patterns between these individuals. Thus one may also find the following subsystems [27]:

1. Spouse subsystem. Its members exhibit interaction for cooperation, expressing affection, handling stress, decisions on obtaining and releasing of members, and utilization of resources.
2. Parent-child subsystem. An intergenerational subsystem of unequal power for the purpose of control and guidance.
3. Sibling subsystem. A peer relationship that provides competition, cooperation, negotiation opportunities, friends (and enemies) for the developing child.

Each subsystem in a family provides a different learning experience in interdependence. The same individual may be a participant in more than one subsystem; thus the boundaries must be very clear, or role confusion emerges and system dysfunction can occur. The parent generally makes it clear that the child does not possess equal power if the child attempts to become too bossy or independent within the home: "As long as you live under this roof. . . . " The child will generally not tolerate a sibling who assumes a parental role: "You are not my mother!"

Each subsystem must be free to function without interference from other subsystems; thus siblings should usually be allowed to settle their own disputes without parental domination. Lines of authority and communication must be especially clear if there is a grandparent in the home. When the boundaries between subsystems are unclear, the system may become overloaded by increased stress levels. This idea fits well with Herman Witkin's limited-domain approach to personality functioning. He observed that the more specialized and clearly delineated are the subsystems, the more efficiently the system is able to respond to the environment. Individuals with a low degree of differentiation are more dependent on other persons for decision making and task accomplishment. Highly differentiated subjects are able to identify their own boundaries and resources and thus can function more effectively.

Families whose subsystems are so enmeshed that boundaries are no longer identifiable function very poorly as a system. Its members are too dependent to execute their tasks efficiently or effectively. There may be conflict stemming from seniority rights or even "juniority" rights (see Chap. 17). On the other hand, if boundaries are too rigid, family members may become too independent and disengage (decrease commitment) from the family system. Chapter 34 explores factors that lead to fractionalized families. The family's health can be assessed by its ability to summon alternative coping patterns and to function flexibly when under stress [27]. Stress is experienced each time a member is admitted to, or lost from, the system because of the need to restructure, reassign tasks, reassess goals, and maintain continuity.

When working with clients, the practitioner must assume an ecological systems approach that includes a concern for the total family as the supportive system.

THE AUTHORS' PERSPECTIVE ON HUMAN DEVELOPMENT

Everyone has his own perspective and ideas about the nature of humanity. The authors—each one in this text—also have theirs. In fairness to the reader, we are sharing the biases of the primary authors with you, although we have attempted to present many other views objectively—even those we disagree with. Our own backgrounds, experiences, and education, and the unique blending of these factors are bound to be reflected in both the content of this text and the emphasis rendered various points.

Some of our viewpoint is already apparent in what has been written in this chapter. We believe that human beings are holistic organisms who can be understood only from an ecological approach. We believe that human potentials are biologically determined, and that the environment can facilitate or hinder the development of those potentials. The functioning of the individual, therefore, is determined by the unique blending of his or her biological potentials, biological maturation, and experiences.

We believe that a person's current behavior is the result of a unique integration of past experiences with anticipation of future events. As such, behavior is an integrated function of all four domains. Early experiences are significant because they must be integrated into all future experiences. A critical experience can continue to influence later behavior, or it can be overruled if a person has several contradicting experiences later in life. From this perspective, development is not complete at age 21; humans continue to develop and change throughout their entire life cycle.

The family system is critical to the continued development of its members—both children and adults. The mother, because she is usually the primary caregiver, is the most significant component in the early biophysical, cognitive, affective, and social development of the child. She provides early education and continues to structure the environment during early childhood.

We believe that the major responsibility of parenthood is to prepare the child for adulthood. Successful adulthood is the ability to cope with the demands of one's culture flexibly and independently. The skills for successful coping are most naturally learned during childhood. These skills are most easily learned when the parents offer good role models and moderate guidance according to the child's developmental level, are consistent in their expectations, and love both themselves and their children enough to enjoy a warm, respectful, affirming relationship.

We believe that every person wants to be his or her best, and that most individuals are capable of higher levels of functioning. We believe that all people have the right to maximize their potentials. We further believe that an individual has the potential for continuous growth from experiences, and, therefore, for gaining satisfaction from a dynamic process of self-realization.

We believe that each reference group defines what is normal for the members of its group, and therefore a wide range of what is normal not only exists but is a subjective criterion. In other words, "normal" people are not all alike. Individuals who are deficient in one or more areas of development still possess potentials that can be developed for fuller living; many individuals only need the opportunity or encouragement, or both, to express their talents and potentials.

We believe that true happiness is found when one finds the balance between personal rights and societal responsibilities, when one masters a challenge, and when one is comfortable with oneself. When one is sure of his or her own identity, there can be self-respect and the offer of true respect to others.

CONCLUSION

In order to reach maximal levels of functioning, each person must be offered opportunities and encouragement by family members and other significant persons (friend or practitioner). The key to offering support is a belief in, and a commitment to, the value of the other person. For some, this means love; for others it is intimate caring. However this commitment is shared or conveyed, it requires the valuing of the other person as strongly as one values oneself. This may be an intangible element, but most of us are intuitively aware of whether or not the other person **really** cares. It is this commitment to others that we hope you will carry with you into your professional contacts with clients, family, and friends. We hope that by exploring the process of human development, you will increase your appreciation of holistic human development.

The rest of this text will present an interdisciplinary approach to the study of the human life cycle. It is hoped that from this study you will better understand both yourself and others. We, the authors, hope that you will find professional satisfaction by helping others to maximize their potentials, for in so doing, you will begin to maximize your own potentials and find richer meaning in life.

REFERENCES

1. Allport, G. W. The Open System in Personality Theory. In W. F. Buckley (Ed.), *Modern Systems Research for the Behavioral Scientist.* Chicago: Aldine, 1968.
2. Anthony, E. J., and Benedek, T. (Eds.). *Parenthood: Its Psychology and Psychopathology.* Boston: Little, Brown, 1970.
3. Bassler, S. F. The origins and development of biological rhythms. *Nurs. Clin. North Am.* 11:575, 1976.
4. Bertalanffy, L. von. General Systems Theory—a Critical Review. In W. F. Buckley (Ed.), *Modern Systems Research for the Behavioral Scientist.* Chicago: Aldine, 1968.
5. Bertalanffy, L. von. General Systems Theory. In B. R. Ruben and J. Y. Kim (Eds.), *General Systems Theory and Human Communication.* Rochelle Park, N. J.: Hayden, 1975.
6. Bertalanffy, L. von. *General Systems Theory: Foundations, Development, Applications* (Rev. ed.). New York: Braziller, 1980.
7. Bloom, B. S. (Ed.). *Taxonomy of Educational Objectives: The Classification of Educational Goals. Handbook 1. Cognitive Domain.* New York: David McKay, 1974.
8. Bloom, B. S. *Stability and Change in Human Characteristics.* New York: Wiley, 1964.
9. Boulding, K. General Systems Theory—The Skeleton of Science. In W. F. Buckley (Ed.), *Modern Systems Research for the Behavioral Scientist.* Chicago: Aldine, 1968.
10. Bredemeier, H. C., and Stephenson, R. M. *The Analysis of Social Systems.* New York: Holt, Rinehart and Winston, 1962.
11. Buckley, W. F. (Ed.). *Modern Systems Research for the Behavioral Scientist.* Chicago: Aldine, 1968.
12. Clausen, J. A. (Ed.). *Socialization and Society.* Boston: Little, Brown, 1968.
13. Colquhoun, W. P., (Ed.). *Biological Rhythm and Human Performance.* New York: Academic Press, 1971.
14. Combs, A. W., Richards, A. C., and Richards, F. *Perceptual Psychology: A Humanistic Approach to the Study of Persons.* New York: Harper & Row, 1976.
15. *Demographic Yearbook, 1980* (32nd issue). New York: United Nations, 1980.
16. Emery, F. E. (Ed.). *Systems Thinking: Selected Readings* (Rev. ed.). Harmondsworth: Penguin, 1981.
17. Hall, A. D., and Fagen, R. E. In W. F. Buckley (Ed.), *Modern Systems Research for the Behavioral Scientist.* Chicago: Aldine, 1968.
18. Hall, A. D., and Fagen, R. E. Definition of Systems. In B. D. Ruben and J. Y. Kim (Eds.), *General Systems Theory and Human Communication.* Rochelle Park, N. J.: Hayden, 1975.
19. Hall, L. H. Circadian rhythms: Implications for geriatric rehabilitation. *Nurs. Clin. North Am.* 11:631, 1976.
20. Horton, T. E. Conceptual Basis for Nursing Intervention with Human Systems: Families. In J. E. Hall and B. R. Weaver (Eds.), *Distributive Nursing Practice: A Systems Approach to Community Health.* Philadelphia: Lippincott, 1977.
21. Ilg, F. L., Ames, L. B., and Baker, S. M. *Child Behavior* (Rev. ed.). New York: Barnes & Noble, 1982.
22. Janchill, M. P., Sr. Systems concepts in casework theory and practice. *Soc. Casework* 50(2):74, 1969.

23. Jenkins, A. H. *The Psychology of the Afro-American: A Humanistic Approach.* New York: Pergamon Press, 1982.

24. Lanuza, D. M. Circadian rhythms of mental efficiency and performance. *Nurs. Clin. North Am.* 11:583, 1976.

25. Lugo, J. O., and Hershey, G. L. *Human Development: A Psychological, Biological, and Sociological Approach to the Life Span.* New York: Macmillan, 1979.

26. Mahler, M. S., Pine, F., and Bergman, A. *The Psychological Birth of the Human Infant: Symbiosis and Individuation.* New York: Basic Books, 1975.

27. Minuchin, S., and Minuchin, P. The Child in Context. In N. B. Talbot (Ed.), *Raising Children in Modern America: Problems and Prospective Solutions.* Boston: Little, Brown, 1976.

28. Mussen, P. H., Langer, J., and Covington, M. *Trends and Issues in Developmental Psychology.* New York: Holt, Rinehart and Winston, 1969.

29. Natlini, J. J. The human body as a biological clock. *Am. J. Nurs.* 77:1130, 1977.

30. Palmer, J. D. *An Introduction to Biological Rhythms.* New York: Academic Press, 1976.

31. Roffwarg, H. P., et al. Ontogenetic development of human sleep-dream cycle. *Science* 152:604, 1966.

32. Shontz, F. C. *The Psychological Aspects of Physical Illness and Disability.* New York: Macmillan, 1975.

33. Sills, G. M., and Hall, J. E. A General Systems Perspective for Nursing. In J. E. Hall and B. R. Weaver (Eds.), *Distributive Nursing Practice: A Systems Approach to Community Health.* Philadelphia: Lippincott, 1977.

34. Smith, D. W., Bierman, E. L., and Robinson, N. M. *The Biologic Ages of Man from Conception Through Old Age* (2nd ed.). Philadelphia: Saunders, 1978.

35. Smuts, J. C. *Holism and Evolution.* New York: Macmillan, 1926.

36. Toffler, A. *Future Shock.* New York: Random House, 1970.

37. Tom, C. K. Nursing assessment of biological rhythms. *Nurs. Clin. North Am.* 11:621, 1976.

38. Tom, C. K., and Lanuza, D. M. Symposium on biological rhythms. *Nurs. Clin. North Am.* 11:569, 1976.

39. Vickers, G. Is adaptability enough? *Behav. Sci.* 4:219, 1959.

40. Werner, H. The Concept of Development from a Comparative and Organismic Point of View. In D. B. Harris (Ed.), *The Concept of Development.* Minneapolis: University of Minnesota, 1957.

41. Werner, H., and Kaplan, B. *Symbol Formation; An Organismic-Developmental Approach to Language and the Expression of Thought.* New York: Wiley, 1963.

42. Witkin, H. A. Heinz Werner: 1890–1964. *Child Dev.* 36:307, 1965.

43. *World Almanac and Book of Facts, 1983.* New York: Newspaper Enterprise Association, 1982.

II
Antenatal Development

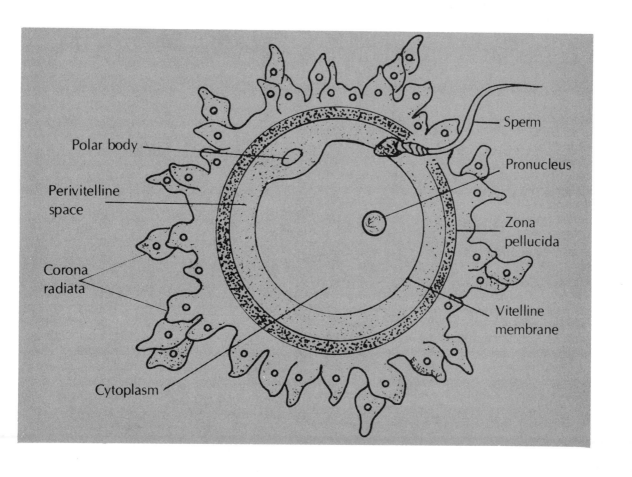

3
In the Beginning

Clara S. Schuster

Insofar as there is a physical and chemical world, life must manifest itself through more or less complicated, more or less durable physiochemical systems.

—L. J. Henderson, *The Order of Nature*

Every living organism begins life as a single cell. Research indicates that it takes only about 44 geometrically progressive divisions (2^{44}) of that cell to transform it into an infant mature enough to sustain life outside the mother's uterus, and only four more divisions to transform the newborn into an adult [5,6]. It is estimated that the adult body is composed of about one hundred quadrillion (10^{14}) cells. If the process has proceeded systematically, the nucleus of each of these cells is an exact duplicate of the original cell, and each cell works in harmony with other body cells to meet both its own needs and the needs of the total system.

Each individual, the end product of this cell division, is strongly influenced by events that occurred before he was ever conceived. At conception, there were potentially 70,368,744,180,000,000,000,000 or $(8,388,608)^2$ different genetic combinations. Each combination provides a different biological base for future development.

The study of the process of human development, to be complete, must begin with those events that occur prior to conception: the preparation of a suitable environment, the formation of parent cells from which the new individual is created, and the hereditary mechanisms that regulate and influence the individual's potentials for growth and development for the rest of the life cycle.

BODY GROWTH

All body growth and functioning occur on a cellular level. An understanding of the inner action of a single cell becomes basic to understanding total body growth and reproduction.

Anatomy Of A Cell

The significant parts of a human body cell include the following: (1) the cell membrane, which identifies the perimeters or boundaries of the cell system and acts as a regulator for the entrance or exit of substances into or out of the cell; (2) the cytoplasm, which carries out the work and maintenance functions of the cell; and (3) the nucleus, which functions as the administrative center for the cell—directing both the activities occurring within the cytoplasm and the reproduction of the cell or total organism. Although the appearance and the function of the nucleus remain constant from body tissue to body tissue, the cell wall and the cytoplasmic portion of body cells differ greatly according to the responsibility of that cell in total body functioning.

CYTOPLASM

The clear fluid part of the cytoplasm contains dissolved amino acids, protein molecules, electrolytes, glucose (sugar), and other elements which become the building blocks and energy sources for cellular activities. The cytoplasm also contains the centrioles, the organelles that become the foci for polar movement of chromosomes during cell divisions.

NUCLEUS

The nuclear sap contains two major structures:

1. Nucleoli. Organelles that are believed to store ribonucleic acid (RNA) until it is needed to control cytoplasmic functions.
2. Chromatin. Long, thin strands composed of nucleoproteins that contain deoxyribonucleic acid (DNA) surrounded by a protein coat. DNA, the functional portion of the chromatin, is responsible for directing all activity of the cell. These strands of chromatin shorten, thicken, and divide to form chromosomes during periods of cell division.

All normal human body cells have 46 chromosomes. The chromosomes are divided into 22 pairs of autosomes and one pair of sex chromosomes, known as "X" and "Y". Each member of a pair is similar in size and shape to its sister chromosome, except for the sex chromosomes. Although the chromosomes are invisible to the naked eye, special staining techniques and microphotography can capture the chromosomes of a single cell during the process of cell division for study purposes [3]. After enlargement, individual chromosomes are cut from the photograph, matched in pairs, and mounted on another paper; they are then grouped and labeled according to the Denver karyotype classification system (Fig. 3–2). The size and shape as well as the unique position of the centromere, a constricted area on each chromosome, are used to sort and identify individual chromosomes.

A karyotype is invaluable to the geneticist who is

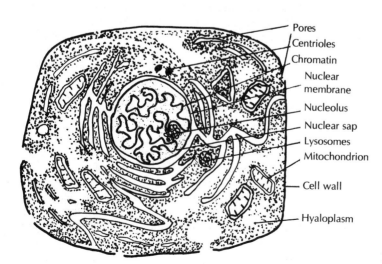

Pores
Centrioles
Chromatin
Nuclear membrane
Nucleolus
Nuclear sap
Lysosomes
Mitochondrion
Cell wall
Hyaloplasm

Figure 3–1. Anatomy of a cell.

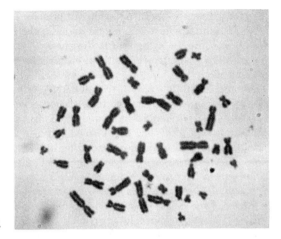

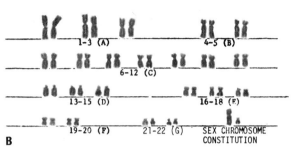

A   B

Figure 3–2. A karyotype. (A) Chromosomes during mitosis. (B) Matched, sorted, and labeled chromosomes from (A). Is this karyotype from a male or a female? Answer pages 57 and 64. (Courtesy Dr. Stella Kontras.)

looking for possible causes of hereditary defects. This process may also be used to identify a person's biological sex to determine eligibility for athletic competition. The individual who has 22 pairs of autosomes and two X chromosomes is a biological female; the individual with 22 pairs of autosomes and one X and one Y chromosome is a biological male.

Cellular Function

Cellular function—in fact, all organismic function—appears to be under the combined action of DNA and RNA. DNA, the structural unit of chromatin, controls the formation of RNA. RNA, which is free to move throughout the cell, controls protein synthesis. Together they effectively direct the characteristics and quantity of all proteins within the cell and, consequently, of the total body. In this way DNA essentially controls both cell and body functions (*Fig. 3–3*).

DEOXYRIBONUCLEIC ACID (DNA)

In 1962, James Watson and Francis Crick were awarded a Nobel Prize in medicine and physiology for their model of DNA structure. Their research indicates that DNA is composed of six basic compounds: phosphoric acid (P), deoxyribose (D) (a sugar), and four nitrogenous bases. Each of the four nitrogenous bases combines with one molecule of deoxyribose (sugar) and one molecule of phosphoric acid to form the four L-shaped nucleotides of DNA. These four nucleotides in turn form the structural units of chromosomes.

The four nucleotides are also the biochemical, functional units of DNA. When these nucleotides chain together in a long strand (template), they leave the

nitrogen base free to combine with a complementary nitrogen base of a second chain. The resultant double strand of DNA assumes the appearance of a ladder, with the nitrogenous bases comprising the rungs and the phosphoric acid and deoxyribose forming the sides or backbone of the DNA molecule [1]. Each chromosome consists of two strands of templates. Watson and Crick's model shows that this ladder is then twisted to form what has become known as the "double helix," approximating the external appearance of a twisted rope or a strand of licorice candy. Each full turn of the helix contains 10 pairs (or rungs) of nucleotides [3]. When the strands become separated, each nucleotide simply attracts its specific complementary nucleotide. This phenomenon is especially significant during reproduction, when exact replication is essential.

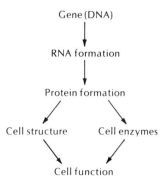

Figure 3–3. General schema by which the genes control cell function. (From A. C. Guyton, *Basic Human Physiology* [2nd ed.]. Philadelphia: Saunders, 1977. With permission.)

Code Words. The secret of control of the functioning of the cell lies in the sequential arrangement of the nucleotides in each strand of the helix. Groups of three nucleotides (triplets) form "code words". The nitrogenous bases of the DNA strand can be arranged in 64 different triplet patterns [10]. When the strands of the helix are split, the nitrogen bases of the triplets are exposed to serve as templates to control the synthesis of proteins. Each triplet pattern indicates a code word for a specific amino acid or action. Since there are only 20 known amino acids, it is postulated that most amino acids have more than one corresponding code word. Some code words are responsible for initiating and others for terminating a synthesis action. A series of triplets is necessary for formation of one protein: One code word will start the action, the next will direct placement of amino acid no. 1, the third will direct placement of amino acid no. 2, and so on until the specific protein is synthesized. The last code word will terminate the synthesis [1].

Genetic Code. The nucleotides of the DNA chains are arranged in specific sequential order to specify not only a particular amino acid but also the sequencing of amino acids within a protein molecule. The sequential arrangement of code words serves as a map to direct the actions of the cell. Each DNA strand or template is composed of multiple code word units known more simply as genes. **Genes** are units of hereditary traits, which specify the formation of proteins [3].

Since DNA is chemically bound within the chromatids of the nucleus, a second mechanism is needed to translate this plan into action. RNA becomes the mediator between the map and the action. The DNA code-word units (genes) act as templates for the formation of complementary RNA code words, or codon units. The RNA codon unit is exactly complementary to the DNA strand from which it was formed. A single strand of RNA may contain several hundred or even several thousand codons, depending on the complexity of the protein it is responsible for synthesizing [4]. It is the genetic code, then, that is translated into action by the RNA codon units.

RIBONUCLEIC ACID (RNA)

There are three basic types of RNA, each of which assumes a unique responsibility in the synthesis of a new protein:

1. **Messenger RNA** (mRNA) obtains the genetic code from the DNA strand through the process of transcription. A strand of mRNA contains the complete plan for the step-by-step production of a protein. The mRNA strand is able to migrate through the nuclear membrane into the cytoplasm to direct the sequential addition of amino acids to the protein under formation.

2. There are at least 20 types of **transfer RNA** (tRNA), one for each amino acid. Each tRNA functions as a carrier of a specific amino acid under the direction of the mRNA codon. The tRNA delivers the appropriate amino acid to the corresponding mRNA codon, thus assuring correct sequencing of amino acids within the protein molecule.

3. **Ribosomal RNA** (rRNA) is found in the ribosomal particles. Each cell is estimated to contain approximately 15,000 ribosomes [10]. It apparently reads the mRNA code and matches it with the tRNA to assure proper and smooth sequencing of amino acid additions.

CELL ACTIVITY

The proteins formed through the coordination of DNA and RNA action essentially control all other chemical reactions occurring within the cell. As seen in *Figure 3–3*, some proteins exist basically for cell growth. Thousands more become enzymes that function as organic catalysts in regulating metabolism and catabolism both within and outside the cell. Enzyme action and levels are known to have feedback and chaining effects, in which one enzyme will activate or inhibit the action of another enzyme or synthesized product. In this way, the cell and the total organism can facilitate growth, maintain homeostasis, or avoid oversynthesis of products that could become toxic in excess quantities.

One postulate offered to explain the growth of cancer cells is that a change in the genetic code has interfered with the normal feedback mechanism, allowing growth to continue unabated [4]. Random mutations or environmentally induced changes in the genetic code may reactivate repressed genes and suppress normally active genes, allowing for undifferentiated, unlimited cellular growth [9]. The abnormal genetic code is passed on to daughter cells along with other codes during cell duplication. The competition for nutrients and space by the rapidly growing cells often means death to normal (starved) cells. If vital functions are grossly disturbed, the total organism may die when it can no longer maintain homeostasis.

Mitosis

A cell can divide or reproduce in two ways. Each method has a different purpose: Cell division by the process of **meiosis** prepares a new cell for the purpose of reproducing the entire organism; this process will be discussed in the section on gametogenesis. Through the process of **mitosis,** a body cell exactly reproduces itself by forming two new or daughter cells. Some cells, such as blood cells, may duplicate themselves as rapidly as every 10 hours [4]. Muscle cells may wait several years between cell reproductions. Nerve cells do not reproduce themselves once a full complement has been established.

It is through the mitotic process that the single cell of conception becomes the complex individual capable of extrauterine survival. It is also through mitosis that the organism grows in size, repairs itself when injured, and replaces cells suffering from wear and tear. This method of cell division and duplication is a continuous process that body cells undergo as long as the life of the organism is maintained. Mitosis is divided into five phases:

1. Interphase. The majority of the life cycle of a cell is spent in this stage. At some point subtle changes begin to occur that herald the onset of active mitotic activity. During this late interphase state, the cell begins to enlarge slightly, and the centrioles begin to be pushed apart from each other by the growth of protein microtubules, or spindle threads, between them [7]. At the same time, the chromatin granules begin to condense into definable threadlike structures known as chromosomes. Since each of the 46 chromosomes produces an exact replica of itself, for a brief period there are actually 92 chromosomes in the cell. Each part of the double chromosome is known as a chromatid. This early phase may take almost 20 hours. The next four stages occur in less than one hour [7].

2. Prophase. During this stage the centrioles move to opposite poles of the cell, the nuclear membrane dis-

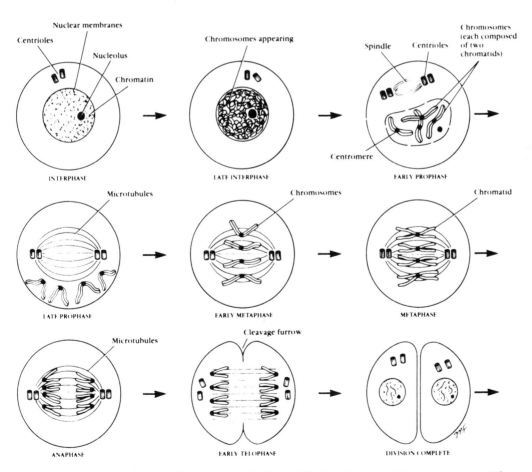

Figure 3–4. The mitotic process. (From R. S. Snell, *Clinical Histology for Medical Students.* Boston: Little, Brown, 1984. With permission.)

appears, and the chromosome structures shorten and thicken by a coiling process.

3. Metaphase. During this, the shortest phase, the double chromosomes line up on an equatorial plane midway between the two centrioles.

4. Anaphase. The microtubules or spindle threads gradually pull the double chromosome apart. One chromatid, or daughter chromosome, goes toward each centriole. In this way each set of daughter chromosomes is an exact duplicate of the other.

5. Telophase. As the chromatids are pulled closer to the centriole, the spindle threads begin to disappear. A nuclear membrane begins to form around the daughter chromosomes. At the same time, the cytoplasm begins to pinch itself off at the equatorial plane, and the centriole replicates itself in preparation for the next active mitotic phase. The daughter cells thus formed enter the interphase.

REPRODUCTION

Each individual begins life as a single cell that is formed by the union of two gametes—a sperm and an ovum (egg). If gametes were produced through the process of mitosis, then each gamete would bring 46 chromosomes to the union, and the new individual would have a total of 92. It is obvious that a different process is needed to ensure that the new individual has only 46 chromosomes. Gametes, or half-cells, are produced in the reproductive system through a specialized process of cell division and chromosome reduction known as meiosis.

Gametogenesis

Production of both the sperm and the ovum is accomplished by the same basic maturational stages—the meiotic process. The meiotic divisional phases are very similar to the mitotic phases, but the process requires two cell divisions rather than one in order to accomplish reduction of the chromosome numbers. The daughter cells will contain only one chromosome from each original chromosome pair.

Immature (primary) germ cells contain 46 chromosomes. During the first meiotic division, the chromosomes duplicate themselves, forming 46 chromatid pairs (92 chromosomes). The sister chromatids remain attached. A nuclear membrane forms around the 23 double chromosomes. This new cell contains 46 chromatids—23 of which are the exact duplicates of the other 23 chromatids.

During the second meiotic division, there is no du-

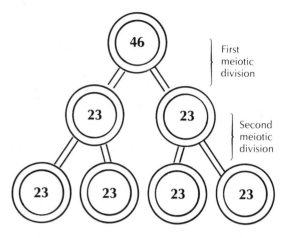

Figure 3–5. The meiotic process.

plication of chromosomes; the chromatid pairs are divided equally between the two new cells, and the meiotic process is then complete. Each original primary germ cell produces four daughter cells, each with 23 chromosomes (haploid cells).

The meiotic process describes the distribution of chromosomes among the new nuclei. However, cytoplasmic distribution is quite different in the gametogenesis of the sperm versus that of the ovum, and thus the two will be given separate attention.

FEMALE REPRODUCTIVE SYSTEM

Anatomy. The female reproductive system consists of four major organs:

1. The ovaries, which produce the ovum or egg and the female hormones estrogen and progesterone.
2. The fallopian tubes, which transport the mature ovum from the ovary to the uterus.
3. The uterus, which protects and nurtures the developing fetus from conception to birth. The three major divisions of the uterus—the fundus (top), body, and cervix (neck)—become most significant during the childbirth process.
4. The vagina, which provides an access route for the sperm and an exit route for the baby.

The ovarian cycle. The ovarian cycle consists of a complex series of changes in the ovary and in the hormonal balance of the female organism. These changes are cyclic in nature and are usually repeated at 21- to

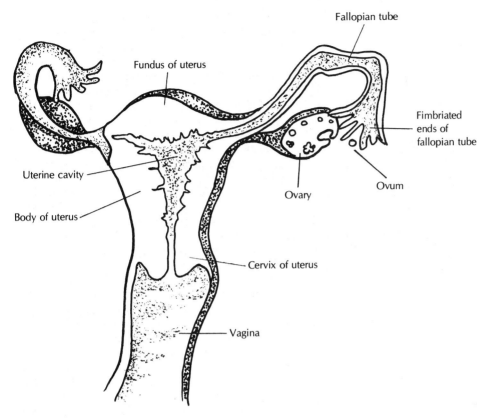

Figure 3–6. The female reproductive system.

35-day intervals for the purpose of reproduction. The cycle consists of two phases, which are distinctly separated by the phenomena of ovulation and menstruation.

Prefollicular Phase. Prior to the onset of the ovarian cycle (at puberty), the female organism has already laid the foundation for the process of reproduction. Before she is even born—in fact, by the fifth month of fetal life—the female organism already has 7 million immature ova [8], all the ova she will ever produce. From this point the number begins to diminish. It is estimated that the female infant at birth has approximately 2 million primary oocytes (immature ova), and the 7-year-old girl has 200,000 [8]. By the time she reaches puberty, only about 100,000 primary oocytes will remain [12]. However, since (usually) only one ovum is allowed to mature per cycle, it is obvious that even this number is more than adequate and that many will never reach maturity. During the reproductive life of the female, only about 400 ova will mature to the stage where fertilization is possible.

It is significant to note that the immature ovum may be present in the body for 20, 30, or 40 years before it matures and may be subject to many misfortunes in the meantime. Consequently, the older the ovum (or the maternal organism), the greater are the chances of producing a defective mature ovum. Very young as well as older mothers experience an increased risk of defective offspring owing to deviations in the meiotic process.

Follicular Phase. The follicular phase is under the control of follicle-stimulating hormone (FSH), which is produced by the anterior pituitary. The pituitary gland is a small reddish body located in the brain just behind the root of the nose. The anterior or frontal section of this gland secretes its hormones directly into the bloodstream. The target organ of FSH is the ovary, and in particular, the immature primary follicle. Under the influence of FSH, 15 to 20 of the primary follicles begin to mature, but by some mechanism that is not yet understood, only one becomes a mature graafian follicle.

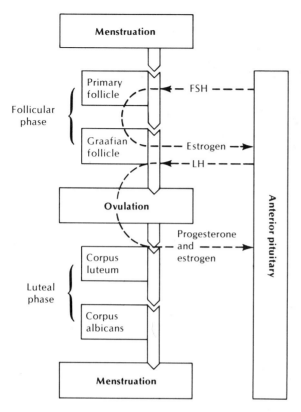

Figure 3–7. The ovarian cycle. Hormonal relationship between the ovary and the anterior pituitary gland.

The **graafian follicle** enlarges as it fills with follicular fluid. The layer of cells surrounding the ovum thickens by developing several layers and gradually moves the follicle toward the surface of the ovary. The inner layer of cells, known as the **theca interna,** secretes the hormone, estrogen, into the follicular fluid [12]. The immature ovum, which has undergone the first meiotic division during fetal life, resumes its maturational process at this time.

Estrogen is absorbed by the bloodstream and enters the general body circulation. It causes growth of the **endometrium,** or lining of the uterus, by thickening and vascularization. Another major target organ of estrogen is the anterior pituitary: Estrogen suppresses the production of FSH by the anterior pituitary. At the same time, estrogen stimulates the anterior pituitary to produce luteinizing hormone (LH). This is only one example of the delicate feedback mechanisms that occur among many organs of the body to maintain homeostasis—normal, rhythmic function of the total body.

Ovulation. The walls of the graafian follicle thin as it continues to expand in size and to move toward the surface of the ovary. At full maturity, the follicle may reach one-half inch in diameter [12]. The stigma, a small area on the center of this swelling, protrudes like a tiny nipple. A large amount of LH is released the day before ovulation; this LH surge appears to stimulate rapid follicular growth [4]. The follicle ruptures at the stigma, causing extrusion or release of the ovum—the phenomenon known as **ovulation.**

Ovulation may be accompanied by **mittelschmerz** in some women. This momentary midpain may be very mild or quite sharp; it may pass unnoticed, or it may cause enough discomfort to awaken the woman from sleep or cause her to gasp and double over momentarily in spontaneous response to the unexpected discomfort. Some women experience vaginal spotting or a dull lower abdominal aching due to a small amount of bleeding that may accompany the rupture of the follicle.

The increase in estrogen levels causes changes in the vaginal secretions and in the mucous plug that blocks the cervix. At ovulation, when estrogen levels are highest, these secretions become thinner, clearer, more copious, and more elastic. Viscosity and pH also change, making the environment receptive to penetration by the sperm and facilitating their entrance into the female reproductive system.

Basal metabolic temperature (the body temperature at rest) elevates after ovulation. If one asks a large group of women how many of them feel cold in a room (temperature about 70°F) and how many feel warm, almost all those who feel cold will be in the follicular phase of the ovarian cycle; those who feel warm will probably be in the postovulatory or luteal phase of the ovarian cycle. Basal body temperature change is due to the presence of progesterone, a hormone secreted during the luteal phase. Changes in body temperature as related to hormonal balance are discussed in greater detail in Chapter 31 in the section on contraception.

After the ovum is extruded from the graafian follicle, it is at the mercy of the unique structure of the reproductive system, since it has no means of propelling itself to the uterus. Three features of the fallopian tubes seem to be significant in transporting the ovum to the uterine cavity: (1) the fimbriated ends, (2) the cilia lining, and (3) the peristaltic movements. The fingerlike projections on the end of the tubes move and appear to set up a current that draws the ovum to it. The cilia move like the oars of a scull boat or like wind blowing over a field of grain. The peristaltic movements are muscular contractions that move in waves down a tube and propel an object before them, like an ostrich swallowing a golf ball, or a snake swallowing a mouse.

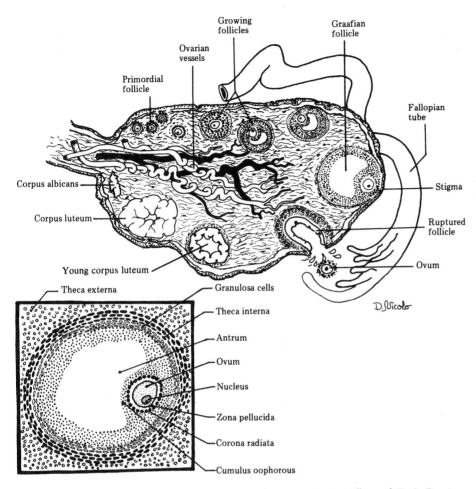

Figure 3–8. Ovarian changes during the ovarian cycle. (From M. A. Miller and D. A. Brooten, *The Childbearing Family: A Nursing Perspective* [2nd ed.]. Boston: Little, Brown, 1983. With permission.)

Luteal Phase. After the extrusion of the ovum, the graafian follicle collapses under the influence of LH and becomes a yellow-colored, solid tissue mass known as the **corpus luteum.** FSH production by the anterior pituitary ceases. The corpus luteum continues to produce estrogen but now also begins to produce progesterone. The corpus luteum has a life span of 8 to 10 days; at this point it begins to deteriorate, and secretion of estrogen and progesterone ceases. LH production by the anterior pituitary also ceases. The yellow tissue of the corpus luteum is replaced by a white connective tissue known as the **corpus albicans.** If the ovum is fertilized and a pregnancy is achieved, the corpus luteum will continue to secrete estrogen and progesterone for 3 to 4 months (see Chap. 4).

Menstruation. One of the major functions of progesterone is to prepare the uterus to receive and to nourish a fertilized ovum. Progesterone causes an increase in the secretions and the depth of the endometrial lining of the uterus. When the secretion of both estrogen and progesterone by the corpus luteum ceases, this endometrial lining begins to degenerate and slough off; this is the phenomenon known as menstruation (see Chap. 25). At this point the entire cycle begins to repeat itself. The anterior pituitary will resume production of FSH until the estrogen levels are once again elevated.

Length of Cycle. One cannot predict the length of the follicular phase (menstruation to ovulation) except to make an estimation based on the history of the individual woman. Although it would be very helpful to know exactly when ovulation will occur, many increases in family size bear testimony to the fact that someone's calculations were in error. The luteal phase (ovulation to menstruation), on the other hand, is predictable because of the life span of the corpus luteum. The luteal phase is 12 to 14 days in length. Because of the variation in the length of the follicular phase, the total cycle varies in length with each woman. Most women start a new cycle every 28 ± 7 days. The day of ovulation can be estimated by subtracting 12 to 14 days from the day menstruation is expected to begin. If a woman normally has a 22-day cycle, then ovulation would probably occur between days 8 and 10 (using the first day of the menstrual period as day 1 of the cycle). A woman who has a 32-day cycle would most likely ovulate between days 18 and 20 of the cycle.

Oogenesis. By the time of birth, the primordial germ cells have already begun the process of meiotic maturation. In fact, they have advanced to a late prophase stage of cell division [5,7]. Maturation of the primary oocyte is held in abeyance at this point. The first meiotic division is not completed until the time of ovulation, when the ovum leaves the graafian follicle as a secondary oocyte. Cellular division is very unequal: The nuclear contents are equally divided, but all the cytoplasmic material goes to one daughter cell. The other daughter cell is known as a **polar body.** The first polar body usually degenerates immediately but may go on to replicate itself during the second meiotic division. The second meiotic division of the ovum does not occur until after the sperm has penetrated the cytoplasm [5,7]. The second meiotic division also produces a nonfunctioning polar body; the cytoplasm remains with the pronucleus, which will join with the sperm's pronucleus.

Through meiosis, one ovum and two or three polar bodies are produced with each ovarian cycle. The ovum is the only one of the four resultant haploid (half) cells that is capable of being fertilized. It has received not only an equal division of the chromosomes, but also a majority of the cytoplasm and nourishment contained in the original germ cell. The polar bodies are of no significance; they may be retained briefly before degeneration.

MALE REPRODUCTIVE SYSTEM

Anatomy. The male reproductive system consists of five major parts and several accessory organs:

1. The testes, which produce spermatozoa and the male hormone, testosterone
   a. The seminiferous tubules, which produce the sperm
   b. Leydig cells, which produce the testosterone
   c. The epididymis, which stores sperm until maturation is complete and the sperm become mobile

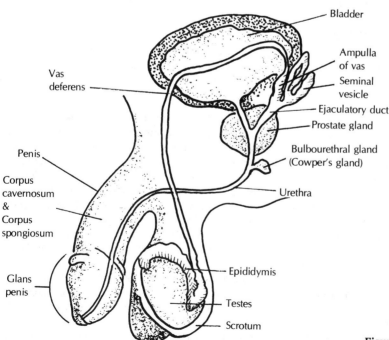

Figure 3–9. The male reproductive system.

2. The vas deferens, which is the excretory duct and storage area for mature sperm
3. The seminal vesicles, which discharge a fluid at the time of ejaculation of sperm that facilitates mobility and provides nutrition for the sperm
4. The ejaculatory duct, which is the excretory duct that allows passage of the sperm to the urethra
5. The penis, which is the male organ for copulation and urinary excretion
   a. The urethra, which provides an exit route for the sperm
   b. Erectile tissue, which, on distention of its large sinuses with blood, causes the penis to become firm and erect

Accessory organs that add fluids to the semen include the prostate gland and the bulbourethral (Cowper's) glands.

Spermatogenesis. Unlike the cyclic production of the single ovum by the female, in the male millions of sperm are continuously in various stages of maturation. Spermatogenesis occurs in the seminiferous tubules of the testes. The inner surfaces of these tubules are lined with both spermatogonia (primary germ cells) and Sertoli cells. As they mature, the spermatogonium cells gradually move toward the lumen of the tubules, the first and second meiotic divisions occurring as they migrate toward the surface. The spermatids produced by the second meiotic division become embedded in the outer surface of a Sertoli cell; here they undergo metamorphic changes that transform them into spermatozoa. The cytoplasmic material gradually dissipates, and a flagellum, or tail, grows at one end. The nucleus of the sperm remains located in its head portion. The anterior portion is covered by the acrosome cap. On completion of the maturational process (a process that takes approximately 3 weeks from spermatogonium to spermatozoon), the sperm are released into the lumen of the epididymis for storage. Spermatogenesis is a continuous process after puberty. Each primary germ cell produces four spermatozoa, each of which is potentially capable of joining with an ovum to create a new life.

Hormonal control. As in the female, the anterior pituitary of the male also produces FSH and LH. These hormones have different actions on the target organs,

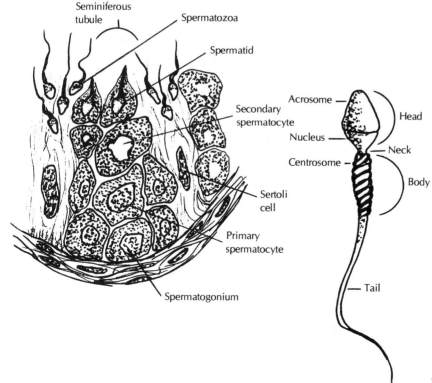

Figure 3–10. Spermatogenesis.

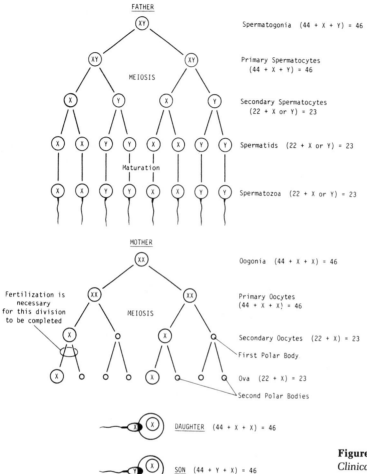

Figure 3–11. Gametogenesis. (From R. S. Snell, *Clinical Embryology for Medical Students* [3rd ed.]. Boston: Little, Brown, 1983. With permission.)

however. LH stimulates the Leydig cells of the testes to produce testosterone, and FSH stimulates the production of spermatozoa. However, each of these gonadotropic hormones potentiates the action of the other. In both the male and the female, the gonadotropic hormone FSH stimulates maturation of the gamete; LH stimulates production of the appropriate gender-associated hormone by the gonad.

Conception

After extrusion from the ovary, the ovum slowly starts its journey through the fallopian tube toward the uterus. Fertilization generally occurs in the outer one-third of the fallopian tube. The acrosome cap of the sperm releases the enzyme, hyaluronidase, which digests the outer protective coat of the ovum to gain entrance. Many spermatozoa may enter the outer coat (zona pellucida); however, only one is allowed entrance through the cell membrane. Once this entrance has occurred, all other sperm are rejected. The fertilized ovum becomes known as the conceptus or zygote.

FERTILITY PERIOD

The ovum is viable, or capable of joining with the sperm, for about 12 to 24 hours. Once the sperm has entered the female reproductive tract, it may be viable for as long as 48 to 72 hours. Therefore, sperm that have entered the reproductive tract as long as 2 days before ovulation may still be able to fertilize the ovum shortly after ovulation. Sperm that have been introduced within 22 hours after ovulation may also result in conception (this figure allows for 2 hours of travel time). Although some women may believe as a result of their personal experience that conception can occur at any point during the ovarian cycle, there are actually only about 90 hours per cycle when intercourse can result in conception. Other points of time during

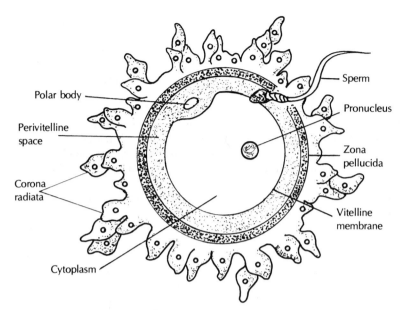

Figure 3–12. Conception.

the ovarian cycle are "safe." However, as mentioned earlier, the crucial factor is still to pinpoint when ovulation will or does occur.

When the male and female gametes join to form a new, complete cell, the ovum immediately repels and prevents the admission of all other sperm; the nuclei join; the chromosomes are paired; the gender of the new individual is determined; and a new life begins. After a brief rest, the new cell begins the mitotic process. This is the only whole cell capable of cell division that will produce a separate individual. Through the process of mitosis, this single cell will become a moving, breathing, crying newborn infant and, eventually, a biologically mature adult capable of repeating the process of reproduction.

GENDER DETERMINATION

The female can only produce ova containing 22 autosomes and the X sex chromosome. Males, because of the XY sex chromosome configuration, will produce sperm with 22 autosomes and either the X or the Y sex chromosome. It is the sperm, therefore, that determines the gender of the new individual, as shown below:

ovum	sperm	new individual
22 + X	22 + X	= 44 + XX = female
22 + X	22 + Y	= 44 + XY = male

Knowing that half of the sperm contain the male chromosome, one would predict that 50 percent of babies would be male; however, for unknown reasons, males have a slightly higher conception and birth rate than females. Nevertheless, a higher male infant and childhood mortality rate results in a greater number of women than men in the world [7].

INHERITANCE

During metaphase of the first meiotic division, each pair of chromosomes is randomly divided, with the two members of each pair migrating to opposite centriole poles. This independent, random division of the 46 chromosomes from each parent offers at the time of union of the gametes a possibility of 8,388, 608 (2^{23}) × 8,388,608 (2^{23}) different chromosomal combinations. Only identical twins (formed from the same fertilized ovum) have the exact same karyotype. This process of chromosomal division, transmission, and mixing accounts for both the continuity and the variations in characteristics found in families and in the human race.

Because of this random selection of chromosomes from the parents, and the difference in physical traits exhibited by the parents, the question arises of what happens when parents display different characteristics for the same trait. It is evident that some rules must govern which special characteristics of a trait the offspring will exhibit. Characteristics are inherited according to specific laws, and the possibility of their occurrence in a new individual can be predicted.

Mendelian Laws

During the 1850s, Gregor Mendel (1822–1884), an Austrian monk, discovered the laws of inheritance by working with pea plants. He noted that certain characteristics were transmitted to the offspring in an orderly, predictable manner. Mendel published his findings in an obscure source in 1866, where they were rediscovered around the turn of the century. Although the intricacies of the process of inheritance are not yet completely understood, Mendel's basic laws of inheritance still form the foundation for the study of genetics today [7].

GENE THEORY

As previously discussed, **gene** is the name given to the section of a chromosome (DNA) that is responsible for the formation of a specific protein [3]. The growth and functioning of cells are the direct or indirect result of protein formation and enzymatic action; consequently, every hereditary trait is under the influence of one or more genes. The genetic code that is responsible for a given trait occupies a unique position or locus on the chromosomes of a pair of matching chromosomes. Re-

searchers have been able to map the location of some of the genes for specific traits through special techniques [5]. Genes that produce alternative characteristics for a specific trait are known as alleles. Alleles affect the same target organ, tissue, or cell.

GENOTYPE VERSUS PHENOTYPE

Alleles become paired when the chromosomes of the gametes join (genotype). Although the target tissue is the same, the genetic code held by one member of the pair may not be the same as the blueprint held by the other allele.

When the offspring receives the same genetic code from each parent for a specific trait, he is said to have a homozygous (matching) genotype. The traits exhibited by the individual (phenotype) will obviously be the same as those carried by the matching genes. When the offspring receives a different genetic code from each parent for a specific trait, he is said to have a heterozygous (mixed) genotype. Only one of the characteristics can be expressed; the one that is exhibited is said to be **dominant**. The gene that is not displayed is said to be **recessive**. These concepts will be explored in the next section with specific examples.

Other factors besides clear-cut recessiveness or dominance of a gene may affect the phenotype of an

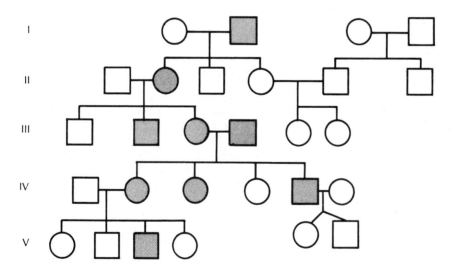

Figure 3–13. Hypothetical model of inheritance of a dominant characteristic, such as polydactyly. Small squares designate males; circles designate females. Horizontal lines connecting a square and a circle indicate matings. Vertical lines indicate offspring. Twins are indicated by an inverted V. Roman numerals along the left-hand side are used to indicate generation. Individuals exhibiting the phenotype are indicated by filling in the circle or the square. Known or suspected carriers are indicated by a dot or by filling in one-half of the gender indicator.

individual. There may be a wide spectrum of characteristics for a trait with various levels of dominance in relation to each other. Traits under the influence of several allele pairs are known as polygenetic: skin, hair, and eye color are good examples. A blending of traits rather than clear-cut dominance will be exhibited.

Rh factor. If an individual receives two genes for Rh-positive blood, he will have an Rh-positive phenotype:

Rh positive (P) + Rh positive (P) = Rh positive (PP)
(genotype)   (phenotype)

But what happens when the offspring receives alternative genetic characteristics for a specific trait, for instance, one gene for Rh-positive blood and one for Rh-negative blood? He is said to be heterozygous for that trait. When an individual possesses a heterozygous genotype, only one characteristic will be exhibited. Mendel discovered that certain characteristics will always be exhibited if the individual carries the gene for that trait. Rh-positive blood is one such dominant characteristic:

Rh positive (P) + Rh negative (n) = Rh positive (Pn)
(genotype)   (phenotype)

A recessive characteristic will exhibit its presence only if both genes are identical for that trait (homozygous):

Rh negative (n) + Rh negative (n) = Rh negative (nn)
(genotype)   (phenotype)

Going back to the original question, what happens when parents display different characteristics for the same trait? The Rh-negative parent is obviously homozygous for Rh-negative blood and therefore can only give a gene for Rh-negative blood to any offspring. If the other parent is homozygous for Rh-positive blood, then all the offspring will have Rh-positive blood. The children will have a heterozygous genotype for the trait, but because of the dominance of Rh positive over Rh negative, they will exhibit a phenotype of Rh-positive blood:

	Rh pos (P)	Rh pos (P)
Rh neg (n)	Pn	Pn
Rh neg (n)	Pn	Pn

If the Rh-positive parent is heterozygous for the blood trait, then 50 percent of the offspring may express the recessive phenotype:

	Rh pos (P)	Rh neg (n)
Rh neg (n)	Pn	nn
Rh neg (n)	Pn	nn

Can two Rh-positive parents have a Rh-negative child? Yes, if they are both heterozygous for the trait. Twenty-five percent of the children may have Rh-negative blood:

	Rh pos (P)	Rh neg (n)
Rh pos (P)	PP	nP
Rh neg (n)	nP	nn

It is significant to note that a recessive characteristic for a trait may pass from generation to generation without ever exhibiting itself and then suddenly "crop up out of nowhere." If such a trait is undesirable, one might like to think that it came from "the other side of the family." However, since a person must possess two genes for a recessive characteristic before it will exhibit itself in phenotype, one gene must come from each parent (see Fig. 3–14).

Sickle cell anemia. Some genes may show incomplete dominance; sickle cell anemia is an excellent example. Fifty thousand to 100,000 Blacks in the United States are homozygous for this trait. One out of 10 Blacks are heterozygous [8]. The red blood cells of the persons who are homozygous for the characteristic exhibit sickling when exposed to lowered oxygen tensions [8]. Persons who are heterozygous for the characteristic may exhibit mild symptoms (sickle cell trait) or no symptoms at all. As a result of incomplete dominance for the characteristic, heterozygous persons usually have some red blood cells that are affected by the characteristic. Blood testing procedures have been developed that allow for identification of carriers.

Sex-linked characteristics. Recessive characteristics carried on the X or Y chromosomes are known as sex-linked. X-linked characteristics will usually show up only in male offspring because there is no dominant gene to mask the effect of the recessive gene for the trait (see Fig. 3–15). Red-green color blindness, muscular dystrophy, baldness, and some types of hemophilia are probably the best known examples [8], although more than 65 different X-linked traits have been described [3]. All female offspring of an affected male will be carriers of the trait; the heterozygous genotype of the female masks the fact that she is a carrier

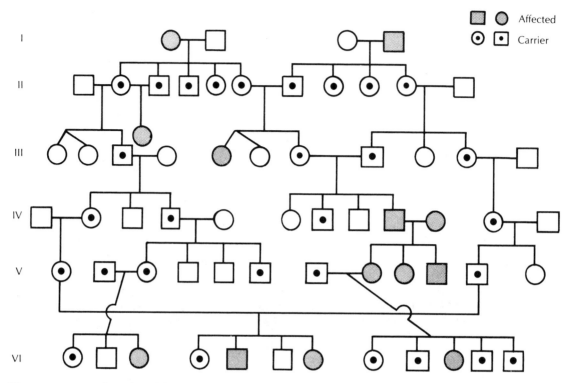

Figure 3–14. Hypothetical model of inheritance of a recessive trait, such as albinism.

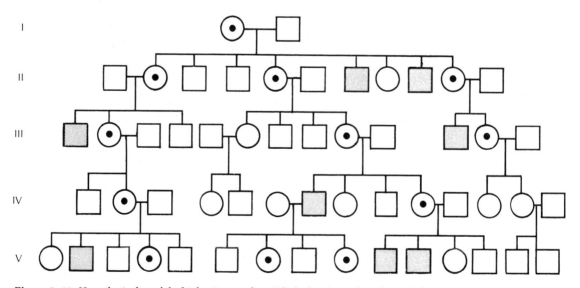

Figure 3–15. Hypothetical model of inheritance of an X-linked trait, such as hemophilia.

for the characteristic. In the following diagrams, X^h stands for a hemophilia carrier chromosome and X^H for a normal chromosome.

		normal male	
	X^H	Y	
carrier	X^H	$X^H X^H$	$Y X^H$
female	X^h	$X^H X^h$	$Y X^h$

$Y X^h$ = affected male

The female offspring of an affected male may also exhibit the trait if the mother is a carrier.

		affected male	
	X^h	Y	
carrier	X^H	$X^h X^H$	$Y X^H$
female	X^h	$X^h X^h$	$Y X^h$

$X^h X^h$ = affected female

Sex-linked traits carried on the Y chromosome are passed directly from the father to all male offspring but never to a daughter. At this time, only the genes for the H-Y antigen and the testis-determining factor are known to be Y-linked [7]. Hypertrichosis, or hairiness of the pinna of the ear, is suspected of being Y-linked, but the interdependence of genes can alter the expression, and clear association with the Y chromosome is not yet established.

Blood type. Codominance is observed with some genotypes; blood typing is probably the best example. Four major blood type groupings are known: A, B, O, and AB. Type O is recessive to both A and B; however, when genes for A and B are received from opposite parents, the blood of the offspring will contain both A and B antigens:

	A	O		A	A
B	AB	OB	B	AB	AB
O	AO	OO	O	AO	AO

	A	O		A	A
B	AB	OB	B	AB	AB
B	AB	OB	B	AB	AB

If both parents are type O, then all offspring will be type O. If both parents have AB blood type, none of the offspring will have type O:

	O	O		A	B
O	OO	OO	A	AA	BA
O	OO	OO	B	AB	BB

Blood typing cannot be used to prove parentage, but it can be used to rule out parentage—a useful piece of knowledge in a court of law.

Mutations. Occasionally mutations will occur. A **mutation** is a random but permanent change in the code of a specific gene and, as such, is transmissible to offspring. Many of these changes are relatively insignificant and may account for the occasional situation in which an unexplainable trait or a dominant characteristic appears in the offspring of parents expressing a recessive phenotype. Mutations can account for many minor variations of phenotype. Other mutations, however, may lead to diseases and malformations. A change in just one codon of a gene will change the corresponding amino acid added to the forming protein chain and thus can produce abnormalities in many organs or even result in the death of the individual [1]. Sickle cell anemia is an example. It is estimated that 10 percent of congenital malformations are a result of gene mutation. Phenotype depends on the genes affected.

Pedigrees

Pedigree analysis can be used to trace the occurrence of a trait through multiple generations. Through such tracings, the geneticist can often identify whether a trait is dominant, recessive, polygenetic, or sex-linked.

Dominant traits are fairly easy to trace, since they show up in every generation. There is a 50-percent probability that the offspring will exhibit the trait if one parent is heterozygous for the characteristic. Polydactyly is a good example of a dominant trait. However, because the extra finger or fingers are usually professionally removed in very early infancy, many family members are unaware that the trait has appeared in their family.

Recessive traits are more difficult to trace. An affected individual will have all normal offspring if the mate is not a carrier; consequently, a trait may skip two, three, or more generations. Carriers can be identified only in retrospect. Because they draw from the same genetic pool, the offspring of consanguineous parents have a much greater chance of exhibiting a recessive trait.

Figure 3–14 shows the inheritance of the recessive trait of albinism, which results from a failure to synthesize the enzyme, tyrosinase [5]. This enzyme is essential to the formation of skin, hair, and eye pigments. Lack of pigmentation allows the color of the blood to be seen through the skin and eyes, giving them a pinkish hue.

Chromosomal Alterations

Inheritance as discussed so far has dealt with the transmission of a single gene—the genetic code for a specific trait as mediated through protein formation. Changes in the genetic code (mutations) can occur without affecting the overall structure of the chromosome. However, structural changes of the chromosome itself may occur during either the mitotic or the meiotic process. Such changes are particularly significant if they occur during the meiotic process, since they can be responsible for major variations in human characteristics or can lead to severe congenital malformations (birth defects). Other changes in chromosome configuration may create such severe disruptions in the catalytic action of RNA as to be incompatible with life.

CROSSOVER

When crossover occurs, the parts of one pair of chromosomes are evenly exchanged during cell division. This crossing often explains the occurrence of blue eyes with black hair or brown eyes with blonde hair. This phenomenon cannot always be identified through karyotype examination. The first generation offspring will be normal, but second generation offspring may have gross abnormalities because of an imbalance of specific genetic material.

TRANSLOCATION AND DELETION

When a piece of one chromosome is broken off and becomes attached to another, the resultant division of chromosomal material between the two centrioles is uneven. One new nucleus contains chromatin material that has been translocated to a new chromosome, resulting in extra genetic material in the nucleus. The nucleus receiving the chromosome with deleted chromatin material will be deficient in genetic material. The effect on the individual depends not only on the amount of genetic material deleted or translocated but also on which genetic codes are so affected. These

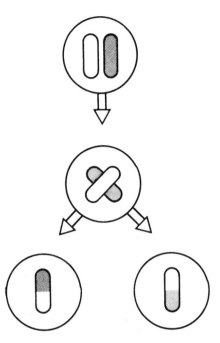

Figure 3–16. Crossover. The chromosomes exchange parts during the process of cell division.

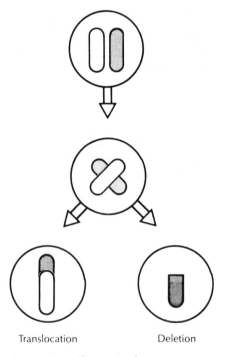

Translocation   Deletion

Figure 3–17. Changes in chromosome structure. Part of one chromosome becomes attached to another during cell division.

phenomena can be identified through karyotype examination.

NONDISJUNCTION

Occasionally during cell division a pair of chromosomes will fail to separate. Both chromosomes will go to only one daughter cell. If this occurs during meiosis, one gamete will contain 24 chromosomes, the other 22 chromosomes. When this gamete joins with a normal gamete, the new individual may have three chromosomes for one pair, **trisomy** (total 47 chromosomes), or only one chromosome for a pair, **monosomy** (total 45 chromosomes). Nondisjunction can occur with either the autosomes or the sex chromosomes. Clinically identifiable syndromes are associated with an abnormal count of specific chromosomes.

A nondisjunction that occurs after conception and during the early days of life can cause the phenomenon known as **mosaicism.** Some of the systems of the body are normal; other systems have an abnormal chromosome count. The effect on the total individual is determined by how many systems are affected by the abnormal chromosome count and which chromosome pair is involved in the nondisjunction.

Down's syndrome (mongolism) may be the result of any of three different phenomena: translocation, meiotic nondisjunction, or mitotic nondisjunction. All three factors result in extra genetic material from chromosome number 21.

CONCLUSION

The growth and functioning of individual cells and of the total body are highly dependent on the genetic code inherited from the parents. The DNA chains comprising the chromosomes of each cell essentially direct all biological functioning of the body, striving to maintain adaptive equilibrium in the healthy body. However, environmental factors can also influence the quality of life. Reasonable health care, particularly good nutrition, is essential to ensure that the body has the essential ingredients available for translating the genetic code into body proteins and enzymes. The chemicals that affect the body through environmental pollution or by ingestion are known to inhibit this process or to initiate mutations and chromosomal alterations. X-rays are a major precipitator of mutations and chromosomal abnormalities. These environmental factors will be discussed in Chapter 4.

An understanding of the genetic inheritance of characteristics can be very valuable in counseling parents, in planning one's own family, or in a court of law. When parents have an impaired child, they want to

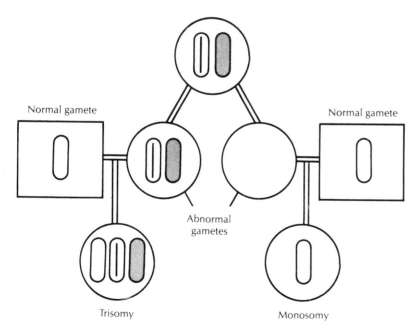

Normal gamete   Normal gamete

Abnormal
gametes

Trisomy   Monosomy

Figure 3–18. Changes in chromosome number. Both members of a pair of chromosomes go to the same daughter cell during cell division.

know the probability of having a second child with the same defect. A pedigree analysis can give valuable information on the inheritance pattern for a particular characteristic or a defect in a family. However, one should keep in mind that inheritance of a particular trait cannot be definitely predicted, except in the case in which both parents exhibit the phenotype of a recessive characteristic. Due to the independent nature of meiotic chromosomal division, the inheritance of any characteristic is based on random probability—not on an established pattern. Students who are interested in pursuing this topic in greater depth are encouraged to take a course in genetics. Those individuals seeking a source for genetic counseling may contact either of the following organizations:

1. The March of Dimes Birth Defects Foundation
   1275 Mamaroneck Avenue
   White Plains, N.Y. 10605
   (914-428-7100)

2. The National Genetics Foundation
   555 West 57th St.
   New York, N.Y. 10019
   (212-759-4432)

REFERENCES

1. Brewer, G. J., and Sing, C. F. *Genetics.* Reading, MA: Addison-Wesley, 1983.
2. Burns, G. W. *The Science of Genetics: An Introduction to Heredity* (5th ed.). New York: Macmillan, 1983.
3. Goodenough, U. *Genetics* (3rd ed.). Philadelphia: Saunders, 1984.
4. Guyton, A. C. *Basic Human Physiology: Normal Function and Mechanisms of Disease* (2nd ed.). Philadelphia: Saunders, 1977.
5. Levitan, M., and Montagu, A. *Textbook of Human Genetics* (2nd ed.). New York: Oxford University Press, 1977.
6. Lowrey, G. H. *Growth and Development of Children* (7th ed.). Chicago: Year Book, 1978.
7. Mange, A. P., and Mange, E. J. *Genetics: Human Aspects.* Philadelphia: Saunders, 1980.
8. Novitski, E. *Human Genetics* (2nd ed.). New York: Macmillan, 1982.
9. Pai, A. C., and Marcus-Roberts, H. *Genetics: Its Concepts and Implications.* Englewood Cliffs, NJ: Prentice-Hall, 1981.
10. Redei, G. P. *Genetics.* New York: Macmillan, 1982.
11. Villee, C. A. *Biology: The Human Approach* (7th ed.). Philadelphia: Saunders, 1977.
12. Ziegel, E., and Cranley, M. S. *Obstetric Nursing* (8th ed.). New York: Macmillan, 1984.

Answer to question in Figure 3–2: The sex chromosomes are markedly different in size, therefore an XY configuration. The karyotype indicates a male genetic makeup.

4
Intrauterine Development

Clara S. Schuster

For no king had any other first beginning;
But all men have one entrance into life,
And a like departure. . . .

—The Wisdom of Solomon, The Apocrypha

In just 9 months, the single-cell fertilized ovum is transformed into a complex system of approximately **15 trillion** (15,000,000,000,000) cells [41] possessing a synchrony of function capable of sustaining life outside the uterus. This physical growth is accomplished by more than simple mitosis. Although the nuclear material is exactly duplicated with each cell division, the cytoplasm and cell membranes differentiate so that each cell, tissue, organ, and system of the body is uniquely constructed to carry out a specific function for the entire organism.

Growth of the biophysical domain is accomplished through two major processes:

1. Hyperplasia. Through the mitotic process, the number of cells increases. The size of the cells remains small.
2. Hypertrophy. The number of cells remains constant, but the size of individual cells increases. The cytoplasmic portion of the cell is free to increase in size, but the nuclear size remains constant.

During the early days and weeks of intrauterine life, hyperplastic growth predominates. Mitosis allows for an increase in body mass, while the genetic code guides the differentiation of cellular structure. Hypertrophic growth begins to predominate during the later days and weeks of intrauterine life. Hyperplastic and hypertrophic growth continue throughout life. Hyperplastic growth during later years allows for replacement and repair of cells, rather than body growth.

The study of prenatal development can help us to understand the normal relationship of body structures and the causes of some malformations. The miracle of creation is awesome if we consider even a fraction of the intricate chemical reactions patterned by deoxyribonucleic acid (DNA) units, acknowledge the chains of reactions mediated by messenger ribonucleic acid (mRNA), and then observe some of the factors that can interrupt those delicate processes!

DEVELOPMENT OF THE CONCEPTUS

The 9-month gestational period is divided into three 3-month periods, known as trimesters. During the first trimester (conception to 12 weeks), cells begin to differentiate through the mitotic process into systems and organs. The new individual undergoes very rapid growth in both number and configuration of cells. All the basic systems are developed, and the biological foundations for life are established. Because of this very rapid growth and differentiation of cells, the organism is extremely sensitive to insults that can stop or alter the growth pattern.

During the second trimester (13 to 24 weeks), the fetus experiences continued growth and further tissue differentiation. There is a gradual increase in the functional abilities of all body structures and systems. The growth in length is rapid, but body mass remains relatively small. At the end of this trimester, the fetus may be able to sustain extrauterine life if provided with intensive medical and nursing intervention.

During the third trimester (25 weeks to birth), the systems and organs continue to develop to a stage where they can function adaptively outside the uterus. Body weight increases more rapidly than body length. The fetus begins to store up fat, iron, and other minerals in preparation for birth and independent living.

Zygote Stage

For the first week after conception, the conceptus is identified as a zygote. The fertilized ovum rests briefly following union with the sperm. Approximately 30 hours after fertilization, the first division or cleavage occurs. Since the two new daughter cells are smaller than the original parent cell, the entire organism does not increase in size. The four-cell stage is reached at about 40 hours, the 12- to 16-cell stage at about 60 hours [15]. The entire solid mass, now known as as morula,

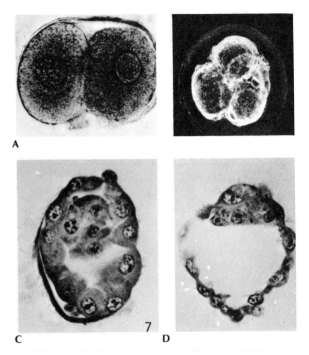

A

C   D

Figure 4–1. Early development of the zygote. (A) Intact two-cell conceptus, showing zona pellucida and two polar bodies. (B) Intact four-cell conceptus. The granular zona pellucida can be distinquished. (C) Section through a 58-cell blastocyst. The zona pellucida is visible on the lower left-hand side where a polar body can also be seen. Peripheral cells are trophoblastic. (D) Section through a 107-cell blastocyst. The blastula cavity is now quite large. The embryonic disc is in the upper portion. Peripheral cells are trophoblastic. (Courtesy Carnegie Institute of Washington.)

still has not changed in total size; there also does not appear to be any differentiation in cells at this point. The cells have merely decreased in size with each cleavage. This fact is significant because the morula must pass through the narrow lumen of the fallopian tube. If the morula were to increase in size, it could easily become wedged in the narrow lumen and never reach the uterine cavity. When this occurs, the conceptus continues to grow for 6 to 8 weeks within the fallopian tube (ectopic pregnancy). Since the tube is unable to expand adequately to accommodate the growing embryo, rupture of the tube usually means death for the embryo.

Approximately 4 days after conception, the morula reaches the uterine cavity. The mitotic process continues at a rapid pace. A cavity forms in the center, and the morula begins to increase in size as it absorbs fluids from the endometrial lining. The conceptus is now known as a blastocyst.

The 4½-day conceptus consists of 107 cells. A cross section shows a ring shape with a cell mass on one side. Eight of the cells (embryoblast) of the inner mass will become the embryo (or baby). The other 99 cells (trophoblast) will form the support structures (e.g., placenta).

Between 5½ and 6 days a slight thickening is noted in the cells closest to the uterine wall [15], and the conceptus begins to attach itself to the endometrium. Secretion of proteolytic enzymes by the trophoblast cells allows the conceptus to erode and to invade the epithelial cells of the endometrium. The uterine mucosa, however, appears to promote production of the enzyme, thus evidencing an interdependent action [15]. By the seventh day the zygote shows a distinct division between the body cell mass, called the embryonic disc, and the trophoblast.

Nidation

The ovum is usually fertilized in the outer third of the fallopian tube. The zygote continues to travel through the fallopian tube to the uterus, a process that takes approximately 3 to 4 days. The zygote, like the ovum, is dependent on the ciliary action of the fallopian tubes for its transportation. During this time, the zygote is bathed by nutritive fallopian fluids, a phenomenon that appears to be essential to its survival.

Meanwhile, the uterus has been preparing for the arrival of the zygote. During the follicular phase of the ovarian cycle, the hormone, estrogen, stimulates the growth of the endometrium to form a thick, spongy mass. The hormone, progesterone, of the luteal phase continues to stimulate endometrial growth and also causes the endometrium to secrete fluids rich in nutritive value for the zygote. The vascularity (blood supply) of the endometrium increases, and it becomes very rich in glycogen (animal starch) content.

Another significant effect of progesterone is to reduce uterine contractions. This role of progesterone is essential to allow for nidation, the implantation of the zygote in the endometrium, as well as to maintain pregnancy. The corpus luteum normally will continue to produce progesterone for only 8 to 10 days. If pregnancy is achieved, another hormonal feedback mechanism goes into effect: The zygote begins to secrete human chorionic gonadotropin (HCG). HCG stimulates the corpus luteum to remain viable and continue to secrete progesterone for another 12 to 16 weeks, at which time the placenta is able to assume the responsibility of providing enough progesterone to prevent undesirable uterine contractions. The mother and the fetus have achieved an interdependent relationship before the new individual is even 2 weeks old.

HCG is the biological basis of positive pregnancy tests. Minute amounts can be detected in the blood and urine samples of a pregnant woman as early as 6 to 8 days after conception (1 week before the menses is due) [4]. However, the reliability of very early tests is still in question. Because of the high error rate, the results must be validated at a later time for accuracy. In-home early pregnancy test kits are available, which report very high accuracy rates with urine specimens obtained 9 days after the menses was due. Many professionals who work with pregnant women feel that

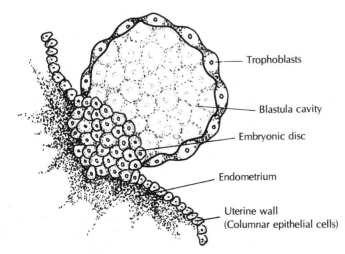

Trophoblasts

Blastula cavity

Embryonic disc

Endometrium

Uterine wall
(Columnar epithelial cells)

Figure 4–2. Seven-day-old zygote invading the endometrium.

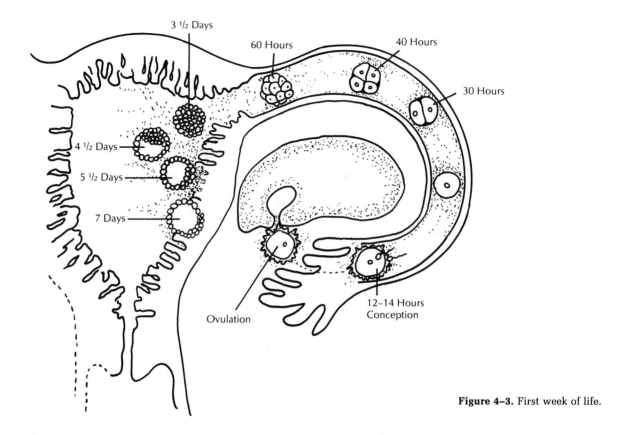

Figure 4–3. First week of life.

HCG may also be one of the major causes of "morning sickness," since women are more likely to experience this reaction when HCG levels are highest.

Nidation occurs 6 to 7 days after conception. The outer cells of the zygote digest their way into the endometrium and begin to obtain nourishment from its rich blood and glycogen supply. The zygote usually implants itself in the upper portion of the uterus. Infants who are attached to the lower portions of the uterus frequently experience difficulty before or during the birth process because the placenta may partially or completely block the infant's exit from the uterus.

Embryonic Stage

During the second through seventh weeks of life, the embryo firmly establishes its home within the uterus and undergoes rapid cellular differentiation that changes its appearance from that of a flat, solid mass of cells to an organism that has distinctly human characteristics.

The differentiation of cells appears to be the result of several factors:

1. Genetic regulation. DNA strands contain regulatory genes that have the ability to regulate the activity of other genes [9].
   a. Some regulatory genes are programmed to activate or inhibit the production of enzymes based on the concentration of specific cellular substances under their control. This sensitive feedback system can function on an intracellular, intratissue, or intraorganismic level.
   b. Other regulatory genes appear to be programmed to activate or to inhibit the production of enzymes based on the time since conception. This is one theory offered to explain why cellular division does not continue where it left off if the conceptus is traumatized.
2. Enzyme regulation. Inhibition and production of enzymes may be directly or indirectly controlled by other chemical substances or enzymes.

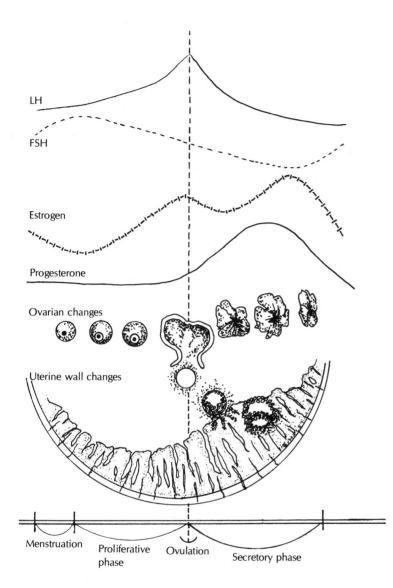

LH

FSH

Estrogen

Progesterone

Ovarian changes

Uterine wall changes

Menstruation   Proliferative   Ovulation
                phase   Secretory phase

Figure 4–4. Endometrial changes related to hormone levels and ovarian changes.

a. Many of the chemical substances formed in the cell have a direct feedback effect on the enzyme that synthesized it [9]. When a threshold level of the substance is achieved, the enzyme is inactivated and synthesis of the product or growth ceases. This process may explain why the liver, when more than half of it is surgically removed, will replace itself to its original size—but no larger [32].

b. Many body tissues depend on the availability of a product that is the result of an earlier enzyme reaction. The genetic code is responsible for the initial enzyme, but subsequent enzyme formation is dependent on a specific sequencing of events. It is the sequencing or the chaining of events that is responsible for continued growth.

SUPPORT STRUCTURES

The structures that support the life of the baby in utero develop mainly from the external portions of the blastocyst (trophoblast). The blastocyst is covered with shaggy, hairlike projections known as chorionic villi. These villi are metabolically very active and will literally digest or eat their way into the endometrial lining of the uterus. This process creates a pool of blood that bathes the conceptus. By the process of diffusion, the embryo is provided with the nutrients needed for rapid growth and development.

Placenta. The villi that are closest to the uterine wall enlarge rapidly and invade the deeper layers of the endometrium. The endometrial surface defect caused by the blastocyst is usually healed by the thirteenth day, and a rich supply of maternal blood begins to suffuse the area. Occasionally the area is not yet completely sealed, and bleeding may occur; the woman may confuse this with normal mentrual bleeding [15]. By the end of the first month of life, these chorionic villi have become the placenta. Tiny blood vessels develop in each of the villi and continue to grow and to branch in a treelike fashion. Each **cotyledon** (branch of the placenta) continues to be immersed in a pool of maternal blood (intervillous spaces). With all the convolutions caused by the branching, it is estimated that the total surface area of a full-term placenta is almost 15 square yards [21]. Contrary to popular belief, the baby and the mother do not share the same blood supply; they maintain completely independent circulatory systems. A thin membrane between the two systems allows for selective admittance and filtering (osmosis and diffusion) of substances passing between the two. This selective processing is known as the placental barrier.

The placenta is the organ of nutrient, oxygen, and waste exchanges between mother and baby. The placenta also functions as an endocrine gland; by the second month of life it is producing estrogen and progesterone. Progesterone levels are maintained at high levels throughout pregnancy even though the corpus luteum ceases to produce progesterone after the third or fourth month. This high progesterone level explains why most pregnant women complain of feeling too warm throughout pregnancy. A decrease in progesterone toward the end of pregnancy, together with aging of the placenta, is one of several explanations postulated for the initiation of labor.

Chorionic membranes. The villi farthest away from the uterine wall degenerate and leave a membrane, known as the chorion, which envelops the developing baby. This membrane is part of the "bag of waters," which helps to protect the baby from bacterial invasion.

The amnion, a smooth membrane arising from the ectoderm (see the next section), lies adjacent to the chorionic membrane. It becomes the lining of the bag of waters. During the early months, the amnion secretes the amniotic fluid, which provides a protective environment for the developing baby by regulating the

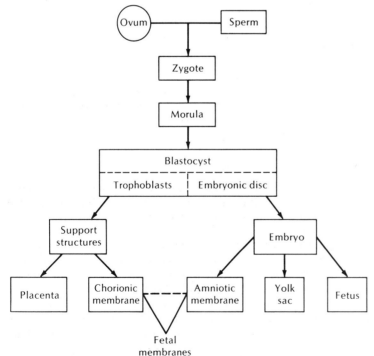

Figure 4–5. Origin of embryo and support structures.

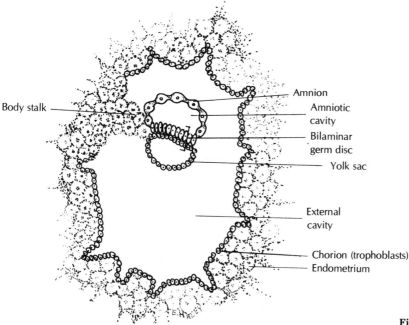

Body stalk

Amnion

Amniotic
cavity

Bilaminar
germ disc

Yolk sac

External
cavity

Chorion (trophoblasts)

Endometrium

Figure 4–6. Sixteen-day-old embryo.

temperature, providing a medium for movement, and protecting the infant from injury should the mother hit her abdomen. The amniotic fluid also contains urine from the immature urinary tract. At term the uterine cavity may contain 500 to 1500 ml of amniotic fluid. The baby swallows this amniotic fluid throughout gestation. Toward the end of gestation, the amniotic fluid is completely exchanged every 3 hours [32]; this feat is accomplished through fetal swallowing and absorption through skin and lungs.

Yolk sac. Humans have a yolk sac during early embryological development. However, it does not provide nutrition for the developing baby. The yolk sac arises from the endoderm (see the next section) and disappears by the seventh week of embryological development. During its short life span, however, it will [20]:

1. Assist in the transfer of nutrients from mother to embryo during the second and third weeks
2. Provide embryological blood cells during the third through sixth weeks until the liver, the spleen, and the bone marrow assume this function
3. Provide the lining cells for the respiratory and the digestive tracts

4. Provide the primordial germ cells that migrate to the gonads to become the primitive germ cells

EMBRYONIC DISC
The major event of the second week of life is the development of the embryonic disc, which enlarges and forms two basic layers: the endoderm (which at this stage of development produces the primitive yolk sac), and the ectoderm, which has started formation of the amniotic sac. The amniotic sac gradually enlarges until it envelops the entire developing baby and intimately contacts the chorionic membrane.

Several other important events occur over the next 7 days. Placental circulation is evidenced by the eleventh to twelfth day of life [15]. By the fifteenth day, when the first menstrual period would be due, the cranial end of the elongated disk has begun to thicken, giving the disk a pearlike shape. By the sixteenth day, a third primary germ layer, the mesoderm, appears between the ectoderm and endoderm. Although all three of these layers originated from the single-cell zygote, the differentiation process now becomes increasingly complex as the embryo develops.

Differentiation of Germ Layers. All future body organs can be traced back to one of the three germ layers, as shown in the following lists:

Ectoderm (outer layer)	Mesoderm (middle layer)	Endoderm (inner layer)
Sensory epithelia of ear, eye	Dermis	Trachea and lungs
Epidermis	Connective tissue	Gastrointestinal tract
Hair, nails	Bones, cartilage	Liver, pancreas
Central nervous system	Muscles	Urinary bladder
Cranial nerves	Dentine of teeth	Pharynx
Urethra	Heart	Thyroid
Upper pharynx and nasal passages	Spleen, blood	Tonsils
Enamel of teeth	Kidneys, ureters	Lining of urethra, ear
Peripheral nervous system	Gonads, uterus	
Mammary glands		

It is significant to note that one system may have organs or tissues arising from more than one germ layer. For instance, the urinary system receives the kidneys and ureters from the mesoderm, the bladder from the endoderm, and the urethra from the ectoderm. Synchronization of growth is essential for proper linkage of these organs that arise from different germ layers. Some congenital anomalies are the result of failure to obtain fusion or linkage during early periods of growth.

Development of Various Body Systems. Cellular differentiation and resultant changes in shape are very rapid and complex following the sixteenth day of development. The development of several of the body systems is of particular interest.

The Spinal Cord and Brain. On the sixteenth day of development, the three germ layers lie flat and are attached to each other. Ectodermal growth is most rapid. On the seventeenth or eighteenth day, a slight dip begins to traverse the longitudinal dorsal aspect of the embryonic disc. The edges gradually heighten and then fold over toward each other. By the twenty-second day, these edges fuse to form the neutral tube, which becomes the spinal cord and the brain.

On the twentieth day, a series of somites, blocks of mesodermal tissue, begins to form on each side of the groove. These somites eventually form the spinal column. Each of the 44 pairs is responsible for the development of a specific segment of the skeletal, muscular, and dermal portions of the body. Spina bifida results from the failure of these segments to fuse properly. The brain cells continue to grow rapidly, causing the cephalic portion of the embryo to fold over by the twenty-sixth day of development.

The Heart. During the early days of growth, the zygote and embryo are able to obtain nourishment through simple diffusion. Subsequently, however, the cell mass rapidly becomes too thick for diffusion. Consequently, the embryo early on has to develop cells to carry oxygen and a transportation system.

Around the eighteenth or nineteenth day of development, a narrow tube appears on each side of the embryonic disc in the mesoderm. These tubes migrate toward each other as the mesoderm folds around a section of the endoderm. The two tubes meet and fuse on the twenty-first and twenty-second days at the same rate that the ectoderm is meeting and fusing to form the spinal cord and the brain [20]. As this single tube continues to grow, it folds, creating two chambers. Tiny blood vessels have already formed enough pathways to provide circulation for the rapidly developing organism. At 22 days, the heart initiates functioning of the first system of the body.

The Face. The facial development of the embryo is fascinating. On the twenty-second day, the eyes begin to form on the sides of the head; each must travel almost 80 degrees to the front of the face to arrive at its final destination. The nose is formed by one tab that grows from the forehead and two others that approach from each cheek. These two cheek tabs also form the upper jaw; evidence of their joining can still be seen in the dip or groove found in the upper lip just below the nose. The failure of these three tabs to fuse results in various degrees of cleft palate, cleft lip, or both. The lower jaw is also formed by tabs approaching from each side of the embryonic face.

The Appendages. The leg and arm buds appear about the twenty-sixth day and grow outward from the body. By the fortieth day, the elbows and knees become apparent, but the fingers and toes are webbed. By the end of the seventh week, the fingers and toes become separate entities.

Fetal Stage

The foundations for all internal and external structures are present by the fiftieth day of life. Since the basic structures for all the body systems are established by the beginning of the eighth week of life, the

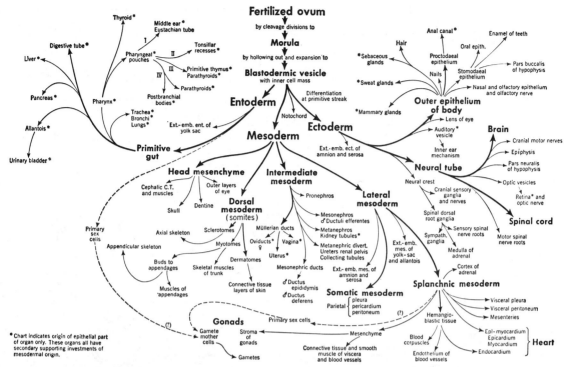

Figure 4–7. Derivation of the various organs and tissues of the body by progressive differentiation and divergent specialization. Note especially how the origin of all the organs can be traced back to the three primary germ layers. (From B. M. Carlson, *Pattern's Foundations of Embryology* [4th ed.]. New York: McGraw-Hill, 1981. With permission.)

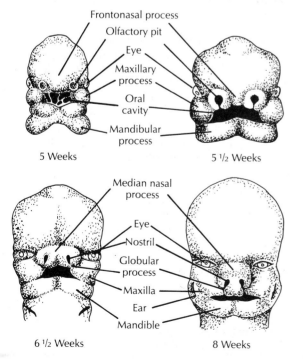

Figure 4–8. Development of the face. Note that the maxillary processes extend from each side and fuse at the midline. Incomplete fusion leads to various degrees of cleft lip, cleft palate, or both.

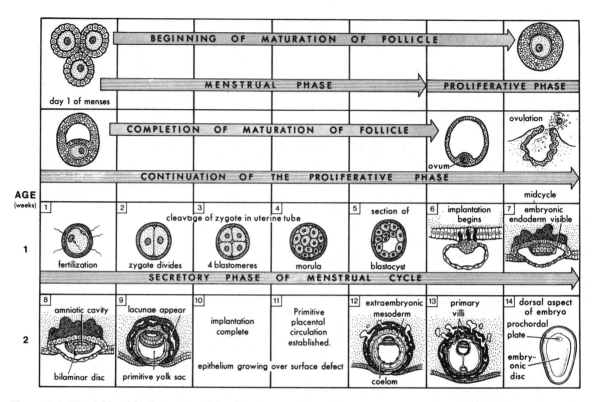

Figure 4–9. Timetable of human prenatal development, 0 to 2 weeks. (From K. L. Moore, *Before We Are Born: Basic Embryology and Birth Defects.* Philadelphia: Saunders, 1974. With permission.)

remainder of the intrauterine period is spent in growth and refinement of body tissues and organs. Although weighing barely 1 gm (1/30 of an ounce) and measuring just over 1 inch in length, the fetus has distinctly human characteristics. The rapid growth of the brain creates a top-heavy appearance; at this stage of development, the head accounts for about 50 percent of the total length of the baby [28]. The stubby tail at the end of the spinal cord that made its appearance about the twenty-sixth day has now disappeared. The heart has already started its arduous task of pumping blood through the body at the rate of 40 to 80 beats per minute [28]. A thin pink skin covers the body. Sufficient skeletal, muscular, and neurological development has occurred to allow primitive movement by the fetus [7, 43].

During the fetal stage, the body begins to lengthen rapidly. By the twelfth week the head accounts for about one-third of the total body length; by birth, it is about one-fourth of the total length. Eyelids form around the ninth week and seal the eyes shut until about the twenty-fifth week. At 12 weeks the gender

of the fetus is easily distinguishable. Although the mother is not usually aware of it, the baby can now move easily and frequently. At the end of the first trimester, the limbs and facial features have become so greatly refined that the fetus now gives the appearance of a delicate 3½-inch bisque-colored doll.

The list given below summarizes the development of the fetus by the lunar month. The weights given are approximate, since authorities vary widely in their figures.

First month (1 to 4 weeks after conception)
Conception, rapid growth
Nidation, symbiotic relationship established
Differentiation of individual from accessory structures
Three germ layers differentiated
Rudimentary body parts formed
Cardiovascular system functioning
Yolk sac begins to diminish

Second month (5 to 8 weeks)
Formation of head and facial features

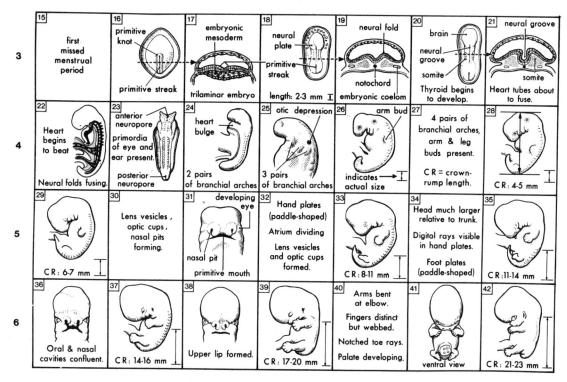

Figure 4–10. Timetable of human prenatal development, 3 to 6 weeks. (From K. L. Moore, *Before We Are Born: Basic Embryology and Birth Defects.* Philadelphia: Saunders, 1974. With permission.)

Very rapid cell differentiation and growth
Beginning of all major external and internal structures
External genitalia present, but gender not discernible
Heart functionally complete
Some movement by limbs
Yolk sac incorporated into the embryo
Weight: 1 gm

Third month (9 to 12 weeks)
Eyelids fused, nail beds formed
Teeth and bones begin to appear
Kidneys begin to function
Some respiratory-like movements exhibited
Begins to swallow amniotic fluid
Grasp, sucking, and withdrawal reflexes present
Moves easily (not felt by mother)
Gender distinguishable
Weight: 30 gm (1 ounce)

Fourth month (13 to 16 weeks)
Much spontaneous movement
Moro reflex present
Quickening—fetal movement may be felt by mother

Rapid skeletal development
Meconium present
Uterine development in female infant
Downy hair (lanugo) appears on body
Weight: 120 gm (4 ounces)

Fifth month (17 to 20 weeks)
Begins to exchange new cells for old, especially in skin
Usual time of quickening
Vernix caseosa appears
Eyebrows and head hair appear
Skeleton begins to harden
Strong grasp reflex present
Permanent teeth buds appear
Heart sounds can be heard with a stethoscope (special equipment may pick up heart sounds earlier)
Weight: 360 gm (12 ounces)

Sixth month (21 to 24 weeks)
"Miniature baby"
Extrauterine life possible (but very unlikely)
Mother may note jarring but rhythmic movements of infant indicative of hiccups

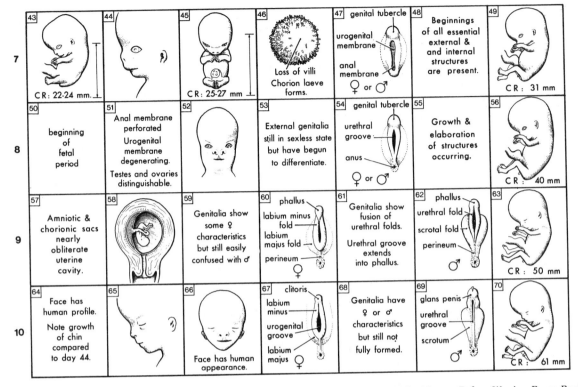

Figure 4–11. Timetable of human prenatal development, 7 to 10 weeks. (From K. L. Moore, *Before We Are Born: Basic Embryology and Birth Defects*. Philadelphia: Saunders, 1974. With permission.)

Body becomes straight
Fingernails present
Skin has red, wrinkled appearance
Alternates periods of sleep and activity
May respond to external sounds
May try to find "comfortable" position
Weight: 720 gm (1½ pounds)

Seventh month (25 to 28 weeks)
Respiratory system and central nervous system sufficiently developed, so that 10% of babies may survive with excellent and intensive care
Eyelids reopen
Assumes head-down position in uterus
Respiratory-like movements
Weight: 1200 gm (2½ pounds)

Eighth month (29 to 32 weeks)
Begins to store fat and minerals
Testes descend into scrotal sac
Mother may note irregular, jerky, "crying-like" movements
Lanugo begins to disappear from face

Skin begins to lose reddish color
Can be conditioned to environmental sounds
Exhibits good reflex development
Good chance of survival if born
Weight: 2000 gm (4 pounds)

Ninth month (33 to 36 weeks)
Continues fat deposits
Body begins to round out
Increased iron storage by liver
Increased development of lungs
May become more or less active due to space tightness
Excellent chance of survival if born
Lanugo begins to disappear from body
Head hair lengthens
Weight: 2800 gm (6 pounds)

Tenth month (37 to 40 weeks)
Lanugo and vernix caseosa both begin to disappear
High absorption of maternal hormones
Skin becomes smooth, plump
Firming of skull and bones
Continued storage of fat and minerals

Ready for birth
Weight: 3200 to 3400 gm (7 to 7½ pounds)

Fetal Circulation

As the fetus enlarges, the need for oxygen and nutrients to meet its growth needs increases rapidly. During intrauterine life, all supplies are obtained and all waste products are excreted through the placenta. The circulatory system is constructed in such a way that with minimal changes after birth, the infant's body can obtain oxygen from the lungs and nutrients from the gastrointestinal tract. At full term, the placenta measures approximately 8 inches in diameter and weighs about 1¼ pounds.

The umbilical cord, connecting the infant with the life-supporting placenta, houses the umbilical vessels in a bluish-white gelatinous substance known as Wharton's jelly. This jelly supports the vessels and helps to prevent their accidental closure by bending, kinking, or pressure. Although the length may vary greatly, the umbilical cord is approximately 20 inches long and about 1½ inches in diameter. Because the single umbilical vein is longer than the two umbilical arteries and the length of the cord [20], it spirals around the arteries, giving the umbilical cord a twisted, knotted appearance.

In addition to the placenta and the three umbilical blood vessels, there are four other distinctive features of fetal circulation:

1. The foramen ovale. A direct opening between the right and left atria of the heart
2. The ductus arteriosus. A fetal vessel connecting the pulmonary artery and the aorta
3. The ductus venosus. The fetal vessel connecting the umbilical vein with the inferior (ascending) vena cava
4. The hypogastric arteries. Arteries that branch off the femoral arteries and become the umbilical arteries after leaving the body and entering the umbilical cord

In tracing the course of fetal blood, it is easiest to speak of oxygenated and unoxygenated blood, although the blood circulating through the fetus is never completely oxygenated. The blood is oxygenated at the

A

B

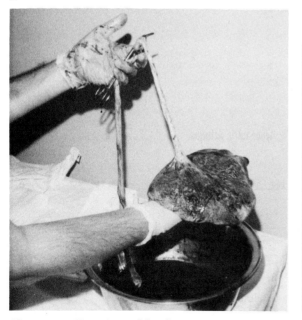 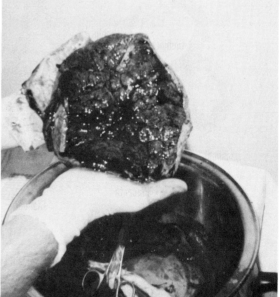

Figure 4–12. Two views of the placenta. (A) Fetal surface and umbilical cord. (B) Maternal surface. Because of the presence of the amniotic membrane, the side of the placenta that faces the infant is smooth and shiny. The umbilical cord usually enters the center of the rounded placental disc, and vessels can be seen radiating out to the cotyledons or branches of the placenta. The maternal surface, resembling a piece of liver, is dull and extremely convoluted where the cotyledons have branched and massed together to conserve space and to utilize maximally the maternal pools of blood.

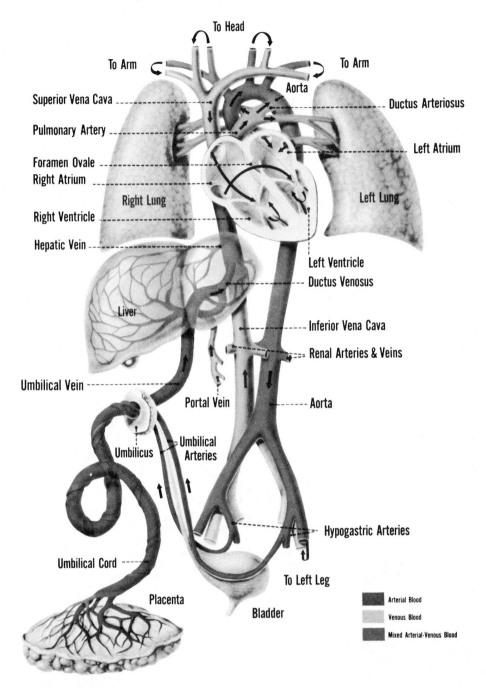

To Head

To Arm

To Arm

Aorta

Superior Vena Cava

Ductus Arteriosus

Pulmonary Artery

Left Atrium

Foramen Ovale

Right Atrium

Right Lung

Left Lung

Right Ventricle

Hepatic Vein

Left Ventricle

Ductus Venosus

Liver

Inferior Vena Cava

Renal Arteries & Veins

Umbilical Vein

Portal Vein

Aorta

Umbilicus

Umbilical
Arteries

Hypogastric Arteries

Umbilical Cord

To Left Leg

Placenta

Bladder

Arterial Blood

Venous Blood

Mixed Arterial-Venous Blood

Figure 4–13. Fetal circulation. (Ross Clinical Educational Aid No. 1. Courtesy Ross Laboratories.)

placenta, circulates through the body, and is returned unoxygenated to the placenta. Some authorities indicate that the oxygen concentration of the blood is as low as 60 percent (in extrauterine life, the oxygen con- centration of aortic blood should be 98 to 100 percent). To compensate for the low oxygen saturation, the fetus produces more red blood cells to carry oxygen to the rapidly growing body. Consequently, the fetus and the neonate have a very high red blood cell count. It is interesting to note that the organs that have first access to the oxygen and nutrient-rich blood are the key organs of the body—the brain, the heart, and the liver.

ASSESSMENT OF FETAL AGE AND MATURITY

When a woman becomes pregnant, both she and the doctor want to know when the baby is due to be born. Rough estimates of fetal age can be achieved through a history of the last menstrual period (LMP). The gestational period, the length of time from conception to birth, is approximately 266 days; this can also be stated as 38 weeks or 9 calendar months. Medical personnel frequently use lunar months (28 days) for calculation. The length of pregnancy is 280 days, 40 weeks, or 10 lunar months when calculated from the first day of the LMP (assuming a 28-day cycle).

The expected date of delivery can also be calculated by Naegele's rule: To the first day of the LMP add 7 days, subtract 3 months, and then adjust the calendar year. This rule assumes a 28-day ovarian cycle with ovulation occurring about day 14; women experiencing longer or shorter cycles would need to adjust the formula accordingly.

If the LMP began on November 8 (eleventh month of the year), the use of Naegele's formula indicates the infant would be due August 15 of the next year, as shown in the following calculations:

8th day	11th month	1987
+ 7 days	− 3 months	
15th day	8th month	1988

If the LMP were February 18, then the infant would be due November 25 of the same year. Fifty percent of deliveries occur within 5 days of the date obtained by Naegele's rule. However, this method is not completely accurate. A woman's menstrual history may be very irregular, making the time of ovulation difficult to determine. Occasionally, a woman experiences enough breakthrough bleeding when the first menstrual period after conception is due that the pregnancy is not suspected; as a result, the calculations may be inaccurate by a full month.

The height of the fundus (top of the uterus) can also give a rough estimate of fetal age. However, a multiple pregnancy will rule out the use of fundal height for estimating age. A multiple pregnancy is usually not identified as such until the third trimester of preg-

nancy (and occasionally not until the birth process is under way!)

Quickening (the first time fetal movement is felt by the mother) also gives an estimate of fetal age. The first movement is usually felt during the fifth month of pregnancy. However, since mothers have various degrees of sensitivity to fetal movement, this phenomenon cannot be used as an accurate guide to gestational, or fetal, age.

A fairly accurate way of determining fetal age is through x-ray. The degree of ossification or bone formation can indicate the developmental stage quite precisely. However, most doctors are quite reluctant to expose the developing fetus to x-rays unless absolutely essential because of the potential negative effects on the mitotic process.

Ultrasonography, the use of ultrasound waves to obtain a picture of the fetus, can indicate fetal size and position. Fetal maturity can be estimated within 4 days of gestational age during the first trimester, within 7 days during the second trimester, and within 14 days during the third trimester.

Fetal age can also be estimated with Hasse's rule, using the length obtained during an x-ray, an ultrasonogram, or after the birth of the infant. The gestational age of fetuses up to 5 months is estimated by taking the square root of the length of the fetus in centimeters.

Lunar month	Length of fetus (cm)
1	1
2	4
3	9
4	16
5	25

After 5 months, division of the fetal length by 5 will give the approximate age of the fetus.

Lunar month	Length of fetus (cm)
6	30
7	35
8	40
9	45
10	50

As the placenta ages, its functional capacity begins to decrease; the adequacy of its functioning can be determined by the amount of estrogen (urinary estriols) found in the maternal urine. Low levels indicate that the placenta has aged to a point where it may no longer

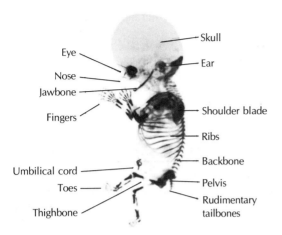

Skull
Eye
Ear
Nose
Jawbone
Fingers
Shoulder blade
Ribs
Backbone
Umbilical cord
Pelvis
Toes
Rudimentary tailbones
Thighbone

Figure 4–14. Two-month-old fetal skeleton. (From R. Rugh and L. B. Shettles, *From Conception to Birth*. New York: Harper & Row, 1971. With permission.)

be able to sustain the life of the infant. This test measures the efficiency of the placenta—not the age of the fetus.

The most accurate (and relatively painless and simple) process for determining the status of the fetus is through amniocentesis [8]. A needle is inserted through the cervix or through the mother's abdominal wall and uterus into the amniotic cavity. A small amount (10 to 30 ml) of clear white amniotic fluid is withdrawn for analysis. Changes in the color of the fluid indicate that the baby may be in difficulty. Inadequate oxygenation will cause the baby to release meconium (bowel movement) into the fluid, turning it a greenish-brown color. Blood incompatibility may be exhibited by a yellow color. The discarded cells found in amniotic fluid can be karyotyped for chromosomal abnormalities.

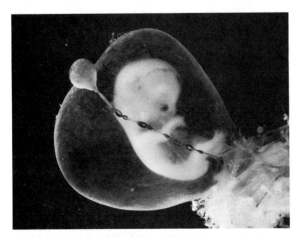

Figure 4–15. The fetus at 40 days' gestation.

One of the most frequent reasons for performing amniocentesis is to determine lung maturity, a fairly accurate indicator of fetal age. The ratio of lecithin to sphingomyelin (L-S ratio) is a very accurate indicator of the ability of the lungs to support extrauterine life. The L-S ratio indicates the ability of the lungs to produce surfactant, a substance that is essential for maintaining lung expansion. Infants who are unable to produce sufficient surfactant develop respiratory distress syndrome, more commonly known as hyaline membrane disease. Many of these infants die from the inability to maintain expansion of the lung tissue. This is a self-terminating disease that is very specific to the newborn during the first 4 days of life. Those infants (usually premature) who survive the first 72 hours generally begin to produce adequate surfactant.

FACTORS AFFECTING DEVELOPMENT

Intrauterine events may prevent survival or may affect the quality of an individal's future life. Research indicates that 50 percent of fertilized ova die before a pregnancy is recognized, either because the zygote is unable to achieve nidation or because early factors in development are incompatible with life [11]. These zygotes are usually excreted as a normal menstrual period. Ten to 25 percent more die before they are able to sustain independent extrauterine life (spontaneous abortion) [11]. A high percentage of these deaths result from chromosomal abnormalities and congenital malformations. Congenital malformations will continue to take their toll in the quality of life of those individuals who do survive the intrauterine period. Chapters 19 and 35 discuss the effect of congenital anomalies on the level of health achieved by the individual and the family. Because of the irreversible effect of these early influences on development, information is presented here as a foundation for promoting high level health through preventive health education. Concerned professionals should attempt to prevent congenital anomalies through education of parents and potential parents.

There are two major categories of factors that affect fetal development: (1) the genetic inheritance or chromosomal factors, and (2) events occurring after conception—environmental or developmental factors.

Chromosomal Factors

To date, little if anything can be done to prevent anomalies due to chromosomal abnormalities except to avoid, when possible, situations that lead to higher incidences of anomalies. Exposure to frequent or high doses of x-rays is associated with higher incidences of both numerical and structural changes of chromosomes. Therefore, women are encouraged to avoid all exposure of the pelvic area to x-rays before and during pregnancy, especially during the first trimester.

Mothers under age 16 or over age 35 also have higher incidences of malformed infants. One explanation given for the increased incidence found among younger mothers is that the primary germ cells are not yet ready to successfully complete the meiotic process; another reason is the inadequate nutritional intake of many adolescent mothers. In the case of the older mother, it must be remembered that the woman has carried the primary germ cells since birth. Consequently, the older the mother, the greater is the chance of producing a defective ovum. Using Down's syndrome (mongolism) as an example of chromosomal abnormality, the incidence is about 1 per 700 births for women in their twenties but rises to 1 per 70 births for women in their early forties [18].

Approximately 3 percent of neonates have a congenital anomaly that requires medical intervention: one-third of these are life-threatening [31]. One-half of the children in hospitals have a prenatally acquired defect. When a baby is born with an anomaly, one cannot say with certainty that it is due to chromosomal, genetic, or developmental causes. Identical malformations may have either a genetic or a developmental origin. A careful history, including pedigree and karyotyping studies, should be taken to try to determine the causative factor. Parents often want to know whether or not a defect is hereditary before conceiving another child. Unfortunately, even careful studies undertaken by competent professionals cannot always determine a definitive cause. Anomalies due to developmental factors are not inheritable.

Developmental Factors

The developing fetus is very dependent on the environment provided by the mother, both positively and negatively. It is estimated that only 30 percent of anomalies are due solely to hereditary factors and that consequently more than 50 percent of congenital anomalies are preventable [28]. Even the most conscientious mother may unknowingly be exposed to factors that can negatively influence the development of the baby. Many substances are known to pass through the placental barrier to retard or arrest the infant's development.

TERATOGENS

Substances or factors that are known to cause congenital malformations are called teratogens. Some may cause alterations in the configurations or structure of chromosomes, thus disturbing the genetic code. Other substances may prevent transfer of adequate nutrients or oxygen to vital areas or can interfere with the enzymatic, catalytic actions of RNA to cause a temporary arrest in cellular division or growth. Since timing is so critical in early fetal development, and a single step in development may be part of a chain of reactions, the ability of a substance to interfere with a single step in mitosis and cellular differentiation can result in either minor or gross anomalies of the individual, depending on the stage of development when the insult occurs and the target reactions arrested. Some arrests in development are incompatible with continued life, resulting in death of the fetus.

Each organ or tissue has its own timetable for maximal growth. Since several organ systems or tissues are developing simultaneously, some defects are frequently found to be paired with defects in other organs that were also at critical points of development when the teratogen was introduced. Thus, ear anomalies are frequently associated with kidney anomalies, and single-artery umbilical cords with gastrointestinal anomalies. Other teratogens appear to have an affinity for specific tissues or organs. Most teratogens exhibit immediate effects by causing growth retardation or or-

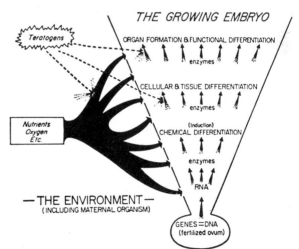

Figure 4–16. Action of teratogens on the developing embryo. Note that the embryo is dependent at all stages on materials coming to it by way of its environment. Teratogens do not appear to be effective in causing recognizable malformations until cellular differentiation has begun. It seems probable, however, that early action may cause death of the embryo before specific local manifestations are established. (From B. M. Carlson, *Patten's Foundations of Embryology* [4th ed.]. New York: McGraw-Hill, 1981. With permission.)

gan deformity. However, some teratogens have a delayed action, and their influences are not apparent until age 7 or even 20 years of age or more, during the final stages of the development of a tissue.

Because specific birth defects are relatively rare, and potential teratogens are unique in their effect on the developing fetus, it often requires years of painstaking detective work to associate the two. A cause-effect relationship is often implied by association rather than by clinical proof; rarely are there enough clear-cut associations to prove causality. Even the teratogenic effects of thalidomide and rubella must be studied in retrospect. No humane researcher would deliberately expose a fetus to a suspected teratogen. Occasionally, experiments (e.g., thalidomide) on animals do not indicate teratogenic effects because of a difference in the genetic code and the enzymes or enzyme sequences responsible for human development versus animal development.

Another point that makes cause by association difficult is that most agents are not 100 percent teratogenic. Although thalidomide and rubella have very high anomaly-producing rates, many infants may still escape damage after exposure. Other teratogens may avoid detection because they are dose-related; effects may not be seen unless the agent reaches a particular threshold. The effects of lower dosages may be so subtle as to go undetected (e.g., alcohol consumption) for years.

Table 4–1 lists potential teratogens and their effects on the fetus.

Although the zygote is not usually susceptible to teratogens because it is not yet dependent on the environment for nutrients [20], the general rule is the younger the conceptus, the greater the susceptibility to teratogens. The embryo is the most susceptible; it is during this period that the most rapid differentiation of cells is occurring and the foundations are being laid for body organs and systems. Multiple malformations may occur because many body systems are developing simultaneously. One teratogen may affect several body systems if it arrests all chemical reactions and mitotic divisions at that point. Arrested development does not resume at a later time. There is a time schedule for development; if a reaction does not occur as scheduled, it is skipped. There are no pauses. If development cannot occur around the missed processes, the fetus will die. If development can continue in spite of the skipped reactions, life continues; the thalidomide babies are a good example of this process. Thalidomide, a tranquilizer, was prescribed for thousands of mothers during the first and second trimester of pregnancy.

A high percentage of these babies were born with abnormal limb formation.

MATERNAL ENVIRONMENT

The infant is affected directly and indirectly by the mother's state of health and nutritional intake. The embryo makes minimal nutritional demands on the mother. The caloric and nutritional elements essential to growth and development increase with fetal size, requiring increased maternal intake to meet the needs of both. Maternal nutritional intake during the last 4 months of pregnancy appears to be especially critical to optimal fetal development.

Nutrition. Mothers who are on diets with restricted caloric intake need assistance in selecting foods that will provide adquate protein, vitamin, and mineral intakes to meet the infant's needs as well as her own. A balanced diet that consists of foods from all four food groups is essential. The pregnant teenager must provide for her own growth and developmental needs as well as those of the fetus; therefore, she needs approximately 300 calories more than the pregnant adult woman.

During World War II, food supplies were cut off to major cities of the Netherlands during the winter of 1944–45. As a result, thousands of pregnant women were exposed to near-starvation conditions for more than 6 months. Birth weights dropped by more than 10 percent, and an increase in congenital anomalies was noted [31].

The fetal cerebrum experiences maximal growth between 26 and 32 weeks of gestation [39]. Research indicates that inadequate intake of protein and calories at this time can permanently reduce the number of brain cells by as much as 40 percent [39]. Improved nutrition following a period of inadequate hypertropic brain growth will not increase the number of cells. Thus, an individual's intellectual functioning for a lifetime can be affected by the nutritional status of the mother. WIC (Women, Infants and Children) and other prenatal health programs emphasize the importance of nutrition and assist mothers in obtaining an adequate diet. Inadequate caloric intake during fetal and early infant development is associated with a child's later passivity, dependency, and anxious behavior irrespective of cognitive effects [2]. Apparently, the child must have adequate energy intake during early infancy for later social-emotional development.

The mother's nutritional state prior to pregnancy can be as significant as the nutritional intake during pregnancy. It is recommended that the mother discuss her

Table 4–1. Teratogenic Agents

Agent	Effect on Fetus
Drugs	
Alcohol	Neonatal addiction, IGR, cleft palate, cardiac anomalie, microcephaly, postnatal growth retardation, cognitive deficiencies, fine motor dysfunction, increased fetal and perinatal death rate, hyperactivity, learning disabilities
Antihistamines (?)	Fetal death, anomalies
Aspirin	Neonatal bleeding
Barbiturates	Neonatal addiction, neonatal bleeding, neurological impairments
Cigarette smoke	Prematurity, IGR, anomalies, spontaneous abortion, delayed cognitive skills
Corticosteroids	Anomalies, cleft lip, IGR
DES	Cancer of reproductive system 20 years later in female; reproductive system anomalies in male
Ergot	Fetal death
Hormones	Masculinization of female infant; feminization of male infant
Insulin (shock)	Fetal death
LSD	Chromosomal damage, anomalies, spontaneous abortion
Marijuana	Chromosomal damage
Morphine	Neonatal addiction, anomalies
Streptomycin	Damage to 8th cranial nerve
Sulfa drugs	Jaundice
Tetracycline	Discoloration of permanent teeth, inhibited bone growth
Thalidomide	Fetal death, abnormal extremities, hearing loss, cardiac anomalies
Radiation	Anomalies, microcephaly, chromosomal damage, leukemia
Maternal diseases	
Cytomegalic inclusion disease	Jaundice, blood dyscrasia, microcephaly, IGR, mental retardation
Diabetes	Large birth weight, stillborn baby, anomalies
Gonorrhea	Neonatal blindness
Hepatitis	Neonatal hepatitis
Herpes virus	Neonatal infection/death, microcephaly, retinal dysplasia
Influenza	Abortion, cardiac defects
Rubella	Abortion, cardiac defects, deafness, blindness, mental retardation, IGR
Syphilis	Fetal death, anomalies, congenital syphilis, prematurity
Toxoplasmosis (carried by infected cat feces)	Blindness, mental retardation, fetal death, cardiac anomalies
Other	
Lead	Fetal death, anemia, hemorrhage
Smallpox vaccination	Fetal vaccinia, fetal death

IGR = intrauterine growth retardation; ? = evidence strong but not conclusive.

nutritional needs with a dietician during the early months of her pregnancy in order to identify and remedy potential deficiencies and thus increase the chances of a successful outcome of the pregnancy. Many physicians encourage mothers to restrict their weight gain to 20 to 24 pounds; however, weight gain recommendations should be individualized according to the unique needs of the mother (see Chap. 32).

Pica. Occasionally a mother will develop pica, an abnormal craving for nonedible materials. Some studies reveal communities in which as many as 55 percent of women exhibit pica during pregnancy [19]. Pica is frequently culturally influenced but often has no apparent rationale behind the inordinate appetite. Women express the ideas that they believe these substances will relieve nausea, prevent vomiting, relieve dizziness, or cure swollen legs and headaches; that they are necessary for the baby's development; or that they will ensure a beautiful baby. Refusal to satisfy a craving may even be thought to cause birthmarks [19]. The craving may be for clay, unprocessed flour, dirt, wood, or many other unusual ingestants. These products may harm the baby because of some teratogenic ingredient or because the mother may actually eat so much of the substance that she fails to have an adequate nutritional intake. Pica is frequently associated with iron-deficiency anemia, and in some cases it appears to be resolved by iron therapy [19].

Maternal Disease. Chronic maternal diseases may contribute to congenital anomalies. The incidence of congenital anomalies is about ten times greater in mothers with diabetes than in mothers without this disease [18]. These babies tend to gain excessive amounts of weight before birth and to become critically hypoglycemic (having low blood sugar) after birth. There is evidence that mothers with cardiac disease or anemia may not be able to supply the infant with enough oxygen to meet its developmental needs or to support the infant through the birth process. These infants are more likely to experience intrauterine growth retardation and anomalies. The babies of mothers with metabolic diseases may develop hypertrophy of the corresponding affected maternal gland, creating metabolic disturbances that can threaten the life of the baby following birth.

Stress. Severe maternal stressors (e.g., illness or the death of a family member, marital discord, war) are known to be potential teratogens. The incidence of malformations in babies of mothers with critical stress during the first trimester is very high compared to those of nonstressed mothers [36]. There is evidence that the biochemical responses associated with emotional reactions to maternal stress can create changes in the electrical activity of the brain of the fetus as early as 8 weeks after conception. Abnormal changes in the electrical activity of the fetal brain correlate highly with low Apgar scores (see Chap. 5), neonatal problems, and neurological abnormalities [3].

An increased number of anomalies were noted during and after World War II in offspring of mothers experiencing emotional stressors even before the nutritional deprivation occurred. Central nervous system anomalies were frequent. A survey of 55 German hospitals showed a 400 percent increase in anomalies from 1930 to 1950 [36].

Several processes appear to be activated by stress. Stress creates changes in the sympathetic nervous system that in turn may cause (1) reduced blood flow to the uterus, and (2) hormonal changes. Reduced uterine blood flow would limit the amount of nutrients and oxygen available for fetal growth. The fetus is known to change activity patterns or to exhibit strong fetal movements in a manner similar to the activity observed in oxygen-deficient fetuses when the mother suffers severe emotional stress [36]. Both adrenaline and cortisone levels are elevated during stress, and both of these hormones can pass through the placental barrier and affect the fetus. Increased adrenaline levels increase fetal activity. Cortisones are known to be teratogenic to body organs, especially to the developing reproductive system. The diagram given below shows the relationship of stress to elevated adrenaline and cortisone levels.

For some women who continue to work during the third trimester, the work may serve as a stressor, as indicated by a reduced birth weight of 150 to 400 gm [22]. However, 95 percent of pregnant women and their babies are able to adjust to continued working without experiencing serious side effects [42].

STRESS
activates
HYPOTHALAMUS
which regulates
AUTONOMIC NERVOUS SYSTEM
to stimulate
ADRENAL MEDULLA
to release
ADRENALINE
which stimulates
ANTERIOR LOBE OF PITUITARY
to produce
ACTH (Adrenocorticotropic Hormone)
which activates
ADRENAL CORTEX
to release
CORTISONE
which enters
MATERNAL BLOODSTREAM
passes through
PLACENTAL BARRIER
enters
FETAL BLOODSTREAM

Drugs. Cortisones and other hormones as well as synthetically prepared drugs repeatedly have been documented as teratogens [30]. The effect of the drug on the infant depends on (1) the kind of drug, (2) the dosage, (3) the gestational stage of the infant, and (4) the specific sensitivity of an organ. Some drugs are known to prevent conception; others may cause anomalies or fetal death.

Mothers should take no drugs during pregnancy unless they are prescribed by the doctor. Occasionally, even drugs thought to be safe have unexpected side effects. The antibiotic, tetracyline, when taken by the mother during pregnancy, inhibits bone growth and causes brown stains to appear on the permanent teeth of the child at 6 to 7 years of age. An increased incidence of cancer of the vagina and the reproductive tract in females, and anomalies of the reproductive tract in males have been found among young people 10 to 24 years of age whose mothers were given diethylstilbestrol (DES), a hormone prescribed to help maintain pregnancy in mothers who threatened to abort [17, 38]. Even one tablet of aspirin increases the bleeding time of both mothers and babies exposed to the drug within 1 week of birth. **Cigarette smoking, a known cause of intrauterine growth retardation and premature birth, is suspected of decreasing the oxygen supply** [14, 33]. Birth weight is reduced by an average of 180 gm, and the perinatal mortality rate is increased by 30 percent [37]. The risk of congenital heart defects and limb reductions is greatly increased in infants born to mothers treated with progestins during the first 4 months of pregnancy [25].

Lysergic acid diethylamide (LSD) is known to cause chromosomal abnormalities. A federal report on marijuana released in 1974 indicates there is strong evidence that marijuana also causes chromosomal and genetic damage [34]. **A strong association has also been identified between alcohol consumption, anomalies, and hyperactivity** [5]. One study, involving 633 mothers, indicates that 17 percent of infants born to mothers who consumed alcohol (at any point during pregnancy) experienced major congenital anomalies [24, 35]. The frequency and amount of alcohol consumed appear to be correlated with the severity and frequency of congenital anomalies, regardless of the maternal nutritional status [24]. The fetus appears to be sensitive to the effects of alcohol throughout gestation, but the brain appears to be most sensitive between 18 to 20 weeks of gestation [27]. The National Council on Alcoholism and the National Institute of Alcohol Abuse and Alcoholism (under the Department of HEW) have issued a warning that just two drinks of hard liquor per day consumed by the mother may cause fetal defects.

An infant born to a mother who is addicted to a narcotic or a barbiturate will also be addicted to the drug. There is an increased incidence of these babies being born either prematurely or small for gestational age (SGA). The babies will go through a withdrawal period and will often require hospitalized intensive care to maintain life. Their maturational potential may be adversely affected if their mothers practiced poor nutritional habits during pregnancy. Because there is less opportunity to bond and to establish attachment behaviors with their mothers, these babies are considered to be at a higher risk of developing psychological patterns that are maladaptive. The social environment following birth may be conducive to the child's use of drugs, but this influence is independent of the original dependence.

Biological Teratogens. Viruses and bacteria can also have severe teratogenic effects on the fetus; many appear to interfere directly with translation and implementation of the genetic code. Rubella (German measles) virus is devastating to the embryo, causing severe eye, ear, brain, and heart anomalies. The affected infant may continue to be a reservoir of the rubella virus to other persons for as long as 1 year after birth. Rubella vaccine is now available, and most school systems require all children to have the rubella vaccination along with other immunizations. This requirement will help protect future children from contracting congenital rubella. The vaccine is usually contraindicated for women of child-bearing age for fear that it may cause fetal anomalies if the woman becomes pregnant within 3 months after receiving the vaccine. Any young woman considering pregnancy should ask her doctor to check her immunity to rubella through a special blood test. Other viruses, including the viral cold, have been associated with birth defects.

Syphilis can be transmitted to the infant after the eighteenth to twentieth week of gestation; before that time the placental barrier is able to prevent its passage to the fetus. Syphilis can cause congenital anomalies, prematurity, or even intrauterine death. Treatment given the mother will also be effective for the fetus. Gonorrhea is not transmitted to the fetus during pregnancy but may be transmitted to the baby's eyes during the birth process. Since methods for detecting gonorrhea are not 100 percent accurate and since a woman could contract gonorrhea after testing, state laws require the immediate administration of medication to the eyes of all newborns as a prophylactic measure to kill the gonorrhea bacillus, which would cause blindness if it were present and left untreated. An active case of maternal genital herpes may also be transferred to the baby during the birth process. Consequently, a cesarean section is generally recommended to protect the infant from contact with this potentially damaging virus.

FETAL FACTORS

Occasionally the chromosomal configuration and the environment provided by the mother are optimal for the growth and the development of the fetus, but the site chosen for implantation or the presence of more than one fetus may present potential threats to maximal development or survival.

Nidation. As mentioned earlier, nidation usually occurs in the upper area of the uterus. A placenta that develops too close to the cervix may block the exit of the baby or may begin to separate prematurely as the cervical area stretches to prepare for birth. Unless facilities are available to assist the baby's safe exit (usually through cesarean section), the baby may not survive the birth process. Implantations outside of the uterine cavity are known as ectopic pregnancies. The zygote may get caught in the fallopian tube if the lumen is too narrow or if the zygote begins to increase in size before reaching the uterus. Most ectopic pregnancies do not survive because they are unable to obtain an adequate maternal blood supply source or room to expand.

Inadequacy of the Placenta. Occasionally the placenta is too small or malformed to support fetal growth and development adequately. Intrauterine growth retardation or death may result.

Twinning. Perhaps the most interesting variation of fetal development is twinning. Twins occur in about one out of 86 births [28]. Identical twins account for about one-third of twin conceptions; these monozygotic twins are formed by the union of one sperm and one ovum. A complete split occurs during one of the early cleavages, or by early subdivision of the inner cell mass of the blastocyst, allowing the freed cells to continue development independently [26]. At birth these twins will share a large placenta. One chorionic membrane envelops both of them; however, each twin develops its own amniotic membrane. Siamese twins are caused by incomplete separation of the inner cell mass; the twins can be attached to each other at any point. Most do not survive.

Fraternal or nonidentical twins are created by the release of two ova, both of which are fertilized by separate spermatozoa, that continue on to form two separate individuals. These fraternal or polyzygotic twins are no more alike than any other two siblings would be.

Twins experience problems not faced by the singleton. Because of the limited intrauterine space, there is

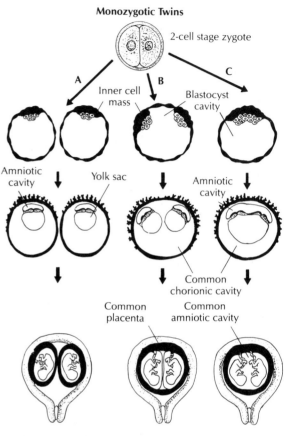

Figure 4–17. The possible relationships of the fetal membranes in monozygotic twins. (A) Splitting occurs at the two-cell stage, and each embryo has its own placenta, amniotic cavity, and chorionic cavity. (B) Splitting of the inner cell mass in two completely separated groups. The two embryos have a common placenta and chorionic sac but separate amniotic cavities. (C) Splitting of the inner cell mass at a late stage of development. The embryos have a common placenta, a common amniotic cavity, and a common chorionic cavity. (From J. Langman, *Medical Embryology* [4th ed.]. Baltimore: Williams & Wilkins, 1981. With permission.)

a higher incidence of prematurity. Twins have a perinatal death rate two to three times higher than that of singletons. The second-born twin is especially prone to difficulty during the birth process. There is also an increased incidence of congenital anomalies in twins, perhaps due to the same factor that originally caused the abnormal division in the blastocyst, or perhaps due to inadequate oxygen and food. Some monozygotic twins experience the fetal transfusion syndrome: The twins share the same placenta, and an extra blood vessel connects the two fetuses. Under this arrangement, blood is shunted from one twin to the other. At birth the donor twin shows marked signs of undernourishment; it is pale and anemic and shows signs of severe intrauterine growth retardation. The recipient twin is fat and red, often weighing twice as much as the donor twin. Both twins are considered to be high risk: the one because of inadequate blood supply and shock and the other because of too much blood and possible heart failure.

PSYCHOSOCIAL DEVELOPMENT OF THE FETUS

It is not yet known whether or not events occurring during intrauterine life directly affect the psychosocial development of the fetus. Our knowledge about prefunctional organization of human behavior is too limited to justify the theory that heredity alone is responsible for the infant's neuropsychological status at birth [40]. Gesell postulates that biophysical development, movement, and responses in utero lay a foundation for reflexive and voluntary movements or responses after birth [7].

Current methods of investigation rule out objective, systematic study of psychological interactions between mother and fetus, let alone the effect of such interaction on the development of the fetus. Available studies are limited to those parameters that can be measured objectively—biological events. Observations of affective events are limited to the subjective interpretation of the mother. Consequently, studies of infant behavior—particularly in the affective domain—are limited to the moment of birth as the point of departure. This is not to deny that prebirth events help to mold affective, cognitive, or language development; it is a recognition of our current inability to assess that development objectively.

The fetus evidences a wide range of activity patterns even before birth. Some fetuses move almost constantly; others establish daily patterns that consist of both peak activity and rest periods; others may be very quiet or exhibit inconsistent sleep-activity periods. Fetuses are known to respond to light and also to maternal activities. Many seem to enjoy the gentle sway of body motion and become active (or agitated?) when the mother lies down to rest. Mothers often indicate that there is a high correlation between the amount of intrauterine and extrauterine activity, but it is not known whether this is genetically or environmentally mediated.

It has been shown that a woman's emotional state can influence fetal motility and that fetal hyperactivity is related to neonatal hyperactivity. Both maternal stress and fetal or neonatal stressors are known to have an adverse effect on affective development. Thus a mother's emotional state during pregnancy may affect the kind of baby she produces [40].

Infants born to stressed mothers during World War II were noted to exhibit disturbed affective behaviors and hyperactivity [36]. Stott discovered in a controlled study that 75 percent of the offspring of mothers experiencing critical stress during pregnancy suffered from a serious illness at some time during the first 3 years of life; only 28 percent of infants of nonstressed mothers experienced similar serious illness [36]. Brazelton notes that infants who suffer intrauterine growth retardation seem to have more difficulty organizing neuromuscular responses and are frequently labeled as "colicky" by mothers [3].

The cochlea becomes functional by the fifth month of fetal life [3]. Fetuses are known to respond to external sound; changes in the fetal heart rate indicate that the fetus is capable of both discrimination of sounds and habituation to a sound. If a man and woman talk simultaneously to a neonate from opposite sides of the room, the infant will turn toward the female voice. Is this an innate preference for higher-pitched sounds, or the result of intrauterine familiarity with the mother's voice? Many mothers who sang or played a musical instrument during pregnancy report that their infants evidenced differential responses to different types of sounds and music before birth and a preference for the same mother-produced music after birth [16]. The infant's preference for the specific music as evidenced by discriminative responses has been reported to occur even with a 3- to 5-month lapse in presentation of the same auditory stimulus after birth and to persist for several years [13, 16].

Fetal hiccups are a common phenomenon, easily felt by the mother. Some mothers indicate that the infant exhibits crying behaviors and may even (rarely) emit sound while in utero. Some fetuses may arch their backs against the side of the uterus when the mother's abdomen is gently rubbed. Fetal activity represents a form of mother-baby communication [3] that helps the mother become attached to the new family member. Some adoptive mothers express a feeling of loss at not having shared this time with a new family member; we do not yet know the reciprocal effect on the infant.

It is established that biological events affect the development of the fetus in utero; these events may have psychosocial sequelae. Sensory apparatuses are intact and functioning even before birth. The effect of conditioning is very real but as yet has been inadequately studied. The fetus and neonate are amazingly resilient and plastic, allowing for many environmental events to occur in the pyschosocial realm without permanent or damaging effects. The use of neonatal and maternal tools for the purpose of establishing and maintaining effective psychosocial development after birth will be discussed in Chapters 5, 8, 9, 14, and 32.

SUMMARY

Growth of the fetus occurs by both hyperplasia and hypertrophy of cells. During the first trimester, the zygote traverses the fallopian tubes and implants in the upper uterine wall. The cells of the embryo undergo very rapid differentiation with the growth of body cells and organs. By the eighth week, all the basic structures for body systems are present. At the end of the first trimester, the infant is distinctly human in all external features, including genitalia. Growth and refinement of body organs and systems continue through the second trimester; continued growth and preparation for the birth process and independent survival are the focus of the third trimester. The fetus is known to respond to external events of light, sound, maternal emotions, and maternal activities.

The period of intrauterine life is one of the most critical phases of an individual's growth and development. The sensitive balance between external and internal environments creates a biological level of health that will influence the rest of the individual's life.

In the United States, about 3 percent of infants exhibit major congenital anomalies at birth [1]. Although genetic influences on development are established at the moment of conception, environmental factors also influence development. These must be controlled to prevent congenital anomalies. Maximal, normal growth of cells can be impeded at any point during development by various teratogenic agents. The effect of the agent depends on the stage of growth when the insult is introduced. Arrest of hyperplastic development cannot be reversed.

Health care for the infant should begin even before conception occurs through good nutrition and avoidance of nonessential exposure to x-rays and drugs. Maximal efforts should be directed toward creating an intrauterine environment that is conducive to optimal growth and development of the potentials present at conception. Amniocentesis can give us some information about the quality of intrauterine life and the readiness of the fetus for extrauterine life.

REFERENCES

1. Aase, J. M.   Environmental causes of birth defects. *Continuing Education for the Family Physician*, 3:29, Sept. 1975.
2. Barrett, D. E., Radke-Yarrow, M., and Klein, R. E.   Chronic malnutrition and child behavior: Effects of early caloric supplementation on social and emotional functioning at school age. *Dev. Psychol.* 18:541, 1982.
3. Brazelton, T. B., Parker, W. B., and Zuckerman, B. Importance of behavioral assessment of the neonate. *Curr. Probl. Pediatr.*, 7(2):1, 1976.
4. Early pregnancy test developed. *Cornell News*, April 1976.
5. Erb, L., and Andresen, B. D.   Hyperactivity: A possible consequence of maternal alcohol consumption. *Pediatr. Nurs.* 7(4):30, 1981.
6. Garn, S. M., et al.   Effect of maternal cigarette smoking on Apgar scores. *Am. J. Dis. Child.* 135:503, 1981.
7. Gesell, A. L.   *The Embryology of Behavior: The Beginnings of the Human Mind.* New York: Harper & Brothers, 1945.
8. Golbus, M. S., et al.   Prenatal genetic diagnosis in 3000 amniocenteses. *N. Engl. J. Med.* 300:157, 1979.
9. Guyton, A. C.   *Basic Human Physiology: Normal Function and Mechanisms of Disease* (2nd ed.). Philadelphia: Saunders, 1977.
10. Hanson, J. W., Jones, K. L., and Smith, D. W.   Fetal alcohol syndrome: Experience with 41 patients. *J.A.M.A.* 235:1458, 1976.
11. Hertig, A. T., Rock, J., and Adams, E. C.   A description of 34 human ova within the first 17 days of development. *Am. J. Anat.* 98:435, 1956.
12. Influence of maternal drug therapy on the fetus-newborn. *Perinatal Press* 1:10, 1976.
13. Jackson, K. H.   Music and the fetus. *Child. Today* 7(6):37, 1978.
14. Kline, J., et al.   Smoking: A risk factor for spontaneous abortion. *N. Engl. J. Med.* 297:793, 1977.
15. Langman, J.   *Medical Embryology: Human Development—Normal and Abnormal* (4th ed.). Baltimore: Williams & Wilkins, 1981.
16. Lind, J., and Hardgrove, C.   Lullabies. *Child. Today* 7(4):7, 1978.
17. Linden, G., and Henderson, B. E.   Genital-tract cancers in adolescents and young adults. *N. Engl. J. Med.* 286:760, 1972.
18. Lowrey, G. H.   *Growth and Development of Children* (7th ed.). Chicago: Year Book, 1978.
19. Luke, B.   Understanding pica in pregnant women. *Am. J. Matern. Child Nurs.* 2:97, 1977.
20. Moore, K. L.   *Before We Are Born: Basic Embryology and Birth Defects* (2nd ed.). Philadelphia: Saunders, 1983.
21. Moore, M. L.   *The Newborn Family and Nurse.* Philadelphia: Saunders, 1981.

22. Naeye, R. L., and Peters, E. C. Working during pregnancy: Effects on the fetus. *Pediatrics* 69:724, 1982.

23. O'Rahilly, R. *Developmental Stages in Human Embryos, Part A: Embryos of the First Three Weeks.* Washington, D.C.: Carnegie Institute of Washington, 1973.

24. Oullette, E., et al. Adverse effects on offspring of maternal alcohol abuse during pregnancy. *N. Engl. J. Med.* 297:528, 1977.

25. Patient brochure for progestins warns against use in pregnancy. *FDA Drug Bulletin* 8:36, 1978–1979.

26. Patten, B. M. *Patten's Human Embryology.* New York: McGraw-Hill, 1976.

27. Renwick, J. H., and Asker, R. L. Ethanol-sensitive times for the human conceptus. *Early Hum. Dev.* 8:99, 1983.

28. Rugh, R., and Shettles, L. B. *From Conception to Birth: The Drama of Life's Beginnings.* New York: Harper & Row, 1971.

29. Sacksteder, S. Embryology and fetal circulation. *Am. J. Nurs.* 78:262, 1978.

30. Shepard, T. H. *Catalog of Teratogenic Agents* (4th ed.). Baltimore: Johns Hopkins University Press, 1983.

31. Smith, C. A. Effects of maternal undernutrition upon the newborn infant in Holland (1944–1945). *J. Pediatr.* 30:229, 1947.

32. Smith, D. W., Bierman, E. L., and Robinson, N. M. (Eds.). *The Biologic Ages of Man: From Conception Through Old Age* (2nd ed.). Philadelphia: Saunders, 1978.

33. Socol, M. L., et al. Maternal smoking causes fetal hypoxia: Experimental evidence. *Am. J. Obstet. Gynecol.* 142:214, 1982.

34. Special: The alarming new evidence about marijuana's effects. *Good Housekeeping* (February 1975) 180:161.

35. Stephens, C. J. The fetal alcohol syndrome: Cause for concern. *Am. J. Matern. Child Nurs.* 6:251, 1981.

36. Stott, D. H. The Child's Hazards in Utero. In J. G. Howells (Ed.), *Modern Perspectives in International Child Psychiatry.* New York: Brunner/Mazel, 1971.

37. Tanner, J. M. *Foetus into Man: Physical Growth from Conception to Maturity.* London: Open Books, 1978.

38. What is the threat to men exposed to DES in utero? *Contemporary Ob/Gyn,* 8(3):53, 1976.

39. Winick, M. Cellular growth during early malnutrition. *Pediatrics* 47:969, 1971.

40. Wolff, P. H. Mother-Infant Relations at Birth. In J. G. Howells (Ed.), *Modern Perspectives in International Child Psychiatry.* New York: Brunner/Mazel, 1971.

41. Woollam, D. H. M. The effect of environmental factors on the foetus. *Journal of the College of General Practitioners,* 8(Suppl. 2):35, 1964.

42. Working in pregnancy: How long? How hard? What's your role? *Contemporary Ob/Gyn* 16:154, 1980.

43. Ziegel, E. E., and Cranley, M. S. *Obstetric Nursing* (8th ed.). New York: Macmillan, 1984.

III
The Neonate

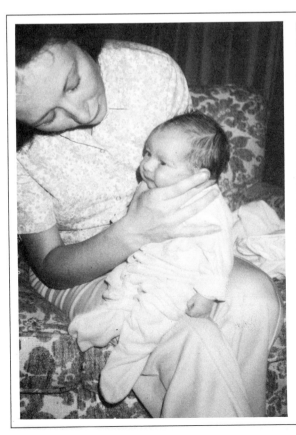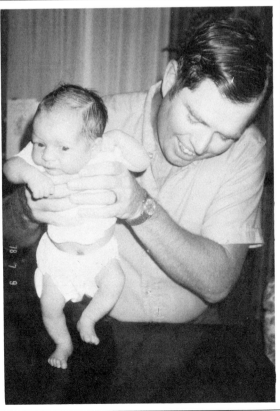

5
Transition to Extrauterine Life

Clara S. Schuster

The world hates change, yet it is the only thing that has brought progress.

—Charles Franklin Kettering

The first 24 hours of extrauterine life are the most tenuous and critical in a person's life. Events occurring during this time can affect the quality of life 7, 18, or even 40 years later. An infant experiences a greater risk of death during the first 7 days than during the next 30 years of extrauterine life [9]. Of the 3.5 million babies born alive each year in the United States [29], approximately 1 percent die within the first 24 hours and another 1 percent die within the first week.

The leading causes of neonatal death are associated with prematurity. Infants who are born before their body systems and organs are mature enough to maintain life independent of the mother require intensive medical intervention. Other major causes of neonatal deaths include asphyxia, congenital malformations, birth injuries, pneumonia, problems of the placenta, hemolytic disease, and infection. From this listing, it is obvious that many of these deaths could be prevented with the proper medical care. It is an embarrassment to the United States that it is not first or even second in the world in terms of survival of newborns, one of the indicators of the quality of a country's health care; rather, it is eighteenth! According to statistics compiled by the United Nations, in 1980 the United States had a neonatal (under 28 days of life) death rate of 13.0 per 1,000 live births. Sweden, which ranks first in infant survival, reported only 7.3 neonatal deaths per 1,000 live births [33]. Many of the preventable deaths are associated with inadequate prenatal care, a factor that should spur all practitioners, regardless of their discipline, to encourage every pregnant woman to seek adequate health care to reduce the incidence of prematurity, birth complications, and neonatal deaths. Some high-risk populations in major United States cities have a mortality rate of 20.0 per 1,000.

Even with the best of care, the process of transition to extrauterine life, which includes both the birth process and the adjustment of the newborn to physiological independence, is potentially traumatic and precarious. In this chapter, we will discuss the major stressors facing the infant and some of the factors that commonly affect the adjustment process.

THE BIRTH PROCESS

For 10 lunar months the infant has been cradled, protected, nurtured, and nourished within the controlled environment of the mother's uterus. Stimuli have been limited; nothing has been demanded of the fetus but to grow. Most fetuses experience no discomfort or pain—only a little cramping of space, yet even this seems to afford security.

Toward the end of the gestational period the irregular periodic uterine contractions (Braxton Hicks contractions) that have been present throughout the entire pregnancy become stronger and frequently are noticeable to both the mother and the infant (as evidenced by increased fetal movement). At some point these contractions suddenly become regular and stronger and begin to cause dilation and effacement (thinning) of the cervix, signaling that labor has begun. The intermittent uterine contractions of true labor gradually propel the infant between the mother's pelvic bones and into the world. This chapter will concentrate on the infant's response to the uterine contractions. The birth process from the mother's viewpoint is discussed in Chapter 32.

Stages of Labor

The birth process is divided into three stages. During the first (and usually the longest) stage, the cervix must thin, and the aperture must open sufficiently to allow the infant to pass through. The presenting part of the infant (usually the head) acts as the dilator of the cervix. This pressure against the presenting part frequently causes bruising and swelling of the infant's tissues. On rare occasions, the baby may actually be injured. Such injuries, which are discussed further in Chapter 6, are usually minor.

Once the cervix is completely dilated, the infant begins to traverse the pelvic passageway. This second stage is not an easy process for the infant, since the

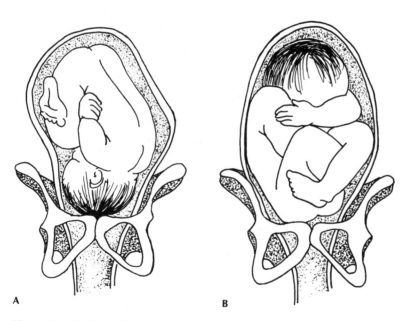

A   **B**

Figure 5–1. Position of fetus at term. (A) Cephalic presentation. (B) Breech presentation.

pelvic passage is not a straight, wide tube. The head, as the largest part of the infant, must accommodate itself to the widest diameters of the pelvis. The narrow, changing diameters and directions of the pelvic passage force the infant to twist, turn, bend, and stretch in order to negotiate the canal successfully. The infant is by no means a passive traveler through the passage. Pressure placed against an infant's head after birth will elicit a stretching, crawling response. It is thought that this same behavior is elicited during the birth process by the contracting uterus and causes the infant to help push himself out of the uterine cavity.

The chorionic and amniotic membranes frequently rupture early in the first stage of labor. If the membranes have not ruptured spontaneously, the physician or nurse in charge of the delivery will rupture them (a painless procedure) at some point during labor or immediately upon the birth of the presenting part of the infant. After the head passes between the muscles of the perineal floor, there is usually a brief pause before the shoulders and then the body emerge from the mother's vagina to the waiting hands of the mother, midwife, or physician.

Even though the infant is safely delivered, all the products of conception must be expelled before the mother can begin the involutional process—the return of the reproductive organs to their nonpregnant state. During the third stage, the placenta and membranes are expelled.

The length of the birth process is influenced by many factors. A small pelvis or an exceptionally large baby may slow it markedly. If the discrepancy is too great, the baby may not be able to traverse the pelvic passageway; in this situation, the baby can be safely delivered by cesarean section. Unusual position of the head or breech presentation also slows the birth process. One of the primary factors influencing the length of labor is the number of previous vaginal deliveries experienced by the mother. It usually takes the first baby about 12 hours to traverse the birth passage. Subsequent babies experience substantially shorter labor: The second and third infants of a mother generally are born after about 4 to 8 hours of labor. Other factors known to increase the length of labor include maternal medication, poor maternal health, and last pregnancy occurring more than 7 years previously. The length of

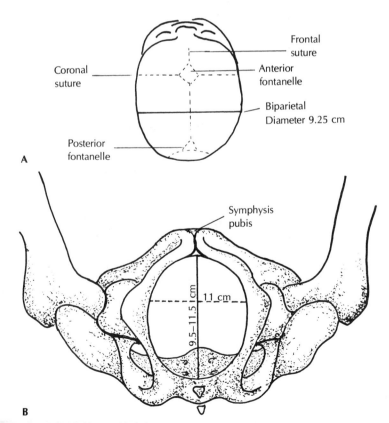

Figure 5-2. Head diameter versus pelvic diameter dimensions. (A) Coronal view of head. (B) Pelvic outlet seen from outlet position.

Engagement, Descent, Flexion

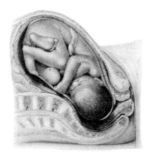
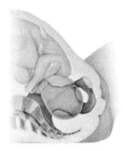
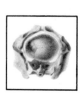

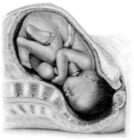
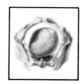

Internal Rotation

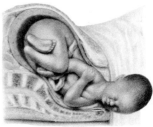
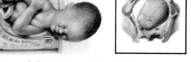

External Rotation (Restitution)

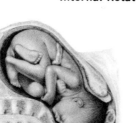
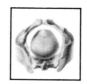

Extension Beginning (Rotation Complete)

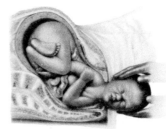
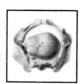

External Rotation (Shoulder Rotation)

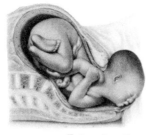

Extension Complete

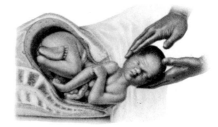

Expulsion

Figure 5–3. Mechanisms of normal labor. (Ross Clinical Education Aid No. 13. Courtesy Ross Laboratories.)

labor does not appear to have a significant effect on the infant's health unless it is accompanied by decreases in oxygen levels.

Fetal Response to Labor

The infant is markedly dependent on its environment for both extrusion and survival. The events that occur during the birth process can present stressors that can leave the infant poorly equipped to make the adjustments essential to successful extrauterine survival. One of the major stressors faced by infants is an irregular oxygen supply. Because of the anatomic structure of the uterus, contractions of the uterine muscles cause a decrease in blood flow within the uterus. Subsequently, the amount of blood filling the intervillous spaces is decreased during contractions, making less oxygen available to the baby. Fortunately, contractions rarely last longer than 60 to 90 seconds. Nature thus provides for a replenishing of oxygen supplies during the 2- to 10-minute rest periods between contractions.

Occasionally, the cord is compressed between the baby and the birth passage. This situation would also cause a decrease in the oxygen available to the infant. Lowered fetal oxygen levels during labor can be identified by medical personnel by monitoring the rate of the fetal heart. The normal range of fetal heart rate is 120 to 160 beats per minute. An acceleration of 15 to 25 beats per minute may occur during contractions. The fetal heart can be externally monitored by a special stethoscope or through electronic microphones. The microphone picks up the sound of the baby's heartbeat through the abdominal wall and magnifies it for medical personnel, the mother, and the father.

A more sensitive and reliable method of monitoring the fetal heart rate is known as internal monitoring. A tiny special electrode is attached to the presenting part of the infant. The fetal heart sounds are amplified if desired, but they are also recorded on a continuous graph paper for identification of patterns of heart rate as compared to the onset and intensity of uterine contractions. A moderate dip in the fetal heart rate with the onset of contractions is a normal phenomenon ac-

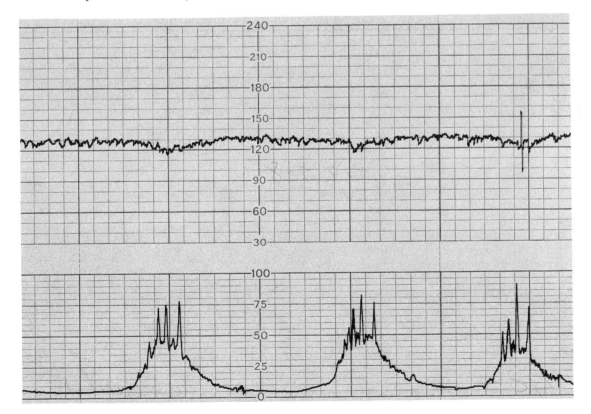

Figure 5–4. Monitor strip from internal monitor. Lower reading is the uterine pressure. Spikes during contractions indicate the mother was pushing down to assist with the descent of the baby. Slight dipping in the fetal heart rate (upper line) is normal during contractions.

companying compression of the baby's head as it presses against the cervix.

All medications given to the mother during labor pass through the placental barrier. A side effect of such medication may be changes in fetal heart rate. After birth, the baby's immature liver and excretory systems may delay excretion of the maternal medications and anesthesia. The postnatal effects of maternal medication are strongest during the first 2 days and gradually decrease over the next 5 to 10 days [3, 23]. A baby who is sedated will have decreased responses to environmental stimuli. The infant may require more vigorous stimulation and assistance to begin breathing and may even need occasional reminding to continue breathing efforts for as long as 2 days after birth. These infants are also sleepier and less responsive to their parents than infants receiving no medication during labor. An underresponsive baby is known to affect the parent-infant relationship negatively—a factor that can have long-range implications (see Chap. 32).

STAGES IN THE TRANSITIONAL PROCESS

The infant faces several critical stressors once the birth process is initiated. Each stage of labor has unique stressors, as do the periods following birth. Any decrease in oxygen supply during the birth process is treated as a medical emergency, requiring immediate intervention and possible cesarean section to maintain the life of the baby.

The infant's skull is composed of eight freely moving flat plates separated by membranous spaces known as sutures (see Figs. 5–2, 6–7). During the compression of the birth process, these cranial bones move, slide, and overlap each other at the edges, decreasing the diameter of the cranial vault. The amount of molding that may occur depends on fetal age and size and on the duration and the intensity of intrauterine pressures as well as the size of the pelvic passage. The molding and edema (swelling) that may accompany the trauma of birth are both normal and temporary. Rarely, an infant may experience intracranial bleeding as a result of the pressures associated with birth; this bleeding can cause temporary or permanent brain damage. The problem occurs more frequently in the premature than in the full-term infant because of the greater fragility of the blood vessels.

The First Thirty Minutes

Every person who is privileged to witness the entrance of a new life into the world experiences an indescrib-

able thrill. As the head is delivered, each witness instinctively takes a breath, tightens, and waits in anticipatory silence for the newcomer to take the first breath. The skin is a deep bluish-gray. The clock slowly measures off time. Each second seems an eternity. You find yourself silently telling the child to breathe—to take a breath—to live. Suddenly that first gasp is drawn and the baby's skin flushes bright pink. The tension is broken. You take a breath. Talking resumes in the delivery room; smiles return to faces. But there is no smile on the baby's face. For the first time the baby is facing light, gravity, and cold air. The newcomer cries and vigorously, much to everyone's delight. Now is not a time for sleep!

ACTIVATION OF THE RESPIRATORY SYSTEM

Establishment of effective respiratory efforts is the most critical and immediate change following birth. Respiratory-like movements of the lungs have been present since about the fourth month of gestation. Although the stimulus for initiating respiratory efforts is not clear, decreasing oxygen levels and increasing carbon dioxide levels of the blood make pulmonary air exchange essential within 1 minute following birth. Theories regarding respiratory initiators include the physical stimulation of the birth process, the sudden release of pressure from the thoracic cavity, and the decrease in blood oxygen levels [25]. Because it is not unusual for an infant to take the first breath and cry before the birth process is completed (especially if minimal or no medications are given to the mother), the last two theories appear invalidated. The sudden change in the baby's environment, the exposure to firm touch, and the cooling effect of air have more support as initiators of respiratory efforts.

The pressure exerted on the lungs during crying helps to expand the alveolar (air) sacs. The newborn frequently cries a total of 1 to 2 hours out of every 24. Respiratory rate may range from 50 to 80 breaths per minute during the first 24 hours. After the first 24 hours, respirations average 40 per minute but may range from 30 to 60 per minute. The chest and abdominal wall frequently rise and fall together. Both respiratory rhythm and depth of breaths may be very irregular. Short, rapid, shallow breaths are frequently followed by a 5- to 10-second pause in breathing. A frequent interspersing of slow, deep respirations may lead the casual observer to believe that the infant is gasping for breath. The occurrence of mild retractions—a drawing in of the soft tissues surrounding the thoracic cavity during inspiration and crying—is not unusual until the alveoli are fully expanded.

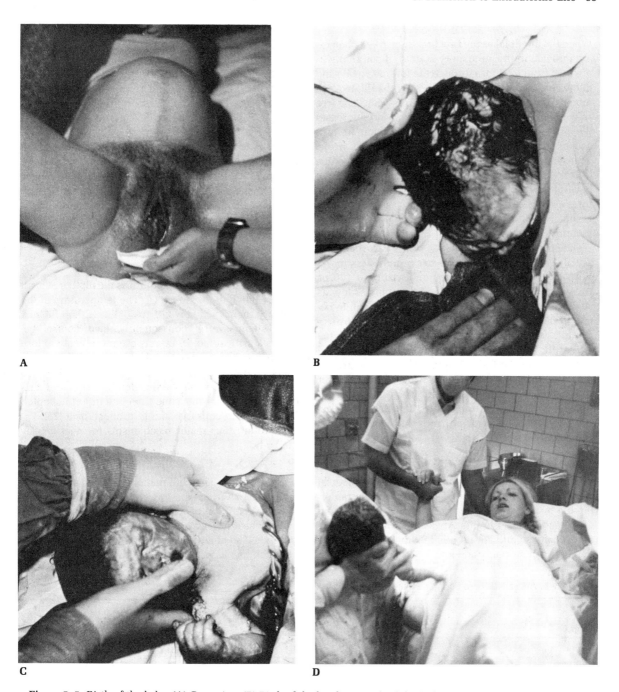

Figure 5–5. Birth of the baby. (A) Crowning. (B) Birth of the head. (C) Birth of the body. (D) Birth process completed; the baby is shown to the mother and the father. (Photographs B and C used with permission of Sandy Eckstrom, Manchester Monitrice Association, Manchester, Connecticut.)

CIRCULATORY SYSTEM CHANGES

When the infant takes the first breath, marked changes are initiated in the circulatory system. Blood that was diverted from the lungs through the foramen ovale and ductus arteriosus now passes through the dilated pulmonary vessels to receive the needed oxygen. The free flow of blood through the pulmonary artery increases the pressure within the left atrium, which in turn causes closure of a flap valve over the foramen ovale. Transient heart murmurs lasting for several days due to leakage of blood through the fetal openings do not have pathologic significance. The four special structures associated with fetal circulation (see Chap. 4) are gradually obliterated during the next few weeks and months.

The pulse rate after the first 24 hours is variable but usually rapid, 120 to 150 beats per minute. It is markedly affected by activity, commonly rising to 170 or 180 when the infant is crying and dropping as low as 90 during deep sleep. Blood pressure is difficult to obtain in the neonate and is highly subject to the instruments used to measure the pressure as well as to the skill of the practitioner. Birth weight is also a critical factor. During the first 12 hours, blood pressure can range from 49/26 to 66/41 [12]. A full-term baby over 24 hours of age averages 80/46 [6]. Sluggishness of peripheral circulation during the first few days of life accounts for the blue color of hands and feet known as acrocyanosis.

APGAR SCORE

At 1 minute and again at 5 minutes after birth, medical personnel assess the infant's adaptation to extrauterine life by use of the Apgar newborn scoring system developed by Dr. Virginia Apgar in 1953 (Table 5–1). Statistically significant correlations have been identified between mortality and low Apgar scores at 1 minute of life; even more significant correlations are found with low 5-minute scores. Infants in the latter category also have a high incidence of neurological defects [22]. The five factors evaluated are color, heart rate, reflex irritability, muscle tone, and respiratory effort. Each factor is rated as 0, 1, or 2 according to the objective criteria. A delay in "pinking" often prevents a perfect score of 10.

Evaluation of the Apgar score is as follows: a score of 7 to 10 is considered good; 5 to 7 is poor—these infants may need assistance to maintain life and have a higher mortality rate; 0 to 4 is very poor—these infants need immediate cardiac and respiratory assistance, and those who survive have a high incidence of neurological defects.

HEAT CONTROL

The baby is the same temperature as the mother at birth (98° to 100°F or 36° to 38°C). The temperature of the delivery room is usually 20° to 30°F less than the maternal temperature; consequently, heat control becomes a critical factor. Infants are more likely to lose heat in a cold room than adults because of the greater proportion of body surface to body weight. They also have less subcutaneous fat (insulation) than older children or adults. At the same time, the infant is limited in the ways to conserve and to produce heat [28].

There are four major mechanisms for heat loss by the body:

1. Evaporation. The chill that one feels when stepping out of a shower or a swimming pool is caused by the evaporation of water from the body into the air. Body heat is used to transform the liquid into water vapor. The newborn is covered with amniotic fluid, which has bathed him for the past 9 months; thus,

Table 5–1. Apgar Newborn Scoring System

Sign		Score		
		0	1	2
Appearance	Color*	Pale	Blue extremities	Pink
Pulse	Heart rate	Not detectable	Below 100	Above 100
Grimace	Reflex irritability	No response	Grimace	Vigorous cry
Activity	Muscle tone	Flaccid	Some flexion of extremities	Active motion
Respiration	Respiratory effort	Absent	Slow, irregular	Good (crying)

*Alternative measures of circulatory adequacy may be used for assessing nonwhite children (such as color of mucus membranes or color of lips, palms, nail beds, and soles of feet).
Source: Modified from V. Apgar et al., "Evaluation of the Newborn Infant—Second Report." J.A.M.A. 168:1988, 1958. Copyright 1958, American Medical Association.

vigorous efforts to the dry the infant are essential to prevent heat loss by evaporation.

2. Conduction. Body heat is lost to cooler objects that are in direct contact with the skin. Most of us shiver at the thought of putting on a jacket that is kept on the back porch in the winter or jumping between cold bed sheets in the evening. The preheating of blankets, towels, diapers, and cribs can help to prevent massive heat loss by this mechanism.

3. Convection. Cool air passing over the body also tends to rob it of heat. Specially heated cribs and infant warmers can heat the surrounding air and block breezes that could add unnecessary stress to the newborn.

4. Radiation. Heat can also be transferred through the air to other, cooler objects and to the walls of the room. Have you ever noticed how much cooler 70°F rooms feel during the winter months than during the summer months? It is not a psychological phenomenon; your body is actually helping to maintain the enviromental temperature by radiating heat to the walls, which are in contact with the cold outside air. Well-insulated houses feel much warmer at 70°F than do poorly insulated ones. There is no way to ensure protection against radiation loss except to insulate the room and to block the loss of heat through layers of clothing. Wrapping the newborn securely in blankets helps to reduce the degree of heat loss from radiation.

From the moment of birth, the neonate should be provided with a neutral thermal environment, a room temperature at which oxygen consumption and caloric expenditure for heat production is minimized [28]. In the neonate, the heat control mechanism of the brain is as yet poorly developed. Few newborns are able to shiver adequately to produce much heat. Newborns do experience an increase in metabolic rate in response to cold, allowing them to produce additional body heat to offset the heat loss. Three other mechanisms of heat conservation and production are available to the normal full-term infant:

1. Constriction of blood vessels. By constricting the blood vessels to the body surface areas, heat can be maintained in the inner parts of the infant's body. Two common side effects are mottled skin and acrocyanosis (bluish-colored hands and feet).

2. Positional changes. By flexing the extremities and back, the infant can bring the body closer to itself, thus decreasing the total amount of exposed skin surface (as in Paul Chabas' painting "September

Morn"). Since the immature neurologic system of the premature infant does not yet allow this defensive behavior, the premature infant is at high risk of pathological heat loss.

3. Metabolism of brown fat. During the last month of intrauterine life, the newborn has been storing in the upper portions of the body a unique type of adipose (fat) tissue, which can produce heat under the stress of cooling. Brown fat comprises about 2 to 6 percent of the neonate's body weight [32]. The rich nerve and blood supply of these special cells give brown fat both its color and its ability to be mobilized, metabolized, and disseminated quickly as heat when needed.

It is estimated that the wet newborn can lose up to 200 calories of heat per kilogram per minute [22]. When one considers that the adult at full compensation can produce only 90 calories of heat per kilogram per minute, the stress of cooling can be put into a new perspective. An increase in metabolism causes an increase in the consumption of both glucose (sugar) and brown fat and in turn increases the need for oxygen.

The impact of the stress of cooling at birth can continue to exhibit its effects through a higher metabolic rate for as long as 7 to 10 days after birth [37]. Energy used for heat maintenance cannot be used to aid in the other adjustments to extrauterine life or for body growth. Moreover, babies who have lost excessive amounts of heat are unable to produce surfactant well. (Surfactant is a thin film of fluid found coating the inner lining of the lungs; this lipoprotein reduces the surface tension of the alveoli, allowing them to expand and preventing their collapse.) Consequently, even though infants need increased amounts of oxygen to meet the demands of increased metabolism, they may not be able to obtain sufficient oxygen due to respiratory distress syndrome—the result of decreased pulmonary surfactant.

It is normal, not pathological, for the infant's temperature to drop 1° to 2°F immediately after birth. In a protected environment, the temperature begins to rise spontaneously and returns to normal by 8 hours of age. Nevertheless, prevention of excessive heat loss, especially during the first 15 minutes of life, is extremely significant to the infant's ability to make a successful transition to extrauterine life.

LeBOYER'S METHOD OF CHILDBIRTH
In 1929 Otto Rank, a psychoanalyst, identified the experience of birth as a major influencing factor in an individual's view of the world as either friendly or hos-

tile. He felt that birth trauma could be so great that it would significantly interfere with an individual's ability to cope with stressors later in life [27]. In the early 1970s Frederick LeBoyer [18], a French obstetrician, developed a new method for handling the newborn during the first 15 to 30 minutes after birth, which he feels reduces the potential trauma inherent in the experience. According to LeBoyer, medical personnel need to pay greater attention to the newborn as an individual in the minutes following birth. He suggests minimizing the stressors facing the neonate by reducing the intensity of new stimuli, such as light, gravity, and coolness. He recommends eliminating all but essential talking, turning down all lights, and placing the baby on the mother's abdomen until the cord ceases pulsating (3 to 5 minutes). During this time the doctor or parent gently massages the baby's back to simulate the uterine contractions. After the cord has been cut, the infant is placed in a warm water bath for 10 to 15 minutes and then wrapped in a warm blanket and placed at the mother's breast for nursing. LeBoyer advocates his method of introducing the neonate to the world as being less traumatic and consequently emotionally safer than the current practice of placing the naked infant in a crib under bright lights. He feels that infants treated by his method experience less crying and are more alert during the first hour of life.

Current observations indicate that gentler treatment of the newborn during this first 15 minutes does result in quieter, more alert infants during the next few days of life. However, pediatricians T. Berry Brazelton and Marshall Klaus disagree with LeBoyer's rationale for providing a water bath, stating that the increased quiet alertness (Wolff's state 4) found during the first 30 minutes of life will be present in any infant who is free of depressant maternal medication and who is kept warm. They advocate keeping the baby with its mother during the first hour. These doctors claim that the new stimuli, especially mild temperature changes, are essential to maintain respiratory efforts. Brazelton and Klaus offer as evidence an experiment in which three normal 2-hour-old infants stopped breathing completely when they were placed in a water bath approximating the mother's temperature [30]. Although infants born by the LeBoyer method tend to have higher scores on the Brazelton Neonatal Assessment (see Chap. 6), there are no observable differences in development or temperament by 8 months of age [25]. Additional observations are needed to identify the critical positive components of LeBoyer's method and the long-range as well as the short-range effects.

The First Three Days

During the first 3 to 4 days of life the newborn continues to take giant steps toward independent physiologic functioning. The stomach, the intestines, and the liver must begin to accept and to metabolize food for the body. The kidneys and the bowel must begin to function as systems for eliminating wastes. Neurological tissues must recover and begin to assume responsibility for controlling respiratory efforts, heat control, and protective reflexes. Most of these physiological changes are covered in Chapter 6. The four factors discussed here represent normal phenomena in the neonate but offer potential threats to survival if they are not adequately anticipated or monitored.

BEHAVIOR PATTERNS

The first 12 hours after birth are usually marked by two periods of intense activity followed by periods of rest. Most babies then begin to fall into a relatively stable pattern of sleeping versus waking behaviors that coincide with feeding times.

The first period of activity immediately follows birth. The infant experiences vigorous, intense activity characterized by outbursts of intense crying and hyperreflexive reactions. The respiratory rate may be as high as 82 breaths per minute during the first hour of life; this rate gradually subsides to 45 to 55 breaths per minute as the lungs expand and adequate ventilation is achieved. The intense stress of the birth process and the adjustment to independent procurement of oxygen also cause a rapid increase in pulse rate. The pulse rate is commonly 180 beats per minute during the first hour of life but gradually decreases as the physical stressors diminish and emotional comfort is offered, stabilizing between 120 and 160 beats per minute. The newborn usually remains alert and active until the period of the first extrauterine sleep, which occurs in the nonsedated baby about 1 to 2 hours after birth. Observations by Klaus and Kennell indicate that neonates will spend the majority of the first period of activity in the quiet alert state if they are kept warm and with the mother [14]. As mentioned earlier, activity and alertness during the first 2 hours can be greatly depressed if the mother has received medication during labor.

After 2 to 4 hours of sleep, the newborn enters a second period of wakefulness, lasting 1 to 2 hours. The baby is temporarily hyperactive to all stimuli and experiences swift color changes, quickly flushing red when crying. Many infants secrete excessive amounts of mucus at this time as a normal protective response to the drying effect of air on the tender lungs. Most infants achieve relative stability with a decrease in hypersensitivity to the environment by 12 hours of age.

STATES OF CONSCIOUSNESS

Wolff objectively divides the activity-sleep state of the neonate into six specific categories [35].

State 1 regular sleep	Regular respiratory rhythm, frequent Moro reflex, no grimacing or eye movement.
State 2 irregular sleep	Erratic respiratory rhythm, decreased Moro reflex, increased limb and body movement; grimacing, smiling, and mouthing; frequent REMs (rapid eye movements).
State 3 drowsiness	Irregular respiratory rhythm, opening and closing of eyes, less Moro reflex than in regular sleep but more than in irregular sleep; activity greater than in regular sleep, less than in irregular sleep.
State 4 quiet alert	Fairly regular respiration; eyes wide open, appearing to focus; increased moisture on eyeball gives "bright" appearance; attends quickly to auditory and visual stimuli.
State 5 active awake	Irregular respirations, nonfocused, dull eye movements; frequent spurts of diffuse activity, grunting, groaning, or fussiness.
State 6 crying	Irregular, forceful respirations; diffuse physical activity.

These states appear to develop by the thirty-eighth week of gestation. Behaviors are less clearly differentiated in gestationally younger babies [8, 26]. The activity periods of the first 24 hours include expressions of states 4, 5, and 6. The quiet, alert babies described by physicians Kennell, Klaus, Brazelton, and LeBoyer are experiencing state 4, the normal activity state of the 5- to 60-minute-old neonate who is kept warm and secure. State 4 is especially significant to mother-infant interaction and to early childhood education.

COMMON PROBLEMS OF THE
TRANSITIONAL PERIOD

Two rather common but transient problems face the newborn during this transitional period. Because breathing is a new experience to the infant and the respiratory center of the brain may not yet be fully operative, some infants may literally forget to breathe. Medicated and premature infants in particular may have this problem. Gently hitting the crib or shaking the baby's leg is usually sufficient to rouse the infant from the too-comfortable state and reinitiate respiratory efforts. More aggressive interventions are occasionally necessary if these measures are inadequate.

Excessive amounts of thick oral mucus can block the respiratory passages. This hypersecretion is apparently a compensatory effort by the body to keep the lung membranes moist and to prevent entrance of foreign material. The presence of excessive mucus coupled with the typically poor coordination of the sucking and swallowing reflexes can lead to difficulty during the first few feedings. Tipping the baby upside down and gently patting the back allows and facilitates the escape of the mucus through the mouth.

EARLY PHYSIOLOGICAL CHANGES

Changes in the Cord. The bluish-white, gelatinous cord is usually cut 1½ to 3 inches away from its juncture with the abdominal wall. The 1½-inch diameter decreases sharply with the collapse of the umbilical vessels. Because of the high water content, the stump of the cord dries and shrinks rapidly, losing its flexibility by 24 hours after birth. By the second day, it is a very hard yellow (dehydrated Wharton's jelly) or black (blood) tag on the skin. Slight oozing where the cord joins the abdominal wall is common and offers an excellent medium for bacterial growth. Parents are encouraged to clean the area with cotton balls and alcohol, or another antiseptic solution, several times daily until the cord has dropped off (6 to 14 days). This frequent cleaning should be continued until the area is completely healed (2 to 3 days after the cord falls off).

Physiological Jaundice. Fifty percent of all full-term newborn infants exhibit some degree of jaundice (yellow coloration) on the second through the sixth day of life. Persons who are not familiar with this normal phenomenon of adjustment to extrauterine life—especially new parents—frequently fear that the child's life is in jeopardy due to a disease, such as hepatitis. An explanation can relieve much anxiety.

Because of the low oxygen concentration experienced during intrauterine life, the fetus produces many immature red blood cells to carry the available oxygen to vital areas of the developing body. After birth, with better oxygen concentrations, this number of red blood cells is unnecessary; consequently, the body begins to hemolyze, or destroy, the excessive and immature red blood cells. The breakdown products circulate in the blood until they are stored, excreted, or metabolized.

Red blood cells break down into heme and globin. Globin, being a protein, is recycled by the body for growth needs. Heme undergoes further breakdown into iron and indirect bilirubin. The iron is stored in

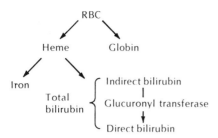

Figure 5–6. Hemolysis of red blood cells. Indirect bilirubin cannot be excreted by the kidneys and will accumulate in the baby's body until it is converted into direct bilirubin.

the liver to be recycled later; the bilirubin, however, is a waste product, which is excreted through the kidneys. Because the indirect form of bilirubin is not water-soluble, it cannot be excreted through the urine. The enzyme glucuronyl transferase, produced by the liver, functions as a catalyst to transform the indirect bilirubin into a water-soluble form, direct bilirubin, which can be excreted [10].

During the first few days of life, when excretory needs are high, the newborn's capacity to convert indirect bilirubin is only 1 to 2 percent of that of the adult [17]. The spillover phenomenon of this buildup of indirect bilirubin in the circulatory system causes the skin and eyes to become a yellow color. Fortunately, this condition is self-correcting. As the liver gradually matures and mobilizes its resources, the bilirubin is converted and excreted. The jaundice usually disappears without treatment between the seventh and fourteenth days of life. It should be noted that jaundice appearing during the first 36 hours of life is considered pathologic. All jaundiced babies should be observed carefully and given appropriate treatment if the blood level of indirect bilirubin becomes too high. Abnormally high concentrations of indirect bilirubin can cause brain damage and even death. Moderately high levels may be associated with hyperactivity, learning disabilities, and behavior problems.

Transitory Coagulation Defects. The ability of the liver to produce substances essential to coagulation of the blood is delayed until the intestine is able to synthesize vitamin K. Consequently, bleeding problems may be experienced between the second and fifth days of life. Many health care agencies give all infants an injection of vitamin K shortly after birth as a prophylactic agent to prevent bleeding problems.

FACTORS AFFECTING TRANSITION

One of the major factors affecting the newborn's ability to adjust to extrauterine life is gestational age. The length of time spent in the uterus directly correlates with the maturity of the organs and their consequent ability to function independently of the mother's support. Just as individuals grow at different rates after birth, the same is true during intrauterine development.

Infants over the ninetieth percentile are considered large for gestational age; those under the tenth percentile are considered small for gestational age. Traditionally, any baby weighing less than 2500 gm (5½ pounds) at birth was considered to be premature. However, it is obvious that the terms **premature** and **small for gestational age** are not synonymous, as Figure 5–8 shows. Intrauterine growth may be affected by both hereditary and developmental factors. Infants of physically small parents are more likely to be smaller than the average baby. However, a birth weight under 2500 gm indicates that growth rate is suboptimal at the time of birth regardless of cause. Recognizing this fact, the World Health Organization gives the following definitions based on 40 weeks' gestation from the last menstrual period (LMP) [17]:

Low birth weight. Under 2500 gm
Premature. Born before the end of the thirty-seventh week
Full term. Born between the thirty-eighth and forty-first weeks
Postmature. Born after the beginning of the forty-second week

Assessment of Gestational Age

Since the due date as calculated by the LMP is not always accurate, gestational maturity is often assessed by external signs of physical and neurological maturity. Figure 5–7 gives one example of a gestational age assessment chart. The major factors that change with increased gestational age are skin color and translucency, body weight, and neuromuscular functioning. Mature functioning of the central nervous system is exhibited by increased muscle tone and coordinated reflexes. Since gestational age is usually more significant than body weight as an indicator of the problems the infant may experience during the transitional period, assessment of external characteristics is essential for anticipating and planning intervention strategies.

GESTATIONAL AGE ASSESSMENT (Ballard)

NAME _____   DATE/TIME OF BIRTH _____   BIRTH WEIGHT _____

HOSPITAL NO. _____   DATE/TIME OF EXAM _____   LENGTH _____

                                 AGE WHEN EXAMINED _____   HEAD CIRC. _____

RACE _____   SEX _____   EXAMINER _____

APGAR SCORE: 1 MINUTE _____ 5 MINUTES _____

NEUROMUSCULAR MATURITY

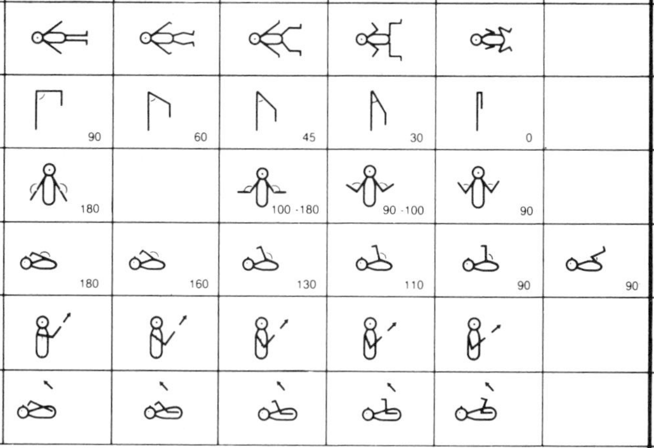

NEUROMUSCULAR MATURITY SIGN	SCORE						RECORD SCORE HERE
	0	1	2	3	4	5	
POSTURE							
SQUARE WINDOW (WRIST)	90	60	45	30	0		
ARM RECOIL	180		100-180	90-100	90		
POPLITEAL ANGLE	180	160	130	110	90	90	
SCARF SIGN							
HEEL TO EAR							

TOTAL NEUROMUSCULAR MATURITY SCORE

PHYSICAL MATURITY

PHYSICAL MATURITY SIGN	SCORE						RECORD SCORE HERE
	0	1	2	3	4	5	
SKIN	gelatinous red, transparent	smooth pink, visible veins	superficial peeling, &/or rash few veins	cracking pale area rare veins	parchment deep cracking no vessels	leathery cracked wrinkled	
LANUGO	none	abundant	thinning	bald areas	mostly bald		
PLANTAR CREASES	no crease	faint red marks	anterior transverse crease only	creases ant. 2/3	creases cover entire sole		
BREAST	barely percept.	flat areola no bud	stippled areola, 1-2mm bud	raised areola, 3-4mm bud	full areola 5-10mm bud		
EAR	pinna flat, stays folded	sl. curved pinna; soft with slow recoil	well-curv. pinna; soft but ready recoil	formed & firm with instant recoil	thick cartilage ear stiff		
GENITALS (Male)	scrotum empty no rugae		testes descending, few rugae	testes down good rugae	testes pendulous deep rugae		
GENITALS (Female)	prominent clitoris & labia minora		majora & minora equally prominent	majora large, minora small	clitoris & minora completely covered		

Reference
Ballard JL, Novak KK, Driver M: A simplified score for assessment of
fetal maturation of newly born infants. *J Pediatr* 95:769-774, 1979.
Reprinted by permission of Dr Ballard and *Journal of Pediatrics*.

TOTAL PHYSICAL MATURITY SCORE

SCORE

Neuromuscular _____

Physical _____

Total _____

MATURITY RATING

TOTAL MATURITY SCORE	GESTATIONAL AGE (WEEKS)
5	26
10	28
15	30
20	32
25	34
30	36
35	38
40	40
45	42
50	44

GESTATIONAL AGE (weeks)

By dates _____

By ultrasound _____

By score _____

Figure 5–7. Clinical estimation of gestational age. (From J. L. Ballard, K. K. Novak, and M. Driver. A simplified score for assessment of fetal maturation of newly born infants. *J. Pediatr.* 95:769–774, 1979. With permission.)

Prematurity

Approximately 8 percent of infants may be classified as premature at birth in the United States [37]. This figure would include babies under 38 weeks gestational age whether over or under 2500 gm. Babies of diabetic mothers frequently are large for gestational age but still may be premature by birth. Multiple-birth pregnancy also increases the frequency of prematurity.

The head of the premature infant characteristically appears to be too large for its body, although this feature depends on the degree of prematurity. Blood vessels can be seen through the delicate, loose, wrinkled skin. The thin arms and legs frequently lie flat on the mattress; this characteristic is in sharp contrast to the healthy full-term infant, who keeps the extremities flexed. Reflex movements and crying are spasmodic and weak in the premature baby. The eyes and abdomen are prominent and the genitalia small. The fingernails are thin, and hair is fine and fuzzy. Lanugo and vernix still cover the body. Many of these infants need vigilant observation because they "forget" to breathe. The shorter the gestational time, the greater is the likelihood that respiratory distress syndrome will develop because of the infant's inability to produce surfactant.

IMMEDIATE PROBLEMS
The problems and prognosis of the premature infant correlate very highly with the degree of immaturity (see Fig. 5–8). Only 45 percent of infants born at 26 weeks survive [11]. Forty percent of surviving infants who weighed under 1000 gms at birth have major handicaps [15]. Essentially normal premature babies who survive the first 72 hours of life usually have a good chance of continued growth and development. The second week of life may present a critical, but avoidable, threat to survival, that is, the danger of infection. The immunologic system of the premature infant is very immature. Even the full-term infant is poorly protected physiologically from bacteria because antibodies are not yet developed to ward off infection. Although the mother does transfer some antibodies to the infant during pregnancy, every effort must be made by all persons having contact with the newborn to avoid transfer of potentially harmful bacteria. Some bacteria that are normally present on the adult body can be controlled and tolerated because of the adult's mature immunologic system; the same bacteria can cause death in the young infant.

Many premature infants who successfully survive the first 2 weeks of life are again threatened during the third month of life. The breakdown of red blood cells following birth, combined with the lack of opportunity to store up sufficient reserves of iron because of the shortened intrauterine period, can lead to anemia or a deficiency in hemoglobin and red blood cells. This anemia in the third month of life that results from inadequate iron reserves can be avoided by consistently adding iron to the infant's diet.

LONG-RANGE PROBLEMS
The long-range effects of prematurity per se are difficult to identify and document because of the close association of prematurity with both prenatal and postnatal complications as well as infant-mother separation [14]. Most long-range effects appear to be due to the complications rather than to the fact of prematurity alone. Prematurely born children do exhibit a higher incidence of mental retardation and abnormal neurologic entities, such as cerebal palsy, convulsive disorders, and learning disabilities.

During the 1940s and the 1950s blindness, specifically retrolental fibroplasia (RLF), was a frequent sequela of prematurity. In 1951 it was discovered that the high concentrations of oxygen given to maintain the life of the premature infant and to prevent brain damage were causing pathological changes in the blood vessels of the eye [17]. The early constriction of the retinal vessels led to architectural changes of the retina that caused the retina to become detached and scarred 1 to 2 months after oxygen therapy was terminated. The result in many cases was total, irreparable blindness. Careful monitoring of the oxygen concentrations of the arterial blood has caused a marked reduction in RLF. Nevertheless, there is a thin line between too much and too little oxygen for the critically ill, premature infant; some newborns still sustain either brain or retinal damage despite the best of medical care.

The other potentially critical effect of prematurity is maladaptive emotional adjustment. Studies in the area of touch and mother-infant separation in the premature baby are still in the early stages. However, such studies do show that the baby who is gently rocked and caressed and is given other appropriate stimuli is calmer and gains weight faster than the premature infant who is cared for with a "hands-off" policy [5, 16]. Parents who have limited contact with their new baby who is ill may feel more like strangers than excited, loving mothers and fathers. Fears of losing the baby, mental retardation, and a myriad of indefinable unknowns coupled with minimal contact and factors, such as financial concerns and family pressure, may

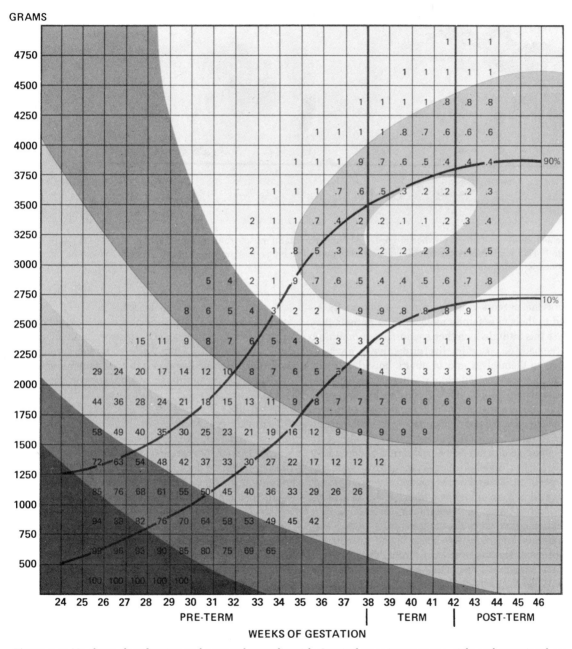

Figure 5–8. Newborn classification and neonatal mortality risk. Survival rates increase as weight and gestational age increase. (From L. O. Lubchenco, D. T. Searls, and J. V. Brazie. Neonatal mortality rate: Relationship to birth weight and gestational age. *J. Pediatr.* 81:814–822, 1972. With permission.)

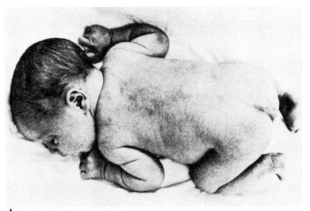 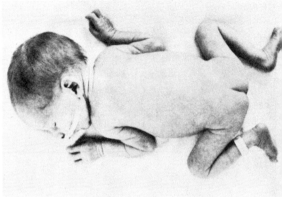

A   B

Figure 5–9. Body positions of newborn infants. (A) Full-term infant; muscle tonus is good. The infant keeps the extremities close to the body. (B) Premature infant; body tonus is poor. The hips and shoulder joints exhibit marked extension. (Courtesy Mead-Johnson Laboratories.)

prevent the parents from becoming emotionally attached to their new family member. The parents may express this attitude by either spending minimal time with the baby or becoming overprotective as a way of denying to themselves and to others how they really feel. An abnormal parent-child relationship is a critical factor in maladaptive behavior. Studies by Klaus and Kennell indicate that parental acceptance of the premature infant and the child's long-range affective and cognitive adjustments are enhanced when health agencies encourage and support early parent-child contact [14]. For more detailed discussion of this issue see Chapters 9, 14, 19, and 32. Maladaptive emotional adjustment is not an inherent characteristic of prematurity, but it may be secondary to maladaptive interactional patterns with the parents.

Premature infants experience a lag in growth and development. Parents frequently put high emphasis on the first recognized social behavior—the responsive smile. When the sustained responsive smile fails to occur at the expected age after birth, this may reconfirm parental fears that the child is retarded and cause them to further separate themselves emotionally from the new baby. Parents should be helped to realize that most of the early developmental milestones, besides being individually determined, are primarily determined by the child's developmental age since conception rather than birth. To obtain a more accurate idea of when certain skills might be achieved, one should use the expected, not the actual, date of birth as the baseline. With appropriate care and stimulation, most premature infants "catch up" with full-term infants in phys-

ical, neurological, and social skills by 2 to 3 years of age (depending on the degree of prematurity). The most critical factors appear to be the sensory stimulation and environmental enrichment offered by the parents [11, 34]. Synchronized responses to the infant's behaviors are essential to facilitate development of the baby's skills.

Postmaturity

Approximately 12 percent of babies are born after the forty-first week of gestation [17]. The characteristics of these infants are dependent both on the length of gestation and on the efficiency of placental circulation. As the placenta approaches 38 weeks, it begins to age, losing some of its efficiency as an organ of exchange. The fetus subsequently may not be able to obtain sufficient nutrients and oxygen to meet continued growth needs; thus, the fetus may begin to depend on fat stores to meet energy needs while in utero. If placental efficiency has deteriorated markedly, it may not be able to support the infant through labor.

The survival and potential quality of life of the postmature infant depend heavily on the sufficiency of the placenta. Seventy-five to 85 percent of the deaths of postmature babies occur during the birth process because of insufficient oxygen [17]; other postmature infants may suffer brain damage because of low oxygen availability. A 24-hour maternal urine sample for estriol levels can be used to evaluate placental efficiency. Low levels indicate inadequate functioning of the placenta and the need for cesarean section to prevent fetal problems during birth.

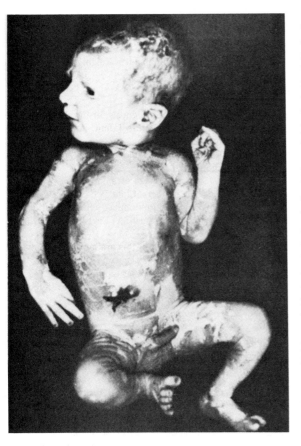

Figure 5–10. Postmature infant. (From S. H. Clifford. Post-maturity. In S. Z. Levine (Ed.), *Advances in Pediatrics*, Vol. 9. Chicago: Yearbook, 1957. With permission.)

At birth, the postmature baby may weigh more than 2500 gm but will show evidence of recent weight loss. The baggy skin dries and cracks quickly after birth because of the loss of the protective vernix caseosa several weeks earlier. Scalp hair is usually thick and long. The fingernails are well developed and may require clipping to prevent facial scratches. The postmature baby is long and thin and often has an alert, wide-eyed appearance. (Because of this increased maturity, a strong, responsive smile can sometimes be elicited from attentive postmature babies—much to the delight of their parents, who are convinced they have a gifted infant.)

Intrauterine Growth Retardation

Some of the causes of intrauterine growth retardation were discussed in Chapter 4. Insults that occur during the embryonic and hypoplastic stages of development can considerably reduce the number of body cells. As a result of interference with mitotic processes, fewer new cells are formed, causing organs to be small and thereby reducing body weight. Insults occurring during the later gestational period (during the hypertrophic stages of development) do not appear to affect the number of cells but rather the amount of cytoplasm present in each cell. Reduced weight is due to the decrease in cellular weight rather than number of cells.

Studies of the effects of maternal nutrition and fetal malnutrition have been conducted for the last 40 years. The results indicate that the last few months of gestation and the first few months of extrauterine life are the most critical periods for hyperplastic brain growth. Severe or continuous malnutrition during these periods may irrevocably reduce cellular quantity and thus permanently impair intellectual capacity. Autopsy on chronically malnourished infants who died during the first few months of life showed a 60 percent reduction in the expected number of brain cells, whereas infants whose malnutrition was confined to the postnatal period exhibited a 15 to 20 percent reduction in the expected number of brain cells for their age [17]. A number of studies have found a significantly higher incidence of brain-wave changes and learning disabilities in children who were small for their age but were full-term infants [31].

SUMMARY

The transition from the relative passivity of intrauterine life to the assertiveness that is essential to survival in extrauterine life is a critical stage of development. The length of time spent in utero affects the infant's ability to draw upon his or her coping skills and to maintain life independently of the mother's protective environment. An appropriate assessment of gestational age and a knowledge of the common problems faced by the newborn can alert health care personnel to potential problems. Ten percent of infants experience some type of illness or difficulty during the transitional period; most of these conditions are self-limiting in nature and cause no permanent effects if appropriate treatment is given immediately. However, it cannot be assumed that the infant who appears to be normal and healthy at birth will easily pass through this period.

When rendering care to the fetus and the newborn, health care professionals must be concerned with survival. Moreover, through the provision of a supportive environment, we must also ensure the new individual's right to maximize his or her potentials and to function as an intelligent, independent, contributing member of family and society.

REFERENCES

1. Apgar, V., et al. Evaluation of the newborn infant—second report. *J.A.M.A.* 168:1985, 1958.
2. Avery, G. B. (Ed.). *Neonatology: Pathophysiology and Management of the Newborn* (2nd ed.). Philadelphia: Lippincott, 1981.
3. Brazelton, T. B. Behavioral Competence of the Newborn Infant. In G. B. Avery (Ed.), *Neonatology: Pathophysiology and Management of the Newborn* (2nd ed.). Philadelphia: Lippincott, 1981.
4. Brazie, J. V., and Lubchenco, L. O. The Estimation of Gestational Age Chart. In C. H. Kempe, H. K. Silver, and D. O'Brian (Eds.), *Current Pediatric Diagnosis and Treatment* (3rd ed.). Los Altos, CA: Lange, 1974.
5. Chaze, B. A., and Ludington-Hoe, S. M. Sensory Stimulation in the NICU. *Am. J. Nurs.* 84:68, 1984.
6. Chinn, P. L. *Child Health Maintenance: Concepts in Family-Centered Care* (2nd ed.). St. Louis: Mosby, 1979.
7. *Demographic Yearbook, 1975* (27th issue). New York: United Nations, 1976.
8. Dierker, L. J., et al. Active and quiet periods in the preterm and term fetus. *Obstet. Gynecol.* 60:154, 1982.
9. Editorial. *Medical World News* 14(19):60, 1973.
10. Gannon, R. B., and Pickett, K. Jaundice. *Am. J. Nurs.* 83:404, 1983.
11. Hayes, J. S. Premature infant development. *Pediatr. Nurs.* 6:33, 1980.
12. Herschel, M., et al. Survival of infants born at 24 to 28 weeks' gestation. *Obstet. Gynecol.* 60:154, 1982.
13. Kitterman, J. A., Phibbs, R. H., and Tooley, W. H. Aortic blood pressure in normal newborn infants during the first 12 hours of life. *Pediatrics* 44:959, 1969.
14. Klaus, M. H., and Kennell, J. H. *Maternal-Infant Bonding: The Impact of Early Separation or Loss on Family Development.* St Louis: Mosby, 1976.
15. Knobloch, H., et al. Considerations in evaluating changes in outcomes for infants weighing less than 1,501 grams. *Pediatrics* 69:285, 1982.
16. Korner, A. Maternal rhythms and waterbeds: A form of intervention with premature infants. In E. B. Thoman and S. Trotter (Eds.), *Social Responsiveness of Infants.* New Brunswick, NJ: Johnson & Johnson, 1978.
17. Korones, S. B. *High-Risk Newborn Infants: The Basis for Intensive Nursing Care* (3rd ed.). St. Louis: Mosby, 1981.
18. LeBoyer, F. *Childbirth Without Violence.* New York: Knopf, 1975.
19. Lubchenco, L. O., Searls, D. T., and Brazie, J. V. Neonatal mortality rate: Relationship to birth weight and gestational age. *J. Pediatr.* 81:814, 1972.
20. Mahan, C. S. When patients ask about "gentle birth." *Contemp. Ob/Gyn* 7(4):51, 1976.
21. Miner, H. Problems and prognosis for the small-for-gestational-age and the premature infant. *Am. J. Maternal Child Nursing* 3:221, 1978.
22. Moore, M. L. *The Newborn and the Nurse* (2nd ed.). Philadelphia: Saunders, 1981.
23. Murray, A. D., et al. Effects of epidural anesthesia on newborns and their mothers. *Child Dev.* 52:71, 1981.
24. Nelson, N. M., et al. A randomized clinical trial of the LeBoyer approach to childbirth. *N. Engl. J. Med.* 302:655, 1980.
25. Nelson, N. M. The Onset of Respiration. In G. B. Avery (Ed.), *Neonatology: Pathophysiology and Management of the Newborn* (2nd ed.). Philadelphia: Lippincott, 1981.
26. Nijhuis, J. G., et al. Are there behavioral states in the human fetus? *Early Hum. Dev.* 6:177, 1982.
27. Rank, O. *The Trauma of Birth.* New York: Harper & Row, 1973.
28. Scopes, J. W. Thermoregulation in the Newborn. In G. B. Avery (Ed.), *Neonatology: Pathophysiology and Management of the Newborn* (2nd ed.). Philadelphia: Lippincott, 1981.
29. U. S. Bureau of the Census. *Statistical Abstract of the United States: 1981* (102nd ed.). Washington, DC: 1981.
30. Vaughan, V. C., and Brazelton, T. B. (Eds.). *The Family—Can It Be Saved?* Chicago: Year Book, 1976.
31. Walzer, S., and Richmond, J. B. The epidemiology of learning disorders. *Pediatr. Clin. North Am.* 20:549, 1973.
32. Washington, S. Temperature control of the neonate. *Nurs. Clin. North. Am.* 23:13, 1978.
33. Wegman, M. E. Annual summary of vital statistics—1980. *Pediatrics* 68(6):755, 1981.
34. Werner, E. E., et al. Cumulative effect of perinatal complications and deprived environment on physical, intellectual and social development of preschool children. *Pediatrics* 39:490, 1967.
35. Wolff, P. H. The Classification of States. In L. J. Stone, H. T. Smith, and L. B. Murphy (Eds.), *The Competent Infant; Research and Commentary.* New York: Basic Books, 1973.
36. Yunek, M. J., and Lojek, R. M. Intrapartal fetal monitoring. *Am. J. Nurs.* 78:2102, 1978.
37. Ziegel, E., and Cranley, M. S. *Obstetric Nursing* (8th ed.). New York: Macmillan, 1984.

6

The Normal Newborn

Clara S. Schuster

I don't know what your destiny will be. But one thing I know; the only ones among you who will be really happy are those who will have sought and found how to serve.

—Albert Schweitzer

A baby is a baby, is a baby. Not so! Look through the window of a newborn nursery and you will begin to see almost as much variation in the characteristics of these initiates to life as among your peers. Ask any new parent—they can (and will) readily share with you all the superior characteristics that individualize their new family member from the other residents of the nursery. Even at this early age, both physiologic and affective differences are apparent. Even with the infant's individuality, however, the neonate (birth to 28 days of life) shares more common characteristics with peers than at any other stage of extrauterine life.

The head appears large compared to the diameter of the thorax (chest) and pelvis (hips); it accounts for about one-fourth of the total body length. The adult's head is only one-seventh to one-eighth of the total body length. Relatively large organ size combined with rather weak musculature causes the abdominal wall to protrude. The relatively short arms and legs are kept in a flexed or semiflexed position. The short legs place the midpoint of the body at the umbilicus rather than at the symphysis pubis, as in the adult (see Fig. 22–2).

At birth the newborn is usually covered with some blood and vernix caseosa, the thick, cheesy coating that protects the skin from the amniotic fluid. Many health care practitioners wash the infant shortly after birth to remove these substances; others prefer to allow the vernix to remain on the skin as a natural lubricant and protection against bacteria and drying and cracking during the first 3 to 4 days of life.

In this chapter we will identify the normal characteristics of the newborn and some of the reasons for variations in those characteristics.

PHYSIOLOGICAL PARAMETERS

The first question the new parent asks is, "Is it a boy or a girl?" After the gender is established, the second question inevitably is, "Is my baby OK?" or "Is my baby normal?" After a few ooh's and ah's and comments on fingers and toes, color and cry, the third big question is, "How much does he (she) weigh?"

Weight

Ninety-five percent of full-term infants weigh between 5½ and 9½ pounds (2500–4300 gm). The average weight for males is 7½ pounds (3400 gm); for females, 7 pounds (3200 gm). Size is influenced by many factors, including placental efficiency, maternal nutrition, size of the parents, and racial characteristics. Caucasian babies tend to be heavier than those of other races. Mothers who have diabetes during pregnancy tend to have much larger babies.

Most infants lose 5 to 10 percent of their birth weight during the first few days of life. This weight loss is generally attributed to the relatively low fluid and food intake combined with the loss of body fluids (urine, stool, and physiological edema) following birth [19]. The weight usually becomes stationary on the third or fourth day and then begins to increase. The birth weight is usually regained between the eighth and fourteenth days of life. Most infants continue to gain at the rate of about 1 ounce (30 gm) per day, or 2 pounds (900 gm) per month, during the first 3 months of life [19].

Length

Ninety-five percent of infants are between 18 and 22 inches in length at birth (46 to 56 cm); the average length is 20 inches (50 cm). Although several studies have been undertaken to correlate birth length with adult height, the results are not sufficiently correlated to use this factor as a predictor. By the time a child has reached 3 years of age, however, one can begin to predict adult height [19].

Characteristics of the Head

The newborn's face is typically round and puffy in appearance. The eyes are closed much of the time, even when the baby is awake—a characteristic that may be frustrating to the parents, who feel they have not really been introduced to their baby until the infant's eyes open and look back at them. Most neonates have eyes of a slate blue color. Some, especially those who will have dark brown or black eyes as adults, may stare out with dark blue or gray-black eyes. True eye color usually does not begin to emerge until about 6 weeks of age. Permanent coloration is generally present by 6 months. Swelling of the eyelids is common in newborns; the most common cause is a temporary reaction to the medication instilled to prevent blindness from gonorrhea. Only about 20 percent of neonates produce tears when crying [35]. Many exhibit strabismus (crossed eyes) and nystagmus (wandering eye movements) due to immaturity of the nervous system and inability to control the eye muscles voluntarily.

The newborn has a flat pug nose and a receding chin. These characteristics help the infant to nurse more easily—a protruding nose and chin would get in the way. The fat cheeks of the infant are created by cheek pads, which consist of solid, round tissue (1 to 1½ inches in diameter) that prevents the cheeks from collapsing with the suction required for nursing.

CIRCUMFERENCE
The measurement of the head circumference provides extremely significant information to medical personnel. The size of the head increases rapidly during infancy. Measurements taken during infancy and early childhood are compared to a baseline taken shortly after birth and can be used to evaluate whether the head is growing too rapidly or too slowly. Early identification of either of these situations should lead to appropriate intervention to prevent brain damage or even death. Ninety-five percent of heads measure between 13 and 14.5 inches (33 to 36.5 cm) at birth; the average head circumference is 13.5 inches (34 cm). The head should measure about 1 inch (2.5 cm) larger than the chest at birth. Eighty percent of children with a head circumference below the second percentile experience some degree of mental retardation [19].

FONTANELLES
Two fontanelles, the anterior and the posterior, are formed where the bony plates of the head meet. These "soft spots" are covered by a tough membrane that helps to prevent damage to the soft brain tissue underneath. Mothers frequently avoid washing the scalp over these areas for fear of injuring the infant; this precaution is unnecessary. The gradual growth of the cranial bones causes closure of the anterior fontanelle by

18 months of age. The posterior fontanelle usually closes during the third month of life (see Fig. 5–2A).

The fontanelles are considered nature's safety valve that allows for the rapid growth of the brain, accommodates the birth process, and reduces undue pressure on the brain if fluid is retained. It is normal for the anterior fontanelle to pulsate with the heartbeat; it also becomes very tense during crying. A tense, bulging anterior fontanelle during periods of relaxation is indicative of increased intracranial pressure and requires immediate medical evaluation. A depressed fontanelle may indicate a state of dehydration.

CHARACTERISTIC FUNCTIONING OF THE MAJOR SYSTEMS

Every system of the body undergoes some adjustment to extrauterine life. Transitory phenomena (e.g., acrocyanosis and mild retractions during crying) are characteristic of the adjustment process but would be considered pathological in the same baby at 1 month of age. Changes occurring in the respiratory and circulatory system were discussed in Chapter 5; other changes are covered here.

Gastrointestinal System

The gastrointestinal system includes the body's entire alimentary tract, from lips to anus. Although the newborn has been swallowing amniotic fluid during intrauterine life, the introduction to, and ingestion of, milk and the passage of the first stool are major milestones.

INTAKE

The infant's mouth is equipped with a shallow, rigid, and hard flat palate and a large tongue for easy grasping and compression of the nipple. During and following nursing, the area around the lips may turn white or even bluish from the effort of sucking. This phenomenon, known as perioral cyanosis, is considered normal when nursing. The lips may also be slightly puffy or swollen after nursing. A large white blister in the middle of the upper lip, known as a labial tubercle, or sucking callus, may be found for about one-half hour after each nursing until approximately 6 months of age.

The boat-shaped stomach stretches easily, causing some babies to overeat. The ready emptying of stomach contents into the duodenum may cause the baby to cry from perceived hunger about 2 hours after eating. Most pediatricians recommend waiting at least 3 hours before refeeding the infant to allow complete emptying of the stomach. However, breast-fed babies may need more frequent feedings than bottle-fed babies because of the easier digestibility of breast milk as opposed to cow's milk [20]. The intestine, which is proportionally longer than in the adult, is poorly equipped with muscular or elastic tissue. Nervous system control is also inadequate. Some digestive enzymes are present, but the infant can digest only simple foods—not complex starches or proteins.

Some health care practitioners recommend waiting about 12 hours before feeding the infant for the first time to allow the infant to adjust to extrauterine life and to begin stabilizing critical functions. Glucose (sugar) water or sterile water is the fluid of choice when feedings are delayed until 12 hours after birth. After the infant is able to coordinate sucking and swallowing, milk is offered. The average total intake is only 45 to 90 cc during the first 24 hours. The amount taken with each subsequent feeding varies greatly with the child's state of alertness and hunger. By the end of the third day, most infants are consuming 2½ to 4 ounces per feeding. The 12-hour baby often plays with the nipple (breast or bottle) and seldom takes more than one-half ounce (15 cc) of fluid. Often this distresses the mother, who may interpret the baby's difficulty with feeding as a rejection of her. If feeding problems continue, she may feel she is an incompetent mother [31].

Other practitioners encourage the mother to nurse the infant immediately after birth, during the first period of activity when the infant is in state 4. Early-fed infants appear to coordinate the sucking and swallowing reflexes more effectively at this point and to experience less weight loss. The infant receives colostrum (precursor to milk) and the early suckling stimulates earlier production of milk by the mother. Some research now indicates that close contact with the mother's normal bacteria and factors in the milk, such as antibodies, help to impart immunity to the infant [15]. Another significant advantage of this approach is the responsiveness of the infant to the mother at this early time, which helps to foster a more positive mother-infant relationship. Therefore, long-range as well as short-range effects may be noted by fostering early contact and breast feeding [17, 25].

Babies who are not breast-fed are usually placed on a cow's milk formula. The manufacturers try to replicate the constituents of human milk as closely as possible; however, some significant differences are as yet unavoidable and warrant brief discussion. Cow's milk contains twice as much protein as human milk. Since it is not as easily digested by the infant, water is added to dilute the protein and to aid in the excretion of waste products. The extra water reduces the number of calories per ounce, requiring the addition of some form of sugar to elevate the caloric value to 20 calories per ounce—the same as breast milk. However, the amount of sugar must be carefully regulated, because too much sugar in a formula can cause loose stools and too little may lead to constipation.

Many mothers will question the wisdom of giving an infant extra water, which supplies no calories for energy and growth. Babies do need extra fluid—especially if the baby is bottle-fed. Because of the low fluid intake of both bottle-fed and breast-fed infants, many experience a transitory fever between the second and third days of life. The temperature may rise to 100° or 101°F. Other symptoms of dehydration may be present—dry skin, flushing, marked weight loss, sunken fontanelle, and decreased urinary output. These symptoms are readily remedied by increasing the fluid intake.

OUTPUT

The newborn will frequently void at birth when the body comes in contact with the cool air. This reaction will persist for several months (to the frustration of the person who just changed a wet diaper!). Failure to void within 12 hours after birth calls for closer observation. An infant who fails to void within 24 hours should be checked carefully for possible congenital malformation or health problem.

STOOL CYCLE

During fetal life, the infant swallows amniotic fluid. The water is absorbed into the infant's bloodstream, while the solid particles and nonabsorbable wastes are passed through the intestines. The swallowed fluid with its lanugo, skin cells, and vernix combines with the mucus, digestive secretions, and bile pigments; together these elements form an odorless, dark green, thick, bowel movement known as meconium. The fetus routinely releases meconium into the amniotic fluid for the first 16 weeks. After 20 weeks, release of meconium would be considered pathological [1]. Babies born in the breech position (buttocks first) or those who experience some distress during labor may pass meconium stool before or during the birth process. Most babies begin excretion of this bowel filler during the first 24 hours after birth. Occasionally, the first sticky movement is accompanied by a 2- to 5-cm, capsule-shaped, rubbery mass that is white or white and green in color, called a meconium plug.

Between 36 and 72 hours of life, the stool will change character as the meconium mixes with the milk. This transitional stool is lighter green, sticky, rather watery,

and contains curds of undigested milk. Its passage is frequently accompanied by the explosive sounds of flatus (bowel gas).

After the first 3 to 4 days, the color and character of the stools depend on the type of milk the infant is fed. The yellow or golden stools of breast-fed babies have a slightly sour odor. At first, the breast-fed infant may have six to eight soft or loose stools per day due to the effects of colostrum, the precursor to human milk. By 4 weeks of age, the breast-fed baby generally has only one or two stools per day; some infants only defecate every other day.

The bottle-fed baby usually has lighter yellow stools, which are more formed than those of the breast-fed baby in spite of adequate fluid intake. The young formula-fed infant has about four to six stools per day. It is normal for the infant to flush and strain, or push, during a bowel movement. The infant should be evaluated for constipation if there is excessive effort and evidence of discomfort or passage of very dry, hard stools.

REGURGITATION

Regurgitation, or spitting up milk, is a frequent occurrence in young infants. Almost all babies will gag and vomit at least once during the first 36 hours because of mucus. Regurgitation frequently accompanies a burp or an air bubble released from the stomach. Even breast-fed babies swallow air while nursing and need to be "bubbled" well during and after each nursing. The baby should be held in an upright position and patted or rubbed **gently** on the back to facilitate relaxation of the cardiac sphincter of the stomach, which allows escape of the swallowed air.

Other common causes of regurgitation are overfeeding, too much physical activity after feeding, or placement of the head lower than the stomach during or after feeding. The baby should be placed on the abdomen or right side after feeding to reduce the possibility of aspiration (inhalation) of the regurgitated milk. The infant who frequently vomits large amounts immediately after feedings should be medically evaluated even in the absence of other symptoms.

Genitourinary System

As mentioned previously, the stimulation of cold air frequently causes the infant to void. Urinary output is small during the first 24 hours—15 to 60 ml. The output gradually increases to 8 or 10 voidings per 24 hours, amounting to about 100 to 400 ml by 3 days of life. In the neonate the bladder is an abdominal organ, since the pelvis is still too small to hold it. Occasionally, uric acid crystals found in concentrated urine may cause a rusty stain on the diaper during the first 2 days of life; these have no known significance.

The vaginal area of female babies is covered with a thin, bluish-white mucus known as smegma. This mucus offers a protective coating for the tissues and helps to prevent fungal and bacterial infections.

UNDESCENDED TESTICLES

The testes should be palpable in the scrotal sac. When the perineal area is cold, however, the scrotum will wrinkle and become smaller due to muscular contractions. The testes may be drawn back and up into the inguinal canal. Testes that have not descended at birth will usually descend within the next 3 months. If they have not descended by 1 year of age, the infant may need surgical assistance. Testicles that remain undescended until the pubertal years will be incapable of producing viable sperm. Surgery is usually performed during the toddler years, because critical emotional overtones may arise when genital surgery is performed during the preschool or early school-age years.

CIRCUMCISION

Many parents choose to have their male infants circumcised. Circumcision (removal of the foreskin of the penis) has special religious significance to some parents. Many persons have adopted the custom for its hygienic value to help prevent infections. Actually there is no proved medical rationale for circumcision, although extra careful attention must be given to hygienic measures when a boy is uncircumcised. Some psychologists are concerned about the subconscious but potentially long-lasting effects of the pain of the procedure and recommend the use of some form of analgesic. When done early and well, the procedure is quick and can be relatively painless. The healthy newborn appears to have minimal physical and psychological response to pain. Plasma arginine vasopressin levels (a physiological response to pain) show no elevation during circumcision [34], but further research is needed. Some infants may even sleep through most of the procedure when given some extra attention, cuddling, and a nipple to suck on. It is worth noting, however, that the infant's sensitivity to pain increases with neurological maturity [8], consequently, the procedure is potentially less traumatic for the 1-day-old than for the 1-week-old infant.

Neuromuscular System

The neurological system is initially evaluated in terms of its effect on the muscular activity of an individual;

thus, the two are frequently approached as one system in the neonate. The nervous and muscular systems of the newborn are extremely immature. As a result, the movements of the neonate appear to be very uncoordinated and weak. Tremors of the extremities or the chin are normal at this stage of life and have no pathological significance; they merely reflect immature myelinization. Because the myelin sheath (which acts as insulation around nerves) is not yet complete, it is not unusual for the newborn to "short-circuit" when touched; for instance, a touch on the foot may elicit a total body response.

At birth the brain is only one-fourth of its adult size [19]. The brain will continue very rapid hyperplastic as well as hypertropic growth during the first 5 months of extrauterine life. However, years will elapse before the anatomical and physiological growth of the system is complete. There are marked differences in maturational rates between the genders. Neurologically, the female neonate is approximately 4 to 6 weeks more mature than the male. The maturational gap widens with age, females reaching terminal physical maturation at approximately 21 years and males at 24 years [2]. On the average, the black infant has greater biological maturity at birth than white neonates [30].

REFLEXES

Much of the newborn's physical behavior appears to be reflexive in nature. As the nervous system matures, these reflexes disappear and are replaced by more purposeful, directed, voluntary, and coordinated movements. The presence or the absence of these early reflexes is an indicator that can be used to evaluate the health state and developmental progress of an infant [27].

Moro reflex. The Moro reflex (also known as the startle reflex) is probably the most significant reflex in terms of evaluating the baby's neurological status. This reflex may be elicited in response to any sudden internal or external stimulus; it is also common during periods of sleep. This reflex is characterized by stiffening of the body and legs with an outward thrust of the arms, followed by a rapid inward movement as if to embrace. The thumb and forefinger form the shape of a C. It is frequently followed by crying. Absence of this reflex in the first 24 hours may be due to brain edema caused by the birth process and has no known clinical significance [29]. A lack of symmetry or a persistent absence of the Moro reflex is indicative of pathology and the need for medical evaluation. This reflex usually disappears by 5 months of age.

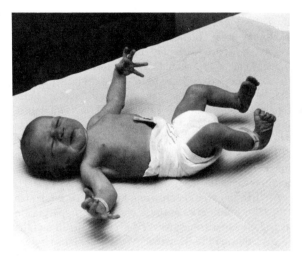

Figure 6–1. The Moro reflex. The infant appears to be reaching outward as if to hook onto something in order to break a fall. Even legs, feet, and toes appear to be embracing. Note the clamped umbilical cord on this 15-hour-old baby.

Tonic neck reflex (fencing position). Turning of the head to the side causes the arm and leg on that side to straighten and stiffen, and the opposite arm and leg to bend and stiffen. If this reflex does not disappear by 3 months of age, motor coordination will be delayed.

Rooting reflex. The rooting reflex was so named because the infant's behavior resembles that of a piglet hunting for roots. When hungry, the baby will turn the mouth in the direction of the cheek that is touched. The baby often breathes rapidly and makes sucking noises with the lips. Mothers frequently make the mistake of trying to push the baby's mouth toward the nipple by pushing against the opposite cheek; this behavior only antagonizes the natural reflex of the infant, causing an attempt to take hold of the mother's fingers with the mouth. This natural reflex can be made to work for the mother if she merely touches the cheek on the side to which she wishes the baby to turn. The rooting response may persist during sleep until 7 or 8 months of age [16].

Sucking, swallowing, and gag reflexes are poorly coordinated at birth. Babies who are fed immediately after birth seem to catch on more quickly and have fewer coordination problems during the next 48 hours.

Palmar grasp and hand-to-mouth reflexes. The full-term newborn will curl the fingers tightly around any small object placed in the palm of the hand. The grasp

is tight enough and can be held long enough to actually support the baby's body weight (briefly). This palmar grasp reflex is often combined with the hand-to-mouth reflex, which causes the baby to direct a curled-up hand to the mouth. When hand, thumb, finger, or held object touches the mouth, the rooting reflex is elicited; this in turn elicits the sucking reflex. This sequence of events can be seen even in the delivery room. It does not take long for the infant to perfect this sequence (or schema, if one uses Piaget's terminology). By the third day of life, the infant often has already established a preference for sucking of thumb versus knuckle versus index or index and middle finger. There is evidence that thumb-and-finger-sucking also occur in utero [28].

Stepping and crawling reflexes. Whether held upright or lying on a flat surface, the baby will make walking movements when the soles of the feet touch an object. This reflex disappears by two months of age and reappears as purposeful, directed movement several months later. Crawling-like movements may be present when the baby is placed on the abdomen. These movements can actually propel the infant forward or

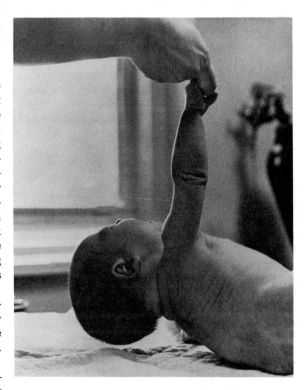

Figure 6–2. Palmar grasp reflex.

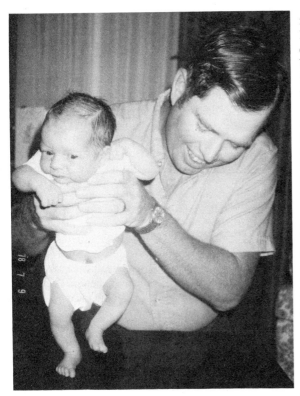

Figure 6-3. Stepping reflex. Note the stump of the umbilical cord, which is still intact on this 7-day-old baby.

backward and should be considered a safety hazard when the baby is placed on a flat surface.

Protective reflexes. The newborn also has a wealth of protective reflexes. Initially the whole body may react, for example, when the foot is pricked with a pin, because the nervous system cannot yet isolate the exact source of the pain. The normal newborn will soon conserve energy, however, and will withdraw only the touched extremity if the procedure is repeated several times [3]. Bright lights, an object that zooms in, or a touch on the eyelid will cause the neonate to blink. A firm touch on the eyelid will cause the baby to squeeze the eyelids shut so tightly that it is almost impossible to force them open. If the head is face down and the airway is occluded, the healthy neonate will turn the head to the side. Some experiments indicate that newborns will hold their breath briefly if placed under water. A small cloth placed over the infant's face will elicit batting motions of the hands and the fists to remove the offending object.

Sneezing, a method of clearing the nasal passages, is frequently elicited by a bright light or some unknown factor and as such is not symptomatic of upper respiratory complications. Yawning expands the lungs. Hiccups appear to be a reflection of an incompetent cardiac sphincter. Many mothers indicate that their babies experienced hiccuping even before birth. Giving the neonate a nipple to suck on frequently stops the symptoms.

The baby doll reflex is another phenomenon of neonates. In states 3, 4, and 5 (see p. 103), the infant will often close the eyes when horizontal and open them when raised to a 30-degree vertical position. This behavior appears to be mediated by vestibular response to positional change [3]. If this reflex persists, however, it may indicate brain damage [7].

PERCEPTIONS OF THE ENVIRONMENT

The neonate, far from being passive or unresponsive to the environment, is amazingly alert to a wide variety of stimuli. The alert, discerning professional can objectively identify and utilize for evaluative purposes many of these subtle but specific responses. The healthy newborn shows strong preference for specific stimuli and quickly adapts to new stimuli. The infant will respond discriminatingly to prolong contact with a pleasant stimulus or to avoid contact with an unpleasant stimulus.

Vision. Because of the neonate's aversion to bright lights and the presence of nystagmus (wandering eye movement), professionals thought for many years that newborns were essentially blind, except to distinguish light from dark. However, many mothers will say, even on the first day of life, that "the baby stares at me as if he knows I am his mother." These mothers are right, at least about the focusing of attention. Recent research indicates that the neonate is able to fixate—to zero in on an object visually. The infant consistently

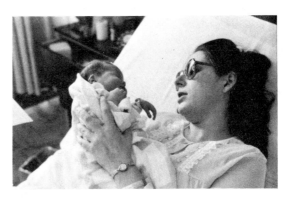

Figure 6-4. En face position. The mother aligns her face with the plane of the baby's face so that their eyes are parallel.

prefers complex patterns to simple patterns, and curved lines to straight lines. Sharply contrasting colors and medium-bright lighted objects are also appealing to the neonate and will elicit a prolonged fixation behavior [9].

The infant also shows a marked preference for the unique pattern of the human face in the en face position, the position in which the mother's and infant's eyes are parallel to each other. In this position, the neonate will maintain interest longer than when the mother's head is turned sideways to the infant. The mother's eyes appear to offer contrast points. Perhaps this is why so many mothers instinctually assume the en face position when holding the newborn; the greater focusing attention elicited from the baby encourages the mother to maintain and repeat her behavior. When fixating, the infant in state 4 will stop or reduce sucking, stop body movement, and elevate the eyelids, giving an alert, bright-eyed appearance.

Within 15 minutes after birth, the infant can see and will visually follow a brightly colored object with the eyes. The infant will even turn the head to track an object, which is moved in a slow 180-degree arc 7 to 10 inches from the eyes [3, 12]. Visual acuity is approximately 20/150, which is adequate to perceive both form and color [12]. However, the infant's eyes are unable to accommodate well for distance, since most infants have a fixed focal length of about 19 cm (7½ inches) [4].

Studies indicate that the infant prefers and will visually follow the human face more readily than other stimuli. Even 7 to 10 minutes after birth, neonates who have never seen a human face (doctors and examiners were masked) consistently fixated and visually followed a pattern of a normal human face significantly more than scrambled facial patterns or a blank face [14]. These results indicate that (1) visual discrimination is present at an early age, (2) fixation and following is an unlearned capacity, and (3) there is an unlearned responsiveness or innate bias toward the design of the human face. At birth, vision is not only a sensory system but a perceptual system as well.

Hearing. The presence of the Moro reflex in response to loud sounds indicates that the infant is able to hear immediately after birth. A newborn will turn his head to sound within an hour after birth [3, 35]. Infants also show distinct preference for particular sounds. The sound of the human heart has a quieting effect (perhaps because of familiarity with a sound associated with intrauterine life). The neonate appears to be predisposed to respond selectively to auditory stimuli (pattern, pitch, volume) that are embodied in human caretakers, especially females [8].

If one listens to a mother talk to her baby and then to an older child or another adult, it will be noted that the mother will instinctively slow her speech and elevate her vocal pitch when addressing the baby. In the middle of a sentence, she may turn to an adult in the room and, without a breath, suddenly drop her voice to a normal pitch; just as rapidly she will exaggerate her words, and reverse the sequence. Interestingly, the newborn prefers and distinguishes higher-pitched sounds more readily than lower-pitched ones [12]. In states 2 and 3, the infant will change breathing patterns, grimace, suck the lips, or twitch an eyelid, which

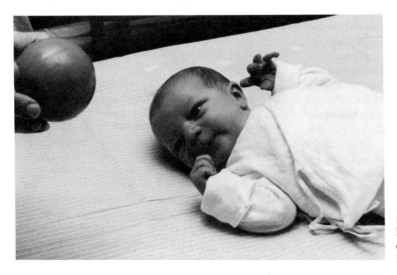

Figure 6–5. Fixation. This 1-hour-old infant is able to look at and follow with her eyes and head movements the course of a small red ball held 7 to 10 inches away from her face.

indicates an acute awareness of sounds in the environment. These subtle facial changes often encourage the mother to continue talking to her baby.

The crying infant is often soothed by the calm, directed human voice. Crying will stop and attempts will be made to locate the source of comfort by turning the head and opening the eyes—again, a strong reinforcement to the mother to vocalize with her newborn. Most mothers appear to have an insatiable desire to talk to their babies, especially to repeat the baby's name frequently, as if to connect the two, to reassure themselves of the reality of this new life in their care—to confirm the miracle. Recent studies indicate that by 3 to 8 days of life the newborn will respond differentially to the mother's voice repeating his or her name as opposed to other words or other voices repeating the name [33].

Condon and Sander have discovered that neonates as young as 12 hours of age exhibit precise and sustained segments of movement that are synchronized with the adult's articulation of words and sentences [6]. Frame-by-frame microanalysis of the infant's response (in state 4) to both taped and live adult vocalization indicates an amazing correlation of the rhythm of the extremities, the eyes, and the mouth with the speed and the pitch of the adult's speech. Disconnected vowel sounds fail to show the same degree of correspondence that is elicited by natural, rhythmic speech. Although the synchrony is often too subtle to pick up easily by merely observing the parent-child interaction, it is apparently this phenomenon that accounts for the mother's comment, "He acts as if he knows what I'm saying." Interactional synchrony may be evaluated in the future as a method of early identification of children with aphasia, autism, schizophrenia, and learning disabilities.

Taste and smell. Taste and smell also appear to be well-developed at birth. The newborn will show a distinct preference for sugar water rather than plain water and for milk rather than sugar water. Studies indicate that breast-fed newborns are able to distinguish the odor of their mother's milk by the tenth day of life [21]. Breast-fed infants often respond differentially to the mother by an increased number of snuggling and rooting behaviors directed toward the mother versus other persons—again, a reinforcement to the mother.

Touch. The newborn is very sensitive to tactile stimulation. In fact, adequate physical contact is essential to optimal growth. A gentle, soothing touch helps the baby to relax, which leaves more energy available for growth purposes. Unpleasant stimuli, such as pain, cold, or a wet diaper, increase activity and energy expenditure, depleting the calories available for growth. Newborns are very uncomfortable on a flat surface without support. Wrapping the baby comfortably in a blanket or turning the infant on the abdomen (a position that gives more surface contact) appears to increase the feeling of security. The cuddled, touched, caressed infant usually responds by relaxation and snuggling behaviors. The lips appear to be particularly sensitive to touch, responding by smacking or sucking movements when touched. These behaviors usually cause the caretaker to repeat the touching activity.

NEONATAL ASSESSMENT

Dr. T. Berry Brazelton has been a pioneer in recognizing the individuality of infants. He postulates that the neonate is not a tabula rasa at birth but, rather, a unique individual already possessing specific unlearned skills that are significant to fostering and shaping the parent-infant interaction [24]. To Dr. Brazelton, the significant point is not just the integrity of the neonate's reflexes, but also the infant's skill in organizing and controlling those reflexes and those reactions to both internal and external environments: the neonate's ability to quiet himself when distressed, as well as the neonate's need for, and attention to, stimulation. The Brazelton Neonatal Assessment Scale, reflecting the range of behavioral capacities of the normal full-term neonate, is based on a competency rather than a neurological deficit approach to assessment. This assessment evaluates the neonate's capacity to (1) organize his level of consciousness; (2) habituate his response to disturbing events; (3) attend to and process both simple and complex environmental stimuli; (4) control motor tone and activity while attending to stimuli; and (5) perform integrated motor behaviors [3]. The evaluation is relatively simple and quick to perform by both medical and nonmedical personnel trained in the assessment skill.

Brazelton postulates that the neonate's ability to selectively use different states of consciousness to maintain control of reactions is a reflection of the integrity of the central nervous system and of the infant's potential for self-organization. As such, this ability is a predictor of individual temperament and measures the baby's potential for response to the environment.

The baby's response to visual, auditory, and tactile stimuli are "tools" for interacting with the environment. The infant uses crying, quieting behavior, and searching behavior to indicate a need for more or less of the stimulus. The clearness and readability of these cues is important for a parent's response to the baby

[11]. If a baby is fussy or has difficulty with state control, it may exert a negative influence and contribute to parent-infant stress [26, 32]. If the infant's cues are not read correctly, then the parent may not be able to establish contingently responsive interactions with the baby [11]. The parent and infant may thus unilaterally or mutually fail to support the continuing development of the other [32].

The Brazelton Neonatal Behavioral Assessment Scale is a valuable parent-teaching tool as well as an infant assessment tool [13]. It can familiarize parents with their infant's unique qualities, facilitate a synchronized communication, and relieve parents of the total responsibility for the interaction. If the baby is difficult, this assessment tool, properly used, can provide guidance for the parents to interact positively for the child's benefit despite poor or weak infant communication skills.

COMMON VARIATIONS

Some characteristics are peculiar to the newborn period of life. If the parents are unprepared for these unique but common variations, they may become unduly concerned about the child's health in terms of both present survival and future functioning. The mother's perception of her infant's health can be in-

timately intertwined with her concept of personal adequacy both as a woman and as a mother. The mother who fears that her child will die or will be retarded may not be able to express the same joy and spontaneity in interacting with the baby. She seems to withdraw and protect herself from the pain of loss she is sure will come. A simple explanation is often all that is needed to help her to experience the joy of motherhood that is rightfully hers.

One mother of healthy premature twins refused to visit the nursery and spent hours crying in her hospital room. A concerned student nurse helped her to express what she was feeling and the reason for her behavior. To everyone's amazement, the mother believed that all premature babies were retarded—and that now she had two retarded children! Within half an hour she was smiling, asking to see her babies, and helping to feed them. Knowledge of the normalcy of common characteristics of newborns can allay many parental anxieties and thus enhance the parent-infant relationship.

Birth Traumas

Many temporary symptoms are a direct result of the stressors experienced during birth. Swelling of the presenting part due to edema (fluid in the tissues) and bruises resulting from breakage of the fine blood vessels are to be expected.

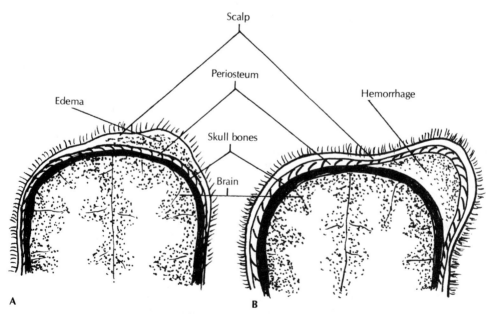

Figure 6–6. (A) Caput succedaneum. Swelling of the soft tissues of the scalp. (B) Cephalhematoma. Bleeding under the periosteum, causing it to separate from the bony plate.

Caput succedaneum is a swelling of the soft tissues of the scalp. It is a soft, boggy mass that causes an elongated appearance of the head. The swelling is not limited to the suture line. The fluid that is present at birth or shortly thereafter is absorbed by 1 to 3 days of age (see Fig. 6–6).

Bruising and abrasions are frequently seen on the head and the cheeks. They are frequently associated with the use of forceps but may also be caused by tightness of the birth passage.

Molding is the shaping of the fetal head to accommodate to the size of the birth passage. This repositioning and overriding of the bony plates of the cranium causes a temporary asymmetry of the infant's head. A normal, round shape is usually assumed within 72 hours, although overriding may occasionally be found in a 2-week-old baby.

Petechiae (small, nonraised, irregular, round, purplish-red hemorrhage spots) are frequently found on the face or scalp (or on the buttocks of breech-born babies). These spots are caused by breakage of the tiny skin vessels when the cervix tightens around the presenting part. Petechiae usually disappear between 3 and 7 days of life.

Subconjunctival hemorrhage may be found in both the mother (as a result of straining during labor) and the infant after birth. The crescent-shaped red patches in the sclera adjacent to the iris are caused by the breakage of vessels on the surface of the eye due to the pressures of the birth process. These hemorrhagic areas may turn brown or yellow before being absorbed spontaneously approximately 3 weeks after birth. There is no clinical significance to this phenomenon, and parents can be assured that it does not cause blindness or other visual problems.

Cephalhematoma, which occurs in about 1 to 2 percent of deliveries [21], is often not apparent until several hours to several days after birth. The pressure of the head against the bony parts of the birth passage can cause a loosening of the periosteum (membrane covering a bone) from one of the bony plates of the cranial vault. This separation causes a breakage of the capillaries and subsequent bleeding. The blood collects between the bony plate and the periosteum, causing a gradually increasing bulge on the scalp. The bleeding is limited to the surface of the specific bone (or bones) involved; therefore, the swelling does not cross the suture line. Since the bleeding is on the outer surface of the bony plate, there is no pressure on the infant's brain. Most of these "blood blisters" will gradually be absorbed without treatment by 6 weeks of age, and in rare instances, they may remain for more than 1 year.

Mothers should be encouraged not to touch the area unnecessarily and to protect it from further injury (see Fig. 6–6B).

Hormonal Influences

During intrauterine life, maternal hormones cross the placental barrier and influence the infant's development. After birth their presence and withdrawal can cause transient symptoms that are not clinically significant.

Engorgement of the breasts may be found in infants of either gender. This enlargement due to estrogen may last several weeks. During the first weeks of life, babies of both genders have a small amount of fluid in the breast, known as **witch's milk** [5]. Eighty percent of these infants may actually secrete some of the fluid [19]. Gentle, regular body cleaning is all the care that is needed.

Genital hypertrophy is found in both sexes. It may be particularly pronounced when combined with the edema that accompanies a breech birth. This swelling also recedes in a few weeks.

Pseudomenstruation occurs in 2 to 3 percent of female babies [19]. During fetal life, the high estrogen levels cause hypertrophy of the endometrial lining of the uterus. At birth, a decline in estrogen levels causes disintegration of the endometrial tissue, simulating the process found in mature females. Small to moderate amounts of blood stain the smegma between the third and fifth days of life. All parents of female infants should be advised of this phenomenon.

Skin Markings

History and folklore offer many stories surrounding the presence or appearance of birthmarks—tales are told of inheritances and kingdoms won or lost on the basis of a skin marking. Some marks appear to be genetically determined, but most are merely quirks of nature.

The common birthmark (pigmented nevus) is usually a single small brown area. It may be slightly elevated and may even have tufts of hair. Since it is a permanent marking and may appear on any body surface, the parents may wish to remove the nevus for cosmetic purposes; otherwise it has no clinical significance.

Freckles—small, multiple, flat patches of darker colored skin—are rarely found on infants. Most tend to appear later in life, especially after exposure to sunlight.

Mongolian spots are nonelevated blue colorations found over the buttocks and occasionally on the back

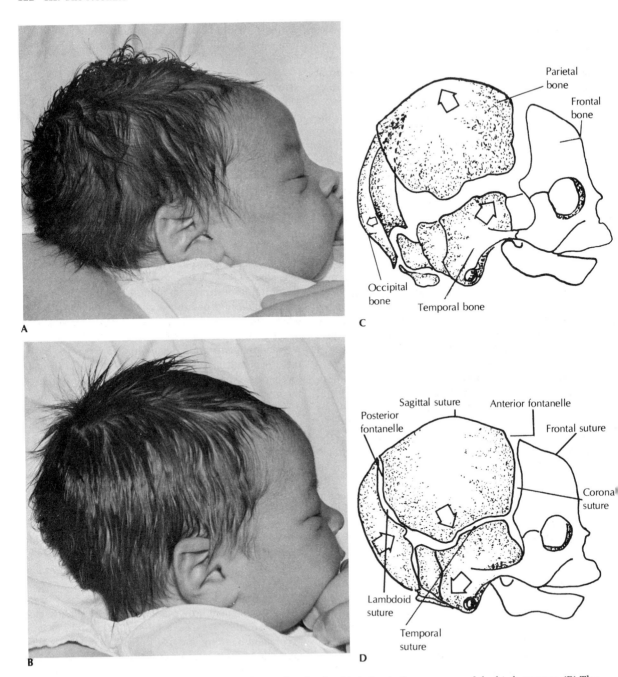

Figure 6–7. Molding. (A) Elongation of the head immediately after birth due to the pressures of the birth process. (B) The same baby 24 hours later; the elongation has receded considerably and the head has assumed a more rounded shape. (From E. Ziegel and M. S. Cranley, *Obstetric Nursing* [7th ed.]. New York: Macmillan, 1978. With permission.) (C) Overlapping and movement of the cranial bones during molding. (D) Return of the bony plates to normal positions.

and outer surfaces of the hands and feet of darker-skinned babies. Since their appearance is very similar to that of severe bruises, it is essential to tell the parents about this birthmark. Difficult situations have arisen from fathers accusing mothers (or vice versa) of child abuse because of the coloration. Mongolian spots generally disappear by the time the child is 5 years old.

Capillary hemangiomas are caused by hyperplastic development of blood vessels; they may be apparent at birth or may appear several months later. Except for the true nevus flammeus, they disappear spontaneously with age. Four types of hemangiomas are commonly found in infants.

A **"stork bite"** (pseudo nevus flammeus) is a flat, pinkish-purple coloration found on the midline of the face, usually above the nose, and the upper lip and on the eyelids. Many infants also have stork bite marks on the back of the neck just above the hair line. Much to the parents' distress, this mark becomes brightly colored when the infant cries. Mothers and fathers are reassured to know that the marks (except those on the nape of the neck) tend to fade after 8 months of age.

A **port-wine stain** (true nevus flammeus) is a flat, irregularly shaped, red to deep purple mark found unilaterally on the face or other parts of the body. The mature nature of the capillaries prevents blanching of the skin when pressed and spontaneous disappearance with age. These marks are present at birth. The parents may be so upset by the child's appearance that a normal parent-child relationship may be difficult; they can be assured that cosmetic preparations and surgery are available. Argon laser beam surgery is also very successful in reducing the skin color [18].

A **strawberry mark** (nevus vasculosus) may or may not be present at birth. The immature capillaries usually become apparent by 4 weeks of age. Any surface of the body may be affected, although the face and neck are the most common targets. Strawberry marks begin to enlarge rapidly once they appear. They are named for their red, elevated appearance. Nevi vasculosi continue to increase in size and color for about 8 to 10 months, leading some mothers to fear the child has a skin cancer. They begin to recede spontaneously around the age of 1 year; most disappear by 3 years of age. More extensive strawberry marks, however, may take 5 to 8 or even 10 years to resolve completely. Treatment is unnecessary unless the growth interferes with vital functioning (e.g., if it presses against the trachea).

Cavernous hemangiomas, which are rare, are very distressing to parents because of their size and appearance. This meshwork of vessels is located in the

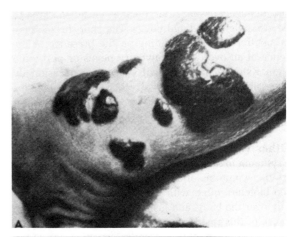

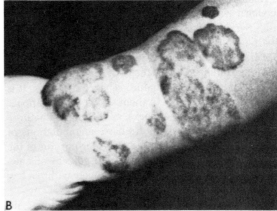

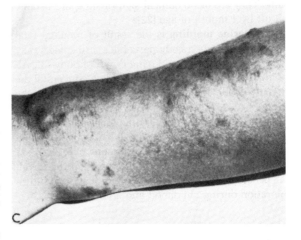

Figure 6–8. The spontaneous progressive involution of a strawberry hemangioma. (A) Age 6 weeks; (B) age 8 months; (C) age 2 years. (From C. F. Burgoon, Jr., The Skin. In V. C. Vaughan and R. J. McKay, *Nelson Textbook of Pediatrics* [10th ed.]. Philadelphia: Saunders, 1975. With permission.)

subcutaneous tissue. A large sinus causes the area to be grossly enlarged and boggy. The skin surface may be neutral or red, depending on the presence or absence of an overlying strawberry nevus or port-wine stain. Extremely rapid growth or bleeding occasionally necessitates surgical removal; otherwise, spontaneous gradual involution can be expected after 8 months of age.

Other Variations

Erythema toxicum neonatorum (newborn rash) mimics the symptoms of a skin infection or allergy. Small red blotches, often with hivelike centers, spread rapidly over the body, and just as rapidly disappear. The cause of this rash is not known; some feel it may be the result of contact of the tender, sensitive skin of the newborn with the harsh fabrics of clothing and bedding. Symptoms may continue to appear during the first month of life.

Milia, pinpoint white spots across the infant's nose, chin, and forehead, are caused by retention of secretions in the ducts of immature sebaceous glands. It is imperative not to squeeze them. Milia will disappear spontaneously in 2 to 4 weeks, as the glands mature.

Epstein's pearls, which are hard accumulations of epithelial cells found over the posterior portion of the hard palate, are present in about 50 percent of newborns. They will disappear spontaneously within a few weeks of birth.

Hymenal tags are frequently found on female infants. They are of no clinical significance and usually fall off by 1 month of age [22].

Intrauterine molding is the result of prenatal fetal position. Misshapen body parts (face, arms, legs) may be caused by the uneven laying down of body fat. Although the appearance may resemble a congenital defect, it will correct itself within the first 4 to 6 months of life.

One other point worth comment concerns **skin color.** Dark-skinned babies are born with light pigmentation; the coloration then darkens over the next 2 to 6 days. The darker skin found around the navel, nail beds, and ear lobes gives some indication of future coloration during childhood and adult years.

SUMMARY

Newborn infants share many common physiological characteristics. Weight is usually within 2 pounds of 7½ pounds, and length falls within a 4-inch range of 20 inches. However, variations in both physical ap-

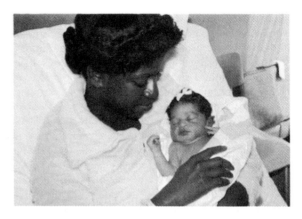

Figure 6–9. This mother and daughter exemplify the pigmentation differences that are evident in newborns of dark-skinned parents.

pearance and attention to the environment make each newborn unique from the start. Many phenomena, although transient in nature, may mimic serious congenital defects. A thorough understanding of the causes and courses of particular characteristics can allay the practitioner's or parents' anxiety.

The newborn is far from a passive piece of clay to be molded by the environment. During the newborn period, temperamental and interactional differences are clearly apparent. Although the four domains are very primitive at this point, the infant is able to skillfully intertwine his or her biological, emotional, social, and cognitive domains into behaviors that enhance interaction with the caretaker.

Students who are interested in further exploration of this period of life are encouraged to take a course in neonatology.

REFERENCES

1. Abramovich, D. R., and Gray, E. S. Physiologic fetal defecation in midpregnancy. *Obstet. Gynecol.* 60:294, 1982.
2. Arganian, M. Sex Differences in Early Development. In J. C. Westman (Ed.), *Individual Differences in Children.* New York: Wiley, 1973.
3. Brazelton, T. B. Neonatal Behavioral Assessment Scale. In *Clinics in Developmental Medicine,* No. 50. Philadelphia: Lippincott, 1973.
4. Brazelton, T. B. Behavioral Competence of the Newborn Infant. In G. B. Avery (Ed.), *Neonatology: Pathophysiology and Management of the Newborn* (2nd ed.). Philadelphia: Lippincott, 1981.
5. Buehring, G. C. Witch's milk: Potential for neonatal diagnosis. *Pediatr. Res.* 16:460, 1982.

6. Condon, W. S., and Sander, L. W. Neonate movement is synchronized with adult speech: Interactional participation and language acquisition. *Science* 183(4120):99, 1974.

7. Cratty, B. J. *Perceptual and Motor Development in Infants and Children* (2nd ed.). Englewood Cliffs, NJ: Prentice-Hall, 1979.

8. D'apolito, K. The neonate's response to pain. *Matern.-Child Nurs. J.* 9:256, 1984.

9. Eisenberg, R. B. Stimulus Significance as a Determinant of Infant Responses to sound. In E. B. Thoman and S. Trotter (Eds.), *Social Responsiveness of Infants.* New Brunswick, NJ: Johnson & Johnson, 1978.

10. Fantz, R. L. Visual Perception from Birth as Shown by Pattern Selectivity. In L. J. Stone, H. T. Smith, and L. B. Murphy (Eds.), *The Competent Infant: Research and Commentary.* New York: Basic Books, 1973.

11. Field, T. M. Interactional Patterns of Pre-Term and Term Infants. In T. M. Field (Ed.), *Infants Born at Risk: Behavior and Development.* New York: S. P. Medical and Scientific Books, 1979.

12. Freedman, D. G. *Human Infancy: An Evolutionary Perspective.* New York: Halsted Press, 1974.

13. Gibes, R. M. Clinical uses of the Brazelton Neonatal Behavioral Assessment Scale in nursing practice. *Pediatr. Nurs.* 7(3):23, 1981.

14. Goren, C. C., et al. Visual following and pattern discrimination of face-like stimuli by newborn infants. *Pediatrics* 56:544, 1975.

15. Grams, K. E. Breast-feeding: A means of imparting immunity. *Am. J. Maternal Child Nursing* 3:340, 1978.

16. Haynes, U. *A Developmental Approach to Casefinding, with Special Reference to Cerebral Palsy, Mental Retardation, and Related Disorders.* Washington, DC: U.S. Dept. of H.E.W., Children's Bureau, 1967.

17. Klaus, M. H., and Kennell, J. H. *Maternal-Infant Bonding: The Impact of Early Separation or Loss on Family Development.* St. Louis: Mosby, 1976.

18. Larrow, L., and Noe, J. M. Port wine stain hemangiomas. *Am. J. Nurs.* 82:786, 1982.

19. Lowrey, G. H. *Growth and Development of Children* (7th ed.). Chicago: Year Book, 1978.

20. Lozoff, B. M. An anthropological approach to infant care. *Birth and the Family Journal* 5:192, 1978.

21. MacFarland, A. Olfaction in the Development of Social Preferences in the Human Neonate. In *Parent-Infant Interaction,* Ciba Foundation Symposium (New Ser.) 33. New York: Elsevier, 1975.

22. McKilligin, H. R. *The First Day of Life: Principles of Neonatal Nursing.* New York: Springer, 1970.

23. Moore, M. L. *The Newborn Family and Nurse* (2nd ed.). Philadelphia: Saunders, 1981.

24. Nugent, J. K. The Brazelton Neonatal Behavioral Assessment Scale: Implications for intervention. *Pediatr. Nurs.* 7(3):118, 1981.

25. Ogra, P. L., and Greene, H. L. Human milk and breast feeding: An update on the state of the art. *Pediatr. Res.* 16:266, 1982.

26. Pantone, J. L. The Relevance of Infant Individuality within the Early Mother-Infant Relationship (Doctoral dissertation, The Ohio State University, 1977). *Dissertation Abstracts International.* (University Microfilms No. 7805902)

27. Prechtl, H., and Beintema, D. *The Neurological Examination of the Full-Term Newborn Infant.* London: The Spastics Society (Medical Education and Information Unit), 1964.

28. Rugh, R., and Shettles, L. B. *From Conception to Birth: The Drama of Life's Beginnings.* New York: Harper & Row, 1971.

29. Scipien, G. M., et al. (Eds.). *Comprehensive Pediatric Nursing* (3rd ed.). New York: McGraw-Hill, 1985.

30. Tanner, J. M. *Foetus into Man: Physical Growth from Conception to Maturity.* London: Open Books, 1978.

31. Taylor, L. S. Newborn feeding behaviors and attaching. *Am. J. Matern.-Child Nurs.* 6:201, 1981.

32. Thoman, E. B. *Disruption and Asynchrony in Early Parent-Infant Interactions.* University of Connecticut, 1979. (ERIC Document Reproduction Service No. ED 180140)

33. Vaughan, V. C., and Brazelton, T. B. (Eds.). *The Family—Can It Be Saved?* Chicago: Year Book, 1976.

34. Waters, C. B., et al. Arginine vasopressin levels during a painful stimulus in infancy. *Pediatr. Res.* 16:569, 1982.

35. Wolff, P. H. Observations on Newborn Infants. In L. J. Stone, H. T. Smith, and L. B. Murphy (Eds.), *The Competent Infant; Research and Commentary.* New York: Basic Books, 1973.

IV
Infancy

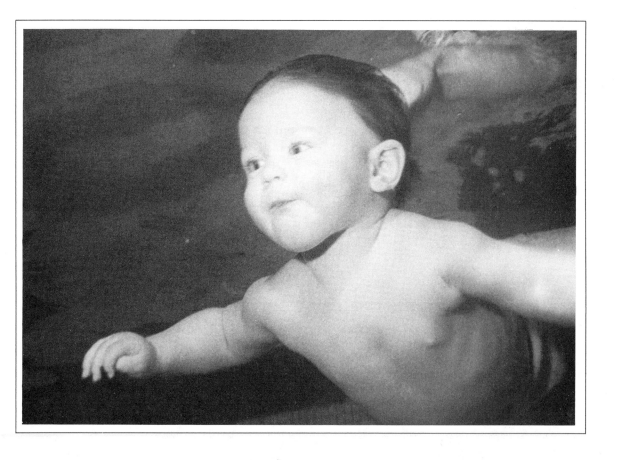

7

Biophysical Development of the Infant

Shirley S. Ashburn

... I look upon your creation in amazement
For we are indeed fearfully and wonderfully made
All its secret, silent machinery—
the meshing and churning—
what a miracle of design.

—Alton Ochsner

Parents rarely need reminding to take pictures of their fast-growing babies, especially during the first 15 months, when so many physical changes are apparent. The average baby gains about 1 inch per month in length for the first 6 months and increases in length by about 50 percent by the end of the first year [30]. The average baby also gains almost 2 pounds per month, or nearly 1 ounce per day for the first 3 months of life [30]. Caretakers should not weigh their babies daily because minimal fluctuations in the baby's weight may cause them to falsely perceive a health problem. Most babies double their birth weight by 5 months. After 6 months, the baby's weight gain decreases to 1 pound per month. Birth weight often triples by the end of the first year. Parents may become overly concerned about the baby's eating patterns during the second year when the monthly increment slows to one-half pound [30]. The important factor is that the baby gains weight steadily over time.

Growth charts have been constructed that present the average weight for gender-age-height groups (see Appendix D). Growth charts indicate **average** physiologic parameters, but **individual** children should be evaluated in terms of health, race, gender, and genetic factors. Premature infants, for example, may consistently lag behind norms because they are actually younger than the full-term infants on whom norms are based. Oriental infants and children tend to be smaller.

especially if born overseas where nutritional intake may not be optimal [49]. Weight measurements for an individual baby usually fall within the same percentile group at sequential ages or change only gradually from one period to another. Although a baby's height and weight often differ in their actual percentile positions, they tend to keep the same general relationships over time. Babies and children whose height and weight measurements fall close to, or outside of, the fifth and ninety-fifth percentiles should be seen by a health professional to rule out growth abnormalities.

SOMATIC DEVELOPMENT

Nervous System

The human nervous system consists of two major components: the central nervous system (CNS) and the peripheral nervous system. The CNS, composed of the brain and the spinal cord, orchestrates control of all body functions. The peripheral nervous system consists of the autonomic (involuntary) nervous system and the somatic (voluntary) nervous system, both of which carry impulses to and from the CNS. Nerve impulses transmitted by the autonomic nervous system control the body's internal organs (e.g., heart, liver, kidneys) without conscious control. The somatic nervous system consists of afferent nerves, which carry sensory impulses (e.g., taste, pain) to the CNS, and efferent nerves, which carry impulses from the CNS to muscle groups.

Nearly one-half the brain's postnatal growth is achieved by the end of the first year [30]. Most of the growth in size occurs in the cerebral cortex (the outer layer of the cerebrum), which is associated with sensation, motor functioning, and cognitive processes (such as storing, processing, organizing, and retrieving information). The brain stem, located at the base of the brain, is relatively well developed by birth compared to the other structures of the CNS. The brain stem primarily controls survival functions, such as reflexes, respiration, digestion, and heartbeat. These vital functions continue to be irregular through the early months of infancy, indicating that brain stem development is incomplete. The cerebellum, located behind the brain stem, shows an increase in weight throughout the first decade [30]. The cerebellum coordinates movement and equilibrium.

MYELINIZATION

A fatty substance called **myelin** grows around the fibers of both the CNS and the somatic nervous system (autonomic nerves do not, in general, become myeli-

nated). This myelin sheath, which initially appeared during the fourth month of intrauterine life [30], functions much like the insulation on an electric wire; it quickens the flow of nerve impulses and directs them to a target organ. The appearance and coordination of selected neurological and motor functionings are correlated with the deposition of the myelin sheath.

At birth the pathways of sensation and equilibrium are myelinated in the brain, as are most of the afferent nerves. This does not mean, however, that the neonate will react to a sensation (e.g., pain) in the same way a neurologically mature individual would. The infant's underdeveloped efferent nerves must mature sufficiently to allow coordinated voluntary movements. Reflexive behavior is thus normal during early infancy but slowly begins to fade as voluntary efferent pathways mature. The corticospinal nerve tract does not acquire myelin until shortly after birth and does not approach completion until toddlerhood. The myelinization of these efferent nerve fibers follows the cephalocaudal and proximodistal principles discussed in Chapter 2. Myelinization explains why the infant first acquires neurological control of head and neck and then trunk, arms, hands, pelvic girdle, legs, bowel, bladder, and so forth. Some nerve tracts are not completely myelinated until several years after birth. Even after they are fully covered, the myelin sheath will continue to thicken for several years [30]. The fibers of the higher centers of the brain (e.g. cerebral cortex, thalamus) are the last to be myelinized.

HEAD CIRCUMFERENCE

During infancy the head grows at a relatively rapid rate. Skull growth closely parallels brain growth. The measurement of head circumference and the assessment of fontanelle status are ways to monitor this growth. The head circumference increases from an average of 34 cm (approximately 13½ inches) at birth to 44 cm by 6 months, and to 47 cm by 1 year [2]. The posterior fontanelle closes during the third month of extrauterine life. The anterior fontanelle may increase in size until the baby is 6 months old; then it begins to diminish and is closed by 18 months.

PERCEPTUAL ORGAN DEVELOPMENT

The perceptual organs of the body help the baby to learn about the world. All these organs as they pertain to the infant are discussed in more depth in Chapter 8.

The Eye. The shape of the eyeball changes throughout life. In the beginning the eye is short, which causes light rays to focus behind the retina (see Chap. 22). The ability of the lens of the eye to accommodate (adjust to different distances) the image viewed on the retina increases rapidly during the first few months of infancy. By 5 months of age, most babies can fixate on a 1-inch cube brought within 1 to 2 feet of their eyes [26]. Because of the immaturity of the eye muscles of the young infant, the eyes may not be able to fixate consistently on an object or may not always appear to be fixating together. Persistent crossing of one or both eyes after 6 to 8 months of age indicates the need for an ophthalmological examination [47].

The Ear. The cartilage which gives the external earlobe its shape does not reach full maturation until late infancy; consequently, it tends to temporarily assume the shape of whatever is pressed against it. The eardrum (tympanic membrane) separates the middle and outer ear. The middle ear is almost adult size at birth, and the three small bones that conduct sound vibrations from the eardrum to the inner ear are well-developed at birth. The inner ear, which facilitates postural equilibrium and transmits auditory sensations to the brain, is well-developed at birth.

Taste Buds. The taste buds, which are present at birth, are more widely distributed about the tongue in the infant and the child than they are in the adult and are especially numerous on the tip of the tongue. Infants prefer sweet-tasting substances.

The Nose. The nose is an important organ for filtration, temperature control, and humidification of inspired air. The olfactory membrane, lying in the upper part of the back of the nose, is almost adult-size at birth. The sense of smell in humans does not develop to the same extent that it does in many other animals. Nevertheless, from birth, the infant begins to learn about the world through the use of smell.

Musculoskeletal System

The tissues that compose the muscular and skeletal systems provide structure and allow movement of the infant's rapidly growing body.

SKELETAL SYSTEM

Bone development follows well-defined steps. In general, cartilage is first deposited and then gradually replaced by mineral salts that aid in the formation of bony tissue. Ossification (bone formation) is explained in more detail in Chapter 22, but it is important to emphasize here that except for the bones of the face and the cranium (which are ossified during fetal life), all other bony structures undergo gradual hardening after birth [7]. If this immature, soft bone is subjected to trauma, "greenstick" or incomplete fractures may result. However, rapidly growing bones heal quickly. While ossification is occurring, bones continue to grow in length and width and, consequently, change in shape. Racial and gender variations are apparent. Black children show more rapid maturation than white children; the bones of girls usually grow and mature faster than those of boys [30, 44].

MUSCLE

The muscular growth of infancy is due mostly to the hypertrophic growth of the already formed muscle fibers, although some hyperplastic growth continues. Of the three types of muscle tissue—voluntary (striated), involuntary (smooth), and cardiac (heart)—the voluntary muscles comprise the bulk of body weight at birth [30]. The growth rate of muscle is about twice as fast as that of bone during the period of time from 5 months to 3 years. During these early years, pituitary growth hormone, thyroid hormones, and insulin all play a role in the growth of muscle tissue. As a muscle grows in size, its strength should increase if adequately exercised. Play activities are critical for developing the potentials of the baby's motor functioning. Table 7–1 summarizes the major gross motor (large muscle) and

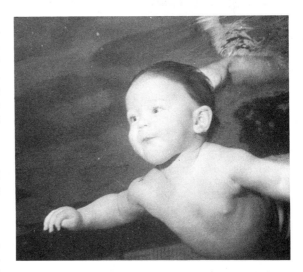

Figure 7–1. Combining exercise with play at an early age can maximize the potentials of the baby's motor functioning. YMCAs and YWCAs offer water orientation classes for infants and their mothers. Some babies learn to swim before they can walk.

Table 7–1. Neuromotor Development during Infancy

Gross Motor Skills	Fine Motor Skills
1 month When prone, may lift head occasionally, but unsteadily. Will turn head from side to side. Will make crawling movements when prone. Is able to push feet against a bare surface to propel self forward. When head is turned to one side, extends arm on the same side and flexes the opposite arm to his shoulder (tonic neck reflex). "Dancing" or "stepping" reflex when held upright. Symmetrical Moro reflex.	Hands are held predominantly in fists. Demonstrates a tight hand grasp. Head and eyes move together. Rooting reflex. Sucking reflex. Shows dorsiflexion of the big toe and fanning of the other toes when sole of the foot is stroked gently from heel to toe (positive Babinski reflex).
2 months When held in sitting position lifts head up but will then bob forward. Can turn from side to back. When prone, can raise head and chest slightly up and off surface on which lying. Tonic neck reflex beginning to fade. Kicks feet alternately.	May hold a toy placed in hand for a brief time. Good palmar grasp. Follows movements of objects or people easily with eyes and head turns. Smiling.
3 months When prone, holds head at 45- to 90-degree angle, some bobbing of head, keeping legs outstretched. Stepping and crawling reflexes absent. When supported, sits with rounded back and flexed knees. May turn from front to back. Tonic neck reflex disappearing.	Plays with fingers and hands. Will reach for bright objects, but will obtain them only by chance. Is able to carry an object from the hand to the mouth. Grasping, rooting, and sucking reflexes beginning to fade.
4 months Uses arms to support self at 90-degree angle when on abdomen. Can turn from back to side. Can sustain part of own weight when held upright. Will sit upright if adequately supported and safely propped. No head lag when pulled to sit. Moro reflex disappearing.	Spreads fingers to grasp. Hands held predominantly open. Will hold on to and shake small objects. Will bring hands to midline and watch them for prolonged periods of time.
5 months Will hold back straight when pulled to sitting position with no head lag. Reaches for objects. Can turn from back to front.	Beginning to use thumb in partial apposition to fingers. Grasps with whole hand ("mitten grasp"), reaches for objects with two hands. Can transfer small object from hand to hand.
6 months Can pull self up to a sitting position. Sits briefly without support if in a comfortable leaning position. Can turn completely over in either direction. Voluntary crawling may appear. May "hitch" (propel self in a sitting position, using arms and legs to move body). When held in standing position, bears almost all of weight.	Bangs object held in hand. Can release an object. Reaches for and grasps an object, usually carrying it to the mouth. Uses all four fingers in apposition to base of the thumb for grasping. Can scoop up a raisin with hand.
7 months Will sit briefly, using arms thrust forward for support. Enjoys bouncing when sitting or held in a standing position. Bears full weight on feet.	Can approach toy and grasp with one hand. Bangs cube on table. Uses the tips of all fingers against the thumb. Will bring feet to midline and watch them for prolonged period of time. May grasp feet and suck on toes.
8 months Sits well alone. Will attempt to flee from an unpleasant event. May stand while holding on. Raises one foot while standing.	Uses index and middle fingers to form a crude pincer grasp with the thumb. Releases objects at will.
9 months Although different children exhibit unique styles, just about all are crawling (infant is prone with abdomen touching floor; body is pulled by arm movement with legs dragging). May "creep" (trunk is above and parallel to floor, with both hands and knees used in locomotion). Pulls self to feet, holding on to something for support.	Complete thumb apposition. Uses pincer grasp (thumb and forefinger) for small objects. Manipulates objects by pushing, pulling, sliding, squeezing. Holds bottle and places nipple in mouth as wanted.

Gross Motor Skills	Fine Motor Skills
10 months Pulls self to feet, holding on to something for support. Can walk sideways holding on to something ("cruising"). May cry when unable to sit down without assistance. Sits by falling down.	Uses index finger to "poke" at objects. Feeds self finger foods (crackers, etc.). Can bring hands together and play "peek-a-boo." Enjoys throwing objects.
11 months Can stand erect while holding on to some form of support with one hand. Will walk holding on to adult hands. Lowers self to floor.	Picks up tiny objects, such as raisins, with very precise pincer grasp. Can hold crayon to make a mark on paper.
12 months Stands alone momentarily. Walks alone (some before this; some after). Climbs onto sofas, chairs. May sit down from standing without assistance.	Positive Babinski reflex fading. Puts one object after another into a container. Can drink holding cup, but needs assistance.
13 months Climbs stairs well on hands and knees. Throws ball with whole body in motion.	Holds caretaker's hand when being spoon-fed. Will position body to assist with dressing. Can turn pages in a book, several at a time.
14 months Steps off one step well. May walk backwards.	Pats pictures in books. Holds spoon to feed, but needs assistance.
15 months Creeps up stairs. Cannot walk around corners or stop suddenly without losing balance. Walks backwards.	Builds a tower of two to three blocks. Opens most boxes, pokes finger into holes. Scribbles spontaneously.

fine motor (small muscle) activities of children from birth to 15 months.

One should keep in mind that an individual baby may differ from the "average." Cross-cultural studies illustrate extreme variability of motor development in young children.

Integumentary System

The integumentary system includes nails, hair, skin, and selected glands that pass through the skin.

SKIN

In addition to its cosmetic function, the skin aids in protecting the body from extreme temperatures, excess humidity, bacterial invasion, and other agents that are harmful. The outer layer of the skin, or epidermis, gives protection against such elements. During infancy, the epidermis is loosely connected to the layer of skin beneath it, the dermis. Because both layers are relatively thin, the infant has an increased susceptibility to blistering and chafing (or "rub burns") [7]. Melanocytes in the skin produce pigmentation (melanin) that protects the body from harmful sun rays. How-

ever, the infant's ability to produce pigmentation is limited, with a resulting sensitivity to the sun. Infants should initially be placed in the sunlight for only 2 minutes, with exposure increased gradually [41]. Black and olive-skinned babies have no more melanocytes than do fair-skinned babies [47].

DERMATOGLYPHICS

Each individual has a distinct set of handprints, fingerprints, and footprints created by epidermal creases and ridges [19]. Many of these patterns, or dermatoglyphics, are formed in the third fetal month. Other explicit wrinkles develop throughout the individual's life cycle. These patterns, unique to each individual, provide cues to possible chromosomal abnormalities as well as clues to personal identification.

GLANDS

During adulthood, the two types of sweat glands (eccrine and apocrine) secrete perspiration in response to emotional stimuli. The eccrine glands, which produce sweat in response to both thermal and emotional stimuli, are present but are not fully functional during early infancy. This may be one way the baby is able to conserve water to meet a relatively high need for fluid [7]. Aprocrine sweat glands (responsible for what is commonly called "body odor") are fully developed at birth but do not begin to function until the prepubertal years [47].

The sebaceous glands, which help to produce the vernix caseosa of the newborn, are distributed all over the infant's body except on the palms and the soles of the feet. These glands actively secrete sebum during early infancy and thus lubricate the baby's skin. The sebaceous glands decrease in activity during childhood and are reactivated during the pubertal period (see Chap. 25). Because of this decrease in active production of sebum, older infants and children may have relatively dry skin in cold and low-humidity environments.

Even though the epidermis and the glands work together to prevent bacterial invasion, infection can still occur because of the extreme sensitivity of the skin to rubbing, heat, or trauma. The routine cleansing and drying of all the body areas is the best deterrent to bacterial growth.

HAIR

The development of the baby's scalp hair often provides a topic for lively discussion among relatives. Some babies are born with a full head of hair and others are bald. Genetic factors affect the appearance of the hair. The texture and color of the hair at birth may be quite unlike the hair the same individual will possess later on. Scalp hair tends to be very fine and thin during infancy and may even fall out and reappear with a different texture, color, or both.

NAILS

Full-term babies are born with fingernails and toenails. Although the nails are very thin, they grow fast and need to be kept clean and neatly trimmed.

Cardiovascular System

The blood and the vessels that transport it as well as the heart that pumps it comprise the cardiovascular system. This system carries nutrients to, and waste products from, every cell of the body.

HEART

The heart of the infant will double its weight by the first birthday [30]. It lies in an almost horizontal position at birth. As the baby grows older, the heart will gradually shift to a permanent, more vertical position. The heart in the infant and the child is situated higher in the chest than it is in the adult. For this reason, the external cardiac compressions of cardiopulmonary resuscitation (CPR) are performed between the nipples on the chest of a baby but are performed much lower on the chest of older individuals.

At birth the left and right lower chambers of the heart (ventricles) are approximately the same size. By 2 months of age, the muscular walls of the left ventricle will become thicker than those of the right ventricle [47]. This differentiation in size is critical because the left ventricle is responsible for pumping blood to the entire body while the right ventricle pumps blood to the lungs. The strength of the left ventricle contraction is reflected in the numerator of the blood pressure fraction (systolic pressure). As the total heart grows larger, the heartbeat will slow and the blood pressure will rise (see Appendix E). Heart murmurs produced by vibrations within the heart chambers or in the major arteries from the back-and-forth flow of the blood are common and not necessarily pathological in infancy.

BLOOD VESSELS

Under the influence of the involuntary nervous system and hormones, the small capillaries in the infant's body contract to conserve body heat and expand to cause heat loss. These abilities, which are essentially absent in the neonate, gradually begin to develop after the first few weeks of extrauterine life [7].

BLOOD VALUES

The blood values of the infant reflect information such as the oxygen-carrying capacity of the red blood cells and the defense abilities of the white blood cells (see Appendix E). During early infancy, the hemoglobin can drop as low as 10 gm per deciliter. This "physiologic anemia" reflects the body's need to decrease the number of red blood cells (and thus the attached hemoglobin) because of the relative overproduction during the fetal period. Under normal circumstances, the baby will not be endangered because the lowered hemoglobin will stimulate the bone marrow to produce more red blood cells. Although the blood values of the average infant are different from those of the adult, the infant is capable of maintaining physiological equilibrium. Lymphoid tissue (a part of which exists in the blood as lymphocytes) grows rapidly during infancy and provides some protection against illness. Lymphocytes are active in the formation of antibodies.

Respiratory System

Although the neonate's initial respiratory efforts expand most of the alveoli, not all are expanded until a few days or even a few weeks after birth [47]. These alveoli increase in numbers and complexity at a relatively rapid rate during infancy [36]. The weight of the lungs is doubled by 6 months and tripled by 1 year [30].

The infant's relatively more rapid respiratory rate is due in part to the large amount of "dead air space," or that portion of the airway where air passes but gases are not exchanged [7]. This anatomical situation combined with the high metabolic rate requires that proportionately more air enter and exit the lungs per minute. The baby is predominantly a nose-breather during the first few months of life and then gradually learns to breathe through the mouth by the third or fourth month [10]. Blocked nostrils (e.g., a cold) will make nursing and swallowing very difficult and will require more time for feeding.

Gastrointestinal System

At birth, the gastrointestinal system of the infant is ready to ingest and digest breast milk or its equivalent. With further growth and development of the child, it is capable of digesting a wide variety of different-textured foods.

MOUTH

Salivation is adequate at birth to maintain sufficient moisture in the baby's mouth. However, the maturation of many of the salivary glands does not occur until the third month of life and corresponds with the baby's learning to swallow at other than a reflex level. The result is a marked increase in the baby's drooling. Swallowing, sucking, and respiration, activities which are adequately developed in the healthy full-term infant, require coordination to prevent aspiration of ingested materials during feeding.

Initially, all foods placed in the infant's mouth are manipulated in the same way that the infant manipulates the nipple. The forward-thrusting movement of the tongue (extrusion reflex) may be misinterpreted by many parents as a dislike for solid foods. This reflex begins to fade at about 4 months. At approximately 6 months of age, control of lateral jaw movements increases, allowing the infant to begin a chewing movement when eating food.

ESOPHAGUS AND STOMACH

The esophagus of the infant differs from that of the adult because the tone of the lower esophageal sphincter is poor, which accounts for the frequent spitting up of foods. The first 3 months of life constitute the most rapid growth period for the stomach. The capacity of the stomach varies among individuals. By the age of 1 month, the stomach's capacity is generally 90 to 150 ml (3 to 5 ounces); at 1 year of age, the capacity is 210 to 360 ml (7 to 12 ounces) [30]. The rate of gastric (stomach) emptying also varies among individual infants. Digestion in the stomach occurs primarily as a result of the secretion of hydrochloric acid and pepsin, both of which aid in the breakdown of protein. This ability, however, is relatively limited throughout infancy. Consequently, many pediatricians advise delay of the introduction of solids until the second half of the first year of life.

SMALL INTESTINE

Most of the digestion and absorption of foodstuffs occurs in the small intestine, which increases its length by 50 percent during the first year. Pancreatic secretions composed of three enzymes (trypsin, lipase, and pancreatic amylase) are released into the small intestine. Neonatal levels of trypsin, which further break down the partially digested proteins that travel from the stomach, are equal in amount to adult levels.

Pancreatic amylase, which digests starch, is secreted at adult levels at 3 months. Lipase, which breaks down fats, also reaches adult level at 3 months, although this does not mean that the infant is capable of digesting all fats by this age. Lipase needs mature bile (secreted from the liver and stored in the gallbladder) to aid in digestion of fat. By the time the infant is 1 year of age, the lipase and bile are working together well enough to approximate adult fat digestion. Polyunsaturated fatty acids (found in breast milk and in infant formulas) are more easily absorbed than saturated fats during the first year of life [18].

LARGE INTESTINE

Although some water is absorbed in the small intestine, more is absorbed into the bloodstream, along with electrolytes, by the walls of the large intestine. Since the intestinal contents move rapidly through the gastrointestinal tract and the large intestine is initially immature in water absorption, the infant's stools during the first year of life contain relatively more water and are consequently looser. This biophysical fact combined with the environmental factor of more adult foods being added to the infant's diet contribute to the stools' becoming more formed and solid in consistency at approximately 1 year of age. While the newborn may have a bowel movement after each feeding, during later infancy the frequency may range from three to six stools per day [20]. The large intestine also plays an important role in the synthesis and absorption of vitamin K, which is necessary for normal blood clotting (coagulation). When the newborn begins to ingest milk or formula, normal bacteria will grow in the intestinal tract and will aid in the production of vitamin K by the second week of extrauterine life [37].

Genitourinary System

GENITALS AND REPRODUCTIVE ORGANS

The baby's genitals and reproductive organs remain relatively immature during infancy. However, the internal reproductive organs do increase in weight in preparation for later functioning. A discussion of the development of these organs is deferred until Chapter 25.

EXCRETORY SYSTEM

The excretory organs (kidneys, ureters, bladder, and urethra) constitute the genitourinary system. The kidneys are responsible for filtering wastes from the blood and maintaining fluid and electrolyte balance; they function in an immature way during the first few weeks of extrauterine life. The ability to form urine involves many factors: among these are the reabsorption and secretion powers of the kidney tubules and the filtering capacity of the kidney epithelium [32]. The tubules, short and narrow at birth, closely approximate adult size by 6 months [47]. At the time of birth, some kidney epithelium is very thick and is therefore less efficient in filtration; it gradually becomes thinner throughout infancy. Thus the young infant's ability to concentrate urine (reabsorb urinary filtrates for body use) gradually improves. Since more urine must pass through the kidneys to excrete wastes, the infant's fluid needs, which are based on body weight, are relatively greater than the adult's. However, if an infant is given an overload of fluid, the kidneys are unable to respond adequately by increasing urinary output [30]. Consequently, a baby can become overhydrated if he is given too much fluid. He needs approximately 2 ounces per pound, or 120 to 160 ml per kilogram, in a 24-hour period (or a comparable amount over a smaller increment of time).

Endocrine System

The endocrine system is composed of glandular structures that are found throughout the body. These glands secrete hormones directly into the bloodstream to affect the functioning of organs in other parts of the body. The immaturity of this system at birth becomes a dis-

advantage if for some reason the infant must adjust to wide fluctuations in water concentration, electrolyte levels, glucose (simple sugar), or amino acids (building blocks for proteins). Mature hormonal control of physiological functions by the endocrine system is not achieved during infancy [7].

GLANDULAR STRUCTURES

The pituitary body (hypophysis), which lies at the base of the brain, produces several hormones. The most important hormone produced during infancy is the pituitary growth hormone (PGH). This hormone, produced by the anterior lobe of the pituitary, aids in the control of extrauterine skeletal growth as well as the metabolism of protein, fats, and carbohydrates. PGH becomes a major factor in growth control after the infant reaches 1 year of age [30].

Adrenocorticotropic hormone (ACTH) is secreted by the anterior pituitary, and antidiuretic hormone (ADH; also referred to as vasopressin) is produced by the posterior pituitary. The functions of both these hormones are limited during infancy. ACTH stimulates the adrenal glands to produce hormones affecting the metabolism of glucose, protein, and fat. ADH acts on the kidneys, so that water excretion through urine is di-

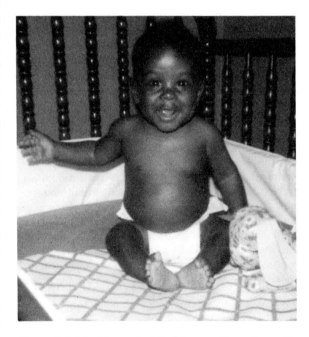

Figure 7–2. Most 8-month-old babies are able to sit steadily unassisted, which frees their hands to engage in other activities.

minished when the body needs to conserve water (e.g., baby with fever). Unfortunately, the infant's kidneys do not respond well to ADH. Furthermore, it is suspected that the pituitary's ability to produce ADH is limited during the first few months of infancy.

The thyroid gland, located in the lower neck in front of the trachea, stores and secretes the thyroid hormones that are responsible for tissue respiration rate and other important metabolic processes at the cellular level. The thyroid function is mature from birth [30]. If the thyroid gland produces too much hormone (hyperthyroidism), the individual will demonstrate symptoms of a rapid metabolism (e.g., extreme nervousness, weight loss). When the thyroid gland produces too little hormone (hypothyroidism), skeletal maturation and central nervous system development are adversely affected. The mental deficiency that results (cretinism) is partially reversible if hormone therapy is initiated before 6 months of age [47].

The parathyroid glands, located in the lower neck near the thyroid, produce a hormone that acts with vitamin D to regulate calcium and phosphorus metabolism, which is vital to the growth and the development of bones.

The adrenal glands, which are located on top of the kidneys, are quite limited in function at birth. The inner part of each adrenal gland (called the adrenal medulla) secretes epinephrine (adrenalin) and norepinephrine (noradrenalin). In a situation perceived as threatening, both of these hormones work to decrease blood flow to tissues such as the gastrointestinal tract (which is not needed in emergency situations), and to increase blood flow to tissues such as the heart and the skeletal muscle, which are usually needed to meet a sudden challenge. These same hormones also aid in the use of fat, increase the basal metabolic rate, and elevate the level of blood sugar. The hormones secreted by the adrenal cortex mediate the metabolism of water, sodium, potassium, protein, fat, and carbohydrate. During infancy, however, the efforts of the adrenal cortex are immature.

The islets of Langerhans of the pancreas manufacture insulin and glucagon, both of which facilitate glucose metabolism. Blood sugar levels may fluctuate widely throughout infancy and childhood. When the child's blood sugar level is too low, he or she will tire easily, become irritable, and interact less effectively with the environment. Too much refined cane sugar may lead to hyperactivity in some children.

The liver, located behind the ribs in the upper right portion of the abdomen, is relatively large at birth. It performs several metabolic functions: converting the blood sugar into glycogen, storing the glycogen, and converting the glycogen again into glucose to be released into the bloodstream as needed. The liver also synthesizes and oxidizes fats, stores some vitamins and minerals, manufactures some blood proteins, and removes toxic substances (e.g., drugs, alcohol) from the blood. Its functioning remains immature throughout infancy.

Fluid and Electrolyte Balance

Body fluid consists mostly of water and dissolved substances. Those substances whose atoms possess an electrical charge (i.e., in ionic form) are called electrolytes. Water and electrolytes transport nutrients and other substances to and from body cells, maintain the blood volume, dilute the products of metabolism, and regulate the pressure of all body fluids (including blood) as well as the acid-base balance and the conductibility of neuromuscular tissue [34].

WATER

Water is more essential to the body than food; it is second only to oxygen in importance for bodily survival. Water comprises the major portion of body structures, serves as a solvent for minerals and other compounds, aids in the transport of food and wastes to and from the cells, and helps to maintain body temperature.

The newborn's body is approximately 75 percent water. By 1 year of age, the total body water content has decreased to 64 percent. **Extracellular water** refers to the water in plasma (the liquid fraction of the blood), and between cells. During infancy, extracellular water comprises a greater proportion of total body water than in older children and adults [34]. Because of the relatively greater proportions of total body water and extracellular water, the infant must consume more water per unit of body weight than adults. The infant is also more susceptible to dehydration than is an adult because his kidneys do not yet conserve water well. **Intracellular water,** the fluid contained within body cells, is less subject to problems of fluid imbalance, but these problems are more serious when they do occur.

Water is lost from the body through several routes. Its excretion in urine is obvious; it is also contained in perspiration where it seeps through the epidermis and evaporates. Perspiration, the amount of water excreted with feces, and the amount that is "blown off" from the lungs during normal breathing all comprise the rather difficult-to-measure insensible water loss (IWL). IWL is relatively greater in infancy than in adulthood, owing in part to the infant's proportionately greater area of body surface, increased respiratory rate, and looser bowel movements. Evaporative water loss is estimated to be approximately 210 ml per day at 1 month of age and 500 ml per day at 1 year of age [18].

Relatively more fluid is required to rinse the body of products left by the infant's high metabolic rate. The term **renal solute load** refers to those solutes that must be excreted by the kidney; this load is affected by the amount of protein and salts in the diet. Infants who are fed formulas receive a slightly higher renal solute load than do breast-fed infants. The renal solute load is generally not a major concern unless the infant receives excessive amounts of protein through improper formula preparation or through overuse of solids at an early age. Infants are particularly vulnerable to water imbalances during illness. Fever, vomiting, or diarrhea can markedly increase fluid losses. Therefore, extra attention must be paid to the fluid requirements of the infant during illness or when fluid intake is poor.

ELECTROLYTES

Sodium and chloride are the primary electrolytes found in extracellular fluids; potassium is concentrated within the cells. A proper balance of electrolytes is essential for the functioning of all the cells in the infant's body. Imbalances in electrolytes become a major concern when losses are increased through gastrointestinal routes (e.g., vomiting, diarrhea), particularly when fluid losses are replaced only by nonelectrolyte fluids, such as water or diluted tea. Boiled milk contains an excess of protein and electrolytes because of water evaporation. Homemade electrolyte solutions that contain salt, baking soda, or sugar are risky because they may be incorrectly prepared. A health professional must ascertain the specific type of dehydration the infant is experiencing to prescribe the proper fluid and electrolyte replacement.

Dentition

The teeth begin to grow during the prenatal months. The first "baby" teeth that erupt are called primary or deciduous teeth; the teeth that a person develops later in life are referred to as permanent teeth. There is wide variation in what is considered a normal time for the emergence of the first tooth. The first one, usually a lower tooth (the primary mandibular central incisor), cuts through the gums at about 6 to 7 months of age. The time of emergence depends on health, heredity, prenatal and postnatal nutrition, race, gender, and other factors; for example, females usually cut their first tooth earlier than males. There will eventually be a total of 20 deciduous teeth that appear at a rate of about one per month after the first tooth emerges until the child is 1 year of age. It is the sequence of these eruptions that is far more important than the age of eruption. An irregularity in the sequence of eruption is likely to cause misalignment of the teeth and to result in poor alignment of the jaws (malocclusion), even affecting the way the permanent teeth will come in.

The second tooth to erupt is usually the second lower mandibular central incisor. By 1 year of age, the four upper maxillary incisors are usually present. A few months may pass before more teeth appear; then in

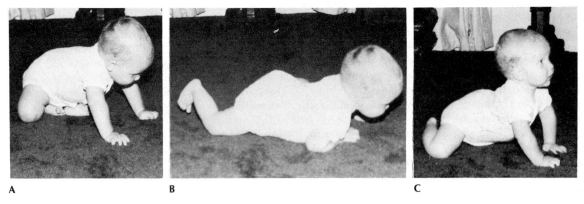

A   B   C

Figure 7–3. One child's sequence of quadruped locomotion. Not all infants follow the pattern of hitching, crawling, and then creeping. Children have different versions of these maneuvers; some may even skip a stage. (A) Hitching. The baby moves backward in a modified sitting position by using the arms and hands to push. (B) Crawling. While prone with the abdomen touching the floor and the head and shoulders supported with weight borne on the elbows, the baby pulls the body and drags the legs as the arms move. (C) Creeping. While the trunk is carried above the floor and parallel to it, the baby uses hands and knees to move forward.

relatively rapid succession, the two remaining lower mandibular incisors and all four first molars emerge. The rest of the deciduous teeth emerge during toddlerhood, and the set is usually complete by 2½ years of age.

MAINTAINING HEALTH

Infancy is the stage in life where the most rapid extrauterine biophysical growth and development occur.

Basal Metabolism

The basal metabolic rate (BMR) is highest during periods of rapid growth, particularly during the first 2 years of life. Basal metabolism is the minimum amount of heat produced by the body in a fasting state while one is awake but at rest. It indicates the amount of energy needed to maintain life processes. The BMR is affected by a variety of factors, including body surface area, gender, age, weight, endocrine activity, and general state of nutrition. Basal metabolic requirements decline gradually during adulthood and old age.

Energy requirements are stated in kilocalories (kcal) per kilogram (kg), or pound, of body weight. A kcal is the amount of energy required to raise 1 kg of water 1°C. Total energy requirements are based on metabolic rates, rate of growth, body size and surface area, and physical activity. The recommended energy intake for children of various ages is given in Appendix E.

NUTRITION

Initial Feedings. Three primary sources are available to meet the nutritional needs of the neonate: human breast milk, modified cow's-milk formulas, or formulas based on soy protein. The formulas have vegetable oils, carbohydrates, and vitamins added. Breast milk and the majority of commercially prepared formulas contain approximately 20 calories per ounce. When provided in sufficient volume, both breast milk and commercially prepared formulas are adequate to meet the protein, caloric, and vitamin needs of the infant during the first 4 to 6 months of life. Breast milk offers, in addition, antibodies and enzymes that may protect the infant against infections. Infants who are fed formulas will require vitamin supplements. Cow's milk, whether whole, 2 percent fat, or skimmed, is not adequate to meet the nutritional needs of the young infant. The protein of whole cow's milk has caused bleeding into the gastrointestinal tract of some infants that in turn has led to iron deficiency anemia [17]. Neither lowfat nor nonfat milk is recommended for in-

fants less than 1 year of age, and nonfat milk is not recommended before 2 years of age. These milks are frequently fortified with nonfat milk solids that increase the load on the young child's maturing kidneys. The infant or young toddler who drinks either nonfat or lowfat milk will not derive enough calories because of low carbohydrate content [38].

Babies cannot remain healthy with milk as the only source of nutrients throughout infancy. Healthy full-term infants have sufficient body stores of iron to meet their needs until 5 to 6 months of age. Supplemental iron in formula or vitamin preparations will help to maintain adequate levels and to prevent iron-deficiency anemia [9, 18]. Iron-deficiency anemia has detrimental effects on growth, immune factors, energy capacity, and learning abilities of young children. The iron available in breast milk is well-absorbed and therefore may be sufficient to meet the infant's requirements if the mother's diet is adequate [17]. However, a number of pediatricians recommend addition of an iron supplement to the diet of the young breast-fed infant (see Chap. 32 for further discussion of breast feeding).

For the first few years of childhood, many pediatricians recommend multivitamin preparations that contain B vitamins as well as vitamins A, D, and C. Babies who are on evaporated-milk formulas require vitamin C supplementation; however, orange juice should not be introduced until 6 months of age, since many younger infants demonstrate an allergic response to it. During the second half of the first year, parts of the baby's skin (usually the palms, the ear lobes, and the soles of the feet) may exhibit a yellow sheen. This condition is due to an excess of carotene (a precursor of vitamin A) that is circulating in the blood and is caused by a high intake of yellow vegetables. It is not pathological and will disappear when carotene sources are reduced. This condition is in no way connected to the jaundice that occurs when bilirubin is elevated (which also causes the sclera, or the firm outer coating of the eyeball, to turn yellow).

Introduction to Solids. The addition of solid foods to a baby's diet is a highly individual matter. Babies are different—some are hungrier than others. Much confusion and misinformation exists regarding the introduction of solid foods to the infant's diet. Most infants will tolerate cereals and other solids even when introduced in the first weeks of life; however, the fact that the foods are tolerated does not mean that it is desirable to offer them at such an early age. In fact, a number of potential problems may result from the too early introduction of solids. The addition of solids at a very early age may result in an inadequate intake of milk, with insufficient or inappropriate vitamin and protein intakes as well as insufficient fluid intake. The addition of solids to an adequate intake of milk may result in overfeeding and obesity. The introduction of certain solids before the infant is 6 months of age also increases the risk of developing certain food allergies; wheat cereals, citrus juices, and egg whites are the most frequent causes of allergic reactions.

A noticeable increase in appetite often indicates that a baby is ready for foods to supplement breast milk or formula. If the baby breast feeds more frequently than every 3 hours or consumes more than 1 quart of formula per day, a need for additional food may be indicated. When an infant who is more than 6 months of age is eating 1½ jars of strained baby food or its equivalent, some homogenized, vitamin D-fortified whole milk can be fed without fear of provoking nutritionally significant gastrointestinal blood loss [18].

The first food introduced is generally rice cereal, since few people are allergic to this grain. The dry cereals generally provide larger amounts of a more readily absorbed form of iron than the wet-packed cereals. The infant should be started on 1 or 2 small spoonfuls of dry cereal mixed with water, breast milk, or formula; this amount can be gradually increased to 2 to 4 tablespoonfuls twice a day. Preparing the cereal with strained citrus juices or vitamin C-fortified juices will increase the bioavailability (the amount absorbed into the bloodstream) of the iron in the cereal [12]. Once the infant has accepted and tolerated cereal, mashed banana and other strained fruits or vegetables may be added. Strained meats are generally added last.

New foods should be introduced one at a time, initially in small amounts and allowing for several days to elapse between each addition of new food. When eggs are introduced, the yolk is commonly fed to the infant first, because it is a good source of iron, and babies are more often allergic to the egg white. If at any time the infant appears to develop a reaction, such as vomiting, rash, or diarrhea, a food should be withdrawn and reintroduced several weeks later. Any new food will cause some alteration in the color and the consistency of the stool; these minor changes do not necessarily indicate an intolerance of the food.

Parents who elect to use commercially prepared baby foods should be advised to read the labels carefully. Mixed-food dinners sometimes contain foodstuffs and additives that could cause allergic reactions in some babies. The food contents are listed on the label in descending order from highest to lowest percentage. Foods that have additives of salt, sugar, and starches should be avoided.

Feeding Schedules. For most infants, a flexible demand-feeding schedule is preferable to a rigid feeding schedule. The infant is fed when hungry, and the tendency to underfeed or to overfeed the infant is minimized. For most infants, a demand schedule may start with as many as eight feedings per day at irregular intervals, but with time the infant generally establishes a 3½-to-4-hour feeding schedule. In the first 3 months of life, the bottle-fed infant requires from five to seven feedings per day because of the smaller capacity of the stomach and the high metabolic needs in relation to body size. By 4 or 5 months of age, the number of feedings generally decreases to four per day. Babies may be ready for three meals per day any time between the ages of 4 and 10 months [41]. Additional fluids and snacks will need to be offered between meals. Many variations exist to these guidelines; Doctor Benjamin Spock's sensible discussion of the matter in his *Baby and Child Care* [41] is recommended. One safety point is critical: Bottles should **never** be propped. The danger of a baby choking or inhaling the contents of a propped bottle is real.

It is important that the caregiver recognize the infant's cues for readiness to feed as well as those for satisfaction. The young infant indicates satisfaction by slowing the sucking activity, falling asleep, turning the head away, or allowing milk to run from the mouth. Cues of satiety provided by the older infant are more direct: The child may clamp down on the nipple rather than sucking, push the spoon or cup away with the hand, or draw the head back. The parent or caregiver should not try to coax the infant to finish solids or formula, since this can lead to overfeeding, discomfort, and obesity.

The baby's rate of growth begins to slow down at the end of the first year of life. At this time many parents become concerned that their child is not eating well. This is a normal process as long as the child continues to make expected weight gains (see Appendix D).

Most babies are eating mashed or junior food preparations by 8 to 9 months. Self-feeding can be initiated by providing small pieces of toast, teething crackers, bananas, and other table foods. The child who is beginning to self-feed should not be left alone, because he or she has a tendency to "bite off more than can be chewed" and may choke. The use of finger foods also allows the infant to explore different shapes and textures. Nuts, raisins, small candies, and popcorn are

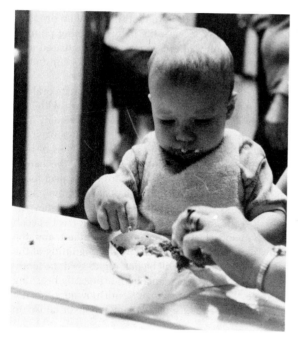

Figure 7–4. During midinfancy, babies enjoy manipulating objects by pushing, pulling, sliding, banging, and squeezing them. They make use of these skills as they attempt to feed themselves.

difficult for the older infant (and toddler and young preschooler) to chew and can cause choking.

At approximately 9 months of age, a training cup can be introduced. The infant will be awkward and messy with the cup at first, but it is important that the opportunity be given to try it.

Weaning an infant from the bottle or the breast to a cup should be a gradual process. The cup can be introduced during meals, with the bottle being reserved for nap and bedtime. Weaning is generally accomplished by 12 to 14 months of age, although some children will continue to need a bedtime bottle or the breast for a short time longer. Adult foods can be gradually added as tolerated. Individual families and cultures vary widely in their perception of an infant's readiness to be weaned and the manner of introducing new foods and textures.

Overfeeding. In recent years the long-term effects of infant overfeeding and obesity have become a concern. A fat baby has a high chance of becoming an obese child. Longitudinal and retrospective studies have demonstrated that 80 percent of overweight children become overweight adults [27]. Other studies,

however, suggest that the majority of fat babies will outgrow their baby fat and will have normal weights in childhood [39]. Studies of the number and the size of adipose (fat) cells in obese and nonobese children and adults suggest that there may be two subgroups of obese children [27]: The group with increased numbers of adipose cells are apt to remain obese while the other group will outgrow their baby fat. Genetic predisposition and family eating patterns also influence the development of childhood obesity. There is some evidence that overfeeding babies may induce an excessive number of fat cells to be produced during this sensitive growth period [44]. This data suggests moderation in infant feeding with alertness to cues of infant satiety [22].

Sleep

The infant's rapidly growing body needs adequate rest for optimal growth, since pituitary growth hormone is excreted mainly during periods of deep sleep [30]. New babies tend to be noisy sleepers; they gurgle, cough, sneeze, sigh, and make other sounds that only a baby can produce. As the baby's nervous system develops and matures, periods of deep sleep and alertness become longer. Every infant has a unique sleep pattern. As he or she learns how to sleep and how to stay awake, the patterns of sleep will change (see Chap. 27 for further discussion of sleep).

By 2 months of age, many babies are beginning to sleep through the night feeding; by 3 months, about 70 percent of babies will sleep most of the night [40]. At 6 months of age, the baby is probably taking two or three naps per day and sleeping a total of 16 to 18 hours out of 24. The baby may again begin episodes of frequent night awakenings at approximately 7 to 9 months [48]. Although some babies wake up because they are teething, many do so because they have been dreaming, a sign of normal neurological development. At about 10 months, they usually sleep 10 to 12 hours at night and take two naps during the day. By 1 year of age, most babies sleep 11 to 12 hours at night and 3 or more hours during the day in one or two naps [40].

Dental Care

Healthy teeth and gums are affected not only by the baby's current intake but also by the prenatal nutritional environment. Fluoride strengthens the enamel of the teeth and increases their resistance to decay. It is especially effective when it is incorporated in the tooth during the formation of enamel (which occurs prenatally and before the tooth has erupted). Prenatal fluoride preparations are available for pregnant women. Infants and children who drink water containing approximately 1 part per million (ppm) fluoride throughout the period when their teeth are forming may have a decrease in tooth decay (caries)[21].

Children who do not have access to fluoridated drinking water should receive fluoride supplements from birth through 14 years. Dosage is based on the child's age and the level of fluoride in the child's drinking water. Prescriptions are written according to recommendations made by the American Dental Association and the American Academy of Pediatrics (refer to Table 7–2).

Because children less than 3 years of age are apt to swallow much of the toothpaste used in brushing their teeth and because there may be 1 mg of fluoride per gram of fluoridated toothpaste, only the smallest amount of fluoridated dentrifice (i.e., no larger than the size of a small pea) should be used each time.

TEETHING

Infants vary in their response to teething. One baby may gnaw on objects, drool excessively, and fret for 3 or 4 weeks before a tooth emerges. Another baby's mother may discover a new tooth without warning when she hears it click against the feeding spoon. Teething sometimes interferes with a baby's sleep patterns or appetite.

During teething, the baby is at the height of incorporating and learning about the environment by way of the mouth. Oral gratification is necessary; providing the baby with a rubbery, chewable object may prove refreshing to teething gums, especially if it has been cooled by being placed in the refrigerator. Increasing fluid consumption at this time is encouraged. Many

caretakers unwisely use products that contain drugs or alcohol, allegedly to ease the baby's teething pain. A rise in body temperature, loose stools, increased salivation, and a rash around the mouth can occur during teething [6].

During the early postnatal months, adequate oral hygiene consists of cleaning the baby's mouth with sips of clear water after feedings. The baby may enjoy having the gums massaged with a moist, clean gauze pad. Massaging the gums removes plaque (patches of bacteria). Toothbrushing should begin when the baby's first tooth has erupted. Proper care of the deciduous teeth is essential to prevent tooth decay and tooth loss; the deciduous teeth maintain spaces for the later permanent teeth and assist in developing correct speech habits. A soft-bristled brush for the infant and the young child is recommended. By the beginning of the second year, the baby will be helping to hold the toothbrush but is in no way capable of efficiently brushing the teeth without assistance. Tooth powders are not recommended because babies may inhale or choke on them.

DENTAL CARIES

Dental caries (tooth decay), which may begin any time after the first tooth has erupted, occur when the normal bacteria (flora) of the mouth digest carbohydrates (sugars) and leave an acid that erodes tooth enamel. The production of this acid begins as soon as sugar in any form (e.g., milk, formula, or juice) is placed in the mouth. Teeth should be brushed after eating sticky foods (e.g., peanut butter, cheese) that allow the acid to remain in contact with the teeth. If no toothbrush is available, a water rinse will help.

One form of tooth decay that is most difficult to treat but relatively easy to prevent is known as "baby bottle mouth" or "nursing bottle mouth syndrome." Often discovered in late infancy, the baby's upper front and side teeth are severely decayed and may be broken off. Inevitably, the parents in these cases admit to putting the baby to bed for naps and at night with a bottle. When the baby nurses slowly at these times, the liquid (e.g., milk, formula, juice) coats the front and side teeth for long periods of time while the tongue, saliva, and nipple protect the lower teeth. Because of these problems, many pedodontists recommend that children be weaned from the night bottle feeding by at least 1 year of age and that they not be allowed to remain at the breast after they have fallen asleep. A pacifier can replace the bottle if the child's sucking needs exceed nutritional needs, but it should never be used to replace essential human contact.

Table 7–2. Supplemental Fluoride Dosage Schedule (mg/day)[a]

Age	Concentration of Fluoride in Drinking Water (ppm)		
	<0.3	0.3–0.7	>0.7
2 weeks to 2 years[b]	0.25	0	0
2 years to 3 years	0.50	0.25	0
3 years to 14 years	1.00	0.50	0

[a]2.2 mg sodium fluoride contains 1 mg of fluoride.
[b]Because breast milk contains only trace amounts of fluoride and fully breast-fed infants consume little or no water, a fluoride supplement of 0.25 mg daily should be prescribed for the infant who is breast-fed exclusively more than 6 months.
Sources: Adapted from Committee on Nutrition, American Academy of Pediatrics. Fluoride supplementation: Revised dosage schedule. *Pediatrics* 63:150, 1979; and Fluoride Compounds. *Accepted Dental Therapeutics* (39th ed.). American Dental Association: Chicago, 1982. P. 349.

Five percent of children less than 1 year of age and 10 percent of children less than 2 years of age develop dental caries [31]. The baby's teeth need to be inspected regularly for a general assessment and to check for caries. Children should be seen by a dentist for the first time during their first year, especially if the baby is considered to be at high risk for dental disease (i.e., a history of developmental disability, nonexposure to fluoride, or a family history of dental disease). All children should be seen by a dentist by 12 months of age if one is concerned about preventive dentistry [31].

Immunizations

Immunity involves the ability of the body to defend itself against substances (e.g., bacteria, viruses) that can cause physical disequilibrium or illness. The purpose of immunization or vaccination is to protect a child from disease by causing the body to produce antibodies for use against these substances. See Chapter 10 for a further discussion of immune system development.

In most cases, the newborn has a temporary, naturally acquired immunity (3 to 6 months) to the following diseases: measles (rubeola), German measles (rubella), mumps, poliomyelitis, diphtheria, and scarlet fever. The infant is not protected from chickenpox, tetanus, whooping cough (pertussis), streptococcal infections, and the common cold. Giving the newborn immunizations will not help since the infant's immature immune system is unable to produce effective antibodies. Table 7–3 gives a recommended immunization schedule for normal infants and children. Research is ongoing to find new immunizations to combat diseases which as yet have no effective vaccines (e.g., chickenpox, scarlet fever).

Under normal circumstances, the adequately immunized adolescent of 14 or 15 years of age would receive an adult tetanus and diphtheria booster (Td) and would be due for another one at 24 or 25 years of age, provided a serious major wound has not been sustained.

Tuberculin skin tests (Tbc) are not immunizations, but they are recommended at 1 year of age. The individual's reaction to Tbc indicates whether or not there has been exposure to the tubercle bacillus, which causes tuberculosis. A positive test requires follow-up investigation by a physician.

Health Assessment

Most neonates are examined several times during their hospital stay and then are scheduled for a follow-up physical examination between 3 and 6 weeks of age. Following the first official checkup, the baby should be scheduled for regular monthly visits. Well-baby checkups are usually scheduled every 3 months during the second year.

In newborns, vision is tested mainly by checking for light perception. A light is shined into the eyes and responses are noted such as pupillary constriction, blinking, following the light to midline, increased alertness, or refusal to open the eyes after exposure to the light. Special tests are available during infancy to confirm blindness.

If a baby's hearing ability is questioned (e.g., the infant does not appear to be soothed by the parent's voice in early infancy), then a hearing test should be arranged. Special tests can document hearing loss in young infants. Poor hearing due to an accumulation of earwax (cerumen) can be prevented by proper ear cleaning. A health professional should be consulted as to how it should be removed.

Parent Education

New parents usually have many questions. In addition to being concerned with the common variations dis-

Table 7–3. Recommended Immunization Schedule for Normal Infants and Children

Age	Vaccines	Comments
2 months	DTP, Polio	DTP: diphtheria, tetanus, and pertussis (absorbed type) vaccine. Polio: trivalent oral polio vaccine (TOPV).
4 months	DTP, Polio	
6 months	DTP*	
15 months	Measles Rubella Mumps	M/R: one dose of measles/rubella (combined) vaccine; or M/M/R: one dose of measles/ mumps/rubella (combined) vaccine (if available).
18 months	DTP, Polio	These doses constitute an important part of the immunization series.
4–6 years	DTP, Polio	

*Another dose of TOPV is optional but may be given in areas with a high risk of poliomyelitis.
Source: Adapted from American Academy of Pediatrics: Report of the Committee on Infectious Diseases, III, ed. 19, Chicago, 1982.

cussed in Chapter 6, they may have various practical questions; for example, they may want to know how to take a baby's temperature. Most health professionals recommend taking it under the baby's armpit (axillary method). Although there is an abundance of well-written baby care literature, such books and pamphlets should not replace the consultation of a health professional who can individualize the baby's care. Information about infant health care is often provided by the local health department or clinic. Community organizations may promote projects to encourage and administer immunizations. Parents can learn how to care for their infants and children more effectively by attending the classes provided by the local chapter of the American Red Cross, the extension service of their state's department of agriculture, the children's service division of the Human Services Department (welfare bureau), or adult education programs. Numerous federal programs have been created to support healthy infants and children.

COMMON CONCERNS WITH INFANTS

Some of the many concerns that cause anxiety in caretakers, especially those who have the responsibility for the first time, have already been mentioned. Three additional entities have been selected for a brief discussion here.

"Spitting Up" and Regurgitation

The return of small amounts of food during or after a feeding is a common occurrence in infancy. It should not be confused with vomiting or other more serious feeding problems. The following terms are defined for clarification:

1. "Spitting up." Dribbling of unswallowed formula from the infant's mouth immediately after a feeding.
2. Regurgitation. The **involuntary** return of undigested food from the stomach, usually accompanied by burping.
3. Vomiting. The forcible **involuntary** ejection of stomach contents, often accompanied by nausea.
4. Rumination. The active, **voluntary** return of swallowed food into the mouth. The food is then rechewed, reswallowed, or expelled. Rumination is often caused by the same factors that precipitate nonorganic failure-to-thrive syndrome (see Chap. 9).

Regurgitation generally resolves at approximately 2 to 3 months of age as the sphincter muscle tone of the lower esophagus tightens. In the interim, caretakers can help many infants with this problem by placing them in an infant seat after feedings to keep their heads higher than their stomachs or by instituting minor changes in feeding routines, such as more frequent, gentle burping during feedings. Some babies regurgitate if they are rocked too vigorously during or after the feeding. A preferred position after feeding an infant is to place the baby on the right side to permit the feeding to flow toward the lower end of the stomach and to allow any swallowed air to rise above the fluid and through the esophagus. Keeping the corners of the infant's mouth dry of formula will decrease the chance of a rash. Regurgitation in infants more than 2 to 3 months or excessive regurgitation at any age should be referred for medical evaluation [8].

Colic

Many individual patterns of colicky behavior exist. In general, a colicky infant is defined as one who either extends the legs and body in a rigid manner or draws the knees up to a distended abdomen and cries persistently for several hours. Some pass large amounts of flatus (gas). Many cases of alleged colic may actually be caused by thirst, hunger, or inadequate feeding techniques. Colicky behavior may also be a symptom of an underlying problem, such as food allergy, malabsorption, or central nervous system immaturity.

The cause of true colic, which commonly begins when the baby is 2 to 6 weeks old, is still subject to debate. Sometimes a nervous caretaker may be the cause of a baby's display of colicky behavior. Meeting the needs of an anxious caretaker may alleviate much of the problem. Colic may be a sign of a sensitivity to cow's milk, thus the elimination of cow's-milk products from the diet of the baby or lactating mother may reduce the symptoms [29]. Unless an underlying disease is found, parents can be reassured that the infant is not ill and will probably outgrow the colic at about 3 months of age [8]. A few babies have colic until they are 6 months old. Despite the indications of colic pain, the baby gains weight.

Treatments for colic vary. Sometimes, especially for bottle fed babies in warm weather, all the infant needs is an extra drink of water. Colicky babies usually appear most comfortable when lying on their stomachs. It is suggested that the caretaker cuddle the baby and place the infant across the lap, over the shoulder, in a front carrier ("snugli"), or even lie down with the baby's abdomen against the caretaker's. Decreasing environmental stimuli (e.g., turning down the volume of the telephone, closing the blinds, feeding the baby in a quiet area of the house) may soothe the sensitive, colicky baby. Some babies seem to fare better with a pacifier. Placing a hot water bottle on the baby's abdomen is not recommended. They are dangerous even if padded with towels, since they may leak or burn. Medication may decrease the infant's ability to attend adequately to the environment, and thus may affect cognitive and socioaffective development.

A major concern is that the colicky behavior will interfere with the establishment of a strong parent-child relationship. Parents should not feel that the infant's behavior is a result of their inadequate caretaking. Parents can be shown how to read their infant's subtle interaction cues, thus facilitating more effective communication with the infant. As the colicky behavior decreases, the parents and the baby will be able to synchronize their responses to each other more quickly.

Respiratory Infections

Many growth and developmental factors predispose the infant to respiratory difficulties in times of illness. The short, wide, horizontal eustachian tube, which connects the middle ear to the nasopharynx, facilitates the traffic of organisms that cause middle-ear infection. The infant's trachea (airway to the lungs) is relatively small in diameter and is surrounded by soft (as opposed to rigid and more supporting) cartilaginous rings. Both of these factors contribute to blockage of air if inflammation or swelling is present [47].

The major path to the right lung (the right main bronchus) is larger than the left main bronchus as well as being more in line with, and at less of an angle to, the trachea. Thus aspirated foreign bodies more often enter the right bronchus and cause obstruction or infection. Relatively large tonsils and adenoids may also cause obstruction even though their purpose is to aid the body in fighting infection. The chest muscles are immaturely innervated, with the result that the infant depends primarily on abdominal muscles and diaphragm to breathe. The relatively large abdominal organs may also impede vital breathing. The infant's small thoracic cavity is cylindrical with horizontal ribs, a factor which limits expansion potentials. All these factors, coupled with a tongue that is not well supported, make the infant's cough less effective and cause fatigue much more rapidly [42]. To compensate, the infant must breathe faster to get the much-needed oxygen. The faster the baby breathes, the more water he loses. The infant who is breathing faster than usual can also upset the body's delicate acid-base balance.

Most infants have at least one respiratory infection during the first year of life, and many babies have more than one [13]. Dressing the baby properly and assuring adequate housing, temperature, humidity, nutrition, hydration, and ventilation promote high level wellness. Babies should not be exposed to tobacco smoke: Studies are pointing to the increased risk of the healthy infant contracting bronchitis or pneumonia in such environments. Tobacco smoke aggravates the condition of the child with asthma and other respiratory difficulties [3].

SUMMARY

Each part of the infant's body grows and develops at its own rate. The infant's motor skills become more complex with the synchronized maturation of the musculoskeletal and neurological systems and the opportunity to exercise them. Most of the baby's senses are well developed at birth, allowing input from the world. Many changes occur in the cardiovascular system that aid in transporting life-giving blood. The gastrointestinal, genitourinary, and endocrine systems meet the needs of the healthy baby in terms of ingestion, digestion, secretion, excretion, and general homeostasis. Under normal conditions, the infant's respiratory system adequately supplies oxygen and removes the necessary amount of carbon dioxide. The baby's delicate skin is most adequate for protecting the body.

As the infant's baby teeth emerge and erupt, and as the body systems continue to grow and mature, feeding habits change. Proper nutrition and feeding schedules are important to provide the necessary ingredients that allow the body to maximize the baby's biophysical potential.

For a few months after birth, the baby retains antibodies received from the mother, which makes the infant immune to several diseases. With so many infants and children contracting infectious diseases, the importance of the baby receiving immunizations according to schedule cannot be overemphasized. Regular health assessment is paramount to high level wellness; this assessment includes not only the baby but also the family and the community in which they live. Necessary intervention, which includes parent education and community involvement, should be identified from such assessment. The infant's biophysical systems are normally well equipped to aid the healthy baby in everyday living. Under stress, however, these systems may need the assistance provided by the intervention of health professionals.

REFERENCES

1. Barnard, M. U., et al. *Handbook of Comprehensive Pediatric Nursing.* New York: McGraw-Hill, 1981.
2. Behrman, R. E., Vaughan, V. C.; Senior Editor W. E. Nelson. *Nelson Textbook of Pediatrics* (12th ed.). Philadelphia: Saunders, 1983.
3. Boldon, D. Personal communication, 1977.
4. Bradshaw, T. W. Teething. *Pediatr. Nurs.* 7(3):41, 1981.
5. Brasel, J. A. The Effects of Feeding Practices on Normal Growth, Failure to Thrive, and Obesity. In L. J. Filer, Jr. (Ed.), *Infant Nutrition: A Foundation for Lasting Health?* Part 2. Bloomfield, NJ: Health Learning Systems, 1977.
6. Carpenter, J. V. The relationship between teething and systemic disturbances. *J. Dent. Child.* 45:381, 1978.
7. Chinn, P. L. *Child Health Maintenance: Concepts in Family-Centered Care* (2nd ed.). St. Louis: Mosby, 1979.
8. Christie, D. L. Gastrointestinal Symptoms Related to Feeding in the First Two Years of Life. In *Problems Related to Feeding in the First Two Years.* Columbus, OH: Ross Laboratories, 1977.
9. Committee on Nutrition, American Academy of Pediatrics. Vitamin and mineral supplement needs in normal children in the United States. *Pediatrics* 66:1015, 1980.
10. Comroe, J. H. *Physiology of Respiration: An Introductory Text* (2nd ed.). Chicago: Year Book, 1974.
11. Cowan, E. B., Bouchard, J. C., and Suarez, M. M. Child health screening for the nurse practitioner. *Nurse Practitioner* 1(3):109, 1976.
12. Dallman, P. R., et al. Iron deficiency in infancy and childhood. *Am. J. Clin. Nutr.* 33:86, 1980.
13. Davidson, M. Normal Gastrointestinal Function in Children up to Two Years of Age. In M. H. Sleisenger and J. S. Fordtran (Eds.), *Gastrointestinal Disease: Pathophysiology, Diagnosis, Management* (3rd ed.). Philadelphia: Saunders, 1983.
14. De Angelis, C., et al. Introduction of new foods into the newborn and infant diet. *Issues in Comp. Pediat. Nurs.* 2(1):1, 1977.
15. De Castro, F. J., Rolfe, J. T., and Drew, J. K. *The Pediatric Nurse Practitioner: Guidelines for Practice* (2nd ed.). St. Louis: Mosby, 1976.
16. Dudding, B. A. Problems related to the common cold. *Issues in Comp. Pediat. Nurs.* 3(2):1, 1978.
17. Fomon, S. J., et al. Human milk and the small premature infant. *Am. J. Dis. Child* 131:463, 1977.
18. Fomon, S. J., et al. Recommendations for feeding normal infants. *Pediatrics* 63(1):52, 1979.
19. Green, M. *Pediatric Diagnosis: Interpretations of Symptoms and Signs in Different Age Periods* (3rd ed.). Philadelphia: Saunders, 1980.
20. Gryboski, J. D. Gastrointestinal function in the infant and young child. *Clin. Gastroenterol.* 6(2):253, 1977.
21. Horowitz, H. S. Community Water Fluoridation. In D. J. Forrester, M. L. Wagner, and J. Fleming (Eds.), *Pediatric Dental Medicine.* Philadelphia: Lea & Febiger, 1981.
22. Infant feeding somatic growth and obesity. *Nutr. Rev.* 35:235, 1977.
23. Iron absorption from breast milk and cow's milk. *Nutr. Rev.* 35:203, 1977.
24. Jeliffe, D. B., and Jeliffe, E. F. P. "Breast is best": Modern meanings. *N. Engl. J. Med.* 297:912, 1977.
25. Johnson, T. R., Moore, W. M., and Jeffries, J. E. (Eds.). *Children Are Different: Developmental Physiology* (2nd ed.). Columbus, OH: Ross Laboratories, 1978.
26. Kempe, C. H., et al. *Current Pediatric Diagnosis and Treatment* (7th ed.). Los Altos, CA: Lange Medical Publications, 1982.
27. Knittle, J. Obesity in childhood: A problem in adipose tissue cellular development. *J. Pediatr.* 81:1048, 1972.
28. Kotlow, L. A. Breast feeding: A cause of dental caries in children. *J. Dent. Child.* 44(3):24, 1977.
29. Lothe, L., et al. Cow's milk formula as a cause of infantile colic: A double-blind study. *Pediatrics* 70(1):7, 1982.
30. Lowrey, G. H. *Growth and Development of Children* (7th ed.). Chicago: Year Book, 1978.
31. Matthewson, R. J., et al. *Fundamentals of Dentistry for Children. Vol. I: A Complete Guide to Comprehensive Dental Care for the Child and Adolescent.* Chicago: Quintessence, 1982.
32. McCrory, W. The Excretory System: Anatomic and Physiologic Considerations. In R. E. Cooke (Ed.), *Biologic Basis of Pediatric Practice.* New York: McGraw-Hill, 1968.
33. McMillan, J. *Iron Sufficiency in Breast-Fed Infants and the Availability of Iron from Human Milk.* Franklin Park, IL: La Leche League International, 1976. (1976 Paul Gyorgy Award)
34. Metheny, N. M., and Snively, W. D. *Nurses' Handbook of Fluid Balance* (4th ed.). Philadelphia: Lippincott, 1983.
35. Montagu, A. *Touching: The Human Significance of the Skin* (2nd ed.). New York: Harper & Row, 1978.
36. Murray, J. F. *The Normal Lung: The Basis for Diagnosis and Treatment of Pulmonary Disease.* Philadelphia: Saunders, 1976.
37. Phillips, C. R. *Family-Centered Maternity/Newborn Care.* St. Louis: Mosby, 1980.
38. Pipes, P. L. (Ed.). *Nutrition in Infancy and Childhood* (2nd ed.). St. Louis: Mosby, 1981.
39. Poskitt, E. M. E., and Cole, T. J. Do fat babies stay fat? *Br. Med. J.* 1:7, 1977.
40. Riley, H. D., Jr., and Berney, J. Infant sleep. *American Baby* 38(12):27, 1976.
41. Spock, B. M. *Baby and Child Care* (4th ed.). New York: Hawthorn Books, 1976.
42. Talabere, L. Personal communication, 1977.
43. Tanner, J. M. Growing up. *Sci. Am.*, 229:34, 1973.
44. Tanner, J. M. *Foetus into Man: Physical Growth from Conception to Maturity.* London: Open Books, 1978.
45. Timiras, P. S. *Developmental Physiology and Aging.* New York: Macmillan, 1972.
46. Tudor, M. Developmental screening. *Issues in Comp. Pediat. Nurs.* 2(2):1, 1977.

47. Valadian, I., et al. *Physical Growth and Development: From Conception to Maturity.* Boston: Little, Brown, 1977.

48. Wenner, W., and Barnard, K. The Changing Infant: Sleep and Activity Patterns during the First Months of Life. In K. Barnard, *The Nursing Child Assessment Sleep/Activity Record.* Seattle: 1979.

49. Whaley, L. F., and Wong, D. L. *Nursing Care of Infants and Children* (2nd ed.). St. Louis: Mosby, 1983.

50. Will a fat baby become a fat child? *Nutr. Rev.* 5(6):138, 1977.

8
Cognitive Development during Infancy

Shirley S. Ashburn and Clara S. Schuster

But understanding alone is not enough. When I understand something but do not put it into action, nothing has been accomplished either in the outside world or within myself.

—Barry Stevens, *Person to Person*

For centuries the question, What goes on in a baby's mind? has been asked by scholars and philosophers, but only in the past 25 years have answers been provided through systematic research. Babies and young children are not only **aware of** stimuli and activities around them but begin to **learn** from such experiences from the first days of life [20, 35, 36, 52]. A young baby who accidentally shakes a rattle may not initially know what caused the experience, but the baby will be aware of it, will respond to the stimulus, and will begin to associate it with his or her own action. Every experience (e.g., the satisfaction of hunger, the hugging of a fuzzy toy) becomes an opportunity for acquisition of knowledge.

One of the leaders in the study and explanation of the process of cognitive (intellectual) development is Jean Piaget. His concept that cognitive development occurs through the interaction of an individual's genetic disposition with environmental experiences has promoted an interest in pacing the experiences offered to infants (and older children) to facilitate the maximizing of potentials. Other researchers, using Piaget's framework, are reexamining the effects of early sensory deprivation on the child's intellectual development [36].

Evidence exists (see Chap. 4) that the fetus is capable of being conditioned in utero [39], giving support to the idea of the existence of a cognitive domain for human beings before the beginning of extrauterine life. **Cognition** is the process of obtaining and using knowledge about the world through the use of perceptual abilities, symbols, and reasoning. Cognition includes the processes by which knowledge is acquired and used; therefore, ideas (concepts or mind symbols) and language (verbal symbols) are two of its tools. Sensory organs receive input about the environment (to experience the world). This normally leads to **perception,** the process of extracting information in such a way that the individual transforms sensory input into meaning. **Learning,** the dynamic process in which perceptual processing of sensory input leads to concept formation and change in behavior, is an integral part of cognition. It should be noted that learning does not necessarily always follow immediately after the reception of sensory input, nor does the change in behavior always have to be such that it can be observed by others.

A person who has a healthy nervous system (in the biophysical domain) possesses the basic tools for meaningful perceptual experiences. The nervous system should contain receptors that detect input accurately, a brain that can interpret the information efficiently, and transmitters that can transport decoded information—all necessary components of cognition and communication (see Chap. 13). Suboptimal functioning of any of the body systems can delay the development of cognitive processes. Human infants differ in their degree of neurological maturity and these differences are critical in producing early individual differences in learning [25].

J. S. Watson was one of the first to point out that babies can subordinate their affective and social domains to their cognitive domain. He discovered that babies quickly learn to initiate and to control parental reactions by providing feedback through cries, smiles, and other forms of infant communication. Dubbed "The Game," Watson observed this form of learning in babies as young as 2 months of age [59]. Other researchers have discovered that babies can give more subtle cues soon after birth (e.g., pause and stop sucking during feeding; turn the head away from the nipple) [32].

Each individual experiences unique interactions among his or her affective, biological, cognitive, and social domains; it follows that each person's cognitive capabilities will differ somewhat from those of another.

DEVELOPMENT OF PERCEPTION

Most theorists consider perception to be an intermediate stage in the transmission of information from sensory end organs to the central process of cognition. We present the human sensory capabilities, with particular emphasis on those of the infant.

Sensory Capabilities

The sensory receptors can be divided into three categories [21]:

1. Exteroceptors ("distance senses")
   a. Vision
   b. Hearing
2. Proprioceptors ("near senses")
   a. Cutaneous (skin) senses, which detect and communicate (transduce) changes in touch (pressure), temperature, and pain
   b. Chemical sense of taste
   c. Chemical sense of smell
3. Interoceptors ("deep senses")
   a. Kinesthetic sense, which transduces changes in position of the body and motions of the muscles, tendons, and joints
   b. Static or vestibular sense, which transduces changes related to maintaining position in space and the regulation of organic functions such as metabolism, fluid balance, and sensual stimulation

SIGHT

Some visual skills are already present at birth (see Chap. 6) [4, 5]. Infants use their vision in combination with other senses to perceive and learn about the world. Brazelton's studies show that an infant less than 1 hour old can fixate on and follow a slowly moving object [7].

HEARING

As soon as amniotic fluid has drained from the outer ear of the newborn (usually just a few minutes after birth), the infant will respond to noise (usually demonstrating a Moro reflex, an eye blink, or turn toward the sound) [57].

During this first few months, infants are sensitive to the frequency, duration, and intensity of sounds [13]. By observing face, motor movement, heart-rate changes, and other communicative efforts of babies, researchers concluded that some newborns can detect the difference between tones of 200 and 250 cycles per second, which is approximately equivalent to one step in a musical scale [8].

Neonates can make pursuit movements toward a sound [7], and by 2 to 2½ months of age, the infant can recognize and locate mother's voice in a noisy room [57]. At 6 months of age, most babies will respond to their name by turning toward the speaker. Long before the end of the first year, the infant is sensitive to minute differences between combinations of sounds and will show recognition of frequently used, meaningful words.

TOUCH

The sense of touch, (discussed further in Chap. 9) is an important perceptual tool. At birth, peripheral sensory receptors are mature and are capable of receiving sensations of pain, pressure, and temperature. An immaturity of the cerebral components that respond to tactile sensations probably accounts for the differences in infant versus adult responses. Infants appear to differ from one another in skin sensitivity [16]. Many people believe that because the nervous system is immature, an infant cannot experience pain. Current research contradicts this [38]. An infant is able to perceive pain before myelinization of the nerve pathways is complete. Even fetuses will move away from a source of pain. During the first month of life, the full-term infant is likely to respond in a diffuse, global manner to pain. The neonate will probably cry immediately, reflexively withdraw an extremity (if that is the source of the pain), and show some degree of generalized body movement. As the infant matures, these responses are replaced by more localized movements.

In general, the sensorimotor aspects of the child's behavior develop slightly earlier than the cognitive aspects and conative aspects (conscious desire to act with or without knowledge of the origin of the drive). Localization is well-established before the child achieves integration of the various neural centers that permit adequate appraisal of the situation and a masterful response. Between 5 and 9 months, most babies begin to develop an idea of the origin of pain [28]. Most babies over 5 months will fuss, cry, or exhibit an individualized withdrawal reaction to pain. The extent to which the sensorimotor aspects both influence and are influenced by the cognitive and conative aspects is difficult to assess and is highly individual.

TASTE

Although the location of taste buds has been mapped, the processes of taste activtion, adaptation, discrimination, and preference are not clearly understood. At birth, babies perceive differences between widely varying tastes, such as sugar and salt. By 2 weeks of age, babies will suck when given sugar water and grimace when citric acid (contained in orange juice) is placed on their tongues. They also stop sucking when salty solutions or quinine water are placed on their tongues.

Taste preferences are influenced by individual cultures. The Eskimo child learns to ask for whale blubber, and the Hawaiian youngster craves poi. Infants are born with many taste buds, enabling infants and very young children to savor the natural flavor of foods (hence, adding sugar or salt to baby's food is unnecessary). During the first 5 years of life, the number of taste buds gradually decreases [3].

SMELL

The newborn who is exposed to olfactory stimuli, such as ammonia or acetic acid, will turn the head away from these unpleasant stimuli. However, infants are

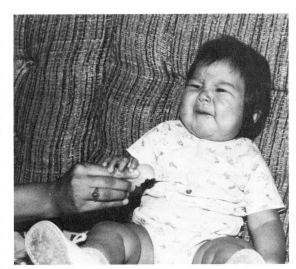

Figure 8–1. Even though the initial physical reaction to a piece of lemon or sour pickle may be strong, many young babies will continue to suck on the tidbit until the flavor is gone and may even cry if it is taken away. Such exposure to new experiences helps children to increase their awareness of the world and their own body.

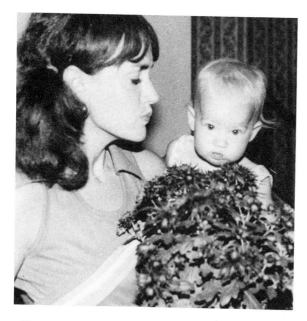

Figure 8-2. Imitation is a form of learning that originates during infancy. This mother's encouragement to sniff the flowers is helping the baby to use the sense of smell to gain more information about the environment.

generally nonreactive to stimuli that older children and adults find disgusting, because they have not yet learned that the culture considers the odors unpleasant. Some odors may provoke increased neonatal activity [41]. Breast-fed babies can smell their mother's milk and often refuse formulas. Locating the source of odors is not very precise in humans, and appears to vary greatly from one individual to another. Nevertheless, the infant's sense of smell can be a valuable tool for learning.

Assumptions about Perception

Perception provides the bridge between the reception of stimuli by the senses and the cognitive processes that organize and use the input for adaptive functioning. Since perceptual skill is an internal event, its presence and development are inferred by changes in overt behavior. Consequently, certain assumptions must be made.

Hierarchical Organization of Perceptual Skills

The views of perceptual development range from "Deity to DNA" [40]. Some perceptual skills appear to be unlearned. This may be the result of genetic bias toward particular stimuli, or innate behavioral systems

that are activated by the presence of a species-specific stimulus [1]. However, whether originally innate or learned, all perception soon entails storage and retrieval of information.

The perceptual process goes through a series of developmental sequences, which can be identified as the **hierarchical organization of perceptual skills.** These steps are as follows:

1. Detecting stimulus energy
2. Differentiating gradients in stimulation
3. Differentiating the world in terms of similarities and differences
4. Distinguishing foreground stimulation from background activity
5. Responding to patterns and wholes rather than to separate details
6. Identifying form
7. Recognizing form and manipulating it in various situations
8. Learning body schemata and orientation
9. Developing space perceptions

Perceptions of any type of stimulus (e.g., visual, tactile) follow this general pattern throughout the life cycle. The tasks that comprise this process to some degree go on forever—a person does not just master each task once and then forget it. Every time a healthy person perceives a stimulus, at least part of the process is used. The more novel the stimulus, the further back (and thus closer to the first tasks) the person must go to conceptualize what is being interpreted. Individual maturation and experience combine to form uniqueness within the pattern.

Infants use this process and often proceed through most of the steps more than once as they come upon new stimuli and learn new things about old stimuli. Sensory factors are dominant in the determination of the lower-order tasks, whereas experiential factors contribute increasingly important effects as higher levels of the perceptual tasks are reached [21].

DETECTING STIMULUS ENERGY
Because the perceptual world of the fetus is still very much a mystery to us, it is difficult to pinpoint the first time an individual becomes aware of a sensory stimulus. A 5-day-old baby sucking on a pacifier may momentarily stop sucking if an object begins to move in the infant's visual field [28]. This is an example of the baby's ability to detect the movement of a stimulus (in this case, a stimulus other than the pacifier).

Table 8–1. Assumptions about Perception

Statement	Explanation/Example
1. Perception includes both the sensing of input and the interpretation of that input.	1. Someone slams a door, and a baby hears the noise (detects an auditory stimulus) and perceives it as uncomfortable (interpretation of the input).
2. Perception is each individual's representation or image of reality.	2. Different people attach different values to different stimuli that are perceived.
3. Perception is selective.	3. Individuals do not perceive accurately, but selectively, choosing to complete the perceptual process by interpreting some input and disregarding other input.
4. Psychosocial as well as neurophysiological factors affect perceptual processes.	4. Physical fatigue as well as emotional stress can affect what a person perceives as a stimulus.
5. Perceptions differ according to past experiences, self-concept, socioeconomic group, biological inheritance, and educational background.	5. Preferences for foodstuffs vary according to culture and geographical location: Orientals find raw fish a delicacy but may at first shun the traditional American fried chicken.
6. Perceptual processes are important to learning and interacting.	6. Perception serves as a selective filter. Through perception, potentially significant events are brought into meaningful focus [40].
7. Perceptual skills gradually become more refined, stable, and integrated.	7. Individuals are able to differentiate and articulate input at increasingly more complex levels with maturation and experience.
8. Perception is a dynamic process, which becomes increasingly adaptive with development.	8. Perceptual input is synthesized and becomes more complex and richly patterned with experience.
9. An individual who is unable to receive sensory input from one modality can learn to depend more heavily on alternative sensory input.	9. An individual who does not have vision can learn to rely heavily on the senses of touch, taste, smell, and hearing.
10. The use of alternative sources for sensory input may affect interpretation and thus perception of the environment.	10. An individual who has partially lost the abilities to taste and smell may prefer foods more highly seasoned than an individual who has normal olfactory senses.

DIFFERENTIATING GRADIENTS IN STIMULATION

Because the 5-day-old baby will look for different amounts of time at stimuli that vary in intensity of brightness, it is inferred that the infant has detected a difference in the stimulus energy. We are not yet able to decipher whether the infant is actually ordering the stimuli according to some criterion or simply responding to something that "hooks" attention.

Fantz [17] has discovered that 1-week-old infants are capable of pattern (shape) perception, which requires that infants differentiate one stimulus in some respect from another. To carry out his experiment, Fantz presented infants with four black and white patterns (horizontal stripes, a bull's-eye, a checkerboard, and a gray patch) in random order. A standard gray field was presented simultaneously for comparison with each pattern. By determining how long a reflected image of each stimulus appeared in the baby's pupil, Fantz measured the differences in response to the patterns. Some researchers have interpreted these results to indicate

that the infant has early sensitivity to, and preference for, contour, complexity, or both.

DIFFERENTIATING THE WORLD IN TERMS OF SIMILARITIES AND DIFFERENCES

There are conflicting theories about when infants first perceive color (detecting stimulus energy) and then discriminate one color from another (differentiating the world in terms of similarities and differences). Some developmentalists maintain that the infant begins to discriminate specific colors at 1 to 2 months of age, when the retinal cones and macula of the eye develop sufficiently [57]. In one experiment, 4-month-old babies were tested to ascertain if they could remember the colors they saw. The babies were shown the same color until they lost interest in it; then that color was brought back later along with an entirely new one. The rationale was that if the babies had "forgotten" the first color, they should have been equally fascinated by both. As it turned out, the new color captured their attention, indicating that babies at this early age had both the ability to discriminate and to remember. The babies also indicated specific color preferences: red was the favorite, followed by blue, yellow, and green [42]. The results of such an experiment might suggest that babies should not be exposed to colorful mobiles until they are 1 or 2 months of age. On the contrary, such toys are essential from the very beginning. Babies probably perceive color earlier than we can prove, and mobiles have other attributes a baby can enjoy, especially if they are attached in such a way that they are set in motion by the baby's activity. Upon mastery of this skill, a person can distinguish objects in terms of distinctive qualities and uniqueness.

DISTINGUISHING FOREGROUND OF STIMULATION
FROM BACKGROUND OF ACTIVITY

The individual must learn to select a pattern to treat it as a separate entity and hold it against the tendency for some other pattern to become a part of the figure.

Bower placed infants in their second week of life upright (to facilitate maintenance of state 4; see Chap. 6) and moved various objects toward their faces [3]. The babies appeared to perceive that the objects were approaching, because they cried, pulled their heads back, and shielded their faces with their hands. If the object was moved farther away, the babies did not demonstrate this behavior. It seemed that the babies could distinguish the moving object from the background and responded as if the object were going to touch them.

Gibson and Walk [26] designed a test of infant depth perception called a "visual cliff." A clear glass-top table had checkered linoleum secured immediately under the glass on one side and 3 to 4 feet below the glass on the other side. The baby was placed on a board just above the line separating the two sides of the table, where the infant could see through the glass to the checkered linoleum on each side. The infant could move onto either side of the glass table top. The researchers discovered that the infant would move only to the table surface that had the linoleum secured immediately under the glass [26]. This experiment, and a later one conducted by Scarr and Salapatek, demonstrated that infants will use depth cues after the age of 7 months [47]. However, **infants must have some crawling experience before they will refuse to get too close to the "cliff."** The young infant who cannot crawl and who is placed on the "deep" side of the table apparently does not experience fear but does perceive some difference, because the infant's heart rate will decrease markedly (researchers believe that this decrease connotes some form of attention) [9].

RESPONDING TO PATTERNS AND WHOLES
RATHER THAN TO SEPARATE DETAILS

Responding to patterns and wholes means that the individual is taking in as many aspects of the stimulus as possible so that increased information is gained. When first beginning to look at pictures, the child tends to point at details with an index finger, attending to eyes or a bright spot of color. As perceptual skills improve, the child will pat the whole picture and respond verbally with "mama" or "kitty," or another appropriate label.

IDENTIFYING FORM

The task of identifying form involves the individual's recognizing similarities in contour and differentiating those essential to the concept. This requires that the individual note and extract distinctive features in order to identify similar stimuli. It is difficult to pinpoint when babies are capable of actual form perception, because we do not really know for sure how they are thinking or why they are responding the way they do. Fantz concluded that if an infant is shown two stimuli with differing amounts of contour and looks longer at one of them, then the infant has detected the difference between them. It is also known that infants will look longest at stimuli that possess a moderate amount of contrast—too much contrast seems to be overwhelming and too little appears not to be perceived.

The individual is gradually able to distinguish the more subtle features of a stimulus with increased development and experience. For example, at approximately 5 months, many infants are noted to be studying faces and to be making visual checking behaviors with the face of their mother in the presence of others.

RECOGNIZING FORM AND MANIPULATING IT
IN VARYING SITUATIONS

Recognizing form in varying situations is an important task to master if one is to identify order in the world. With development, the perception of a stimulus becomes separated from the context in which it is presented. This skill helps in the recognition of a bottle even though it may be handed to the baby upside down. It will later help a person to recognize, in a novel setting, a person who usually wears a uniform and is seen only in a specific setting or that the food on a plate is a variety of potato—whether it is baked, mashed, or french-fried.

Bower studied shape constancy in human infants between 50 and 60 days of age. By using very precise experimental manipulations, he concluded that these young infants already possessed a perceptual corrective mechanism with which they could recognize an object presented to them in a new orientation [4].

Several studies suggest that young infants perceive a grossly overpopulated world of objects. The infants may perceive one object as a different object when it is moved to a new location. If so, it is possible that babies would not know they each had just one mother but would think that each time mother left and returned, she was a new person! Bower performed some research that supports this theory: He used mirrors to create the illusion that there were three of the baby's own mother in the room with the baby. He found that 3-month-old babies reacted with pleasure to three mothers, whereas those who were 4 months old tended to cry and to exhibit disturbed behaviors. From this experiment he suggested that babies less than 5 months may think that they have many identical mothers [5]. **Object constancy** is the ability to **recognize** that an object or a person in the bedroom is the same as that in the kitchen or that mother-from-a-side-view is the same as mother-from-a-front-view. This concept is to be distinguished from Piaget's concept of **object permanence,** which entails **remembering** an object or a person when the child is no longer in direct contact (usually visual) with the object or person. The skill of object constancy develops from the need to conserve cognitive effort in the overpopulated world of objects.

Object constancy is one of the first required skills in the ability to categorize. As the child begins to remember more objects, people, and events, information overload occurs. The ability to categorize is crucial to continued cognitive development. This grouping, or structuring, of information facilitates generalization and encourages further differentiations through attention to details [33]. Some children with learning disabilities continue to have difficulty with object constancy, categorization, and differentiation skills all their lives.

LEARNING THE SCHEMATA OF THE BODY AND ORIENTATION
The individual forms schemata, or mental pictures, of his own body; the body then becomes a stable reference point from which to view and to relate all the experiences and observed phenomena of life. Opportunities for the development of gross and fine motor skills are essential to aid the child in developing body image and spatial awareness. As the child moves, he or she begins to identify the self as a separate entity, developing a sense of individual physical potentials and relationships to other objects. While children are learning a new skill, they must consciously think about

which parts of the body to move and how to restrict movement to the critical muscle groups. The very young infant has to learn how to move hands and eyes at will. When a neonate visually fixates on an interesting object, mouth, hands, and arms will open as well as eyes as if to engulf the object.

Body schemata are continually being changed, especially during childhood. Perceptions of the self and the world change dramatically as the child successively advances from a supine position to sitting, standing, walking, running, jumping, and so forth.

DEVELOPING SPACE PERCEPTION
The mastery of this task is critical for the individual's orientation to the environment and mobility within it. Blind persons experience much difficulty mastering this task. Our spatial perception enables us to make assumptions about the world. We can, for example, judge distance by picking up cues from texture, brightness, clarity, shadows, and so forth.

The idea of space will emerge gradually—first, the space between oneself and various objects, and, later, the space between objects. The first primitive concept of space is called the "action-space concept" because the baby is aware only of the area being experienced at a particular moment. Several "spaces" exist for the infant under 4 months of age (e.g., visual space, au-

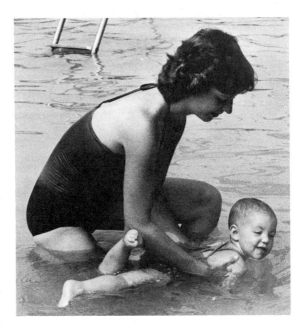

Figure 8–3. When given the opportunity, many babies are able to swim before they are able to walk.

ditory space); after that time the baby begins to cognitively map (mentally organize) various spaces into a more holistic environment or gestalt (see Piaget's sensorimotor substage III for further explanation).

Infant Tools

The quality of the early caretaker-infant relationship is critical to the maximal development of the cognitive domain [50]. Early interaction between babies and their primary caretakers is facilitated through the use of "innate" tools on the part of both the caretakers and the infants. The term **innate** is qualified in its use at this point, since it is not yet known whether the infant's tools are truly innate or are learned in utero. Nevertheless, when they are functioning optimally, the reciprocal use of these tools leads to, and reinforces, an intense, mutually satisfying relationship that facilitates the development of the cognitive domain (see Chap. 9 as well as the section on parent-infant bonding in Chap. 32).

Infants use both the senses and sensorimotor devel-

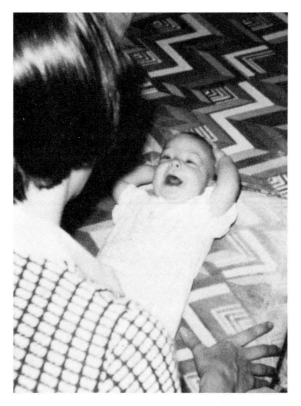

Figure 8–4. The infant learns early in life that smiling and laughing will "capture" the caretaker and prolong interaction time.

opment as tools to make social contact with others. Although infants have a variety of tools, the possession of those mentioned in the following section appears to be the most critical in facilitating a positive response from caretakers [48].

SMILING

Smiling in our culture is indicative of happiness, relaxation, and acceptance of others; thus it becomes an essential tool in positive interactions. Mothers have been telling us for years that their babies can smile from birth. Medical personnel and psychologists have hypothesized that one form of smile from the newborn is merely a "gas bubble." Research now identifies two distinct kinds of neonatal smiles that may occur as early as the seventh month of fetal life. The gas-bubble smile is accompanied by tensing of the body and grimacing, indicating that the baby has intestinal discomfort. Another more relaxed type of neonatal smiling is "eyes-closed" smiling [24]. At first the neonate tends to turn up the corners of the mouth fleetingly, with the muscles of the eyes not being used until after the first week of life. The neonate looks very content—it is this smile that new parents often interpret as a sign of approval of the caretakers. Wolff, who has painstakingly researched smiles in babies, categorizes neonatal smiling as either (1) "spontaneous" smiling, which occurs without known external causes, or (2) "elicited" smiling, which appears to be caused by external stimulation (e.g., high-pitched voices, tickling, bright lights) [61]. It must be remembered that the state of consciousness appears to affect variations of smiling responses.

The smile of the human infant has caught the attention of other researchers [55]. Many views have been offered, but not all are supported with evidence. John Bowlby, a noted child psychologist, has offered the following observations [6]:

1. The "motor" pattern of a smile is instinctive.
2. Smiles can be elicited by many types of stimuli, but, because the human organism is biased from the first, some stimuli are more effective than others.
3. Effective stimuli are initiated more by the mother figure (primary caretaker) than by anyone or anything else.
4. By the process of learning, effective stimuli become restricted to those of human origin, often the human voice and face.
5. With increased learning, smiles are elicited more promptly and more intensely by a familiar voice. It does not take the baby long to figure out that parental attention—a reinforcer to the baby—can be re-

tained through continuing to smile in the parents' presence.

Sullivan has said that by mid-infancy, the baby has learned the patterns of "postural tension" of the face that are culturally reinforced. He goes on to say that the most important of these learnings is smiling. Although facial postures and their meanings vary from culture to culture, infants soon learn that they are the rudimentary aspects of interpersonal relations. When infants later combine smiles with vocalization, they have an effective tool for social control of the environment.

Developmentally, volitional and sustained smiling is a milestone. Parents will compare their baby to others by asking, "Has your baby begun to smile yet?" Prolonged delay in the onset of social smiling in a full-term baby can indicate the need for further examination. Babies who do not demonstrate a social smile by the age of 2 months, for example, warrant a neuro-developmental examination [10]. If infant smiling is delayed, the environment in which the infant lives may need to be altered (see Chap. 9 for further information on smiling).

CRYING

All new babies cry. Even the newborn can effect a beneficial change in environment by crying. When a baby cries, all heads turn and each person (externally or internally) reaches out to shut off the cry—whether altruistically motivated to decrease the infant's distress or because the sound is an unpleasant stimulus. When the infant cries, the caretaker is stimulated to perform activities, such as holding and rocking. Almost always the crying then ceases and the caretaker is reinforced; the infant's tension is decreased and the infant also is reinforced. Gradually the infant can learn to control the environment through crying (or vocalization with greater maturation).

It takes time for novice parents to differentiate among the various types of cries that their child gives forth. When the baby is hungry, a unique pattern of crying can be observed. This pattern has been noted to develop within one-half hour after birth and with some variation, it lasts at least until 6 months of age. Wolff describes the typical hunger cry as consisting of "the cry proper (mean duration 0.6 second), followed by a brief silence (0.2 second), a short inspiratory whistle (0.1 to 0.2 second) of higher fundamental frequency than the cry proper, and another brief rest period before the next cry proper begins"[62].

Some babies have been known to introduce their "pain" cry as early as 1 to 2 days after birth. Wolff observed such a cry during the obtaining of a blood sample by heel prick [62]. Infants differ in breathing patterns during pain cries.

Many babies have their own special "anger" cry. Sometimes fatigue is the cause, and the baby needs an environment conducive to sleep. Other babies seem to get lonely and want some company; still others tend to be more irritable in nature and possess a different temperament than their peers. Some babies become quite distressed at a wet or dirty diaper and therefore voice their opinion. Many babies become upset when too warm, too cold, or when some other external factor makes them uncomfortable.

Another type of crying exists in infants: the unexplained episode of crying. It occurs in most healthy infants—not necessarily in infants of an "irritable nature"—and continues even after the caretakers have exhausted their efforts in making the environment pleasant and comforting (e.g., position change, offering a new toy or a bottle.) This type of crying, unless it becomes a pattern or occurs for extensive periods of time, does not hurt the baby. In most cases, it should be considered a healthy outlet and is just another form of cathartic exercise. It is not unusual for a baby to have 1 to 2 hours of "fussy time" daily during the early months.

Wolff found that after an infant is 5 weeks old, even a "fussy" baby may stop crying upon hearing a human voice or seeing a human face. This finding has implications for quieting a crying baby, since speaking to a mildly crying baby at this age can arrest the crying of some babies as long as they can see the face belonging to the voice. Other babies need more than this: They need a gentle, warm hand placed on their back or their chest in addition to the soothing voice. Infectious crying may also be observed in babies: When one baby starts crying, others often follow suit (see Chap. 9 for further discussion of crying).

LOOKING

The infant's ability to look directly at a face is a tool highly prized by parents. Mothers frequently say that they have not seen their baby until he or she opens the eyes and looks back at them [48]. The state 4 alertness that is present during the first hour after birth is an optimal time for mother-infant introduction. The sleepy baby who does not meet his mother until 6 or even 12 hours after delivery often does not appear interested—which can be a detriment to the relationship. An alert baby elicits adult attention.

FIXATION

Fixation, or the ability to visually zero in on an object, is a form of looking that is deemed very special by many caretakers. Since the infant shows a marked preference for the unique pattern of the human face (especially when the head is held on the same plane as the infant's), the baby's fixating on the caretaker's face can be a great thrill, both for the caretaker, who usually exclaims, "He (or she) is looking at **me**!" and for the baby, who is reinforced by the caretaker's apparent excitement. When fixating, the infant will also stop or reduce sucking, will elevate the eyebrows, and may stop other body movements. This adds to the import of the episode because all these behaviors give the baby an alert, "bright-eyed" appearance, which makes many caretakers feel that they are truly the object of the baby's affection. This kind of feedback may be critical for maintaining quality interaction between a parent and an infant.

HEARING

The infant's ability to hear is another effective tool for learning and establishing interpersonal relationships. The infant's tendency to turn the head toward the source of sound as the caretaker enters the room or speaks can be most endearing. The synchronous response of the baby's body movement to the articulation, the pitch, and the speed of the caretaker's voice [11] accounts for the comment, "He acts like he understands what I said to him!"

SELECTED REFLEXES

The **palmar grasp** and **hand-to-mouth** reflexes also endear the baby to caretakers. ("He's holding my hand." "She already knows how to suck her thumb.") Interpreting these behaviors as infant trust and intelligence, caretakers may begin to stimulate the infant further and thus augment the baby's learning.

Sucking, another reflex, is the method by which the infant receives nourishment for growth. The psychoanalytical school places high emphasis on this skill, stating that the infant equates food with the mother and that the mother in turn equates the infant's acceptance of food or feeding as an acceptance of herself. New parents (especially breast-feeding mothers) express great anxiety if the neonate nurses poorly and elation when the baby eats vigorously. These verbal expressions indicate a dual concern: that the infant may not get enough to eat, and that the infant does not like them. The infant who nurses well helps the parents to relax, to smile, and to enjoy feeding time with the baby. If the mother is breast-feeding, this relaxation aids with the "let-down" of milk—another reinforcer for good sucking.

General physical appearance should not be ignored as a tool for enhancing interaction and learning. The "cute" baby elicits more interactional behaviors from the primary caretakers and from others. The general appearance of an infant seems to elicit universal responses from adults, but sustained attention is related to the adult's perception of the infant's "cuteness" [31]. Characteristics such as rounded cheeks, pleasing coloration, fuzzy hair, and petite proportions appear to elicit a desire for adult interaction, which takes the form of touching, caressing, holding, and talking to the child—all excellent ways for the baby to begin learning about the world. Studies on variations in infant's behavior indicate that the infant's appearance influences adult expectations and can therefore result in differential treatment [1, 31]. If the infant is premature or malformed in some way, the parents may experience difficulty in establishing positive feelings toward the child, a factor that may lead to behavioral and personality disorders in later childhood [31]. Acquaintances and strangers also tend to interact more positively with the cute baby—a reinforcement to both the infant and the parents.

SIGNIFICANCE OF TOOLS

The primary caretaker (usually the mother) also possesses critical tools that facilitate caretaker-infant social and cognitive interaction (see Chap. 32 for a discussion of parental tools). As the baby uses a tool, the caretaker ideally reciprocates with a reinforcing tool that encourages the infant to repeat the behavior or to continue the interaction.

If the child's innate tools are weak or missing, it can interfere with the mother-child bond and the quality of maternal interaction with the infant [49, 50]. The quality of the home environment or the ability of the mother to draw out the "weaker" infant can change the outcome for the infant. Those infants whose developmental functioning places them at risk for continued delays will often exhibit normal functioning at 2 years of age when they are offered an appropriately stimulating home environment [50]. Early intervention programs have positive long-range results, in part because children and their parents establish early healthy patterns or forms of interaction that resist change [15].

As children learn to control a particular behavior, they identify the effect on the environment. Behaviors that produce the desired outcome are strengthened; behaviors that cannot be associated with an outcome or that produce an unpleasant or less desirable result are weakened. Infants begin to anticipate a result from their actions; thus they will kick their feet to cause the crib mobile to move, smile at mother to get her to speak, or let go of the nipple to hear the air bubbles rise in the bottle. Chapter 12 discusses the effect on child development when there is no response to the infant's smile and when there is an absence of manipulative, stimulating toys.

DEVELOPMENT OF COGNITION

Concept Formation

We structure reality and deal with the world by forming concepts. Many theorists suggest that concept formation, which includes symbolizing, categorizing, and generalizing, is characterized by the formation of a common response to several stimuli [19]. This association could be made on the basis of some arbitrary characteristic of a stimulus (e.g., if an animal meows, it must be a cat) or on the common elements possessed by several stimuli (e.g., car, bicycle, bus, and train all have wheels; therefore they can all move from one spot to another).

In 1958 D. O. Hebb, an experimental psychologist, postulated the concept of "cell assemblies" and "phase sequences." The development of cell assemblies, or the neurological building blocks of the brain, depends on adequate exposure to sensory experiences during biologically determined critical periods. Hebb maintained that the neurological building blocks remain undeveloped and the neural network unconnected if inadequate sensory experience is provided. He reported that animals reared in the dark experience marked visual disabilities, and offered this information to confirm how the lack of early experience may be related to perceptual disabilities [29].

Cognitive theorists continue to debate the maturational versus the constructionist view of early infant development [51]. In general, according to maturationist theory, the psychological structures that involve perceptual and motor skills will emerge according to maturational schedule regardless of the quality of the environment or the child's interaction with it. Piaget, however, maintained that in the first 18 months of life (or more), infants actively participate in creating or constructing their cognitive structures and developing and coordinating actions into an organized "schemata of action" (or "sensorimotor schemata"). During the latter part of the sensorimotor stage, the infant begins to categorize events (e.g., smoke from a cigarette and steam from coffee mean "hot"). This coordination of

stimuli is one form of Piaget's early "representational thought." True representational thought depends on the child's ability to represent one thing by another and originates from the sensorimotor schemata [58]. The older infant who pokes a finger into steaming hot chocolate and then observes an adult adding cold milk to it may request that cold milk be poured over a "steaming" ice cube!

Researchers have only recently begun to explore whether or not qualitative differences exist between Western thinking and that of other societies. Experiments indicate that different **means** of thought can lead to the same cognitive **ends** [27]. Children in two diverse cultures may arrive at the same answer when presented with the same problem even though they think in different languages, value divergent concepts, and have a different concept of time [27].

Piaget's Sensorimotor Stage

The young child does not use the same discriminators as those used by older children or adults to categorize their world. During Piaget's sensorimotor stage (birth to 24 months), the infant changes from operating primarily at a reflex level to consciously organizing sensorimotor activities in order to understand and to exert control on the environment. Piaget observes that the baby's activities progress from organized reflex action to trial-and-error learning and then to systematic solving of relatively simple problems. During this period of time, the baby becomes goal-oriented and attempts to devise ways to get what is wanted. This activity requires that the infant become aware of where the boundaries of the body end and where those of the world begin. This is a lot of work—biophysically, cognitively, and psychosocially—for such a young individual to master!

A brief review of Piaget's definitions and assumptions (see Appendixes B and C) may be helpful to the reader before proceeding to the following sections concerning the substages of the sensorimotor stage.

SUBSTAGE I: REFLEX ACTIVITY (BIRTH TO 1 MONTH)
Piaget says that the neonate exists in a state of complete egocentrism. This cognitive state is one in which the neonate perceives the world from a single point of view without the knowledge that any other viewpoints exist [19].

When the neonate is stimulated, the reflexes respond. When an object is put into the neonate's mouth, it is sucked; when an object is placed on the neonate's palm, it is grasped. Piaget presents no evidence that the infant in this substage can differentiate between objects; thus it would seem that most activity during this first month is assimilated, or incorporated, into a very primitive schema. Because reflexive behavior can enable the neonate to survive, it is adaptive. Piaget believes that these reflexes constitute the foundation of all subsequent sensorimotor and intellectual development, because the repetitive nature of the reflexes is the beginning of associations between an act and a sequential response.

SUBSTAGE II: PRIMARY CIRCULAR REACTIONS (1 TO 4 MONTHS)

During substage II, the early reflexes are modified as a function of experience and neurological maturation. The emphasis is on the infant's circular reactions, or a series of repetitions of sensorimotor actions. These primary circular reactions are active efforts made by the infant to reproduce a behavior that was previously achieved by chance (through random activity). A very good example of such a response is one that tends to bother many parents—thumb-sucking. Building on the reflexive sucking action, an infant may discover that inserting the thumb in the mouth brings real pleasure. So it is done again—and again. Furthermore, the baby will suck on almost anything if it provides sucking pleasure. When doing so, the baby will assimilate each object into a sucking schema.

The baby also shows an awareness of objects, or "object concept," that was not present during substage I. The baby will demonstrate this awareness by looking at the breast or feeding bottle and expressing eager behavior on its presentation. Already, the perception of more than one stimulus (both visual and olfactory) is being combined with a motor behavior. During substage II, the infant will repeat his or her own behaviors, especially if an adult mimics the baby's vocalizations, but will not imitate a novel behavior or vocalization.

SUBSTAGE III: SECONDARY CIRCULAR REACTIONS (4 TO 8 MONTHS)

During substage III, the infant's behaviors become increasingly oriented toward objects and events in the environment. Previously, the infant's behavior was directed primarily toward the self and was elicited by internal stimulation (e.g., hunger, wet diaper, fatigue). Many five-month-old babies begin to learn to "control" their environments by making use of visually directed reaching (sighting an object, reaching for it, and making contact with it)—something the infant could not accomplish neurologically until this stage.

Piaget says that actions during this period are secondary because they are "intentional," that is, the behavior is initiated to obtain results on an external object (e.g., cry to get mother). Secondary circular reactions develop new goals for motor responses that already exist. A young baby will express delight at kicking a crib mobile over and over again. In this substage, a behavior is repeated and prolonged for the response that results—grasping and holding now become shaking, banging, and pulling.

Piaget also views secondary circular reactions as leading the way to the infant's ability to classify objects (e.g., a mobile is to kick, a rattle is to shake, a teething ring is to bite). Piaget underscores how fundamental secondary circular reactions are by showing that adults, when faced with a new situation, may resort to them again (e.g., smile to attract someone's attention, or hit the side of a malfunctioning television). During substage III, the infant will imitate the behavior of others if the skill is already within the infant's repertoire.

SUBSTAGE IV: COORDINATION OF SECONDARY SCHEMATA AND THEIR APPLICATION TO NEW SITUATIONS (8 TO 12 MONTHS)

By using those responses that have been previously mastered, the infant can now solve simple problems and begins to use the responses as means to achieve ends that are not immediately attainable in a direct way. The infant will begin to use one object or action (means) to achieve a specific goal (end). An unwanted toy, for example, will be moved out of the way to reach a more desirable one. By this substage, changes have occurred in how the baby approaches the solving of a problem. Earlier, the baby would simply run through a repertoire of schemata, in any order, whether or not they were appropriate. By the end of this substage, the baby uses only those actions based on his past experiences that are likely to work. This suggests the baby possesses some form of memory.

The substage IV infant evidences the concept of **object permanence,** or the knowledge that an object exists independently of one's own actions and current perceptions. During the early part of substage IV, the goal (the desired toy) must be partly visible behind the obstacle before the infant will seek it; this restriction disappears later in substage IV. There are researchers who take issue with Piaget as to when an individual first evidences the concept of object permanence. T. G. R. Bower [5], for one, found that babies as young as 20 days appeared to know that an object still existed even when it was hidden, but short memory and attention span prevent sustained search efforts for the hidden object.

Piaget says that the baby who is 8 to 10 months old will start to search for objects that disappear. Try an experiment similar to an observation that Piaget made with one of his own children. First, hide the child's rattle under a blanket while the child is watching you do so. The baby should easily retrieve the toy by reaching under the blanket, demonstrating a knowledge that objects still exist when they disappear from view. If you refined this experiment by sequentially hiding the rattle under a pillow, you would discover that the baby's concept of object permanence is still limited because the baby will look under the original blanket. The infant at this age still does not always search for objects where they have disappeared but, rather, where they were found the last time.

The infant also shows clear signs of anticipation of events during this substage, recognizing certain signs as being associated with certain actions that follow the sign. This partially explains why the 9- or 10-month-old infant cries when seeing mother pick up her pocketbook or when another person comes to the home (interpreted by the baby as "Mother is about to leave").

Piaget says that it is during substage IV that the shape and the size of objects become stable concepts for the infant. He attributes much of this stabilization to the coordination or synthesis of perceptual experiences. This stabilization is reflected in more controlled movements; for example, the infant sees the upside-down bottle, reaches out, and turns it around into the correct position, thus judging distance and attributing a fixed shape to a permanent solid.

During this substage, for the first time the infant will show awareness that objects (besides the self) can cause activity. An 8-month old baby may laugh gleefully as the mother winds up a musical swing. When the swing begins to slow and come to a standstill, the baby may try to reach for the winding crank, realizing that the crank starts the fun all over again. During substage IV, the infant will imitate the behaviors of others if the skill is similar to skills already mastered.

SUBSTAGE V: TERTIARY CIRCULAR REACTIONS—THE DISCOVERY OF NEW MEANS THROUGH ACTIVE EXPERIMENTATION (12 TO 18 MONTHS)

During substage V, the infant continues to make accidental discoveries of pleasing activities, but instead of repeating them in exactly the same way, the infant chooses to vary them. By using this type of experimentation, the infant is actually intentionally accommodating to find new solutions to old problems. The infant at this time will also approach a new object with old familiar responses and then develop variations of the old patterns of response.

During this substage the infant will search for objects in the area of the last visible displacement. If a toy originally hidden in place A is now hidden in place B while the baby is watching, the baby searches for the toy in place B; the substage V baby does not hunt first at place A as would have been done in the previous substage. The handling of "invisible displacements," or unseen spatial displacements, does not occur until substage VI (which is considered to be well into toddlerhood in this text, see Chap. 11). In terms of cognitive development, substage VI is of special importance: Piaget says the infant's behaviors become "intelligent" because the child acquires the ability to solve new problems [43]. In other words, the child is able to manipulate events mentally before acting. The infant in substage V will physically manipulate events to test their effect but does not evidence the ability to mentally manipulate the event before it happens.

The infant at this time realizes that other objects can not only be a source of actions, but they can also affect an activity. Many infants will look to an adult in the room to fetch a remote object for them; they consciously communicate to the adult through pointing, crying, grunting, or using a word. They are now making a new use of their knowledge that other people can affect activity, too. In previous substages, the infant was learning how sensations and movements interrelate, but tended to focus on just those two entities; at this point, however, the infant is capable of noticing the relationship between objects in different spaces and the different ways that modalities can be used to obtain or send information about the objects. During substage V, the infant will atttempt to imitate novel behaviors exhibited by others in the immediate environment.

A summary of Piaget's six substages and examples of infant behavior in each substage are given in Table 8–2.

Learning

We can begin to make inferences that infants are learning almost from the minute they are born by observing their increasing repertoire of behaviors. Attention to external stimuli appears to be facilitated when affective needs are met. High levels of anxiety preclude attention to significant events or stimuli in the environment.

Table 8–2. Summary of Piaget's Sensorimotor Stage

Substage	Developmental Unit	Approximate Age	Behavioral Example
I	Exercising the ready-made sensorimotor schemata	0–1 month	Baby demonstrates neurological reflexes (e.g., rooting, sucking, swallowing) that become more useful and efficient.
II	Primary circular reactions	1–4 months	Baby repeats simple acts; may use repetitive kicking, continues hand play (e.g., fingering of an object placed in or near hand; sucking for a long period of time); may modify use of a reflex (e.g., adjusts swallow to different textures of food). Coordinates certain reflexes for more efficient use (e.g., sucking and swallowing, reaching and grasping).
III	Secondary circular reaction	4–8 months	Infant shows intentionality by repeating those acts that produce novel, pleasing, and interesting results (e.g., may repeat an action over and over again that brings laughter from caretaker, prefers to kick a musical toy instead of just a blanket). There is further coordination of efforts that have been previously unrelated (e.g., mouthing objects in environment by combining grasping and sucking). Makes brief search for an absent object.
IV	Coordination of secondary reactions (schemata) and applications to new situations	8–12 months	Infant consciously uses an action that is a means to an end (e.g., uses reaching ability to obtain many new and interesting objects); begins to solve simple problems, such as initiating an active search for an absent object.
V	Tertiary circular reactions	12–18 months	Child will show trial and error experimentation; is capable of more complex problem solving and can modify and vary movements to suit purposes; will search for a hidden object where last seen; if the child sees an object put under a cloth, will lift the cloth to find it, but if it is shifted to an adjacent cloth without the child's knowledge, will continue to look only under the first cloth.
VI	Invention of new means through mental combinations	18–24 months	Child can be seen solving "detour" problems; can predict effects from observing causes, and can also infer a cause when only the effect is seen; is able to follow an invisible displacement.

Source: Adapted with permission from M. S. Brown and M. A. Murphy, A child grows. *Pediatric Nursing*, Vol. 1, No. 3, p. 9, May/June 1975.

CRITICAL ISSUES IN THE LEARNING PROCESS

Selected studies pertaining to a child's learning process have centered on perceptual learning, observational learning, attention, and memory. Individual cognitive styles do appear to exist, but the search for special and common factors and their correlation with the learning process still continues.

Attention. Peter H. Wolff, in his study of the development of attention, identified the baby's arousal state as an important factor that influences the infant's response to stimuli (see Chap. 5). Stimuli that violate the infant's expectations, or are novel, may capture attention. The attention span in infants is variable: One baby will look at an object for several minutes, whereas another will be easily distracted. Much emphasis has been placed on studying the baby's visual abilities: visual scanning; visual fixation (choice of target, length, frequency); and the bodily accompaniments of attending to an object (demonstrated by cardiac and respiratory deceleration, pupillary dilation, and decrease in body movements). The reverse of these indicators of attention is also significant. The infant's ability to "habituate" (to become familiar with a certain stimulus and thus decrease response to it or shut it out) demonstrates three things: the infant (1) can detect changes in environment; (2) can discriminate among stimuli; and (3) appears to remember a stimulus (at least for a short period of time). There is still disagreement among researchers as to whether habituation is a form of actual learning or merely a decreased response due to fatigue of the sensory receptors [53]. Habituation is one reason why an infant can fall asleep in the midst of loudly playing older brothers and sisters, when the television is on, or in the middle of a lively ball game.

Memory. Human memory plays a major role in learning. Learning cannot occur without the retention and recall of past experience. Memory is necessary for conceptualizing, whether it serves the simplest assimilation or the most complex accommodation. An individual's conceptual system may be activated by using the observed properties of a stimulus and scanning the more extensive data stored in the memory bank for "linkages with past stored knowledge" [25]. As the memory bank becomes filled with more data, these associations become more complex.

Obviously, the young infant has limited use of the scanning mechanism of the memory bank. The infant also possesses a relatively small amount of data. It has been stressed that those experiences the young infant does have are not yet tied together through a symbol system, such as language. Language helps to "cluster memories together so they can be retrieved as a single bundle, rather than one at a time"[25].

Elkind stresses that "memory of previous experiences affects current behavior" [14]. This statement applies to infants as well as to older persons, although the question of when memory becomes effectively operative is still undecided. Memory plays an important role in the acquisition of object permanence.

It is helpful to distinguish two different forms of memory. Elkind states that the most elementary type of memory (and therefore the most prominent in infancy and early childhood) is called sensorimotor memory. This involves, as one might expect after having read Piaget's theory, the retention of sensorimotor coordinations that are learned as the individual adapts to the immediate environment. It is this type of learning that includes the retention of motor coordinations practiced in infancy and early childhood (e.g., swimming, dancing). The memory traces left by such sensorimotor activities facilitate relearning of the same unpracticed coordinations years later. When a person gives directions, the eyes are frequently closed to picture the route, the body position is redirected, the arms are used to indicate turns, and so forth; this represents adult functioning at a sensorimotor level.

"Representative memory," or memory involving the retention of certain means-end relationships, makes its appearance in midinfancy. An excellent example of this type of memory is demonstrated when the infant seeks an object that is hidden from view. An adult may see a flower or a unique color or hear a song that is reminiscent of an earlier event; an object or symbol is used to represent a part of an earlier experience. Sensorimotor and representative memory develop more fully through experience and maturation of cognitive structures.

ASSESSMENT OF DEVELOPMENTAL LEVELS

Some tests have been devised that lean heavily on the work of Arnold Gesell, and his original Gesell Developmental Schedules are still widely used. These schedules include an infant assessment tool, which evaluates the child from 4 weeks to 1 year of age in four areas: motor, adaptive, language, and personal-social. Information is obtained through the observer's noting the baby's response to the kit materials (e.g., does the baby merely stare at the bottle and pellet or does the baby attempt to do something with them?), as well as through reports from the infant's mother about what her baby usually does at home.

A raw score is calculated and is then converted into a percentile for all four areas of development tested. A fifth, overall score is called the **developmental quotient** (DQ). The term "developmental quotient" is used to distinguish this evaluation from the **intelligence quotient** (IQ), which measures a different type of intellectual behavior in older children and adults. DQ and IQ are two separate items and should not be confused with each other. A more detailed discussion of IQ is found in Chapter 23.

The Bayley Scale of Infant Development is designed to evaluate children between the ages of 6 months and 30 months in three areas: mental, psychomotor, and behavioral development. They are composed of many tasks that are similar to the pioneer work of Gesell. Several factors are tested: postural development, motor development, perception, attention span to objects and humans, language, object manipulation, understanding commands, and problem solving. The Bayley Scale provides a raw score, which is converted to an estimated mental age. The Bayley Scale of Infant Development is standardized for all sociocultural levels existing in the United States.

Subscribing to the notion that all behavior has both an affective and a cognitive aspect, Uzgiris and Hunt have developed a novel approach to the assessment of psychological development in infants up to the age of 18 months. Greatly influenced by Piaget, these researchers devised scales that permit ways of comparing the levels of cognitive organization achieved by different infants, and a way of determining the influence of various combinations of environmental circumstances on early development [56].

One of the most widely used screening tests for assessing a young child's development is the Denver Developmental Screening Test (DDST) (see Figure 8–5). The test is divided into four components that screen personal-social, fine motor-adaptive, language, and gross motor skills. It is applicable for children from birth through 6 years of age. On the score sheet, each task to be tested is represented by a horizontal bar; various points on these bars represent the ages at which 25, 50, 75, and 90 percent of children master the task.

An abbreviated form of the DDST was devised in 1979 for those practitioners who wanted to save time and not expose the young child to any more testing than necessary [23]. If all items are passed, the child receives no further testing at that time. However, if one or more items are failed or refused, the full, nonabbreviated DDST is administered.

In 1981 Frankenburg et al. revised the still much used DDST [23]. Both the original DDST and this revised version (DDST-R) have been subjected to several reliability and validity tests and have been found to yield results that correlate with psychometric tests, such as the Cattell Infant Intelligence Scale and the Revised Bayley Infant Scale. One weakness of the DDST testing is its limitations in terms of predictive validity with lower socioeconomic groups.

A person who wants to use any of the DDST testing should be adequately trained and checked for reliability before beginning to administer a test routinely. (DDST forms and instruction manuals are available from LADOCA Publishing Foundation, East 51st Ave. and Lincoln St., Denver, CO 80216.) Any improvising on the examiner's part will invalidate the test (for example, if the baby had difficulty picking up the block, the observer should not pick up the block and place it in the child's hand!). It is important for the child's parents to understand before the test begins that the DDST is not an IQ test, but rather, a developmental screening device used to estimate the child's level of maturation in the use of language, body, and selected social activities, and also used to identify areas needing an indepth assessment.

Many other assessment tools exist for developmental evaluation of individual children. Their major value is in the early detection of developmental delays, for the development of appropriate habilitation plans. Although the usefulness of screening tests should be respected, it is important to remember their limitations. Once a lag is suggested by the testing, arrangements should be made for additional, more specific examination and consultation for the individual child (and perhaps the family).

MAXIMIZING THE COGNITIVE POTENTIAL OF THE INFANT

How important is "good mothering" or "good parenting" in the development of a child's intelligence? What helps (or hinders) a child to develop full learning potential? Questions such as these led to an extensive research project initiated by psychologist Burton L. White in 1965. The research method of his Harvard Preschool Project is described in Chapter 14, but the results of this study merit emphasis here: The period in a child's life that is most decisive for the development of intellectual potentials appears to be the time from birth to 1½ years of age [46]. This conclusion is not meant to imply that stimulation and interaction after this period are insignificant; what it does emphasize is that the attributes necessary for effective later learning are established before the child is a toddler and are very strongly influenced by infant-caretaker interaction.

Infant Stimulation

Crucial to a baby's successful learning, as well as ultimately successful living, is a climate in which the baby will receive stimulation and opportunity to grow. Such a climate is greatly aided by a setting in which the baby feels loved and appreciated. Many books are available that discuss infant stimulation and child-rearing. Caretakers should use caution in trying to apply all that they read from such sources. Although environments that are devoid of problems to solve reduce the interest to do so in the infant, environments in which situations are too difficult for the infant precipitate frustration. A professional person who is familiar with the individual baby and the family is the best resource in assessing the most effective ways to maximize the baby's cognitive potential. We especially recommend Burton L. White's *The First Three Years of Life* [60] to the interested reader. Dr. White divides the first 36 months into seven successive development stages. For each of these phases, he describes characteristic biophysical, socioaffective, and cognitive developments that caretakers should be aware of in their children. He then includes a list of guidelines concerning child-rearing practices and strategies. Dr. White even suggests toys and other equipment that will help the young child to grow holistically.

The goals of infant stimulation programs should be based on two major assumptions: (1) that services to enhance a child's development should be available as early in the child's life as possible, and (2) that services to caretakers should enable them to guide their chil-

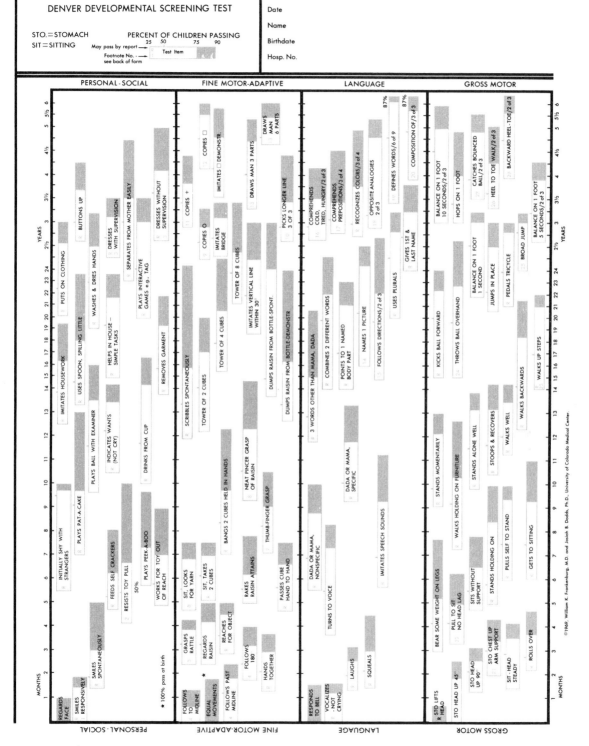

Figure 8–5. The Denver Developmental Screening Test (DDST). (Courtesy W. K. Frankenburg, M. D., and J. B. Dodds, Ph.D., University of Colorado Medical Center, 1969.)

1. Try to get child to smile by smiling, talking or waving to him. Do not touch him.
2. When child is playing with toy, pull it away from him. Pass if he resists.
3. Child does not have to be able to tie shoes or button in the back.
4. Move yarn slowly in an arc from one side to the other, about 6" above child's face.
   Pass if eyes follow 90° to midline. (Past midline; 180°)
5. Pass if child grasps rattle when it is touched to the backs or tips of fingers.
6. Pass if child continues to look where yarn disappeared or tries to see where it went. Yarn
   should be dropped quickly from sight from tester's hand without arm movement.
7. Pass if child picks up raisin with any part of thumb and a finger.
8. Pass if child picks up raisin with the ends of thumb and index finger using an over hand
   approach.

      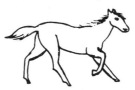

9. Pass any enclosed form. Fail continuous round motions.

10. Which line is longer? (Not bigger.) Turn paper upside down and repeat. (3/3 or 5/6)

11. Pass any crossing lines.

12. Have child copy first. If failed, demonstrate

When giving items 9, 11 and 12, do not name the forms. Do not demonstrate 9 and 11.

13. When scoring, each pair (2 arms, 2 legs, etc.) counts as one part.
14. Point to picture and have child name it. (No credit is given for sounds only.)

   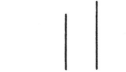   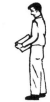

15. Tell child to: Give block to Mommie; put block on table; put block on floor. Pass 2 of 3.
    (Do not help child by pointing, moving head or eyes.)
16. Ask child: What do you do when you are cold? ..hungry? ..tired? Pass 2 of 3.
17. Tell child to: Put block on table; under table; in front of chair, behind chair.
    Pass 3 of 4. (Do not help child by pointing, moving head or eyes.)
18. Ask child: If fire is hot, ice is ?; Mother is a woman, Dad is a ?; a horse is big, a
    mouse is ?. Pass 2 of 3.
19. Ask child: What is a ball? ..lake? ..desk? ..house? ..banana? ..curtain? ..ceiling?
    ..hedge? ..pavement? Pass if defined in terms of use, shape, what it is made of or general
    category (such as banana is fruit, not just yellow). Pass 6 of 9.
20. Ask child: What is a spoon made of? ..a shoe made of? ..a door made of? (No other objects
    may be substituted.) Pass 3 of 3.
21. When placed on stomach, child lifts chest off table with support of forearms and/or hands.
22. When child is on back, grasp his hands and pull him to sitting. Pass if head does not hang back.
23. Child may use wall or rail only, not person. May not crawl.
24. Child must throw ball overhand 3 feet to within arm's reach of tester.
25. Child must perform standing broad jump over width of test sheet. (8-1/2 inches)
26. Tell child to walk forward, ⚬⚬⚬⚬➝ heel within 1 inch of toe.
    Tester may demonstrate. Child must walk 4 consecutive steps, 2 out of 3 trials.
27. Bounce ball to child who should stand 3 feet away from tester. Child must catch ball with
    hands, not arms, 2 out of 3 trials.
28. Tell child to walk backward, ⬅⚬⚬⚬⚬ toe within 1 inch of heel.
    Tester may demonstrate. Child must walk 4 consecutive steps, 2 out of 3 trials.

DATE AND BEHAVIORAL OBSERVATIONS (how child feels at time of test, relation to tester, attention
span, verbal behavior, self-confidence, etc,):

Figure 8–6. The DDST score sheet offers simple guidelines on how to administer portions of the assessment. (Courtesy
W. K. Frankenburg, M. D., and J. B. Dodds, Ph.D., University of Colorado Medical Center, 1969.)

dren's growth effectively. Many enjoyable interactions (for both baby and caretaker) have been suggested by these programs. For example, since 2-month-old babies like to listen to musical sounds, watch moving objects, and smile, the caretaker should give the baby opportunities to watch mobiles, listen to music, and interact with smiling adults. Since 5-month-olds like to shake, feel, and bang things, sit with support, and roll over, caretakers are advised to give the infant rattles and other infant toys; to encourage sitting with support; and to provide opportunities to explore new textures. Some babies may begin to enjoy "pat-a-cake." These activities, in addition to many others, aid the infant in mentally coordinating different sensory impressions of the biophysical and socioaffective world.

Safety

Regardless of how much cognitive prowess we attribute to the infant, we must be constantly aware of the infant's need to be placed in a safe environment. The infant is not capable of self-discipline or predicting outcomes in a potentially dangerous situation. The adult must think for the baby, who still lacks experience, memory, and problem-solving skills.

Accidents are a principal cause of injury and death to infants. Since the newborn is incapable of extensive head lifting or turning from one side to the other, many caretakers are unconcerned with safety precautions during this time. However, even a newborn placed on the abdomen on a particular spot in a crib can be found

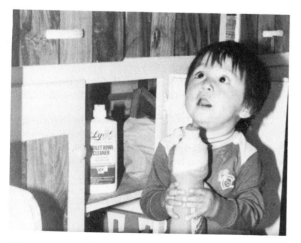

Figure 8–7. An increasing repertoire of motor skills, an insatiable curiosity, and a lack of self-discipline make it imperative that poisons, electrical sockets, and other potentially harmful items are made inaccessible by parents and caretakers.

minutes later in a different location. A newborn can roll and fall from an unguarded table, a bed, or a couch. It is therefore of paramount importance that safety precautions be instituted immediately after birth. The use of an infant car seat—from birth—is now mandatory in many states. Consistent use will establish an early pattern for the child of being restrained while riding in a vehicle and will make it easier later to restrain an active toddler or preschooler.

The 4-month-old baby may attempt to reach out for things and practice palmar grasp. Several safety implications should be apparent from an awareness of this developmental milestone. The infant should not be placed close to potentially dangerous heat sources, especially shiny, bright (but hot) water faucets or anything with a flame. Realizing that the young infant will try to place almost anything into the mouth should be a reminder to keep small items, diaper pins, sharp-edged objects, deadly plants, and other toxic or inhalable materials away from the infant's "action space." As the baby becomes more mobile, opportunities to explore (and to get into danger) increase. The knowledge of what the baby can do today and the anticipation of what might possibly be attempted tomorrow are important aspects of baby-proofing an environment. The infant has the biophysical skill to perform activities that experience and cognitive reasoning processes cannot as yet warn the child are unsafe.

The infant can begin to learn the fundamentals of accident prevention by meaningful interaction; this can be accomplished by becoming accustomed to the safety measures implemented by the caretaker. The baby will soon learn that the caretaker is displeased when a behavior is demonstrated that may lead to harm. Many helpful pamphlets and supplementary literature are provided free of cost by the U.S. Consumer Product Safety Commission (Washington, DC 20207). Local chapters of the American Red Cross are involved in child safety programs. The Shriners' Burns Institute, 51 Blossom St., Boston, MA 02114, has excellent resources on fire and burn prevention. Health professionals and county extension agencies are also active in suggesting safety tips.

CONCLUSION

Those who are involved in an intimate, long-time relationship with one or more children become acutely aware of how much information we as adults take for granted. These little ones have a lot to learn in a very short period of time. As we begin to understand both how and what babies know about their world, we can

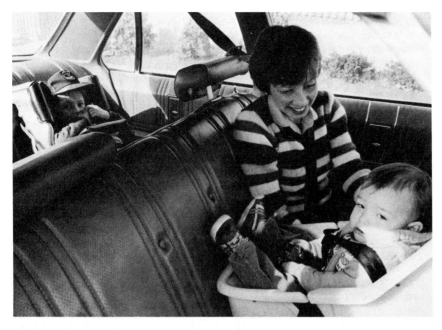

Figure 8–8. Safety is an integral part of maintaining biological integrity. Establishing an attitude of safety early in life can foster maximization of potentials.

aid them in coping with, and learning from, that world. At this point, the keys to maximizing the potentials of an infant appear to be: (1) a warm, secure caretaker relationship that frees the child to attend to external stimuli; (2) adequate sensory stimulation, to enable the child to develop neural networks, appreciation of various perceptual modalities, or motor meaning of events; (3) a sensitive, responsive environment and persons who can help the child to experience control of some events; and (4) a sufficient consistency of experiences to allow the child to see relationships and to predict the outcome of his or her own behaviors as well as the behaviors of others.

REFERENCES

1. Adams, G. R. Physical attractiveness research: Toward a developmental social psychology of beauty. *Hum. Dev.* 20:217, 1977.
2. Ainsworth, M. D. S. Object relations, dependency, and attachment: A theoretical review of the infant-mother relationship. *Child Dev.* 40(4):969, 1969.
3. Bellam, G. Personal communication, 1972.
4. Bower, T. G. R. Slant perception and shape constancy in infants. *Science* 151:832, 1966.
5. Bower, T. G. R. The object in the world of the infant. *Sci. Amer.* 225:30, 1971.
6. Bowlby, J. *Attachment and Loss, Vol. 1: Attachment.* New York: Basic Books, 1969.
7. Brazelton, T. B. Neonatal Behavioral Assessment Scale. *Clinics in Developmental Medicine,* No. 50. Philadephia: Lippincott, 1973.
8. Bridger, W. H. Sensory habituation and discrimination in the human neonate. *Am. J. Psychiatry* 117:991, 1961.
9. Campos, J. J., Langer, A., and Krowitz, A. Cardiac responses on the visual cliff in prelocomotor human infants. *Science* 170:196, 1970.
10. Capute, A. J., and Biehl, R. F. Functional developmental evaluation: Prerequisite to habilitation. *Pediatr. Clin. North Am.* 20(1):3, 1973.
11. Condon, W. S., and Sander, L. W. Neonatal movement is synchronized with adult speech: Interactional participation in language acquisition. *Science* 183:99, 1974.
12. Cratty, B. J. *Perceptual and Motor Development in Infants and Children* (2nd ed.). Englewood Cliffs, NJ: Prentice-Hall, 1979.
13. Eisenberg, R. B. The organization of auditory behavior. *J. Speech Hear. Res.* 13:461, 1970.
14. Elkind, D. Cognition in Infancy and Early Childhood. In Y. Brackbill (Ed.), *Infancy and Early Childhood: A Handbook and Guide to Human Development.* New York: Free Press, 1967.
15. Elkind, D. Cognitive Frames and Family Interactions. In

V. C. Vaughan and T. B. Brazelton (Eds.), *The Family—Can It Be Saved?* Chicago: Year Book, 1976.

16. Escalona, S. Emotional Development in the First Year of Life. In M. J. E. Senn (Ed.), *Problems of Infancy and Childhood.* New York: Josiah Macy, Jr. Foundation, 1953.

17. Fantz, R. L. Pattern vision in young infants. *Psychol. Records* 8:43, 1958.

18. Feetham, S. L. Acute and chronic pain in maternal-child health. *Matern. Child Nurs. J.* 9(4):249, 1984.

19. Flavell, J. H. Concept Development. In P. H. Mussen (Ed.), *Carmichael's Manual of Child Psychology* (3rd ed.). Vol. 1. New York: Wiley, 1970.

20. Flavell, J. H., and Ross, L. (Eds.). *Social Cognitive Development: Frontiers and Possible Futures.* Cambridge: Cambridge University Press, 1981.

21. Forgus, R. H. *Perception: A Cognitive-Stage Approach* (2nd ed.). New York: McGraw-Hill, 1976.

22. Frankenburg, W. K., Kamp, B. W., and Van Natta, P. A. Validity of the Denver Developmental Screening Test. *Child Dev.* 42:475, 1971.

23. Frankenburg, W. K., et al. The newly abbreviated and revised Denver Developmental Screening Test. *J. Pediatr.* 99:995, 1981.

24. Freidman, S., and Vietze, P. The competent infant. *Peabody J. Educ.* 49:314, 1972.

25. Gallagher, J. J. Perception. In J. J. Gallagher (Ed.), *The Application of Child Development Research to Exceptional Children.* Reston, VA: Council for Exceptional Children, 1975.

26. Gibson, E. J., and Walk, R. D. The visual cliff. *Sci. Am.* 202:64, 1960.

27. Greenfield, P. M. On Culture and Conservation. In J. S. Bruner, et al., *Studies in Cognitive Growth: A Collaboration at the Center for Cognitive Studies.* New York: Wiley, 1966.

28. Haith, N. M. The response of the human newborn to visual movement. *J. Child Psychol. Psychiatry* 3:234, 1966.

29. Hebb, D. O. The motivation effects of exteroceptive stimulation. *Am. Psychol.* 13:109, 1958.

30. Hershenson, M. Visual discrimination in the human newborn. *J. Comp. Physiol. Psychol.* 58:270, 1964.

31. Hildebrandt, K. A., and Fitzgerald, H. E. The infant's physical attractiveness: Its effect on bonding and attachment. *Infant Mental Health Journal* 4:3, 1983.

32. Hill, V., and Eriks, J. Turn-Taking in the Caregiver-Infant Interaction System. In *Nursing Child Assessment Training Learning Resource Manual.* Seattle, WA: 1979.

33. Hupp, S. C., and Mervis, C. B. Acquisition of basic object categories by severely handicapped children. *Child Dev.* 53:760, 1982.

34. Johnson, O. G., and Bommarito, J. W. *Test and Measurements in Child Development: A Handbook.* San Francisco: Jossey-Bass, 1976.

35. Kaye, K. *The Mental and Social Life of Babies: How Parents Create Persons.* Chicago: University of Chicago Press, 1982.

36. Martin, W. E. Rediscovering the Mind of the Child, A Significant Trend in Research in Child Development. In I. B. Weiner and D. Elkind (Comp.), *Readings in Child Development.* New York: Wiley, 1972.

37. McGraw, M. B. *The Neuro-Muscular Maturation of the Human Infant.* New York: Hafner, 1969.

38. McGuire, L., and Dizard, S. Managing pain in the young patient. *Nursing '82,* 12(8):54, 1982.

39. Montagu, A. *The Direction of Human Development* (New and rev. ed.). New York: Hawthorn Books, 1970.

40. Munsinger, H. *Fundamentals of Child Development* (2nd ed.). New York: Holt, Rinehart & Winston, 1975.

41. Mussen, P. H., Conger, J. J., and Kagan, J. *Child Development and Personality* (6th ed.). New York: Harper & Row, 1984.

42. Out of the minds of babes. *Family Health/Today's Health* 8(11):27, 1976.

43. Piaget, J. *The Origins of Intelligence in Children.* Translated by M. Cook. New York: International Universities Press, 1952.

44. Piaget, J. *The Language and Thought of the Child.* Translated by M. Gabain. New York: Meridian Books, 1969.

45. Piaget, J., and Inhelder, B. *The Psychology of the Child.* Translated by H. Weaver. New York: Basic Books, 1969.

46. Pines, M. A child's mind is shaped before age 2. *Life* 71(25):63, 1971.

47. Scarr, S., and Salapatek, P. Patterns of fear development during infancy. *Merrill-Palmer Q.* 16:53, 1970.

48. Schuster, C. S. Relationship of Neonatal Characteristics to Specific Learning Disabilities and Behavioral Disorders of Early Childhood. Unpublished paper, 1977.

49. Schuster, C. S. The Relationship of Prenatal and Perinatal Factors to the Mother's Perception of Her One-Month-Old Infant. Unpublished doctoral dissertation, The Ohio State University, 1981.

50. Siegel, L. S. Infant tests as predictors of cognitive and language development at two years. *Child Dev.* 52:545, 1981.

51. Simillie, D. Rethinking Piaget's theory of infancy. *Hum. Dev.* 25:282, 1982.

52. Starkey, D. The origins of concept formation: Object sorting and object preference in early infancy. *Child Dev.* 52:489, 1981.

53. Stevenson, H. W. *Children's Learning.* New York: Appleton-Century-Crofts, 1972.

54. Sze, W. C. *Human Life Cycle.* New York: Jason Aronson, 1975.

55. Trotter, R. J. Baby face. *Psychology Today* 17(8):14, 1983.

56. Uzgiris, I. C., and Hunt, J. M. *Assessment in Infancy: Ordinal Scales of Psychological Development.* Urbana, IL: University of Illinois Press, 1975.

57. Valadian, I., and Porter, D. *Physical Growth and Development: From Conception to Maturity.* Boston: Little, Brown, 1977.

58. Wadsworth, B. J. *Piaget's Theory of Cognitive Development: An Introduction for Students of Psychology and Education.* New York: David McKay, 1971.

59. Watson, J. S.   Smiling, Cooing and "The Game." In L. J. Stone, H. T. Smith, and L. B. Murphy (Eds.), *The Competent Infant; Research and Commentary.* New York: Basic Books, 1973.

60. White, B. L.   *The First Three Years of Life.* Englewood Cliffs, NJ: Prentice-Hall, 1975.

61. Wolff, P. H.   Observations on the Early Development of Smiling. In B. M. Foss (Ed.), *Determinants of Infant Behaviour, IV.* New York: Wiley, 1963.

62. Wolff, P. H.   The Natural History of Crying and Other Vocalizations in Early Infancy. In L. J. Stone, H. T. Smith, and L. B. Murphy (Eds.), *The Competent Infant; Research and Commentary.* New York: Basic Books, 1973.

9
Psychosocial Development during Infancy

Clara S. Schuster and Shirley S. Ashburn

We are molded and remolded by those who have loved us; and though the love may pass, we are nevertheless their work, for good or ill.

—François Mauriac

The psychosocial realm (a combination of the affective and social domains) includes the intrapersonal and interpersonal responses of an individual to external events. It includes how one feels about oneself and subsequently how one relates to others. **Personality,** a term frequently used synonymously with the psychosocial realm, may be defined as "the integrated totality of the characteristic habits, attitudes, and ideas of the individual and the distinctive organization of his responses to social stimuli" [61].

Most theories of development contend that the early mother-child relationship is pivotal to the quality of social relationships in later life. According to learning theory, any interaction, whether positive or negative, will influence the psychosocial development of an individual. Other theories are based on observation of adult pathologies that seemed to have the common component of a poor mother-child relationship in earlier years.

Inadequate attention to the affective and social domains have serious consequences. The biophysically normal infant who suffers even minor deprivation may experience negative effects in the development of cognitive, biophysical, and social potentials.

King Frederick II, a thirteenth-century monarch of Sicily, wanted to know which language children would speak if they were never spoken to during early childhood [53]. He ordered a group of foster mothers and nurses to feed and bathe their charges, but stipulated that they were never to communicate verbally or to play with the infants. All the children died. Consequently, the king's question was never resolved. Some stimulus necessary to sustain life was missing.

From the first minute of life, each infant is uniquely individual in response to the environment. The infant is an active and reactive participant in the social process, sometimes the recipient of an interaction and at other times the initiator. Individual differences in infant activity level and temperament can be observed at birth, before environmental factors have had time to produce any effect [11, 16, 17]. These differences elicit qualitatively and quantitatively different responses from the parents. The baby's ability to accept and to use comforting to control his state will frequently influence the mood and quality of care administered by the baby's principal caregiver. The quality, quantity, and consistency of the caregiver's reactions to the baby's crying will in turn help to mold their relationship and will affect in part the way the baby will interact in social environments [5, 55, 58].

The biological mother of the child may not always assume the traditional mothering role; therefore, the terms **mother, parent, caregiver,** and **caretaker** are used interchangeably to indicate the primary person whose actions and interactions are associated with the nurturing role.

THE PROCESS OF ATTACHMENT

For centuries artists have attempted to capture on canvas the essence of the mother-infant relationship. During the past century, psychologists and social scientists have attempted to describe and to explain this relationship through theory and research. **Attachment,** a term coined by Bowlby in 1958, refers to the emotional ties one person (in this case the infant) has for another person or persons, a pet, or even objects [55]. This focused relationship develops over time while the child experiences repeated contacts with a person(s). **Attachment behaviors** are those activities that serve to obtain or to maintain contact or proximity with the attachment object (e.g., visual tracking, grasping, reaching, smiling, babbling, clinging, crying).

The concept of bonding implies a selective attachment [18] that persists over time even during periods of absence. This selective attachment is generally present by 6 months [23, 55]. Bonding gives the child a security base, which at first provides a source of strength and identity, and later, a point of detachment or separation. It is a paradox of development that the most securely attached child finds it easiest to move away from the attachment object. Most infants form multiple attachments. Although attachments are similar in quality, they differ in intensity and are not freely interchangeable [55]. When the child is under stress, a hierarchy of relationships appears as the child seeks comfort and security from the person nearest the top of this pyramid.

An adequate attachment of the child to the caregiver is seen as the cornerstone of all future development because early attachment facilitates:

1. Differentiation between self and others
2. Exploration of the environment
3. Development of a conscience
4. Attainment of cognitive potentials
5. Development of perceptual skills
6. Development of logical thinking
7. Coping with stress and frustration
8. Self-reliance
9. Reduction of fear and anxiety
10. Dissipation of jealousies and rivalries
11. Development of autonomy
12. Attainment of self-confidence
13. Development of self-acceptance
14. Development of later social and emotional relationships

Sensitive Period

"Imprinting," a concept of attachment that has originated from animal research, occurs only during the critical period following birth. The animal infant (such as a duck or goat) attaches to, and follows, a selected object, usually its mother. In one experiment, Konrad Lorenz [37] became the attachment object of incubator-hatched geese who saw him before seeing an avian mother. The little birds followed him about with great vigor. They ran toward Lorenz for comfort when frightened (even if their biological mother was present). As the goslings matured, they demonstrated courting behaviors toward him. No evidence supports the phenomenon of imprinting in humans. However, infants more than 5 months of age who change caretakers (e.g., due to maternal illness, return to work, or adoption) evidence extreme stress [23, 55]. This behavior indicates that selective attachment has been established during the first 6 months of life. Even though disruption of a relationship is traumatic, once a child has learned to trust and attach to one person, it is easier to bond to a second person. Children who have never attached to another person experience great difficulty with this process [23, 55].

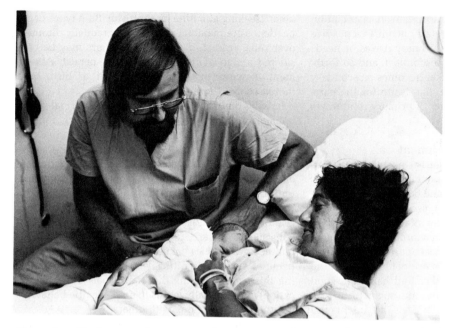

Figure 9–1. The best start for a neonate is two parents who genuinely care. (Courtesy of the Department of Medical Photography, Children's Hospital, Buffalo, N.Y.)

Need Satisfaction

Early theories emphasized physiological need satiation as the basis for the infant's development of attachment to, and meaningful relationships with, others. In 1958 Harry and Margaret Harlow proved that there is more to attachment behavior than just being fed adequately [27]. They raised infant monkeys in cages with two very different surrogate mothers. One "mother" was covered with soft terry cloth; the other was composed of hard wire mesh and had a feeding apparatus. The baby monkeys did not spend much time with the wire surrogate mother that fed them but clung to the cloth surrogate that did not feed them at all. The "need theory" was shattered: The provision of food was not the basis for attachment; comforting potential was much stronger.

When the infant monkeys in Harlow's experiment reached adulthood, they demonstrated marked social difficulties and sexual maladjustment [27]. Research with well-cared-for institutionalized children who experienced as many as 50 to 80 caretakers indicates that inadequate bonding experiences in infancy lead to excessive attention-seeking and indiscriminate friendliness by 4 years of age [70] and to impaired relationships with peers and adults during school years [71]. Inadequate, inconsistent, or nonresponsive attachment objects in infancy prevent adequate socialization.

Theories of Attachment

Human infants become attached to a primary caretaker who provides a source of consistent, intimate interaction. Several theorists offer explanations of the process. Freud based his theory of attachment on instinctual drives, viewing the infant as a narcissistic organism who attaches to those perceived as persons who can reduce one's tensions and meet one's needs (object relationship).

Mary Ainsworth indicates that attachment is influenced by the continuous, sensitive feedback between infant and caretaker. She notes that the frequency and intensity of attachment behavior (e.g., clinging, crying when mother leaves) decreases as the infant increases in ability to use verbal language [1, 2].

Jacob Gewirtz, a behavioral learning theorist, suggests that differential reinforcement leads to attachment [24, 25]. He suggests that attachment is a specific pattern of response that evolves as a result of the infant and caretaker learning to exert control over one another's behavior, each focusing energies toward the other (a positive stimulus and reinforcer). However, even in the face of severe maltreatment and severe punishment, attachment behaviors may be exhibited by infants and young children [55].

Robert Sears, a developmental learning theorist, equates attachment with dependence. He calls attachment a "secondary drive," arising from association with primary drives. The caretaker acquires a positive value as he or she meets the primary drives or needs of the infant: hunger, thirst, discomfort, and so forth. At the same time, the caretaker becomes a secondary general reinforcer; therefore, the desire for the caretaker's nearness as a dispenser of primary reinforcers results in attachment [41].

Bowlby's Theory of Attachment

John Bowlby, a child psychiatrist, postulates that attachment is the result of interaction between adaptive predispositions in the infant and behaviors of the caretaker. He believes that certain types of stimulation elicit certain types of behavior in the infant, and that infant behaviors elicit particular behaviors in the caretaker. For example, a mother may speak more frequently and lovingly to a baby who smiles or babbles in response to her efforts. Since the mother and baby feel good about this, they repeat the act and begin to form a meaningful relationship. Bowlby feels that infants use sucking, clinging, following, crying, and smiling to elicit parental caretaking and attachment behaviors. In contrast with some theorists, he states that feeding plays only a minor role in the development of attachment [10]. Sensitive social reciprocity is a more critical component.

Bowlby strongly differentiates between the terms **dependence** and **attachment,** which are considered synonymous by some theorists. He states that dependence refers to the extent to which one individual relies on another for existence. Dependent behaviors may be exhibited toward anyone. Two categories are identified: instrumental (seeking help or assistance) and emotional (seeking attention or approval). Both types of dependence are maximal at birth and gradually diminish over time. In fact, dependent behaviors may be considered a sign of immaturity if they persist. Attachment, however, is altogether absent at birth, and increases over time.

Bowlby discusses four phases in the normal development of attachment that have overlapping boundaries. He labels phase one as "orientation and signals without discrimination of figure." He believes that the infant's ability to discriminate one person from another either is absent or is extremely limited from birth until the age of 2 or 3 months (note that more recent research by Brazelton indicates that this skill is present at 2 or 3 weeks [12]). Unfavorable conditions (e.g., inconsistency of care, neglect, abuse) may extend this phase. Bowlby does acknowledge that the baby is capable of eliciting significant responses in others during this time (by using the infant tools of communication) and gradually learns to emit specific behaviors to prolong interactions with others.

The infant first begins nonselective social smiling between 2 and 8 weeks. This response is characteristically elicited by both stationary and moving visual stimuli (even the pendulum on a clock). Other stimuli (e.g., auditory, tactile) may also be used in conjunction with visual stimuli to elicit the smile. Smiling occurs whether the stimulating face is familiar or unfamiliar.

During phase two (3 to 6 months), "orientation and signals directed towards one or more discriminated figures," the infant begins to behave toward the mother figure "in more marked fashion" than toward others. However, Brazelton has observed that infants begin to respond discriminately to mother versus father versus stranger by 3 weeks of age [12]. During this phase, the various components of full facial smiling become integrated. Massive, total body activity also emerges around this age.

Selective social smiling usually emerges before 20 weeks and overlaps with its nonselective predecessor. Between 3 and 5 months, the securely attached infant will visually explore the face of a stranger and then visually "check" the parent's face, as if comparing and analyzing the similarities and differences between the two. This visual-checking behavior is usually continued during the first 18 to 24 months. Selective social smiling coincides with the baby's increasing fear of, or caution with, strangers and anxiety when separated from primary caretakers. At approximately five months, many babies display sobriety or cry at a stranger's friendly smile. Some babies will deliberately avoid eye contact with strangers.

Table 9–1. Bowlby's View of Attachment versus Dependency

Factor	Attachment	Dependency
Specificity	1 person	Anyone
Duration	Over time	Transient
Developmental level	All ages	Immature only
Affect	Strong, intrinsic passion	Minimal or no emotional involvement
Proximity-seeking	Focused toward specific person	Contact with anyone who can meet/relieve need
Acquisition	Learned over time	Unlearned Maximal at birth; should diminish over time

During Bowlby's third phase of attachment formation (7 to 36 months), "maintenance of proximity to a discriminated figure by means of locomotion as well as signals," the infant demonstrates extreme discrimination between the mother figure and others. The infant tends to become less friendly to others, except for a select few, and often demands constant contact with, or close proximity to, the mother figure—a situation some mothers find difficult while fulfilling their other responsibilities. Some infants who have had little contact with a stable mother figure may not begin this phase until after 12 months of age.

Scary situations (e.g., encountering Halloween masks) and alterations of the human face (e.g., sunglasses or beard) usually will not evoke crying in an infant until the end of the sixth month. If a **familiar** face becomes altered, however, crying may occur in an even younger baby. One 4-month-old baby girl began to cry in terror when she first saw her mother wearing a turban towel wrapped around her just-washed hair. However, not all distortions of the familiar face will provoke an adverse response. For instance, the removal of glasses from the mother's face when the baby is accustomed to seeing her with glasses might provoke crying, but the addition of glasses to a mother's face that is usually seen without glasses may not evoke crying [76].

Around the first birthday, the child begins to understand that the mother figure is an independent person who tends to behave in predictable ways. The child's view of the world becomes more realistic, more sophisticated, and potentially more flexible. This is the beginning of Bowlby's fourth phase, called "formation of a goal-directed partnership." Under healthy circumstances, this new-found but vacillating security lays a foundation for the child and the mother to develop a more complex, interdependent relationship with each other [9, 10].

THE SEPARATION–INDIVIDUATION PROCESS

The psychological birth of the human infant, unlike the readily observable biological birth, is a slowly unfolding intrapsychic process [38, 39]. During the first 2½ to 3 years of life, the young child gradually becomes more aware of the separateness of self and significant others. This awareness leads to the development of a body image, a sense of self, a rudimentary understanding of object relationships, and the reality of the external environment. The development of object permanence and constancy (see Chap. 8) appears to be a prerequisite for developing a sense of self. It is possible to think of oneself as a coherent and lasting entity only when one is aware that both self and others are entities that remain in essentially the same form (object constancy) and continue to exist, although not seen all the time (object permanence).

Mahler's Psychological Birth of the Infant

Margaret Mahler, a psychoanalyst, theorizes that every individual gradually establishes a sense of separateness from, yet an awareness of, a relationship to the world of reality. This process involves recognition of the separateness of one's own body and will from that of the primary love object [39, 40] (see Table 9–2).

Mahler postulates that the major achievements of this process are accomplished between the fourth or fifth month to the thirtieth or thirty-sixth month of life. Although the processes of separation and individuation are closely related and intertwined, they are not identical. **Separation** is the recognition of biological disjunction and consists of the child's emergence from a symbiotic fusion with the mother. **Individuation** is the recognition of affective and social disjunction and consists of those achievements marking the child's assumption of individual characteristics [39]. Both processes deal with the infant's gradual emancipation from a "mass," or "fused," ego identity, a process that may continue throughout life in other relationships (see Chap. 30) [8, 40].

ANTECEDENTS OF THE
SEPARATION-INDIVIDUATION PROCESS
Before the infant can begin to differentiate between self-nonself and good-not good, psychosocial equilibrium must be attained. This equilibrium depends on the ability of the mother and infant to establish communication. A mutual cuing begins, with the caretaker focusing on the infant's needs and responses; gradually over a period of several months, the situation evolves to a more balanced sharing of feelings and needs between the caretaker and the child.

Normal autism. According to Mahler, the early weeks of life are characterized by absolute primary narcissism. The infant is unaware of the role of the mothering agent in satisfying needs. The mother protects the neonate from extremes of stimulation in order to facilitate physiological growth. Since the infant's natural tendency is to spend considerable periods of time in Wolff's states one, two, or three (see p. 103), the mother's ministrations not only help to maintain phys-

Table 9–2. Mahler's Intrapsychic Separation-Individuation Process

Phase	Age	Characteristics of Child
Forerunners of process		
Normal autism	Birth–1 month	"Absolute primary narcissism." Lack of awareness of mothering agent. Unaware of self-other differentiation. "Primitive hallucinatory disorientation." Physiological rather than psychological processes dominate behaviors. Energies focused toward physiological need satisfaction and maintenance of homeostasis. Minimal response to external events.
Normal symbiosis	1–5 months	"Socio-biological interdependence." Primary narcissism now includes mothering agent. Sees mother as a part of self—a dual unity with a common boundary. Dimly aware that he cannot meet his own needs. Beginning to be aware of and attend to external events, but unable to distinguish between internal and external experiences.
Subphases of process		
Differentiation	5–9 months	"Lap baby." Specific bond between the infant and his primary caretaker emerges. Explores her face and body. Begins to distinguish and differentiate between own and mother's body, self–nonself, and mother–not mother. Molds to body of caretaker. Begins to alter behavior in response to mother's cues. Curiosity and wonderment with novel experiences. Much visual inspection of both people and the environment.
Practicing Early (crawling) Late (walking)	9–14 months	Elated investment in his own burgeoning physical autonomy. Begins to move away from mother physically. Becomes absorbed in own activities, but mother needs to be present as an anchor for safe exploration of the environment. Many "emotional refueling" behaviors. May have a transitional toy or object.
Rapprochement	14–24 months	Uses mother as an extension of self. Recognizes own physiological separateness from mother. Wants to share each new accomplishment with her. Shadowing and darting away behaviors. Stranger shyness and adverse reactions to separations may be due to a growing sense of vulnerability. Increased "emotional refueling" behaviors.
Consolidation	24–36 months	Establishment of affective object constancy—ability to separate from mother without extreme anxiety. Emergence of core gender-identity. Play becomes more purposeful and constructive. Symbolic play emerges. Able to wait for need gratification.

Source: Extracted from M. S. Mahler et al. [39].

iological homeostasis but also help to increase the neonate's "sensory awareness of and contact with the environment" [38, 40] by increasing the amount of time spent in state four.

Gradually the neonate develops a dim awareness that needs cannot be satisfied without assistance. Innate skills and reflexes begin to be used as tools to obtain wished-for pleasures and to achieve homeostatic equilibrium. Movement to the symbiotic phase is facilitated by the increased responsiveness to external stimuli found in state four (if the caretaker has previously responded consistently and in synchrony with the baby's needs and behaviors).

Normal symbiosis. According to Mahler, from the second month of life until the fourth or fifth month, the infant develops a "dim awareness of the need-sat-isfying object." The infant no longer responds only to physiological needs and perceptions but begins to exhibit conscious attempts to control stimuli in the environment. During this time, the infant perceives the self and the mother figure as one, "a dual unity with one common boundary." Self-nonself is not yet differentiated. The infant appears to experiment with obtaining and maintaining the appearance of mother's face, touch, and voice in much the same way as the infant experiments with the limited movements of his or her own body to create a desired effect. This observation is consistent with Piaget's description of the infant in substage II (see Chap. 8).

Symbiosis is optimal when enfolding, caressing, and en face behaviors are freely used by the caregiver, and when the caregiver responds contingently to the infant, and allows the infant time to respond with cooing, body movements, and smiles. Although internal versus external experiences are only vaguely differentiated, this ability to begin to invest oneself emotionally in another person lays the foundation for all subsequent human relationships [10, 38, 40].

MAHLER'S SEPARATION–INDIVIDUATION PERIOD

Differentiation. Differentiation, the first subphase of the separation-individuation period, begins at the peak of normal symbiosis (7 to 8 months). The infant's more alert state enables more learning about the external world through increased use of the senses. Visual and tactile exploration of faces, watches, eyeglasses, and so forth aid in gaining information about objects and lay the foundation for the intellectual ability to compare objects never before seen with a more familiar object. The infant "learns how to learn" during this first year. Children of this age spend much time in close contact with mother. Touching the mother's face and other parts of her body allows the infant to make comparisons with the corresponding parts of the infant's own body and the bodies of other people. Naming the parts of the body as the baby touches them fosters language development. Pat-a-cake, itsy-bitsy-spider, and other games foster reciprocal and cooperative interaction. This "lap-baby" period may be critical to the ability to engage comfortably in intimate physical relationships later in the life cycle.

Practicing. The differentiation period is overlapped by the "practicing" subphase. The beginning part of this subphase incorporates the infant's earliest ability to move away physically from the caretaker (e.g., crawling, climbing) while the latter part includes the actual use of upright locomotion. Exploration of inanimate objects becomes paramount; the baby can often be seen fingering, tasting, shaking, and smelling objects in the environment. Three important skills are gained: the infant (1) increases familiarity with, and knowledge about, the world, (2) begins perceiving, recognizing, and enjoying the mothering person from a greater distance [39, 40], and (3) begins synthesizing sensory input. **Emotional refueling** is evidenced by a baby during this phase and continues into the toddler and preschool years. It takes great courage and emotional energy for the newly separating infant to venture forth to explore the environment independently. Consequently, the infant makes frequent physical and visual contact with the mother before continuing exploratory

and play activities. The baby who crawls across the room from the mother may find it necessary to travel back to her side and lean against her briefly before again venturing forth. In new or strange situations, the child will cling to the mother or hide behind her legs. The physical contact appears to give the baby the security and the emotional power to go out into the world again (even if it means only traveling to the other couch, or waving "bye-bye" to a departing visitor).

Mahler's third and fourth subphases, which normally occur during the toddler and preschool years, are discussed in Chapter 12.

Erikson's Basic Trust versus Basic Mistrust

Erik Erikson's theory of infant psychosocial development is complementary to Mahler's model. Erikson states that the degree to which the infant develops self-trust as well as trust in other people and the world in general depends on the quality of care the infant receives during the early months. He feels that the most significant developmental task of infancy is to resolve a crisis between a "sense of basic trust" and a "sense of basic mistrust." The consistency and quality of parent-infant interaction have a direct impact on the development of the infant's ego-identity, or self-concept. Erikson views this time as a foundation for all psychosocial development, especially the acquisition of a sense of hope, which should permeate the entire life cycle [21].

The neonate has come from a warm, protective intra-uterine environment in which all needs were met and no demands were made. Birth presents a new world with which to cope. Comfort and protection are no longer guaranteed. The baby needs feeding, sucking pleasure, warmth, comfort, sensory stimulation, and many other ministrations to extend the sense of love and security. The consistency with which these needs are met enables the infant to begin to predict responses to needs and to develop trust in the parents. Erikson is quick to point out that the amount of trust an infant derives from early experience "does not seem to depend on absolute quantities of food or demonstrations of love, but rather on the **quality** of the [maternal] relationship" [21]. It is the manner (not necessarily the technical skill) in which these needs are met that is fundamental. If care of the infant is inconsistent, inadequate, or rejecting over a period of time, a sense of mistrust develops. This mistrust, according to Erikson, imparts an attitude of suspicion and fear toward oneself, other people, and the world in general. A sense of mistrust will prevent or delay cognitive development and the achievement of other stages of psychosocial development.

EARLY INCORPORATIVE STAGE

Erikson views the infant's first 6 months of extra-uterine life as a time when the infant is capable of, enjoys, and learns from "taking in" the external world. Erikson goes beyond Freud's emphasis on the infant's use of the mouth to explore and includes the infant's visual abilities to incorporate the "world." He calls this first stage the "incorporative mode," when the infant takes in everything offered [22]. Erikson emphasizes that the primary caretakers must coordinate and offer stimulation in appropriate degrees of intensity at the right time (synchronized interactional exchange), lest the infant's willingness to accept quickly be converted to either a defensive schema or lethargy [22]. Too much stimulation will be overwhelming; the infant may "tune out" stimuli as a defense against the environment, and integration of the experiences for cognitive and affective growth may become impossible. The consistency of synchronized, positive sensory stimulation helps the infant to trust the environment as well as his or her own abilities to predict outcomes of behavior. The infant begins to associate the primary caretakers with relief, comfort, and the pleasurable sensations of being picked up, caressed, rocked, and fed. Erikson associates the psychosocial domain with the biophysical domain when he concludes: "The first demonstration of social trust in the baby is the ease of his feeding, the depth of his sleep, the relaxation of his bowels" [21].

ADVANCED INCORPORATIVE STAGE

The second stage of Erikson's incorporative mode emerges about the time the first teeth erupt [41]. The infant has now learned to control the environment to some extent. The infant discovers that more can be learned about an object by placing it in the mouth, and that biting can relieve some of the pain that accompanies teething. The baby begins to coordinate oral, olfactory, visual, auditory, and motor skills with neuromuscular maturation and experience [41]. The older infant gradually coordinates touching and grasping with visual, auditory, and tactile stimuli to learn more about the environment.

During infancy the individual needs to feel that the world is a safe, happy place that will meet basic needs and provide sufficient novelty to stimulate interest beyond self. The infant needs protection to feel secure in attempting new skills, exploring new objects, or making a new acquaintance. Each situation helps to produce expectations of new experiences. Situations

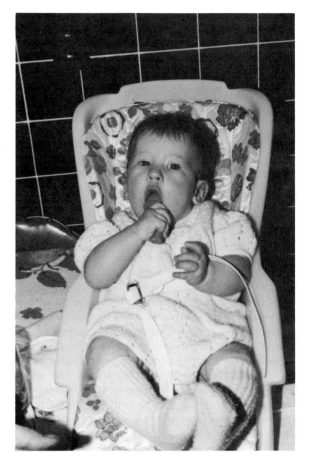

Figure 9–2. During Erikson's advanced incorporative stage, the baby's mouth, instead of sucking in a relaxed way, may be found clamped onto many different types of objects. It is the satisfaction of such needs that gives the baby a sense of the world as a good, stable, pleasant, and somewhat predictable place to be—all of which is necessary for the formation of basic trust.

eliciting mistrust should also occur. The infant needs to learn to trust feelings of mistrust—fear of heights and strangers can be healthy.

The problem of basic trust versus mistrust is not resolved once and for all during infancy, but occurs again at each successive stage of development. Each new relationship goes through a period of developing a deep trust or mistrust [21]. If the basically trusting child is lied to by someone whom the child respects and admires, a sense of mistrust can develop. On the other hand, a very suspicious child or adult who becomes part of a meaningful relationship may eventually be led to experience a sense of trust. An overview of Erikson's theory is given in Appendixes B and C.

Sullivan's Need-Anxiety-Satisfaction

Harry Stack Sullivan emphasizes the importance of interactions between people. Like Mahler and Erikson, he believes that the nature of early social relationships between the infant and the mother are critical in the child's personality development. Sullivan hypothesizes that people are constantly trying to reduce tensions that are the result of biological needs and social insecurity. He defines **tension** as "a potentiality for action for the transformation of energy in the various activities of life" [46]. When a biological need (e.g., food, water, rest) is met, Sullivan postulates that satisfaction is achieved. As long as basic needs are met, the infant is in a state of euphoria or well-being; if they are not met, anxiety or a fearlike state occurs. Sullivan believes that an infant may display increased anxiety by a difficulty with sleeping or feeding and by crying excessively.

Sullivan indicates that anxiety may be felt on a continuum of levels. Mild anxiety serves as an incentive, or a "power motive," for action. When the state of helplessness is discovered, the infant soon discovers tools (e.g., crying) to gain some attention and relief. Sullivan describes infants as being extremely sensitive to the attitudes of others toward them. He believes that a mother can easily communicate her emotional mood (positive or negative) to her infant while meeting the infant's physical needs. Children understand the feelings before the content of a message.

SULLIVAN'S MODES OF EXPERIENCE

Early infancy is described by Sullivan as being very primitive, or "prototaxic." The young infant is unable to differentiate or categorize various experiences. Each experience is responded to as a separate, isolated, unrelated event. Sullivan indicates that at this point, the infant responds nondiscriminatingly and globally to all stimuli.

With the ability to discriminate by organizing and drawing meaning from experiences, the infant moves to the "parataxic" mode—the ability to predict the next event. Visual and auditory cues help the infant to understand causal relationships (e.g., "Milk follows the sight of the bottle"; "Daddy is smiling, so he's going to pick me up and hug me"). Complete transmission to the parataxic mode is achieved with the acquisition of language.

Sullivan emphasizes that the infant's early "personifications" (mental images) of the mother are not realistic but are often perceptions of the interactions experienced between the two (he suggests that the infant initially thinks of mother as a "nipple" because of her nurturing role). Sullivan postulates that in later infancy the baby perceives the mother as a person who is sometimes good (or tender and approving) and sometimes bad (or disapproving and anxiety-provoking). The infant at this point gradually begins to make some discrimination between self and the world, although the child still cannot connect experiences logically as adults do. The more consistent the baby's environment and the more congruent the sequences of life events, the easier it is for the infant to form a secure view of the world and the self. Sullivan contends that the child experiences events primarily through the parataxic mode during the second year of life and that this form of experience continues to occur throughout life [47].

In Sullivan's third and highest type of experience, the "syntaxic" mode, the child learns the meanings and use of the symbols (i.e., gestures, words) that are collectively shared by others in the environment. This enables the child to test subjective perceptions against those of others. Since a child usually begins the syntaxic experience as a toddler, this concept is discussed more fully in Chapter 12.

SULLIVAN'S PERSONIFICATIONS

Sullivan believes that two personifications develop in the baby, the "good-me" and the "bad-me," which eventually fuse and form the essential self. Good-me feelings occur when the baby senses satisfaction; bad-me feelings are aroused when the baby experiences anxiety in an interaction with the caregiver. The fusion of good-me and bad-me occurs at approximately 18 months of age [47]. Which "me" is dominant can change with each situational or maturational crisis. Frequent anxiety can lead to a basic perception of self as bad, to depression, and to feelings of inferiority.

A third personification, "not-me," may be caused by intense anxiety; it represents the individual's attempt to escape the negative feelings evolving from intense or continuous bad-me perceptions. There is a tendency to project the anxiety or bad behavior onto another person or object and to ignore or to deny true feelings. Much of Sullivan's not-me concept pertains to later schizophrenic tendencies, which are beyond the boundaries of a text about normal growth and development. Sullivan also proposes that an infant who suffers intense anxiety over a period of time may drop into an apathetic, sleeplike state called "somnolent detachment." If somnolent detachment is used frequently or for long periods of time, Sullivan predicts that permanent physical or psychological impairment or both could occur.

CAREGIVER ROLE

The parental role, then, is to help the child achieve a state of contentment. This does **not** mean that the parent protects the child from all discomfort or meets the child's needs before they exist (e.g., continuously offering food before the child is hungry). A sense of trust emerges from the child's ability to discern the cycle of arousal/relaxation (need-displeasure-satisfaction-quiescence-recurrence of need). The consistent relief of the unpleasant state by the caregiver is the key to feelings of trust, security, and attachment [23]. All through life, a person must confront challenges head-on before refining discriminations and responses. Successful encounters with these challenges fosters self-confidence and self-respect. In the infant, this is exhibited in the confidence displayed while communicating needs to the caregiver. The consistency of the caregiver's response is critical to the development of trust and self-confidence, thus:

1. Need exists
2. Infant gives generalized behavior
3. Caregiver responds
4. Need satisfied
5. Need recurs
6. Infant predicts caregiver response
7. Infant repeats previous behavior
8. Caregiver's response consistent
9. Need satisfied
10. Infant trusts caregiver
11. Need recurs
12. Infant confident that behavior will elicit appropriate caregiving

Anxiety in the Infant

The theories previously discussed acknowledge that some form of insecurity or anxiety occurs in the infant. During the second month of life, some babies appear to experience a feeling of "being left" and cry when a meaningful object (mother figure) is removed from sight. Babies between 2 and 3 months usually will not cry when a parent leaves as long as another person is present. If that person leaves, however, the baby will frequently cry as hard as when left alone by the parent, which suggests that the infant is beginning to recognize a dependence on adult ministrations but shows nonspecific attachment to the parent figure.

The terms **separation anxiety** and **stranger anxiety** are often used interchangeably but are not synony-

mous. Separation anxiety is the insecurity experienced by a young child when removed from a familiar person, object, or environment. Regardless of the culture or ethnic group studied, the majority of children 10 to 24 months of age will cry following a significant experience of separation [48]. Stranger anxiety is the tension felt by the young child when introduced to an unfamiliar person. The infant may display the same behaviors (e.g., screaming, attempting to withdraw, refusing to cooperate) when experiencing either of these forms of anxiety.

The infant becomes most securely attached to the person whose behaviors or responses can be predicted, that is, a parent or a permanent parent substitute. Separation anxiety peaks when the child is beginning to feel secure in the ability to predict events (approximately 8 to 10 months) and again when the child begins to realize the ability to control some events (18 to 24 months). When children are separated from known persons, toys, environment, or routines, they can no longer predict events, a situation that increases the amount of energy that must be expended in order to process stimulus input.

Although stranger anxiety has been reported to occur as early as 3 months [15], most researchers indicate that wariness of strangers begins at approximately 5 to 6 months, peaks about 12 to 18 months, and then gradually decreases. Because many babies begin to exhibit negative responses to strangers a few months after specific attachments have begun, this behavior has been termed **eighth-month anxiety.** This anxiety is demonstrated in various ways by individual babies, including sober examination of a new face, cessation of smiling, or physical withdrawal and crying.

Learning theorists observe that each mother-infant dyad establishes a unique communication system. Both mother and infant make significant contributions to the relationship by mutually eliciting and reinforcing each other's behaviors. Social interaction is dependent on the infant's ability to identify cues, to form schemata, and to respond discriminatingly. The infant may not be able to predict a stranger's responses. The novel stimulus of a stranger becomes a source of anxiety; the infant is not yet able to generalize discriminatory cues or response behaviors with the new person. When separation occurs, the baby's communication partner is lost. We can equate the experience to travel in a foreign country with a limited knowledge of the language. The child is unable to generalize the communication system or to anticipate the contingencies about a second person until there have been more experiences with persons other than the primary caretaker to facilitate generalization [73]. The number of adults with whom a baby is familiar influences the baby's degree of anxiety with strangers. Infants with limited contact with persons outside the home may have anxiety intensified or prolonged [59].

Cognitivists such as Yarrow believe that attachment is based on the infant's ability to structure perception of the environment and to respond discriminatingly. Attachment occurs because the child develops a schema for "mother" and prefers stimuli that are only mildly discrepant from known stimuli or schemata. Other persons provide different stimuli that do not fit into the child's "people-behavior schema," thereby eliciting stranger anxiety [78]. Some infants may develop stranger anxiety or wariness toward their fathers during the second half of the first year; this is especially likely to occur if minimal time is spent with one another because of the father's work schedule and the baby's sleep schedule. Babies in day care environments may become attached to the surrogate caretaker and respond with anxiety when picked up at the end of the day by their parents.

The appearance of stranger anxiety in the baby reflects an emerging awareness of differentiation of self from others and an awareness of need or love for a significant other. It is also a clear demonstration that the baby is able to discriminate among people and to identify to whom he or she belongs—all positive steps in psychosocial development. However, if reactions are severe and prolonged, professional intervention is appropriate.

What are the practical implications of this anxiety toward strangers and fear of separation? First, a baby should not be separated from the mother for extended periods of time. When a person first approaches a baby, it is wise to keep a safe distance, as defined by the baby's behaviors. Since primary caretakers are sometimes absent necessarily, it is helpful to build other attachments. The baby should be introduced gradually to new situations so that sudden stimulus changes are minimal, and their novelty can be fun. Separations should be avoided if anxiety is acute or when anxiety reactions are at their peak. Hospitalization of either the infant or the primary caretaker should be postponed during such times if possible, or else the dyad should be allowed to remain together in the hospital. If separation must occur during peaks of anxiety, the baby can be provided with a favorite toy or a personal possession of the person to whom the child is attached. Fostering attachment to a transitional object (e.g., Linus's "security blanket") can facilitate the child's separation from mother and serve as a source of emotional

refueling in her absence. Although we have referred consistently to mothers, fathers and siblings are also recognized as significant contributors to the infant's early development.

FACTORS INFLUENCING PSYCHOSOCIAL DEVELOPMENT OF THE INFANT

There has been a gradual shift in the concept of parenting from doing things for the baby to parenting as a process of reciprocal interaction [55]. Sensitive responsiveness appears to be the one factor most likely to foster secure bonding. A secure reciprocal relationship will change in balance and characteristics as the child grows.

Multiple Caretakers

The attachment theory initially assumed that the only person essential for the infant's mental health was the mother. The supporting evidence was indirect because early studies were based on motherless children reared in institutions.

MULTIPLE MOTHERS

Margaret Mead, a well-known anthropologist, was one of the first to question the prevailing view that care by a single, continuous mother figure was a necessary condition for healthy personality development [67]. She studied arrangements that appeared to be successful in other cultures and suggested that children who grow up "mothered" by many women in the tribe are more secure than those who have had an exclusive, intense relationship with only one woman. She observed that the loss of an individual mother would be less traumatic when the child could easily and comfortably turn to someone else. In cultures where multiple mothering is an accepted practice, the children are happy and thrive and behave in a socially acceptable way for the culture.

DAY-CARE CENTERS

Although cross-cultural studies suggest no harmful effects of multiple mothering, critics have questioned whether these findings can be generalized to the infant in a day-care center in the United States. Several studies have found no significant differences (physically, cognitively, emotionally) between infants in competent day-care centers and those from psychologically intact homes [13, 31, 56]. However, when the home environment is poor, there is documented evidence that early day-care experiences increase cognitive competency and social skills [13, 51]. Burton L. White notes that until adequate outcome criteria are identified, research indicating no significant difference may be misleading [75]. Along with the Robertsons of England [52], White strongly hypothesizes that most children get a better start in life when they spend the majority of their waking hours with one or both parents, since most parents are more intensely involved and responsive to the child's burgeoning skills.

It is of primary importance in child-care arrangements that infants be cared for consistently by someone with whom they are comfortable. Ideally, the infants' caretakers, whether at home or at a day-care center, should subscribe to the same principles that the parents deem important in guiding a child to maturity. Day-care centers need to provide adequate equipment and a positively oriented, well-trained staff and not just child watchers who keep the children safe and out of mischief [49].

FATHERS

In Western cultures, infants form attachments to both parents even if the father spends relatively little time with the child [19, 36]. However, these relationships differ in quality, and under stress, the infant preferentially seeks the mother for comfort [19, 31, 36]. Most mothers and fathers interact quite differently with infants. Fathers tend to play vigorously with the infant, whereas mothers engage in more care giving, soothing, and containing modes of play [4, 34]. Studies indicate, however, that the father can be as sensitive to infant cues as is the mother [6, 36, 50].

The characteristic, culturally influenced differences between maternal and paternal interactional styles ensure that mothers and fathers will have distinct and independent yet interdependent influences on their infants' development [36]. Differentiated paternal responses appear to be a major influence in sex-role socialization [35, 36]. The indirect effects of fathers can include financial support, which frees the mother to devote herself to childrearing, and emotional support, which provides a warm, nurturing relationship with the mother and the child [36]. The most sociable infants are the ones who are securely attached to both parents [42]. Fathering may be as crucial a factor in a child's development as mothering. (The concept of fathering is further explored in Chap. 32.)

Interactional Styles

Interactional styles are heavily influenced by individual temperament, memory traces (of earlier life events), the immediate stimulus of the external and internal en-

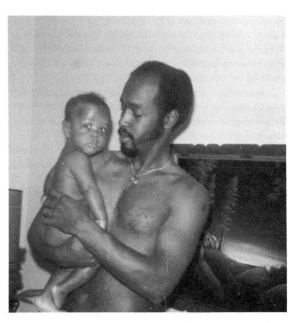

Figure 9–3. This father is providing sensory as well as affective and social stimulation for his infant.

vironment, hierarchical family relationships, level of emotional development, cognitive functioning level, and culture. Consequently, each relationship is unique even within the same family. Since most studies to date have assumed that it is usually the mother who creates the milieu for the first social interactions, an analysis of the mother-infant dyad is presented here. The reader is reminded that the actual primary caretaker who provides nurturing is not always the child's biological mother.

THE MOTHER–INFANT DYAD

The individual differences of temperament in mothers rather than in infants may actually be the major contributor to infant temperament [57]. Mothers who are subjectively rated by researchers as loving, skillful, attentive, and involved tend to have babies who reciprocate with accelerated mental and motor maturity. These mothers, in turn, are described as being emotionally involved with their infants. On the other hand, mothers who tend to be abrupt in their movements involving the baby, who respond indifferently to the child's distress, and who are assessed as having a somewhat low level of affective involvement, tend to have infants who display "hostile demandingness," a factor that appears to reinforce a negative picture of low maternal self-esteem [66].

Louis Sander's research indicates that the early mother-infant relationship is a sequence of adaptations focused around specific interactional tasks. At each level, the child's burgeoning skills demand an adjustment in the mother's responses for synchrony to be maintained. If the pair experiences difficulty coordinating responses at one level, it subsequently interferes with comfortable adjustment at the next. Sander's epigenesis of interaction involves five stages [58]:

1. Initial adaptation (birth to 3 months). Centers around achieving stability of regulation of biological processes (eating, sleeping, elimination). Mother learns to read infant's cues, and infant gives some sign of preferential responsivity to mother.
2. Establishing reciprocal exchanges (4 to 6 months). Reciprocal play activities develop around spontaneous smiling. Infant begins to participate more in feeding and diapering.
3. Early directed activity (7 to 9 months). Baby begins to initiate bids for attention, play, exploration, and to indicate preferences. Mother facilitates success or provides interference that helps to shape direction of baby's behavior.
4. Focalization (10 to 13 months). Locomotion skills enable child to seek own entertainment and maintain desired amount of proximity to mother. Previous maternal availability and consistency determines child's confidence in exploring versus clinging behaviors.
5. Self-assertion (14 to 20 months). The child assumes increasing initiative to determine own activity and amount of contact with mother. Reciprocity of interaction with mother increasingly balanced with environmental interaction.

Mothers who encourage the child to gradually assume more initiative in determining the direction of energy expenditure (toward or away from her) find that the child gradually uses her more as a resource for knowledge, direction, and reinforcement. Mothers who continue to maintain full responsibility for the direction of the child's energy expenditure or who ignore the child's cues will experience increasing frustration with parenting as the child either withdraws from initiating activities, clings to her, or aggressively asserts autonomy without regard for her directions [58]. Sensitive reciprocity is the key to effective parenting and healthy early psychosocial development.

Spoiling. Contrary to popular belief, picking up the infant and giving attention to his or her needs (especially the crying infant) will not "spoil" the child. Bell and Ainsworth found that a mother's prompt response to the crying infant with close, comforting, physical contact is associated with fewer and shorter bouts of crying in the baby's first year [5]. Using Mahler's theory, mutual focusing on the infant's needs lays a foundation for later individuation. Therefore, spoiling is impossible in the first few months. However, continuation of the intensely focused, infant-directed relationship into the late symbiotic and separation-individuation phases delays the child's ability to differentiate between self and others, which interferes with progression toward a realistic perception of the external world. Thus minor delays in the meeting of needs and mild frustrations as the infant grows older aid the infant in learning how to differentiate between self and nonself, encourage him or her to meet personal needs, and force the infant to recognize the needs of others.

Feeding. Sylvia Brody, who extensively researched patterns of mothering, found feeding to be a rich source for data collection. She postulated that the success of the feeding process (both psychosocially to mother and baby and biophysically to the infant) was more a product of the mother's attitude than of the infant's neuromuscular skill [14]. On the other hand, babies demonstrate many different feeding patterns and behaviors that affect the mothering person's attitude about the feeding regimen. The child's degree of adjustment during the feeding process is considered by Bettelheim to have a larger impact on the developing personality than any other human experience [7].

Tactile Stimulation. Around 1920, the infant mortality rate in various foundling institutions throughout the United States was nearly 100 percent [44]. Much earlier, when Dr. Fritz Talbot was visiting the Children's Clinic, in Dusseldorf, Germany, he noticed a "fat old woman, named 'Old Anna,'" who apparently made the babies very happy by carrying them around on her hip as she went about her duties. Whenever the clinical personnel felt everything had been done for a baby medically, and the child still failed to thrive, the infant was turned over to her. "Old Anna" was reported to have always been successful, that is, she always "pulled the child through" [44].

Mahler observed that children separated easily or with difficulty from their mothers, depending on how each child perceived the mother's holding on to them both physically and emotionally [39, 40]. Some babies tend to cuddle more than others. Emerson and Schaffer concluded in one of their studies that there are no apparent reasons why some babies appear to resist physical contact and suggested that one reason may be an innate predisposition [67]. Yarrow emphasizes that the quantity of parental physical contact is not as important as its quality. He found that an appropriate, flexible, and consistent response on the part of the parents to their baby's communications (whether in the form of crying or cooing) was more important than the amount of physical contact they had with the child [77].

These observations have implications for a caretaker who does not feel well or who is subject to a prolonged amount of stress. Having someone else help with housework or child care on a short-term basis or decreasing whatever is causing the severe anxiety or both can influence the direction of the parent-child relationship.

SOCIOECONOMIC AND CULTURAL DIFFERENCES
The attitudes toward parent-child relationships, child-rearing goals, discipline, and life in general vary among different socioeconomic classes and cultures. An important determinant of how the young child will be handled is the parents' belief about the basic nature of children and their personal theory of how one shapes a child into the ideal adult. These differences obviously affect the personal development of each individual. One example is holding an infant. In some American families the parents hold the infant frequently, whereas others limit their caretaking primarily to meeting basic needs. In many nonwestern cultures, babies are maintained in almost constant contact with their mothers, which often includes sleeping with them during the night. Babies may be strapped to cradle-boards and kept vertical or horizontal most of the time. Even the process of bathing varies greatly; it may involve submersion in a tub, bathing with one or more persons in the same vessel, or never being placed in a container of water. With different methods of stimulation, it is presumed that different norms of behavior and development will evolve.

Expressions of Individuality

TEMPERAMENT
To better understand the individuality of personality, researchers have studied the concept of **temperament,** the style of behavior that a child or person habitually uses to cope with the demands and the expectations

of the environment. Thomas and Chess identified nine temperament variables present in infants [70]:

1. Activity level. Refers to how active the infant is
2. Rhythmicity. Reflects how regular a schedule the infant has for feeding, sleep, or bowel movements
3. Approach-withdrawal. Refers to the infant's initial response to a new stimulus
4. Adaptability. Reflects how easily the infant adapts or adjusts a routine to fit a new situation
5. Intensity. Refers to the degree to which the infant expresses self
6. Threshold. Reflects how much stimulus is required before the infant reacts to a given situation
7. Mood. Refers to the amount of happy versus unhappy behavior
8. Attention-persistence. Reflects the length of time a given activity is pursued by the infant and continuation of an activity in spite of obstacles
9. Distractability. Reflects how easily the infant's behavior or attention can be diverted

Thomas and Chess further observed different patterns among the children. The most common were:

1. Easy-child pattern. High rhythmicity, positive mood, positive approach, high adaptability, high intensity
2. Difficult-child pattern. Low rhythmicity, negative mood, withdrawal, low adaptability, high intensity
3. Slow-to-warm pattern. Low activity, withdrawal, low adaptability, negative mood, low intensity

The characteristics displayed by each infant in the Thomas and Chess study correlated with the child's behaviors 5 years later [70]. Being placed in a particular category does not make a child good or bad. Rather, it is the degree of fit between the infant's temperament and the caretaker's ability to respond and positively adapt to it that determines if the parent-infant relationship is at risk.

BRAZELTON'S DIFFERENCES
IN INTERACTIONAL STYLES
From the very moment of birth, and perhaps before, differences in infant behaviors become apparent (e.g., some babies kick more than others in utero). Brazelton indicates that a baby also tends to adopt the characteristics of one of three interaction styles. In his book, *Infants and Mothers: Differences in Development,* he describes the antics, trials, and tribulations of "average" Louis, "active" Daniel, and "quiet" Laura from

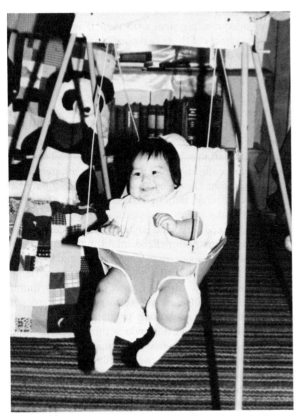

Figure 9–4. From the moment of birth, babies vary immensely in temperament. Parents can better adapt to meeting their child's individual needs and adjusting to their own new roles as caretakers if they recognize and accept these differences.

the moment they are formally introduced to their mothers in the delivery room through their first 12 months of life [11]. They all laugh, cry, sleep, and eat in very different ways. The temperament of these three babies dramatically affects the tenor of parental response and the foundation on which further relationships will be built. Some infants have reactions that are scattered in all three categories. Brazelton's observations are supportive in helping parents to recognize the strengths of their individual babies.

TENSIONAL OUTLETS OF INFANCY

Crying is only one way in which the infant releases tension. Each baby has a unique way of "letting off steam," as well as receiving a sense of security from various comforting behaviors. These behaviors may take the form of hair twisting, presleep rocking in the

crib, or even masturbation in older infants and young children.

Around 6 months of age, infants begin to decrease reliance on the parents by increasing reliance on comforters [65]. A **comforter** is any object or behavior that recreates a physical stimulus that was psychosocially nurturing during early infancy. This increase for the need of comforters is concurrent with the developing separation-individuation process. Transitional objects such as security blankets may also be thought of as comforters, although they serve more as parent substitutes to facilitate extension of self into the environment. Thumb-sucking, an oral comforter, is a response by infants as young as 2 months of age to distress caused by psychological factors, especially by "being left" [76]. Thumb-sucking is most likely to begin around 3 or 4 months of age. The baby may seek continued oral pleasure by sucking the thumb immediately after a feeding. Later the urge spreads to other times of the day and night. Babies who do not suck their thumbs probably have their sucking needs satisfied during feedings. It is important to note that babies who suck their thumbs and those who do not may be equally normal, healthy, and loved.

Thumb-sucking often reaches a peak around 7 months of age, since the infant is enthralled with hand-mouth behaviors at that time. After this period, much variation in the amount of thumb-sucking occurs; it will often recur during toddlerhood and can remain a precious comforter until the preschool years.

The long-range effects of thumb-sucking are still controversial. It may assist the baby to get through teething much more easily than the baby who does not thumbsuck. Almost all 4-month-old infants engage in thumb-, finger-, and hand-chewing. Prolonged sucking of the thumb may push the upper front baby teeth forward and the lower teeth back, marring the shape of the mouth and facial features (see Figure 15–5A). The American Academy of Pediatrics suggests that if a thumb-sucking habit persists beyond age 4 the caretaker should consult a pedodontist or general dentist for advice. Misalignment of the baby teeth can change the child's mouth movements and lead to articulation problems. Variables such as how often and in what position the thumb is held, as well as the general structure of the child's mouth, may be additional significant factors.

Most specialists in child behavior advise that the least traumatizing way for parents to intervene if they are disturbed by the thumb-sucking is to substitute another object for the thumb rather than to pull the thumb directly out of the mouth; this could be done by encouraging the baby to hold a toy or to suck on a pacifier. Pacifiers usually are given up more easily than the thumb [65]. An intervention during the peak of a thumb-sucking period (or during a crisis, such as the birth of a new sibling) will be least effective and perhaps traumatizing to both the infant who wants some form of comforting and the parents who want peace and quiet.

Another mode of intervention is to modify the length and the nature of each infant feeding. The caretaker should make sure that bottle feedings last at least 15 to 20 minutes even if it means changing the nipple so that the bottle contents flow more slowly (one must remember that the baby **needs** to suck). Breast-fed babies should also be kept at the breast for the same amount of time. When satiated, the infant may be switched back to the empty breast for sucking satisfaction. It is not just the length of a particular feeding but also the frequency of feedings that may be significant to a particular infant for adequate sucking. One survey indicates that young babies fed every 3 hours do not suck their thumbs as much as babies who are fed every 4 hours [65].

PSYCHOSOCIAL DEPRIVATION DURING INFANCY

The infant's need for a primary caretaker is absolute. However, the primary caretaker's need for the infant is relative [40]. The validity of these statements becomes apparent when for some reason the caretaker does not or cannot provide the physical or psychosocial nurturing the infant needs. When basic physical needs are not met, the infant perceives that the environment is hostile and may learn to distrust those around him or her. When the infant's attachment behaviors are not consistently responded to and encouraged, they are eventually extinguished. The child begins to consume large amounts of energy meeting self-needs; weight loss and developmental delays may be the result.

Two interrelated yet different terms are used in speaking of psychosocial deprivation. **Psychosocial separation** refers to the physical loss of the maternal figure—the love object. It does not necessarily imply a loss of mothering or a loss of physical care, since this can be provided by the father, a sibling, a surrogate parent, or another person. The term **psychosocial deprivation** is reserved for the emotional loss of a warm relationship. It does not necessarily imply a loss of the maternal figure, but it frequently is accompanied by loss of adequate physical care [54]. It is difficult to study the effects of these two conditions separately because they often occur together and are combined with many variables.

Factors Affecting Infant Response to Separation from the Primary Caretaker

The **age** of the child when the separation occurs is a significant variable, affecting the infant's response to separation or deprivation. Before differentiation of a specific mother figure occurs, any caretaker may be readily substituted, although the lack of consistency in response to the infant's interactional cues may cause delays in the cognitive and psychosocial processes. For instance, the institutionalized infant may show developmental delays as early as 2 months of age [54].

The **gender** of the infant as a significant variable needs more study. Although few studies have found any significant differences, Rutter states that recent studies on young subhuman primates as well as on children indicate that the male is more vulnerable to separation experiences than the female [54]. Girls who experience nonmaternal care exhibit more maternal proximity-attaining behaviors than boys [28].

Infant **temperament** affects how the baby will react to separation. Active infants will usually not become as developmentally retarded as their passive peers when placed in a depriving environment; they will demand attention.

If the **previous mother-child relationship** has been a comfortable one, short-term separation does not appear to cause undue infant stress. Babies whose parents work and who are therefore accustomed to another caretaker in their absence may adapt to new caretakers better than those babies who are used to only one primary figure.

To say that **previous separation experiences** make successive ones easier is not necessarily true. Closely related to how well a child adjusts to separation experiences are how well the child adjusted to earlier ones, how long the separation lasted, and how intensely the separation was perceived.

The other **people** who are **present** at the time of the separation may be a significant variable. Familiar people, such as siblings, can help to reduce stress in children placed in a strange environment. The **approval and caretaking style of the surrogate mother** may also be a decisive factor in the child's adaptation to separation. A warm, nurturing person who knows how and when to respond to the infant's cues can facilitate adaptation to separation and reduce the child's perception of deprivation.

Failure-to-Thrive Syndrome

The term **failure-to-thrive** (FTT) is used to describe infants and children whose weight (and sometimes height) fall below the fifth percentile for their ages (See Appendix D). These children are characterized by lack of physical growth, malnutrition, and retardation of motor and social development. FTT is divided into two categories: organic FTT, which is caused primarily by a physical factor, and nonorganic FTT, which is frequently associated with disturbances of parenting and of family organization [29]. The mothers generally are less affectionate, initiate fewer positive interactions, use physical punishment readily, and hold negative feelings toward their children [79]. The mothers have noticeably failed to establish a synchronized relationship with these children.

The mechanism linking emotional deprivation with failure-to-thrive is unclear. It appears that the increased tensions arising from unmet psychosocial (and physical) needs interfere with sleep patterns. Abnormal sleep patterns may inhibit secretion of growth hormone from the anterior pituitary, thus decreasing hyperplastic cellular growth. The potential for long-range effects is obvious.

Increased tension levels may also correlate with increased vomiting and diarrhea. Ingested calories are not retained, and weight loss results. Restlessness in the form of rocking or spasticity reduces the calories available for growth. Many tense infants experience anorexia—an aversion to food. This behavior may continue into the adult years when some individuals will find it difficult to eat when under stress (others will use food to cope with stress). These children begin to show developmental delays, apathy, irritability, and even self-destructive behaviors [79].

Therapy for children with FTT must include the mother figure [43]. The best programs offer in-home programing or live-in facilities for the infant-mother unit. The mother figure is taught how and when to respond to her infant's cues for interaction. An effective program results in weight gain for the baby and a more satisfying relationship for both mother and child [30].

The Effects of Separation or Deprivation on Development

Two classic studies have been carried out on infants separated from their mothers. The effects of separation on the child were greatly influenced both by age and by the previous mother-infant relationship. Both studies were performed in institutions where separation of the infant from the mother was the rule. Because of the results of these studies, marked changes have been made in the institutional care of infants.

SEPARATION DURING THE FIRST 6 MONTHS

During World War II, John Bowlby [9] studied children in orphanages who had experienced no contact with their natural mothers and had received little nurturing from the multiple caretakers available. He noted that the infants exhibited four behaviors directed toward the caretakers: following, smiling, clinging, and crying. When these attachment behaviors were unrewarded, severe psychological and physiological results occurred.

By 3 months of age, these children no longer made attempts to communicate (e.g., neither cooing nor babbling). They did not adapt or mold their posture to the caretaker when held. Although their joints were movable, they remained stiff and unresponsive. Gradually these children began to refuse contact and lost interest in the environment. Smiles were rare; facial features became unresponsive or rigid. Motor development was retarded, and symptoms of FTT were present. The children suffered from insomnia and restlessness and exhibited poor resistance to infections. Many became so severely depressed both physically and psychosocially that death ensued. Many of the survivors never fully recovered from the effects of the deprivation; they continued to show delays in social, cognitive, and language developments even though their environment was altered.

SEPARATION DURING THE SECOND 6 MONTHS

René Spitz, a psychoanalyst who studied under Sigmund Freud, discovered an institution housing young women and their babies [64]. The infants received both physical and psychosocial nurturance from their own mothers for the first 6 months of life. The infants all exhibited happy, outgoing behaviors. Six months later, the mothers left the institution, leaving the infants to be cared for by other residents and staff while they reestablished themselves in the community. Although the babies received adequate care, they exhibited depression through crying and withdrawal. Spitz observed that this "anaclitic depression" followed a predictable pattern. It is of interest that infants who had previously had a poor relationship with their mothers experienced milder symptoms.

The first month was characterized by weepy, demanding, and clinging behaviors—an attempt to regain mothering by force. During the second month, the infants exhibited intense grief that was evidenced by inconsolable wailing, weight loss, and arrests in cognitive and psychosocial development. During the third month of the separation, the infants lost hope and the desire to reinvest themselves in others. They refused human contact and would lie wide-awake for hours in a prone position on their cots. They refused food, developmental delays became more pronounced, and illness was common. After the third month of separation, lethargy and apathy became the dominant mode of interaction, but the children no longer refused adult attention, and whimpering replaced weeping. The rigidity of their faces and their lack of affective responses indicated that the infants had developed a defensive shell against outside intrusion and reinvestment.

Spitz observed that if the mother was restored after 3 months but before 5 months of separation, the child experienced marked recovery. However, Spitz felt that the recovery was never complete, and emotional scars were left. Those who remained separated 5 months exhibited increasingly serious deterioration with irreversible damage to the psyche. These children became severely retarded, participating in bizarre posturing and finger movements. Like King Frederick's infants, many of the long-term institutionalized infants in Spitz's study died.

IMPLICATIONS
When an infant must be separated from the mother figure, either temporarily or permanently, the child's care should be assumed by one person insofar as this is possible. Adoption or placement in a foster home is preferable to a group setting. Maintaining similar routines and known foods can help to reduce stress. The surrogate parent should be warm and sensitive to the infant's unique communication style and flexible enough to allow the infant to set the pace of their interaction.

If a child is hospitalized, it is important to include the significant parent in the child's care. Many hospitals have a rooming-in program that allows the parent to stay with the infant or the infant with the ill parent. This arrangement can greatly reduce the infant's anxiety, facilitate recovery, and strengthen the parent-infant relationship.

SUMMARY

Over the past two decades, there has been a gradual shift in the concept of parenting. It has evolved from doing things to and for the baby to providing reciprocity of interaction. This change has been influenced by research on neonatal skills and attachment.

During the first 6 months of life, the parent and child are getting to know one another. They begin to establish a primitive communication system. Consistent, sensitive responsivity on the parents' part is critical to the child's ability to develop a sense of trust in the adults and to be able to anticipate the adults' responses. It is also the foundation of secure personal bonding.

The young child usually develops several attachments, but these are not equal in strength, nor freely interchangeable. Fathers, siblings, grandparents, and nonfamily caregivers may all be included as attachment figures. Under stress, the child will seek the comfort of the closest attachment figure.

Attachment bonds persist over time, even when there is no contact with the specific attachment person. The child may undergo a dramatic grief process if separation is prolonged. Once a child has formed a healthy attachment to at least one person, it is easier to transfer that attachment to a second person or to form additional attachments.

Research indicates that as poorly attached children mature beyond infancy, cognitive development is impeded, logical thinking is constricted, ability to cope with frustration and stress is reduced, conscience development is impaired, and social behaviors are disrupted. The mother's presence is not sufficient to foster attachment or to serve as a security base. The mother must be **emotionally available** to respond to the cues of the child for help or encouragement before the child has the permission or the strength to explore the opportunities offered by the environment [62].

The apparent purpose of bonding is to facilitate one's identity as a separate, valued individual and to serve as a foundation for exploring one's capabilities and the environment. It is a paradox that the most securely attached children are those who separate the most easily from their parents to explore the environment [55], enjoy the company of peers [20], and interact more comfortably with strangers. They have learned to trust. This trust dissipates fear, and extends to a general trust in new situations.

Although much research indicates that the infant contributes highly to the quality of the interaction by the strength, consistency, and clarity of signals of need and feeling, a heavy burden still falls on the parents to orchestrate meaningful environmental responses to the child's cues [58]. Thus, the parents of an atypical baby (i.e., premature, post-mature, or disabled) will carry more of the burden for establishing a synchronous interaction [3]. Fortunately, when provided with a normal expected environment, most babies and parents are eventually able to establish a mutually nurturing relationship. Even when the parents and/or the baby get off to a difficult start, the marvelous resiliency of the infant will usually act as a buffer against any long-range detrimental consequences of a single traumatic episode or a poor interaction during the first few months of life [3].

REFERENCES

1. Ainsworth, M. D. S. *Infancy in Uganda: Infant Care and the Growth of Love.* Baltimore: Johns Hopkins Press, 1967.
2. Ainsworth, M. D. S., and Bell, S. M. Attachment, exploration, and separation: Illustrated by the behavior of one-year-olds in a strange situation. *Child Dev.* 41:49, 1970.
3. Bakeman, R., and Brown, J. V. Early intervention consequences for social and mental development at three years. *Child Dev.* 51:437, 1980.
4. Bealsky, J. Mother-father-infant interactions: A naturalistic observational study. *Dev. Psych.* 15:601, 1979.
5. Bell, S. M., and Ainsworth, M. D. S. Infant crying and maternal responsiveness. *Child Dev.* 43:1171, 1972.
6. Berman, P. W. Are Women More Responsive than Men to the Young? A Review of Developmental and Situational Variables. In S. Chess and A. Thomas (Eds.), *Annual Progress in Child Psychiatry and Child Development.* New York: Brunner/Mazel, 1981.
7. Bettelheim, B. *Dialogue With Mothers.* New York: Avon Books, 1971.
8. Bowen, M. *Family Therapy in Clinical Practice.* New York: Jason Aronson, 1978.
9. Bowlby, J. M. *Maternal Care and Mental Health.* New York: Schocken, 1966.
10. Bowlby, J. M. *Attachment and Loss,* Vol. 1: *Attachment.* New York: Basic Books, 1969.
11. Brazelton, T. B. *Infants and Mothers: Differences in Development* (Rev. ed.). New York: Delta, 1983.
12. Brazelton, T. B. *Early Parent-Infant Reciprocity.* In V. C. Vaughan and T. B. Brazelton (Eds.), *The Family—Can It Be Saved?* Chicago: Year Book, 1976.
13. Brock, W. M. *The Effects of Day Care: A Review of the Literature.* Los Alamitos, CA: Southwest Regional Laboratory for Educational Research and Development, 1980. ED 195–348
14. Brody, S. *Patterns of Mothering: Maternal Influence During Infancy.* New York: International Universities Press, 1956.
15. Bronson, G. W. Infants' Reactions to an Unfamiliar Person. In L. J. Stone, H. T. Smith, and L. B. Murphy (Eds.), *The Competent Infant: Research and Commentary.* New York: Basic Books, 1973.
16. Chess, S., and Thomas, A. Temperament in the Normal Infant. In J. C. Westman (Ed.), *Individual Differences in Children.* New York: Wiley, 1973.
17. Chess, S., Thomas, A., and Birch, H. *Your Child Is a Person: A Psychological Approach to Parenthood Without Guilt.* New York: Penguin, 1976.
18. Cohen, L. J. The operational definition of human attachment. *Psychol. Bull.* 81:107, 1974.
19. Cohen, L. J., and Campos, J. J. Father, mother, and stranger as elicitors of attachment behavior in infancy. *Dev. Psychol.* 10:146, 1974.
20. Easterbrooks, M. A., and Lamb, M. E. The relationship between quality of infant-mother attachment and infant competence in initial encounters with peers. *Child Dev.* 50:380, 1979.
21. Erikson, E. H. *Childhood and Society* (2nd ed., rev. and enl.). New York: Norton, 1963.
22. Erikson, E. H. *Identity: Youth and Crisis.* New York: Norton, 1968.
23. Fahlberg, V. *Attachment and Separation.* Lansing: Michigan Dept. of Social Services, 1979.
24. Gewirtz, J. L. A Learning Analysis of the Effects of Normal Stimulation, Prevention, and Deprivation on the Acquisition of Social Motivation and Attachment. In B. M. Foss (Ed.), *Determinants of Infant Behavior.* London: Methuen, 1961.
25. Gewirtz, J. L. (Ed.). *Attachment and Dependency.* Washington, DC: Winston, 1972.
26. Grossman, R. W. A Role the Basic Orientation System May Play in Infancy. In S. H. Bartley, *Perception in Everyday Life.* New York: Harper & Row, 1972.
27. Harlow, H. F., and Harlow, M. Learning to Love. In P. H. Mussen, J. J. Conger, and J. Kagan (Eds.), *Readings in Child Development and Personality* (2nd ed.). New York: Harper & Row, 1970.
28. Hock, E., and Clinger, J. B. Behavior toward mother and stranger of infants who have experienced group day care, individual care, or exclusive maternal care. *Genet. Psychol.* 137:49, 1980.
29. Homer, C., and Ludwig, S. Categorization of etiology of failure to thrive. *Am. J. Dis. Child.* 135:848, 1981.
30. Hufton, I., and Oates, K. Nonorganic failure to thrive: A long term follow up. *Pediatrics* 59(1):73, 1977.
31. Kagan, J., Kearsley, R. B., and Zelago, P. R. The Effects of Infant Day-Care on Psychological Development. Paper presented at a symposium on "The Effect of Early Experience on Child Development," American Association for the Advancement of Science, Boston, Feb. 19, 1976.
32. Korner, A. F. Individual Differences at Birth: Implications for Early Experiences and Later Development. In J. C. Westman (Ed.), *Individual Differences in Children.* New York: Wiley, 1973.
33. Korner, A. F., and Thoman, E. B. The relative efficacy of contact and vestibular-proprioceptive stimulation in soothing neonates. *Child Dev.* 43:443, 1972.
34. Lamb, M. E. Interactions Between Eight-Month-Old Children and Their Fathers and Mothers. In M. E. Lamb

(Ed.), *The Role of the Father in Child Development.* New York: Wiley, 1976.

35. Lamb, M. E.   The development of parental preferences in the first two years of life. *Sex Roles* 3:495, 1977.

36. Lamb, M. E.   Paternal influences on early socio-emotional development. *J. Child Psychol. Psychiatry* 23:185, 1982.

37. Lorenz, K.   Companionship in Bird Life. In C. Schiller (Ed.), *Instinctive Behavior.* New York: International Universities Press, 1957.

38. Mahler, M.   On the first three subphases of the separation-individuation process. *Int. J. Psychoanal.* 53(Part 3): 333, 1972.

39. Mahler, M. S., Pine, F., and Bergman, A.   The Mother's Reaction to Her Toddler's Drive for Individuation. In E. J. Anthony and T. Benedek (Eds.), *Parenthood: Its Psychology and Psychopathology.* Boston: Little, Brown, 1970.

40. Mahler, M. S., Pine, F., and Bergman, A.   *The Psychological Birth of the Human Infant: Symbiosis and Individuation.* New York: Basic Books, 1975.

41. Maier, H. W.   *Three Theories of Child Development* (3rd ed.). New York: Harper & Row, 1978.

42. Main, M., and Weston, M.   The independence of infant-mother and infant-father attachment relationships: Security of attachment characterizes relationships, not infants. In press.

43. Mira, M., and Cairns, G.   Intervention with interaction of a mother and child with nonorganic failure to thrive. *Pediatric Nursing* 7(2):41, 1981.

44. Montagu, A.   *Touching: The Human Significance of the Skin* (2nd ed.). New York: Harper & Row, 1978.

45. Morgan, G. A., and Ricciuti, H. N.   Infants' Responses to Strangers During the First Year. In L. J. Stone, H. T. Smith, and L. B. Murphy (Eds.), *The Competent Infant: Research and Commentary.* New York: Basic Books, 1973.

46. Moss, H. A.   Sex, age, and state as determinants of mother-infant interactions. *Merrill-Palmer Q.* 13:19, 1967.

47. Mullahy, P.   *Psychoanalysis and Interpersonal Psychiatry: The Contributions of Harry Stack Sullivan.* New York: Science House, 1970.

48. Mussen, P. H., et al.   *Psychological Development: A Life-Span Approach.* New York: Harper & Row, 1979.

49. National Association for the Education of Young Children. How to choose a good early childhood program. *Young Child.* 39(1):28, 1983.

50. Parke, R. D., and Sawin, D. B.   The father's role in infancy: A re-evaluation. *Fam. Coordinator* 25:365, 1976.

51. Ramey, C. T., Farron, D. C., and Campbell, F. A.   Predicting I.Q. from mother-infant interactions. *Child Dev.* 50:804, 1979.

52. Roberts, A. R. (Ed.).   *Childhood Deprivation.* Springfield, IL: Thomas, 1974.

53. Robertson, J., and Robertson, J.   *A Baby in the Family: Loving and Being Loved.* New York: Penguin Books, 1982.

54. Rutter, M.   *Maternal Deprivation Reassessed* (2nd ed.). New York: Penguin Books, 1981.

55. Rutter, M.   Maternal deprivation, 1972–1978: New findings, new concepts, new approaches. *Child Dev.* 50:283, 1979.

56. Rutter, M.   Social-emotional consequences of day care for preschool children. *Am. J. Orthopsychiatry* 51(1):4, 1981.

57. Sameroff, A. J., Seifer, R., and Elias, P. K.   Sociocultural variability in infant temperament ratings. *Child Dev.* 53:164, 1982.

58. Sander, L. W.   The Longitudinal Course of Early Mother-Child Interaction: Cross-case Comparison in a Sample of Mother-Child Pairs. In B. M. Foss (Ed.), *Determinants of Infant Behavior IV.* London: Methuen, 1969.

59. Schaffer, H. R., and Emerson, P. E.   Patterns of Response to Physical Contact in Early Human Development. In L. J. Stone, H. T. Smith, and L. B. Murphy (Eds.), *The Competent Infant; Research and Commentary.* New York: Basic Books, 1973.

60. Schwartz, J. L., and Schwartz, L. H. (Eds.),   *Vulnerable Infants: A Psychosocial Dilemma.* New York: McGraw-Hill, 1977.

61. Smith, W. C.   *The Stepchild.* Chicago: University of Chicago Press, 1953.

62. Sorce, J. F., and Emde, R. N.   Mother's presence is not enough: Effect of emotional availability on infant's exploration. *Dev. Psych.* 17:737, 1981.

63. Spitz, R. A.   *The First Year of Life: A Psychoanalytic Study of Normal and Deviant Development of Object Relations.* New York: International Universities Press, 1973.

64. Spitz, R. A., and Wolf, K. M.   Anaclitic Depression: An Inquiry into the Genesis of Psychiatric Conditions in Early Childhood. *The Psychoanalytic Study of the Child,* Vol. II. New York: International Universities Press, 1946.

65. Spock, B.   *Baby and Child Care.* New York: Pocket Books, 1976.

66. Stern, G. G., et al.   A factor analytic study of the mother-infant dyad. *Child Dev.* 40(1):163, 1969.

67. Stone, L. J., et al.   The Social Infant. In L. J. Stone, H. T. Smith, and L. B. Murphy (Eds.), *The Competent Infant; Research and Commentary.* New York: Basic Books, 1973.

68. Sullivan, H. S.   *The Fusion of Psychiatry and Social Science.* New York: Norton, 1971.

69. Thoman, E. B.   Some consequences of early infant-mother-infant interaction. *Early Child Dev. and Care* 3:249, 1974.

70. Thomas, A., and Chess, S.   *Temperament and Development.* New York: Brunner/Mazel, 1977.

71. Tizard, B., and Hodges, J.   The effect of early institutional rearing on the development of eight-year-old children. *J. Child Psychol. Psychiatry* 19:99, 1978.

72. Tizard, B., and Rees, J.   The effect of early institutional rearing on the behavior problems and affectional relationships of four-year-old children. *J. Child Psychol. Psychiatry* 16:61, 1975.

73. Watson, J.   Perception of Contingency as a Determinant of Social Reponsiveness. In E. B. Thoman and S. Trotter (Eds.), *Social Responsiveness of Infants: A Round Table.* New Brunswick, NJ: Johnson & Johnson Baby Products, 1978.

74. White, B. L. *The First Three Years of Life.* Englewood Cliffs, NJ: Prentice-Hall, 1975.

75. White, B. L. Should you stay home with your baby? *Educ. Horiz.* 59(1):22, 1980.

76. Wolff, P. H. The Natural History of Crying and Other Vocalizations in Early Infancy. In L. J. Stone, H. T. Smith, and L. B. Murphy (Eds.), *The Competent Infant; Research and Commentary.* New York: Basic Books, 1973.

77. Yarrow, L. J. Research in dimensions of early maternal care. *Merrill-Palmer Q.* 9:101, 1963.

78. Yarrow, L. J. Attachment and Dependency: A Developmental Perspective. In J. L. Gewirtz (Ed.), *Attachment and Dependency.* Washington, DC: Winston, 1972.

79. Yoos, L. Taking another look at failure-to-thrive. *Matern.-Child Nurs. J.* 9:32, 1984.

V
The Toddler and the Preschooler

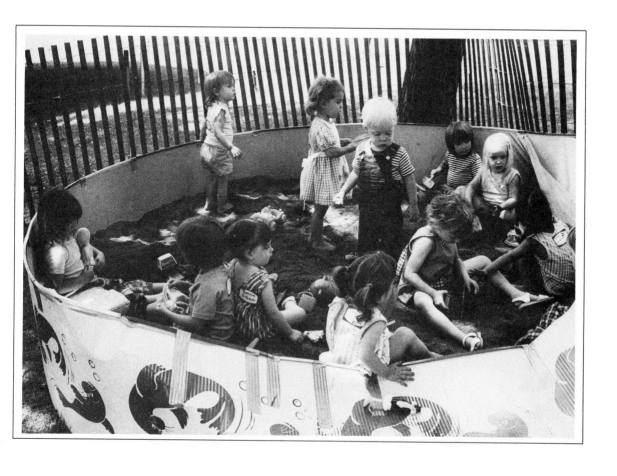

10
Biophysical Development of the Toddler and the Preschooler

Shirley S. Ashburn

A short period of rest acts as an injection of adrenalin for a baby this age. Remarkable resilience in such tiny packages.

—T. Berry Brazelton, *Toddlers and Parents*

It is exciting to watch the metamorphic process that changes the infant into a toddler. The toddling child goes walking about with a new-found enthusiasm that facilitates learning about the world. Biophysically, toddlerhood encompasses the period from 16 through 30 months; preschoolerhood evolves from this period and continues until the child's sixth birthday, although these age demarcations are only arbitrary. Biophysical growth during these years is relatively slow as compared to the infant period. The most significant biophysical change of this period is that the horizontal infant becomes a vertical person. Skills become refined in all areas.

The alterations in the child's body proportions create striking changes in appearance. In the beginning, the toddling baby has a top-heavy appearance that is accentuated by a relatively long trunk and perhaps a bulky diaper that causes the buttocks to appear to be closer to the floor than they really are. As the child begins the second year, the legs begin to grow much faster than the trunk. This change, coupled with erect posture, makes the child resemble in some ways a miniature adult. The abdominal musculature is not as well developed in the toddler as it is in the child of 4 years or more, and this contributes to a "potbelly" appearance. As the toddler first learns to walk, a compensating convex lumbar curve (in the small of the back) begins to develop. The potbelly disappears as the child's muscles strengthen.

From the child's first birthday to the sixth, height will progress from an average of 30 inches to approximately 46 inches. More than two-thirds of all children will stay within 1.5 to 2 inches of the average height for their ages. By age 4, the preschooler will double his or her birth length [15]. Gender differences in height during this time are minimal, although males are generally slightly taller than females of the same age (see Appendixes D and E).

After the child's second birthday, the rate of weight gain will average about 5 pounds yearly until the ninth or tenth birthday. This means that beginning with the second year, the child may gain only one-half pound per month, with many plateaus interspersed throughout this span of time [15]. The accumulation of adipose tissue declines greatly during the preschool years; it begins to increase again at approximately six years of age [7]. Black preschoolers are neurologically more advanced than Caucasian preschoolers during these years, and most Black children have less subcutaneous fat than Caucasian children but are taller and heavier by 2 years of age [22].

SOMATIC DEVELOPMENT

Nervous System

The gradual maturation of the nervous system accounts for many of the behavioral changes observed in toddlers and preschoolers. Electroencephalograms (EEG), which record brain activity and can help to measure the maturation of its different areas, demonstrate that some rhythms associated with the mature adult brain begin to emerge [15]. The changes in neural organization that underlie the appearance and the further development of these impulses are unknown, but they suggest a complex pattern of maturation, and perhaps the key to increased attention span (which is needed for formal schooling).

THE BRAIN
The brain continues to grow during the toddler and preschool years, but not as rapidly as it did during infancy. By the time the child has reached 3 years of age, the brain is three-quarters of its adult size [15]. The cranial vault reaches 87 percent of its adult size by the age of 2 years [29]. The increasing maturation of the brain, combined with opportunities to experience more of the world, greatly contributes to the child's emerging cognitive abilities. The temperature-regulat-

ing center in the brain is becoming more mature, so that the child is less subject to the temperature fluctuations that were common in infancy.

Various areas of the cerebrum develop at different rates. Because the young toddler's immature nervous system cannot handle more than one incoming stimulus at a time, the introduction of a second stimulus will intensify and prolong the action that has resulted from a first stimulus. For example, when the hand of a 16-month old is slapped for touching a forbidden object, the child's grasp (a result of the first stimulus) momentarily tightens, or is prolonged, instead of releasing the object. The child's inability to respond immediately to the parents' command is, in part, physiological, not just a refusal to cooperate [24].

MYELINIZATION
Although most of the myelinization of nerve fibers is complete at about 2 years of age, some myelin sheaths continue to develop, and the number and the size of nerve endings within and between cortical areas continue to grow at least until adolescence. By 2 years of age, one of the toddler's major motor pathways, the corticospinal tract, is myelinated enough to allow the child to refine movement of the lower extremities. By 4 years of age, the fibers that connect the cerebellum to the cerebral cortex are mature enough to allow refined voluntary hand and finger movements for drawing pictures and reproducing simple shapes. Further refinement of these movements will occur with increased myelinization, cognitive development, and appropriate experiences.

PERCEPTUAL ORGAN DEVELOPMENT
The sensory organs continue to refine their abilities during these early childhood years. The concomitant factors of an increased attention span and an improved cognitive discrimination heighten the child's ability to select and to study details and to coordinate schemata (see Chap. 11).

The Eye. Several aspects of visual development have been discussed in preceding chapters. The specific biophysical development of the eye is covered in Chapter 22. Depth perception continues to develop through preschoolerhood, but because of the child's lack of motor coordination, overshooting and undershooting of extremities may lead to poor eye-hand coordination. This in turn leads to many spills, poor art work, or even falls from furniture or climbing equipment.

Dimness of vision without any apparent disease of the eye can occur in approximately 4 percent of children who are not yet in the first grade [2]. Functional amblyopia ("lazy eye") is usually the result of not using an eye in order to avoid the discomfort of double vision that is often caused by imbalanced eye muscles (strabismus) and neural inhibition in the visual pathways in the brain. The exact cause of functional amblyopia is unknown. The child with amblyopia has no way of knowing that he or she is not seeing properly, but the vision is decreased by the fact that the child is allowing one eye to do most of the work. With a diagnosis of amblyopia, treatment may include patching the stronger eye (often for several months) to encourage use of the affected eye, wearing glasses, doing eye exercises, and occasionally eye-muscle surgery may be necessary. The younger the child when treatment is begun, the greater is the possibility of the success of treatment. Strabismus may interfere with learning to read.

It is therefore important that caretakers and other responsible adults be aware of the signs of possible eye problems in the young child. Some of these behaviors include the child's rubbing the eyes or blinking excessively, squinting, appearing irritable when playing games that require good distance vision, shutting or covering one eye, and tilting the head or thrusting it forward when looking at something. If any of these behaviors are present, the child should be examined by an ophthalmologist.

The Ear. The external ear canal in the child who is less than 3 years of age approaches the internal canal at an oblique upward angle. (For this reason, when ear drops are instilled in a child this age, the pinna should be held down and back to straighten the external canal and thus facilitate the flow of the medication [26]). Occasionally, either a middle ear infection or inflammation may occur; such a condition must be treated because it can cause reduced hearing or, in some cases, permanent deafness. Sometimes the middle-ear becomes filled with a serous fluid, which is caused by blockage of the eustachian tube and consequent negative pressure in the middle-ear cavity. In most cases, decongestants prescribed by a physician will aid in resolving the condition [4]. When a middle-ear infection has been caused by pathological bacteria (usually traveling through the short, wide eustachian tube after causing an upper respiratory infection), the doctor may prescribe an antibiotic. If the condition persists and the fluid becomes viscous, the tympanic membrane (eardrum) may need to be surgically incised to facilitate drainage of the fluid. When drainage is insufficient, polyethylene tubes are inserted through the membrane to aid the drainage and thus facilitate healing [26]. These tubes remain in place for several weeks; then, at the discretion of the pediatrician, they are either removed or are simply allowed to fall out spontaneously.

The Taste Buds. The taste buds become more sensitive to the natural flavors of foods during these years. Cognitive processes aid in discrimination of various flavors. By toddlerhood, children are already learning which foods they prefer and which tastes are preferred by those whose culture they share. Preschoolers soon volunteer their advice (and thus assert their initiative) by asking for something that tastes "yummy" and requesting that something else be totally removed from their presence because it tastes "yucky."

The Nose. The capacity to smell, which is closely linked to taste, is also influenced by voluntary control, cultural attitudes, and cognitive development. Usually young children do not mind and may even like body odors. Gradually, they assume the attitudes of the family and the culture toward these odors. Some cultures find body odors quite acceptable while others consider them to be unpleasant or even offensive. Children may initially respond to odors in an uninhibited manner as they learns the taboos, but not the social graces, for handling the situation. They may make faces, laugh, tease, act sick, hold their nose, or rebuke the offender (to the embarrassment of any adult in the situation).

Musculoskeletal System

Many of the changing body proportions mentioned earlier are the direct result of growth of the child's musculoskeletal system. The child's appearance is slowly becoming more adultlike.

MUSCLE

Muscle grows faster than bone during the toddler and preschool years. Actual muscle strength (the amount of force exerted by a contracting muscle) appears to be correlated with the amount of muscle tissue (mass) [29]. Genetic inheritance, nutritional intake, and the opportunity to use the muscles all play a role in how strong a child will be.

SKELETON

Ossification slows after infancy but continues until early adulthood. From infancy to 4 years of age, the child's long-shafted bones contain red marrow, which is capable of blood cell production. From 4 to 7 years, this active marrow is gradually replaced by fatty tis-

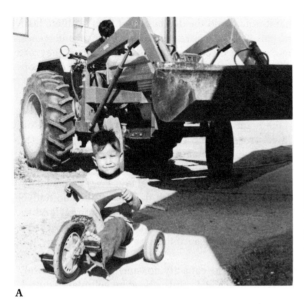

A

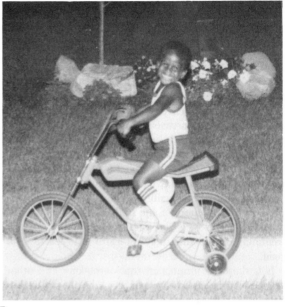

B

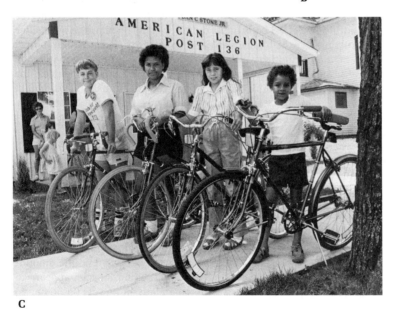

C

Figure 10–1. The progress of motor control is apparent when one compares (A) the young toddler resting on a mini-cycle and (B) the older preschooler steering a bicycle (note that this child still has training wheels). (C) Once the skills are mastered, they are further refined and become a tool for socialization.

sue, eventually leaving red marrow only in pelvic bones, the sternum (breastbone), vertebrae, and some skull and short-shafted bones [15].

CHEST
The child's chest has become less cylindrical by 1 year of age and approximates the adult thoracic shape at age 6 years [15]. This change greatly aids the child's ability to expand the lungs fully when taking deep breaths.

LEGS AND FEET
The legs and the feet of toddlers and preschoolers grow more rapidly than their trunks. A bowed appearance of the legs, which is common in infancy, will probably be noticeable if the baby walks before 1 year of age. It

is usually during the second year that the small-shafted bones rotate and gradually straighten the toddler's legs [3]. Surfaces such as padded playpens and shag carpeting may contribute to awkward stances, gaits, and walking habits in toddling babies. Such surfaces cause babies to separate their feet, turn them outward, and rest on the medial sides of the feet.

To facilitate balance, the infant just learning to walk generally rotates the whole foot outward and keeps a wide distance between the feet. Some infants have a pronounced longitudinal arch before they walk; others who appear to have no arch before walking later develop a normal arch during the toddler years [15, 26]. To decrease the possibility of flatfoot, a youngster should not be urged to walk until he or she is able to pull to a standing position (and thus not strain the developing arches). Walking barefoot during these early years can help to develop the foot arch [15, 28]. There is some evidence that indicates the wearing of shoes is unnecessary until the baby is walking [21]. Even after a child is walking, Spock states that there is real value in leaving the child barefoot much of the time when the weather is warm and the walking surfaces are safe [28].

Properly fitting footwear is essential to aid growth and development of the child's lower extremities, posture, and walking habits. Socks, booties, and shoes should be at least one-half inch longer than the toes. There should also be one-quarter inch between the edge of the little toe and the lateral edge of the shoe when the heel is snug against the back of the shoe. Infants and very young children ordinarily need no heel lift; it is usually not until school age that the child requires a one-half-inch heel [8]. High-top shoes are not necessary to support the walking child's ankles and may in some cases actually impede the child's mobility. But in some cases they may be desirable because it is difficult to fit the heel snugly enough to prevent slipping without at the same time making the shoe too tight [15].

As a child learns to walk, the toes may turn in for several different reasons. The upper long-shafted bone (femur) may still be internally rotated if the walking baby is under 1 year of age. If the baby begins to walk after the age of 15 months, toeing-in may be the result of internal torsion of the same bones that cause bowing [3]. Orthopedic consultation is needed for most cases of toeing-in or "pigeon-toeing." As the child grows taller, the knees are brought nearer together. If at the same time the lower ends of the short-shafted bones or ankled joints (malleoli) rotate externally to give the child a wider base, developmental knock-knee

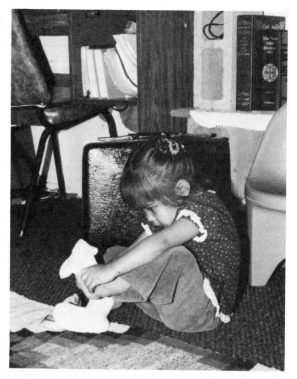

Figure 10–2. Although not yet able to tie, zip, snap, or button, the toddler takes great pride in his or her ability to put on socks and shoes.

(genu valgum) is the result. The incidence of knock-knee is at its peak between 3 and 3½ years of age, which can lead to frequent stumbling and falling. The ankle joints begin to reverse this rotation during the fourth and fifth years. Spontaneous correction is seen in many children between the ages of 5 and 7 years [3].

Most babies learn to walk during the first half of the second year. Children who have not begun to walk unaided by the age of 18 months should be assessed by a team of health professionals. Walking encourages the child's sense of autonomy and expands the opportunities to learn about the environment.

MOTOR FUNCTIONING
Although walking is a major developmental milestone, it is only one of the many motor functions acquired during the toddler and preschool years. Table 10–1 gives examples of the normal sequence of various gross and fine motor skills.

Table 10–1. Neuromotor Development during the Toddler and Preschool Years

Gross Motor Skills	Fine Motor Skills
18 months Runs, with less falling; climbs; pulls toys and large objects, followed soon by pushing them; throws small balls, with minimal directionality; walks up or down stairs with adult holding hand; rolls large ball on floor.	Puts blocks in large holes, rings on peg, or beads into bottle; scribbles and may attempt straight lines; can drink from a cup without much spilling; still has frequent spills in getting spoon contents properly inserted into mouth; unzips large zipper; unties bow by pulling string; builds a tower of four to five blocks.
2 years Tries to jump; can walk up and down stairs, without adult help, holding on to a handrail or using wall for support; sits self in small chair; puts on coat with assistance; throws large ball with both hands.	Can line blocks horizontally to make a train; can turn reachable doorknobs; can imitate a vertical stroke while scribbling; can drink from a small cup, using only one hand; still spills liquids (e.g., soup, milk) from spoon when eating; turns pages of a book one at a time; unbuttons large button; builds tower of six to seven blocks.
2½ years Rides various forms of "kiddie" cars; can stand on one foot alone for at least 1 second; can throw a large ball about 5 feet; can walk on tiptoe; jumps in place; can pick up objects from floor without losing balance; gets down from adult chair without assistance; catches soft object with both arms and body.	Is able to make a tower of nine large blocks; still likes to fill containers with objects; will disassemble objects; can take off socks and other easy-to-manipulate clothing; zips large zipper with help; snaps large snap; buttons large button; moves fingers and thumb separately in imitation games; twists caps off bottles; places simple shapes in correct holes.
3 years Pedals a tricycle; jumps from a low step; can go to toilet unaided; can get undressed in most situations; can go up and down stairs using alternating feet without holding on; throws large ball with one hand; can put on own coat without assistance; catches soft object with both arms.	Begins to use blunt scissors; strings large beads on shoelace; can copy a circle; can help with simple household tasks (dusting, picking up); can wash and dry hands, with some wetting of clothes; can brush teeth, but not adequately; can imitate a bridge made of three blocks; can pull pants up and down for toileting without assistance.
3½ years Skips on one foot; hops forward on both feet; runs well without falling; kicks large ball; twists upper body while holding feet in one place; uses hands to get up from floor; catches soft object with hands; catches large ball with arms.	Can cut straight lines with scissors without tearing paper; manipulates pieces into position for simple puzzles; can weave yarn randomly through a card; places small pegs in pegboard; unbuttons small button; can eat from spoon without spilling.
4 years Jumps well; hops forward on one foot; may catch a large bounced ball with hands; walks backward; catches soft object with one hand; catches small ball with arms.	Cuts around pictures with scissors; can copy a square; can button small buttons; may bathe self, with assistance; folds napkin into a triangle or a rectangle; outlines a picture with yarn.
5 years Can jump rope; runs lightly on toes; alternates feet to skip; gets up without using hands; catches small ball with two hands.	May be able to print own name; copies a triangle; dresses without assistance; may be able to lace shoes; can put toys away neatly; bathes self; threads small beads on a string; eats with fork.

HANDEDNESS

Whether a child's hand preference (handedness) is hereditary or the result of training and social conditioning has been debated for many generations. Scientists are still trying to piece together the relationship among handedness, cerebral dominance, and the ability of the individual to read, to write, and to speak. Does a right-handed person have an advantage in these areas? If so, why? How and when do the left and right sides of the cerebrum develop? Why does it appear, on the basis of the design of their primitive tools, that the people of the Stone Age had no preferred hand? Why are so many people right-handed today? These and many other related questions are still the subject of research. Between 2½ and 3½ years of age, many children demonstrate bilaterality in the use of their hands. The predominance of the unilateral function of the body (which includes handedness) is usually fully established by about 4 years of age. Left-handed children need to have appropriate tools available for their use—especially scissors. Children should be encouraged to use their dominant side, since coordination is usually better. Children also need to develop the motor coordination pathways during preschool years so that they can concentrate on the end product rather than the use of the hands per se.

Integumentary System

The skin, as a sensory and a protective organ, continues to develop during the toddler and preschool years. Children enjoy closing their eyes and identifying different objects by their various shapes and textures (stereognosis). Contact with different textures, positions, and temperatures all help the child to become more aware of body shape and body space. Most toddlers and preschoolers still like to be near to, and hugged by, significant others if they are in the mood, and especially when they need to "refuel" (See Chap. 12). Rubbing the child's body with powder or lotion and drawing simple shapes on the child's back with a finger can help with perceptual discrimination.

The child's skin is not as soft as it was during infancy, since it is changing from a delicate tissue with a high water content to a tougher, more resistant type of skin. A decrease in skin rashes may be noted. The frequency of eruptions due to contact irritants (e.g., harsh detergents) also declines during toddlerhood. A minimal amount of sebum is secreted during toddlerhood and preschoolerhood, making the skin rather dry. Baby lotion may be especially helpful in maintaining the integrity of the skin when it is exposed to drying weather conditions. On the other hand, the skin is better protected from the harsh rays of the sun during the preschool years because the activity of the melanin-forming cells has increased compared to their production during infancy [29]. During the preschool years, the hair grows thicker and may lose some curliness, and it often darkens. Fine hair appears on the lower arms and legs.

Respiratory System

As the lungs grow in size, their volume, and thus the capacity for oxygenation, increases. The respiratory rate decreases because the lungs are relatively more efficient than they were in infancy. Respirations remain primarily diaphragmatic until the child's fifth or sixth year [15]. The bifurcation of the trachea (airway) into the smaller bronchi (branches of the airway) is situated farther down in the chest, so that choking on food particles that could potentially lodge in this part

of the airway while eating is less likely to occur. The epiglottis, a flaplike, cartilaginous structure that closes over the opening to the trachea when the child is swallowing, also slowly descends after infancy. The epiglottis is so high in the chest during infancy that it can be seen through the baby's open mouth [15]. The tonsils and the adenoids increase in size but do not need to be removed so long as they are functional (protecting the child from serious infections) and are not causing obstruction or pressure.

Cardiovascular System

THE HEART

By the time the child is 5 years old, the heart has increased its weight fourfold [15]. The decrease in heart rate (pulse) that normally occurs during early childhood is generally thought to be closely related to the increase in the size of the heart. The larger heart can pump blood with more force and more efficiency than it could when the child was younger. As the pulse decreases, the blood pressure changes (see Appendix E). Through all these maturational changes, both toddlers and especially the preschoolers increase their capacity for more continuous and strenuous physical exercise.

THERMOREGULATION

As the child grows, the capillaries (small blood vessels) become more efficient by constricting in response to cold and dilating in response to heat. Shivering is now much more effective in producing body heat than it was during early infancy. It is also during this time that neural control becomes more integrated so that the child is capable of independent, self-help activities (e.g., taking off a coat, getting under the covers, asking for mittens).

BLOOD VALUES

As long as the child consumes a proper dietary amount of iron during the toddler and preschool years, adequate levels of hemoglobin will be maintained. These hemoglobin needs increase slightly above the levels required in late infancy. Thus, a slightly higher red blood cell count is needed in spite of the more efficient pumping action of the heart. Conversely, the number of white blood cells needed has decreased because their quality has improved. Therefore, the child's natural ability to fight infection and disease is increased.

Immune System

To understand how resistance develops, it is helpful to review the normal functioning and development of the immune system. The immune system must first recognize "self" from "non-self" and then initiate responses to eliminate the "non-self," (antigens or foreign substances) from the body. Antigens are usually protein in nature and are viewed by the body as an attacking force. When the body is attacked by antigens (e.g., bacteria, viruses, substances that elicit allergic responses), it has three ways of defending itself: the phagocytic immune response, the humoral (antibody) immune response, and the cellular immune response.

The first line of defense, the phagocytic immune response, involves the white blood cells, which have the ability to ingest and digest foreign particles. These phagocytes can move to the point of attack to destroy the foreign agents. This form of immunity is often called a nonspecific immune defense because the phagocytes are activated on exposure to **any** foreign substance. The other two mechanisms of defense are specific immune responses because they have the ability to recognize specific antigens and respond selectively.

Humoral immunity, which is the major protective defense mechanism of the body, is involved with antibody production. The primary cell involved in antibody production is the B-lymphocyte. The exact site of B-lymphocyte production in humans is unknown, although some evidence suggests that it is in the bone marrow. B-lymphocytes, when challenged by an antigen, produce and secrete large quantities of antibodies specific to the antigen. Five types of antibodies, or immunoglobulins, have been identified: IgG (gamma G), IgM, IgA, IgD, and IgE.

When initially exposed to an antigen, the B-lymphocyte system begins to produce antibodies, predominantly IgM, which appear in 2 to 3 days. This process is called the primary antibody response.

With subsequent exposure to the same antigen, a secondary antibody response occurs. Antibody, chiefly IgG, is produced in much greater quantities within 1 to 2 days. The immune system can thus recognize the same antigen for months, years, or indefinitely.

IgG is the only class of immunoglobulin capable of crossing the placental barrier and does so at an increased rate toward the end of gestation. IgA is the predominant immunoglobulin in colostrum and breast milk. When an antibody reacts with an antigen, they bind and form an antigen-antibody complex, a compound that is more readily destroyed by phagocytes.

A third protective response, the cellular immune response, is a function of the T-lymphocyte, so named because it is produced in the thymus gland. In contrast to humoral immunity, which can be transferred from one person to another by plasma transfusions, cellular immunity depends on the presence of immune cells.

The cellular immune response is initiated when a T-lymphocyte is sensitized by an antigen. In response to this contact, the T-lymphocyte releases lymphokines, which eventually kill the antigen. One type of lymphokine, interferon, is currently being researched as a treatment for selected types of cancer.

The defense mechanisms of the toddler and preschooler, especially the phagocytes, are much more efficient than they were in the infant. IgG reaches adult levels by the time the child is 2 years old. IgM attains adult levels during late infancy. Levels of IgA, IgD, and IgE gradually increase, reaching adult values in later childhood.

Gastrointestinal System

SALIVARY GLANDS

By the end of the second year, the child's salivary glands are adult-sized and have reached functional maturity [7]. The child is capable of chewing food, so that it stays longer in the mouth, and the salivary enzymes have an opportunity to begin breaking down the food. The saliva also covers the teeth with a protective film that helps prevent decay [29]. The drooling that began in infancy should no longer be present after 2 years; by this time the toddler should have learned to swallow saliva and to keep the lips closed when not speaking or eating.

STOMACH

The secretion of hydrochloric acid continues to increase during early childhood, raising the acidity of the child's gastric juices, but adult levels are not present until puberty [7]. The acidity of the stomach contents has a protective function in that it destroys many types of bacteria. The child's stomach is able to hold approximately 500 ml (almost 17 ounces) by 2 years of age, and 750 to 900 ml (25 to 30 ounces) in later childhood [15]. These increases allow the child to assume a schedule of three meals a day. However, between-meal snacks are very important to prevent low blood sugar due to prolonged fasting.

BOWEL

Sometime during the child's second or third year, the child becomes physically ready to control the eliminative functions of the bowel and the bladder. This physical readiness for toilet training is discussed later in this chapter.

Genitourinary System

GENITALS

The genital organs continue to increase in size but not in function during the early childhood years. The seminiferous tubules of the testes develop their passageways (lumens) and increase in size during childhood. Immature sperm are also experiencing both hyperplastic and hypertrophic growth during these years [15].

It is not uncommon for girls between the ages of 2 and 6 years to have skin adhesions between the inner lips of the vagina (labia minora). These adhesions may be caused by irritation, mild infection, or a nonpathological delay in hormonal influence [15]. Consistent, thorough cleaning and perhaps an occasional separating of the labia minora (usually by the caretaker) may resolve the problem.

A bubble bath can serve as an irritant to the urethra of the young female, causing inflammation that may quickly lead to an infection. It is not uncommon for females under 5 years of age to complain of itching and burning, especially on urination, in the genitourinary area when this infection is present. In such cases the child should be seen and evaluated by a doctor, especially since the infection can spread to the rest of the urinary tract as well as to the vagina [30].

KIDNEYS

By the child's second birthday, the kidneys are able to conserve water under normal conditions and to concentrate urine on a level that approximates adult capabilities [29]. This efficiency is due in part to the filtering membranes of the kidneys, which have become thinner and are therefore more mature. The kidneys are now capable of adequately responding to antidiuretic hormone (ADH) and are producing a more concentrated urine. Since the urine composition does not change significantly once the child becomes a toddler, and because, among other things, it reflects kidney functioning, a urinalysis (chemical examination of the urine) should be initiated at this time and continued periodically through the lifetime.

BLADDER

The capacity of the bladder to hold urine increases during toddlerhood. At 2½ years of age, the average bladder will hold approximately 85 ml (3 ounces) [11]. The child will only experience and respond to a feeling of bladder fullness. The ability of the child to remain dry for at least 2 hours during the day indicates readiness for the toilet-training process. A further discussion of toilet training can be found later in this chapter. Occasional accidents still occur after toilet training is complete because the child, engrossed in play, is not aware of the signs of a full bladder until it is too late.

URETHRA

Under certain conditions, bacteria can ascend the urethra and cause an infection in any portion of the urinary tract. In males, the length of the urethra usually proves to be effective in preventing such infections. In females, however, the urethra is less than 2 cm in length [26], and it opens directly into an area that can easily be contaminated by poor hygiene practices. Females of all ages should wipe themselves from front to back, toward the rectum. Education to prevent contamination is essential. Diapers (even the disposables) and panties (including any soiled clothing) should be changed when wet. Swimming or playing in heated pools and hot tubs for prolonged periods of time may predispose young females to irritation or infection. Cleanliness and prompt drying of the genital area decrease the incidence of infection. Panties with a cotton crotch aid the circulation of air to this area and thus decrease the susceptibility to infection.

Endocrine System

GLANDULAR SECRETION

The endocrine system continues to increase its functioning during the early childhood years. The secretions of the pancreas and the liver, which aid in the digestive process, are functioning at an adult level. Variations in blood sugar still occur because of the labile production of insulin and glucagon. As the child grows, the ability to cope biophysically with stress is increased by more effective adrenal medullar secretion.

Several hormones are vital to normal growth and development during these years; among these are the thyroid hormones and pituitary growth hormone (PGH). The production of hormones, especially aldosterone, by the adrenal cortex remains relatively limited. The adrenal cortex, however, does increase production enough to give the toddler and preschooler more protection against fluid and electrolyte imbalance than during infancy.

FLUID AND ELECTROLYTE BALANCE

By the end of the second year, the total body water of the child is approximately 60 percent of body weight [19]. Although this figure approximates the adult percentage, the distribution of intracellular and extracellular fluids is different. During toddlerhood, about 35 percent of this water is contained within the cells and about 27 percent is outside the cells (compared to 47 and 20 percent, respectively, in the adult) [21]. The toddler is still vulnerable to fluid volume deficits because of the relatively greater extracellular fluid to exchange. The high metabolic rate results in large amounts of wastes to be excreted, and the endocrine system is still not functioning at maximal capacity. The child, therefore, requires more fluid per unit of body weight in a 24-hour period than does an adult. By the time the child is 5 years old, the electrolyte blood concentrations are essentially equal to those of an adult.

Dentition

When the child is between the ages of 18 months and 2 years, the sharp-pointed canine teeth (cuspids) erupt. The last four deciduous teeth to appear are usually the second molars, and they do so shortly after the second birthday. Their appearance completes the set of 20 deciduous teeth. Teeth are like icebergs: much goes on underneath the surface—in this case, within the gums. The mere emergence of a tooth does not mean that its development is complete. The root of the tooth is still growing and developing for several months after its emergence [29].

At the end of the preschool years, the deciduous teeth begin to loosen and fall out; the central incisors are usually the first to go. Premature loss of deciduous teeth may affect the alignment of permanent teeth; therefore, dental consultation should be sought.

MAINTAINING HEALTH

Nutrition

The total caloric intake of toddlers and preschoolers when compared to adult norms is relatively low. Approximately 1300 calories per day are needed by the toddler, and 1800 calories are required by the preschooler. The actual amount of calories needed per unit of body weight decreases during these years because toddlers and preschoolers are growing less rapidly than they did as infants. However, since several portions of the body (e.g., muscles) are still growing quite rapidly, protein needs remain high. The 1 to 3-year-old requires 1.8 gm of protein per kilogram of body weight per day; the 4 to 6-year-old needs 1.5 gm per kilogram. One-half of this protein should be of animal origin to ensure adequate intake of amino acids, B-complex vitamins, vitamin D, iron, and calcium.

Calcium recommendations for these growing children are 800 mg per day, or two to four times the adult daily intake. Both calcium and phosphorus are important for this age group, owing to the increased mineralization taking place within their teeth and bones. Although milk is also a good source of protein, phosphorus, and calcium, too much milk will decrease the child's appetite for other foods and can thus lead to anemia.

The actual portion sizes of foods that a child this age should consume daily do not directly correspond to the popular adult servings of the basic four food groups. Table 10–2 lists realistic portions of food needed by toddlers and preschoolers to promote nutritional high level wellness during early childhood. Food habits vary from one child (and one family) to another. Few children conform to eating three meals per day; preschool children eat an average of five to seven times per day [23].

Pediatricians and other health professionals vary in their opinions as to whether or not toddlers and preschoolers should take daily vitamins. The child who is not consuming an adequate daily diet should certainly take them, but a vitamin pill should not be an excuse to replace good eating habits. Some doctors believe that a child should remain on a daily vitamin pill (often with iron or fluoride supplementation) until completion of the "too-busy-to-eat" toddlerhood years.

The child's liver has been capable of storing fat-soluble vitamins (e.g., vitamins A and D) since infancy. Consequently, excess quantities may lead to toxicity or poisoning; therefore, multiple doses of vitamins should not be given to a child even if the child is a picky eater. Water-soluble vitamins—the B vitamins and vitamin C—are not stored in excess in the body. It is thought that large amounts of water-soluble vitamins are merely passed from the body, primarily in the urine [23].

Some children experience adverse effects (such as headaches or hyperactivity) when they ingest cane sugar or artificial color. Such foods would be considered an allergen and should be removed from the diet. (See Chap. 22 for a discussion of allergies).

Vitamin supplements come in tasty chewable forms and as fruit-flavored liquids but should be treated like all other forms of medicine: They should have child-proof caps and should be placed out of the reach of climbing, curious children.

Dental Care

Since infants and young children do not have the manual dexterity necessary to clean their teeth thoroughly, their parents must assume responsibility for their oral hygiene. The task of cleaning the oral cavity can be divided into four steps: staining, brushing, flossing, and inspection [13].

Table 10–2. Average Food Intake for Young Children[a]

Food	Portion Size	Number of Portions Advised	
		2–4 yrs	4–6 yrs
Milk and dairy products			
Milk[b]	4 oz	3–6	3–4
Cheese	½–¾ oz	May be substituted for 1 portion of liquid milk	
Yogurt	¼–½ cup	May be substituted for 1 portion of liquid milk	
Powdered skim milk	2 tbsp	May be substituted for 1 portion of liquid milk	
Meat and meat equivalents			
Meat,[c] fish,[d] poultry	1–2 oz	2	2
Egg	1	1	1
Peanut butter	1–2 tbsp		
Legumes (dried peas and beans)	¼–⅓ cup cooked		
Vegetables and fruits			
Vegetables[e]		4–5, including 1 green leafy or yellow	
Cooked	2–4 tbsp		
Raw	Few pieces		
Fruit		1 citrus fruit or other vegetable or fruit rich in vitamin C	
Canned	4–8 tbsp		
Raw	½–1 small		
Fruit juice	3–4 oz		
Bread and cereal grains			
Whole grain or enriched white bread	½–1 slice	3	3
Cooked cereal	¼–½ cup	May be substituted for 1 serving of bread	
Ready-to-serve dry cereals	½–1 cup		
Spaghetti, macaroni, noodles, rice	¼–½ cup		
Crackers	2–3		
Fat			
Bacon	1 slice	Not to be substituted for meat	
Butter or vitamin A-fortified margarine	1 tsp	3	3–4
Desserts	¼–½ cup	As demanded by caloric needs	
Sugars	½–1 tsp	2	2

[a]Diets should also be monitored for adequacy of iron and vitamin D intake.
[b]Approximately ⅔ cup can easily be incorporated in a child's food during cooking.
[c]Liver once a week can be served as liver sausage or cooked liver.
[d]Should be served once or twice per week to substitute for meat.
[e]If a child's preferences are limited, use double portions of preferred vegetables until appetite for other vegetables develops.
Source: Adapted from P. L. Pipes, *Nutrition in Infancy and Childhood*. St. Louis: Mosby, 1981.

STAINING

A disclosing agent is helpful in identifying those areas of the teeth where plaque accumulates. It also helps to motivate children to clean their teeth because plaque is otherwise difficult to see.

BRUSHING

It is important to encourage the child to become involved with personal oral hygiene early. The child less than 6 to 8 years of age should be given the opportunity to practice using the toothbrush, but the parent should inspect and provide additional cleaning where needed. During the period when both primary and permanent teeth are present, the child may hesitate to clean the teeth thoroughly because of the discomfort associated with cleaning the spaces created by lost teeth. Brushing after every meal is ideal. It is best to brush each time the child is given liquid medication since most of these preparations contain large quantities of sugar to make them more palatable [31].

FLOSSING

Careful brushing will not clean the areas where the teeth are in contact with one another; these areas can only be reached with dental floss. Again, parents must assist young children with this procedure. It should begin as soon as two teeth are side-by-side. Some dentists claim that unwaxed floss cleans most effectively because its fibers separate to spread over a larger surface and there is no danger of depositing wax during the flossing procedure.

INSPECTION

Inspecting the teeth is the final step performed (usually by a parent) to ensure that all plaque has been removed. Good lighting is essential.

Sleep

Toddlers and preschoolers expend a great deal of energy in growing, learning, and just acting their age; thus, adequate rest and sleep are essential for high level wellness. The toddler requires an average of 12 hours of sleep each night in addition to a daytime nap. Preschoolers need 11 to 12 hours of sleep in a 24-hour period. It is important for parents to realize that preschool children vary widely in the amount of sleep they require. Some children function well with 8 hours of sleep while others require 14 hours [9, 10].

The younger preschooler may not want to sleep during naptime, especially if the child slept well the previous night. Many need a quiet period of rest, however, to give them the necessary energy to carry out their daily activities. This period of rest might include the child's lying quietly and listening to favorite music or reading a preschool book. Without adequate rest periods during the day, the child can readily become fatigued, which may lead to irritability, poor resistance to infection, and restless nighttime sleep.

Exercise, Practice, and Instruction

The emergence of many of the child's motor skills are largely a matter of growth and development, but the child needs the opportunity, the environment, and the encouragement to engage in sufficient gross motor and fine motor activities to learn how the body works and what can be done with it. Children without this experience have a poor concept of body boundaries, body space, or spatial relationships. Many simple movements (e.g., jumping and running) require little instruction or coaching.

Other more complicated motor skills (e.g., swimming, skating, gymnastics, dancing, playing a violin or piano) require more formal instruction. Many older preschoolers are enrolled in such activities. Although early exposure to, and practice of, these more complicated skills may give children an advantage in their

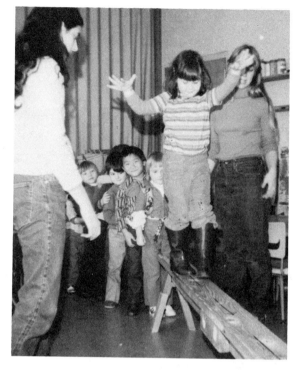

Figure 10–3. Exercise promotes biophysical growth and can aid the child in acquiring a sense of initiative.

performance, it is important for parents to remember some important concepts about the child's motor skills, feelings, and interests that are essential for the child's bio-psychosocial wellness:

1. The child must have achieved a minimal physical size and neurological maturity.
2. The child should be interested in the subject. The parents should not be reliving their childhood days or trying to realize their own unfulfilled dreams.
3. The child must possess enough motivation and self-discipline to "stick with it," and should not be forced or frequently bribed to participate.
4. The child should be given frequent periods of rest if the activity requires intense performance, whether physical, cognitive, or psychosocial in nature.
5. The parents should be familiar with the health and the safety policies of the program [27].
6. The parents should ascertain the goals and the qualifications of the adults in the program [27]. It is helpful to observe the behavior of these adults with the children: how they reward behavior, give guidance, and interact with the children in general.

Health Assessment

Periodic health assessments are a necessity for young children. The child from 18 to 30 months of age should visit a health professional every 3 months. Checkups scheduled every 6 to 12 months are usually sufficient during the preschool years. The child's ability to hear should be tested during these sessions; testing methods vary from technical audiometric methods to whispering to ascertain how well the child hears.

The Snellen charts with letters of different sizes are used to determine visual acuity. Visual acuity refers to the ability to see near and far objects clearly. The Snellen charts consist of nine lines of letters in decreasing size. Each line is given a value; for example, line eight has a value of 20. The individual to be tested stands 20 feet from the chart and reads each line. If line eight can be read, then the person has 20/20 vision, the accepted standard for normal mature acuity. If only line two can be read, the person has 20/100 vision. This individual can see only at 20 feet what the individual with 20/20 vision can see from 100 feet. Younger children may simply be asked to indicate which direction the three legs of the letter E are pointing (using the Snellen illiterate E chart). The National Society for the Prevention of Blindness recommends the following criteria for referring children when using the Snellen charts [32]:

1. Three-year-old children with vision in either eye of 20/50 or less (inability to read the 40 foot line)
2. Children 4 years of age and older with vision in either eye of 20/40 or less (inability to read the 30 foot line)
3. Children with a one-line difference or more between the two eyes, even if visual acuity is between passing standards
4. All children who consistently show any of the signs of possible visual disturbances regardless of visual acuity

The Rader Visual Acuity Screening Chart uses "happy face" and "sad face" to assess the visual acuity of the younger preschool child. Several other tests exist for screening infants and toddlers for visual acuity, fixation, squinting, and strabismus.

Motor functioning and reflex performance are also tested during health visits. One of the reflexes that persist throughout life is the popular knee jerk, which is elicited by tapping the knee with a medical hammer. The child's pupils should constrict when a flashlight is beamed into the eyes [7]. Several other assessments are performed on the child, since every human function—biophysical, cognitive, and psychosocial—is controlled by neural impulses.

Every child 3 years of age and older should have the blood pressure taken at least annually [26]. In the United States, high blood pressure is being diagnosed in children of all ages with an increasing frequency. The problems that lead to high blood pressure may be prevented by teaching the child and counseling the parents on stress reduction, weight control, salt intake, and exercise.

The child should visit the dentist again when all 20 deciduous teeth have emerged. It is best that the child meet the dentist and see the dental equipment while the child is feeling no pain. The child should receive a simple explanation from parents on what to expect before this visit and each subsequent dental checkup. There are several colorful picture-story books written especially for children that describe what to expect when they go to the dentist. The early visits are a time for an assessment of the oral hygiene practices followed at home. Dental visits are encouraged every 6 months after the initial checkup. There are dentists who specialize in the care of young children (pedodontists); other dentists may be highly recommended to parents as being able to work well with children.

The American Foot Care Institute recommends that the sock and shoe sizes of a child who is 2 to 6 years old be carefully checked every 1 to 2 months [8]. Since one foot is often significantly larger than the other, both feet should be measured. The rapid growth of the child's feet may require the purchase of new shoes every 3 to 4 months.

COMMON CONCERNS IN EARLY CHILDHOOD

Feeding and Eating Habits

Most parents worry if their child does not appear to eat much. Some caretakers are concerned about the nutritional content of the foods that the child consumes, while others emphasize a concern for developing appropriate eating habits. All of these concerns, when combined with the normal decrease in appetite and food intake of the developing child, can potentially precipitate both situational and maturational crises. A situational crisis can arise if caretakers force foods and eating habits on a nonconforming child. This situation, in turn, if handled inappropriately over a period of time, can stifle and distort the child's desire for independence and assertiveness. An understanding of the normal sequence of a child's growth and development can aid immensely in assisting the parents to help the child to establish acceptable eating habits. Parent education, caretaker patience, and time are all that is usually needed to prevent major crises.

STRATEGIES THAT ENCOURAGE
NUTRITIOUS EATING

Eating can become an excellent medium through which the child tests the boundaries of what is deemed acceptable behavior. A knowledge of normal growth and development can be used to maximize the eating habits of the toddler and preschooler. For example, the child who is walking is capable of seeking his or her own food, which has implications for the caretakers: It means that foods such as raisins, bananas, and cheese squares can be made available for young children to find (as opposed to mints in candy dishes or bowls of potato chips). Giving the child a cup that is half full will lessen the probability of spilling (and thus the possibility of a feeling of shame in the child). Pieces of meat should be relatively moist (not extremely well done, since this makes the meat tougher to chew) because the deciduous teeth (or lack of them) are not as capable of grinding as are the permanent teeth. Some 4-year-olds begin to develop the skill of cutting their food into bite-size pieces, but they still need assistance for a period of time [23]. Sandwiches cut into quarters are popular with children. Soup can be drunk from a cup or thickened for spooning to make eating a more positive experience for the child.

Many of the strategies that help adults to enjoy eating are effective with children. Most children are more likely to eat foods with which they are familiar; it is therefore advisable to introduce new foods one at a time in smaller portions. Simple pieces of raw vegetables are easier to manipulate in the beginning than salads with drippy dressings. Children, like adults, enjoy a variety of foods, including varieties of texture, flavor, and color, although extremes in tastes are not palatable to the young child, who has an acute sense of taste. Natural fruit juices should be offered to the child rather than sweetened, colored, and artificially flavored drinks.

PATTERNS OF EATING

Idiosyncratic eating patterns or "food jags" are common throughout early childhood. The child may indicate a dislike for a food he or she appeared to relish yesterday. Rituals often become important to the child's eating; for example, one special bowl may be preferred by the child when eating a certain brand of cereal. Both the toddler and the preschooler frequently eat differing amounts of food at each meal. The child may eat virtually nothing (in the parents' estimation) during one meal. The evening meal, usually the time of much social interaction, can be a time when the child has difficulty combining the eating of adequate amounts of food and conversing at the same time. Since this social interaction is beneficial to growth, it is wiser to decrease boisterous frivolities at the table than to eliminate totally the social gathering for the evening meal.

The length of intervals between meals varies from one child to the next. Most growing children need a nutritious snack to tide them over between meals and perhaps at bedtime. However, it is not wise to allow a child to eat a rich or a heavy snack when a regular meal is scheduled within the next hour.

Young children, especially toddlers, tend to dawdle during their eating. As a result, they should be allowed at least 30 to 40 minutes to consume a meal, no matter what time of the day it is (or in how much of a hurry the parents are).

Sleep Routines

Establishing healthy sleeping patterns in the toddler and preschooler may also become a major concern for caretakers. The young child is reluctant to give up an exciting day's activities and to depart from loved ones to go off to a darkened room and do nothing but lie down and remain still. By age 2, the child may have perfected subtle skills of protest against going to bed at night (and perhaps against taking a nap as well). The child may want to hug the parent again and again while sitting on his or her lap or may want one more drink of water. The sky is the limit as to what a child can conjure up to avoid somnolence.

By age 2½, the child may add a ritualistic repertoire to the bedtime performance. These rituals range from simply desiring to take a favorite toy to bed to kissing family members good night in a certain order and only if they are sitting in their "assigned" seats when the kissing is done. Some parents are more patient than others and some children are more demanding than others. Parent-child tensions may increase at the bedtime hours unless a satisfactory balance is found. Anticipating the child's demands and meeting as many of them as possible (within limits) will usually decrease the length of the bedtime preparation (e.g., giving the child a favorite toy, offering a few sips of water, taking a trip to the bathroom, turning on a night light, putting on a quiet record, and perhaps leaving the bedroom door ajar to prevent feelings of isolation).

Children respond to parental firmness and soon

learn that they must go to sleep. Occasionally, parents simply have to allow the child to cry. In his *Baby and Child Care* [28], Spock offers hints for helping youngsters to sleep. Brazelton's *Toddlers and Parents* [6] also provides enjoyable and informative reading about this topic.

By the time a child is 4 years of age, many of the bedtime difficulties have disappeared. The child usually has graduated to a big bed. Many preschoolers fall asleep with relative ease if they are allowed a quiet time before they sleep (some prefer to be alone, others enjoy a brief interaction with a family member). However, even with quiet-time preparation the child may not fall asleep immediately after going to bed.

At 4½ to 5 years of age, nightmares often become intensified. Toddlers and preschoolers normally have fears, especially of the dark and later of monsters and wild animals. (This topic is discussed more fully in Chapter 11.) These fears can lead to nightmares and may be the cause of an awakened, anxious child crying out in the night. Generally, being told that everything will be all right and that the parents are near are the major reassurances the child needs in such situations. A bottle of cologne, renamed "monster spray or repellent," can work miracles in bolstering a child's confidence in a darkened room. Children with sleeping problems resistant to these approaches might benefit from a neuromuscular relaxation program. Helping such children learn head-to-toe relaxation may facilitate their falling asleep at bedtime and may decrease nighttime wakefulness [25].

TOILET TRAINING: A COORDINATION OF DOMAINS

Caretakers in different cultures vary tremendously in when and how they teach their children to acquire control of body functions. The reason for this variance is ascribed to different attitudes regarding cleanliness, self-control, and the question of who should teach the child. The variety in timing and methods of toilet training found among cultures is also present among individual families in different subcultures. Caretakers in the families of some socioeconomic classes in the United States think that a child should be completely trained by the second birthday—a most difficult expectation for many children to meet. As with any other type of learning, the biophysical, socioaffective, and cognitive areas of development must all have matured enough in the individual child to allow mastery of the new behavior. When these interdependent domains

have reached adequate levels of maturity, they are capable of aiding the child in meeting both short-term goals (e.g., not wetting the pants, telling mother he or she has to "go") and may influence long-range behaviors (e.g., the degree of self-assertion in future, social relationships of giving and receiving).

The child's mastery of total training occurs over a period of time. Bowel control is usually achieved first, gradually followed by daytime bladder control, with nighttime bladder control being last. Daytime bladder control rarely occurs with much success before the age of 2 years [33]. As in other areas of development, children express a wide variety of individual behaviors, all of which are normal. Some children may take longer than others to become "totally" trained; some may experience relapses in the process due to their own fears and misinterpretations of what is happening and what is expected (much of which can be alleviated or avoided by an informed caretaker who has a positive attitude).

Physical Readiness for Toilet Training

No two children are ready for toilet training at exactly the same time. Caretakers should not begin toilet training until the child is mature enough physically, cognitively, and emotionally to cooperate in the social skill of controlling the time and the location of elimination of body wastes.

In our culture, some method of toilet training is expected to be initiated by the time the child has reached late toddlerhood. The child should want to assume some responsibility for toileting; he or she should also know what the need to go to the bathroom feels like and what to do about this feeling.

For the child to be ready for toilet training, the nerves and muscles that control the urinary and anal sphincters must be mature. These sphincters operate at a reflex level until there is sufficient myelinization of the neural pathways to allow voluntary control. A child is capable of controlling the sphincters voluntarily between 12 and 18 months; between 18 and 24 months, the child is physically capable of knowing that the bladder is full or the bowel needs emptying. A child usually possesses the head and trunk control to sit on a toilet seat by 2 years of age. The ability to walk to and to get down from a chair are the other skills necessary for toilet training.

Neurological maturity is essential before the child can feel the sensations that indicate a full bladder or bowel and can voluntarily control the muscles that retain or release the contents. These physical signs of readiness, however, do not necessarily imply that the

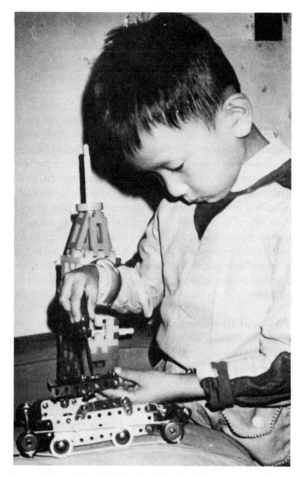

Figure 10–4. Preschoolers develop their fine motor and eye-hand coordination skills as they work on intricate toys and puzzles.

child is ready for toilet training in the other domains. To maximize individual potential, the child must be prepared in all domains.

Signs of Cognitive and Psychosocial Readiness

The child must also be ready cognitively and psychosocially for this important event. As the toddler becomes aware of the feeling of fullness in bladder or bowel, he or she learns to indicate this knowledge by doing things, such as pulling at the diapers, grasping the genital area, squatting on the spot where he or she is standing, and eventually repeating a word or phrase that has come to be associated with the feelings being experienced. Many children have learned the difference between "wet" and "dry" if the caretaker has en-

couraged such fundamental symbolic thought in caring for the child previous to toilet training (e.g., "Your orange juice spilled on the floor. Before it spilled the floor was dry; now it is wet").

Anyone who has cared for a toddler will recall that before toilet training the child eliminates regardless of where he or she is, what time it is, or who is holding the child. Gradually, the child learns that this behavior is socially unacceptable and that it makes the caretaker happier when he or she makes use of facilities expressly made for such purposes. The child learns to accept these values best through gentle and consistent reinforcement. In addition, around 2 years of age the toddler's desire to please significant others emerges, and the child begins to learn that sometimes it is "more blessed to give than to receive." Not all the toddler's altruistic efforts, however, revolve around "offering" a bowel movement in the potty to mother (a Freudian interpretation). This is the age at which many a photographer has also captured a toddler's tiny fingers clutching a freshly plucked dandelion as an offering of love to a mother. It is important to emphasize that although this desire to please is apparent, it is not as much a sign of readiness for toilet training as it is a symbol of the child's striving for independence and mastery of self [34]. The fact that children, beginning in their second year, become fascinated with things that can be placed in containers has been offered as another sign of readiness to deposit body excretions into the potty [35].

There are times when the family is not ready for the child to initiate such learning. Crises such as illness of the caretaker, a new baby or a child joining the family, the death of a family member, or a family move from one location to another warrant the delay of actual toilet training until the family stressors are reduced.

How To Begin

DEVELOPING BOWEL CONTROL
Many children move their bowels at approximately the same time each day. Since eating stimulates bowel action, evacuation frequently occurs shortly after a meal. Therefore, the training process is facilitated if the caretaker observes the child's habits and places the child on the potty at the time a movement is expected. This action accustoms the toddler to sitting on the potty and to evacuating the bowels there. Sometimes, after a few weeks of this form of conditioning, an infant or young toddler may discover the ability to "push" and to evacuate the bowels whenever the child is placed on and feels the potty. This ability does **not,** however, indicate

that the young toddler is trained. The child has not indicated to anyone a desire to "go"; he or she has not gone to the potty alone or pulled the pants down. It indicates that the primary caretaker has been successful in "catching" the child when he or she had to "go." Spock acknowledges that this form of early conditioning may help both baby and caretaker through the early stages of actual toilet training **if** the baby is regular enough to be "caught" and **if** the mother does not condition the baby by using punishment, extreme sternness, or her own frustration to elicit the results. The caretaker should accept the fact that some perfectly normal babies do not move their bowels daily and that the use of enemas or any other form of medication without the guidance of a pediatrician is potentially dangerous both physically and psychologically.

When toddlers are placed on the potty, they should be told in a positive manner why they have been placed there. They should not be required to sit there until they eliminate lest they experience feelings of frustration, shame, or doubt because of their inability to please someone they love very much. Giving toys while the child sits on the potty may only divert attention from the task at hand. Spock suggests that in some cases the caretaker should sit with the child (as long as the experience does not become an expected social occasion). This strategy may prove especially helpful with the child who is somewhat anxious because of what a movement feels like. Sitting with the child who is starting toilet training may also help if the child is apprehensive about the toilet itself. In such a situation, it is especially useful to use a less threatening child-size potty chair or a toilet that allows the child to sit comfortably and more securely with the feet on the floor or a footstool. Having the feet on the floor also gives the child better control in "pushing" and thus in evacuating the bowels. Because many young children are afraid of the sound of a toilet flushing and because some do not understand why their caretaker wants to discard immediately the much-wanted product from their bodies, it may be better to empty the potty and flush the toilet after the child is either off the large toilet (if it was used) or out of the bathroom completely.

Sometimes reading a book to the child written for children about toilet training contributes to motivation and aids the learning process. These illustrated books usually reinforce the process by praising the child who acts like a "big girl" or a "big boy." Changing from diapers to training pants makes some children feel more responsible in assuming some control of their elimination. If the child does not respond to, or thoroughly protests against, any of these training tips, he

or she may not be ready for bowel training, and all attempts at training should be discontinued for several weeks.

Toddlers, by nature, like to explore and "mess." Playing with and smearing of feces, however, must be restricted because (1) it is unsanitary and (2) it causes arousal of disgust in others that might be interpreted by the toddler as self-deprecating. The best way to handle such activity is to direct the child in a consistent and nonpunitive way to a more constructive form of activity (e.g., self-wiping; or indulging in finger painting, squeezing clay, or even crayoning) without calling much attention to the initial socially unacceptable action. However, the opportunity to explore the "product" once or twice under supervision may satisfy the child's curiosity and thus the tendency to explore feces at a less opportune time and in a less opportune fashion when the parent is not present.

DEVELOPING BLADDER CONTROL

Many of the strategies used in promoting effective bowel training also apply to helping a child establish bladder control. Bladder training, although it indirectly begins at the same time as bowel training, usually takes much longer to achieve. Even when the child's bladder is physically capable of holding urine for more than a 2-hour period, the average child may still not be ready cognitively or psychosocially for bladder training. It is often around the age of 12 to 18 months that the child notifies the primary caretaker **after** he or she has already wet. When this point is reached, it will not be long until the child will come to interpret the full bladder as a time to signal the caretaker that he or she needs to "go," and the child will then gradually learn to inform the caretaker before the act has occurred. But even at this point, there may not be time to get to the toilet. The child may be too busy to notice a full bladder and will have accidents. As a matter of fact, many children up to 5 years of age sometimes have to be reminded to take a trip to the bathroom.

Little boys vary in their wish to sit or to stand when urinating (usually they can master going to the bathroom alone and stand to urinate by 3½ years of age). Little girls who have had the opportunity to observe members of the opposite gender void may try to imitate their behavior by standing over the potty; this generally proves to be a frustrating experience that quickly extinguishes itself. An understanding caretaker is essential. To the child, learning about bladder control is a very serious experience.

Nighttime control of the bladder usually comes after

daytime control has been established. Children vary in the age at which they are able to stay dry for the duration of the night. In most cases, the establishment of such control occurs simply because the child's bladder has matured sufficiently to hold a larger amount. Girls tend to gain such control earlier than boys; "relaxed" children tend to stay dry throughout the night more than "high-strung" children [35].

Doctors and researchers do not always agree on the age at which enuresis (bed-wetting) becomes abnormal. Limiting fluids in the evening and getting the child up to go to the bathroom before the parents retire for the night are two supportive measures. If a child continues to wet the bed when most of his or her peers are remaining dry, the caretakers should seek the advice of a health professional. It may be that the child is experiencing anxiety in some domain of life (e.g., too rigid toilet training, inability to make friends, arrival of a new baby in the family). Such anxiety needs to be identified and dealt with. The child's delay in remaining dry throughout the night may also be due to a physiological or a health factor.

No matter when an individual child's total toilet training is considered to be complete, there will be times when relapses or "accidents" occur. When this happens, the caretaker should handle the situation in a manner that promotes healthy toilet training. Lack of parental empathy coupled with harsh discipline are felt by some to foster an obsessive, meticulous, rigid personality. It is the caretaker's calm and patient reassurance that helps the child to establish pride in this new responsibility, instead of shame and doubt about the ability to function in an independent, acceptable manner.

the various orifices (e.g., nose, ear, vagina) of their often self-examined, growing bodies.

Active, systematic stimulation of the senses allows the child to become more aware of the environment and his or her place within it. Many of the toddler's and preschooler's internal physical systems mature sufficiently to allow the child to maintain physiological homeostasis. Under stress, however, they function in a less adaptive manner.

A child is not **biophysically** ready to begin toilet training until late toddlerhood. But, the child must also be ready in the cognitive and psychosocial domain before toilet training is initiated.

The feeding interactions and eating patterns established during early childhood affect the direction of the child's growth in the four domains of life. The toddler and preschooler years are the critical periods in which parents can help the child to establish good eating habits: The child can be encouraged to consume nutritious foods and snacks instead of eating junk foods that contain high levels of saturated fats, salt, and sugar. These early years are also the optimal time for establishing habits of oral hygiene. Similarly, the way in which parents guide the child's sleep routines can have a profound effect on physical, socioaffective, and cognitive realms of development. Adequate sleep, rest, and exercise promote a healthy toddler and preschooler. Clothes and shoes should fit so that the child can comfortably engage in physical activity and have room to grow.

Regular medical checkups are essential. The young child's developing immune system is greatly assisted in fighting infection if he or she is receiving immunizations according to the recommended schedule.

SUMMARY

Many factors contribute to the increased complexity of the motor functioning of young children: increased muscle size, continued myelinization of the neural pathways, and the opportunity to practice a skill. As the various components of the nervous system grow and develop and as the neuromuscular and skeletal systems also become more mature, the young child's movements come under greater conscious control and allow for more refined movements. Stronger bones and a tougher skin help to protect the child from serious injury when experiencing the many tumbles and spills associated with learning and perfecting new skills. Curious toddlers and preschoolers must be observed carefully and taught not to place foreign bodies into

REFERENCES

1. American Academy of Pediatrics Committee on Nutrition. Salt intake and eating patterns of infants and children in relation to blood pressure. *Pediatrics* 53:115, 1974.
2. . . . And don't forget the eyes. *American Baby* (December 1977):34.
3. Asher, C. *Postural Variations in Childhood*. Boston: Butterworth, 1975.
4. Behrman, R. E., Vaughan, V. C. (Eds.); senior editor, W. E. Nelson. *Nelson Textbook of Pediatrics* (12th ed.). Philadelphia: Saunders, 1982.
5. Brunner, L. S., and Suddarth, D. S. The Immune System and Immunopathology. In L. S. Brunner and D. S. Suddarth, *Textbook of Medical-Surgical Nursing* (4th ed.). Philadelphia: Lippincott, 1980.
6. Brazelton, T. B. *Toddlers and Parents: A Declaration of Independence*. New York: Dell, 1974.

7. Chinn, P. L.   *Child Health Maintenance: Concepts in Family-Centered Care* (2nd ed.). St. Louis: Mosby, 1979.

8. Damerel, P.   How to choose shoes that fit your kids' feet. *Family Health/Today's Health* (August 1976):36.

9. Esslinger, P. N.   The Preschooler. In M. J. Smith et al. (Eds.), *Child and Family: Concepts of Nursing Practice*. New York: McGraw-Hill, 1982.

10. Haxton, R.   Personal communication, June, 1982.

11. Horner, M. M. E., and McClellan, M. A.   Toilet training: Ready or not? *Pediatric Nursing,* 7(1):17, 1981.

12. Inglis, S.   The nocturnal frustration of sleep disturbance. *Am. J. Matern.-Child Nursing* (September/October 1976):280.

13. Kilmon, C., and Helpin, M. L.   Update on dentistry for children. *Pediatric Nursing* 7(5):41, 1981.

14. Larsen, E.   Katie's eyes are normal now. *Parents' Magazine* (August 1977):87.

15. Lowrey, G. H.   *Growth and Development of Children* (7th ed.). Chicago: Year Book, 1978.

16. Marlow, D. R.   *Textbook of Pediatric Nursing* (6th ed.). Philadelphia: Saunders, 1985.

17. McCallum, C.   The Contingent Negative Variation as a Cortical Sign of Attention Span. In C. R. Evans and T. B. Mulholland (Eds.), *Attention in Neurophysiology*. London: Butterworth, 1969.

18. Menkes, J. H.   The Neuromotor Mechanism. In R. E. Cooke (Ed.), *The Biologic Basis of Pediatric Practice*. New York: Blakiston Division, McGraw-Hill, 1968.

19. Metheny, N. M., and Snively, W. D.   *Nurses' Handbook of Fluid Balance* (4th ed.). Philadelphia: Lippincott, 1983.

20. Nysather, J. O., et al.   The immune system: Its development and functions. *Am. J. Nurs.* 76:1614, 1976.

21. O'Brien, D.   The management of fluid and electrolyte problems in childhood. *Pediatric Basics* 17:1, 1977.

22. Owen, G. M., and Lubin, A.   Anthropometric differences between black and white preschool children. *Am. J. Dis. Child.* 126:168, 1973.

23. Pipes, P. L.   *Nutrition in Infancy and Childhood* (2nd ed.). St. Louis: Mosby, 1981.

24. Ramsey, N. L., and Haugan, B.   The Toddler. In M. J. Smith et al. (Eds.), *Child and Family: Concepts of Nursing Practice*. New York: McGraw-Hill, 1982.

25. Schumann, M. J.   Neuromuscular relaxation: A method for inducing sleep in young children. *Pediatric Nursing* 7(5):9, 1981.

26. Scipien, G. M., et al. (Eds.).   *Comprehensive Pediatric Nursing* (2nd ed.). New York: McGraw-Hill, 1979.

27. Smith, N. J.   Medical issues in sports medicine. *Pediatrics in Review* 2(8):229, 1981.

28. Spock, B. M.   *Baby and Child Care* (4th ed.). New York: Hawthorn Books, 1976.

29. Valadian, I., and Porter, D.   *Physical Growth and Development: From Conception to Maturity*. Boston: Little, Brown, 1977.

30. Wehe, R. A., M. D.   Personal communication, 1978.

31. Wei, S. H.   Nutrition, diet, fluoride, and dental health. *Pediatric Basics* 30:4, 1981.

32. Whaley, L. F., and Wong, D. L.   *Nursing Care of Infants and Children* (2nd ed.). St. Louis: Mosby, 1983.

33. Ilg, F. L., Ames, L. B., and Baker, S. M.   *Child Behavior* (Rev. ed.). New York: Barnes & Noble, 1982.

34. Juntti, M. J.   Determining Training Readiness. In M. J. Juntti, et al. (Eds.), *Total Toilet Training*. Baltimore: University Park Press, 1979.

35. Spock, B.   *Baby and Child Care* (rev.). New York: Pocket Books, 1977.

11

Cognitive Development of the Toddler and the Preschooler

Shirley S. Ashburn and Clara S. Schuster

It is awesome and responsible to consider one's world as one's representation. Then I am responsible when the world gets mean and small, angry or guilty. I am not only my brother's keeper. I am my brother.

—Wilson Van Dusen, *Person to Person*

Introduction

Cognition
   Piaget's substage 6 of sensorimotor intelligence
   Piaget's semiotic (symbolic) function
   Piaget's preoperational stage
   Cognitive concepts of early childhood
   Fantasy

Learning
   Attention
   Memory
   Development of cognitive skills
   Assessment of developmental level

Maximizing the Cognitive Potential of the Toddler and the Preschooler

Summary

Boundless energy and seemingly indefatigable drive burst forth from the miniature frame of the toddler. The child's insatiable curiosity and quest for new experiences are probably greater during toddlerhood than at any other period of life [19]. Burton White views this time as "the second half of the most important period" for educating a child [35].

This inquisitive behavior is carried over into the preschool years and is greatly facilitated by the increased refinement of neuromuscular skills. The ability to coordinate the use of the senses to learn about the environment increases as the young child matures. A child will shake, sniff, and visually examine an unfamiliar object to determine its qualities and functions. Every sensory modality may be called upon to enable the child to "know" an object or person completely. The integration of alternative ways of identifying an object leads to a considerable increase in the effectiveness of the child's perceptual abilities and knowledge about the world [36]. The child is continuing the process of learning how to learn, becoming a teacher of self through these thorough explorations.

However, the ability to synthesize and to interpret stimulus input is not fully perfected during these early years. One 5-year-old (informing his father about his brother's encounter with a skunk) exhibited a classic mixing of the senses when he said, "You ought to see Jimmy—he smells so bad you can hear him!" Other socioaffective sensations (e.g., pleasure, discomfort, anger) and the meanings they have for individual children are also subject to various interpretations (for example, "I'm so mad my hand wants to hit you!" or "I'm so happy that I taste like chocolate cake!"). The complex mechanisms that enable an individual to identify and to control emotions effectively are not fully developed during these years, but a foundation is laid. As children become more verbal, they become capable of sharing with others the volume and the complexity of thoughts that flow through their very active minds.

COGNITION

Piaget's Substage 6 of Sensorimotor Intelligence

Toddlerhood places the young toddler at the end of the sensorimotor period of cognition (Piaget's substage 6: the invention of new means through mental combinations). It is during this stage (18 to 24 months) that the toddler makes the transition from the sensorimotor level of intelligence to representational intelligence (which includes the ability to picture an event in the mind). Thoughts are becoming symbolic, enabling the child to "play out" in his mind the sequence of a behavior rather than actually having to participate in the event physically or to manipulate the physical aspects of the event. In substage 5 (see Chap. 8), the infant attained new means for solutions to problems through laborious trial and error experimentation. In substage 6, because many solutions can be "tried out" in the mind, the child is capable of inventing new means much more quickly. Furthermore, the child can remember the actions of others no longer present and imitate them as well (delayed imitation).

This new cognitive accomplishment is reflected in the child's advanced concept of objects. He or she can now find an object hidden by invisible displacement (i.e., searching for, and finding, objects that the child has not observed being hidden). The child knows that objects are permanent and that they (as well as significant people) exist even though they cannot be seen. The child can recall some previous hiding places and will search them first, doing his or her best to hunt for the object until it is found.

Through the use of this new capacity for mental representations, the toddler can begin to predict many cause and effect relationships accurately. For example, a child who is trying unsuccessfully to open a door may attribute failure to the door being locked. He or she may or may not be correct; nevertheless, these new mental abilities increase an awareness of causality.

Upon completion of the sensorimotor stage, the child is on the threshold of the next level of cognitive development. Intellectual development will continue primarily within the symbolic realm, as opposed to working through sensorimotor experiences. Sensorimotor experiences continue to be important, but thoughts and actions are dominated by representational activities.

Piaget's Semiotic (Symbolic) Function

When the child is approximately 1½ to 2 years old, the cognitive process appears that is fundamental to the development of language, mental imagery, and symbolic gesture. This process, called the semiotic (or symbolic) function, consists of the ability to represent something (a "signified" something: object, event, conceptual schema, and so forth) by means of a "signifier," which is differentiated from other objects and serves a representative purpose [28] (see Fig. 11–1).

The essential difference between a child who is in the sensorimotor stage and one who is at an advanced level of cognition is the latter's increased ability for mental manipulation of symbols that represent the environment [23]. The foundations of symbolic activity are laid during the sensorimotor stage. "Motor meaning" develops in substage 3 when the infant begins to imitate an object by reproducing a simple action that is associated with its presence, for example, banging the high chair tray with the hand instead of a spoon. In substage 4, "symbolic meaning" takes place when the "actions" consist of complex neural patterns that serve to represent the object, and the overt responses are not to the sensory input itself (the glass, the keys) but to its symbolic meaning (milk, mother's departure).

Piaget says that although true mental representations do not exist in the early sensorimotor substages, young babies do begin to recognize **significates**—the actual object, event, action, or behavior that is immediately present in the real environment [28]. Receptive intelligence is dependent upon memory of previous contact or experience. The baby may identify some salient feature or part of the significate as an indicator (index or signal) that the schema is present. An **index** or signal is usually undifferentiated from its significate (or that which is signified), so a young baby who sees an *orange* ball (the significate I) and focuses on the color (the signal) may immediately perceive that it is *orange* juice (the significate II). The baby's specific-to-specific association that all orange objects are orange

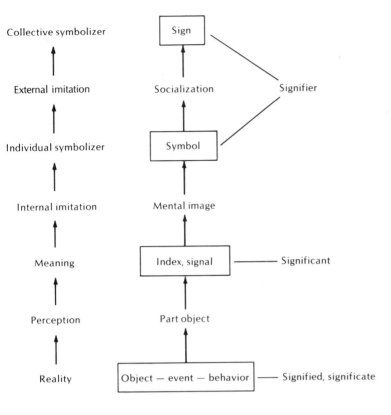

Collective symbolizer

External imitation

Individual symbolizer

Internal imitation

Meaning

Perception

Reality

Sign

Socialization — Signifier

Symbol

Mental image

Index, signal — Significant

Part object

Object — event — behavior — Signified, significate

Figure 11-1. Differentiation between signified and signifier (semiotic function). A system of ready-made collective signs is inadequate and hard to master for the young child; consequently these signs are acquired over a period of many years. In the early months, only concrete, time-limited reality has any meaning to the child. Gradually the child recognizes a significant part of the phenomenon as an indication that the significate is present or is soon to be present. Marked advance in cognitive structuring is evidenced when the child is able to retain or to recall a mental image of the significate. Eventually, this idiosyncratic, personal significant is accommodated to the culturally accepted gestural (e.g., sign language) or verbal symbolizer. It is not until the child has a fairly good concept of verbal or gestural collective symbolizers that he or she is able to comprehend and to accept the even more abstract concept of written collective symbolizers.

juice is an example of transductive reasoning, which is more fully described later in this chapter (see Fig. 11-2).

Piaget does not believe, however, that the child is thinking in truly representative fashion until he or she can internally evoke some word or image in the mind without some form of external cue. Piaget believes that, beginning at some point close to the last substage of the sensorimotor period, the child demonstrates several behaviors that can be inferred to aid in the establishment of recognizing a sign for something that everyone in the child's culture understands (a collective symbolizer). To do this, the child must first be able to imitate a schema in its presence and then must imitate the schema when it is absent. This delayed imitation in itself is proof that the child can internally represent or form a mental image of the selected schema (internal imitation). The most common example of using collective signs is the use of language to represent an object that is not immediately present. When a child learns to write, he or she learns that written signs in addition to verbal signs can represent objects, events, or concepts. Each level of symbolic

representation is one step more abstract than the previous level. It also becomes obvious that the steps are sequential, since they build on each other. Therefore, inadequate sensorimotor experience may delay or prevent formation of adequate indexes and thus the ability to develop more abstract representation of an object.

The attainment of symbolic function manifests itself in several ways when the child is between 2 and 4 years of age (Fig. 11-2). The child can change mental symbols to words to communicate with others (although this can lead to confusion if the child is still at a level where the meaning of the word used is still very personal and is not known to the person with whom the child is conversing!). The child may also use one object to represent another in "make-believe" or symbolic play because the two objects have some common feature that is used as an index for both objects. The child distorts reality by taking into account only the characteristics of objects that meet immediate needs. The index may be shape, color, movement, or any other salient feature the child uses to categorize an object, an event, or a person. Consequently, a shell may become a cup, a cap, or a fan with equal facility; it may

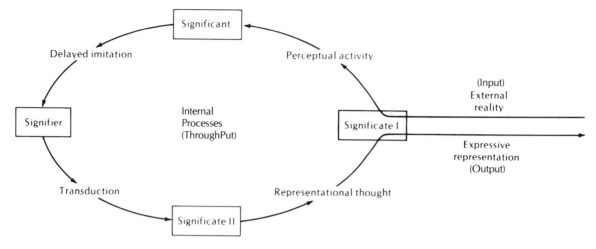

Figure 11–2. Operational dynamism of representational thought, symbolic function, or symbolic play. **Significate I:** actual object or event (becomes representative for Significate II through representational or symbolic thought). **Significate II:** signified object or event. "As long as egocentric assimilation of reality to the subject's own action prevails, the child will require symbols; hence symbolic play or imaginative play, the purest form of egocentric and symbolic thought, the assimilation of reality to the subject's own interests and the expression of reality through the use of images fashioned by himself" [27]. **Perceptual activity:** incomplete accommodation of present significate. Egocentric distorting, or receptive assimilation. **Delayed imitation:** evokes symbol of earlier accommodation. **Transduction:** representative assimilation, centration on significant specific-to-specific association. **Representational thought:** (1) ludic (play) symbol—expressive assimilation, symbolic play; (2) conceptual activity—representative imitation; (3) beginning of representative adaptation, which is early cognitive representation leading to conceptual representation or primitive conceptual framework.

also be a boat, a flower, or even a telephone, depending on the child's skill at specific-to-specific association, which is essential to conscious representational thought and symbolic play (see Fig. 11–2).

Piaget's Preoperational Stage

During Piaget's preoperational stage (2 to 6 years of age), new cognitive processes allow the child to use mental symbols to think about events of the past, to anticipate the future, and to think about what might be going on somewhere else at the present moment. In the beginning, the child will probably call every night in the past "last night" and every day in the future "tomorrow" and will love to ask if other boys and girls are getting up to eat breakfast just as he or she is preparing to do.

The preoperational stage is divided into two substages: preconceptional thought and intuitive thought. Because most children during the first 4½ years or so base their thinking heavily on the concrete perceptions and actions of their immediate environment, Piaget labels their thinking "preconceptual" [3]. Until a child is halfway through the preschool years, he or she is unable to form true concepts. Up to that time, the child

inconsistently assigns one word to several rather similar actions instead of using one word to identify just one class of objects (for example, "Daddy" describes any male voice on the telephone; "Nanny" is any woman with white hair and glasses).

Piaget says that a period of "intuitive" thought builds from preconceptual thinking (extending from about 4½ to 7 years of age) [3]. The differences between preconceptual and intuitive thinking are extremely fine. The intuitive child can more efficiently differentiate between signifiers (mother getting her pocketbook) and significates (mother going out to the car), realizing that the pocketbook does not necessarily have to be associated with mother leaving or going for a ride. During the intuitive substage, the child begins to be able to give reasons for beliefs and a rationale for actions. The logic, however, remains one-sided and opinionated. Intuitive thinking enables the child to internally represent, relive, and reshape events.

Flavell identifies the following as major characteristics of the preoperational stage [6]:

1. Egocentrism
2. Centration

3. Focus on states
4. Action rather than abstraction
5. Irreversibility
6. Transductive reasoning

Early preoperational thought is dominated by all these conceptual schemes. These characteristics often serve as obstacles to what is commonly referred to as "adult logic."

EGOCENTRISM

The thoughts of the toddler and the preschooler are greatly influenced by what is seen, heard, or otherwise experienced at a given moment. The preoperational child is not able to take the role or to see the viewpoint of another person. The only thought in mind is, "This is how the world looks to me." As a result, the preoperational child never questions subjective perceptions or viewpoints because they are, as far as the child is concerned, the only thoughts possible and consequently must be correct. If asked to point to a picture that replicates what can be seen on an actual table, the preoperational child can accurately choose a picture that represents objects in the same spatial relationship as he or she is viewing. However, if asked to choose a picture that represents how a person in another position at the table would see the same objects, the child is unable to do so with accuracy. Piaget says that it is not until the child's thoughts and those of peers conflict in verbal exchange (usually around 6 or 7 years) that the child begins to accommodate to others; egocentric thought may give way under social pressures at this time.

CENTRATION

Another characteristic of preoperational thinking is evidenced when the child tends to "center," or focus on one aspect of a situation, so that he or she neglects to process information from other aspects of the same situation. The child is aware of much less in a situation than is a cognitively more mature person. This inability to explore all the other aspects at the same time (or the child's incapacity to "decenter") often limits the preoperational child's ability to solve what adults would consider the most simple of problems. When solving a puzzle, the child may concentrate on only one detail of the piece, trying to force that segment into any similar space. The child may be able to follow only one direction at a time. The ability to follow two directions in sequence emerges gradually.

FOCUS ON STATES

The preoperational child who is observing a sequence of changes or successive states does not understand how a transformation from one state to the next occurs. Consider a preschooler watching an apple being eaten. The child will center on each of the various in-between states as they occur but will be unable to reconstruct the series of events in terms of a beginning-to-end relationship. If asked to draw what was seen, the child would probably attempt to draw only a whole apple (the initial state) and an apple core (the transformed state). He or she can only attend to one mental event at a time. As a result, some successive conclusions will contradict one another (for example, "Only mommies can have babies." "Men can have babies if they are married."). The child throughout these early years feels no need to justify a rationale (and even if an attempt is made, the child would cognitively be unable to reconstruct the steps that led to the conclusions). Because the preoperational child is unable to order all the sequences of an event realistically, he or she will exhibit a lack of consistent direction in thinking.

Adult: Tommy, what happens when it rains?
Child: The sky cries.
Adult: How does it happen?
Child: Because we cry.
Adult: What makes it rain?
Child: Because we have tears.

The fact that raindrops precipitate from above and that tears fall from our eyes is sufficient reason, Tommy believes, to make the statements he does. In addition, the child at this cognitive level attributes life and feeling to inanimate objects and believes that natural phenomena (e.g., lightning) are made and controlled by human beings.

ACTION RATHER THAN ABSTRACTION

The preoperational child who is experiencing symbolic mental representations simply "runs through" the symbols for an event as if actually participating in the event itself. Everything is viewed vicariously. Even the body movements of the child—especially the hands—can be observed to mimic those of the person whom the child is watching. This concreteness is ever-present during the preoperational stage (as opposed to the analyzing and synthesizing that adults ordinarily do). Since the egocentric child can only think about things in terms of the subjective meanings attached to them, he or she cannot understand and will become angry when others do not understand his or her concrete, idiosyncratic speech and thoughts.

IRREVERSIBILITY

Irreversibility is characteristic of all the cognitive activities of the preoperational child. Since the child cannot reverse thoughts, then a line of reasoning cannot be followed back to its beginnings. Because every logical or mathematical statement *is* reversible, it is no wonder that toddlers and preschoolers often become confused and frustrated; they reason so differently from the adults in their world.

One of the best examples to illustrate the irreversibility of thought that is present at this age is to ask a 5-year-old if he or she has a brother. The child will answer, "Yes" (assuming the child does indeed have a brother), but when asked if that brother has a brother, the child will answer, "No." By the age of 7 years, more than one-half of all children will solve this kind of problem correctly [24].

TRANSDUCTIVE REASONING

During the sensorimotor stage, the infant gradually begins to develop an idea of causality. Piaget sees transductive reasoning as a transition between sensorimotor causality and adult reasoning. Transductive reasoning is also synonymous with "specific-to-specific" thinking. If two things are alike in one aspect, the child reasons that they are alike in all aspects; thus a child who sees Daddy turn on the water to shave may reason that Daddy is going to shave again the next time father is seen to turn on the same source of water. With experience, the child will learn that expectations do not always prove to be true. Nevertheless, reasoning from particular to particular rather than from particular to general (inductive thinking) or from general to particular (deductive thinking) reigns supreme throughout these early childhood years.

Cognitive Concepts of Early Childhood

CLASSIFICATION

Children in the preoperational stage tend to group objects and experiences on a perceptual or sensorimotor basis rather than by abstract qualities. Classification activities involve, first, the **matching** of identical objects. Gradually, the child is able to match two objects based on a specific common quality, such as color, shape, name, or use. Eventually, a transitional classification activity, called **chaining,** emerges. The child lines up several objects that bear some relationship to one another (e.g., same color or shape). However, the

index used to match A and B may be different from that used to match B and C, since only one dimension is considered at a time and each matching is independent of the previous matching. Gradually, the child is able to maintain a constant index for a large group of objects. The child will then be able to **sort** a large number of objects into separate piles based on prespecified indexes. Early classifications are based on concrete indices, such as use. In time, the child is able to make more refined distinctions and to use more abstract qualities, so that gradually, the child is able to coordinate two indices at the same time, such as color and shape. More abstract classification indices (weight, size, tonal pitch) appear later as the child begins to make quantitative comparisons of the same index. Objects can then be placed in order according to height, tonal quality (musical scale), color shade, and so forth in the process known as **seriation.**

CONSERVATION

During the preoperational stage, children usually cannot "conserve," or hold one dimension invariant, when changes occur in the other dimensions of a schema. For example, if a row of six pennies is suddenly altered in such a way that the spaces between the pennies are made larger, there are still six pennies; that is, the number of pennies does not change when an alteration is made in another irrelevant dimension (the length of the row in this case). However, the early preoperational child believes the number of pennies does change in this situation because the child is incapable of conserving the concept of number. By the end of the preoperational period (which corresponds to the school-age child of 7 years), some forms of conservation (there are several) are usually developed. A continuing discussion of conservation is found in Chapter 23.

ANIMISM

Toddlers and preschoolers, because of their limited experience and knowledge, tend to believe that inert objects possess consciousness and can think and function with intent. Thus, when these children fall and injure themselves, it is the rock or the door frame that "hurt me on purpose. That is a bad rock (or door frame)." They may afterward treat the injuring object as an enemy. Other objects can assume a positive valance by their presence during a positive event.

One of the most comprehensive and well-known studies of animistic thinking was made by Piaget, who concluded that children's animistic thinking evolves through the following four stages [26]:

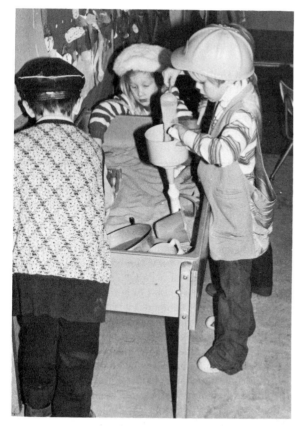

Figure 11–3. Fluid materials such as sand are responsive to the child's actions. Even though these children are motivated to experiment with the sand by pouring it into containers of assorted shapes and sizes, none of them will be able to conserve a given quantity of it until the school-age years.

Stage I Child believes that all objects, whether animate or inanimate, are alive.

Stage II Child believes that everything that moves (e.g., wagon, car, pendulum clock) has life.

Stage III Child believes that objects that can move on their own accord (e.g., sun, wind) are alive.

Stage IV Child believes that both plants and animals, or maybe just animals, possess life.

For further discussion, see Chap. 20.

TIME

Toddlers do not have an adult concept of time (e.g., afternoon, Wednesday, 3 o'clock); instead they relate to the predictable concrete activities of their ritualistic everyday schedule ("We will go shopping after your nap"). By the time the child becomes a preschooler, time words begin to be associated with everyday events. Many 5-year-olds know the days of the week; some begin to recognize units of time as being coincident with the placement of the big and little hands on the clock. As with all concepts, experience with the concept of time and reinforcements to the child's interpretation of time will aid in a correct understanding of it.

Fantasy

Young children, observing how adults can make things happen with such ease, often miss the action that caused the event. They attribute the result to magical powers—thoughts and wishes alone can make it happen. Often the parents, anticipating the child's needs, meet them before the child expresses them, lending power to the concept that parents can read minds or have magical powers of thought. The preoperational child begins to believe that personal wishes, thoughts, gestures, and noises command the universe. The child is a magician who stands midway between two worlds: the preverbal egocentric world of magic and the world of reality [8].

Through the use of fantasy or mental play, the child adapts to the tensions, the anxieties, and the fears experienced about self and the surrounding world. From the beginning of toddlerhood, the child believes that a magical power of thought is the cause of all events: This is the belief that wishing something will make it so. Sometimes a child believes that personal wishes actually caused some tragic event (e.g., the death of an unliked relative or the loss of a parent by divorce) and will need consistent reminding to understand that wishes alone do not cause events. Toddlers and many preschoolers feel supremely powerful and responsible for happenings, but are also vulnerable to feelings of shame, self-doubt, and guilt. Since toddlers especially do not distinguish clearly between fantasy and reality, they need patient and understanding parents as they live out their fantasies.

FAIRY TALES

Bettelheim maintains that a child's cultural inheritance endows his or her life with meaning and knowledge [4]. He indicates that one of the best ways to obtain this information is through children's literature. For a story to capture and hold a child's attention, it must not only entertain but must arouse curiosity. To enrich the child's life, stories must stimulate the child's imagination, help develop intellect, clarify emotions, reflect anxieties and aspirations, and give full recognition to frustrations while suggesting solutions to the problems that perturb the child.

How can fairy tales meet all these criteria? Bettelheim feels that fairy tales provide the rich fantasy necessary for expressing the total personality—both conscious and unconscious. Studies based on Jung's theory that the unconscious plays a vital role in living also support this view [10]. Fairy tales and their meaning, like other forms of art, will be interpreted differently by each individual and by the same child at various times in life. Depending on the concerns and needs of a given moment, a child may extract from the story of Cinderella the idea that "good" people don't get to go to parties (perhaps he or she had chickenpox and was not allowed to go to a birthday party). The child may return to this fairy tale at a later time, searching to enlarge on the same meaning or literally to reconstruct it. The healthy child will extract only those parts of a fairy tale that can be handled and will not be frightened to the point of hysteria (as adults sometimes think) when the witch threatens to eat Hansel and Gretel. Parents who participate with their children by reading and telling fairy tales as well as attending plays or puppet shows are rewarded by establishing closer and more positive family relationships through the shared experience.

BELIEFS

Santa Claus and Friends. Most American families promote the idea that Santa Claus, the Easter Bunny, and often the Tooth Fairy exist; most toddlers and preschoolers accept such beliefs with enthusiasm. Although the concept of Santa Claus is rather vague, the 3-year-old is most interested in hearing stories about Santa (especially the part about the gifts!). The average 4-year-old believes in Santa Claus and enjoys hearing about every detail. It is the 5- and 6-year-old child, however, who possesses an unshakable and dedicated belief in Santa [12]. The 6-year-old delights in printing requests to Santa and will deny any suggestion that Santa is not "real." This loyalty usually reaches a peak just before the child's seventh birthday and is slowly replaced by a growing skepticism that parallels the child's ability to use more logical thought processes in analyzing the world. First, the belief that Santa travels over the entire world may be questioned; then the child may ask how all those toys could fit in one sack. This process continues until, usually around 8 or 9 years of age, the child is able to accept the concept of Santa Claus as a symbol of love and sharing rather than an actual physical entity. Most people feel that the joy that

most children derive from an early belief in Santa Claus is worth the minimal disillusionment that may occur later "when they find out the truth" [12].

Belief in a Deity. The opportunity for religious experience that parents provide for their children is an individual and personal matter. As a child matures, the cognitive and emotional abilities to accept religious teachings will grow. How the parents live their beliefs is as important as what they tell the child. Unless one's concept of God includes that of a personal relationship, this concept, like the belief in Santa Claus or the Easter Bunny, will begin to fade into an intellectual exercise or cultural myth along with the other traditions of the culture and the family. It will become merely the symbol of interpersonal love.

Ilg and Ames have studied many aspects of the factual (as opposed to the reverential or subjective) side of a child's concept of a deity. They found that it is usually around the age of 4 (when the child seems to begin every other sentence with "Why?" "Who?" "Where?") when a religious sense is evidenced. Many parents of deep religious persuasion share that their children are sensitive to concepts of God and to their basic beliefs about interpersonal and spiritual relationships during the second year of life. Church school attendance augments but cannot replace the values taught by parents. Children learn best from that which they see in everyday life.

One kind of religious concept that exists in the young preschooler is what Piaget calls the "religion of the parents." Because the small child sees parents as all-knowing, all-powerful, and living forever, the child may equate them with a Supreme Being.

The most important thing for parents to remember throughout the early preschool years is to answer the child's questions without giving so much information that the child becomes confused. Both 4- and 5-year-olds can memorize short prayers, although it is questionable whether they can attribute the same meanings to their recitations as can older children or adults.

Interestingly, Ilg and Ames found many 5-year-olds critical of what they deemed "God's mistakes" (e.g., "God made a mistake when He made mosquitoes. Give me one good reason why He should have made a mosquito") [12]. Such statements imply that the level of religious and spiritual comprehension is still limited in a 5-year-old child.

Similar to the course he takes in expressing belief in Santa Claus, the 6-year-old may become extremely interested in hearing about the adventures of God (as well as the activities of an opposite entity—the Devil). Many deeply religious family members may become distraught if this enthusiasm later turns to skepticism. It may be of some comfort to them if they realize that this skepticism is, in part, a healthy questioning that feeds into a fundamental sense of identity. Those families who do not adhere to traditional religious affiliations may be frustrated by their 6-year-old's avid interest in God. Piaget says that this interest may be inspired by the child's discovery that the capacity of humans is limited; the child thus attributes the quality of omnipotence to a supreme being alone and begins to see the vulnerability of self and others—especially the parents (see Chap. 20).

Throughout these early years, the child's overall religious beliefs will be a reflection of the kind and the amount of religious teaching received in the home environment.

DAYDREAMING

Daydreaming, a form of mental fantasy, differs from regular make-believe or dramatic play (see Chap. 15). The child engaged in dramatic play is more likely to "play out" activities and concerns related to daily living, whereas the child who is daydreaming is more often pretending to be either a hero or a martyr (depending on the child's adjustment in the socioaffective domain) and is often startled when the daydreaming is interrupted. Well-adjusted children who are successfully accomplishing their psychosocial developmental tasks tend to daydream more about becoming very important people in real life (e.g., an expert in some field or endeavor). On the other hand, if a child is adjusting poorly, daydreams may predominantly revolve around being a misunderstood martyr or a long-suffering invalid. Without doubt, the daydreams of all children, regardless of their psychosocial adjustment, may be influenced by the mass media. Daydreaming may begin during the preschool years, especially if the child is relatively more quick to learn than some of his or her peers. This form of mental play reaches a peak during early adolescence. Daydreaming is a way to attain omnipotence by warding off feelings of vulnerability. It can be a very positive, adaptive response, especially at this stage of development and again during adolescence.

Too little daydreaming may be as detrimental to a child's (or any individual's) socioaffective development as too much of this form of retreat and entertainment [29]. The healthy child will usually resort to daydreaming when bored or unable to participate in some other form of play. The poorly adjusting child, on the other hand, may frequently substitute day-

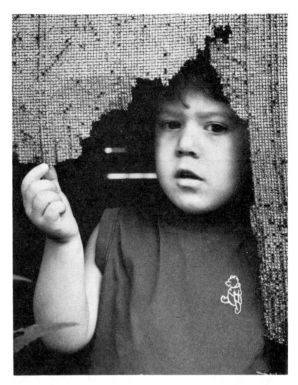

Figure 11–4. The toddler possesses a remarkable curiosity that observes and searches for causes. As preschoolers seek causes for phenomena that cannot be accounted for within their limited, pragmatic experiences, they turn to the use of "magical" powers of thought.

dreaming for other forms of age-appropriate play. A teacher or any other adult who observes a child consistently daydreaming (especially if the child expresses tendencies to daydream of being inferior or wronged) should refer the child and the family to professional guidance. Daydreaming can be a constructive activity when used to expand and understand one's world, but it may become very destructive when used to retreat from the realities of life.

UNTRUTHFUL FANTASIES ("WHITE LIES")

The toddler and the preschooler often appear to have little regard for the truth itself. They may recognize it as something that appears to make their parents happy, but their attempts to adhere to it are frustrating, intrusive, and quite often, because of their limited concept of cause and effect, confusing. Many "white lies" are told by children during these years. In contrast to the untruths and the falsehoods told by persons who reason at a higher cognitive level, the child's white lie is not intended to deceive others; children share what they **want** to be the truth and actually believe what they are saying (e.g., "Kitty tell me she break glass Mommy"). Other white lies stem from daydreaming, when children review things they would like to be doing in real life. "I fly airplane yesterday, Daddy." The frequency of white lies tends to peak around 4 to 5 years, and begins to decrease in frequency as the child makes cognitive advances. Some children will tell a white lie as a means of trying to justify an event, because they think it is what the adult wants to hear, or because it will make the adult feel better. They may even feel they are protecting a cherished adult. For others the white lie may be the externalization of a fantasy. Because they do not realize the inconsistencies or implications, further problems may arise.

The way in which significant others in the child's life react to this form of fantasy can also affect its extinction as well as the child's self-concept. Encouraging white lies by acting overly amused (e.g., "How cute! Say that again for Aunt Mary!") will only serve to reinforce such behavior. This reaction does not help the child begin to understand the value of telling the truth or to perceive the world as it really exists. On the other hand, to assume that the child is actually lying and to punish him or her may only make the child feel guilty and ashamed of inner wishes. This reaction will not help the child to form a positive self-concept and may decrease the desire to be creative. A child will benefit from an adult's reaction to white lies when the reaction consists of acceptance followed by guidance to ascertain what, why, and how something really occurred:

Mother: So, Kitty said she wanted to go out and eat hamburgers?
Child: Uh-huh.
Mother: How did she tell you that?
Child: She open her mouth and say 'meow'!
Mother: And you think that means she wants to go out and eat hamburgers?
Child: Kitty only say 'meow.' But **I** want go out, eat hamburgers!

During the period of conscience development, children are most sensitive to the behavior and examples set by adults. They therefore need to live (and love) in an environment where trust and truth are a mutual basis for interpersonal relationships.

IMAGINARY PLAYMATES
"Mommy, you shut the car door on Marie's fingers!" cried Jenny as her mother walked toward the house. In actuality, no such person was still sitting in the car and experiencing excruciating pain. But as a compan-

ion and confidante, Marie did very much exist (and therefore her fingers were turning blue) in the creative mind of 4-year-old Jenny.

Similar experiences are not uncommon with many children who are approximately 3 to 6 years of age. Imaginary playmates are invisible to the adult; sometimes their presence is apparent if the child chooses to bestow such magical honors on a pet or a stuffed animal. Whatever form they take, and whether or not they are seen and heard by adults, their creation has special significance to the child. An adult can often infer the basis of a child's need for an imaginary playmate by listening to the child's "discussions" with a newfound friend. Imaginary playmates have been known to replace a next-door friend who moved away, an older sibling who started going to school, or a significant other who died. In some instances, imaginary playmates have been "born" when the child wants extra attention from parents or needs an outlet for a creative mind. Preschoolers may use imaginary friends to talk to so they can express their innermost feelings and find out more about themselves. In addition to all these functions, imaginary playmates occasionally take the blame for a misdemeanor, such as spilled milk or clothes put on the wrong way.

Imaginary friends are created more often by the child with an above-average intellectual potential. Constructing an imaginary companion involves increased mental activities and energy. Bright children, even in a stimulating environment, may be lonely and thus may have the time as well as the motivation to conceive such a fantasy. One normal and healthy gifted child created a whole community of imaginary friends, who married, gave birth, built houses, gave plays, and even died as part of a fantasy that extended over a 2-year period. (This same child, at the age of 12, wrote a delightful six-chapter fantasy tale, and at 16, a whole novel!) Most imaginary playmates, however, are not adults, but may possess the adult characteristics of power, strength, knowledge, or authority.

A child who is experiencing a fractionalized relationship within the family (e.g., newborn brother or sister, hospitalized parent, or actual child abuse) also has a tendency to construct an imaginary character. The Sullivan school of thought maintains that children who cannot, for some reason, obtain "cooperation" from the significant others in their lives are likely to "multiply the imaginary personifications that fill their minds and influence their behavior" [21].

It is important to emphasize that happy children who are accomplishing their psychosocial developmental tasks appropriately may still envision imaginary playmates during the preschool years. Imaginary friends constitute a normal, constructive phenomenon of early childhood. Not all children may share their imagination with adults, however. Since having an imaginary friend can, if continued over a lengthy period, alienate the child from other children and encourage an exaggerated egocentrism, caretakers need to accept the fantasy while trying to work through and decrease the need for its existence. When the child's needs are met, it is not uncommon for the child to announce, for example, that "Marie went to live somewhere else and isn't coming back." The child who needs professional intervention is the one who would rather stay in a fantasy world than play with peers or engage in activities that would help master the environment at increasingly complex levels.

FEARS

Fear is a normal, and often necessary, phenomenon. It is a way of alerting one that danger is present and that something may need to be done to protect oneself. Therefore, there are some fears that a child should have, but they should exist only to the point of aiding the child in averting absolute trauma. A child, for example, should be cautious with a strange dog because of the possibility of harm, but this prudence should not become an immobilizing threat every time the child sees a dog or views a picture of a canine.

The toddler or the preschooler has much to learn about the world and often misinterprets situations. It takes time, experience, cognitive growth, and loving guidance for the young child to understand that a screeching siren means someone is receiving help or that the dark makes it easier to sleep. Because children of this age readily absorb the fears held by significant others in their lives, it is appropriate for these other persons to work through their fears and recognize the attitudes they may be passing on to the child.

Since every child is unique, so will be the child's fears and the way they are formed. One young child may fear television sets because his mother shouted at him while she was listening to the television. Another child may have been handled roughly during an x-ray and thus is afraid of sitting still to have her picture taken. Some children will adjust to their fears more quickly than others; nevertheless, some fears tend to be characteristic of certain age levels. Examples of such fears are as follows: fear of loud, sudden noises at age 2; fear of animals at ages 3 and 4; fear of the dark at ages 4 and 5; and fear of the dark and being lost at age 6.

Children demonstrate fear in many ways. They may not always be capable of verbalizing their fears. They may regress (e.g., by resuming thumb-sucking, whining, wetting their pants) in either the presence or the expectation of the feared object or situation. Other tensional outlets (see Chap. 12) may also begin to appear: The child may become cruel (both physically and verbally) toward other people, animals, or toys; or he may be restless or irritable. Although such behaviors can be symptomatic of other things besides fear, they warrant investigation.

A child will frequently attempt to "play out" fears. For example, a 4-year-old who tries to put a Band-Aid on the family dog may actually be working out how he feels about receiving his immunization in the doctor's office earlier in the day. This action is a way of making the situation more familiar through dramatic play and thus serves as a strategy for handling fear. Important guidelines must be followed if dramatic play for therapeutic purposes is to be successful. Petrillo and Sanger offer some excellent suggestions for allowing a child to play through feelings and fears [22]. Although geared toward health professionals, their ideas can be used by those in any child care setting. However, these approaches do not replace guidance from a child psychologist for a severely disturbed child.

After a young child has been in a fearful situation, he or she may want to have especially close contact with the caretaker. The child may also want the caretaker to listen over and over again to his or her perception of what happened.

Recognizing that each child is an individual, and that any general advice is sometimes of limited value, Ilg and Ames have composed a list of "dos" and "don'ts" in assisting the child who is afraid [12]:

Don't make fun of the child's fears.

Don't humiliate him or her in front of others because the child has a fear.

Don't force the child to confront the fear (an unknowing parent may throw a hysterical child into a swimming pool to "get him (her) over fear of the water").

Don't call the child a "baby" because he or she has a certain fear.

Do realize that with time the child will outgrow the majority of his or her fears.

Do allow the child a respected period of withdrawal from the object or situation that evokes fear before gradual attempts to adjust to it are made (for example, if the child is afraid of cars, allow the child, first, to sit with you in a car that is not moving, and so on).

Do try within reason to avoid situations that scare the child so much that he or she just cannot cope.

Do be familiar with the common fears that most children naturally experience at various ages.

With a gradual introduction to potentially frightening situations, the young child will begin to cope with fears and to learn how to master new situations by small steps instead of withdrawing from them.

DREAMS

Vivid imaginations become more active when children are left alone at night. Shadows on the wall take on strange forms; the rustle of leaves outside a window may suddenly become mysterious footsteps. At this age, the child is learning to distinguish fantasy from reality and may still be confused about the reality of a dream. Frightening experiences of the day may be blown out of proportion, causing the child to wake up feeling that something terrible is about to happen. Perhaps the child witnessed two cars running into each other and later had a dream related to the same situation, or perhaps he or she felt the need to express feelings through a temper tantrum just before going to bed and continued this impulsiveness in the form of a dream. Another possibility is that some of the common fears of early childhood take control while the child is sleeping. Not all childhood dreams are unpleasant, however; on the contrary, many children report having a "fun time" while dreaming.

Just when dreams first appear is open to question. Occasionally, a baby's "smiling" while asleep has been interpreted by parents to mean that the infant is experiencing a pleasant dream. Some researchers believe that even premature babies may dream. However, Piaget reports that he and his associates have been unable to "find evidence of authentic dreams" until the child is able to talk and communicate with adults. Piaget goes on to say that the youngest age at which he observed definite proof of dreaming was in the range between 21 months to 2 years of age. These children talked in their sleep and gave an account of their dreams when they awoke [25]. This would indicate that dreams do not occur until the child is able to mentally manipulate events (Substage 6).

Piaget was less interested in when dreams first occur, however, and more interested in the type of symbolism present in childhood dreams. The question he asked was whether or not the manifestations of symbolic thought in childhood dreams became more complex as the child developed cognitively. He found that indeed they did become more complicated, although

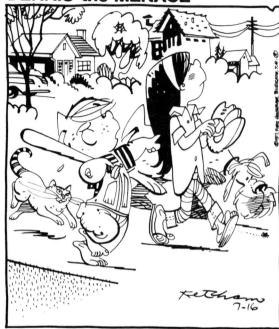

DENNIS the MENACE

"HOW COME YOU DON'T REMEMBER MY DREAM? YOU WAS IN IT ENOUGH!"

Figure 11–5. Reprinted courtesy of *Dennis the Menace.* Copyright Field Newspaper Syndicate, T.M.®.

the construction of play is much more "deliberately controlled" than that of dreams, which contain schemata from the unconscious [25].

The frequency of dreams as well as their content tends to change from one life phase of human development to the next. The younger 3-year-old may be awakened by a dream, for example, but may not appear to be very disturbed by it. In contrast, the older 3-year-old who experiences a nightmare may require some comforting after calling out in the night that he or she is frightened (see Chap. 12 for a discussion of quieting the frightened child at night). If the child's dreams are frightening, they often have a theme related to the common fears the child experiences when awake. Dreaming appears to increase in quantity when the child approaches 5 years of age. He or she may have considerable difficulty in going back to sleep after a nightmare and needs the caretaker's calm and reassuring presence until falling asleep again. Ilg and Ames suggest that caretakers may help children who have trouble waking from a frightening dream by carrying them into another room or washing their faces gently with cool water [12].

Pleasant dreams occur more often as preschoolers grow older (perhaps with more experience they have learned that some things can't always harm them). In his studies, Piaget categorized different dreams according to their content: wish fulfillment, painful experience recalled but given a happy ending, real nightmares, punishment or autopunishment, and dreams that are a "straightforward symbolic translation of an immediate organic stimulus" (e.g., a child with a stomachache may dream of eating a pebble) [25]. It might be noted that Freudian psychology places heavy significance on the content and meaning of dreams, theorizing that dreams are an essential part of coping with life. The symbolism of dreams is used by psychoanalysts to help individuals understand problem areas in their lives.

No matter what the true significance of dreaming is to a child, it is important to realize that dreams are probably related to unconscious symbolic thought and are soon forgotten by the child who experiences them.

BODY CONCEPT

Throughout childhood (and throughout life), the image of one's body and the affective significance of that image are in a state of continual change. Even in infancy, the child's clearest concepts of self as an entity are based on stimuli from the body. Arms and legs, hands and feet, skin, and gastrointestinal tract all continue to experience sensations and provide functions that help the child further construct a body image [34]. Nevertheless, the toddler is not always aware of the whole body or the distal parts and might even consider feet or other distal parts as something only peripherally related to self.

Usually around 3 or 4 years of age, the child's attempts to draw a human figure become recognizable to most adults. These illustrations usually consist of the head (with features such as eyes, nose, ears, and so on being added as the child grows older) and the arms and the legs (drawn as four or more lines issuing from the head). This does not mean, however, that a concept of the inner body is lacking in the young child. An extensive study of 96 hospitalized children, for example, found that, contrary to traditional belief, even 4-year-olds could name appropriate items contained within their bodies. They tend to conceive that their inner bodies contain elements, such as food, beverages, bowel movements, urine, and blood. Some children also become aware of components, such as bones, heart, nerves, and stomach [9]. By 4 years of age, some

children are aware that the brain is an internal body part associated with an array of distinctly mental acts [15].

BODY INTEGRITY

As preschoolers become more aware of themselves as individuals, they become more concerned about body integrity and intactness. The sense of vulnerability that accompanies growing self-awareness is often manifested in specific fears or anxieties and increased awareness of the potential dangers in the environment. The child's fears may or may not be realistic, since they are often related to the child's difficulty in distinguishing fact from fantasy.

The more conscious the child becomes of self as a separate person, an "I," the more he or she appears to fear physical injury and seeks assistance and consolation when injured. The child's "wholeness" as a personality seems to be closely related to the completeness and integrity with which he or she views the body. The

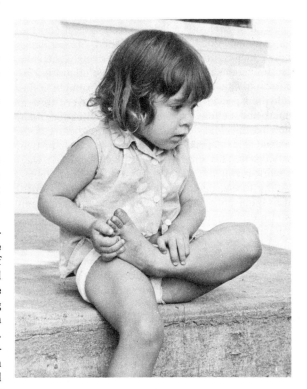

Figure 11–6. The preschooler's concept of body is constantly changing in accordance with daily experiences. Preschool children are well-known for their conscientious concern about the intactness of their bodies—every scratch and scrape is a crisis.

child values the body because within it is the source of feelings of self (the psychic "I"), and it is also the source of pleasure (the physical "I"). It is understandable, then, that during late toddlerhood or the early preschool years (around age 3), children begin to show greater concern for the safety and intactness of their bodies. During this time, many children exhibit concern about minor cuts and scratches. For the 2- to 3-year-old, a box of Band-Aids is a treasured gift. The child who is extremely upset by a minor bruise or scratch is frequently "restored" with a Band-Aid and feels "whole" again [8].

LEARNING

Attention

Attention is fundamental to discrimination learning. Unless a child attends to the stimulus, he or she will be unable to isolate the properties or indexes that differentiate one stimulus from another [31]. Attention span depends on the nature of the material being attended to as well as on the intellectual level and the self-confidence of the individual child. Studies have shown that children can learn surprisingly difficult discriminations if they are given guided opportunities to learn to attend to relevant cues. For example, if the child is expected to point to a square every time a square and a circle are seen in a given situation, then showing the child the square in isolation before each test will help the child to discriminate between the two test objects. This strategy represents a simplistic way of emphasizing the differences between stimuli by attending to one cue. The importance of such experiences is that once a child learns to attend to the relevant feature of a stimulus, he or she can learn to transfer or to generalize what has been learned to other, more difficult tasks (e.g., pointing to a striped square in a situation that also contains a striped circle).

The concept of attention in late preschoolerhood has been used to explain why children in different cultures acquire various concepts at different ages. In such studies researchers have been puzzled as to why children of the same chronological age answer questions about problem solving in a way that implies that they are at different levels of cognitive growth. Bruner [5] feels that the slower group needs to be taught how to increase the attention paid to selected perceptual features involved in the problem. Once they develop this skill, they are capable of giving equivalent answers. This concept forms part of the foundation for Montessori's educational materials and for a behaviorist or

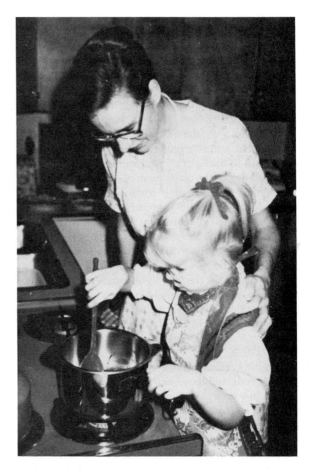

Figure 11–7. In guiding preschoolers through a new learning experience, it is usually beneficial to assign one task at a time. Their short attention span is thus optimally utilized when directed toward the mastery of individual, sequential steps especially when mastery of these short-term tasks results in immediate and desirable products.

systematic approach to teaching young children. Inhelder and colleagues state that the ability to shift attention from one perceptual feature or action to another more important one or to a more inclusive schema (the ability to generalize) is the key to the problem-solving process [14]. Whatever the reason, and no matter how closely related these two interpretations are, they both recognize the importance of attention in cognitive growth.

Some children between the ages of 14 and 24 months exhibit "dual focus," or the ability to maintain concentration on nearby work and simultaneously monitor or be aware of what goes on around them, usually in a busy environment (e.g., nursery school). The same ability is present in many 3- to 6-year-olds [35]. Researchers do not know how to train a child to do this, but White cautions that encouraging children to become involved in more than one task at a time before they are ready to do so will only interfere with their capacity to do either task well.

Memory

The rate at which the young child progresses in both cognitive and language development attests to a maturing memory. Information gained through selective attention to the environment is placed in the child's long-term memory (see Chap. 23).

Representative memory, which involves the child's retaining a mental image (see Chap. 8), appears in early toddlerhood. It is aided by verbal mediation in that a new word initially may serve as a symbol to prolong the image (words actually replace the image later in older children and become a sign used collectively). Representative memory assists the preschooler to remember where he or she put a box of crayons last month or to recall with vivid detail an event that occurred last year.

In discussing the memory processes of infancy and early childhood, Elkind says that rote memory appears as the child's language skills develop. He states that this form of memory involves the repetition of heard language sequences that "may but usually do not have an adaptive function" [5]. The child may be able to count to 10 or 20 but cannot tell you how many blocks are on the table. Toddlers will also use the second person pronoun or even use a question format when expressing a need, since they repeat, in rote fashion, what they have heard before they can creatively and flexibly construct their own ideas in words. For example, a child may say: "Do you need to go potty?" meaning that he or she needs to go.

Development of Cognitive Skills

It is appropriate at this time to present some of the cognitive behaviors that are typical of the average healthy toddler and preschooler. Table 11–1 lists chronologically the expected emergence of cognitive skills. Many of these behaviors are not **initially** examples of representative thought but are the behaviors of a child imitating the environment.

Assessment of Developmental Level

The most common test of intelligence in the United States is the Stanford-Binet, which measures what the individual has learned. This test includes several verbal and performance items. For example, at the 4-year-old level of the Stanford-Binet, the child is asked to name pictures that illustrate a variety of common objects, to name objects from memory, to discriminate between geometric forms (circles, squares, triangles), and to define words, such as "hat" and "bat." The test is scored in terms of mental age as a ratio of mental age over chronological age multiplied by 100. For example, a child whose third birthday occurs the day the test is taken and who scores a mental age of 3 years and no months would be given an intelligence quotient (IQ) of 100.

Another common intelligence test used with preschool-aged children is the Wechsler Preschool-Primary Scale of Intelligence (WPPSI), which also has a verbal scale and a performance scale. There are subtests within each scale, and each subtest is scored in terms of the mean for the age group. The IQ is derived from the total scores on all subtests. There is high correlation between IQs derived from the Stanford-Binet and from the WPPSI even though there are differences in the test items given and the methods of computation.

The newly revised Gesell Preschool Test [2] measures four aspects of early childhood development: motor, adaptive, language, and personal-social in children ages 2½ to 6 years (compare to DDST explained in Chapter 8). The kit contains developmental schedules for the easy charting of each child's behavioral age in the four areas. This Gesell test makes use of a variety of play materials that assess (among many other factors) eye-hand coordination, ability to follow directions, maturity of visual perception, understanding of words, elementary concepts of space, ability to hold information in short-term memory, ability to work out sensible solutions to social-problem situations, adaptability, and attention span. It is described by its creators as being valid for all children because it is "culture-free" and "culture-fair." The Gesell Preschool Test may be used for assessing and determining placement in preschools and kindergartens, for meeting the Child Find requirements of Public Law 94–142 (refer to Chap. 19), and for prescriptive and diagnostic purposes by qualified practitioners.

MAXIMIZING THE COGNITIVE POTENTIAL OF THE TODDLER AND THE PRESCHOOLER

Conscientious parents and caretakers are searching their local libraries or bookstores to obtain texts that contain the condensed results from recent child learn-

Table 11–1. Cognitive Skills of Early Childhood

Average Age	Expected Behaviors	Average Age	Expected Behaviors
18 months	Begins many questions with "what"	3 years	Asks many "Why" questions
	Uses some words and many gestures to indicate needs		Talks in sentences using four or more words
	Imitates anyone and anything in the environment		May talk about fears
			Can give first and last name
	Is beginning to understand that something else besides the present exists		May explore environment outside the home if given the chance
	Understands space only from the activity of moving through it		"Chains" objects using subjective attribute for categorizing (e.g., red block next to yellow block next to yellow crayon)
	Begins to follow simple, one-part directions		
	Begins to use "magical" power of thought		May retain urine through a night's sleep and wake up dry
	Will infer causes from observing effects		May use profane language if older children or adults heard using it
	Will explore extensively		
	May indicate wet pants		Counts to three
2 years	Is beginning to learn about time sequences (e.g., "after lunch")	4 years	Begins many questions with "Where"
	Will attempt new solutions to old problems		May talk with imaginary playmate
	Increases use of "magical" power of thought		May threaten to "run away from home"
			Can count to 5 and is learning number concepts
	May arrange several words together in grammatically incorrect two- and three-word sentences		Can name color of three objects
			Can give opposite of up (down), and hot (cold)
	May demonstrate a beginning cooperation in toilet training by anticipating a need to "go"		Can associate familiar holidays with the season in which they occur
			Completes 8- to 10-piece puzzle
	Matches simple shapes and colors		Understands 4 to 6 prepositions
	Names three body parts on request		"Magical" power of thought at a peak
2½ years	Is beginning to understand "tomorrow" and "yesterday"	5 years	May begin many questions with "How"
	Often talks by abbreviating grammatical adult speech (e.g., "Mommy eat")		Asks the meaning of words
			Knows days of the week
	Tends to talk in monologue (as though not expecting listener feedback)		Can count to 10
			Talks "constantly"
	Is beginning to think about the consequences of behavior		Can identify coins correctly
	May sort objects (blocks, dolls) and pretend they are members of a family (e.g., big block is head of the family)		May need to be reminded to eat and to go to bathroom because attention is so externally focused, may not recognize subtle internal cues
	Names six body parts on request		Can follow a three-step direction in proper order
	Understands 2 to 3 prepositions		Capable of memorizing own address

ing studies. Most of these writings suggest guidelines that can be applied in the home. As long as these guidelines are not carried to extremes, they can be very supportive. However, many caretakers do not know when they are encouraging an extreme [11]. Another problem may be that equally competent professionals recommend opposing approaches. Guiding a child's learning should be individualized. The child's individuality should not be stifled because of a preference for drawing with a large crayon while the caretaker thinks he or she should advance to the use of a new medium; nor should a child be punished because he wants to sketch a spider when his pilot father thinks he should be playing with plastic airplane models.

Since no two children have precisely the same cognitive abilities or exactly the same opportunities to learn, no two children will have identical concepts. However, children experiencing similar training and living in situations where there is an adherence to similar values will have similar concepts. The question then arises as to whether or not children can be taught selected concepts (e.g., conservation, classification) before actually discovering them for themselves. The child who is experiencing a transitional cognitive period at the time such training is introduced may be accelerated; however, the actual benefit of such acceleration remains to be proved. **It is more important that the environment keep pace with the child than to**

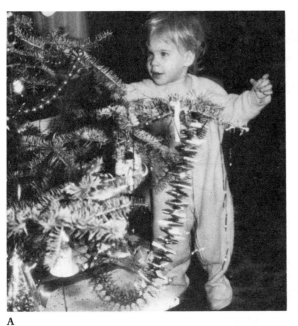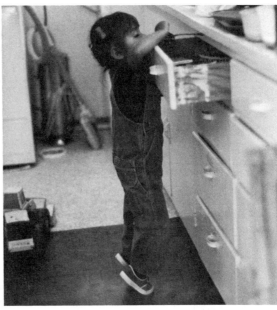

A   B

Figure 11–8. (A) The inquisitive toddler must be carefully watched by caretakers as the child examines the beautiful but potentially dangerous decorations of Christmas and other busy holidays. (B) The curiosity of the preschooler may prompt the opening of many containers that should remain safely closed and untouched by little hands.

force the child to keep pace with the environment. The child's interests and motivations should always be kept in mind.

Memory is one of the earliest and most important processes to develop in children [20]. Since many studies demonstrate that mentally retarded children have poor memories, efforts are being made to study the use of strategies for organization of information for memory. Such information could also help the intellectually superior child to maximize the rate of cognitive development.

Another type of learning necessary to the individual child's well-being is the concept of safety. More than one-half of all childhood deaths are caused by accidents. Many of these involve motor vehicles. Three out of four nonfatal accidents to young children occur in the home or in areas nearby [33]. Of these accidents, 90 percent have been estimated to be preventable.

Prevention must take the form of continued supervision as well as education. By toddlerhood the child is cognitively ready to understand the meaning of "hot," "sharp," "hurt," and "no" (although such words must be repeated for some time from one situation to another).

Young children do not always understand events in the way adults think they do. No matter how much learning adults may think has transpired, nothing should be taken for granted. The toddler's insatiable curiosity easily overrides parental admonitions about "not getting into things." For that reason, all potential poisons (including cosmetics) should be kept out of the reach of ingenious youngsters who have learned how to pull drawers out, use them as steps, and climb. Young children should be warned about appliances that burn, and they should never be left alone when such equipment is in operation. Matches are a terrible temptation to many toddlers; young children **must** be taught the dangers of playing with matches. Sharp-edged objects, such as razor blades or scissors, are a potential hazard to anyone and should be stored in safe places. No sharp object should be carelessly tossed aside into a wastebasket where a young child may discover and examine it. Any babysitter should be informed of all the precautions and safety rules of the household so that the rules can be enforced when the primary caretakers are not present.

Children are not as safe in their own yard as is often thought. Poisonous plants that look "good enough to eat" should be removed. In addition to "childproofing" the yard, the caretaker should make sure that the

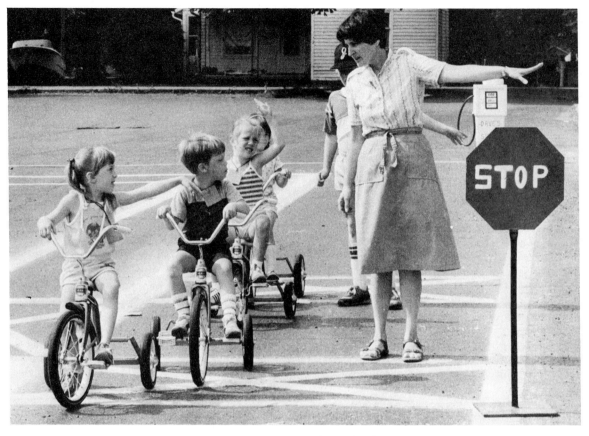

Figure 11–9. The preschool years are an excellent time to start teaching vehicular safety rules.

child understands the boundaries of the play area and should check frequently to make sure the child remembers. Children should be taught to use caution with all animals, no matter how much they think animals like them.

Even before preschoolers are old enough to cross the street alone, they should be taught how to do so and what will happen if they do not cross carefully. Caretakers can illustrate this safely and graphically with toy trucks.

The safest place for any child riding in an automobile is usually in the back seat; the child is **least** safe when held in the arms of a person in the front seat of a car. Special equipment (e.g., car seats, harnesses) can be purchased that has been especially devised to protect the child who weighs less than 40 pounds. Instructions on how these safety devices should be used accompany the product or can be obtained from the manufacturer. Most children who weigh over 40 pounds are able to use a standard seat belt. Car doors

should always be locked and the windows rolled up to a safe height. Children should **never** be left alone in a car—not even for a few minutes. They need to be protected not only from their own curiosity but also from vulnerability to strangers. These rules should be enforced from the beginning. Riding in a car can be fun for children who are taught activities, such as naming the things they see, identifying their colors, counting them, and so on.

Most young children love water and for this reason may be given swimming lessons very early. Even after children have learned to swim, they must have constant adult supervision (and that adult should be an accomplished swimmer). Sprinklers are safer than pools for young children. A full forward fall into just 3 inches of water may so frighten a young child that he or she may not be able to raise the head out of the water for air.

Why do young children sometimes disobey the rules? A variety of factors interplay: Perhaps they become too busy and forget; perhaps they have a greater need to assert self-will; perhaps they are confused about the caretaker's expectations in the first place. Frequently a child has to see if the caretakers really mean what they say. It is possible that the theory that the child's left brain (which handles mostly logical and analytical problems, including the following of directions) does not mature sufficiently until he or she is chronologically beyond the preschool years has some validity [18]. Whatever the major reason turns out to be, some basic premises about early childhood learning remain. Young children learn by doing. Sometimes a mistake can be a way of learning; the caretaker can encourage the child to feel that it is all right to attempt a realistic goal, and that failure does not make the child "bad." A negative result is not a "failure" but an opportunity for another learning experience.

Ames and Ilg feel that the main prerequisite is that everyone involved in the learning situation (both caretakers and child) be relaxed. If the child is provided with an environment of love and sharing; friendly, interested people; creative materials, books, and toys; and pleasant trips and excursions with significant others, then the healthy child will "learn as naturally as he grows and breathes" [1].

SUMMARY

Selma Fraiberg has dubbed the toddler-preschool period as the "magical years." And indeed they are for both children and their parents. Children are enchanted by the world around them. Each new object and event has a magical drawing power on the child who stares in wide-eyed wonderment at events as simple as a chicken pecking at grains in the gravel or as complex as the Rose Bowl parade. Each new object is explored and reexplored with all the senses and from every angle. Even emerging motor skills become events to explore and to repeat ad infinitum until the novelty wears off, mastery is assured, and the skill is incorporated into the repertoire of tools used by the child for further exploration of the environment. Through all these experiences, children are refining and expanding their schemata or bases of knowledge.

The parents are equally caught up in the child's joy of learning. They provide new experiences and challenges and are rewarded by the child's obvious infatuation with, and enthusiasm for, the event. They are amused by their child's observations, questions, and conclusions, often recalling comparable experiences from their own early years. This can be a thrilling, enriching period of family life as the parents share the culture and its rules, values, and accoutrements with the child.

A major theme of these years is the discovery of cause-effect relationships. Toddlers and preschoolers do not possess the same concept of these relationships as do adults. Their processing of information is rarely logical and may lead them to false or unsafe conclusions. Their observations of the ease with which adults make things happen may lead them to believe that all adults have magical powers—events occur because of the power of thought. Consequently, they may express as "truth" those events they would like to have happen, or they may feel responsible when a catastrophic event occurs during a period when they are angry or "feeling bad thoughts."

Gradually the child begins to differentiate between internal feelings and external behaviors and to separate internal images from external events. The increased ability to use symbols and signs facilitates both the child's internal thought processes and communication with others.

Children become fascinated by their own learning processes. They actively seek new information and try to identify relationships during these years. Children learned how to learn during infancy, but as Ralph Waldo Emerson observed, during these toddler and preschooler years the child's mind becomes aware of itself. During toddler and preschool years children learn how to teach themselves through the development of systematic exploration, trial and error, repetition, and experimentation.

REFERENCES

1. Ames, L. B., and Ilg, F. L.   *Your Four-Year-Old: Wild and Wonderful.* New York: Delacorte Press, 1980.
2. Ames, L. B., et al.   *The Gesell Institute's Child from One to Six: Evaluating the Behavior of the Preschool Child.* London: Hamish Hamilton, 1980.
3. Beard, R. M.   *An Outline of Piaget's Developmental Psychology for Students and Teachers.* New York: New American Library, 1972.
4. Bettelheim, B.   *The Uses of Enchantment: The Meaning and Importance of Fairy Tales.* New York: Knopf, 1976.
5. Elkind, D.   Cognition in Infancy and Early Childhood. In Y. Brackbill (Ed.), *Infancy and Early Childhood: A Handbook and Guide to Human Development.* New York: Free Press, 1967.
6. Flavell, J. H.   *The Developmental Psychology of Jean Piaget.* Princeton, NJ: Van Nostrand, 1968.
7. Flavell, J. H.   Concept Development. In P. H. Mussen (Ed.),

Carmichael's Manual of Child Psychology (3rd ed.), Vol. 1. New York: Wiley, 1970.

8. Fraiberg, S. H. *The Magic Years: Understanding and Handling the Problems of Early Childhood*. London: Methuen, 1968.

9. Gellert, E. Children's conceptions of the content and functions of the human body. *Genet. Psychol. Monogr.* 65:293, 1962.

10. Helson, R. Through the pages of children's books. *Psychology Today* 7(6):107, 1973.

11. Hymes, J. L. *Teaching the Child Under Six* (3rd ed.). Columbus, OH: Merrill, 1981.

12. Ilg, F. L., Ames, L. B., and Baker, S. M. *Child Behavior* (Rev. ed.). New York: Barnes & Noble, 1982.

13. Inhelder, B., and Piaget, J. *The Early Growth of Logic in the Child*. Translated by E. A. Lunzer and D. Papert. New York: Humanities Press, 1970.

14. Inhelder, B., Sinclair, H., and Bovet, M. *Learning and the Development of Cognition*. Translated by S. Wedgwood. Cambridge, MA: Harvard University Press, 1974.

15. Johnson, C. N., and Wellman, H. M. Children's developing conceptions of the mind and brain. *Child Dev.* 53(1):222, 1982.

16. Juntti, M. J. Determining Training Readiness. In M. J. Juntti, et al. (Eds.), *Total Toilet Training*. Baltimore: University Park Press, 1979.

17. Katz, L. Interracial awareness and acceptance. *Parents Magazine* 56(7):94, 1981.

18. Lease, C. A. Mind reader: Children can be too young for discipline. *Columbus Dispatch* (Ohio), p. D-1, Dec. 23, 1977.

19. Missildine, W. The toddler and motivation. *Feelings and Their Medical Significance* 18(4):19, 1976.

20. Moss, J. W., and Mayer, D. L. Children with Intellectual Subnormality. In J. J. Gallagher (Ed.), *The Application of Child Development Research to Exceptional Children*. Reston, VA: Council for Exceptional Children, 1975.

21. Mullahy, P. *Psychoanalysis and Interpersonal Psychiatry: The Contributions of Harry Stack Sullivan*. New York: Science House, 1970.

22. Petrillo, M., and Sanger, S. *Emotional Care of Hospitalized Children: An Environmental Approach* (2nd ed.). Philadelphia: Lippincott, 1980.

23. Phillips, J. L. *The Origin of Intellect: Piaget's Theory* (2nd ed.). San Francisco: Freeman, 1975.

24. Piaget, J. *Judgment and Reasoning in the Child*. New York: Harcourt, Brace, 1928.

25. Piaget, J. *Play, Dreams and Imitation in Childhood*. Translated by C. Gattengo and F. M. Hodgson. New York: Norton, 1962.

26. Piaget, J. *Six Psychological Studies*. Translated by A. Tenzer. New York: Vintage Books, 1968.

27. Piaget, J. *The Psychology of Intelligence*. Translated by M. Piercy and D. E. Berlyne. Totowa, NJ: Littlefield, Adams, 1976.

28. Piaget, J., and Inhelder, B. *The Psychology of the Child*. Translated by H. Weaver. New York: Basic Books, 1969.

29. Segal, J. The gentle art of daydreaming. *Family Health* 7(3):22, 1975.

30. Spock, B. *Baby and Child Care* (rev.). New York: Pocket Books, 1977.

31. Stevenson, H. W. *Children's Learning*. New York: Appleton-Century-Crofts, 1972.

32. Wadsworth, B. J. *Piaget's Theory of Cognitive Development* (2nd ed.). New York: Longmans, 1979.

33. Wegman, M. E. Annual summary of vital statistics—1980. *Pediatrics* 68(6):755, 1981.

34. Wenar, C. *Personality Development: From Infancy to Adulthood*. Boston: Houghton Mifflin, 1971.

35. White, B. L. *The First Three Years of Life*. New York: Avon Books, 1978.

36. Zaporozhets, A. V. The Development of Perception in the Preschool Child. In *Cognitive Development in Children: Five Monographs of the Society for Research in Child Development*. Chicago: University of Chicago Press, 1970.

12

Psychosocial Development of the Toddler and the Preschooler

Shirley S. Ashburn

To stop playing is not to grow up; it is to cease living authentically.

—William A. Sadler, Jr.

Introduction

Separation-Individuation during the Toddler Years
    Mahler's rapprochement subphase
    Erikson's autonomy versus shame or doubt
    Sullivan's syntaxic mode
    Expressions of autonomy

Separation-Individuation during the Preschool Years
    Mahler's consolidation subphase
    Erikson's initiative versus guilt
    Gender identity
    Significant relationships
    Tensional outlets

Development of Self-Control

Psychosocial Deprivation during the Toddler and Preschool Years
    Response to illness and hospitalization
    Child abuse

Conclusions

The ability to walk presents the child with new challenges in all four domains. The world and its relationships take on new perspectives and meaning. As the experience of children broadens, they become more aware of self and family within a larger social context. Children are confronted with increasingly complex conflicts, challenges, and fears as they struggle to identify themselves and their individual places in their ever-expanding social world.

During the toddler years, self-knowledge and progressive differentiation of self from the environment are gradually integrated into an emergent self-image. As children are increasingly able to regulate their own behavior, they begin to think and act on their own. This process, begun in infancy, continues during the preschool years. The establishment of independence is the major theme of toddlerhood.

Once the child is established as a separate, autonomous individual, the ability to interact with others is enhanced. As contacts with other children increase during the preschool years, elementary lessons of give and take may be learned in preparation for the social adjustments that are essential to school and to life outside the family (see Chap. 14). Weaning from a relatively great dependency on the mother and other family members is well under way. The beginnings of cooperative behavior are made as the child's concentration of interest on his or her wishes and impulses is gradually superseded by more controlled interactions. The child begins to assume responsibility for both the self and his or her world. Culturally acceptable social behaviors have their beginning in early childhood; their roots are found in the family.

The establishment of a personal and social identity is highly complex. Interrelated aspects include the following: (1) aggression/cooperation, (2) autonomy/shame or doubt, (3) initiative/guilt, (4) dependence/independence, and (5) gender role identity. Each aspect exerts a modifying or regulating influence on the child's personality and, as such, lays a foundation for future development.

Robert Havighurst [15] identifies eight developmental tasks for this period (see Appendix C); each task accommodates both individual needs and societal demands. These behaviors are those that an individual must develop in order to be judged reasonably happy and successful by self and others. Havighurst's concept assumes an active learner interacting with an active social environment. Some tasks arise mainly from physical maturation (e.g., learning to walk); others arise primarily from cultural pressures, such as learning to eliminate body waste at socially acceptable times and places. A third source of developmental tasks is the personal values and the aspirations of the individual. Examples of early childhood tasks arising from this source include beginning to learn "right" from "wrong" (which overlaps the tasks arising from cultural pressures).

Havighurst's concept clearly demonstrates two major principles: (1) that all areas of growth and development are interrelated, and (2) that the process of development, while similar for all children, is also unique to each child. The child who feels a sense of accomplishment in mastering Havighurst's tasks will experience a sense of independence.

SEPARATION-INDIVIDUATION DURING THE TODDLER YEARS

The separation-individuation process described by Margaret Mahler [20] (introduced in Chap. 9) continues throughout early childhood as the child establishes an awareness of and a sense of separateness from his or her relationship to mother and significant others. The interrelated processes of separation and individuation emerge from the symbiotic fusion the infant experienced with the primary caretaker. The toddler years roughly correspond to Mahler's third subphase, the period of "rapprochement," that extends from

about 15 to 24 months. Her fourth and final subphase is described as "consolidation of individuality and beginning of emotional constancy." This subphase represents the period of separation-individuation, which occurs primarily during the third year of life. Although the process of identifying one's own individual characteristics continues throughout life, it is during this period that the child recognizes the ongoing reality of self and others and begins to realize that he or she can function adaptively without the constant presence of the primary caretaker.

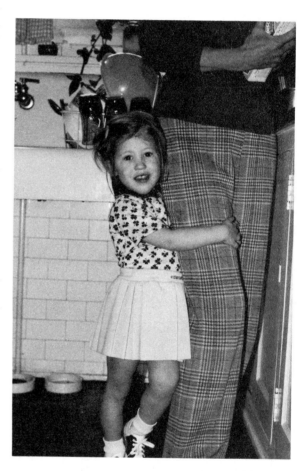

Figure 12–1. The phenomenon of "refueling" continues for several years when novel situations arise and may be displayed in various ways by each individual child. It provides the child with the necessary affective energy for independent exploration of, and interaction with, the environment, or to face an anxiety-provoking situation (in this case, a stranger with a camera).

Mahler's Rapprochement Subphase

With the increase in locomotion as well as cognitive and language skills, the stage is set for the child to emerge as a separate, autonomous person. Mahler postulates that as independent locomotion begins, the child becomes more aware of physical separateness from the mother. According to Mahler, this new freedom to move away from her freely creates both a pleasure in mastery, which differs in degree with different children, and a feeling of separation anxiety. With an increasing awareness of physical separation, the child begins to lose the previous resistance to separation, yet appears to become even more concerned about the mother's whereabouts. As he or she becomes more aware of a growing ability to move away, the toddler seems to develop a heightened desire and need for the primary caretaker to share every new experience and skill that is acquired. The contact with novel experiences, objects, and events appears to require more energy than the toddler has to expend. The child "refuels" by physically approaching the primary caretaker or by making eye contact before returning to the world of reality with renewed vigor.

As the child becomes more aware of separateness, he or she tries to cope with it by alternately moving away from and toward the mother. The child's degree of pleasure in independent functioning and desire to venture into an expanding environment seem to be proportionate to the ease of eliciting the caretaker's continued interest and participation. The toddler's growing awareness of personal vulnerability heightens the need to seek protection to control the environment through eliciting the mother's attention and assistance at times of anxiety.

The child's need for the mother as a "love object" and the return of the "object's" love become paramount. The child actively approaches the mother figure each time stress or a threat arises. Signs of directed aggression begin to emerge, along with a growing possessiveness and ambivalence. Many toddlers become jealous of anyone or anything (even the telephone!) that competes with them for the mother's attention. The child's calm acceptance of knocks and falls begins to disappear. The toddler appears to become more easily frustrated and demands more assistance, especially from the mother, when faced with frustration. During this period, the toddler's need is specifically for the mother (or primary caretaker); substitutes are not easily accepted, particularly for physical or comforting contact.

Sometime between the ages of 18 and 24 months, the rapprochement struggle reaches a peak in what Mah-ler terms the **rapprochement crisis.** The child's clamoring for omnipotent control, the extreme expressions of separation anxiety, and the ambivalent demands for closeness and for autonomy become intensified. The child appears to use the mother as an extension of self. Gradually, as individuation proceeds, this crisis becomes integrated and resolved. The child begins to find an optimal distance from the mother, a distance at which he or she can function well without the necessity of the mother's physical presence. At first, physical contact is essential for refueling, but gradually eye contact becomes sufficient. Some children eventually will be satisfied with carrying an object around with them that belongs to or represents the mother (transitional object). With the resolution of this final stage of the "hatching process," the toddler reaches a first level of identity, that of being a separate entity. A "self" is established [20].

Erikson's Autonomy versus Shame or Doubt

The rapprochement phase of separation-individuation described by Mahler complements Erikson's description of the toddler's developmental phase: acquiring a sense of autonomy [8]. According to Erikson, if the infant has developed an early sense of basic trust in the primary caretaker, the environment, and the way of life, the child begins to discover that events can be predicted and thus controlled to some degree. The mastery of motor skills and language, together with expanding cognitive powers, allows the child to differentiate self, both physically and emotionally, from the primary caretaker and the environment. Two psychological processes seem to be related to this enhanced self-awareness. Some awareness grows out of the action and the feelings that correspond with particular activities. As the child meets and masters problems, there is a feeling of being competent and "good." Awareness also comes from the child's expanding ability to recognize other people's reactions to what he or she does: Thus if mother is proud of the toddler's accomplishments, the toddler takes pride as well. Throughout toddlerhood, then, much of the energy of children centers on asserting that they are human beings with minds and wills of their own. As they develop a sense of autonomy—the feeling that they are independent human beings—healthy toddlers also recognize that they still need and are able to use the help of others.

Toddlers insist that they be allowed to explore and to do things for themselves (or at least to try). Allowing safe activities is critical to the emergence of a sense of autonomy. The child experiences an inner urge to express will and mobility while also feeling an inherent reluctance to experiment with potential capacities. Erikson considers these conflicting pulls, to assert the self and at the same time to deny the right and capacity to assert the self, as major themes during this phase; thus the child's struggle between the need for help and the urge to acquire independence becomes paramount. The favorable solution to this problem is to establish a sense of self and of self-control without loss of self-esteem. Erikson feels that this stage is decisive in determining the individual's capacity for, or balance between, love and hate, cooperation and willfulness, and the freedom of self-expression or its suppression. This means parents need to provide protection from physical and emotional harm while allowing the child as much independent activity and as many choices as possible. The parents can maintain control by predetermining the alternatives (e.g., giving the child a choice of orange juice or apple juice). Unfair criticism, lack of opportunity, or the child's inability to master tasks that foster a sense of autonomy can result in feelings of shame in the child and a lasting sense of doubt about self and others [8].

Erikson considers the stage of autonomy extremely important because "in it is played out the first emancipation, namely from the mother." The child's desire for expanded autonomy may find expression in negativism toward the mother and others. In situations where the mother has been the primary caretaker, the father assumes increasing significance as the child's world expands and he or she begins to explore and to develop more meaningful relationships with others in the family. Autonomy contributes to an eventual identity formation by giving the child courage to choose and to guide personal actions and the future. The child learns the conviction, "I am what I can will freely" [9].

Throughout this process of separating the self from the primary caretaker and identifying the self as an independent entity capable of asserting some control over self and the environment, several classic struggles emerge.

One of the most dramatic manifestations of developing autonomy is negativism, a form of behavior that occurs as the child becomes frustrated with blocks to any expressions of autonomy. With guidance and assistance, the child gradually learns socially acceptable methods of handling frustrations during the preschool years [33]. Negativism reaches a peak sometime during the second or third year and then gradually declines throughout the preschool years as the child learns (1) to control behavior and (2) that to cooperate with others is sometimes advantageous. Mahler relates the negativistic behavior to the child's attempts to disengage the self from symbiotic ties with the mother [19].

The toddler becomes easily frustrated when adult authority prevents the pursuing of an urgent need or a wish and requests that the child change an activity or suggests a novel experience. Toddlers perceive most activity as being urgent; postponement of such urgent wishes (activities) requires so much exertion that they have to summon all their energy reserves to oppose the wish. Usually a 2-year-old cannot summon enough opposition when urges are very strong; the adult must help the child with redirection and self-control. As a result, age 2 is often a very difficult age for the family [10].

The toddler's negativism is often expressed in a variety of ways. Stereotyped gestures and expressions of "No," going rigid all over, kicking, biting, hitting, throwing, breath-holding, and severe temper tantrums are characteristic of many children at some time during toddlerhood. This behavior is so universal that some writers refer to the toddler period as the "terrible twos." Negative behavior indicates, however, a major step in the child's progress from initial passivity and relative dependence to the assertion of an autonomous will. Negative behavior in the context of how children learn to deal with frustration is discussed in more detail later in this chapter in the section on the development of self-control.

Sullivan's Syntaxic Mode

Harry S. Sullivan indicates that a child first experiences the highest form of relating to others, or the syntaxic mode, between the twelfth and the eighteenth month [34]. It is during this time that the young child becomes capable of using some gestures or words that indicate the same meaning to the child as they do to others. It is this ability to "consensually validate," or to check that the message sent by the encoder was received and accepted by the decoder, that distinguishes syntaxic operations from the prototaxic or parataxic ones discussed in Chapter 9. The ability to consensually validate thoughts and actions clarifies communication with others and facilitates interpersonal relationships throughout the life cycle. As the young child recognizes the signs of approval or disapproval of behavior and as he or she experiments with how much the behavior of others can be manipulated, the child learns more about the ability to control personal desires and behaviors. If there is an excess of parental disapproval during these years, the child may come to view the world in negative and hostile terms [34].

Many of the young child's interactions with others

do not transpire in the syntaxic mode. Often a caretaker's actions are not communicative (for example, either "Do it because I say so" may be the only explanation the child gets, or the caretaker may use words in an explanation that the child does not understand), or a young child's defiant behavior (ranging from saying "No" to doing the opposite of what he or she is told) blocks most of the communication process.

As the child's command of the language increases, so does the opportunity to experience the syntaxic mode. Since true communication is a two-way process, however, caretakers must ever be mindful of the need to consensually validate their communications with the child. Since the child is still learning what words and gestures symbolize and perceives the world at a different cognitive level from adults, caretakers should remember to find out just what the young child is saying and what it **means to the child**. Successful communication through the spoken word and body language supports the child's developing sense of autonomy and lays a foundation for initiating experiences.

Expressions of Autonomy

The words "I," "me," and "mine" begin to have great affective significance as the child's sense of autonomy deepens and the knowledge of physical structures and boundaries progresses. Learning to control urination and defecation is in part a function of the child's expanded self-awareness.

The toddler should be able to point to major facial features and body parts on request. The body becomes a tool for experimentation. The young "researcher" may dabble in whatever appears interesting, such as cereal, mud, the cat box, or his own feces, although afterward he or she is likely to demand clean fingers. Toddlers try vigorously to use their bodies and mobility to do everything on their own: to feed themselves, to walk, to open and shut things, and to dress (or, more often, undress) themselves.

Because the body is a proud possession, the toddler may resist being handled by adults, particularly when held in a passive position, such as when being dressed or diapered. The toddler may not even like to be hugged or kissed at times. Thus the child's enhanced self-awareness significantly affects autonomous development during the separation-individuation process.

AMBIVALENCE

Ambivalence, or finding something simultaneously attractive and repulsive, is characteristic of the child's struggle to achieve autonomy. The toddler must learn

to coordinate a number of highly conflicting action patterns characterized by "holding on" and "letting go" [8]. The child becomes preoccupied with activities of retaining and releasing in all areas of functioning: perception, interpersonal relationships, desires, and manipulative objects. Ambivalence can be clearly seen in the child's attempts to hold on and to let go with the eyes, mouth, hands, and eventually the sphincters because of inner conflict—the desire to return to old dependence situations while also wanting to try new experiences. Psychoanalytical theorists feel that the anal zone is extremely important in the child's expression of the conflicting desire for dependence and autonomy. Experiences during bowel and bladder training provide a major test for the child's growing concept of self-regulation or self-control versus control by others [21] (see Chap. 10).

The child soon transfers the meaning of this struggle between self-control and control by others, the vacillation between dependence and independence, into other areas of life. Social behavior often reflects patterns of holding on and letting go. Activities such as collecting, hoarding, and piling up rather than putting things away become pronounced. Mahler describes toddler behavior of "shadowing" the mother versus darting away with the expectation of being chased and swept into her arms as being a major characteristic during rapprochement [20]. The term **shadowing** refers to the child's incessant watching and following every move of the caretaker. As individuation proceeds and the child exercises it to the limit, he or she becomes more aware of separateness and begins to employ numerous mechanisms in order to deny the actual separateness. The toddler experiences rapidly alternating desires to push the caretaker away and to cling to her—to hold on and to let go. When on a walk, the toddler may plunge off in pursuit of an interesting animal or activity only to stop short and come hurtling back into the caretaker's arms. The child may strike out alone and then burst into tears with the discovery of being surrounded by strangers. Every mother has experienced how a toddler will snuggle close to her one minute and ruthlessly push her away the next. Just when children are vigorously asserting autonomy, they may suddenly want to be helped, carried, babied, or cuddled.

The toddler's ambivalent behavior becomes compounded if the parents are also ambivalent about the growing autonomy. Most parents take pride in each new step forward and yet may lament the child's increasing independence and separateness. Parents may feel unsure of how much to trust the child's developing

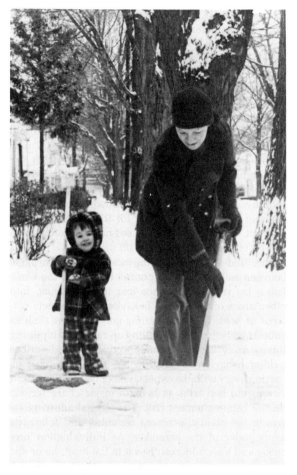

Figure 12–2. Toddlers and preschoolers, in their striving for independence and competence, need to feel that their efforts are appreciated. Imitation of adult behaviors is very common during these years. Parents can set limits as to how much the child can "help."

competence, when to keep hands off, and when to intervene. The child's insistence on autonomy may be aggravating to the parents. "A moment ago you did not want me to help. OK! Do it yourself!" may be the mother's response. Shame and doubt may begin to creep in. Parental support and tolerance of ambivalence are extremely important to assist the child in meeting the demands of burgeoning autonomy without creating a feeling of shame or doubt.

SEPARATION ANXIETY

The rapprochement phase is characterized by the toddler's renewed sensitivity to the parents' presence. An enhanced awareness of separation and an ambivalent push toward more independence, together with egocentric thought processes, leave the toddler particularly vulnerable to separation, especially if the separation is prolonged. The child's intense desire to function independently occurs at the point in development when the child's own feelings and wishes versus those of the caretaker are still poorly differentiated. The toddler's wish to be autonomous—to let go and to leave the mother—means to him or her that mother might also wish to leave. This fear may be compounded when the mother reacts adversely to her separating, individuating toddler. Thus one finds a powerful resurgence of the stranger reaction, especially toward people who earlier may have been regarded as friends. Difficulties with leavetaking itself begin to emerge, and the child may desperately cling to the caretaker and cry if she attempts to leave. The toddler may enjoy "darting away" but does not like to be passively left behind [20]. Separations can be well-tolerated if the child initiates them, but the child may "fall apart" when the parent initiates them. It is important to apprise children about imminent separations and reunions, even though they may protest vigorously. In this way, they are able to predict even though they cannot control the events; the trust relationship with adults is enhanced, and they are afforded the opportunity to develop elementary coping strategies.

Activities such as peek-a-boo, disappearance-and-return games, and the shadowing and darting-away behavior described by Mahler assist the child to overcome the anxiety experienced with separation. By repeating disappearance and return over and over under conditions he or she can control, the child is helped to overcome the anxiety that accompanies separation. The child can thus be assisted in learning to manage small amounts of discomfort and frustration. Empirical findings show that the developmental course of separation anxiety seems very similar for day-care and home-reared children. These studies have found (1) that day-care children develop emotional bonds in much the same way as children do at home and (2) that these secure attachments are usually with the parents as opposed to the day-care staff [29].

PLAY DURING TODDLERHOOD

Play assumes a special importance during toddlerhood. It provides a "safe island" in which autonomous development can proceed within the child's own set of boundaries [21]. The activities of eating, dressing, bathing, locomotion, and active exploration can all become forums for play. Even periods of negativism often have a playful quality. It is during this stage that the beginnings of dramatic play are seen—the imitation or acting out of scenes and events of everyday life. Through dramatic play, the child tries out roles and begins to identify with the adult models he or she is exposed to. The child's recognition of separateness as well as the similarity between self and others is expressed in play as the child shows a greater desire to have and to do what another child (or adult) had or did. In other words, the child has a desire to mirror and to imitate and thus begins to identify with the other person [20]. The first dramatic play of the toddler is episodic and is confined to simple, unelaborated themes. Much of this play reveals early identification with the parents; the toddler may trail the mother around the house imitating her activity (see Chap. 15).

LIVING WITH A TODDLER

Living with a toddler can be exceptionally pleasant and, at the same time, quite frustrating. The beauty and frustration of living with a child who is discovering the limits of autonomy are sensitively described by Fraiberg [10].

Everyone complains about the two-year-old. His parents complain about his willfulness, his stubbornness. His older sister complains about his peer group integration. "He won't share. He wants everything for himself!" If there is a younger brother or sister, an infant, he adds his lamentations to the chorus. In rare moments . . . when silence descends upon the household, the intuitive mother tenses herself in expectation of a shriek of pain which will certainly come in a moment from the direction of the baby's room. Everyone complains. But the family dog does not complain. When the two-year-old comes after him with playful cries, this sensible beast takes off to his sanctuary under the couch.

But miraculously, out of these ominous beginnings, a civilized being begins to emerge. For we have painted a dark picture, the two-year-old as his worrying parents see him. There is another side of the two-year-old which holds the real promise for the future.

He loves, deeply, tenderly, extravagantly, and he holds the love of his parents more dearly than anything in the world. To be fair about it, he also loves himself very, very much, and this conflict between self-love and love of others is the source of his difficulty at this age. But when put to the test, it is love for his parents which wins out . . . He wants to be good so he can win their love and approval; he wants to be good so that he can love himself.

SEPARATION-INDIVIDUATION DURING THE PRESCHOOL YEARS

As the toddler moves into the preschool years, the dual processes of separation and individuation continue. Mahler's fourth subphase centers around a twofold task: (1) the beginning of a lifelong consolidation of individuality or self-identity, and (2) the attainment of emotional constancy [20].

Mahler's Consolidation Subphase

The establishment of emotional-object constancy, in Mahler's sense, is based on the child's heightened cognitive powers, the concept of "object permanence" that began to develop during infancy, and on numerous other aspects of the child's personality, such as reality testing, greater tolerance for frustration, and so forth.

As used by Mahler, **object constancy** describes the "gradual internalization of a positively cathected, inner image of mother" [20]. This process was begun in infancy (see Chap. 8). The 3- to 4-year-old child is able to maintain a mental representation of the loved one and thus can periodically "refuel" from a mental image (a photograph can help some children to bridge the gap between physical presence and mental image).

The preschooler, then, develops an ability to remember the "object," the mother, and recognizes that needs can be satisfied even though the mother may not be present. The child gradually becomes able to accept separation once again, as happened during the practicing subphase. This ability leads to a greater tolerance of temporary separation experiences and appears to be a common point of readiness for nursery school. Thus the preschool child makes a slow transition from the ambivalent love characteristic of toddlers, which exists only as long as needs are satisfied, toward the more mature, mutual, give-and-take relationships seen in the school-age child and the adult [20].

Mahler postulates that during the fourth subphase (24 to 36 months) a stable sense of self-boundaries is attained, along with consolidation of gender identity. Verbal communication, which began during the third subphase, develops rapidly and replaces other modes of communication, although gestural language and mobility remain evident. Play becomes much more purposeful and constructive with a beginning of fantasy play, role playing, and make-believe. Observations about the real world become more detailed and are included as a predominant theme in the child's play. There is an increasing interest in playmates and other adults. The child's rapidly expanding cognitive capacity also assists him or her to tolerate greater delays in gratification.

The fourth subphase, then, is enhanced by the unfolding of complex cognitive functions. Individuation proceeds rapidly. This subphase is not a subphase in the same sense as the first three; Mahler describes the process as being "open-ended." As the child learns to recognize and deal with physical and emotional separation from the primary caretaker, a new level of self-awareness is attained. The preschool child achieves individuality as perceptions and responses to a rapidly expanding environment lead the child to a gradually solidifying adaptive style. He or she begins to learn to deal with life's successes and disappointments in an individual manner [20].

Individuation proceeds so rapidly during the preschool years that it is difficult to speak of specific or characteristic traits in the manner used to explore infancy and toddlerhood. Personal style becomes more salient. Some styles can be defined in terms of orientation, such as "leader," "follower," "participant," or "onlooker." Other dimensions, such as bold versus timid, hostile versus friendly, and independent versus dependent, become more individually characteristic [19].

Erikson's Initiative versus Guilt

Erikson's major developmental alternatives of the preschool years, "initiative" versus "guilt," closely correspond to and complement Mahler's separation-individuation framework. The child, having reached a measure of autonomy and recognizing him- or herself as a separate person, begins to question and to explore in order to find out what type of person he or she may become. The preschool years are a period of rapid fluctuations between dependence and independence, competence and ineptitude, maturity and infantilism, growing affection and antisocial destructiveness. This fluctuation is understandable in light of the child's continued striving for individuality and the rapid cognitive and motor advances that occur during this period. The child of 5 or 6 years of age is very different from the 3-year-old child; however, just as a toddler retains many infantile characteristics, the young preschool child is, in many respects, similar to the toddler.

Erikson and Mahler correlate psychosocial development with the child's growing facility with motor, language, and cognitive skills. These skills aid in the resolution of the preschooler's initiative versus guilt crisis in various ways. First, as the child masters skills, such as walking, running, and skipping, he or she is able to move about more freely and develops a wider

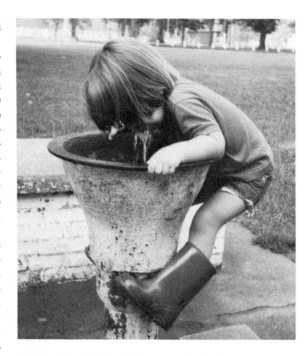

Figure 12–3. As the healthy preschooler develops a sense of self, he or she becomes more independent when faced with the realities of everyday life.

radius of activity and attainable goals. Once locomotion skills have been mastered, the child can concentrate on a more constructive goal, or on what can be **done** with these skills. Second, the child gradually is able to understand and to express more thoughts through the medium of language. The use of adjectives and adverbs allows for finer discrimination between, and expression of, ideas. The child begins to question everything and everyone incessantly and likes to predict or to control the answers. Third, reaching out with both locomotion and language skills permits children to expand fields of imagination. They may even frighten themselves with some of their ideas. They feel and fear, "I am what I can imagine I will be" [9, 20]. Separation of reality and fantasy may be difficult.

Having achieved some measure of autonomy and conscious control over self and environment, preschoolers move forward to master new challenges in ever-widening social and spatial spheres. Healthy preschoolers exhibit initiative or planning for events in more areas of life; the social environment challenges them to make more choices, to be more purposeful and active in goal setting. They are able to begin to assume some responsibility for self and others (e.g., their bodies, their toys, their pets, other children). Children search for and create fantasies about the kind of person they would like to become. They may now begin to visualize themselves as "grown-ups" and try to comprehend possible future roles or, at least, to understand what roles are worth imagining. Role models become critical to this process. This joyful spontaneity and the characterizations of adult life can be delightful to observe. Because play in all forms is so intimately related to the child's psychosocial identity, the reader is referred to Chapter 15 for a more thorough discussion of this topic.

Preschool children "intrude" into the spheres of others and imitate their behavior to learn how to understand other people as well as to learn who they themselves are and what they can become. This behavior includes: (1) intrusion into space by vigorous locomotion; (2) intrusion into other people's minds by the aggressive voice; (3) intrusion into the unknown by consuming curiosity; (4) intrusion upon or into other bodies by actual physical attack; and (5) intrusion upon other people's time by requests for a play companion or assistance with a task.

This new behavior causes considerable feelings of discomfort and guilt because it negates, to some extent, the trusting relationship previously formed with caretaking adults. This is also a period when the conscience (superego) begins to function as an inner censor of behavior (see Chap. 18). Erikson, in fact, refers to the conscience as the "great governor of initiative." Faced with the universal crisis of separating from a psychological attachment to the parents, the child begins the slow process of becoming a "parent" as well.

The first step in becoming a parent involves the preschooler's ability to begin to supervise him- or herself in the place of the parents. The child hears the "inner voice" of self-observation, self-guidance, and self-punishment and increasingly assumes the supporting and controlling functions of significant adults in the environment. The child's conscience, however, can be primitive, cruel, and uncompromising and often tends to conflict with what the child fantasizes he or she is or wants to be.

The crisis, then, according to Erikson, is to test one's own will without an overwhelming sense of guilt about one's actions. Actions, such as speaking first, asking for a drink, completing a puzzle, or running after a ball, need to be reinforced frequently. When guidance is critical to safety, the child's goal should be acknowledged as desirable while the dangers are explained in such a way as to maintain self-esteem and to minimize guilt. The positive outcome is a sound sense of initiative that is guided and modified by a growing sense of conscience and reality [9, 21].

Many writers, including Erikson, have spoken of the preschool years as a "first adolescence." It is a time for the first identity formation, as the child prepares to move away from the family into the world of school, peers, and practical achievement. The child invests a great deal of energy in refining muscular activity, accuracy of perception, assessment of others, and communication skills. The healthy preschooler is an eager learner who directs effort toward defining a purposeful existence and a sense of self-identity, which gradually begins to modify the child's egocentricity [21].

The child needs to learn to respect limits without

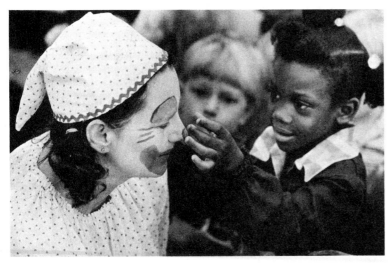

Figure 12-4. The toddler and the preschooler need multiple sensory experiences to help them to integrate perceptual information.

being made to feel guilty or that he or she is being punished for bad wishes. The child needs to be assured that feelings of anger and disappointment are normal and to be given words and behaviors appropriate for expression of those feelings. The child who in anger wishes father to die must learn that having bad wishes will not make the wishes come true. Parents can help the child in two ways: They can view the child's frustration, fury, and fear sympathetically and, at the same time, convey silently the reassuring message, "I will not let you carry out your fearful wishes." This attitude is very important to the preschool child because some primitive thinking still dominates certain areas of his or her life, and the child may anxiously fear that "terrible wishes" will come true. During the preschool years, then, the child moves from being the center of the universe to assuming a modest place in human society; he or she achieves what Erikson has called a "realization of purpose."

Three sources of fear or anxiety predominate the preschool years; fears about the body and body mutilation, fears about death, and fears associated with loss of self-control. These specific sources of anxiety are related to the child's growing identity, concern for the body, and the crisis of initiative versus guilt. The reader is referred to Chapter 11 for a discussion of other fears encountered during this period of development.

Gender Identity

Freudian theory proposes that the child has no clear concept of "boy" or "girl" until he or she makes the first observations of genital differences between self and others. For most children, this observation occurs sometime during the third or fourth year of life, depending, of course, on the child's contact with parents, siblings, and other children. These first observations of genital differences may produce reactions of surprise or shock. Direct observation of small children indicates that the discovery of genital differences may be disturbing and painful; there is evidence that the discovery may lead to infantile fantasies of body damage and mutilation. Freudians state that as parents provide the necessary support and information to correct primitive thought, the little boy can begin to recognize that nothing has been taken away from the little girl and that nothing will be taken away from him. Gradually the child can begin to take pride in his or her own gender because the child is made like a beloved parent. However, this process of education takes a long time, and even during the preschool phase of development, some elements of this primitive theory of gender differences will survive [10].

Toddlers become aware of gender differences; preschoolers consciously begin to learn and to practice their roles as male or female in an expanding social realm. The child begins to learn how gender influences feelings and behavior in relation to others, and how it may influence career and social potentials [21].

The preschool child's increasing interest in sexuality is simply an extension of a curiosity about all phases of living. This vivacious little person, not yet fully concerned with the feelings of others, is actively interested in toilet activities and innocently unaware of adult standards of modesty (although many young preschoolers sporadically display episodes of false modesty). Preschoolers want to watch others use the toilet, are full of "bathroom humor," and want to look at and touch breasts and bottoms (both their own and those of others).

The young child's interest and curiosity in sexual differences is expressed in many ways. The child begins to question, "Who am I?" "Where did I come from?" The little boy or girl may be observed to slouch in front of a mirror to simulate the "big tummy" of pregnancy. Some children may ask to bathe with the parents or to touch their bodies; others may simply burst into the bathroom or bedroom when parents or other siblings are attempting to maintain privacy.

Sex play with other children also occurs, often in the form of assuming roles (e.g., mother-father, doctor-patient). Parents are often concerned about how to handle sex play and masturbation and the preschooler's consuming curiosity related to gender differences, because they know that excessive shame or anxiety connected with the genitals can seriously disturb the child's personality development and adult sexual functioning. Parents must respect the child's curiosity and actions as being normal without judging the child or the activity as wrong or bad. At the same time, parents must decide on limits of privacy for themselves and others. This is the age to help the child begin to learn about "public" self and "private" self. Masturbation and toileting are natural activities involving the "private" self. Such clarification sets limits without criticism, thereby reducing the potentially damaging emotional undertones. Such clarification also lays a foundation for prevention of sexual abuse.

When parents discover their child involved in sex play with other children, it is best simply to ask the children to dress and find something else to do. The parents of both children can talk privately with them about the incident at a later time. Talking privately helps each child to maintain a sense of dignity. Children are often ashamed or worried about their games even though they cannot control their curiosity; at times they even appear to arrange the situation so the caretaker can "find out." In talking with the child, it is important to point out (1) that interest in how boys and girls are made is natural, but the child cannot get all the answers to questions by looking or playing games, and (2) that the child can ask mother or father everything he or she wants to know. In this way, the child is not made to feel ashamed or frightened. Curiosity can be satisfied within the context of the parents' moral philosophy while helping the child to set more socially acceptable limits on behavior. In instances where the child is cared for by another person in the parents' absence (e.g., if both parents work), the babysitter should be informed how to handle sexual curiosity on the part of the child.

Other forms of sexual curiosity should be handled in a similar manner. Questions should be answered simply and truthfully without elaborate explanations. Preschoolers can accept straightforward answers, even though they may not understand them completely. They gradually learn the basic anatomical structures and functions of their own body and those of the opposite gender as well as simple facts about conception, pregnancy, and the birth process. Preschool children can be told that a baby grows for about 9 months in a special place inside the mother and that there is a special place for the baby to come out when it is ready to be born. Information must be modified according to the child's cognitive skills at a particular stage of development. Numerous books are now available to assist parents in teaching their children.

During these early years, the child must realize and accept the fact that parents have a private life together from which he or she is excluded. The parents' bedroom can become a symbol of such privacy. Many parents exclude the child from the dressing, toileting, and bathing of the parent of the opposite gender. (Other parents do not feel strongly about this, or may feel strongly about **not** hiding everyday activities of personal hygiene.) In any case, the child should learn very early that mother and father belong to each other and that the quality of their love for each other is different from, but does not eclipse, the quality of their love for the child.

Significant Relationships

The role of the family, especially the parents, is discussed either directly or indirectly in almost every chapter of this text. Family relationships lay the foundation for all future interactions. Family experiences provide the opportunities for a child to become aware of the emotions of others as well as his or her own. Beginning in toddlerhood, the child is capable of experiencing sympathy toward family members, although this is partly an imitation of the attention and ministrations offered to the child at times of stress. (Paradoxically, a child of this age who has been the victim of child abuse may attempt to soothe a frustrated abuser when sensing that there is again a danger of being harmed.)

RELATIONSHIPS WITH SIBLINGS
Chapters 17 and 32 discuss the effects of birth order and sibling rivalry on the psychosocial development of the individual. Siblings offer constant challenges to the development of interpersonal relationships. Some preschoolers prefer playing with younger siblings in order to protect or to help them. Such relationships can foster a sense of responsibility and self-worth in the preschooler. Obviously, not all children experience these feelings toward their siblings, nor does any one child possess generous thoughts all the time; such thinking would be contrary to human nature and especially to the egocentrism of the normal preschooler. Young children may or may not be included in the play of their older siblings. If they are "allowed" to play, they are not always happy with the roles they are assigned (e.g., "baby" when playing house). Other young children do not seem to mind what roles they play as long as they are included; they willingly become the sibling's servant in exchange for the privilege of participation.

RELATIONSHIPS WITH GRANDPARENTS
The influences of grandparents on the developing child vary with the personality structure of the persons involved as well as the social structure of which they are a part. When grandparents engage in a mutually fun-seeking relationship, the child usually looks forward to their times together (although the grandparents may be a threat to the parents' rules of discipline in such situations). The grandparent who is in some way distant when he or she interacts with the child may teach the child that some people can serve as objects of indifference. In such situations, the child may learn that material goods serve as tokens of recognition or as substitutes for more meaningful relationships. Separation or infrequent visitation need not be synonymous with indifference if the quality of relationship is rich and meaningful to both when they are together.

Those grandparents who serve as surrogate parents may affect the child's development as strongly as if they were the child's real parents. If the grandparents live in the home with the parents and child, the three-way relationship may become very complex, since discipline and values may be sources of conflict. Many families still reside within extended family groups where any member may hold the reins of power. In some Native American cultures, for example, the grandmother, not the parent, has authority over the grandchildren (to the point of being consulted if the child needs a consent form signed for surgery). The lines of authority and responsibility should be clearly defined in each multi-generation family to prevent frictions resulting from role confusion.

RELATIONSHIPS WITH AGE-MATES
In studying the interaction patterns of young children, it has been noted that infants show relatively more responsiveness to active, mobile, adult caretakers than they do to their infant age-mates who do not supply as many stimuli [14]. Toward the middle of the second year, however, many young toddlers become curious and attend positively to their peers.

The older toddler's first reaction to the distress of an age-mate (other than a sibling) usually takes the form of bursting into tears. This is probably a display of "empathetic participation" rather than actual sympa-

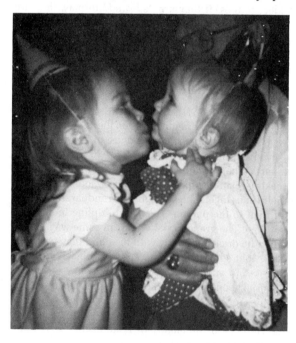

Figure 12–5. Sometimes toddlers fear that whatever is harming a crying baby may also harm them. To reduce the possibility of such an occurrence, they will attempt to comfort the baby, thus reflecting poorly differentiated boundaries between the baby's feelings and their own.

thy, and such behavior probably reflects poorly differentiated boundaries between the child's feelings and those that are expressed by others.

True sympathy to the feelings of others, which in the beginning is sporadically displayed for sometimes questionable reasons (e.g., guilt, wanting to be in charge), begins to appear later in the preschool years.

RELATIONSHIPS WITH PETS
Many adults have fond memories of their childhood pets. Having a pet who loves a child unconditionally gives the child a sense of self-worth. With guidance, young children can learn the facts of life and death, gentleness, compassion, and sharing by having animals in the environment. An only child may value a pet both as a playmate and as a prized possession to "show off" when others come to visit. Being introduced to various animals by an understanding adult can help a child overcome fears of certain animals. At the same time, the adult approach to an unfamiliar animal can teach a child to be cautious in relating to animals. Animals have been effectively used in school classrooms, including nursery schools, to accomplish these same goals. Children who have never visited a farm or a zoo can profit from such a learning experience. Disadvantaged children can learn to appreciate the lives and purposes of other living beings when a thoughtful teacher brings an animal to school.

Many parents who concede to a preschooler's request for a pet will do so principally because they believe that the pet will teach the youngster to be responsible. Such parents are likely to be disappointed. A sense of responsibility cannot be acquired overnight; it develops gradually.

In choosing an animal for children, the parent or teacher should consider the temperament and habits of the animal as well as its compatibility with the family and their life-style. Some types of dogs, for example, do not adapt well to suburban restrictions. Veterinarians, a reliable pet dealer, and the library are valuable sources of information. Responsibilities should be determined beforehand (e.g., the schedule and the type of feedings the animal requires, walking the animal, cleaning up accidents, bathing, doctor's visits) in order to balance the assets and liabilities of pet ownership. Above all, a family with both a young child and a pet must continuously assess their ability to live safely under the same roof.

Tensional Outlets

As discussed in Chapter 9, many factors influence the child's ability to deal with the painful aspects of separation-individuation. The child's age, temperament, and the previous parent-child relationship are all important factors. Each child will respond uniquely. Separation will cause a degree of anxiety and tension for all toddlers, particularly during the rapprochement crisis, but some are able to deal with separation better than others.

Some degree of anxiety is both normal and necessary for growth. It functions as an energizer—an impetus for problem solving, decision making, or skill performance. When tension becomes more marked, the excessive energies may be released through physical activities (motor discharge). Many parents discover that their toddler or preschooler develops what appear to be "bad habits," or at best, "very strange behavior" during this stage of development. These behaviors may include rocking, head banging, masturbation, thumb-sucking, and so on. Bizarre as these behaviors seem to the adult, they may simply reflect the child's individual pattern for dealing with tension or may provide the child with a predictable, soothing form of self-stimulation. The majority of the time, the child will outgrow these behaviors. Repeated attention to the behavior can reinforce its use since it secures coveted parental attention. A child may develop a favorite method (or methods) for relief of tension; some behaviors may gradually decrease and later reappear.

Some behaviors that begin during infancy may persist through the early years and well into the school-age period of development. Ilg and Ames found that the exacerbation of a tensional outlet fluctuates with age. They feel that 2½, 3½, and 5½ to 6 years are ages that seem to harbor more tension than others. Many parents may be able to accept these behaviors during infancy but may consider them to be signs of insecurity, unhappiness, or maladjustment as the child grows older, reasoning that "normal children don't behave this way." A parental attitude of calmness, relaxation, and acceptance will help to reduce tension and thus will benefit the child [16].

These behaviors may also be used by the child simply because they provide pleasurable sensations. Thumb-sucking as a form of tension relief often reaches a peak during late infancy or early toddlerhood. This form of behavior, along with practical suggestions for dealing with it, is discussed in Chapter 9.

The use of security objects or transitional objects is common during toddlerhood. The toddler (or infant) begins to utilize inanimate objects provided by the caretaker, such as car keys, a stuffed toy, or a bottle, to assist the transition during the separation-individuation process. Separation from the mother may seem less intense to the young child who is able to cling to an object provided by her. Some toddlers may carry a

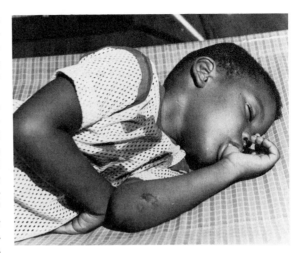

Figure 12–6. This youngster, revealed in all his innocence, is still very much a baby. Many children continue to suck their thumbs through their toddler and preschool years.

blanket with them at all times; others may use a security blanket only at bedtime when they separate from the activities of a busy day or when they are unusually distressed. Security objects are often used in conjunction with thumb-sucking or other forms of tensional outlets. The specific object and use of that object is unique for each child.

Some toddlers and preschoolers may engage in rocking, particularly at bedtime or during sleep. Rocking generally starts out as a perfectly natural developmental behavior. At approximately 25 weeks of age, before the infant can creep or crawl, an infant may get up on the hands and knees and begin to rock. Usually this rocking subsides once the child is able to creep; however, this normal behavior may persist for several years. If rocking behavior does not stop during infancy, it often reaches a peak around 2½ to 3½ years and then gradually fades away. Although rocking is essentially harmless for the child, it may be troublesome for the parents. Since rocking during toddlerhood occurs primarily at bedtime or during sleep, parents may try several things to minimize the behavior and the noise such behaviors may create: Cribs can be padded and tightly screwed together, and a rug can be placed under the crib. These measures will reduce noise and movement, so that the rocking behavior may not be as reinforcing for the child. Sometimes a prolonged bedtime routine that involves pleasurable, quiet activity may reduce tension and minimize presleep rocking. Older children may cease this normal form of rocking when they are moved to a larger bed that they feel is their own.

Head banging is similar to rocking; it is often more frightening for parents, since it may result in actual bumps or welts on the child's forehead. The child simply selects a hard surface (e.g., bed frame, wall, stove) and bumps the head against it. This form of tensional outlet usually begins in infancy and disappears before 3 years of age as language skills increase.

Head banging is common enough to be listed as a variation of development; this view can be reassuring for parents. Except for welts and bruises, it is uncommon for the head banger to do any real damage to himself. Parents can assist the head banger by picking the child up and comforting him or her without drawing attention to the behavior. Distraction with music, a toy, or some other device is also helpful. As a rule, scolding and punishing are completely ineffective. The professional and the parent would be wise to reassess the environment from the child's perspective and make attempts to reduce stressors and provide a more responsive, appropriately stimulating but safe environment.

Masturbation is another tensional outlet of early childhood. A child becomes aware of genital sensations in infancy, but the genitals generally do not serve as a primary focus for pleasure until after 3 years of age. Young children may masturbate before they sleep, or when they are fatigued or bored. Masturbation serves the child as a form of self-love when lonely, self-employment when bored, and self-consolation when tired.

According to the psychoanalytical view of development, specific organs become the focus of awareness because of the greater amounts of tension that accompany their functions. As mentioned in Chapter 9, the organ of concentrated pleasure for the infant is the mouth. During the second year, the child becomes aware of tension and relief sensations that accompany evacuation. It is easy to see how the anus achieves importance, at least for a short period of time. Late in the first year, the male infant may discover genital sensations; the genitals, however, do not become an important focus of pleasurable sensations until the third year and later. At this time, one can observe an increased interest and more frequent handling of the genitals by the child. From the third year on, the genitals assume more importance for the child because they have become special organs of pleasure.

Children of 2½ to 3 years old are often very casual in the way they handle themselves. When his or her hands stray to the genitals, the young child is not concerned about the presence of others. One should keep in mind that masturbation does not have the same connotation for young children as it does for adults. The caretaker may provide something else for the child to do with the hands or gently remove the hands and pick up the child. As the child grows older, he or she begins to internalize adult standards and thus tends to masturbate only when alone.

Although childhood masturbation may comfort the child, it can cause conflicts for many parents. The manner in which parents respond to this behavior can significantly affect the child's developing awareness of his or her own sexuality and feelings about the self. If a parent strongly forbids this behavior, a child may feel extreme guilt or shame when, for example, half asleep, he cannot keep himself from doing what is forbidden. Experts differ in suggestions for dealing with masturbation. A realistic and objective assessment of how much masturbation is occurring is essential. The occasional or before bedtime variety is usually considered normal, but continual masturbation to the exclusion of other activities needs to be treated. Many psychologists feel that excessive parental efforts to prevent masturbation may be psychologically harmful and suggest ignoring the behavior when it occurs [10, 12, 16]. They suggest that parents may exert mild pressure to eliminate the behavior, but the emphasis should be to assess and to improve the child's life in general so that the child will feel less tension or will find other means of satisfaction. Personal achievements and relationships should be the child's main source of satisfaction. Intervention should be individualized to the age of the child, the type of masturbation, and the parents' feelings about this activity.

Frequent and open masturbation by the school-age child does not have the same meaning as the casual touching characteristic of toddlers. Persistence of this type of masturbation in older children may indicate unresolved anxieties; it may become a "too ready consolation" for mishaps, failures, or feelings of discomfort. In fact, a child who touches the genitals repeatedly throughout the day, or a boy who hangs onto his penis, usually derives no pleasure from this behavior; it restricts the ability to become fully involved in more productive behaviors, and it may begin to interfere with social relationships. Parents may want professional assistance in evaluating or handling such behavior in a child.

Sleep disturbances are common during the toddler and preschool years. Busy parents may not realize that overscheduled life-styles may breed sleep problems in their children. When the separation-individuation struggle is at its peak during toddlerhood, falling asleep may represent an experience of another separation. Mild sleep disturbances of a transitory nature are a normal phenomenon in children 15 to 30 months of age [12]. The sleep disturbance is often related to an anxiety dream in which a frightening experience in waking life (particularly a separation experience) is repeated over and over. When reexperiencing the anxiety in a dream, the child will awaken with frightened cries, both as a reaction to the dream and a summons to the parents. The toddler may resist sleep even if the parents come to comfort him or her.

In infancy and early childhood, a dream is considered a real event; it is usually not until the third or fourth year that a child knows what dreaming means. The child is convinced that there really was a "tiger in the bed." (A more detailed discussion of fears and dreams is found in Chapter 11.)

If preschoolers have older siblings who stay up later, they may rebel at bedtime and not sleep well because they exaggerate what they may be missing. For all young children, sleep disturbances may be triggered or intensified by illness, moving to a new home, the arrival of a new baby, a prolonged separation from the mother, staying up to watch television, or overstimulating movies. Even waking up to find a strange babysitter may be traumatic enough to disturb a toddler's sleep for several weeks. A consistent bedtime ritual is helpful.

The child who suffers from sleep disturbances and wakens with anxious, fearful cries should, of course, be reassured by the mother or father. The parents should try to reassure the child in his or her own bed. Many psychologists believe that if the parents offer the child too many special satisfactions and pleasures, such as prolonged rocking, a bottle, toys, or the opportunity to come to bed with them, they may inadvertently provide another motive for waking—the motive of pleasure gain. The parents should go to the child in an unhurried manner and talk in a quiet voice. The diaper should be checked and changed if necessary. If very young and unduly upset, the child may be held for a few minutes but then should be put back to bed again, even though still awake. An older child can be patted and talked to reassuringly. After the child has had time to awaken fully and to absorb the reassurance, he or she will usually go back to sleep. Some parents feel that children who have developed the habit of awakening in the middle of the night may have to "cry it out" for several nights before they realize that the previous reinforcers of their waking-up behaviors are no longer available. Other parents find this solution too punitive and prefer to live with the situation until it resolves itself.

The child who has severe anxiety at bedtime, wakes up several times at night, and clings desperately to the mother or the father needs more support. This type of severe sleep disturbance indicates an excessive reaction to separation or fears that the child has developed. Parents may need to seek professional assistance in determining the source of the child's anxiety and in modifying daily routines so that the child's anxieties become more manageable. If the child has been recently hospitalized or otherwise separated from the caretaker, extra attention before bedtime may be helpful. The parent may put the child to bed but stay with the child to read or to sew, thus providing additional reassurance. A night light frequently proves beneficial to children.

The process of growing up is rarely a smooth one. Sleep disturbances are merely a reflection of the fears and anxieties that occur normally as the child develops. The home atmosphere is extremely important in minimizing sleep disturbances. Development of mutual respect in all aspects of child-rearing will help the child to overcome the problems that have resulted in sleep disturbances, while fostering sound mental health [10, 31].

DEVELOPMENT OF SELF-CONTROL

Learning self-control—how to handle frustration and aggression—is one of the most crucial components of psychosocial development during the toddler and preschool years. Aggressive impulses may occur as the child experiences some form of frustration. Aggressive behavior is a normal part of early social development and has a definite place in the acquisition of independence. However, the child must learn to control and to use aggression constructively to avoid infringing upon others or depriving them of their rights [3, 10, 21].

Socialization, the acquisition of culturally acceptable standards of behavior (which includes restricting some forms of impulses, wishes, and aggressive behavior), is achieved through the laws of learning theory. The child acquires self-control as the parents set and enforce limits. **Patterns of parental control during these early years serve as patterns of self-control in later years** [13].

Spitz [33] observes that there is a developmental sequencing of four behavior patterns in response to the frustration of self-will. The first response to limits is usually passivity. For example, when a toy is removed from an infant or the infant is told "No" when touching the television knob, the child is generally quiescent and cooperative. As the child matures, the parents begin to ask the child to delay immediate gratification (experienced during infancy) and to socialize his or her behavior. The phase of passivity soon changes into active physical aggression or resistance. This shift indicates a major step forward and creates a new method for the child to deal with the environment and self. The young toddler becomes physically aggressive, frequently striking out at the adult or the object seen as the source of frustration. This form of behavior is necessary for the child's progress from relative dependence toward an increasing autonomy, self-assurance, and initiative [10, 37].

Temper tantrums become a symbol of the toddler's response to frustration and are an example of active physical aggression. With increased maturity and language skills, the child's physical aggression gradually gives way to a somewhat more sophisticated form—verbal aggression, particularly the aggressive "No!" that becomes characteristic of older toddlers and early preschool children [33].

The toddler's ability to show aggression verbally by saying "No" indicates the memory of parental prohibition and the fact that the child is identifying with significant adults. The child may aggressively resist, but at the same time he or she is trying to do what the beloved parents want. It is not uncommon for toddlers to utter parental prohibitions to themselves. For example, a toddler may walk over to a stove or an electric outlet, knowing it is out of bounds, and begin to play with the forbidden object while mumbling, "No, no, hurt, no" to himself. Thus language makes it possible for the child to incorporate parental verbal inhibitions,

and it is indispensable to conscience formation during the preschool years. This process of incorporating parental inhibitions to attain self-control requires several years [10].

Verbal aggression expands during the preschool years (as physical aggression decreases) into name-calling, "bathroom" talk, and four-letter words.

The young child, then, moves from passivity to physical aggression to verbal aggression, and finally to acceptance of limits and more socialized forms of impulse control and frustration. Wolfgang points out that the preschooler who yells, "You're a poopy pants" to a peer who has stolen his or her toy may not appear to be any more mature than the preschooler who retaliates with outward physical attack. However, this child's initial use of language will lead to the more socialized response, "That's mine. Give it back," and eventually, perhaps, "That's mine, but I'll share it with you if you share with me" [37]. It is important to note that the child's transition is not smooth. Children will fluctuate in their ability to control themselves for many years, and it is not uncommon to see the preschooler physically attack a peer, even though the child has the ability to use words instead.

Clara Schuster, in her work with preschool-aged children, has observed that each of Spitz's four stages of response to frustration is comprised of three or four overlapping substages, which appear to emerge sequentially, but may be resolved quickly by the normally developing child. Emotionally or behaviorally disturbed children may fixate at one or more substages, requiring adult guidance that is designed to help them progress through the stages toward cooperation rather

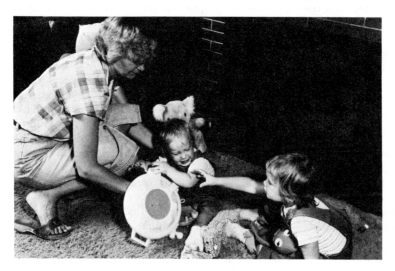

Figure 12–7. Healthy children express their egocentrism, aggression, and unwillingness to share in many ways. Those who have not yet become sufficiently socialized to adopt culturally approved ways of discharging their affective energy will physically attack other children, adults, or objects. Constructive direction by an adult may be needed.

than using intervention aimed only at extinguishing the undesirable behaviors and eliciting compliance. These stages are:

I. Passive Acceptance
   A. Naiveté
   B. Bewilderment
   C. Protest
   D. Noncompliance
II. Physical Aggression
   A. Toward others (bite, hit, pinch, kick)
   B. Toward self (grab hands, bite arm)
   C. Toward inanimate objects (throw, hit)
   D. Generalized energy expression (run, foot stomp)
III. Verbal Aggression
   A. Overt toward people
   B. Overt toward inanimate
   C. Overt to self
   D. Covert to self
IV. Socially Acceptable Behavior
   A. Alternative means
   B. Bargaining
   C. Alternative goal
V. Cooperation

The child who realizes the ability to control events through alternative means or goals or through bargaining eventually develops internally mediated, mutually cooperative behaviors with other persons. However, the child who is unable to utilize alternative strategies for dealing with frustration may comply with externally enforced behaviors without developing alternative means or goals for dealing with frustrations. Cooperation retains the self-respect, the self-control, and the autonomy of the child. Compliance extinguishes them, even though on the surface the adult may obtain the same behavior. Cooperation is growth-inducing; compliance is growth-inhibiting.

Parents, through the limits they set, play a major role in the child's ability to learn self-control. Limit setting for young children should not be considered as punitive but rather as a vehicle for caregiving that enables the child to balance maturing capabilities with an expanding world and the social restrictions imposed by others. The setting of firm limits helps to develop self-control, character, orderliness, and efficiency.

It is not advisable for parents to respond to the blows of the physically aggressive child by striking back. This might serve only to reinforce the child's physical behaviors [13]. The parents should stop or restrain the behavior while describing to the child other ways in which to express anger. If parents deny their child the right to express anger in any way, the child may feel that the emotions themselves are unacceptable and become a person who feels so guilty about experiencing quite normal feelings that true feelings are rarely expressed later on in life. This same child may also grow up believing that any anger expressed toward a loved one will result in alienation. It is essential for parents to learn forms of discipline that facilitate socialization.

The child's education in self-control takes many years. Although improved control can be expected by the end of the third year, the child is still a pleasure-loving little person, and lapses in control are frequent. Without consistent parental discipline, a child is inclined to remain on a more primitive discharge level because it is easier. Without limits, the child will experience heightened anxiety, tension, and ambivalence during a critical stage of social development. Many parents find limit setting very difficult; they may be afraid that they will not be liked by the child if they exercise control. However, discipline, periodic physical separation, and opportunities for independent functioning are just as important for the child's mental health as are love and security. The child cannot experience the pride of mastery unless there is a challenge to overcome. This is as true in the social domain as in the physical domain. Parenting requires the ability to attach as well as to let go at the appropriate times. If parents earnestly accept this responsibility, they are rewarded by the excitement of seeing their child reach the point of saying "I'm in control!" [3, 10].

PSYCHOSOCIAL DEPRIVATION DURING THE TODDLER AND PRESCHOOL YEARS

Some children are able to maximize their potentials **because of** their families; others, it seems, do the same **in spite of** their families. In our modern society, young children depend on their families to help them cope with numerous situational crises. The toddler who is a child of divorced parents, for example, must often adjust to new rituals, deal with the anxiety of separation from a parent, and be helped to work through self-doubt and shame. The preschooler in the same situation, in addition to mastering the same problems encountered by the toddler, must be helped to overcome guilt that he or she is being punished for past misbehavior and/or has caused the divorce.

Response to Illness and Hospitalization
Much has also been written about the stresses of short- and long-term separation and the resulting effects on child development. Hospitalization may present one of

childhood's most fearful experiences, particularly for children less than 6 years of age. When a child is hospitalized, the energy normally used to attack and to master the daily tasks of development must be reinvested by the child in efforts to cope with the added physiological and psychological stresses inherent in the hospital setting. Illness and hospitalization present additional tasks for the child to master.

Regression to earlier levels of social and emotional adaptation may be seen to some degree in all children who are ill. Due to the lack of verbal skills, the young child's adaptation to stress must be assessed through nonverbal behavior responses. The following types of behavior have been observed in hospitalized preschool children: increased crying; changes in patterns of eating, sleeping, and toileting; restlessness, hyperirritability, hyperactivity, and aggression; withdrawal, immobilization, and depression; and increased use of primitive gratifications (thumb-sucking, rocking, masturbation). Although these regressive behaviors are adaptive coping maneuvers that may be "normal" for a child during an acute crisis, they are not positive adaptive responses in a developmental sense unless they are used only temporarily as the child mobilizes the strength to deal with the stressor in a better way [2, 25].

The hospitalized child experiences separation from significant others, familiar environment, and everyday routine; unconscious perception of threat to life or body integrity; regard of illness as punishment; painful procedures; fears of mutilation or disfigurement; loss of independent activity; and the anxiety of parents or other caretaking adults that is communicated to the child. One or more of these stressors, when associated with hospitalization, may be sufficient to produce a significant degree of anxiety or tension. The age of the child and the child's relationship with the parents may be crucial variables in determining the extent to which the child can successfully cope with these stress-producing situations [36]. The toddler and the young preschooler are particularly sensitive to separation from parents during hospitalization (see Chap. 20 for discussion of protest, despair, and detachment/denial).

Parents play a major role in promoting the young child's adjustment and psychological health both during and after hospitalization. The mere presence of parents may offer support as the child attempts to cope with stress (unless they are so anxious that they communicate their anxiety to the child). Children with the most successful adjustments to the stressors involved in hospitalization are those with the most satisfying relationships with their parents [25].

A child normally copes with stress and anxiety

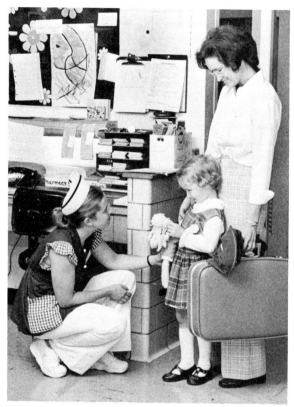

Figure 12–8. Personnel who understand the growth and development of children can aid hospitalized children in coping with the separation from their family. (Courtesy of the Department of Medical Photography, Children's Hospital, Buffalo, N.Y.)

through continuous interactions with the parents; the fundamental basis for personality development is the sense of trust that results from parent-child interactions. This sense of trust may be jeopardized following the child's hospitalization. In the child's mind, the parents may have allowed or caused the traumatic events to occur; the parents may feel that they are dealing with a different child. Thus parent-child relationships and interactions must be reestablished. The relationships that develop may positively or negatively affect the child's physical recovery and future mental health.

If the parent-child interaction can be sustained while the child is hospitalized, the physical and emotional involvement of the parents will be increased. If, on the other hand, the parents cannot be present during much of the child's hospitalization, alternative measures must be taken by the hospital staff to preserve the child's sense of security as well as autonomy and initiative. Assigning the child to a small group of the same people to administer care may help the child to maintain a trust in people, to predict events and responses, and to express feelings.

Child Abuse

Child abuse is a comprehensive term that includes physical abuse or neglect, emotional abuse or neglect, or sexual abuse. The exact cause of child abuse is not known but three major factors appear to be necessary in order for a child to become a victim: specific abuser traits, categorical environmental conditions, and selected child characteristics.

The person who has the potential to abuse shows one common characteristic: He (or she) has little emotional energy to cope with the usual task of child rearing and is extremely vulnerable to additional crises of any nature. The person strikes out at the child as a method for the release of frustration and anxiety. (Spitz, level two) The environment is typically one of chronic stress, including long-term illness or disability, divorce, extramarital relations, financial deficit, unemployment, alcohol or drug addiction.

There are several characteristics that predispose a child to abuse. The child's temperament, ordinal position in the family, additional physical needs, activity level, and sensitivity to parental needs all in some way contribute to being a victim of abuse. Often the precipitating factor for the abuse is something that would not upset a well-adjusted parent who is familiar with normal childhood growth and development. But the person with the potential to abuse cannot cope with the ordinary daily tasks of child rearing (from caring for the totally dependent infant to guiding the child in self-help skills, speech development, toilet training and so forth). When considering the characteristics of the normal toddler and preschooler—the quests for autonomy and initiative, minimal self-control, intrusive behaviors, temper tantrums—it is easy to understand why they comprise the most highly abused age group.

The separation-individuation process is seriously interfered with as a result of the abusive parent-child relationship. This interference results in delayed object relations and the belief that no one can be trusted, a feeling that is characteristic of both the abuser and the abused.

The incidence of child abuse is increasing. We must be concerned with protecting the child and helping the abuser to learn how to cope positively with stress. To speak fully to the issue of child abuse and to discuss how the vicious cycle of abuse (abused children often grow up to be abusers) can be broken is beyond the scope of this text. Readers should refer to the chapter reference list for further readings. The effect of abuse on the child is further explored in Chapter 14, and the effect of abuse on the family is discussed in Chapter 34. Further characteristics that predispose individuals to child abuse are described in Chapter 35.

CONCLUSIONS

The parents of toddlers and preschoolers need to be flexible. They must grow and expand in their ability to relate constructively to their child as he or she grows and expands in spheres of activity. Many excellent resources (e.g., books, parent-child classes, health professionals) are now available to assist the parents' understanding of their child's needs and capacities.

Parental wisdom in the conduct of feeding, toilet training, sex education, and discipline is vital to developing the child's self-esteem. These practices can support the child's self-esteem by promoting love and confidence in the parents and by strengthening the child's own ability to regulate body needs and impulses.

Quality day-care centers do not appear to disrupt positive emotional bonds between children and their parents [29]. The very process of development itself requires the child to meet and to master anxiety-producing and sometimes painful situations successfully. There is no growth without challenge or frustration. Each stage in human development has its own crises.

Even the most ideal early environment does not eliminate all anxiety or remove the hazards that exist everywhere in the child's world. One cannot help the child avoid all fears and frustrations—nor is this desirable. Nearly all toddlers have simple tantrums, and most preschool children develop occasional anxiety dreams. Healthy psychosocial development depends on the child finding the solutions to problems that are created by growth. The ways in which young children are helped to manage frustrations determines the course of their socioaffective development. The ultimate outcome of achieving a sense of autonomy is the attainment of an overall feeling of self-control and willpower; the eventual goal of achieving a sense of initiative is the acquisition of a prevailing inspiration for direction and purpose.

REFERENCES

1. Berelson, B., and Steiner, G. A. *Human Behavior: An Inventory of Scientific Findings.* New York: Harcourt, Brace and World, 1967.
2. Bowlby, J. Grief and mourning in infancy and early childhood. *Psychoanal. Study Child* 15:9, 1960.

3. Brazelton, T. B. *Infants and Mothers: Differences in Development* (Rev. ed.). New York: Delta Books, 1983.

4. Campbell, C. E., and Mead, J. J. *Child Abuse and Neglect: An Educator's Handbook.* Brea, CA: For Kid's Sake Press, 1983.

5. Chadwick, B. J., Pflederer, D., and Ray, M. A. Maintaining the hospitalized child's home ties. *Am. J. Nurs.* 78:1360, 1978.

6. Critchley, D. L. Therapeutic group work with abused preschool children. *Perspect. Psychiatric Care* 20(2):79, 1982.

7. Do you have a spoiled child: An interview with Dr. T. Berry Brazelton. *Harper's Bazaar* (July 1977):89.

8. Erikson, E. *Childhood and Society* (Rev. ed.). St. Albans [Eng.]: Triad/Paladin, 1978.

9. Erikson, E. *Identity: Youth and Crisis.* New York: Norton, 1968.

10. Fraiberg, S. H. *The Magic Years: Understanding and Handling the Problems of Early Childhood.* London: Methuen, 1968.

11. Gesell, A. L., and Ilg, F. L. *Infant and Child in the Culture of Today.* New York: Harper & Row, 1974.

12. Ginott, H. G. *Between Parent and Child: New Solutions to Old Problems.* New York: Avon, 1971.

13. Hammer, D., and Drabman, R. J. Child discipline: What we know and what we can recommend. *Pediatr. Nurs.* 7(3):31, 1981.

14. Hartup, W. W. Peer Interaction and Social Organization. In P. H. Mussen (Ed.), *Carmichael's Manual of Child Psychology* (3rd ed.). New York: Wiley, 1970.

15. Havighurst, R. J. *Human Development and Education.* New York: David McKay, 1965.

16. Ilg, F. L., Ames, L. B., and Baker, S. M. *Child Behavior* (Rev. ed.). New York: Barnes & Noble, 1981.

17. Isaacs, S. S. *Social Development in Young Children.* New York: A.M.S. Press, 1979.

18. Kando, T. M. *Sexual Behavior and Family Life in Transition.* New York: Elsevier, 1978.

19. Mahler, M. On the first three subphases of the separation-individuation process. *Int. J. Psychoanal.* 53:333, 1972.

20. Mahler, M. S., Pine, F., and Bergman, A. *The Psychological Birth of the Human Infant: Symbiosis and Individuation.* New York: Basic Books, 1975.

21. Maier, H. W. *Three Theories of Child Development* (3rd ed.). New York: Harper & Row, 1978.

22. Monea, H. E. Psychosocial Development of Children: Holistic Care-giving Approaches. In I. M. Burnside, P. Ebersole, and H. E. Monea (Eds.), *Psychosocial Caring Throughout the Life Span.* New York: McGraw-Hill, 1979.

23. Piaget, J. *Judgment and Reason in the Child.* Translated by M. Gabain. New York: Harcourt, Brace, 1928.

24. Piaget, J. *On the Development of Memory and Identity.* Translated by E. Duckworth. Worcester, MA: Clark University Press, 1968.

25. Prugh, D., et al. A study of the emotional reactions of children to hospitalization and illness. *Am. J. Orthopsychiatry* 23:70, 1953.

26. Robertson, J. *Young Children in Hospital* (2nd ed.). London: Travistock Publications, 1970.

27. Rosenberg, N. M., et al. Prediction of child abuse in an ambulatory setting. *Pediatrics* 70(6):879, 1982.

28. Rubenstein, J. L., et al. A two-year follow-up of infants in community-based day care. *J. Child Psychol. Psychiatry* 22(3):209, 1981.

29. Rutter, M. Social-emotional consequences of day care for preschool children. *Am. J. Orthopsychiatry* 51(1):4, 1981.

30. Schumann, M. J. Neuromuscular relaxation—A method for inducing sleep in young children. *Pediatr. Nurs.* 7(5):9, 1981.

31. Sperling, M. Sleep Disturbances in Children. In J. G. Howells (Ed.), *Modern Perspectives in International Child Psychiatry.* New York: Brunner/Mazel, 1971.

32. Spitz, R. A. *The First Year of Life: A Psychoanalytic Study of Normal and Deviant Development of Object Relationships.* New York: International Universities Press, 1973.

33. Spitz, R. A. *No and Yes: On the Genesis of Human Communication.* New York: International Universities Press, 1966.

34. Sullivan, H. S. *The Interpersonal Theory of Psychiatry.* New York: Norton, 1953.

35. Vernon, D. J. Changes in children's behavior after hospitalization. *Am. J. Dis. Child.* 111:581, 1966.

36. Wolff, S. *Children Under Stress* (2nd ed.). Harmondsworth [Eng.]: Penguin, 1981.

37. Wolfgang, C. H. *Helping Aggressive and Passive Preschoolers Through Play.* Columbus, OH: Merrill, 1977.

VI
Life Span
Developmental
Concepts

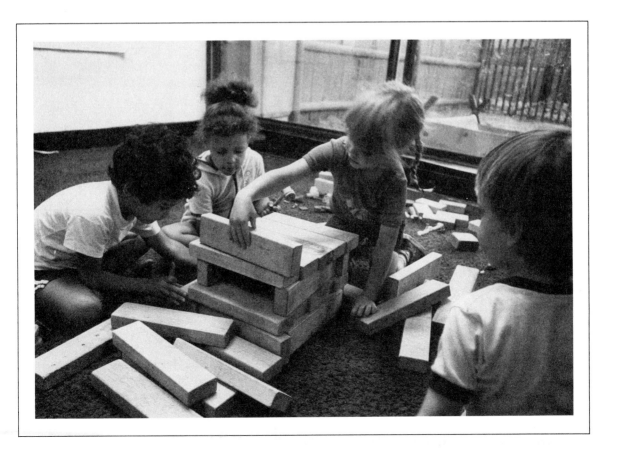

13
Language Development during Childhood

Shirley S. Ashburn, Clara S. Schuster, William A. Grimm,
Sheila M. Goff

Words are the mind's attempt to order itself.

—Richard D'Ambrosio, *No Language But a Cry*

The world's creatures communicate with others of their own kind and, to a lesser extent, with other species. Some animals, such as dolphins, employ highly sophisticated modes of communication that scientists are now attempting to comprehend. Others, such as parrots or mynah birds, mimic human speech. Chimpanzees, possessing a capacity for manual manipulation, have been taught to use the hand signs of deaf persons to communicate with one another and with humans. Other chimpanzees have learned to use pictures (e.g., Bliss symbols) or plastic tokens to represent words and ideas. But among the various species, the human being is unique in the ability to use a symbolic code to communicate abstract ideas. Humankind is not limited to barking, whining, or growling but has created a highly refined verbal language.

Biophysically, humans are endowed from birth with the physical equipment that enables us to employ verbal and nonverbal behaviors for purposes of communication. We are capable of considerable variation in the sounds we can produce. These variations of sound are mentally categorized and combined to form units of meaning. We can also control the pattern of inhalation and exhalation to provide power for speech, while simultaneously meeting our need to obtain oxygen. The combination of brain, neural system, and vocal tract physically sets the human being apart from other animals. We can remember what we said in the past and can verbalize what we will do in the future. We can teach our children by using the written word as well as the spoken word. Early speech development is highly dependent on the quality of the caretaker-infant relationship and is mediated by the child's cognitive development [52].

There are a number of theories that attempt to explain the Hows and the Whys of language development. The theory expressed by Chomsky [19] and the research performed by Condon and Sanders [21] indicate that infants are born with a propensity for responding to spoken language. During the months of infancy, the child begins to develop a comprehension of one of the world's 3000 languages. During the toddler years, children begin to use language symbols to represent adroitly and accurately their concerns, activities, and events. The period from 18 months to 4 years of age is probably the most critical time for the development of expressive language. During the preschool years, the child refines these skills in preparation for school.

PROCESSES OF LANGUAGE ACQUISITION

Growth in the affective, social, and cognitive domains is evidenced by an increased awareness of the environment and changes in behavioral patterns. Concomitant with this growth, the individual develops the unique capacity for verbal comprehension, retention, language expression, and usage. As the individual progresses through the various stages of the life cycle, each developmental phase requires increasingly complex communication abilities and skills.

Principles of Communication
Thoughts, needs, desires, and feelings are communicated through the use of a system of codes. A code may be defined as "an agreed transformation, or set of un-ambiguous rules, whereby messages are converted from one representation to another" [17]. The code, or language, may consist of either nonverbal or verbal symbols or signs [1]. Regardless of whether the message is encoded verbally, nonverbally, or in various combinations, exact meaning cannot be conveyed by one person to another because in the encoding process, people are bound by the limitations of the code. For example, some things can be said in French that cannot be translated into English. Other examples include trying to explain to another person the intensity of love felt for someone or the depth of a spiritual experience.

Language utilizes a system of codes or signals understood by two or more people [32]. For instance, an English-speaking person may use the spoken word "chair," which is comprised of the verbal sounds that form a code word for a piece of furniture on which to sit. A policeman's sharp blow on a whistle is a nonverbal code in this country that signals "stop." If communication is to be effective, the code used by two persons must be understood by both the speaker and the listener; that is, they must understand the rules of the communiqué. The nonverbal hand signal that means "goodbye" in one culture may signify "come here" in another.

This chapter will concentrate on the acquisition of verbal communication. A simple schematic representation of the verbal communication process is presented in Figure 13–1. Although the model can be expanded greatly, the one presented is adequate to illustrate the general levels of verbal communication that are discussed in this chapter. In this communication model, the speaker must first encode the message. **Encoding,** which is primarily a function of the brain, is the mode through which the message is organized and formed for the listener. The transmission process begins by emitting air and then modulating and trans-

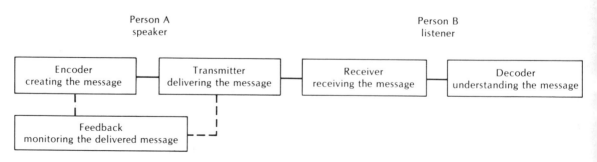

Figure 13–1. Communication model demonstrating the ability of humans to exchange information between parts of the system as well as between the system and its physical and social environments.

forming the airstream into predetermined patterns of sound codes that represent the language.

An important but often ignored aspect of this process is the auditory feedback loop, which is used to monitor the transmitter in terms of what the encoder intended. In other words, people listen to themselves as they speak. Occasionally the transmitter is found to be faulty, and immediately after an utterance the error, perhaps a misplaced word (slip of the tongue), is detected. This monitoring process is so crucial that when the process is altered, the fluency of a person's speech can be destroyed. Researchers have demonstrated and measured the importance of the feedback process by creating dysfluencies when varying the length of the delayed auditory feedback [8]. Some educators believe that children with specific learning disabilities experience an impairment in this feedback process.

In effective communication, the listener is just as active a participant in the process as the speaker, because the coded messages that have been transmitted by the speaker must now be received and interpreted by the listener. The receiving process (in terms of verbal language) is accomplished by the ear and the neural pathways to the brain. Distortions of the signs imposed by the ear can influence the signals forwarded to the listener's decoder (brain). For example, hard-of-hearing persons are likely to miss some sounds. The decoder is involved in an active process: The listener not only makes use of the signals received but also utilizes knowledge of known rules of the language, including the statistical frequency of occurrence of words and phrases, to fill in (predict) the missing parts of a communication that were not received adequately [9]. The listener dips into a well of language experiences by utilizing the clues perceived to determine what was probably said and to predict what will probably be said next. For example, if the word "fun" is used, the listener at a distance from the speaker may not hear the "f" sound. With the information available from the context and the sound "un," the listener (decoder) assumes that the word should be "fun," as the attempt is made to give an adequate response.

Theories of Language Acquisition

The gift of human language is often taken for granted by those who are not conscious of its complexity. The phenomenon of language acquisition has yet to be explained satisfactorily. Recently, increased attention has been applied to the processes involved in how language is acquired. Two main theories influence language research today: one is described in B. F. Skinner's *Verbal Behavior* [56], and the other is discussed in Noam Chomsky's *Syntactic Structures* [20]. Although these theories are incompatible in many aspects, each attempts to explain how a child acquires a set of language rules [53].

B. F. SKINNER'S THEORY

B. F. Skinner proposes that language is learned through operant conditioning (also called behavior modification and stimulus-response conditioning). He believes that verbal behavior is selectively reinforced by one's environment. Initially, an infant makes verbal sounds that are spontaneous or imitative, or both. Parents encourage those sounds that resemble adult speech, and thus the child is reinforced to use them. Gradually, the caretakers shape these approximations to adult speech

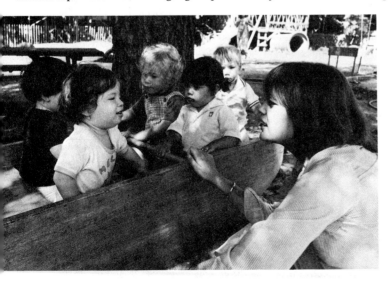

Figure 13–2. The adult who wishes to communicate effectively with a young child must understand the individual youngster's cognitive abilities. It is also helpful and less threatening to the child if the interaction occurs at eye level.

(for example, if the baby says "ba," a ball is given to the baby) until the child is readily able to come forth with everyday language that is complete with "correct speech responses" [58].

NOAM CHOMSKY'S THEORY

Psycholinguists, among them Noam Chomsky, take issue with many of Skinner's statements on language acquisition. They contend that his emphasis on stimulus-response training does not afford total appreciation of the vast potentials of the human organism.

Chomsky's views on language acquisition are well known to linguists and have challenged traditional theories based on stimulus-response and social learning concepts [22]. Chomsky affirms that something more than reinforcement and imitation is needed for a child to develop language acquisition. He recognizes the importance of these factors but maintains that, in addition, the child must have the ability to process the language data heard from other individuals, so that inferences can be made from the data about accurate, acceptable, grammatical forms [18]. Chomsky suggests that humans innately possess a number of complex linguistic mechanisms that compose a "language acquisition device" (LAD). He believes that this device is not actually an organ, but that it is somehow universally present and is thus responsible for human language acquisition throughout the world. Chomsky bases his ideas on (1) observations of the ease and the rapidity with which children acquire their native languages, (2) the similarity of stages of acquisition across different languages, and (3) the influence of what appears to be a critical period of language acquisition. All these factors are evidence, he maintains, that a child has some form of built-in, "prewired" system to process language [22]. Chomsky says that the child "analyzes" language, induces rules about it, tests hypotheses about what rules to use, and thus derives a theory about the native language.

Chomsky's theory is supported in part by neurological research that has shown that language acquisition is related to the increasing specialization of the neural structure and functioning of the human brain. Nevertheless, no one theory has proved to be satisfactory in explaining how children accrue the complex ability to understand and speak the everyday language of their environment.

Cognitive Processes and Language Development

The interrelationship of cognition and language is a subject that has long been and continues to be disputed among psychologists, educators, linguists, and speech pathologists. One of the earliest and most extreme views is found in the writings of John B. Watson, who wrote in the early decades of this century. Watson believed that thought is a form of "subvocal" speech, and that thoughts themselves could actually be seen as tiny movements in the larynx (voice box) [22].

The influence of language on thought has been explored by anthropological linguists. The Sapir-Whorf hypothesis, for example, states that the language spoken by an individual directly determines the major aspects of the individual's thought [57]. For example, use of verbal tenses may affect one's conceptualization of time. The "standard average European" languages (so called by Whorf) conjugate their verbs into tenses basically equivalent to past, present, and future. In contrast, the Hopi Indians of Arizona do not use tenses for their verbs. The Hopi think in terms of things either existing **now** or in a state of **becoming.** For example, a Hopi who begins to weave a rug may put it aside, not really concerned with when it is to be completed. In such an instance, peers do not consider the person lazy because they believe that the craftwork will become a rug whenever "nature so ordains" [61]. One must ask, however, whether the Hopi's concept of the world determined the construction of language symbols or whether the reverse is true.

Cromer's broad research in child language has led him to identify two separate issues involved in analyzing the cognitive process underlying language: (1) language development is greatly dependent on developing "cognitions" (thoughts, intentions, and meanings themselves), and (2) cognitive "structures" result in particular thoughts and perhaps make language acquisition possible at different developmental levels [22]. This second issue is supported by Piaget's theory.

JEAN PIAGET'S APPROACH TO LANGUAGE

Piaget, who proposes that symbolic life develops through interaction with one's world (see Chap. 11), believes that the formation of symbols is aided by, but is not dependent on, the use of language [59]. Piaget views the development of language and thought as parallel processes that become closely interrelated around 7 or 8 years of age when verbal language is used more precisely to express inner thoughts [47, 49].

Piaget contends that the infant is not a passive recipient of the language heard spoken but is quite actively interacting with the environment. During infancy, the individual constructs "sensorimotor accounts" or "actors, actions, and objects of actions, as well as the consequences of specific actor-action object arrangements, before he either comprehends or produces linguistic codes" [53]. Before children can manipulate symbols (language is one form of symbol), they must be able to manipulate the objects these symbols represent [16, 48]. From midinfancy until about 7 or 8 years of age, the child will appear to delight in repeating or mimicking the sounds and then the words or the phrases made by others (echoing) [47]. (The reader should refer to Appendix C for an overview of Piaget's theory of cognitive development and to Figure 11–1 for a summary of the sequential development of symbolic thought.)

During Piaget's preoperational stage (approximately 1½ to 7 years of age), the child's use of language continues to be egocentric. During the toddler and preschool years the child can be observed to engage in thinking aloud or talking in a monologue. Sometimes the child will use monologue speech in the presence of another person, appearing to use this audience as a stimulus to vocalization (dual monologue). The importance of language at this time, according to Piaget, is that the child learns to manipulate the symbols for the **meanings** of objects and events. A schema for the preoperational child is now symbolic (whether or not the logic used helps the child to order the world as an adult would). Although the child's schemata are symbolic, the words and the images are not necessarily organized into well-defined concepts and rules [44]. Such ideas are not well formed or firmly articulated until Piaget's concrete operational years, roughly corresponding to the ages of 7 to 11 years. Until this time, Piaget says that the child can only think egocentrically (seeing the world only from a subjective perspective), and this is reflected in language. During the concrete operational years, the child becomes able to represent a series of actions mentally and, depending on experience, to label and to discuss them. When the child actually becomes capable of placing the self at the point of view of the hearer, the child begins to engage in "socialized speech." This form of speech, according to Piaget, prompts true dialogue [47]. Finally, from approximately the age of 12 years, and during Piaget's formal operational years, the individual's thinking is capable of being rational and systematic. Because a person at this stage is much more aware of thoughts, he or she can discuss (or "intelligently communicate," in Piagetian terms) hypothetical events as well as past, present, and future events with others. For a much more detailed analysis of Piaget's research on cognition and speech, the reader is referred to his book *The Language and Thought of the Child* [47].

COMPILATION OF RESEARCH
Verbal ability facilitates thinking and problem solving, but the growth of cognitive processes is not dependent on language. Many deaf children, for example, who are delayed in verbal communication, may solve problems as well as their peers who hear. The deaf child's cognitive development travels the same course as that of the hearing child, although in some instances the rate of development may be slower.

Luria, a contemporary Russian psychologist, presents a view in distinct opposition to that of Piaget. He maintains that language and thought are closely interdependent in early childhood, but that thinking becomes much more independent of language as the child grows and develops. His thoughts have promoted the importance of the concept of "verbal mediation" in language acquisition [33].

Verbal mediation occurs when a child can use primarily internal, subvocal speech to control actions and responses to external stimuli [28]. A word thus serves as a verbal mediator, for example, when a child is told that something tastes like chocolate and promptly takes a bite of it. Because most children like chocolate, the child is apt to act in the same way toward any substance labeled "chocolate." Although verbal mediation appears to be an essential factor in learning, it may not be essential to knowledge acquisition [27]. It is evident that verbal mediation facilitates memory, but it may not be necessary to enable a child to recall an event. Verbal mediation certainly is not present when a child is able to remember unfamiliar scenes and objects that he or she cannot label [44]. It would appear, then, that humans possess some unique, efficient system of symbols even more fundamental than language itself that helps them to organize and label their world. Whatever this system may be, it appears to become the foundation for the acquisition of language.

Vocalization and Hearing
Infants have all the essential apparatus for producing vocal sounds and for hearing the utterances made by both themselves and others. In vocalization, air from the lungs is forced through the oral cavity or nasal passages by constricting the rib cage and the diaphragm during exhalation. Vocal sound results when the moving air causes the vocal folds to vibrate as it exits from the trachea (see Fig. 13–3). Pitch and volume control also occur at this point. The vibrated air, when impeded at the velum, results in an oral vocal quality or timbre; however, when the air is not impeded, it enters the nose and the vocal quality becomes nasal. The sinus cavities serve as resonance chambers, thus affecting tone quality and projection. The tongue, the lips, and other articulators (jaw and velum) assist the oral cavity to make rapid changes in shape and size, adding greatly to the potential variety of vocal features.

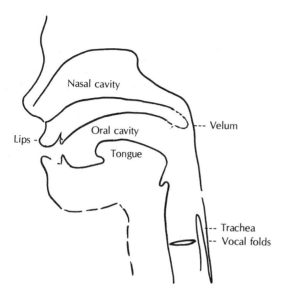

Figure 13–3. Model of the vocal mechanism. Articulators within the oral cavity as well as in proximity to it aid in creating the uniqueness of each human vocalization.

The pinna, or outer ear, collects the moving pressures of air from a sound source and directs them through the ear canal to the tympanic membrane (eardrum, see Fig. 13–4). The air pressure, now concentrated, causes the membrane to be displaced. Other displacements occur beyond the membrane. The ossicles (bones) of the middle ear transmit the vibrations to the cochlea of the inner ear, where they are converted to nerve impulses and sent to the brain by way

of neural networks for processing. Pitch, loudness, and duration of sound are integrated by the brain and translated into meaning.

Early Nonverbal Communication

Humans, in the later stages of fetal development, have the capacity to hear [43]. During the intrauterine period, the fetus experiences the pulsations of the mother's heart and vocalizations as well as the other sounds within this restricted environment. The capacity of the fetus to hear, combined with intrauterine experiences, may enable the infant to perceive categorical differences between sound features shortly after birth. For example, 1-month-old infants will suck a pacifier at a different rate when they are presented with the sound /pa/, after becoming accustomed to the sound of /ba/ [24]. From this type of research, it has been concluded that a baby may be capable of the precise auditory discriminations that are essential in acquiring human language. After birth, the infant will respond with synchronized body movements to normal speech rhythms but not to randomized sound units [21].

The urge to communicate is evident even at an early age. Before an infant is capable of using verbal language, innate nonverbal skills are used to convey needs and feelings (see the section on infant tools in Chap. 8). The baby may cry to indicate discomfort, smile to indicate pleasure at the caretaker's presence, or raise the arms to indicate a desire to be picked up. Even steady eye-to-eye staring, mouth opening and closing, and hand opening and closing are significant forms of communication for the very young infant. The par-

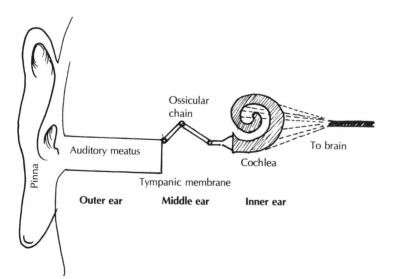

Figure 13–4. Model of the ear. Hearing is a mechanoreceptive sense because the ear responds to the vibration of sound waves in the air. These frequencies are translated into meaningful sounds when they are received by the brain.

ent's ability to respond sensitively to these early nonverbal messages helps the child to learn how to initiate a conversation and to learn the basic rules of reciprocity. The baby less than one week old can and will engage in nonverbal and vocal "turn-taking" communication with the adult who pauses between vocalizations. These vocal and bodily actions become the media for the baby's acquisition of nonverbal language. The infant learns the rules for encoding and transmitting messages nonverbally from hearing and observing the communications of other persons. As the infant matures, he or she comprehends and begins to imitate the verbal and nonverbal communication symbols in the culture.

PROSODY

Prosody is the expression of meaning and emotion through pitch, loudness, tonal quality (or timbre), inflection, and duration of vocalization. Even before children begin to talk, they use prosodic communication features effectively to express themselves or to communicate with others. The 15- to 20-month-old child frequently emits long vocal exchanges with a very serious demeanor. Distinguishable words may not be present, but changes in inflection, pitch, and timbre indicate that the child is intentionally attempting to share thoughts and feelings or pretending to communicate the way the adults in the surrounding environment share ideas. The young child imitates the rhythms and pacings of verbal communication: The Southern drawl, the Irish brogue, or the Texas twang is identifiable in the young child's vocalizations.

The infant learns much about the voice—how to alter it and how to achieve an effect—long before talking. Discomforts, such as hunger, a wet diaper, pain, or fright, elicit vocalization in the form of cries. Research indicates that these infant cries are qualitatively differentiated to communicate the nature of the problem. During the second half of the first year of life, the baby begins to experiment with vocal inflections—the sharp staccato of demand, the legato of intimacy, the duration of caressing—all heard previously in the caretaker's voice. When transmitting vocal messages early in life, the infant is also becoming more aware of the nature of his or her communicative powers. The adult's response to the infant's efforts may reinforce the child's efforts, shape them, or extinguish them.

Knowledge about prosodic messages builds over time. Infants observe prosodic features in the voices of others and learn their meanings. They hear the different ways in which the mother says "No," the sound of approval in her voice, and the overlay of mood on her words. As the baby approaches the first birthday and begins to talk, he or she both understands and uses many prosodic features when sending messages. The difficulties of developing a prosodic competence are obvious for the infant who is born deaf or is hard of hearing. The prosodic features of a language can be elusive to a person entering another culture.

KINESICS

Kinesics is the expression of meaning and emotions through bodily movement. Features of kinesics are facial expressions, hand and arm movements, gestures, and body stances. The infant progresses from random motor behavior to controlled use of the limbs. Vision brings to the infant an awareness of the movements of others. Gradually, the child builds a knowledge of the rules of meaning associated with movements. The shoulder shrug, the wink of an eye, a frown, or even a clenched fist all begin to assume meaning. From early infancy, the child observes the face for signs of attention, loving concern, or anger. The child watches the way others hold their heads when talking, the hand movements that accompany messages, and how to send a greeting across a crowded room. Soon the child's own prowess enables him or her to imitate these cultural codes. Infants who are born blind or partially sighted have difficulty developing a knowledge of kinesic features.

Infants soon learn the limitations of pure nonverbal communication. How does one ask for a drink, or indicate a need for the blue ball rather than the red one? Frustration wells up inside the child; it is this frustration that may serve as an impetus to learn to use the language code.

DEVELOPMENT OF VERBALIZATION

The acquisition of verbal language is a complex process. Factors that support or prevent optimal development in this area may be present prior to birth and even prior to conception. Congenital factors, such as deafness, cleft palate, or mental retardation, can delay the development of meaningful language. Many insults can occur during fetal life that may cause a decrease in language-learning potential. For example, poor nutrition, a disease such as rubella, or an injury during the birth process may adversely affect the cognitive potential necessary for language development. Primary prevention of language problems, therefore, begins prior to conception and centers around the production of a healthy newborn infant.

Language development is a dynamic process, which extends beyond infancy and can continue throughout the entire span of life. The fetus develops presets for language reception and expression; the infant coos and babbles; the child begins to "talk" the language of the environment; the young person tries to master correct grammar and increase vocabulary; and in old age one may continue to add new words and meanings to the vocabulary that was learned previously.

All four domains—biophysical, cognitive, affective, and social—contribute interdependently to the development of the ability to comprehend and to use language. To ignore the complex relationships and contributions of all the developing domains to the child's ability to talk leads to unrealistic expectations for achievement. In judging the adequacy of a young child's knowledge of language, one must consider both the age of the child and the rules of the subculture in which he or she resides, rather than just the middle-class adult standard of the "King's English."

Prelinguistic Period

Hearing permits the unborn baby to receive an input of sound and the particular vibrations of the mother's language. The Italian-speaking mother, therefore, gives her unborn child a unique rhythm and set of vibrating patterns that the infant will continue to hear after birth; the English-, Hebrew-, or Japanese-speaking mother each provides a different stimulation that is characteristic of her language. It is not yet clear what effect this experience has on the child's language and cognitive development. There are some who would contend that teaching can actually begin before birth.

At birth the infant enters a new environment. The cries that the baby emits during the weeks after birth are strident reflections of both an emotionally laden message and a physically changing vocal tract. After 3 or 4 months, the infant begins to increase the proportion of noncrying vocalizations. Concomitant with this change toward more purposeful vocalizations, the physical movements of the infant also begin to show similar modifications; that is, they become less random and more specific. Gradually, the movements become more controlled and discriminately responsive to specific stimulation.

Linguistic Period

DEVELOPMENT OF PHONEMES

A **phoneme** is the smallest unit of distinctive sound features (or finite sets of mutually exclusive classes of speech sounds) that can be recognized by speakers of the language as being the same sound; examples are /p/ and /k/. The classic general American dialect of the English language is usually based on 42 phonemes. Phonemes are used in sequence to form words. In attempts to describe any speech event, linguists are occupied with phonology, which analyzes both phonemic and prosodic patterns of speech [5].

Phonemes are not single, uncomplicated sounds; rather, considered alone, they are bundles of events or features. The role of distinctive features is one of contrasts. For example, features can be either voiceless or voiced. Some sounds are determined by the use of the vocal folds, whereas others are determined by the positioning of the articulators within the oral cavity. A phoneme may be enhanced by vocal characteristics, such as loudness, pitch, rhythm, and duration, all of which must be considered separate from distinctive features.

Just one feature of a given phoneme may be responsible for making the distinction between it and another phoneme. For example, when one changes from voicelessness to voicing, the phoneme /p/ becomes /b/. The phoneme /p/ is (1) voiceless, (2) made in the front of the mouth by the lips, and (3) made by a complete stoppage of the airstream followed by a sudden release; /b/ shares all the features mentioned for /p/ except that is is voiced rather than voiceless. Another phoneme, /k/, shares the above features with /p/ with the exception of the place in the mouth where it is produced. When one changes the tongue from the front position to the back position, /t/ becomes /k/.

The child appears to produce some contrasts earlier than others. Voicing is thought to be the first feature acquired; a later feature is the place of articulation [23, 38]. A feature-by-feature analysis of a child's phonemes may reveal that the nature of the pronunciation errors is expected for the child's age or level of language development. Saying "to" for "shoe," for instance, is normal for 4-year-olds. A child's ability to extract the rules of phonology as well as to refine the movements of speech apparatuses will affect the manner in which the child pronounces early words. Until all the rules governing features in phonemes are acquired, the child will experience articulation difficulties. Articulation skills emerge in sequential order (see Table 13–1).

The mastery of phoneme production at the adult level of intelligibility occurs roughly between 3 and 7 years of age. A child usually has the English vowels mastered by the age of 3 or 3½ years. Consonants emerge as mastered phonemes in a hierarchical fashion between 3 and 7 years of age. Since the consonants "s,"

Table 13–1. Average Age at Which Vowels and Consonants Are Mastered

Age (yr)	Phonemes Acquired
3 or before	All vowels
3	/b/ /m/ /n/ /f/ /w/ /h/
4	/p/ /d/ /g/ /k/ /l/ /t/
5	/v/ /s/ /z/
6	/j/

Source: From B. S. Wood, *Children and Communication: Verbal and Nonverbal Language Development.* Englewood Cliffs, NJ: Prentice-Hall, 1976. (Adapted from P. Ményuk, *The Acquisition and Development of Language,* copyright 1971). Reprinted with permission of Prentice-Hall, Inc.

"l," "r," and "th" are not mastered until about 7 to 8 years of age, substitutions and omissions can still be identified during the school years.

Vowels appear to be easier to master than consonants. Vowels are phonemes that tend to be musical to the ear and can be held or sung; these acoustical sound units can be sustained over a period of time. The mouth must open in different amounts as the tongue and lips shape the sound. Consonants are made with the closures that interfere with the outgoing breath; the resultant sound is aperiodic and noisy. Some consonants are more difficult to produce than others and are mastered later on as the child matures. The vocalizations of very young infants generally consist of vowel sounds. By 3 to 4 months, consonant sounds begin to emerge. The importance of the auditory feedback loop becomes apparent even at this age. The deaf infant, because of inadequate feedback, decreases babbling by 5 to 6 months of age.

Knowledge of the complexity of phoneme production can create greater appreciation of the child's frustration in moving from the various levels of baby talk to adult-approved pronunciation. It is apparent that role models facilitate the direction of a child's language development. Unfortunately, some relatives and friends may think the baby's pronunciations are "cute" and may encourage so-called baby talk to prevail beyond the time when the child is able to speak more maturely.

MORPHOLOGY

Morphemes are the smallest form of sound units that possess symbolic meaning [5]; they are composed of one or more phonemes. A morpheme that can stand alone meaningfully is a "free" morpheme and is considered a word. A vocabulary of free morphemes is acquired early in life (e.g., "ma," "hi," "bye"). The in-

fant's first words will probably be free morphemes because the child has many opportunities to hear them spoken at home. They serve as concrete referents and are usually the major meaning-unit of the mother's sentences [45]. Adults tend to emphasize these words and help the infant to focus attention on them. When a mother says, "The book is on the table," her voice and manner teach **book** and **table** more obviously than the relationship words.

A "bound" morpheme is one that cannot stand alone but must be attached to a free morpheme as a prefix or a suffix (e.g., the "un" in "undress," or the "ger" in "bigger"). Indicators of possession, number, and markers of tense are other examples of bound morphemes. Bound morphemes are rule-based and are acquired only after a basic vocabulary has been established.

Acquisition of Free Morphemes. Infants understand many words before they speak. As early as 8 or 10 months, many infants appear to comprehend the major meanings of the caretaker's speech. Most infants speak their first words at about 10 to 12 months of age; some infants begin talking earlier. The first words are usually nouns—names given to people or things in the baby's immediate environment. During infancy (and beyond) one word may stand for a whole group of objects and actions (e.g., all men are "dada," or all four-footed animals are "kitty"). Some theorists refer to these first words as simple labels for objects and actions in the individual child's world; others speak of these utterances as being entire sentences embedded in the structure of a single word (holophrastic speech) [35]. "Cookie," for example, may mean "I want a cookie" or "I see a cookie." Each word has a much broader and more diffuse meaning for a child than it does for adults. Children often use gestures and varying voice patterns to accompany their holophrases in order to give meaning or intent to what they are trying to communicate.

Of the 20 to 100 morphemes spoken by 18 months of age, almost 75 percent are unintelligible to the casual listener due to the inability of the child to articulate precisely [7]. Fortunately, most of these morphemes are nouns and can be understood by observing the child and deciphering his or her speech intention from a meaningful context. Thus the child's caretaker may extract the child's message (e.g., "daw" means "dog"), whereas the casual listener understands nothing.

By 2 years of age, morphemes may exceed 200 to 300 in number; they are predominantly nouns with a few verbs and other word classes and are at least two-thirds intelligible to persons other than parents. The number of free morphemes increases rapidly, as does their intelligibility—more than 900 words at 3 years with 90 percent intelligibility, and more than 1500 words at 4 years with between 90 and 100 percent inte"ligibility [5]. After the child is 3 years old, verbs predominate. Nouns, pronouns, adjectives, and other classes of words increase in usage as the child grows cognitively and gains more experience.

Acquisition of Bound Morphemes. A competence for the rules governing bound morphemes is acquired by normal children as they are exposed to speech in their environment. This acquisition of bound morphemes is also based on an understanding and usage of rules. Of the bound morphological markers, suffixes are learned before prefixes. Morphological rules are stored by the child in the memory and retrieved as the child attempts to alter the meaning of free morphemes. For example, by 4 years of age the child attempts to attach /s/ or /z/ to spoken free morphemes to show plural meanings or possessive meanings or to show the tense of a verb class morpheme. The child can also attach /t/ or /d/ to indicate past tense. Other endings, such as ing, are acquired as early as 4½ to 5 years of age. The comparative er, as in smaller or larger, is acquired about age 5. Other more difficult markers may be added to the child's repertoire of bound morphemes at a somewhat later time.

Errors are heard frequently in the preschool child's grammar because the child has either failed to apply rules or has failed to learn the exceptions to them. For example, when a child says "There are two house" or "Sheeps say baa," the errors are obvious to adults. In an environment that reinforces the correct use of standard English, these errors normally diminish as the child approaches school age.

Regular rules are mastered before irregular rules. A regular rule governing the choice of /s/ (for example, when "top" becomes "tops") is acquired early. Exceptions to rules are particularly difficult for children and are learned separately and later. One 5½-year-old girl proudly told about helping to care for a baby by saying, "First I fed him, then I drinked him!" Misapplications of regular rules (e.g., "He goed [as opposed to went] home") continue to occur in the early months of the child's first school experience and, it is hoped, are faced by teachers and parents as normal errors for the age of the child.

SYNTAX

Children must acquire rules that enable them to sequence morphemes into phrases and sentences. As very young children hear phrases and sentences spoken around them, they are able to observe and extract rules of syntax.

As vocabulary increases, a child between 18 and 24 months is faced with the social desire and the communicative need to sequence words. The child progresses from the holophrase stage into two- and three-word utterances, the beginning of syntax [34]. These utterances are predominantly various combinations of nouns and verbs, although some other forms of grammar may also occur. These combinations may consist of an agent and an object ("mommy car"), an agent and an action ("mommy ride"), or an action and an object ("ride car"). How the child processes sequential morphemes or "word strings" is not understood fully. One theory suggests that a child employs a familiar and functional word as a pivot on which to hook incoming new words, thus producing a string [12, 13]. One might hear "bye-bye dada" or "bye-bye milk" to connote that someone or something is no longer visible; or perhaps the order of words used by the child is a result of the child's cognitive awareness of relationships [10, 11]. Children require sensitive interpretations of their efforts [14]. To interpret the child's words, for example, "mama shoe" or "that dada," requires intelligent observation of the child in a set circumstance.

This stringing of words is referred to as "telegraphic" speech because it resembles the reduced sentences that are used for telegram transmission (i.e., words, such as articles, prepositions, and auxiliary verbs, are omitted) [15]. Regardless of how and why they are acquired, two-word strings are usually acquired by 2 years of age, and three-word strings follow shortly thereafter. Of course, there are variations from child to child; many children begin earlier than the norms would indicate.

The need for more discriminating forms of communication continues to guide the child toward the acquisition of new rules and words. The simple imperative statement is mastered (e.g., "No!"); when this is found to be inadequate, new rules are added (e.g., "I don't want to!"). The child later discovers that the simple imperative statement can be transformed by rules to become a question (e.g., from "No!" to "Why do I have to?"). Other sentence rules follow as the child matures.

SEMANTICS

Semantics is the study of the special meanings of a language. It includes the relationships among language, thought, and behavior [6]. Morphemes frequently have many meanings, since they have both concrete and implied referents. Most adults associate "dog" with the canine species, or "cow" with a bovine on the farm. However, the relationship of words and meaning is not so simple that a one-to-one relationship exists. One child may think of dog as "cuddly fur," while another thinks of "a bite." Words do not relate directly to specifics but, rather, to the areas into which one organizes a view of the world. One speaker's meaning could differ greatly from that of another using the same word. The way a person views the world is greatly dependent on personal experience and cognitive developmental level; thus, the situation in which a word is used can result in one word's having a host of meanings.

It is evident that word meanings change over the months and years of one's life. A surprising observation is that although an infant appears to understand the word "mama" very early, the infant may use it to address both parents; later "mama" may be used to mean all women. Interestingly, some investigators have endeavored to link "mama," uttered by so many babies over the world, to an easy sound that has derived from the shape of the lips that results from sucking [6]. Piaget suggests that the baby may soon learn that this sound brings a soothing caretaker to meet his or her demands. Whatever the valid explanation is, direct referents and words may not connect immediately in the child's mind. The connecting influences may be the strong emotions associated with "parental" words and the situation in which a parent and infant interact. It is certain that the child's need to communicate may be greater than the short supply of words; thus the words the child uses play many roles, or they have as many meanings as the situation or the circumstance provides.

Until 2 years of age, children operate to identify features of their environment, and their words are tied to the concrete objects they experience (e.g., when asked, "What is a chair?" the child will point to one). Between ages 2 and 7, the child goes beyond using only concrete objects that are present in the immediate environment and is capable of bringing to mind a representation of an absent object or an event (see Chap. 11). From 7 to 11 years of age, children develop an understanding of more complex relationships; however, their language remains on a descriptive and concrete level (e.g., "A chair is to sit on"). After 11 years of age or more, a child can think more abstractly and logically and can use language abstractly to aid in the reasoning process (e.g., "A chair is a piece of furniture that can be used in many ways").

Initially, children may identify only the very general meaning of a language code but will learn more precise or specific meanings later on. Word meanings may change or may carry connotations that a child will acquire later in life. For example, children are often unaware at first that "run," an action for them, may mean a flaw in mother's hose as well.

COMMON VARIATIONS OF LANGUAGE DEVELOPMENT

Although the "King's English," or a standard dialect in the United States, is often alluded to as a desirable goal to achieve when speaking, there appear to be al-

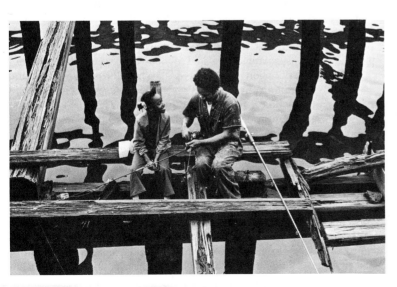

Figure 13–5. The amount and the content of the conversation that takes place between child and parent will affect the child's vocabulary size, fluency, and language style. It will also influence the child's attitude toward the use of speech.

ternative forms of speaking that are acceptable within various subcultures of the population. In recent years there has been emotional concern surrounding the issue of establishing a standard of speech or grammatical form in the United States. However, the standard of one group may serve as a variant for another. Moreover, an individual may use different rules, depending on the circumstances of the moment. For example, one standard is used in a formal speaking situation, but another may be used during informal gatherings of friends. The difference between a "formal" and a "personal" language is more marked in French, German, and Spanish than in English.

Variations in Phonology

Variants in articulation occur concomitantly with those that govern the rules of phonology. The variations may result from the learning that takes place within a dialect or subcultural group, from individual differences in mode of speaking based on personal style, from a biophysical difference (a child may make acceptable sounds that are slightly different from the way others produce them due to some physical difference), or from the various causes of defective speech.

The point at which a variant in speech becomes classed as deviant or defective is not well-defined. The Southerner who moves to the North should be regarded as having different speech, not defective speech. The 3-year-old child who does not articulate the sounds /s/, /r/, or /l/ should not be considered developmentally delayed. It is only when the speech of an individual deviates significantly from the expected mode of the regional-cultural-developmental norm, or when it interferes with communication, that the speech may be considered deviant or defective [65]. A child or an adult having a variation of expected speech patterns should be evaluated and advised by a speech/language pathologist for deviance or defect [67].

Variations in Dialects

Variations in speaking, for the most part, are a result of geographic, social, or stylistic differences. These variations of pronunciation, vocabulary use, and grammar are differences learned from the environment. Of course, there are also biophysically mediated differences in speech that contribute to individual differences. Each human being has unique characteristics or peculiarities; one can identify Grandma on the telephone, associate a neighbor with her unusual vocal resonance, or pick out Crosby's voice on a recording because of the unusual quirk known as a vocal callus.

Widely held variations in speaking, called dialects,

result from a mode of communication that has evolved from persons speaking English as a second language or from the early settlers of an area of the country. A "speech community" is established, and the speakers within the community produce and expect to hear from others their way of speaking. The fewer the contacts outside this community, the more similar are the speech patterns of persons within the community. Children who learn rules of phonology, morphology, syntax, and semantics from their parents learn the rules peculiar to their community. Examples of differing phonological patterns are found in Brooklyn ("a nice goil" [girl]) and in southeastern Ohio ("poosh" [push]; the "boshes" [bushes]; "deesh" [dish]). There are morphological, syntactical, and semantic differences as well. The speech patterns of similar homogeneous groups within the geographical setting will become identifiable.

The speech of educated persons may be as marked as the speech of minimally educated persons; thus, professional persons are generally differentiated in speech from laborers. Often the speech patterns adopted by those of higher socioeconomic status prevail as a standard within a geographical area. Community leaders are usually well educated and their speech patterns are more likely to cross geographical boundaries because of the opportunities associated with education, business, or leisure activities. A wider range of contacts with other groups throughout the country leads to a more homogeneous, "standard American" speech.

Socially determined patterns of speech can apparently change with education. Children born to parents of lower social status may change by becoming "bidialectal"; through education they speak both the patterns of the home and the patterns of higher social groups. If the differences are stylistic, the variations in speaking are related to an awareness of differences in occasion and in people. When the setting for communicative interaction is informal, speech is informal; when a formal setting is recognized, the sytle shifts appropriately. When persons are considered special (e.g., strangers or superiors) the style of language differs from that used for old friends or "good buddies." Older children may have one pattern of speech for adults and another for their peers. They often learn to shift communication patterns early in life.

BILINGUAL HOMES

Children who are reared in a home where two (or more) languages are spoken must learn two sets of formal linguistic rules. Few of these children are truly bilingual, however, since they are usually more adept in the use of one language than in the other. A child may, for example, be able to speak more than one language but may write only one language well. Another child may be able to understand more than one language but may speak only one of them. Many combinations of bilingualism exist. The bilingual child must be able to shift from one language code to another as the need requires. A point of view prevalent among educators is that these children are fortunate to have the mental stimulation of expanded linguistic exposure. In homes where more than one language is spoken, the children have been observed to shift easily from communication with one linguistic speaker to another. Children in European countries are often exposed to two or more languages as a normal part of their life experience. In Switzerland, for example, the economy depends on the successful handling of numerous languages by its natives.

The child who is expected to learn two languages simultaneously must learn to differentiate between them, which some authorities feel may lead to confusion, since the child must learn at least two different words for every object and action. Furthermore, the child must learn two sets of grammatical forms, which often conflict with one another. In addition, the bilingual child must learn how to pronounce the same letters or letter combinations differently. Even when the second language is begun after the child has learned to speak the first one well, there may still be a tendency to confuse the two distinct language systems and misuse them.

However, research by Piaget on bilingual children in Geneva indicates that if the child speaks the second language consistently with one person or in one environment, the confusion is reduced and the bilingualism does not interfere with cognition, language acquisition, or learning to read.

Relatively little information exists to correlate the effects of bilingualism with the child's ability to form concepts. The popular notion is that bilingualism is detrimental to personality integration and emotional adjustment. For example, the child may feel inferior because of using the wrong word at the wrong time, or the second language is viewed as being socially unacceptable in a given situation. However, the bilingual child may actually be at a cognitive advantage because of the experiences of mentally manipulating numerous symbols to represent an object or an event and the cognitive organization that must accompany that process in order to communicate effectively. The child may also have a social advantage because of the ability to communicate with a wider group of people. Since these two factors can enhance self-esteem, bilingualism is more likely to facilitate affective and social adjustment than to interfere with it.

OTHER CULTURAL INFLUENCES

An individual's language performance is greatly influenced by the culture. Evidence exists that mothers in the lower socioeconomic classes, when speaking to their children, use short, restricted sentences that refer to things and actions [4, 29]. Such communications verbally emphasize "the communal rather than the individual, the concrete rather than the abstract, the substance rather than the elaboration of processes, the here-and-now rather than the exploration of motives and intentions . . . "[4]. Because of this tendency, the disadvantaged child may experience difficulty in using abstract language concepts when the object or action is not concretely present. Middle-class mothers put more emphasis on the use of language in socializing and disciplining their children. Such interaction

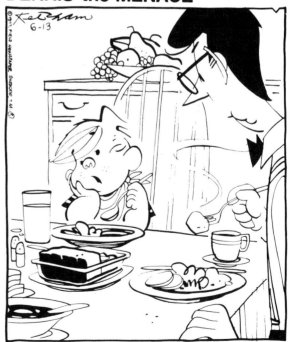

DENNIS the MENACE

"SOME OF THE KIDS' MOTHERS WAS WONDERIN' WHERE YOU GET SOME OF THE EXPRESSIONS I USE."

Figure 13–6. Reprinted courtesy of *Dennis the Menace.* Copyright Field Newspaper Syndicate, T.M.®

influences: (1) the language used by the children, and (2) their ability to think conceptually.

It is necessary to make a distinction between language **performance** and language **competence**. It may be true that middle- and upper-class children can demonstrate superiority over lower-class children in all the traditional measures of language ability (vocabulary knowledge, sentence structure use, sound discrimination, and articulation) [60]. However, more detailed linguistic analyses have demonstrated that the language of children whose dialect differs from standard English (as spoken by the average American middle-class white person) possesses "highly structured grammatical systems through which they can express both emotional and logical thoughts" [44]. Such children are not necessarily deficient in the ability to learn to speak standard English, nor are they necessarily cognitively inept; they are merely the product of their socioaffective environment.

Actually, children often become "bilingual" in that they may be expected to speak one "language" at school and another dialect in their respective neighborhoods. Children whose speech style is very different from the writing style of their books may have difficulty learning to read [55]. The children may have to translate the written word into their own language or dialect before comprehending it [26]. This interesting dilemma is providing controversy among educators, many of whom attest that Standard English is not the only medium through which teaching and learning can occur [30]. Teachers and other authority figures who are critical toward a given child's dialect may have a profoundly negative effect on the child's self-concept [36].

It might prove helpful for those who believe that certain dialects are deficient to study both the structure of the dialect and the history of how it evolved. The **meaning** intended by a word's use is often more important than its variation in phonology or syntax [36]. Many of the sound variations of various dialects are often substitutions that have come about from a person's original language or that of immigrant parents. For example, Ebonics, or Black English, uses "dis" for "this"; or the Appalachian uses "hit" for "it." The /f/ substitution for /th/ in Ebonics (e.g., "birfday" for "birthday") has been traced to a typical sound of Gullah, the language of black speakers in the Carolina Sea Islands [55]. A trained linguist can quickly identify the Celtic English foundation of the Appalachian dialect.

Ebonics is a variation of American English as modified by the African heritage. Rules of logical syntax appear to govern what was long regarded by many American speakers as being merely sloppy or uninformed use of language. Some examples of Black English are as follows: the omission of /t/ in expressions such as "best ever" and of /d/ in "good boy"; the pronunciation of "pest" as "pes," "task" as "tas," and "rasp" as "ras"; and the omission of the final phoneme in "kind" and "hold" [67]. Other interesting features are morpheme selection and how it affects verbal tense in expressions such as "I be busy" or "I done finished," and the omission of "is" in "She going." In the rule system for Ebonics, not all verbs in a given sentence need to indicate past or present tense as long as one of them, or some other word, identifies the time as being either momentary or continuous. "My daddy sick" means that he is ill, but not for long, whereas "My daddy be sick" connotes a long-term illness [61]. In certain plural forms, the /s/ and /z/ markers are omitted, as is the case for the /t/ and /d/ past tense markers. Possessive markers may also be missing, as in "the girl hat." All these examples have a rule at the base of their usage. Whether Ebonics is a distinct dialect or a truly separate language as some theorists contend, it is a patterned way of communicating among a significant number of Americans.

A study of the various words used in different regions of the United States to describe the same object or concept can be both informative and entertaining. A child requests "soda" in the Southeast; a Midwestern counterpart wants "pop"; in New England it is "tonic." The more one understands about other language codes and rules, the easier it will be to communicate with the many persons one comes into contact with daily. Understanding can dissipate prejudice and confusion—essential factors in today's multilingual world.

Variations in Rhythm

In the process of learning language, children may use rhythmic patterns that differ from those of adult speech. However, these differences should be considered normal for the language learning period; they should not be labeled "deviations" or cause undue anxiety among parents.

Practically all children go through periods of dysfluency that resemble stuttering. Such a period usually begins between 2 and 4 years of age (when a child starts incorporating newly learned words and rules of phonology, morphology, syntax, and semantics). This form of dysfluency consists more of phrase repetitions than of sound and syllable repetitions. The child may, however, repeat those sounds and syllables that give trouble in an effort to improve articulation. As such, this dysfluency, or normal stuttering, is inconsistent—sometimes it will occur and sometimes it will not, unlike the abnormal form of stuttering, which occurs regularly in a given situation or with a certain word.

Drawing attention to any dysfluent behavior may tend to aggravate or to reinforce that behavior. When any child is learning to speak in a socially acceptable way, it is important that the child learn to speak at his or her own speed. Many well-meaning caretakers anticipate the word the child is about to use and quickly say it before the child can do so. Other well-meaning parents may correct speech patterns and articulation instead of listening to the child's message. This type of pressure may serve to decrease the child's self-esteem and make conversation less than pleasant for him or her. Correction, when given, must be gentle and inconspicuous.

In some cases, the child may actually stop talking because of the fear of parental criticism. Some children do **not** talk during toddler and preschool years because the parents have not given them any reason to use language. The parents meet all the children's needs before they can verbalize them; the parents speak for the children, or they allow the children to continue to use nonverbal language (pointing, grunting) to identify needs. There is a delicate balance between offering appropriate motivation and assistance and protecting or challenging children beyond reason for their age.

There are instances in which rhythmic deviations exist that are not an acceptable part of normal development. In these instances, the deviations are characterized by the addition of marked tension on the part of the child. Professional advice by a speech pathologist for parental guidance is indicated. The majority of children who demonstrate dysfluencies between 2 and 4 years of age attain normal speech without therapy [65].

Professionals do not agree as to the cause of extreme dysfluencies. However, many do agree that even normal children experience difficulty in storing and retrieving rules of phonology, morphology, syntax, and semantics. In the process of retrieving and applying the linguistic rules for a specific situation, children may exhibit hesitations and repetitions in their speech rhythm. Parents can assist children during this period of development by providing an enriched language opportunity in a relaxed atmosphere. It is hoped that this action will reduce the chance of unnecessary tensions that can mar the pleasures of learning to talk. In this way, some of the extreme problems of dysfluency can be prevented.

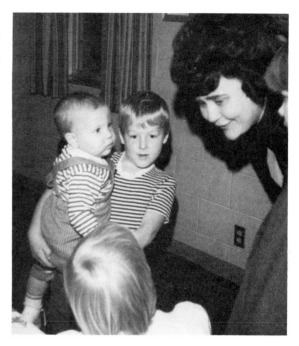

Figure 13–7. In an environment in which others are interested in what he or she has to say, the child may be encouraged to continue to use language to express the self and to interact with others.

Variations in Phonation

Normal variations in voice include differences in pitch, loudness, timbre, and inflectional patterns. These differences are due to biophysical, sociocultural, and emotional factors. Differences reflect both the cognitive intent and the emotional state of the individual. For example, a mother uses a different "voice" when speaking to her child endearingly as opposed to that used when she is distracting the child from playing in the trash can. Age, gender, and size also account for some individual differences. Children normally have higher pitches than adults; men have lower pitches than women. Opera singers are noted for their timbre or vibrato. Normally, adolescents experience a change in vocal pitch. Girls make gradual, smoother changes from childlike voices to mature voices, whereas boys may experience such changes more abruptly. For boys, the abrupt change is closely related to sexual maturity: Tommy Jones becomes Tom or Thomas Jones.

Emotional distress may be reflected in harsh, strident, or piercing voices. The voice of the deaf person is distinct—it is monotone, devoid of inflections. It may be too loud or too soft for the situation. Blind persons may also experience difficulty, using a "broadcast voice" instead of a focused voice that directs sound for direction and distance.

MAXIMIZING COMMUNICATION POTENTIALS

A child does not acquire language in a vacuum. The child must be provided with a rich, responsive linguistic environment. Although the urge to communicate may be present from infancy, the child requires the stimulation of, and interaction with, loving persons who respond to and motivate the child at each stage of development to acquire the skills and the rules necessary for achieving communication competence.

It is important to provide the child with a responsive environment from the first days of life. Communication is a two-way process. It involves "turn-taking":

Parents need to talk to the baby (using slow, exaggerated words), but they also need to provide pauses, rest spots between phrases that allow the baby an opportunity to respond. The neonate may open the eyes, move the mouth and the tongue, and gently open and close the hands. That is responding for a neonate! As the parent resumes talking, the infant will become quiet and search the parent's face with his or her eyes. If parents talk too much or do not allow pauses that provide an opportunity for the baby to respond, the baby will become irritable and struggle to turn away to "turn off" the bombardment.

On the other hand, the baby will attempt to draw the adult into "conversation" if the adult is too quiet, or merely stares at the baby. If the efforts are not rewarded, the baby will give up, usually becoming puzzled and irritable in the process. So even during the first weeks of life, the parents are helping the child to

Table 13–2. A Child's Normal Development of Language and Speech

Average Age	Expected Behaviors
Birth to 1 month	Reflexively vocalizes to given stimuli (e.g., hunger, cold, pain). Responds to social stimuli (eye contact, talking) through mouth and hand opening, throat sounds.
1 to 6 months	Baby "invents" new noises (squeals, "oohs," etc.) and appears to experiment with them. Cooing usually begins around 2 months and occurs especially when the baby appears to be happy (e.g., during or after eating, observing a smiling face, observing or touching objects of interest). By 4 or 5 months, babbling occurs (sequences of alternating vowels and consonants, such as "bababa," that serve as motor practice for true speech)
6 to 9 months	Advances to the **lalling** stage (period in which baby begins to repeat heard sounds or sound combinations)
10 to 12 months	Attempts to imitate all and any sounds, using sounds learned during lalling stage; will select those that help communicate wants or are amusing. Near the end of the first year, the baby's intonation becomes more like adult speech
12 to 18 months	Begins to "talk" (intentionally uses a word, and behavior indicates that the baby understands the meaning of the words appropriate to the situation). Usually begins with a monomorpheme or dimorpheme (e.g., "ma, mama, pa, papa, nana")
18 to 24 months	At 18 months, usually uses 20 to 100 words. Child's one-word sentences are 25% intelligible. Child will use proper vowel inflection but will display uncertainty and inconsistency in saying almost any word. Child's voice will often become high-pitched and appear strained as control is learned. Child will experiment with voice control and will begin to repeat morphemes or words in a playful, but sometimes unconscious, manner. By 24 months, should be using a noun and some verbs to communicate needs
24 to 36 months	Child uses 200 to 300 words in phrases and two-word sentences with 66% intelligibility and has better pitch control, although a "squeaking" voice is common. Child may repeat a word or a phrase and may precede it with a repeated or prolonged "uh"
36 to 48 months	Child's vocalizations are often characterized by repetitions, hesitations, and prolongation. During this period learns to use approximately 900 words (with an increasing number of nouns, pronouns, and adjectives) in three-word sentences that are 90% intelligible. Words are often shortened when pronounced, with many medial consonants being omitted or substituted. Voice is usually well-controlled. By 48 months, child should have a vocabulary of about 1500 words used in short sentences of 90 to 100% intelligibility. By 48 months, pronunciation of more words is well-established (exceptions: some words containing "r" and "l" sounds are mispronounced; medial sounds of "t," "d," and "th" may be omitted). Vocal inflections may be quite dramatic and playful around 48 months. By 48 months, if repetition of a word or phrase occurs, it should be sharply reduced in frequency as compared to previous repetitions

learn the basic rules of effective communication—that of turn-taking.

Closely aligned to the concept of turn-taking is that of taking the initiative or sharing the responsibility for communication. This requires that the parent learn to respond and listen to the infant's early attempts to communicate. This reciprocity needs to continue throughout the early years. Children need to know that their efforts are respected (even when the parent does not understand the toddler's long sound chains). Such sensitive responsiveness encourages the child to put ideas and needs into words.

Many parents do not realize that comprehension of language is far greater than expression. In their eagerness to get children to perform, they bombard them with questions: "What's this?" "Who did you see?" "Where are we going?" Children may feel as if they are having an oral examination. The ensuing tension will reduce performance level and often leads to undesirable behaviors. Children who are pressured into producing sounds ahead of their developmental level may develop dyslalia (articulation problems), revert to using infantile speech, or refuse to talk (elective aphasia). Another problem with the "quiz show" is that it retains control of the topic in the parental field and thus effectively prevents the child from using initiative or sharing the responsibility for an interaction. This has serious social/emotional implications.

Children generally are more comfortable when the parent gives full attention to what the child is saying, responds contingently, and repeats what the child says. When repeating a child's sentence, the parent should model the correct (1) pronunciation of a word, (2) usage of a word, (3) form of verb tense, and (4) structure of a sentence. This process is called expanding a sentence. When children hear the correct grammatical form, they gradually extract the rules and incorporate them into their own vocalizations.

On the other hand, parents need to be sure the child has adequate opportunity to talk. If they identify the child's needs before the child has an opportunity to verbalize them, then language can be delayed. As the child reaches toward the parent to be picked up, modeling the word "up" and pairing it with picking up the child helps with the comprehension phase. Gradually the parent will say, "What do you want?" as the child reaches upward. When there is no response, then the parent may prompt. This prompt gradually is relinquished as the child uses language spontaneously. Immediate responses to the child's use of language also encourage the use of language rather than negative behaviors to obtain attention or to express needs.

As parents are teaching language, they usually start by pairing the object with its name (e.g., "bottle," "ball," "Mama," "doggie"). The child gradually begins to associate the sound code with the visual object. One object may have many names (e.g., pocketbook, purse, handbag, clutch; or sofa, couch, davenport, settee). As in all teaching situations, confusion is reduced and learning enhanced if the same two stimuli are consistently paired. Consequently, parents should stick to one word to represent the object or action. When the child evidences understanding of the first word to identify an object, then a second word can be paired in tandem with the first word when the object is presented. Gradually the second word can be used by itself, and the first word added only as a prompter if the child does not recognize the word. If the two words are used interchangeably from the beginning, confusion is prolonged and learning delayed.

Children love to play with the sounds and rhythms of language. Nursery rhymes and simple songs and poems are valuable adjuncts to helping the child to learn language. However, parents are cautioned that this is a cognitive exercise, not a communication ex-

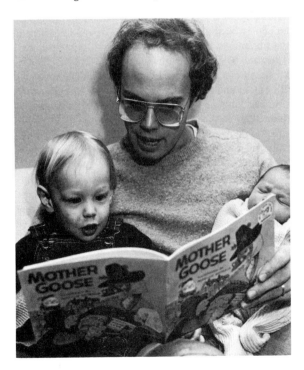

Figure 13–8. Reading aloud to the young child is a form of reinforcing the importance of written language. Children learn rules underlying a particular language when they hear it spoken.

ercise. The most critical factor in learning to communicate is the reciprocal exchange of a meaningful message. For the adult, this means **listening** as well as talking to the child. Communication is the intersect of the biophysical, cognitive, affective, and social domains!

CONCLUSION

The importance of the linguistic environment is obvious when one notes that a baby born to French-speaking parents grows up speaking French; an Italian baby, Italian; and an English baby, English. A baby born in a certain area of the United States to parents who speak a particular dialect learns to speak that dialect also. Rules underlying a particular language and its dialect are learned from the speakers during the baby's most intimate contacts. Exposure to talk or spoken language must occur early and continue throughout the early years of life because the capacity for discriminating sound into categories may begin within hours after birth. The vocabulary of the language, the rules for grammar, and the special meanings that are embedded in the language are usually acquired spontaneously by the normally developing child. Learning the phonemes, morphemes, syntax, and semantics of a second language becomes more difficult with age; those who learn a second language after puberty usually retain an accent even though it may become their primary language for communication for the rest of their lives.

Although frustrations are experienced by children in trying to retrieve and to apply the rules of language, they eventually discover the rewards that contribute to rich social and personal experiences. Through language, children can open doors to more meaningful relationships, to self-realization through self-expression, to exciting exchanges of ideas, to the limitless reaches of learning, and to experiences that are supportive to both affective and cognitive maturation. Higher levels of communication are mastered gradually (i.e., the ability to manipulate language through reasoning, to express vocally substantive thought for others to comprehend, and to employ efficient orthographic symbols through reading and writing of ideas).

Anyone who works with children or their families soon discovers that not all children develop the ability to talk according to normal expectations. Many children have abnormalities that make talking difficult for them; others have environments that are different in affect or in language models.

Speech/language pathologists can provide evaluative and remedial procedures; audiologists and other specialists can evaluate hearing and provide training in sensory perception. These specialists are found in university speech and hearing clinics, public school programs, departments of public health, hospitals, and private clinics. The American Speech and Hearing Association sets the standards for the training and certification of professional persons in these areas. Information regarding the location of qualified persons to advise and to assist the child or the adult with a speech, a language, or a hearing disability in various communities in the United States can be obtained through the state departments of education or health. Talking to infants may seem to be a futile activity (on a par with talking to pets) for a person who is not knowledgeable about language development. However, children who have learned the value of language and how to communicate during these early months and years will find the new language skills of reading and writing to be rewarding and human relationships to be reinforcing. Language is the key to memories of the past, control of the present, and planning for the future.

REFERENCES

1. Allen, R. R., and Brown, K. L. (Eds.). *Developing Communication Competence in Children.* Skokie, IL: National Textbook, 1976.
2. Anastasiow, N. Language: the convergence of developmental interactions. *Infant Ment. Health J.* 4:32, 1983.
3. Bannatyne, A. *Language, Reading and Learning Disabilities: Psychology, Neuropsychology, Diagnosis and Remediation.* Springfield, IL: Thomas, 1971.
4. Bernstein, B. A Sociolinguistic Approach to Socialization: With Some Reference to Educability. In F. Williams (Ed.), *Language and Poverty: Perspective on a Theme.* Chicago: Markham, 1970.
5. Berry, M. F. *Language Disorders of Children: The Bases and Diagnosis.* New York: Appleton-Century-Crofts, 1969.
6. Berry, M. F., and Eisenson, J. *Speech Disorders: Principles and Practices of Therapy.* Englewood Cliffs, NJ: Prentice-Hall, 1956,
7. Biehler, R. F. *Child Development: An Introduction* (2nd ed.). Boston: Houghton Mifflin, 1981.
8. Black, J. W. The effect of delayed side-tone upon vocal rate and intensity. *J. Speech Hear. Disord.* 16:56, 1951.
9. Black, J. W. *Lectures in Speech Sciences.* Muncie, IN: Ball State University Press, 1976.
10. Bloom, L. *Language Development: Form and Function of Emerging Grammars.* Cambridge, MA: M.I.T. Press, 1970.
11. Bloom, L. Why not pivot grammars? *J. Speech Hear. Disord.* 36:40, 1971.

12. Braine, M. D. S. On learning the grammatical order of words. *Psychol. Rev.* 70:323, 1963.
13. Braine, M. D. S. Children's First Word Combinations. *Monographs of the Society for Research in Child Development*, Vol. 41, No. 1, Serial No. 164. Chicago: University of Chicago Press, 1976.
14. Brown, R. *A First Language: The Early Stages.* Cambridge, MA: Harvard University Press, 1973.
15. Brown, R., and Fraser, C. The Acquisition of Syntax. In C. N. Cofer and B. S. Musgrave (Eds.), *Verbal Behavior and Learning.* New York: McGraw-Hill, 1963.
16. Bruner, J. S. The course of cognitive growth. *Am. Psychol.* 19:1, 1964.
17. Cherry, C. *On Human Communication: A Review, a Survey, and a Criticism* (3rd ed.). Cambridge, MA: M.I.T. Press, 1980.
18. Chomsky, N. A review of "Verbal Behavior" by B. F. Skinner. *Language* 35:26, 1959.
19. Chomsky, N. *Language and Mind.* New York: Harcourt, Brace, Jovanovich, 1972.
20. Chomsky, N. *Syntactic Structures.* The Hague: Mouton, 1978.
21. Condon, W. S., and Sanders, L. W. Neonatal movement is synchronized with adult speech: Interactional participation in language acquisition. *Science* 183:99, 1974.
22. Cromer, R. F. The Cognitive Hypothesis of Language. Acquisition and Its Implications for Child Language Deficiency. In D. M. Morehead and A. E. Morehead (Eds.), *Normal and Deficient Child Language.* Baltimore: University Park Press, 1976.
23. Dale, P. S. *Language Development: Structure and Function* (2nd ed.). New York: Holt, Rinehart & Winston, 1976.
24. Eimas, P. D., et al. Speech perception in infants. *Science* 171:303, 1971.
25. Irwin, J. V., and Duffy, J. K. *Speech and Hearing Hurdles.* Columbus, OH: School and College Service, 1955.
26. Jansky, J. J., and deHirsch, K. *Preventing Reading Failure: Prediction, Diagnosis, Intervention.* New York: Harper & Row, 1972.
27. Kagan, J., et al. Memory and meaning in two cultures. *Child Dev.* 44:221, 1973.
28. Kendler, T. S. Development of Mediating Responses in Children. In J. C. Wright and J. Kagan (Eds.), Basic cognitive processes in children. *Monogr. Soc. Res. Child Dev.* 28:33, 1962.
29. Krown, S. *Threes and Fours Go to School.* Englewood Cliffs, NJ: Prentice-Hall, 1974.
30. Labov, W. Academic ignorance and Black intelligence. *Atlantic Monthly* 229(6):59, June 1972.
31. Lee, B. S. Artificial stutter. *J. Speech Hear. Disord.* 16(1):53, 1951.
32. Lenneberg. E. H. *Biological Foundations of Language.* Malabar, FL: R. E. Krieger, 1984.
33. Luria, A. R. The Role of Language in the Formation of Temporary Connections. In B. Simon (Ed.), *Psychology in the Soviet Union.* Stanford, CA: Stanford University Press, 1957.
34. McNeill, D. Developmental Psycholinguistics. In F. L. Smith and G. A. Miller (Eds.), *The Genesis of Language: A Psycholinguistic Approach.* Cambridge, MA: M.I.T. Press, 1966.
35. McNeill, D. *The Acquisition of Language: The Study of Developmental Psycholinguistics.* New York: Harper & Row, 1970.
36. Markham, L. R. De dog and de cat: Assisting speakers of Black English as they begin to write. *Young Chn.* 39:15, 1984.
37. Ményuk, P. *The Acquisition and Development of Language.* Englewood Cliffs, NJ: Prentice-Hall, 1971.
38. Ményuk, P. *The Development of Speech.* Indianapolis: Bobbs-Merrill, 1972.
39. Moerk, E. L. *Pragmatic and Semantic Aspects of Early Language Development.* Baltimore: University Park Press, 1977.
40. Moffitt, A. R. Consonant cue perception by twenty- to twenty-four week old infants. *Child Dev.* 42:717, 1971.
41. More, J., Wilson, W., and Thompson, G. Visual reinforcement of head-turn responses in infants under twelve months of age. *J. Speech Hear. Disord.* 42:328, 1977.
42. Morse, P. A. The discrimination of speech and non-speech stimuli in early infancy. *J. Exp. Child Psychol.* 14:477, 1972.
43. Murphy, K. P., and Smyth, C. N. Response of fetus to auditory stimulation. *Lancet* 1:972, 1962.
44. Mussen, P. H., et al. *Child Development and Personality* (6th ed.). New York: Harper & Row, 1984.
45. Olson, D. Language and thought: Aspects of a cognitive theory of semantics. *Psychol. Rev.* 77:257, 1970.
46. Piaget, J. *Comments on Vygotsky's Critical Remarks Concerning the Language and Thought of the Child.* Translated by A. Parsons. Cambridge, MA: M.I.T. Press, 1962.
47. Piaget, J. *The Language and Thought of the Child.* Translated by M. Gabain. New York: Meridian Books, 1969.
48. Piaget, J., and Inhelder, B. *The Psychology of the Child.* Translated by H. Weaver. New York: Basic Books, 1969.
49. Piaget, J., and Inhelder, B. The Semiotic or Symbolic Function. In H. E. Gruber and J. J. Vonèche (Eds.), *The Essential Piaget.* New York: Basic Books, 1977.
50. Pulaski, M. A. S. *Understanding Piaget: An Introduction to Children's Cognitive Development* (Rev. and expanded ed.). New York: Harper & Row, 1980.
51. Rebelsky, F. G., Starr, R. H., and Luria, Z. Language Development: The First Four Years. In Y. Brackbill (Ed.), *Infancy and Early Childhood.* New York: Free Press, 1967.
52. Ringler, N. M. From prespeech to language: The influence of caregiver-child interaction. *Infant Ment. Health J.* 4:43, 1983.
53. Ruder, K., Bricker, W. A., and Ruder, C. Language Acquisition. In J. J. Gallagher (Ed.), *The Application of Child Development Research to Exceptional Children.* Reston, VA: Council for Exceptional Children, 1975.
54. Sander, L. W. The Longitudinal Course of Early Mother-Child Interaction—Cross-Case Comparison in a Sample of

Mother-Child Pairs. In B. M. Foss (Ed.), *Determinants of Infant Behavior IV*. London: Methuen, 1969.

55. Seymour, D. Z. Black Children, Black Speech. In F. Rebelsky and L. Dorman (Eds.), *Child Development and Behavior* (2nd ed.). New York: Knopf, 1974.

56. Skinner, B. F. *Verbal Behavior*. New York: Appleton-Century-Crofts, 1957.

57. Slobin, D. I. *Psycholinguistics* (2nd ed.). Glenview, IL: Scott, Foresman, 1979.

58. Staats, A. W., and Staats, C. K. *Complex Human Behavior*. New York: Holt, Rinehart & Winston, 1963.

59. Stevenson, H. W. Learning. In J. J. Gallagher (Ed.), *The Application of Child Development Research to Exceptional Children*. Reston, VA: Council for Exceptional Children, 1975.

60. Templin, M. C. Certain Language Skills in Children, Their Development and Interrelationships. *Institute of Child Welfare Monographs*, Series No. 26. Minneapolis, MN: University of Minnesota Press, 1957.

61. Thomson, D. S. *Language*. New York: Time-Life Books, 1975.

62. Tillis, C. H., and Grimm, W. A. Evaluation of the localization auditory screening test in children 6–18 months of age. *Am. J. Public Health* 68(1):65, 1978.

63. Trantham, C. R., and Pedersen, J. K. *Normal Language Development*. Baltimore: Williams & Wilkins, 1976.

64. Trehub, S. E. Infants' sensitivity to vowel and tonal contrasts. *Dev. Psychol.* 9(1):91, 1973.

65. Van Riper, C. G. *Speech Correction: Principles and Methods* (6th ed.). Englewood Cliffs, NJ: Prentice-Hall, 1978.

66. Williams, F., Hopper, R., and Natalicio, D. S. *The Sounds of Children*. Englewood Cliffs, NJ: Prentice-Hall, 1977.

67. Williams, R., and Wolfram, W. *Social Dialects: Differences vs. Disorders*. Rockville, MD: American Speech and Hearing Association, 1977.

68. Wood, B. S. *Children and Communications: Verbal and Nonverbal Language Development* (2nd ed.). Englewood Cliffs, NJ: Prentice-Hall, 1981.

14
Preparation for School

Clara S. Schuster

Imitation is natural to man from childhood, one of his advantages over the lower animals being this, that he is the most imitative creature in the world, and learns at first by imitation.

—Aristotle, *Poetics*, 1448^{b}6

Entrance into first grade constitutes a major change in a child's lifestyle. He or she is introduced to (or confronted with, depending on the child's developmental readiness) new friends, new experiences, and new goals and responsibilities. The greater part of the day is now spent away from home; thus the child experiences a change or broadening of orientation to the environment and the culture. The teacher becomes another significant role model, and peers begin to influence strongly the child's perceived desires and needs as well as behavior patterns. As the child is introduced to other lifestyles and becomes more independent of the parents, he or she may begin to question family rules and regulations, standards, and goals. The child also frequently begins to challenge parental authority.

The child who is progressing normally is ready to tackle Erikson's next core problem—industry versus inferiority. Success in mastering this task is dependent not only on the experiences and support offered during the school years, but also on how well the child has been prepared for school by past experiences.

Preparation for school begins the day an infant is born. Its foundation for success is laid in the parent-child relationship. An enormous amount of learning must occur before the child ever enters school. It all seems very simple to adults looking back from their college years, but it was not simple at the time; each new schema took effort to form. Sensitivity and responsiveness on the part of the parents toward the child's developmental level are essential to facilitate the child's cognitive growth from the basically reflexive activities of the neonate to the sensorimotor thought of the toddler and then to the prelogical thought processes of the preschooler. As the parents structure the environment, they must alternately provide enough security, challenges, frustrations, and successes, so that the child begins to make discriminations; to see relationships; to explore independently; and to master cognitive, affective, social, and physical skills.

EXPECTATIONS OF THE FIRST-GRADE TEACHER

The six-year-old has learned much since birth, but it is only a beginning. The child is not yet ready to face the world alone. Formal education is geared toward helping children to gain the skills essential to cope with adult responsibilities. Although it is recognized that many children may not possess all of the following skills when they enter first grade, success in school is greatly facilitated if they have developed the competencies discussed in the following sections.

Academic Skills

Some skills are prerequisites for learning to read and to write because they involve the child's ability to use language symbols to represent concrete objects, actions, or events. Reading takes the child one step farther away from concrete reality, thereby requiring higher levels of representational thought. The skills discussed in the following sections indicate that lower-level concepts and representational thought have been mastered.

KNOWLEDGE
Progress in first grade is facilitated if the child knows the alphabet before beginning school; this includes knowing the sequence of the letters and the ability to recognize each letter. Teachers frequently find that children know the alphabet song but are unable to identify the corresponding letter. The child who can print the letters and identify the major sound (phoneme) associated with the letter is at a great advantage in beginning to read, especially by the phonetic approach. This ability also involves auditory discrimination skills. Some children are able to recognize the letters and their major sounds but are not able to re-

create that symbol on paper. Being able to print a letter has little to do with phonics; it is a reflection rather of the child's visual-motor coordination skills.

Children who are able to write and to recognize their own name in print have already been introduced to the concept that a written sign represents a verbal symbol, which in turn represents a concrete object—"me." The ability to recognize one's own name among several other names or words fosters discriminatory skills, supports a sense of mastery, and encourages recognition of individuality and self-identity.

Most 6-year-olds are able to count to 10. They should also be able to recognize the written sign for the numbers, but more importantly, they should know the meaning of the number (i.e., the child should be able to identify "3" pencils or "5" stars). This skill is a prerequisite for early mathematics—both addition and subtraction. An understanding of concepts such as "more" and "less" is also basic to first grade mathematics (see Fig. 14–1).

The ability to recognize the colors of the rainbow or the colors in a basic crayon box is also very helpful. Color is frequently used in the early grades to identify a specific book or as part of the directions for an assignment.

UNDERSTANDING
One of the basic concepts the first-grader should know is the concept of direction, especially the ability to distinguish right from left. Children who experience difficulty with this skill frequently have difficulty in reading from left to right and may show word or letter reversals.

The ability to understand position words is also essential to comprehending directions. Words, such as above-below, on-beside, under-over, inside-outside, are common in directions given to the first-grader. Direction words are more abstract than words representing concrete objects and thus may present more difficulty to some children, especially those with learning disabilities.

Activities involving classification skills comprise a large proportion of first-grade work: Is the child able to identify things that are alike and things that are different? Differences in size and basic shapes (triangle, square, rectangle, and circle) are usually learned during the preschool years. Discrimination or comparative activities require the child to identity which object is largest, smallest, shortest, or longest. Higher levels of classification require the child to match objects that have similar usage. Discrimination and classification

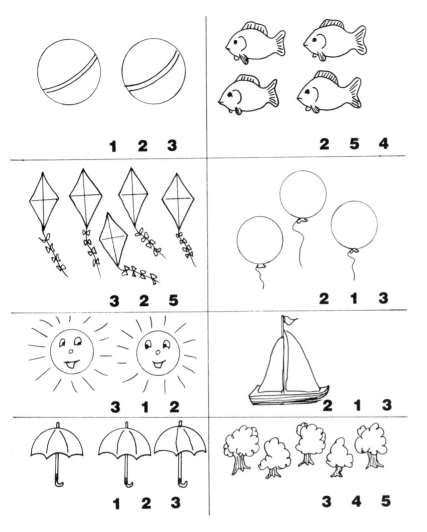

Figure 14–1. Typical counting exercise for first graders.

skills are also challenged by asking the child to match pictures with rhyming words (Fig. 14–2). Although to adults these activities seem simple and fun, to the first-grader they may present major challenges to emerging skills and a sense of mastery. The inadequately prepared child may experience repeated failures.

Physical Skills

Particular physical skills are helpful, if not essential, in helping the child to maintain a feeling of independence, personal integrity, and a positive self-concept in the classroom. Some of these skills are critical to

independent self-care; others are indirectly related to competence in completing assignments.

PERSONAL CARE

The teacher obviously cannot provide personal care for 30 or 35 children. The children should be able to feed themselves, attend to their own toileting needs, and wash their hands independently. Occasionally first-graders need assistance with buttoning clothing or putting on coats or boots. In these instances, the children should be encouraged to help and teach each other, which is a relief for the teacher, a source of pride

Figure 14–2. Typical rhyming-word exercise for first graders.

to the helper, and a peer role model and thus a stimulus for the child who is helped.

COORDINATION

Successful coordination of gross motor skills is evidenced by the ability to hop on both one foot and two feet, to do a jumping jack, to skip, and to walk unassisted on a balance board. Many teachers indicate that children who are unable to perform these skills frequently cannot write well. It appears that lack of adequate gross-motor experience correlates highly with the development of the fine-motor skills necessary for writing. Some contend that prerequisite motor pathways have not been established.

Children should be able to hold a pencil properly[10]; the position is identical to that for holding tableware properly for eating. They should also be able to turn individual pages, a skill that is usually developed during the third year of life. Many children may still have

some difficulty with scissors, but some skill in their use is essential to success in classroom assignments. Research by de Hirsch and associates indicates that the ability to match a tapped-out rhythm and to draw a picture of a person correlate highly with the reading and spelling skills achieved at the end of second grade [10].

Psychosocial Skills

Most children are very excited and eager to start school; it represents a big step in "growing up." The child entering school will need to be able to tolerate separation from mother. Some children have not adequately resolved the separation-individuation process [21] and thus find that they still need copious amounts of emotional refueling in order to face the world. Erikson theorizes that a deep sense of "inadequacy may be caused by an insufficient solution of the preceding conflict [initiative]; he may still want his mummy more than knowledge. He may still rather be the baby at home than the big boy in school" [13]. The child who is unable to tolerate separation from mother may have inadequate energy levels or inadequate motivation to master school assignments.

The first grader needs to know how to share with peers; this includes the sharing not only of objects but also of the teacher's attention and time. An only child may have particular difficulty in this area. Self-reliance, self-entertainment, patience, empathy, and the ability to tolerate frustration of one's goals are all subskills for this area of competence.

Although attention span appears to be affected both by age and by experience, the ability to listen effectively is a skill that is reinforced or extinguished by experiences. The parent-child relationship is a critical factor in this area; parents who ignore the child's attempts to communicate will often find that the child, in turn, will ignore them. Synchrony of communication is mutually reinforcing. The first-grader must be able to listen to two- or three-part instructions and then follow directions accordingly. This skill is obviously closely related to the child's comprehension of language symbols but is also related to the motivation to attend to, to remember, and then to follow directions—a point to be explored further in the section on learned helplessness.

Children listen to guidance and respond most positively when they respect, but do not fear, authority. Fear may cause them to listen, but it may also immobilize them for action. On the other hand, lack of respect leads to chaos in the classroom and academic confusion due to inattentiveness. Children who are most likely to do well in the primary grades are those who have learned how to harness, organize, and focus their energies toward a goal. They are self-confident, participate actively with the environment, enjoy mastery for its own sake, and seem to have an advanced state of ego organization [10].

The mature first-grader has enough self-discipline to modify his or her goals to the rules of the classroom or to the desires of others. The child is able to sit still long enough to attend to assignments and complete them and to restrict talking to appropriate times. Most 5- to 6-year-olds want to "be first," but the combination of burgeoning self-discipline, sharing skills, and the knowledge of social protocols encourages them to begin to take turns—to learn politeness and respect for the rights, feelings, and human dignity of others.

General Knowledge

Thus far, three major skill areas have been discussed in which the child should develop specific competencies prior to entrance into first grade in order to facilitate mastery of the curriculum and the social environment at school. Although skills in these areas are critical to adjustment, a **good** teacher can still help the child who is weak in one or more skills to achieve mastery and progress successfully in school. Although it appears that there may be critical times for learning some skills, the skills can still be learned at a later time

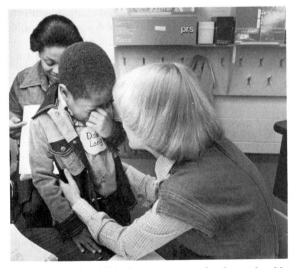

Figure 14–3. The child who is entering school must be able to tolerate separation from the parent before adequate affective energy is available to invest in cognitive and social activities.

with a properly individualized and prescribed program. However, children who are weak in the area of general knowledge may be so handicapped that they cannot be successful in a regular classroom unless extensive remedial assistance is given.

A family who accepted a 5½-year-old girl and an 8-year-old girl as foster daughters is illustrative of this point. Before coming to their foster parents, the girls had apparently spent much time without adult supervision in a small house trailer devoid of running water and electricity. The single bed was shared with their mother. The transient nature of residence in various locations prevented both the establishment of familial attachment and provision of supportive services to the family. The girls were removed from the home as an emergency measure when they failed to attend school and the mother was critically ill. The paucity of their general knowledge, the shortness of their attention span, their inability to remember, their lack of curiosity, and the absence of play activities were astounding. The normal curiosity that begins during the toddler years had literally been extinguished. The girls could not identify the food on their plate or give common names of zoo animals. They did not understand simple commands (e.g., "Sit down," "Open the door," "Pass the potatoes, please"). They did not know the alphabet, nor could they count to 10. The younger girl could not remember three letters in succession.

Since it was summer, the foster parents immediately began an enrichment program. A jungle gym was purchased, and the nearby school playground offered opportunity for gross motor activities. The girls were encouraged to assist in cooking and housekeeping chores. Much guidance, encouragement, and praise was offered for small tasks—jobs they could see they had done. Musical records appropriate for toddlers were played during quiet time and at bedtime. A picture dictionary expanded the world to objects and events the family could not provide in the home or by day trips. The major enrichment technique was communication. The foster parents talked about what they were going to do, what they were doing, and what they had done; they attempted to give the girls a sense of time, planning, and involvement. Each girl was given her own bed, her own toys, her own responsibilities—and her own private time with both the mother and the father.

At the beginning of first grade (the 8-year-old had never attended school), the girls were given assignments, such as those in Figures 14–1, 14–2, and 14–5. But when general knowledge is so weak, how can one be successful at rhyming or identifying initial conso-

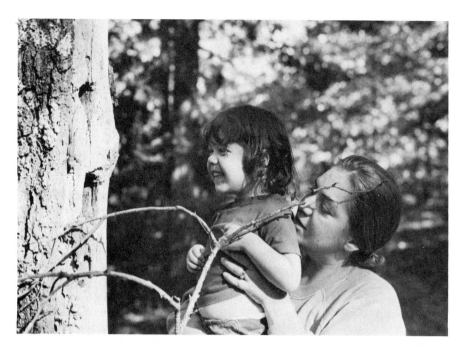

Figure 14–4. Many activities are available to parents and children that can be mutually enjoyed while increasing the child's general knowledge about the world.

nant sounds? These girls, like many others from disadvantaged environments, did not possess the prerequisite skills.

Sara Smilansky's research [35] indicates that severely disadvantaged children experience repeated failure in grade school in spite of extensive enrichment and remedial assistance at school. In this case, after 2 years both of these girls were able to work at their proper grade level. The key difference between Smilansky's research and this situation was the dramatic change that occurred in the girls' home environment. Even though school and peers are very important to the development of the school-ager, the family still remains the key influence in the child's life.

These girls were returned to their natural mother after marked improvements were evidenced in their original home environment. They have continued to function at grade level—with enthusiasm—into their high school years. The cycle of perceived inadequacy had been broken.

THE INADEQUATELY PREPARED CHILD

The previous example was presented so that this chapter might be read with the realization that even though the family environment is critical to fostering maximal

development of the child's potentials, a child who receives a difficult start in life is not necessarily on a failure course. Many factors can change; intervention later in life can help the individual to grow to higher levels of cognitive, social, and emotional maturity. However, the younger the child, the more susceptible he or she is to both permanent damage from overwhelming negative factors and successful remediation by synchronized positive factors.

The Significance of the Parent

Human behavior is so complex and is exposed to so many different variables during the developmental years that the identification of a single correlating variable between early and later development is extremely unlikely and consequently is very significant when found. Research is still in the early stages, but evidence is beginning to accumulate that indicates that the child's primary caretaker is the key to the child's approach to, and mastery of, the environment. Most of the research has centered on the mother-infant/child relationship. However, the gender or the legal relationship of the caretaker is insignificant. The consistency and quality of the interaction are the determining factors.

The Harvard Preschool Project, headed by Burton L.

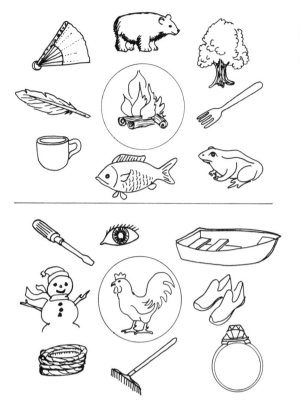

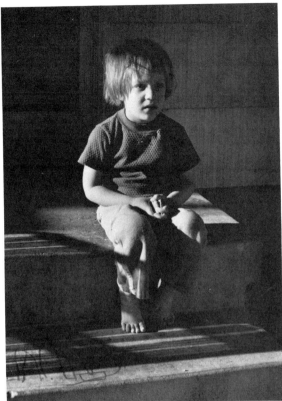

Figure 14–5. Typical initial consonant exercise for first graders (for "f" and "r" sounds).

Figure 14–6. Children left on their own in a barren environment may become bored. This situation, combined with a lack of predictable events (e.g., bedtime, mealtime) or predictable adult responses, can lead to the helplessness syndrome.

White, identified competency characteristics of "A" (high adaptability or flexibility to function well in a variety of living conditions) and "C" (low adaptability) children 3 to 5 years of age [26]. White discovered that the distinguishing characteristics of the two groups were already clearly identifiable by the age of 3 years. White and his associates then went into the homes of infants and toddlers to track down the point at which the paths of "A" and "C" children began to diverge. They discovered that at 18 months of age the path was already predictable. It was not until they studied children as young as 10 months that the behaviors identified as significant discriminators began to merge. Based on their intensive and extensive observations within the home setting, they concluded that the critical variable in the child's development was the mother's approach to the interaction [26].

The research team discovered that "A" mothers seldom gave their babies undivided attention for more than 10 percent of the waking day and did not engage in preplanned formal teaching—quite the opposite of

what the lay person (and even the researchers) would predict. The "A" mother was discovered to be superbly effective in two ways: (1) indirectly, as an organizer and designer of the child's environment, and (2) directly, as a consultant to a busy, exploring, curious, active child. She encouraged and reinforced the child's exploration and independence in a safe environment. When the child met an obstacle, frustration, problem, or novel object or experience, she would verbalize the phenomenon, give directions for resolving the discrepancy with the skills available to the child, or teach him or her new skills. Sometimes the mother "set the stage" for problem solving, but at the child's level of development. She supported and shared the joy of self-discovery and self-accomplishment, offering assistance merely as a backup support system. Thus through these 10- to 20-second episodes scattered throughout the day, the child learned both independence and how to use the adult as a resource—prerequisites for Erikson's initiative stage. This kind of intervention is synchronized intervention because it is responsive to the child's needs and offered at the child's pace.

The "C" mothers, on the other hand, "protected" their children by restricting their freedom to explore. Although they were gentle and loving, gave good physical care, and were patient, these mothers failed to "tune in" to the child's world. They did not share the child's excitement of discovery or verbalize events. They failed to transform the routine diaper change or bath into an intellectually stimulating game of peek-a-boo or water play. White's research indicated that fewer than 10 percent of the children were provided with an environment that would provide maximal opportunities to develop their potentials or to get a really good start in life [40].

Sylvia Krown, doing research in Israel, similarly identified very marked differences in the social and cognitive skills of "advantaged" versus "disadvantaged" 3-year-old children. The characteristics found in these two groups of children are summarized in Table 14–1. Krown found that although the mothers of deprived children were interested in their children's progress and showed much physical affection, they did not understand their child's unique communication system. These mothers were themselves very disorganized and basically passive, and they seemed to lack faith in their ability to control their own world [19]. The mothers were frequently so concerned with their own needs or roles that they failed to communicate to

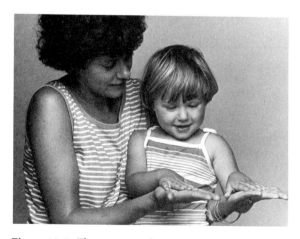

Figure 14–7. The most mundane activities of daily living can become focal points for warm, meaningful, synchronized interaction between parent and child. (Photo by Ed Slaman)

their child a sense of being a separate, special, protected individual. Krown observes that as a result, the children were unable to predict what would happen from one event to the next, had minimal knowledge of language, had difficulty remembering events, and had a greatly decreased curiosity about the world [19]. Competent parents treat their young child as a capable, resourceful person. They are warm, positive, and consistent in their interactions while assisting the child with problem solving [22].

Krown developed a very comprehensive preschool program for these children, which included parent training. At the end of 2 years, there was a marked decrease in the contrast between the two groups, but residual effects, especially in the area of socialization, were still evident.

Both Krown and White found that the child's skills correlated highly with the interactional milieu provided by the mother. White looked for factors facilitating competence, whereas Krown was looking for factors causing incompetence, but their observations support each other. The most significant finding of the Harvard Preschool Project was that differences in later academic competence were identified by 10 months of age.

T. Berry Brazelton has made numerous analyses of mother-infant interactions during the first month of life. He has discovered that the infant's responsiveness to the mother is determined by the infant's ability to organize the stimuli offered by the mother (see Neonatal Assessment, Chap. 6). True reciprocity of interaction is established only if the mother is able to read the infant's cues for boredom and overstimulation [3]. When the mother does not offer the infant enough stimuli, the infant may temporarily seek more attention but may quickly turn attention to other things or may change from state 4 (see p. 103) to another state less conducive to attending to the environment. If the mother offers too much stimuli, the infant becomes "flooded" and retreats in self-defense until he or she is once more able to organize the stimuli and respond. The infant may become so overwhelmed or flooded by the attention that the child begins to behave very irritably or to cry vehemently. The mother who is sensitive to the infant's cues can establish a synchrony of interaction that can sustain the infant in state 4 for prolonged periods of time. Learning is most effective in state 4, since interaction with the environment is at its peak during this state.

Research indicates that synchronized parental responsiveness reduces crying in neonates and young infants. According to Bell and Ainsworth, "spoiled

Table 14–1. Characteristics of Disadvantaged versus Advantaged 3-Year-Olds

Category	Characteristics	
	Disadvantaged Children	Advantaged Children
Physical factors	Clothing about same as advantaged children	Sloppy to new clothes
	Often sent to school ill, with fever	Kept home if ill
	Open, neglected sores; runny noses	Good hygiene
	No breakfast	Fed before school
	Tense posture; guarded movements	Moves with ease and abandon
	Depressed, angry eyes	Alive, alert eyes
	Rigid, unsmiling facial expression	Head up, smiles easily
	Bears pain in silence	Demands attention when hurt
Activity	Constant motion; short attention span	Directed enthusiasm
	Haphazard activity; touches everything	Purposeful activity
	Lacks enthusiasm for exploring	Interested in new experiences
	Disinterested, aimless, wandering	Inquisitive about environment
	Repetitive, stereotyped play	Creative play
	Needs prodding into activity	Exhibits initiative
	Unaware of danger	Avoids hurting self
Mode of thinking	Afraid to tackle new tasks	Interested in new things and information
	Confused sense of time, place, order	Classifies many items
	"In a fog"	Fascinated by surrounding world
	Difficulty remembering concrete events	Talks about events freely
	Does not know how to discriminate	Enthusiastic, curious
	Difficulty with cause-effect relations	Experiments with things around him or her
	Difficulty with sequencing	Follows directions easily
Relationships with people	Withdrawn, shy, suspicious	Friendly, open, outgoing, trusting
	Frequently does not respond	Expresses feelings
	Uneasy with adults	Uneasy when teacher is not near
	Does not address teacher	Seeks attention of adults
	Is a "loner"	Aware of other children
Frustration tolerance	Physical aggression	Controlled, directed behavior
	Impulsive behaviors	Predictable emotional reactions
	Gives up quickly	Seeks teacher's help
Language	Uses isolated words and phrases	Tells stories
	Unable to identify colors, body parts, familiar objects, animals	Rich, expressive vocabulary
	Unable to listen to whole story	Loves story time
	Phonation and enunciation problems	Enjoys speaking and sharing

Source: Extracted from a study by Sylvia Krown [19].

infants" are those whose mothers ignored their cries or delayed in responding to them. Maternal responsiveness in the early months promoted confidence in the environment and fostered greater independence at the end of the first year of life [1]. This decrease in crying behavior can also be empirically identified by the third day of life. Infants who are picked up and talked to each time they cry during the first 3 days of life cry less and are more alert at the end of 3 days than infants who are allowed to cry for prolonged periods (a common practice in some hospital nurseries) [37].

Some extremely interesting data have been collected by Marshall Klaus and John Kennell and their associates. Their research indicates that when infants are kept with their mothers during the first 1 to 2 hours of life, and for 15 extra hours during the first 3 days of life, there are significant differences in maternal behaviors at 1 month and 1 year after birth [17, 18]. These mothers were more attentive and responsive and exhibited greater synchrony of responses (ability to read infant cues) than mothers who experienced standard hospital exposure to their infants (introduction 6 to 12 hours after birth and exposure for 30 minutes every 4 hours for feeding). At 1 year, the early-contact infants exhibited more curiosity and less stranger anxiety than the delayed-contact infants. Follow-up research on the same infants at 2 years and 5 years indicated that the children of early-contact mothers had statistically significant higher intelligence quotients (IQs) and more advanced scores on two language tests [29, 30]. The implications of these studies are that significant preparation for school may actually begin during the first hours of life by sensitizing the mother to the infant's cueing skills.

Whether one takes a Piagetian view of cognitive development (in which intellectual skills evolve from one stage to the next through reorganization or internal structural changes that incorporate lower-level skills) or a behaviorist view (in which cognitive skills evolve through successive approximations, or shaping, to higher-level skills) is insignificant at this point. The skills of children evolve as the environment gives them the opportunity to "try their wings," or the skills may be elicited by an enticing environment. The fact remains that the skills of the neonate are not the same as those of the young school-ager; the skills of the child have evolved sequentially under the combined influence of innate potentials and environmental influences or opportunities. White suggests that during the first 8 months of life, the child's progress is assured by nature as long as he or she is provided with a normal amount of love, attention, and care [40].

Research with twins and adopted children indicates that heredity is very important in determining IQ [16, 33]. However, it is not a fixed entity. Obviously, potentials are limited by neurological maturity, but skills appear to be limited to those that are encouraged, allowed, or supported by the environment. IQ can be influenced by motivation, exposure, and experience. J. McVicker-Hunt postulates that any one individual could have a difference (range) of 75 IQ points, depending on the environment experienced during the early years of life [15, 27]. (Consider the pseudoretardation that stems from severely deprived environments versus the high skill levels that emerge from highly synchronized environments.). It is the unique combination of heredity and environment that determines the child's proficiency; it is the parents who structure the environment, and therefore contribute to either maximizing the child's potentials or hindering them.

Learned Helplessness

Research by Martin Seligman has opened a new door for viewing incompetence in early childhood. His theory is based on a behaviorist approach to mastery of the environment but also includes the psychoanalytical concept of inferiority and the humanistic concept of motivation. Seligman's basic theory is that inadequacy is the result of learned helplessness [33]. As discussed previously, the behaviorist view of learning basically states that an individual will increase or strengthen those behaviors that elicit a desired response from the environment. Behavior, therefore, is elicited, controlled, or molded by the contingent response of the environment. Expectation of a certain response is the basis of motivational, cognitive, and emotional deliberation to perform a behavior ("I act because I will be rewarded"). When an individual believes or learns that behavior and outcome are independent of one another or that events are uncontrollable, the psychological state of helplessness results [33]. If a person believes that his or her actions will not affect the environment, the likelihood of a voluntary response decreases ("Why bother? It won't make any difference").

Learned helplessness is characterized by both cognitive and affective disturbances. If the child learns early in life that outcomes are independent of responses, cause-effect relationships are not learned. It becomes more difficult to learn later in life that response can produce an outcome. Helplessness becomes a self-perpetuating phenomenon; the perceived independence of events interferes with the learning of the interdependence of behavior-outcome contingencies. The need to control or master the environment appears to be a basic drive of life. Anxiety, frustration, or fear is induced, therefore, when the individual realizes an inability to control events [33]. For most people, these emotional responses can be useful, since they maintain the search for alternative responses. However, if a person believes that the outcome or trauma cannot be controlled, Seligman postulates that fear is replaced by depression. Learned helplessness, therefore, undermines a person's motivation to respond, retards the ability to perceive success and to learn that responding works, and results in heightened emotionality due to anxiety and depression.

According to Seligman, "Notions of ego strength and competence are related to mastery over events" [33]. Motivation and emotion are heavily influenced by the environment. Lack of environmental contingencies can create a child who believes he or she is helpless and cannot succeed. Children who believe that they are helpless will perform inadequately, regardless of IQ. The result can be a falsely low IQ score (pseudoretardation) due to inadequate effort. Seligman observes that children who believe in their own competence "can outperform a more talented peer who lacks such a belief" [33]. Unfortunately, helplessness learned in one situation is frequently transferred to other settings.

The **helplessness syndrome** is characterized by the symptoms given below. The first three symptoms are universal; the last three are found only as the depth of perceived helplessness increases.

1. Reduced incidence of initiation of voluntary responses—psychomotor retardation.
2. Negative cognitive set—difficulty learning or accepting that responses will or can produce the desired outcomes.
3. Aggression is attenuated; passivity is exhibited.
4. The effects of helplessness following a single uncontrolled crisis will dissipate with time, but these effects may persist after multiple uncontrollable events.
5. Depressed appetite for food, sex, and socialization; avoidance of self-care or stimulus input, especially if expenditure of energy is required.
6. Physiological change—weight loss, hormonal imbalances, and norepinephrine depletion.

A person may exhibit mild to severe symptoms of the helplessness syndrome (see Chap. 42), depending on age, the quality of previously developed coping skills, the number of other stressors the person faces, and the significance of the uncontrollable events.

According to Seligman, "A child's or an adult's attitude toward his own helplessness or mastery has its roots in infant development. When an infant has a rich supply of powerful synchronies between his actions and outcomes, a sense of mastery develops. Responsive mothering is fundamental to learning mastery" [33]. Each new challenge requires that the child predict an outcome, and outcome is inferred from experience. Therefore, the earlier a child experiences control or lack of control, the more critical and long-lasting is the effect of such experience. Seligman believes that at every opportunity the infant analyzes (on a primitive level) the relationship between his or her behaviors and their outcomes. If a high or low correlation exists, then the child will alter behavior (use of tools for communication) toward obtaining or maintaining the desired environment. If a correlation is not identifiable, the helplessness syndrome results [33]. Stern observes that the maternal responses must occur within 3 seconds after the neonate's behavior to serve as a reinforcer [36]. Helplessness is disastrous to the infant who is laying the structural foundation for cognitive, affective, and motivational development.

The helplessness syndrome can result from absence of the mother, from stimulus deprivation, from nonresponsive mothering, or from a combination of these factors. The result of Bowlby's and Spitz's studies on young infants (see Chap. 9) are classic examples of the helplessness syndrome during infancy. Individuals experiencing reactions to grief and loss also exhibit symptoms of the helplessness syndrome. Increased anxiety around strangers is observed when parents fail to warn the young child that they are leaving him or her with a babysitter. If the parents do not give the child adequate cues or warning signals about their impending departure, the child becomes extremely anxious at inappropriate times. The child cannot predict what will happen and therefore experiences helplessness. The same may occur with the dispensing of medication in the doctor's office, at the hospital, or even at home. The child's excessive fear is frequently the result of inadequate communication or signals from the parents. The child needs to know that the parents can be trusted—that a situation is safe if the parents say so. This view blends with Erikson's concept of basic trust. The child learns to recognize environmental cues. Parental honesty and consistency are essential to learning this trust and thus mastery. Cues are consistent with events; therefore, the child learns to predict and thus to master his or her internal environment. Children can deal with unpleasant events (e.g., the parents are leaving, the injection will hurt) better in the long run if they are given a warning and an honest explanation.

Through the alternating use of maternal and infant tools, the mother and infant inaugurate a synchronized ballet of interaction. Through this mutually reinforcing interchange, the infant strengthens reflexive responses into preplanned, voluntary behaviors. The infant learns to master the self and to obtain the desired pleasure from the environment—the mother's response. The infant whose mother is nonresponsive is thereby deprived of control over stimulation. On the other hand, the mother who is overresponsive to the infant and does not balance the intensity or frequency of her responses to those emitted by the infant is also out of synchrony. Lack of contingent responsiveness leads to helplessness. The key to the infant's mastery, then, is the sensitive, synchronized response of the mother; this is the same conclusion drawn by White, Krown, Kennell, Klaus, Brazelton, and many others studying the behavior of the neonate. The children in Krown's study were suffering from rather marked cases of helplessness syndrome, whereas White's "C" infants exhibited mild cases. The mothers of the "A" infants were able to read the infants' cues, and responded appropriately to them. They did not intrude when uninvited or ignore the child's communication efforts. Consequently, "A" infants exhibited mastery of the environment—high level cognitive and affectional

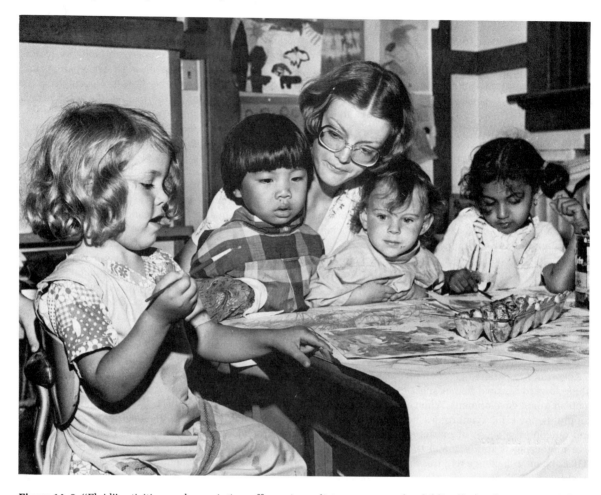

Figure 14–8. "Fluid" activities, such as painting, offer an immediate response to the child's efforts. These activities along with a warm, attentive audience can heighten the child's sense of control and self-esteem—an effective immunization against the helplessness syndrome later in life.

functioning that spilled over to the social and biological domains as well.

FOSTERING POTENTIALS

By now the authors' position is quite clear: The child is born with cognitive potentials that are determined by heredity; the environment will determine how much of the individual's potential will be realized.

Infant Stimulation

Much concern has arisen in recent years about providing adequate stimulation to young infants to help them maximize their potentials at an early age. Detailed manuals have been written for both profession-

als and parents on activities and stimuli that will facilitate the development of the growing infant. Most of the programs are highly geared to (1) increasing sensory stimuli through the provision of appropriate toys, and (2) facilitating neuromuscular development through active and passive physical exercises that are specifically geared to the infant's skill level.

Many parents and some professionals hope that early stimulation of this type will increase the child's adaptive and cognitive functioning levels. Current evidence indicates that well-planned and well-executed programs do accelerate development during the first year. However, developmental differences in stimulated versus nonstimulated infants tend to disappear by 3 years of age, unless the mother is actively involved and

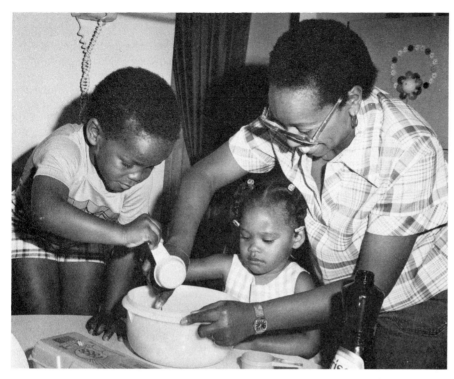

Figure 14-9. First-hand experiences help the child to build up a repertoire of knowledge that serves as a foundation for concepts taught at school.

enrichment activities are continued. The significant effect may lie in Seligman's theory. If the child learns early to master the environment, this sense of control may increase the child's resiliency when minor setbacks or frustrations occur. The increased motivation that accompanies mastery may help the child to persist at a task longer until a new skill is mastered. The child's attitude toward the environment and learning may make a significant difference in achievement.

It should be noted that sensory stimuli and physical exercises are not really the critical factors in infant stimulation programs. As stated before, the critical factor is the synchrony of communication established between the parent and the child. If interaction is asynchronous, then extra stimuli and physical exercises still may not prevent the helplessness syndrome. However, most parents who attend infant stimulation classes and participate in the suggested activities also begin to assess the infant's skill level and communication style fairly realistically in order to individualize their approach and establish a mutually satisfying relationship. Synchronized infant stimulation can maximize developmental potentials and prevent develop-

ment of the helplessness syndrome, which may be more devastating to functional independence than actual retardation [39].

Role of the Parents

Parents are the most significant persons in the developing child's life. They structure and organize the environment, establish the contingencies, and offer the opportunities for development. Parents also serve as role models. The young child is frequently compared to a videotape—recording all that is seen, heard, and felt about the environment. Observed behaviors are emulated in later episodes, either in play or in work. Parents who provide encouragement and foster closeness, perseverance, mastery, and independence have children with functionally higher intelligences [6].

READING READINESS

Parents can help to prepare children for reading activities. The most basic activity is to provide them with a wide variety of experiences that will increase their general knowledge about the world. The more concrete, first-hand experiences children have the greater the number of schemata they will have to draw upon for both verbalization activities and reading. New experiences are easier to assimilate and accommodate if a closely related schema is already present in the child's cognitive structures. The more first-hand experiences children have had, the more indexes they will be able to call upon and to use in more abstract or representational thought processes (see Chaps. 8 and 11). The child needs opportunities for both large and small motor activity: Running, climbing, throwing, working with clay, building with blocks, coloring, and constructing puzzles all give the child an opportunity to see what his or her own body can do and to gain a sense of independence and satisfaction in mastery.

Reading readiness starts with simple verbal synchrony games with the infant. The reciprocal cooing and babbling is the very beginning of identifying cause-effect relationships. Word-object relationship comprehension can be facilitated by presenting the word and object together and restricting the name used to one word; "pocket-book," for instance, may also be handbag, clutch, wallet, or purse. Multiple names should not be used until the first is clearly associated with the object; then a second term should be added in tandem to the first until both are associated with the object.

Communication efforts gradually become more sophisticated and may include simple nursery rhymes and stories with frequent repetition of phrases, such as "The Three Little Pigs" or "The Three Bears." Very young children love these stories because they can predict what will come next. Brief pauses before key words or sentences encourage the child to participate in telling the story. Songs are usually next in the hierarchy of skills and can be performed entirely by the child. Picture books and short stories that can be read aloud or "self-told" also help to prepare the child for reading. The child is becoming interested in what books have to share. Some educators encourage parents of preschoolers to have the children draw pictures and make up their own stories about these pictures; the parent can write the words on each picture and then tie them together as a book. This technique gives the child the idea that what one experiences or thinks can be put into words and shared, and that words in turn can be put into signs and shared again. Written signs begin to have meaning as a form of communication [11]. This activity also helps to encourage the child's growing need for initiative. Sharing, listening, discussing, and experiencing are all significant factors in preparation for reading.

Adequate opportunity for activities that allow dramatic play is also a prerequisite for reading readiness [35]. Through dramatic play, the child is able to use representational thought and to explore alternatives for symbol usage or problem solving. Exposure to educational television is also a very valuable preparatory activity. However, teachers report that children who watch too much television may be bored by school; the child may feel a need to be entertained rather than to participate in activities. This passive approach to life may also be due to lack of adequate opportunity for dramatic and sociodramatic play if television absorbs too much of the waking time activity.

Parents frequently ask whether or not the child should be taught to read before starting school. There are many opinions on each side. The most important factor is the child's attitude toward reading. If the child really wants to learn to read and is already beginning to pick up some words, then the opportunity should not be denied. However, a child should not be forced to learn to read before school or belittled when errors are made. All teaching should be done in a warm, supportive environment. Those children who do know how to read may create some difficulty in the classroom if they feel the skill makes them superior to the other children. The child who reads early should be treated as if this skill were a natural event. The teacher can give the child extra reading and can either concentrate on other activities in which the child may be less skilled or have the child read to other children.

DISCIPLINE

Although an entire chapter is devoted to discipline (see Chap. 18), a brief discussion is in order here because of teachers' concerns. It was mentioned earlier that children need to respect, but not fear, authority; this means, in part, that the child knows the meaning of "No." Unfortunately, many children of permissive or inconsistent parents have not learned the meaning of "No" prior to first grade, so that school becomes more difficult for both the child and the teacher.

Children also need to know how to assume responsibility, which calls for a measure of self-discipline. If the child has not learned how to follow through with responsibilities at home, this will often carry over into the school setting and affect the ability to function independently. The child's lack of self-confidence prevents him or her from working by and for the self. White [40] and Seligman [33] both offer the idea that parents need to provide resolvable frustration and conflict experiences for the developing child. Such experiences help the child to gradually learn to cope with anxiety and frustrations with an increased sense of effectiveness and self-discipline.

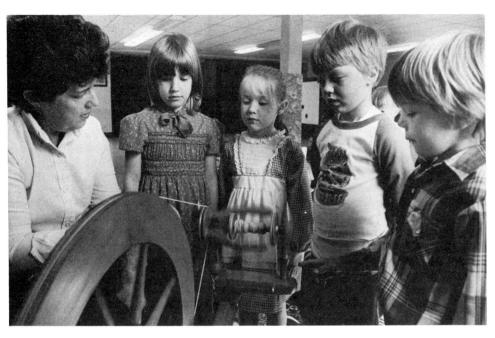

Figure 14–10. Young children enjoy learning about their heritage and the crafts or skills of their forebears.

Nursery Schools

Many parents choose to send their 3- to 5-year-old children to nursery school. Nursery schools usually meet for 2 to 3 hours three to five times a week. They supplement, but do not replace, the home. The major goal of such schools is to offer children peer experiences in order to help them learn to share attention. Exposure to peers offers opportunity for sociodramatic play, competition, comparison, and cooperation, all of which are essential to development. Nursery school also allows the child to relate to someone besides the parents—an aid to the separation-individuation process and to the resolution of Erikson's task of autonomy.

Head Start Programs

In the early 1960s, the United States government recognized that children who grow up in Level I and Level II families (very disorganized, helpless families; see Chap. 34) tend to do poorly in school. This finding has been supported by Krown's and Smilansky's research, and Seligman's theory of learned helplessness now helps to explain this phenomenon. Parents who experience the helplessness syndrome transmit the same attitude to their children by a lack of responsiveness to their children's behaviors: They mutually extinguish

one another's proactive behaviors. Although the parents may be concerned about their children's welfare and may display affection toward them, the attitude of hopelessness toward life's events fosters detachment from the environment, which in turn decreases attentiveness and learning. The children enter school with a weak general knowledge and are unprepared to master either the internal or external environments. Regardless of background, children start school expecting to get good grades. This may be the first time the children have been placed in a competitive situation with peers. When the expectations are not matched and they once again feel out of control, the self-preservation response is to discredit the grades [7]. A pattern of failure is established, and the cycles of helplessness and poverty are perpetuated for another generation.

Project Head Start, a federally sponsored preschool educational program for children 3 to 5 years of age, was started in 1965 as a massive social experiment to break the cycle of poverty. The program is jointly funded by federal and local sources. Services are offered to children free of charge. The major goal is to help each enrolled child to develop a good self-image in order to give him or her the ego-strength to face school tasks successfully. Although Project Head Start served over 7.5 million children and their families during the first 15 years, this represents approximately only 20 percent of those who were eligible [14].

COMPONENTS OF HEAD START PROGRAMS

Although the curriculum of Head Start programs has become more structured since its inception, the basic components have remained unchanged.

Health. Children who are reared in poverty frequently experience suboptimal health status because of inadequate money to provide care and proper nutrition or because of the helplessness syndrome, which prevents the parents from seeking care and providing proper nutrition even if money is available. Recognizing that poor health can interfere with learning, the program provides a complete medical examination to every child. The medical checkup is frequently the first one the child has had since discharge from the hospital as a neonate, even though free child health clinics are available in the community. Each child is given visual and hearing tests and dental examinations. Follow-up services are offered in the form of immunizations and referrals when needed.

Nutrition. The hungry child cannot learn; low energy reserves prevent participation in physical activities and shorten the attention span for other activities. The half-day program provides one snack and one hot meal per day. Many programs also offer the parents an opportunity to learn how to prepare well-balanced meals.

Education. The educational component is structured (1) to introduce the child to her- or himself, and (2) to introduce the child to the surrounding world. Individualized guidance and group experiences encourage the child to learn how to control and to use physical and social skills adaptively. Self-reliance, self-confidence, and self-esteem are fostered through experiences with toys, games, and special equipment. Teachers help each child to identify, to label, and to express in a socially acceptable way the feelings evoked by experiences. Special visitors, field trips, and special activities at the school encourage the children to expand their general knowledge.

Parent Involvement. The planners of Head Start recognized that they could not help the child in isolation from the family; therefore, all programs are required to involve parents in the planning and the operation of the centers. Parents are offered the opportunity to serve in nonprofessional positions (both paid and volunteer) and are welcomed into the classroom at all times. They are encouraged to share goals for their child and to observe what children can do. Classes are provided for parents in areas, such as food purchase and preparation, child care, child development, home improvement, language arts, and first aid. Since each Head Start center is autonomous, the local policy council can determine the programs that best meet the needs of its families.

Social Services. Because of the number of families functioning at Level I and Level II, Head Start provides

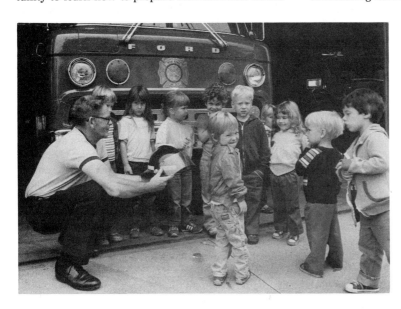

Figure 14–11. Preschoolers are introduced to community helpers, such as firefighters or police officers, in order to help them understand the protective, cooperative role of local agencies.

referral and counseling services as needed. They assist trouble-ridden families to obtain services, such as housing, financial assistance through ADC (Aid to Dependent Children), clothing, medical care, counseling, education, and food stamps from local agencies.

Curriculum. Each Head Start center is free to develop and to implement its own curriculum. Consequently, there is a wide range in the scope and the depth of programs offered. Schools are encouraged to individualize the program to the needs of the community while fostering the development of the gross-motor, fine-motor, self-help, language, cognitive, and social skills of the individual child. Staff members are provided with preservice and inservice training that helps them to understand child development and to learn how to develop effective classroom strategies for groups or individual children. Since approximately 10 percent of enrollment opportunities are reserved for educationally/physically handicapped children, classes and assistance are also offered in individualized program planning and implementation.

Although each center's curriculum varies slightly from the next, some common components can be identified. Language skills are encouraged through listening activities with records and at story time and through expression with puppets, flannel boards, books, and the relating of events. Curiosity is stimulated through questions and simple experiments. Gross- and fine-motor activities are encouraged to refine physical skills. Children also learn to assume and to share responsibilities through cleanup activities, care of toys, and serving food. A major component of the program is to recognize and express inner feelings appropriately; this is encouraged through social modeling, painting, and singing as well as dramatic play with dolls, blocks, kitchen equipment, and dress-up clothes. Children are encouraged to empathize and sympathize with others. All children are offered an opportunity to develop the cognitive skills involved in differentiation and classification. Older children are assisted in learning the alphabet and number concepts.

Although the program usually matches the academic year provided by the local school district, some centers also offer an 8-week summer program for children starting school in the fall.

Studies indicate a "consistently favorable impact on the lives of the children and their families who participate in well-designed early intervention programs" [4]. The greatest success is realized when parents are actively involved in the child's education. Although IQ scores are increased [23], the major change appears to be one of motivation [41]. The children exhibit higher self-esteem, and there is an increase in the vocational aspirations of the mothers for their child [20]. Reading [31, 32] and math [20] skills are higher during the primary grades, children are more likely to be promoted with their age-peers [20], fewer are placed in special educational classes, and a larger percentage are graduating from high school [8]. Since poor school performance is correlated with adult crime and welfare dependence, this prophylactic approach is considered to be cost-effective [8, 32]. It appears that early success in mastering the environment can serve to immunize the individual against helplessness later in life.

Television

Studies show that by the time most children enter school, they may have spent more than 4000 hours watching television—more hours than they will spend attending the first six grades of elementary school [34]. "Television impedes children's normal development by giving them no chance to respond actively and creatively to the stimuli imposed on them, no opportunity to exercise their imaginations, think their own thoughts, or play their own games" [25]. The active manipulation of, and experimentation with, materials and the repetition of experiences and stimuli that are presented at the child's pace are essential for children to make the transformations in cognitive structures and to coordinate sensory input. Children with inadequate "hands-on" experiences may thus demonstrate difficulty with eye-hand coordination, perceptual integration, problem-solving skills, and other reading readiness skills. These children may establish a passive-onlooker rather than active-participant mentality.

Commercial television programs are designed to sell the sponsors' products; they are not designed to provide education. The vast majority of commercial television programs have little or no real educational value; what is learned is only incidental. The television programmer's first allegiance is to the commercial producer who is paying to have the product advertised; faithfulness to reality and truthfulness in presenting real-life situations and solutions are low on the list of the programmer's priorities. Older and more mature viewers are able to discern what is true to life and what is not, but young children cannot do this. Their limited cognitive skills and their inexperience in separating fact from fantasy can lead them to accept as reality whatever they see on television.

Dramatic programs present the problem, the possible answers, and a final solution in less than 1 hour. This type of presentation may condition young viewers in the belief that any problem, regardless of how big or how serious, can be worked through to a solution in a very short span of time—a simplistic way of thinking.

Common stereotypes are perpetuated on television. The white American male is the most visible figure; he is usually young, middle-class, and unmarried. Nurses are frequently shown as cold, impersonal, and totally dominated by the male doctors with whom they work; librarians are seen as quiet, unmarried women; policemen are shown as clever and unfeeling; husbands and fathers are often seen as weak and insecure. The presentation of relationships between men and women is superficial and exaggerated. Sex between unmarried adults is portrayed as a positive and expected part of all male-female relationships. Even crime may be glorified. Children want and need to know about normal, healthy patterns of adult relationships.

Children's cartoons depend on brief, episodic scenes and fast-paced action for their popularity. Children are led to believe that violence is to be laughed at and not to be taken seriously, that it is better to be sadistically clever than to be sensitive or compassionate. The television presentation of violence and its consequences has very little relation to the cause-effect relationships experienced in the real world. Educators and many other adults are concerned about the amount of sex and violence that children see on television. Many investigators believe that watching violence and crime on television tends to blunt the child's sensitivities to suffering and injustice in real life. In 1972 Surgeon General Steinfeld stated before a Senate hearing that "my interpretation is that there is a causative relationship between televised violence and subsequent antisocial behavior, and that the evidence is strong enough that it requires some action on the part of responsible authorities, the television industry, the government, and the citizens" [38]. Several court cases in the late 1970s involved the effect of television on eliciting juvenile crime or offering models for it.

As educators became aware of the potential positive uses of television as well as its negative aspects, they began to consider production of television programs specifically for the education of younger viewers. Educators were also concerned about helping the culturally or socially disadvantaged child to be more successful when he or she enters the educational system. In response to this need, the Children's Television Workshop was created in 1968 to produce a series of daily, hour-long television programs that would provide a useful preschool educational experience for 3- to 5-year-old children, paying special attention to the needs of disadvantaged urban children [12]. The program produced in this experiment in educational television is "Sesame Street." Since it was already known that young children enjoy the style of television commercials, the program was patterned in this manner; that is, the scenes were brief, lively, and to the point.

The major behavioral goals of "Sesame Street" are to promote the intellectual, social, and cultural growth of preschool and kindergarten children. This includes an understanding of (1) symbolic representation (letters, numbers, geometric forms); (2) cognitive organization (perceptual discrimination and organization, relational concepts, classification); (3) reasoning and problem solving (problem sensitivity and attitudes toward inquiry, inferences and causality, generating and evaluating explanations and solutions); and (4) children and their world (self, social units, social interactions, the human-made environment, and the natural environment) [12].

A study of children who had viewed "Sesame Street" for 1 year indicated that these children were more familiar with numbers than with letters. More than one-half of the 4-year-old children showed receptive comprehension of the numbers 1 through 5 as well as the ability to name numerals on presentation. In addition, many children were able to count out objects when the amount totaled less than 5 [28].

The goals of "Sesame Street" have been expanded to include sight vocabulary, addition, subtraction, multiplication, and division. With these additions, the program endeavors to teach basic facts, problem solving, and relationships that lay a foundation for the development of concrete operational cognitive skills [2]. Children who view "Sesame Street" for more than 1 year do not appear to be significantly improved in school readiness, since the programs are repetitious [12].

"Sesame Street" also helps to reduce cultural and racial prejudices because it includes Spanish- as well as English-language episodes. It helps children to see that others can be different from them and their families but can still be OK people.

Children usually are not tested on what they see and learn through television, but parents and teachers are aware that today's children know more about the world outside of their immediate community than their parents did at the same age. Television has a great potential for educating children, but most of the programs that are broadcast for, and viewed by, children today are of entertainment value only. Parental guidance and concern for what children are watching and discussions of programs with children help to explain or to reinforce any television message [5]. The parents' group, Action for Children's Television (ACT), is trying to improve the quality of the programs available for children.

Kindergarten

Kindergarten is required in many states and is optional in others. Although children are taught the basic academic skills mentioned earlier in the chapter, the major goals are to help them learn how to cooperate with peers, to develop good work habits, and to like school. Kindergarten helps the child to develop listening skills, to play and to work independently, and to refine gross- and fine-motor skills. Most teachers feel that kindergarten is essential preparation for a successful first-grade experience. Children's perceptual, motor, and language development should be assessed during kindergarten to determine readiness for first grade. Those who exhibit maturational lags should be offered a "transitional class" program, which can match the educational approach and content to the specific needs of the child. Such extra help for a few weeks to a full year can help the child get off to a good educational start and can avert the need for remedial measures later as well as the emotional frustrations that accompany repeated failure [10]. In 1802 Johann Pestalozzi astutely observed, "Thus, to instruct men is nothing more than to help human nature to develop in its own way, and the art of instruction depends primarily on harmonizing our messages and the demands we make upon the child with his powers at the moment" [24].

SUMMARY

Preparation for school begins with the earliest interactions between parent and neonate. The early establishment of synchronized interaction lays the foundation for cognitive and social structuring. The child who is not offered a synchronized or contingently responsive environment does not learn how to predict and then to control, or to master, the environment—a situation that leads to learned helplessness. Children who feel that behaviors and responses are unrelated are not motivated to learn cause-effect relationships; they begin to withdraw cognitive and affectional investment in both people and the external environment. Although intellectual potential is not decreased, marked retardation may be observed in cognitive, affective, social, and physical adaptation. Prematurely born children frequently exhibit affective, perceptual, and motor delays in kindergarten [10].

These may be due to inadequate synchronized stimulation in early infancy, neurological immaturity, minimal brain damage, or to another, as yet unknown, factor.

Infant stimulation programs need to concentrate on the significance of timing and the intensity of interaction as well as appropriate sensory input and physical exercise. Nursery schools can supplement the developmental opportunities offered at home. Head Start offers intensive remedial and supportive services both to the child and to the family, helping them to realize and to actualize their potentials. Kindergarten helps children to prepare academically and socially for first grade.

Although many resources are available to assist in the preparation of a child for school, the single most critical factor, in the author's opinion, is the interaction between the parent and the child. This point should be emphasized in parent education classes and in high school classes on preparation for family living. Parenthood is an awesome but exciting opportunity for the sensitive, prepared adult.

REFERENCES

1. Bell, S. M., and Ainsworth, M. D. S. Infant crying and maternal responsiveness. *Child Dev.* 43:1171, 1972.
2. Bogatz, G. A., and Ball, S. Some things you've wanted to know about "Sesame Street." *Education* 7(3):11, 1971.
3. Brazelton, T. B., Koslowski, B., and Main, M. The Origins of Reciprocity: The Early Mother-Infant Interaction. In M. Lewis and L. A. Rosenblum (Eds.), *The Effect of the Infant on Its Caregiver.* New York: Wiley, 1974.
4. Calhoun, J. A., and Collins, R. C. A positive view of programs for early childhood education. *Theory Into Practice* (Spring 1981) 20:135.
5. Charren, P., and Sandler, M. Is T.V. turning off our children? *Redbook* (October 1982): 68.
6. Cohler, B. J., et al. Child-care attitudes and development of young children of mentally ill and well mothers. *Psychol. Rep.* 46:31, 1980.
7. Coleman, J. J., et al. *Equality of Educational Opportunity.* Washington, D.C.: U.S. Government Printing Office, 1966.
8. Comptroller General of the United States. *Early Childhood and Family Development Programs Improve the Quality of Life for Low-Income Families* (HRD-79-40). Washington, D.C.: U.S. Government Printing Office, 1979.
9. Consortium for Longitudinal Studies. *Lasting Effects After Preschool, Summary Report.* A report by the central staff of the Consortium for Longitudinal Studies under the supervision of Irving Lazar and Richard Darlington (DHEW Publication No. (OHDS) 80-30179. October, 1979). Washington, D.C.: U.S. Government Printing Office, 1979.
10. de Hirsch, K., Jansky, J. J., and Langford, W. S. *Predicting*

Reading Failure: A Preliminary Study of Reading, Writing, and Spelling Disabilities in Preschool Children. New York: Harper & Row, 1966.

11. Francis, M. Getting ready to read. *American Baby* 36(8):10, 1974.

12. Gibbon, S. Y., Jr., and Palmer, E. L. *Pre-Reading on Sesame Street. Final Report, Volume V of V Volumes.* New York: Children's Television Workshop, 1970.

13. Hauser, S. T., and Kasendorf, E. *Black and White Identity Formation: Studies of the Psychosocial Development of Lower Socioeconomic Class Adolescent Boys* (2nd ed.). Malabar, FL: Krieger, 1983.

14. *Head Start in the 1980's: Review and Recommendations.* U.S. Department of Health and Human Services. Office of Human Development Services. Administration for Children, Youth and Families. Head Start Bureau (HHS-393). Washington, D.C., Sept. 1980.

15. Hunt, J. M. The psychological development of orphanage reared infants: Interventions with outcomes (Teheran). *Genet. Psychol. Monogr.* 94:177, 1976.

16. Intelligence: Genes or environment? *Intellect* 103:422, 1975.

17. Kennell, J., et al. Maternal behavior one year after early and extended post-partum contact. *Dev. Med. Child Neurol.* 16:172, 1974.

18. Klaus, M., et al. Maternal attachment: The importance of the first post-partum days. *N. Engl. J. Med.* 286:460, 1972.

19. Krown, S. *Three and Fours Go to School.* Englewood Cliffs, NJ: Prentice-Hall, 1974.

20. Lazar, I., and Darlington, R. Lasting effects of early education: A report from The Consortium for Longitudinal Studies. *Monographs of the Society for Research in Child Development* 47(2–3, Serial No. 195), 1982.

21. Mahler, M. S., Pine, F., and Bergman, A. *The Psychological Birth of the Human Infant: Symbiosis and Individuation.* New York: Basic Books, 1975.

22. Mondell, S., and Tyler, F. B. Parental competence and styles of problem-solving/play behavior with children. *Dev. Psychol.* 17:73, 1981.

23. Palmer, F. H., and Anderson, L. W. Long-Term Gains from Early Intervention: Findings from Longitudinal Studies. In E. Zigler and J. Valentine (Eds.), *Project Head Start: A Legacy of the War on Poverty.* New York: Free Press, 1979.

24. Pestalozzi, J. H. *Education of Man, Aphorisms.* New York: Greenwood Press, 1969.

25. Piers, M. W., and Landau, G. M. *The Gift of Play: And Why Young Children Cannot Thrive Without It.* New York: Walker, 1980.

26. Pines, M. A child's mind is shaped before age 2. *Life* 71(25):63, 1971.

27. Pines, M. Head start in the nursery. *Psychology Today* 13(4):56, 1979.

28. Reeves, B. F. *The First Year of Sesame Street: The Formative Research, Final Report, Volume II of V Volumes.* New York: Children's Television Workshop, 1970.

29. Ringler, N. M., et al. Mother-to-child speech at 2 years—Effect of early postnatal contact. *J. Pediatr.* 86(1): 141, 1975.

30. Ringler, N. M., Trause, M. A., and Klaus, M. Mother's speech to her two-year-old: Its effect on speech and language comprehension at 5 years. *Pediatr. Res.* 10:307, 1976.

31. Rosenberg, L. A., and Adcock, E. P. *The Effectiveness of Early Childhood Education: Third Grade Reading Level Interim Report, Dec. 1979, ESEA Title IV C Longitudinal Evaluation Program for Selected Early Childhood Education Programs.* Maryland State Department of Education, 1979.

32. Schweinhart, L. J., and Weikart, D. P. *Young Children Grow Up: The Effects of the Perry Preschool Program on Youths Through Age 15.* Ypsilanti, MI: High/Scope Press, 1980.

33. Seligman, M. E. P. *Helplessness: On Depression, Development, and Death.* San Francisco: Freeman, 1975.

34. Sesame Street asks: Can television really teach? *Nation's Schools* 85:58, 1970.

35. Smilansky, S. *The Effects of Sociodramatic Play on Disadvantaged Preschool Children.* New York: Wiley, 1968.

36. Stern, D. Rhythms of Maternal Behavior During Play. In E. B. Thoman and S. Trotter (Eds.), *Social Responsiveness of Infants.* New Brunswick, NJ: Johnson & Johnson Baby Products, 1978.

37. Thoman, E. B., Korner, A. F., and Beason-Williams, L. Modification of the responsiveness to maternal vocalization in the neonate. *Child Dev.* 48:563, 1977.

38. U.S. Congress, Senate. *Hearings before the Subcommittee on Communications of the Committee on Commerce.* Washington, D.C., March 1972.

39. Weisz, J. R. Learned helplessness in black and white children identified by their schools as retarded and nonretarded: Performance deterioration in response to failure. *Dev. Psychol.* 17:499, 1981.

40. White, B. L. *The First 3 Years of Life.* Englewood Cliffs, NJ: Prentice-Hall, 1975.

41. Zigler, E., et al. Is an intervention program necessary in order to improve economically disadvantaged children's I.Q. scores? *Child Dev.* 53:340, 1982.

15

Developmental Concepts of Play

Clara S. Schuster

Children who play life discern its true law and relations more clearly than men.

—Henry David Thoreau

Introduction

Theories of Play
Play versus work
Definitions

Function of Play
Enculturation
Effect of play on the development of the
individual

Classifications of Play
Themes of play
Content of play
Structure of play

Factors Affecting the Quality and Quantity of Play
Parent-child interaction
Other cultural influences

Maximizing Individual Potentials Through Play
Preparation for school
Preparation for adult responsibilities
Maintenance of mental health
Parent teaching
Adult play

Summary

Although play is an essential element in the development of healthy individuals, it is a highly abstract, elusive concept. Defining play presents an enigma to the psychologist or educator; while each of us intuitively knows what play is (or is not)—at least for ourselves—a precise definition is virtually impossible. Even Webster's unabridged dictionary, after two full columns of fine print, is forced to reduce the definition of "play" to a series of synonyms rather than a precise, observable, measurable definition. The only common element to be found among the various attempts to define this construct is that play is an activity voluntarily engaged in for pleasure.

Theorists offer differing views on the significance of play. In 1795, Schiller defined play as a form of art because of its creative, imaginative quality [26]. Herbert Spencer believed that play serves merely to drain off surplus energy. Spencer, who did not view play as constructive, could not explain why a child continues to play even though he or she is exhausted. Stanley Hall looked on human play as a recapitulation of the activities of ancestral primates, since the sensorimotor play of very young human infants does have elements in common with the play of higher-order mammals [15]. However, as children grow and develop, their play activities far surpass those of animals. In 1915, Karl Groos proposed that play provides early training for adult life. However, Groos did not believe play to be a

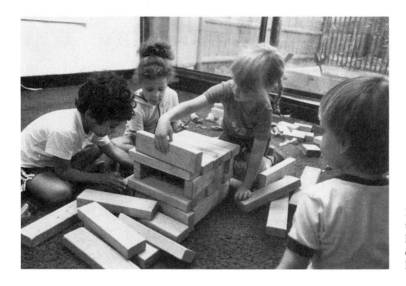

Figure 15–1. Play activities may serve to use up surplus energy. Play also allows a child to repeat a behavior and to experience the joy of mastery, which leads to proficiency.

constructive end in itself but thought that it was merely instinctual, and he did not recognize that a child's level of competence in all four domains affects the type of play in which the child participates [18].

THEORIES OF PLAY

Play Versus Work
To help put play into perspective, one must first look at the differences between the definitions of play and work. It is commonly felt that work is the antithesis of play. However, the same activity can be either work or play, according to the meaning of the activity to the individual; one person's play may be another's work, and vice versa. Tending a garden, sewing, or even engaging in sports may be viewed as being in either category. Harlow speculates that play involves work because it requires both thinking and use of energy. Elizabeth Hurlock and Brian Sutton-Smith propose that when the end takes supremacy over the means, the activity leans toward work, but when the means is more important than the end product, the activity may be categorized as play. Piaget takes issue with this point, indicating that the activity itself may be an end product to the child so engaged, since the same activity may be work at one stage of a person's life and play at another stage.

Learning any new activity, such as riding a bicycle, knitting, reading, pouring from one container to another, or picking up a small object with the pincer grasp, can be either work or play, depending on the individual's stage of development. The learning pro-

cess requires concentrated effort. Once the activity has been learned, the individual tends to repeat it frequently for the pure joy of mastery. It must be kept in mind that both external and internal environmental conditions can change an individual's motivation or ability to participate in a formerly pleasant or play activity, so that the activity may once more become work. Health deterioration, time limitations, or incompatible social or emotional circumstances (e.g., extreme competition) can limit or prevent an activity from being perceived as play per se.

Anna Freud indicates that the ability to work evolves gradually through an individual's developing pleasure in achievement through play activities. Individuals are able to work when the ego acquires the ability to (1) control, inhibit, or modify id impulses; (2) delay gratification; (3) carry out preconceived plans, even when frustrations intervene; (4) neutralize the energy of instinctual drives through sublimated pleasures; and (5) be governed by the reality principle rather than the pleasure principle [6]. Piaget also observed that there is a decrease in play activity as the child "progressively subordinates the ego to reality" [21].

Definitions
The psychoanalytical school, represented here by Anna Freud, Lili Peller, and Erik Erikson, defines play as the attempt of the ego to deal with the pain of reality [20]. Their major attitude toward play appears to be consistent with the basic presupposition of Freudian psychoanalytical theory—that the unattractive id impulses must be socialized and brought under control by the ego. Play serves as the vehicle through which the child

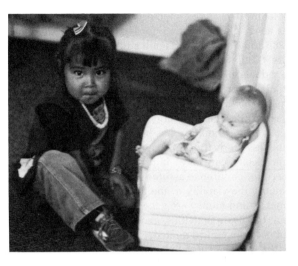

Figure 15–2. Play activities may enable the child to learn to deal with reality and to direct impulses into socially acceptable behaviors. This girl is proud of her "baby's" toilet training success.

learns to deal with the pains caused by frustration of the unexpressed or ungratified id. The fragile ego, as the moderator between the id and society, finds ways to inhibit or sublimate these impulses through voluntary play. Anna Freud suggests that fantasies (pretend play and daydreams) are essential for resolution of anxieties.

Play activities synchronize the bodily impulses with social expectations and experiences, putting the ego in active control of behaviors [4]. These ego expressions are all under the governance of the pleasure principle. When a behavior becomes governed primarily by the reality principle, then the activity is no longer play but work [6]. Peller indicates that play behavior may also be emitted in order to confirm one's control and power over life's experiences, or to repeat a gratifying experience [20]. The ego engages in action that attains or restores a compatible, gratifying balance between self, society, and the requirements of the superego. In succinct form, then, "play is the sublimated expression of the child's various instincts" [26].

Smilansky, with her interest in the sociodramatic play of the preschooler, defines play as "pretended behavior," that is, behavior imitative of life around the child [26].

Hurlock feels that any voluntary activity engaged in for the purpose of enjoyment may be classified as play. Such classification is based on the individual's attitude toward the activity rather than the activity per se. Hurlock recognizes both active and passive expressions of

play, corresponding respectively to neuromuscular versus predominantly cognitive activities [9]. Vicarious experiences, such as reading, watching, television, and attending sports events, would fall into the latter category.

Piaget offers the simplest, most holistic, and yet most complex definition of play. It forms an integral part of his theory of cognitive development. In fact, he states that play and cognitive development are inseparable and include both overt behaviors and daydreams. According to Piaget, the cognitive domain develops through the two processes of assimilation and accommodation (see Appendix B). Assimilation occurs when perception of stimuli is distorted to fit what the individual already knows or can do (schema); accommodation, on the other hand, is imitation of reality or the changing of one's schema or behaviors to adapt to reality. Play, then, is defined quite simply as being pure assimilation—the repetition of a behavior or exercise of a schema solely for the pleasure of feeling virtuosity or power over the skill [21]. With this more narrow definition of play, the accommodation behaviors preceding mastery are classified as work rather than play, even though casual observation may record the same activity. Piaget often used the child's facial expression

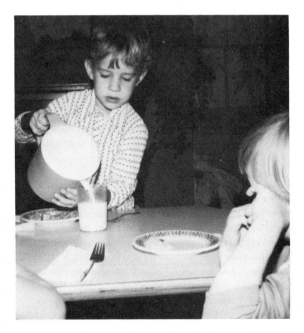

Figure 15–3. The serious face and tense body tone of this boy indicate that he finds pouring milk to be work rather than play. He is still working on mastery rather than proficiency of the skill.

to distinguish when the transformation from work to play occurred: The child still involved with accommodating activity furrowed the forehead and eyebrows and maintained body tension, whereas the child engaged in assimilatory behaviors (ludic behaviors) would smile and have a more relaxed facial and body tension level.

Play in some form occurs throughout the life cycle. This chapter will focus on the play of children; the healthy coping of the individual and adult recreation will be discussed in the chapters dealing with psychosocial development during the adult years.

FUNCTIONS OF PLAY

The functions of play have been hinted at and even stated in the definitions. Because of a particular bias, each theorist views play from a different perspective. However, neither the definitions nor the identified functions of play can be removed from the cultural or subcultural context. The family and educational systems with which the child has the most intimate contact provide the models for behavior, goals and values, tools, time-space perspective, opportunity, reinforcement systems, and so forth.

Enculturation

Culture is transmitted through the imitating and adapting by each succeeding generation of the skills and particular values held by the preceding generation. Play activities allow children to practice the behavior patterns associated with significant roles in their culture and to add their own variations to the scenarios. Games with rules provide socially acceptable "arenas within which to address issues of love and hate (teammates vs. opponents), cooperation and conflict, and symbolically, life and death" [31].

CULTURAL DIFFERENCES
Sutton-Smith has observed that the different types of games engaged in by people are systematically related to cultural variables. Games of strategy appear in cultures that have a hierarchical structure, that emphasize diplomacy, or that engage in warfare. When survival conditions are tenuous, games of chance are more pronounced. Industrialized societies stress product-oriented play. American culture is designated a capitalistic society; perhaps our enjoyment of "Monopoly" and "Trivial Pursuit" supports Sutton-Smith's theory that "the primary function of play is the enjoyment of a commitment to one's own experience" [27].

Cultural systems that include parents who are "adult-

oriented," or "work ethic-oriented," usually view play as being a waste of time for both children and adults [28]. Some examples of adult attitudes in such societies are, "Children are to be seen and not heard," and "Individuals must prove their worth through a productive contribution to society." Children are given substantial responsibility early in life, even during the preschool years; little time or energy is left for active play.

As Western culture has become more technological and less product-oriented and as the standard of living and health care have improved, there has been less need for children to assume a responsible role in maintaining the viability of the family system. More time, energy, and money are generally available for the pursuit of leisure activities, and parents have time to become more child-oriented.

Many researchers have noted that socially deprived children do not follow the same developmental play patterns as more privileged children. Lacking reinforcement for spontaneous play activity in the home setting, these deprived children may actually need to be taught how to play [12, 19, 28, 30, 34]. In the same sense, the product-oriented parent may be very supportive of academically oriented preschool activities, such as learning to recognize letters and to count, but may only tolerate or may even be resistant to activities such as block play, singing, or dressing up [22, 27]. Professionals intervening in such situations may initially find these children to be either hostile or apathetic toward more creative or structured endeavors, especially when group participation is expected.

ADULT ROLES
The years of childhood are spent in preparation for the years of adulthood. Play, especially in early childhood, is the most significant medium through which the developing child learns to adapt to the realities of life in his or her culture. It was probably someone from a work-ethic framework who coined the phrase, "Play is a child's work"; nevertheless, it is true. Through play, children are afforded the opportunity to explore, to master, and to strengthen competencies in all four domains at their own pace and free from many outside constraints.

Although each theorist views the role of play in the development of the individual from a different perspective, all would agree that a child is not transformed into an adult socially, cognitively, physically, or emotionally by one giant step or with the onset of the eighteenth or twenty-first birthday. Each theorist expresses in some way that play is the medium through which the child learns how to cope with the reality of the culture. Through play activities, the child gradually adopts and adapts to more mature ways of functioning.

The preschool years are seen as being particularly critical in the development of social skills and the preparation for adult roles [22]. Through sociodramatic play (strongest from 3 to 6 years of age) the child "tries on" many hats, acting out both family and career roles. Through play activities that mix both fantasy and reality in the child's own formula, the preschooler is able to enter the exciting world of adults [26].

Effect of Play on the Development of the Individual

Play is both the product and the pattern of humanity's biological heritage and culture-creating capacity [7, 31]. Play specifically aids in the development of all four domains, as discussed in the following sections.

BIOPHYSICAL DEVELOPMENT

Almost every imaginable play activity involves the biophysical domain in some way. Piaget, Freud, Erikson, and many others identify the first signs of play activity as participating in the repetition of pleasurable body movements purely for the joy of repeating an event and for self-control. For instance, sounds are repeated for the auditory feedback, but the child is also learning fine

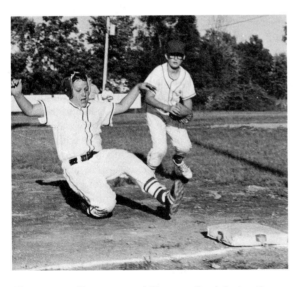

Figure 15–4. Gross-motor skills are refined during the preschool years and strengthened during the school-age years. When combined with the cognitive ability to remember and to use rules, they become the basis of many competitive games.

control of lip, tongue, vocal cord, and diaphragm movements for emission of an exact vibration, pitch, and volume—all precursors to talking.

Play aids in the development of both gross- and fine-motor activity. The coordination and refinement of neuromuscular movements achieved through hitting out at a dangling noisemaker, shaking a crib toy, or repeating a verbal sound after the mother both give pleasure to the baby and make replication of these activities easier at a later date. The joy of gross-motor activity in the infant is obvious. Once the child has learned to perform a physical skill, it will be repeated over and over (to some adults' annoyance) for the joy of mastery until saturation is reached or a new skill emerges for practice. Once crawling, walking, or running has been mastered, there is no backtracking—the child is constantly moving purely for the joy of moving. He or she will run from one spot to another for no other purpose than to run, frequently looking to the significant adult for approval and encouragement at the end of each episode (refueling).

As children continue to learn what their bodies can do through play, they gradually incorporate more and more complicated skills. Children move from scribbling to marking, then to coloring, then to drawing and tracing, and finally to the writing of alphabet letters and numerals. Art forms become more refined and reality-oriented (in some cases) through an increased experience in the use of art materials and the refinement of fine-motor skills.

Gross-motor skills practiced individually during the preschool years become the basis for the group competitive games of the school years, such as tag, Red Rover, baseball, and relay races. Throwing a ball, swimming, and riding a bicycle all involve the same principles of learning body control at a more complex level. The use of the body for progressively more complex activities, such as crawling, running, jumping, climbing, tumbling, and swinging, can eventually lead to extremely refined movement, such as that found in Mary Lou Retton, Peggy Fleming, Doug Flutie, or Rudolf Nureyev. Through play, children learn what the body can do and what they enjoy doing. The degree of refinement of gross-motor skills in the four athletes and dancers mentioned was first identified through play and then maximally refined through concentrated practice (which could be classified as either work or play, depending on the intrinsic meaning to the individual involved). Through play, then, children learn to master a skill, to practice the skill until it becomes a natural part of their repertoire, and then to refine the skill so that it can be used purposefully to accomplish a given goal. Physical activities can also help to use up the excess energy of children, thus freeing their minds to concentrate on academic pursuits. Chemicals and enzymes released during physical activity help to maintain high-level physical, cognitive, and affective wellness.

Although the reader is undoubtedly aware of this phenomenon, it bears repeating at this point that unused muscles will waste (atrophy) and eventually cease to function. Recent emphasis on physical-fitness programs attests to the fact that development of the physical domain through exercise (and play) is a critical national concern. The physical exercise of play can help to maintain high level biophysical functioning and health throughout life.

COGNITIVE DEVELOPMENT
Piaget is very explicit in his viewpoint that play activities are essential to cognitive development. He notes that the type of play activities engaged in are closely related to the child's attained level of cognitive development. Once accommodation of a schema has occurred, further experience with the schema becomes assimilative. Through continued reenactment of the schema—whether motoric, verbal, or symbolic—the event or object can assume new and stable relationships to other schemata. The child learns spatial and temporal relationships, creates classification systems, and develops facility in inductive and deductive reasoning. Through play activities, the child can learn internal manipulation of external objects or events. Play becomes critical in balancing subjective conceptions of reality with the objective quality of reality. Representational thought is enacted through dramatic, symbolic play; one object is used in the place of another. "Pretend" activities strengthen symbolic or representational thinking.

Representational or fantasy play moves through four stages during the preschool years as the pretending gradually becomes less dependent on the immediate stimulation [5]:

1. Reality play. Object is used for intended purpose
2. Object fantasy. Entirely new identity attributed to object
3. Person fantasy. People qualities are actively represented
4. Announced fantasy. Theme is announced before acting out

The child is able to produce novel combinations, to learn to solve problems spontaneously, and to be creatively flexible through play activities [28]. In today's expanding, rapidly changing world, these adaptive skills are highly desirable. Studies show that children with deficient play experiences are not prepared to cope with the demands of a formal academic curriculum and consequently may experience failure despite the concentrated efforts of the teaching staff and the concern of parents [26]. It appears that these children are programmed for failure before they ever start going to school (see Chap. 14). Perceptual skills can be heightened through play. Maria Montessori developed a number of play activities for increasing discrimination skills for all five senses [17].

The value of play in the development of language cannot be overestimated. Once language has been acquired, children can begin to form stable concepts that are shared with others in the culture [26]. Through play, children can test these concepts against those of others—thus organizing their interior language. Through language, children can communicate their needs and reconstruct or create an experience. Play, especially the sociodramatic play of the preschool years, motivates children to organize their thoughts in order to communicate them to others. This type of play also helps to lay the basis for social relationships.

The corrective influence of the concrete experiences offered in play activities leads the child to acquire a broader and more accurate concept of the environment and his or her role in controlling the environment. A young child is often seen repeating an experience in an attempt to comprehend it fully or to establish a cause-effect relationship. Young children will walk alternately on a sidewalk and on grass to test the effect on ease of mobility and balance; they will mix two and then three or more colors of paint to see the result; they will push a bicycle bell with various degrees of strength to assess the effect on tone quality. A child may spend long periods of time grouping and regrouping objects for the pure fun of classification. Table games aid the child in preplanning strategies and their alternatives to achieve a desired end; thus play aids in the development of abstract thought processes. Through play, then, the child's world gradually expands from concrete, self-centered thought and activities to symbolic, object-centered activities and finally to abstract, concept-centered activities. Play helps the child to "comprehend and control the world in which he lives and to distinguish between reality and fantasy" [9].

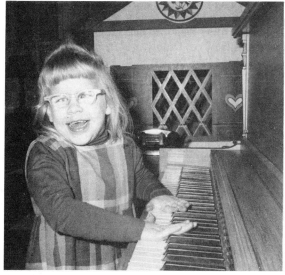

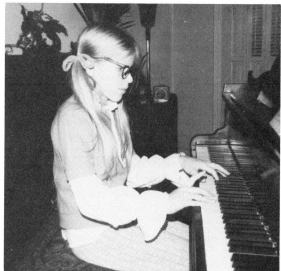

A

B

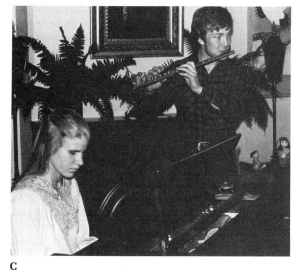

C

Figure 15–5. Imitative play activities (A) gradually become the foundation for systematic work (B). In play, the child assimilates schemata; in work, the child accommodates. (A) During the early years (age 3 years here), the child concentrates on sensorimotor stimuli. (B) In later years (age 11 years here), the child concentrates on cognitive stimulation. Note the marked difference in fine-motor control and facial seriousness. (C) During adolescent and adult years, these skills are further refined and serve as tools for high-level cognitive and social skills.

AFFECTIVE DEVELOPMENT

It is difficult to separate clearly the social and affective domains of development, since they are reflective of each other and are frequently merely expressions of the same phenomenon—the social aspects being external, the emotional ones being internal.

Through play activities, the infant learns to trust both the constancy and the continuity of the external environment (mother, textures, schedules, primitive causal relationships) and the internal environment (awareness of urges, ability to remember and to predict). The consistency and continuity of inner and outer worlds allow the infant to begin to correlate and to predict events, which provides a sense of trust and a rudimentary sense of ego identity [4, 19].

As children mature physically and emotionally, they begin to desire more control over their inner and outer worlds. They begin to experiment with correlations and predictions they have learned to trust. (Can these inner urges and outer events be made to occur at will?) At the same time, social restrictions try to modify some of their experiments. If children are provided with appropriate play materials, they can enjoy autonomy without fear of reprisal or feelings of shame regarding their behavior. Anna Freud observes that the type of play activities that accompanies the toddler period involves actions with play materials that symbolically represent the actions of body cavities, such as filling-emptying, opening-shutting, filling-removing, and messing. Activities involving mobility (e.g., push toys, small cars) and construction-destruction activities (blocks) also allow for symbolic autonomy of action [6]. The child thus learns self-control without loss of self-esteem.

Erikson's stage of initiative versus guilt corresponds to the preschool years (ages 2½ through 5). The play activities of this age enable children to set and to work out goals as they assume various roles. Both Piaget and the theorists of the psychoanalytical school stress the importance of play as an outlet for ego expression. Through play, children can express emotions forbidden in normal social situations without fear of reprisal; they can learn to cope with the environment without repercussions of reality if errors are made. This is especially true of dramatic and sociodramatic play, in which children can reenact events that were confusing or traumatic and can "make" people and events. Peller observes that when children are confronted with a stressful situation in real life, they can use sociodramatic play to (1) change the roles, (2) change the outcome, or (3) become an active rather than a passive participant in the dramas of life [20]. Sociodramatic play allows the child to take the stress in small doses without loss of control or self-esteem.

During play, the child can relive an experience at his or her own pace or change the result to one that can be accepted. The child can also change roles and become the aggressor instead of the aggressed upon or passive observer. The planning of strategies for resolution of the event can help the child to adapt successfully to similar situations in the future. As children gain mastery over different situations, they develop the ego strength and the self-confidence that enable them to participate more freely and fully in real life; thus the ego integrates individual emotionality and social reality through play activities.

Through play activities, the child can learn to control frustrations, which arise when impulsive behaviors or wish fulfillment are blocked (see Spitz-Schuster, Chap. 12). The child who exhibits an arrest or delay in impulse control can be assisted through guided play activities that afford the child the opportunity to gain mastery over the self through gaining mastery over the activity [35]. Ego identity, ego development, and ego strength are thus facilitated through play.

During the school years, the normally developing child begins to become more concerned with reality and a product rather than the expression of physical and social skills for pure pleasure [4]. The focus changes to constructive types of activities, which require more diligence to complete. During this period, one finds children engaging in activities that are halfway between work and play, such as hobbies, competitive sports, and the development of special interests and talents [6]. These "play" activities can lead to a feeling of increased self-esteem and ego identity (or, if success is not achieved or respected, to feelings of inferiority or ego deterioration).

According to Erikson, successful accomplishment of each of these psychosocial stages is essential for the child to emerge from the childhood years with sufficient self-confidence and ego identity to face the responsibilities and social relationships of the adolescent and adult years. Through play, the child learns, experiments with, coordinates, and applies confidently the "rules" of the external and internal worlds. According to Erikson, "Child's play is the infantile form of the human ability to deal with experience by creating model situations and to master reality by experiment and planning" [4].

SOCIAL DEVELOPMENT

Infants and young children are very egocentric; by nature and necessity they are self-centered, or narcissistic. The young child begins life unable to distinguish between self and others [6, 19, 21]. Gradually, through play, the child begins to relate to others—first as an extension of self, then as inanimate objects. Other people are gradually viewed by the child as assistants to aid in completion of a task, and finally they are seen as true and equal partners to be trusted, respected, and afforded human dignities [6]. Through play, then, children learn how to interact with other people; they learn how to get their needs met and how to meet the needs of others; and they learn to find a balance between sharing, giving, and taking.

Parten identifies sequentially emergent degrees of social involvement and awareness as exhibited through the play activities of children 2 to 6 years of age [19]:

1. In **unoccupied behavior,** the child spends time primarily in autostimulatory behavior and restless, ran-

dom movements and activities or wanderings while looking sporadically at others.

2. **Solitary play** is characterized by engrossed, independent play with toys. Minimal attention or regard is given to the proximity or play activities of others.

3. In **onlooker behavior,** the child will closely observe the activities of peers and may even communicate through questions and suggestions with the play participants but will not actively join the activity.

4. Children imitate each other in **parallel play.** Two or more children are seen to play with toys or to engage in activities similar to those of nearby peers. Occasional interaction may occur. Although the children are compatible, they are essentially still in solitary play and are not cooperative in activities.

5. The next level, **associative play,** finds the child still centered on his or her own interests, but within a group. Much borrowing and lending of toys may occur, but no group goals are established.

6. In the final stage, **cooperative play,** highly organized activities are centered around group goals. There are usually one or two leaders.

Through cooperative play activities, the child can learn to cooperate when appropriate, to compete subtly, to sacrifice for peers, to become sensitized to the moods and the feelings of others, to develop friendships, and to control aggression. Through play, then, the autocentric infant gradually develops social competencies that enable him or her to be reciprocally responsive to others in the environment. Flexibility is essential for the establishment of compatible, successful social relationships. Social play activities allow the child to gain this adaptive capacity for varied behaviors [28].

Hurlock and the theorists of the psychoanalytical school feel that children also learn gender-appropriate roles and behaviors in keeping with cultural expectations through play prior to kindergarten. These gender-role behaviors are learned by observation and

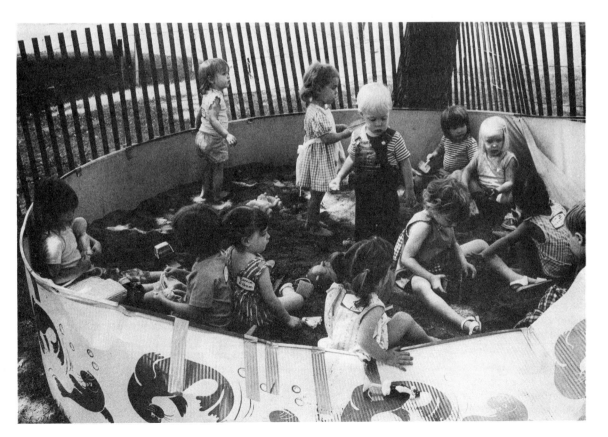

Figure 15–6. Toddlers and preschoolers exhibit many levels of social involvement and awareness through their play activities. How many levels can you identify in this picture?

practice, and through reinforcement. There is evidence that gender differences are observable in play activities as early as the first year of life [9]. However, whether the propensity of boys for gross-motor activity and that of girls for fine-motor activity is biologically or socioculturally determined is a factor not yet clearly established through empirical research. One might theorize that it is a combination of the two—genetic endowment and the unique, subtly influencing quality and quantity of parent-child interaction.

Through play, children gradually develop a sense of moral responsibility, insight into adult roles, and concern for others [4]. They learn to submerge anger and to work cooperatively. Identification with significant adults "permits the dream of early childhood to be attached to the goals of an active adult life" [4]. One reason why young boys may choose strong heroic roles to imitate (fireman, policeman) is because they do not know enough about their own fathers' careers to imitate them in a play setting [22]. Inadequate contact with significant adults may hinder the child's identification with traditional roles or cultural values and the desire to emulate them [14]. Play, then, is the key to successful social adjustments during the childhood years and also serves as a foundation for adult functioning within the culture.

CLASSIFICATIONS OF PLAY

Gender, culture, health, available materials, and environment influence the type of play engaged in by children. Theorists have attempted to identify a core thread that supersedes all of these factors; age is seen as being the most significant factor. By applying a basic theory of play to the activities of children of various ages, each theorist offers a developmental sequencing of play behaviors. The core threads can be further consolidated under theories that emphasize the theme, content, or structure of play. Although approximate ages are shared by some theorists for the emergence and the duration of particular play behaviors, all the ages are flexible and the emergence of play behaviors is heavily influenced by environmental factors.

Themes of Play

Theorists focusing on the theme of play include the three from the psychoanalytical school: Anna Freud, Erikson, and Peller. As mentioned earlier, play serves as a mechanism for the ego to gain mastery over the id and reality. The psychoanalytical school views all behaviors as being libidinal or sexual in origin. The

particular expression of sexuality is sequentially dependent on biological maturity as well as experiences with reality.

THE THEORY OF ANNA FREUD
Anna Freud [6] divides the oral period (birth to 15 months) into three stages. During stage 1, the infant is completely egocentric and views the self as a biological unity with the mother. There is no awareness of separateness. This constitutes a narcissistic milieu (meeting the mother's needs as well as the infant's). Mahler terms this stage autistic. All stimuli are perceived as being a part of, or for, the enhancement of self. Play activities are autoerotic; any activity yielding erotic pleasure is participated in as play. The infant's own body, then, is the focus of play activity. This is evidenced by the infant's obvious fascination with the hands during this stage.

During stage 2 the child begins to distinguish between self and mother or other objects. Mahler states this is a symbiotic (mutually dependent) relationship. Gradually the infant begins to play with the mother's body as if it were a part of the infant's body; but at first there is no distinction between the two (a dual unity).

During stage 3 the infant develops object constancy: when the mother is not seen, she is still remembered. The child will frequently play with, and achieve some comfort in, a soft, cuddly toy as a substitute for play with the mother. This toy may be given the same love as given to the mother in her absence. As mentioned previously, Piaget sees object notion as essential before the bodies of others become realities that children can recognize as being comparable to, but not identical with, their own [21]. Transfer of play behaviors extends to other soft toys. People may also be treated as toys, with pinching, biting, tasting, or pushing behaviors. Mahler theorizes that this stage is significant in the separation-individuation process of the mother-child relationship. Peek-a-boo is a common game that aids the child in the separation process. Since the child often equates food with the mother, feeding play as well as feeding difficulties can give clues to the mother-child relationship [6].

Stage 4 is synonymous with the pre-Oedipal or anal period (16 months through 30 to 36 months) and corresponds to toddlerhood. Cuddly toys begin to disappear except at bedtime, or as transitional objects during separation from mother. Manipulative toys and toys that can be used symbolically to represent body cavities predominate in play activities. Others, especially peers, are still seen as inanimate objects but are gradually incorporated into play activities—if they can help accomplish a task the child wants to accomplish. According to Anna Freud, "Play material serves ego activities and the functions underlying them" [6]. Finger painting has been viewed by those adhering to the psychoanalytical school as a desire to smear one's feces.

Stage 5, corresponding to the phallic period, incorporates the preschool years (2½ to 3 through 5 years of age). This period is also known as the object-centered or Oedipal stage. During this stage, love for self, which had begun to include the mother, now becomes centered on winning the love of the parent of the opposite gender. Play materials and activities come to be used as expressions of libidinal energy or sexuality either in solitary play or for exhibition to the Oedipal object [6]. This orientation combined with greater contact with peers leads to group play in which themes can be expressed through imaginative play. Others become partners in play and can aid in sublimating Oedipal impulses. Gymnastic activities of this period are also viewed as expressions of sexuality (especially masculine) and symbolic enjoyment of phallic activities [6].

Stage 6 includes the primary school years (6 through 10 years) and is referred to as the latency or post-Oedipal period. Children in this stage demonstrate an increased mutual respect toward peers. Sexual drives are latent, with pleasure in finished products taking supremacy over object relations. Play includes hobbies and other constructive behaviors leaning toward work.

Stages 7 and 8, the preadolescent and adolescent years (age 11 and older), include activities that can be defined, according to Freud, more as work than play, even though these activities may be voluntary and occupy leisure time.

To summarize the theories of Anna Freud, play activities are used to transform autoerotic love into constructive work activities through the medium of toys.

THE THEORY OF ERIK ERIKSON

Erik Erikson [4] concentrates more heavily on exploring the sequencing of psychosocial development than the developmental evolution of play. He discusses play as a sequential unfolding of psychosocial relationships.

In stage 1, Erikson's autocosmic stage, infants center on their own bodies. Stage 1 is subdivided into two phases. In phase 1, the self is the center of exploration. Vocalizations are repeated, and the child attempts to repeat or to recapture kinesthetic sensations and sensual perceptions. In phase 2, the exploration extends to other people and objects. The infant's focus is still on sensual pleasure. Different vocalizations and cries may be attempted in order to ascertain the effect on the mother's appearance (perhaps a variation of peek-a-boo, or Freud's stage 3).

In Erikson's stage 2, the microsphere stage (which corresponds to Freud's stage 4), the toddler uses small toys and objects to work out themes. He or she learns to manipulate and to master the world on a micro level.

Gradually the child enters the macrosphere stage of nursery school age (stage 3), in which the world is shared with others. At first other children may be related to as objects, inspected, or even treated as toys, but gradually with time and experience this attitude expands to more cooperative role playing.

To Erikson, play is the vehicle for transforming the egocentric individual into a socialized, other-centered person.

THE THEORY OF LILI PELLER

Lili Peller [20] theorizes that play is instigated by the ego in an attempt to compensate for anxieties and frustrations. She centers her theory on object relationships. Her group I and group II play themes overlap in chronological unfolding, but the focus differs.

In group I play, children are concerned with their bodies, feeling that they cannot control them or perform a desired action. Play enables the child to fantasize and to gain control of desired actions. According

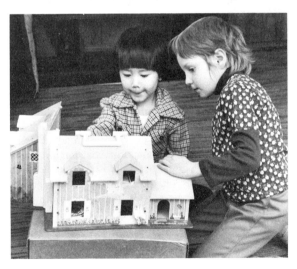

Figure 15–7. Microsphere play activities offer the child the opportunity to manipulate and to master the world on the microlevel. Play therapists frequently use microsphere play as a tool for reaching and understanding the young child and helping him or her to deal with stressors.

to Peller, the child is frequently forced by society to substitute tools and materials for body play or use (such as clay versus feces or shovel in place of hand). Functional pleasure is achieved with increased body skill and mastery of tools.

Group II play behaviors evolve from the child's relationship to the mother and anxiety because of her. Fantasies and games involving control of loss and retrieval aid the child in gaining emotional mastery of the fear of loss. Although other children may occasionally participate in play with the child, the primary focus is toward the mother. Play with dolls is a symbolic exchange of roles between child and mother.

In group III, new anxieties arise in the child with the appearance of the Oedipal period. Children recognize differences between their own world and the adult world and devalue themselves because of this perceived inability to compete for, and win the affection of, the parent of the opposite gender; they fear losing that love. Play, then, serves as a medium for the child to adapt to, and fantasize about, adult roles and relationships. In many homes today, little boys are encouraged to play with dolls in the hope that they will master the tenderness as well as the logistics associated with the mothering role. Colorful, imaginative fantasies emerge as dramatic make-believe play; some complex fantasies require cooperative play with peers who are equally caught up in the drama of their own fantasies.

In Group IV, with entrance to school, the child becomes more reality-oriented and looks to group attachments rather than the Oedipal focus of the previous period. New and intense relationships are formed with peers, including secret clubs. Collecting and hobbies are viewed by Peller as being anal sublimations of a higher order. Group affiliation offers protection from unknown assailants; adherence to group rules, orders, and roles also offers protection against anxieties arising from the superego. Competition exists on an equal footing, in contrast to the previous two levels, where the competition was either unknown or unequally matched. The child learns loyalty to the group through peer relationships.

Peller's view, then, indicates that play activities enable the child gradually to expand relationships and to transfer libidinal energies from self to mother, to other family members, and then to peers—all preparing the way for mature adult relationships in later life.

Content of Play

Some theorists categorize play activities according to the type of activities focused on during each stage of development. These classifications are more descriptive than theoretical, but they can offer some insight into the play behaviors of children.

THEORY OF HURLOCK

Elizabeth Hurlock [9] offers very loose descriptive categories. Stage 1, the **exploratory stage,** is divided into two substages. From birth to 3 months the child explores through the visual mode and through random movements. Once voluntary control of the upper extremities is attained, children are able to coordinate movements for a more thorough exploration of their own bodies and of objects.

Stage 2, the **toy stage,** begins somewhere around 1 year of age and extends into the school-age years, peaking at about 7 to 8 years of age. During the toddler years, the child anthropomorphizes objects with the dramatic use of toys. This dramatic make-believe play will continue into the early school years, peaking around 5½ years of age. Constructive use of toys begins about age 3, with gradually increasing complexity and preplanning of activity that eventually leads to productive constructions through hobbies. Collecting also begins at about 3 years of age; anything and everything is brought home—and forgotten. The child's collections gradually become more refined and discriminating. During the school years, collections can serve as socializing agents and status tokens.

Stage 3, the **play stage** of the school-ager, overlaps stages 2 and 4. Toy play continues here in the more refined form of productive constructions and hobbies. Games with rules and sports replace the spontaneous muscular activity of earlier years. Reading skills learned in school are used for pleasure, especially by bright children.

In stage 4, a decrease in gross-motor activities accompanies the rapid growth and subsequent decline of energy and the increase in body changes accompanying the pubertal period. The **daydreaming** that replaced make-believe play at about 7 years of age now reaches its peak. Daydreaming provides quiet rest for the growing body while allowing integration of past and future, fantasy and reality. Reading becomes a favorite pastime for the same reasons.

According to Hurlock, play allows the child to meet personal needs while adjusting to the demands of the social milieu.

THEORY OF SMILANSKY

Sara Smilansky [26] defines four stages of play, which because of their descriptive nature, may overlap or run parallel to each other or may even continue into adult-

Table 15–1. Evolution of Play Behaviors—Theme of Play

	Birth	4 mo	8 mo	15 mo	2 yr	3 yr	6 yr	7 yr	10 yr	13 yr
Psychoanalytical period	Oral			Anal		Phallic		Latency		Genital
Anna Freud	Stage I: Biological Unity	Stage II: Part Object	Stage III: Object constancy	Stage IV: Pre-Oedipal		Stage V: Oedipal		Stage VI: Post-Oedipal	Stage VII: Pre-adolescent	Stage VIII: Adolescent
Margaret Mahler		Autistic / Symbiotic	Separation-individuation							
	Own body	Mother's body	Toys →			Play with peers →		Work →		
Erik Erikson	Basic trust vs. mistrust			Autonomy vs. shame		Initiative vs. guilt		Industry vs. inferiority		Identity vs. role confusion
	Autocosmic exploration			Microsphere		Macrosphere				
	Self		Others	Small toys		Other people				
Lili Peller	Group 1			Group II		Group III		Group IV		
	Anxieties about body			Fear of maternal loss		Oedipal conflicts		Post-Oedipal play		
	Solitary play			Play with mother, toys		Co-play, shared fantasies		Organized, competitive play, games		Continues into adult years

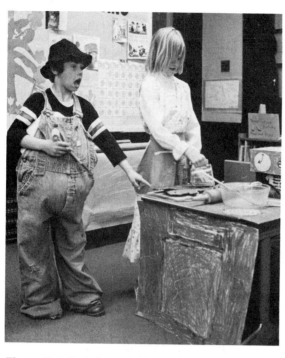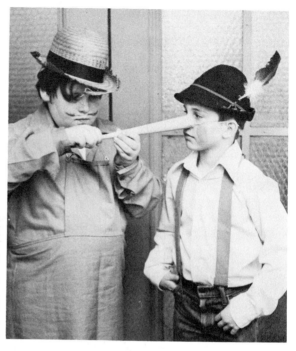

Figure 15–8. Sociodramatic play activities (macrosphere play) carry over to the school-age years but assume a more reality-based, preplanned character.

hood. However, one stage appears to dominate the others at any given point in time. Smilansky's most significant contribution is to the understanding of sociodramatic play.

Functional play includes all simple muscular activities, both behavioral and verbal, that are engaged in for the purpose of manipulation of form. Children try new actions, imitating themselves and others. Play allows them to learn their own physical capabilities, to explore, and to experience the immediate environment.

In **constructive play,** children rejoice in the creation of form. By learning to use materials, they see themselves as the creators of events.

Dramatic play, beginning at about 2 years of age, is symbolic play used to display physical prowess, creative ability, and social skills. By combining reality with magic to fulfill wishes and needs, children are able to connect their own world and the adult world. The two main elements of dramatic play are (1) imitation of an adult (reality), and (2) imaginative or make-believe play (nonreality).

The highest form of dramatic play is **sociodramatic play,** which generally emerges at about 3 years of age.

This voluntary social-play activity involves at least one other child. The target child pretends to be someone else by imitating their speech and actions. This make-believe element of sociodramatic play relies heavily on verbalization and provides for richer reproductions of real life. Words are used to (1) declare a role, (2) identify an object's imaginary identity, (3) substitute for an action, and (4) describe the situation. Thus sociodramatic play encourages verbalization in order to (1) interpret an activity, (2) plan and develop a plot, (3) maintain cooperation, (4) solve problems, and (5) bridge the gap to reality [26].

Sociodramatic play has six elements: (1) imitation of a role, (2) use of make-believe objects, (3) use of make-believe actions and situations, (4) persistence for at least 10 minutes, (5) interaction between two or more children, and (6) use of verbal communication related to the plot. Elements 1 through 4 are components of dramatic play; the addition of 5 and 6 is essential for sociodramatic play. Recent research indicates that participation in sociodramatic play is critical to cognitive development [8, 26].

Smilansky's fourth stage, which begins during the school years and continues through adulthood, involves the playing of **games with rules.** An individual must be able to control behavior, actions, and reactions to participate effectively in group games.

Smilansky's theory states that play activities are essential to adequate preparation for life. If the child does not participate in all levels of play, it will seriously impede his or her social and cognitive development. Sociodramatic play is especially critical to coordinating experiences and forming workable concepts during the preschool years.

THEORY OF SUTTON-SMITH

Brian Sutton-Smith [27, 28] offers a third approach to categorizing play activities according to content. He draws heavily from the theories of others while combining cross-cultural studies to develop his own unique approach to describing play activities. He identifies six major types of play: exploration, self-testing, imitation, construction, contesting, and sociodramatic [28]. He has found the first three types to be universal; the second three, however, are greatly influenced by cultural differences. Since he sees play as the medium through which children gain experience in various behaviors, children may need to be taught how to participate in all six types of play in order to protect them from adaptive deficits in our culture [28].

Sutton-Smith further consolidates his identified types of play into four categories, which overlap heavily. All four types are found concurrently in the 4-year-old child.

Imitative Play. During the first year, the child will repeat what he or she can already do. Perceptual and cognitive skills enable the child to imitate other people during the second year. By 18 months the child may delay the imitation for several hours or days to a time when it is more convenient to repeat a behavior. During the third year, the deferred imitation extends to copying the total person—pretending to be that other person through role playing. During the fourth year, role playing is blended with imagination for imaginative sociodramatic play. Roles and leadership positions are exchanged and shared by the group members.

Exploratory Play. Exploration activities (systematic manipulation of materials for discovery of their sensory value and action potentials) are seen as serious activities for learning. Exploratory play, to observers, may seem to be identical to exploration activities. However, since learning about the object or skill has already transpired, the same activity is engaged in purely for the pleasure of contact with the stimulus.

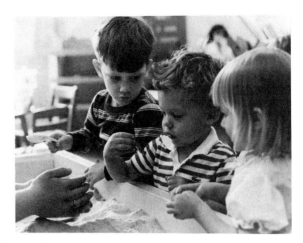

Figure 15–9. Young children must explore the properties and characteristics of materials thoroughly before they can begin to use them constructively.

Attention is focused toward active involvement in the materials or toys and does not degenerate into random, perseverative activity. Exploratory play may begin as early as 6 months, with the tongue and fingers being used as tools. During the second and third years, the activity increases and becomes more complex. Novel verbal combinations used for sound effect and elicitation of responses from others fall under this category. Verbal exploration continues into the school-age years, with jokes, riddles, and exploration of homonyms.

Testing Play. Testing play includes self-assessment of both physical and social prowess. During the second year, children concentrate on large-motor skills. Increased physical skill and social opportunity lead to complex approach-avoidance games during the school years, such as hide and seek, dodge ball, or Space Invaders. Through such activities the child learns and strengthens physical and social skills. He or she increases self-awareness through observation and attention to sensations but also learns to control both memory and impulses.

Model Building Play. Model building play begins at about 4 years of age, with the child imaginatively creating houses, cities, parties, and so on for the purpose of play, often to accompany dramatic or sociodramatic activity. Sutton-Smith comments that observations indicating that today's children spend less time in constructive activities than children of the past may reflect the lack of creative adult examples rather than an increased number of realistic toys [27].

The types of activities that children engage in are unequivocally determined both by innate interests and skills and by environmental opportunities. Sutton-Smith's theory emphasizes that children's participation in play is essential to learning how to enjoy life. "Without the ability to enjoy life, the long years of adulthood can be dull and wearisome" [27].

Structure of Play

A third approach to the categorization of play activities is through the structure of play. Piaget, while recognizing both the themes and the content of play, focuses on the increasing cognitive complexity of play activities beginning with the elementary sensorimotor games and extending to advanced social games [21]. Although there is overlap of these play activities, they are sequentially emergent with very clear delineations between them.

Practice games are the first to appear. They include any skills that are exercised for the pure pleasure of functioning—whether repeating a vowel sound or jumping a narrow stream. These games, described in the outline below, first appear in stage 2 of the sensorimotor level of cognitive development.

1. Pure sensorimotor practice
   a. Mere practice
   b. Fortuitous or "accidentally produced" combinations (includes destruction of object)
   c. Intentional combinations
2. Mental exercise
   a. Mere practice (i.e., "Why?")
   b. Fortuitous combinations (putting words together)
   c. Intentional combinations (making up stories)

Symbolic games first appear in substage 6 of sensorimotor development. The transition from practice games is very subtle, and externally they may appear to be identical. However, in symbolic games the element of make-believe is added. Elements of absent objects or characteristics of objects or persons are represented by distorting reality. The child subjectively links a "signifier" with the "signified" (see Figure 11–2). Thus a small stick may become a car or an old curtain a wedding gown; an empty chair may be inhabited by the Easter Bunny or "whimsy."

As the child engages in more social contacts, the previous two categories can be further combined singly or together into **games with rules.** The content may be identical with the previous stages, but the addition

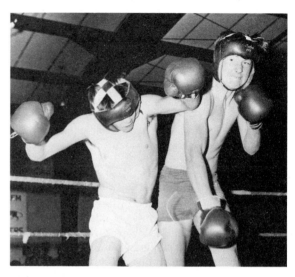

Figure 15–10. Play activities may once more veer toward work activities as children identify and systematically strengthen their physical skills.

of rules complicates mental organization and operations. Games with rules are games with sensorimotor or intellectual combinations in which there is competition between individuals, regulated by either a temporary agreement or a code handed down from earlier generations [21].

A fourth category is identified by Piaget, although he specifies that it does not rightfully occupy its own space. **Constructional games** are found in all three structural types but occupy a position "half-way between play and intelligent work, or between play and imitation" (e.g., hobbies, competition, dramatic presentations) [21].

To Piaget, play and cognitive development are inseparable and interdependent; each supports the growth of the other. Any time a new skill is acquired and the individual practices the skill purely for the sake of practice accompanied by pleasure at mastery, play is the result. Table 15–3 describes Piaget's view of the sequential growth of play activities according to the child's cognitive level of development.

FACTORS AFFECTING THE QUALITY AND QUANTITY OF PLAY

Since play is an essential element in the healthy development of individuals, it is important to look closely at the factors influencing its emergence.

Table 15–2. Evolution of Play Behaviors—Content and Structure of Play

	1 mo	4 mo	8 mo	12 mo	18 mo	2 yr	3 yr	7 yr	11 yr
Elizabeth Hurlock	Exploratory ⟶					Toy	Anthropomorphizing → Dramatic play	Play ⟶ Daydream	
	Random movement	Voluntary						Games ⟶	
	Visual							Sports ⟶	
								Hobbies ⟶	
Sara Smilansky	Functional				Constructive		Dramatic play Symbolic, solitary → Socio-dramatic group	Games with rules ⟶	
Brian Sutton-Smith	Imitative ⟶		Exploratory (physical and verbal)				Dramatic play		
					Testing → Model building			Approach and avoidance games ⟶	
Jean Piaget	Practice games ⟶				Symbolic games ⟶			Games with rules ⟶	
	Stage I 0–1 mo	Stage II 1–4 mo	Stage III 4–8 mo	Stage IV 8–12 mo	Stage V 12–18 mo	Stage VI 18–24 mo	Symbolic games		
							Imaginary friends, symbolic combinations		
	Sensorimotor period 0–2 yr						Preoperational 2–7 yr	Operational 7–11 yr	Formal 11–15 yr

Table 15–3. Piaget's View of the Evolution of Play Activities

Types of Games	Average Age Range	Activities
Practice games		
Substage I Pure reflex adaptations	0–1 mo	No differentiation between assimilation and accommodation. Exercising reflex schemas does not constitute "real play"
Substage II Primary circular reactions	1–4 mo	Slight differentiation between assimilation and accommodation. Repetition of schemata and self-imitation, especially vocal and visual
Substage III Secondary circular reactions	4–8 mo	Differentiation between assimilation and accommodation, both still overlap. Repeating action on things to prolong an interesting spectacle
Substage IV Coordination of secondary schemata	8–12 mo	Clear differentiation between assimilation and accommodation. Application of known schema to new situation. Schemata follow one another without apparent aim. Ritualism of activity for play—the means becomes an end in itself
Substage V Tertiary circular reactions	12–18 mo	Ritualistic repetition of chance schema combinations. Accentuating and elaborating rituals, experimenting to see the result
Substage VI Invention of new means through mental combinations	18–24 mo	Beginning of pretense by application of schema to inadequate object. A symbol is mentally evoked and imitated in make-believe. Reproduction of behavior—primitive symbolic play. Symbolic schema is reproduced outside of context; transition between practice play and symbolic play proper
Symbolic games		
Stage I	2–4 yr	
Type I		Generalizing symbolic schemata (isolated imitations of schemata)
Subtype A		Projection of symbolic schemata onto new objects
Subtype B		Projection of imitative schemata onto new objects
Type II		Symbolic games (assimilation of one schema to another)
Subtype A		Simple identification of one object with another
Subtype B		Identification of the child's body with that of other people or with things
Type III	3–4 yr	Symbolic combinations (construction of whole scenes)
Subtype A		Simple combinations (includes imaginary friends). Reconstruction combined with imaginary elements
Subtype B		Compensatory combinations (materializing fears). Reconstruction with compensatory transpositions
Subtype C		Liquidating combinations (intensifying powers, subordinate threat) in pure reconstruction of situations
Subtype D		Anticipatory symbolic combinations (questioning, orders, and advice). Reproduction of reality with exaggerated anticipation of consequences
Stage II	4–7 yr	Increased orderliness; more exact imitation of reality; use of collective symbolism
Stage III	7–12 yr	Decline in symbolism; rise in games with rules and symbolic constructions
Games with rules		
Stage I	2–4 yr	Rare
Stage II	4–7 yr	Some
Stage III	7–11 yr	Peak
Adulthood		Continue to develop
Constructional games	2 yr–adulthood	Imitation of reality or new combinations. Gradually become more complex and unique to the individual

Parent-Child Interaction

The infant's caretaker, usually the mother, is extremely important in the structuring of an external environment that encourages and facilitates play activities. Such encouragement begins in the minutes and hours after birth as the parent touches, talks to, and looks at the baby. The play activities with the neonate help to alert the infant to the environment and encourage him or her to begin discriminating among stimuli present in the environment [19]. Infants of parents who offer consistent auditory, visual, and tactile contact are able to identify and respond discriminatingly to the mother through voice by 5 days of life, through smell by 7 days of life, and through vision by 2 to 3 weeks of life [1]. The parent who talks to, holds, and rocks the infant will maintain the infant in an alert state (which facilitates visual scanning and learning) for longer periods of time than the infant who receives minimal attention [11]. The cumulative effects of parental attention become clearly distinguishable by the time the child is 10 months old [23]. The author is able to objectively identify differences in quality of parental attention by four weeks of age through assessment with the Brazelton Neonatal Assessment Scale. Infants whose parents have played with them in the course of everyday events (e.g., playing peek-a-boo during diaper changing, or using bath time for water play and retrieval of floating objects) can be objectively identified as being more alert, responsive, and interactive with, and on, the environment.

So significant is play to the very young infant that inadequate play experiences or ineffectual interaction with the parent can lead to physical failure-to-thrive and even to death (see Chap. 9). The dynamics of this phenomenon are unclear; one explanation is that anxiety and stress levels are increased to the point where energies for growth become depleted; anxiety may also decrease the amount of REM sleep during which growth occurs. Here, the social, emotional, and physical domains become closely intertwined in the phenomenon of play. It might be noted that infants with failure-to-thrive syndrome also exhibit cognitive delays.

The interactional framework established with the parents in the early years continues to influence the child's perception of the freedom to explore and to manipulate and the ability to control the environment as well as the child's responsiveness to events and objects. A disorganized home environment is correlated with a decrease in organized, satisfying play activities in preschool children [12, 19, 26, 33]. Sears reports that the degree of maternal warmth, as evidenced through acceptance, nurturance, and supportive responses, is directly related to the child's desire to emulate adult roles through play activities [25]. Smilansky reports that children who fail to participate in sociodramatic play activities (mainly enactment of adult roles) have extreme difficulty with both the social and academic requirements of formal schooling [26]. Schaefer and Bayley coined the word "circumplex" to describe the complex, circular interaction between mother and child that leads to the child's positive or negative adaptational patterns to life. Variances in the child's behaviors do not appear to be related to socioeconomic status but to the interactional framework offered by the parents [24, 30].

Other Cultural Influences

A multistimulatory approach is especially critical during infancy to encourage alertness and responsive interaction with the environment. As children become older, they appear to prefer accoutrements from the adult world instead of specially designed toys. Thus the box and wrappings become more interesting than the doll; kitchen pots and pans hold more interest than the pull toy. Preschoolers and school-agers become even more creative in their imaginative use of raw materials to suit their own ends. Play with these samples of the adult world serves to introduce the child to the tools and equipment of the culture.

Marked cultural differences are found in construction activities, competition games, and the quality and the quantity of sociodramatic play [13, 28]. These play activities are highly dependent on what the caretaker allows or encourages, which in turn is strongly influenced by the values and mores of the given culture.

MAXIMIZING INDIVIDUAL POTENTIALS THROUGH PLAY

Even though each theorist approaches the concept of play differently, certain core ideas begin to emerge. Play activities are unanimously viewed as behaviors engaged in for pleasure. All theorists also acknowledge that play activities prepare children for successful adult living in their culture.

Although Smilansky develops her thesis more extensively than the other theorists around the significance of sociodramatic play, they all acknowledge its value. Piaget and the theorists of the psychoanalytical school—two views of human development that on the surface appear to be most opposed to each other—are amazingly compatible at this point. Piaget expresses the idea that fear can be neutralized through play by "doing in play what one would not dare to do in reality." He states that the function of symbolic play is to assimilate and consolidate the whole of reality to the ego, while "freeing the ego from the demands of accommodation" [21]. The two views are indeed well blended here.

Preparation for School

Unlike other animals, humans rely more on learning than on instincts for survival [14]. Much of the behavior that contributes to our well-being depends on learning.

Smilansky and Krown noted that children who had inadequate play activities during the preschool years experienced difficulty with academic subjects. This difficulty was noted particularly in children who had not participated in sociodramatic play (a symbolic reenactment of adult roles). It appears that this lack of experience in representational thinking, using symbolic processes, hinders the development of the more abstract forms of thought essential to the use of the verbal and written signs of language communication. This would agree with Piaget's ladder of representational thought, which leads from concrete to abstract thought experiences (see Fig. 11–1). Montessori [17], Krown [12], and Weikart [32] all offer preschool curricula that are structured to facilitate cognitive development; structured, guided play activities are the focus of these methods. Through play the child can learn to attend, to discriminate, to manipulate, to classify, and to symbolize—all essential prerequisites for formal schooling.

Preparation for Adult Responsibilities

The sociodramatic play of the preschool years finds children imitating adult roles. Through sociodramatic play, the child can "try on" the role of a parent, a policeman, a paper girl, a television character, or an animal. "What does it 'feel like' to be a. . . . ?" Although many roles may be tried, preschool-age children tend to identify with and thereby emulate the behaviors of adults within the home or the behaviors associated with "what I want to be when I grow up." Identification with and enactment of these behaviors give children a feeling of mastery or power through play [10]. Brian Sutton-Smith observes that even in our "role-enlightened" era, preschool-age children tend to stick to gender role-stereotyped activities during the preschool years.

A most significant ramification of play is its potential for preparation for life, particularly in the present technological world. With the rapidly moving technology of today, the environment—in terms of expectations, resources, numbers of persons one has contact with, skills needed, and so forth—is expanding at an astronomical rate. Toffler states that we are living in a world that is becoming rapidly obsolete—a throwaway society [29]. What the new generation needs is not product-oriented skills, but process-oriented skills. It has been interesting to note the explosion in the number of computerized games available for children, even for preschoolers. Some kindergarten programs are finding that computers can help to bridge the gap between play and study [3]. Children can learn flexibility through play activities, in particular through sociodramatic play in which many roles can be attempted and each role can have many alternative approaches. Group games, whether table games or sports, also lead to the development of alternative strategies. Individuals who have learned alternative ways of approaching problems adjust to unique experiences more easily than persons with limited experience in problem solving and strategy development. A wide variety of play experiences during childhood, particularly sociodramatic play and games of strategy, facilitates adult adjustment to novel experiences and expectations.

Maintenance of Mental Health

If, as the psychoanalytical school believes, play is the outlet for ego tensions, then play becomes essential in maintaining affective equilibrium or positive mental health in both the child and the adult. This hypothesis is the basis for play therapy programs [1]. Children who are experiencing emotional conflict with parents, peers, or others are given the opportunity to express these fears and hostilities through play experiences in the microcosmic sphere, using dolls and other accoutrements. Under the guidance of a trained specialist, children can express and resolve conflicts in this microworld, releasing energies for more successful adaptation or coping in the real world. Many hospitals have play programs to help children not only to fill their time during hospitalization, but also to understand how equipment works, to project anger onto representative and appropriate play objects (e.g., doll figures, punching bags, modeling clay), and to reenact what is happening to themselves. By providing an accepting, secure environment, the play therapist offers children the license to explore toys, self, and relationships as fully as possible in order to gain the necessary tools and the confidence to understand, to accept, and to realize their own potentials for maturity, independence, control, and self-direction [1]. Effective use of such programs can make any experience one of personal growth rather than trauma and regression for the child.

Parent Teaching

If play is indeed essential to the development of all four domains and to adaptive living in a rapidly changing society, then parents need to provide opportunities for children to have adequate experiences in play. Descriptions of play activities for each age are insufficient; parents need to know how and why each play activity facilitates development. They also need to know how to assess their child's individual needs and interests. Classes on child development should be included in all high school curricula, and students should be made aware of the necessity of play in maintaining mental health at all ages. If potential parents are not reached during the high school years, they are often missed entirely, since the ones who need parenting information the most usually do not attend the parenting classes offered by the American Red Cross or other community agencies. Parents who expect the child to meet their needs rather than encouraging and assisting the child to master his or her own needs are setting the child up for potential adjustment problems in adult life—if not before. Children should be seen **and** heard. Children need parents who play with them from infancy on; they need private time to explore and to express their feelings and moods without interference or reprisals; and they need peer experiences to learn social skills and realistic goals.

Children also have the right to engage in safe play. Since they are not always cognitively aware of the hazards of some types of play or play materials, parental guidance in some form is essential to ensure emotional and social safety as well as physical safety.

Adult Play

Opportunities for play continue to be critical for maintenance of mental health throughout the lifespan. Although activities considered to be play may vary from individual to individual, and from culture to culture, the goal remains constant: Play provides relief and release from the humdrum, drudgery, or intensity of everyday living. It acts as an oasis for the refreshment and the renewal of affective and cognitive energies. Hobbies, whether constructing models, refinishing furniture, raising horses, or creating handcrafts, serve to break the monotony of life's responsibilities and to provide a source of pride and accomplishment. Play, whether physical or mental, provides a pressure valve, or an energy reserve, for both individuals and for groups of persons or families. The members of families who regularly enjoy mutually satisfying experiences together (e.g., car washing, swimming, vacations, table games, hobbies, sports) are provided with a buffer against more difficult mutual experiences (e.g., death, illness, disability, unemployment). The communication patterns and friendly feelings generated during times that are not stressful facilitate communication and feelings of optimism during periods of high stress.

SUMMARY

The complexity of the play process and the fact that it is difficult to formulate concrete definitions for the term **play** create discrepancies among theorists as to when play activities actually begin and which activities can be classified as play. The core definition of "play" includes any activity engaged in for pure pleasure.

The main type of play activity characteristic of each age changes over time:

1. Early infancy. Self-centered, self-exploratory, learning to control own body and vocalizations.
2. Middle infancy. Beginning to reach out into the environment to explore parent. Imitate self.
3. Late infancy. Beginning to reach out into the environment to compare self and parent, to explore toys and objects. Imitate others.
4. Early toddler. Learning to manipulate small toys, to control gross- and fine-motor activity.
5. Late toddler. Beginning microsphere symbolic solitary play.
6. Early preschool. Beginning macrosphere symbolic play (parallel to other children).
7. Late preschool. Sociodramatic symbolic play with other children.
8. Early school age. Continued gross-motor and linguistic development. Games with simple rules.
9. Middle school age. Rules become more complex; hobbies are added.
10. Late school age. Much complex diversity: gross-motor sports, reading, hobbies, table games.
11. Early adolescence. Continuance of preferred medium of play expression with addition of daydreaming.
12. Late adolescence and adulthood. Wide diversity, but usually continues to offer a challenge to at least one domain with a sense of pleasure coming from mastery.

From a cultural context, "play has two faces: a social-public one, which addresses social-emotional needs and helps the individual to become assimilated into the protective social network; and a personal-interiorized one, which is more closely associated with ideational needs and is primarily responsible for the generation of new direction in thought and behavior" [31]. Through play, the child learns to manipulate and to master body, mind, emotions, and relationships. Such mastery is essential to cognitive development, strong ego development, and good mental health. The flexibility and the optimism that develops through creating alternative approaches to problems in play is essential to the effective adaptation of the individual to the rapid changes of a technological society.

REFERENCES

1. Axline, V. M. *Play Therapy.* New York: Ballantine Books, 1969.
2. Brazelton, T. B. "The Neonate's Behavior and How It Shapes His Environment." An address delivered at the conference, An Interdisciplinary Approach to the Optimal Development of Infants, held by the Association for Infant Mental Health, Ann Arbor, MI, March 25, 1977.
3. Burg, K. The microcomputer in the kindergarten: A magical, useful, expensive toy. *Young Child* 39(3):28, 1984.
4. Erikson, E. H. *Childhood and Society* (Rev. ed.). New York: Norton, 1963.
5. Field, T., DeStefano, L., and Koewler, J. H. Fantasy play of toddlers and preschoolers. *Dev. Psychol.* 18:503, 1982.
6. Freud, A. The Concept of Developmental Lines. In A. Freud, *Normality and Pathology in Childhood: Assessment of Development.* New York: International Universities Press, 1965.
7. Garvey, C. G. *Play and the Developing Child.* Cambridge, MA: Harvard University Press, 1977.
8. Golomb, C., and Brandt Cornelius, C. Symbolic play and its cognitive significance. *Dev. Psych.* 13:246, 1977.
9. Hurlock, E. B. *Child Development* (6th ed.). New York: McGraw-Hill, 1978.
10. Isaacs, S. S. F. *Social Development in Young Children.* New York: A. M. S. Press, 1979.
11. Korner, A. F., and Thoman, E. B. Visual Alertness in Neonates as Evoked by Maternal Care. In L. J. Stone, H. T. Smith, and L. B. Murphy (Eds.), *The Competent Infant.* New York: Basic Books, 1973.
12. Krown, S. *Threes and Fours Go to School.* Englewood Cliffs, NJ: Prentice-Hall, 1974.
13. Leacock, E. At Play in African Villages. In J. S. Bruner, A. Jolly, and K. Sylva (Eds.), *Play—Its Role in Development and Evolution.* New York: Basic Books, 1976.
14. Lorenz, K. The Enmity Between Generations and Its Probable Ethological Causes. In M. W. Piers (Ed.), *Play and Development; A Symposium.* New York: Norton, 1972.
15. Lowenfeld, M. *Play in Childhood.* New York: Wiley, 1967.
16. Mahler, M. S., Pine, F., and Bergman, A. *The Psychological Birth of the Human Infant: Symbiosis and Individuation.* New York: Basic Books, 1975.
17. Montessori, M. *Dr. Montessori's Own Handbook.* New York: Schocken Books, 1965.
18. Munsinger, H. *Fundamentals of Child Development* (2nd ed.). New York: Holt, Rinehart, & Winston, 1975.
19. Parten, M. B., and Newhall, S. Social Behavior of Preschool Children. In R. G. Barker (Ed.), *Child Behavior and Development.* New York: McGraw-Hill, 1943.
20. Peller, L. E. Libidinal Phases, Ego Development and Play. In *Psychoanalytic Study of the Child,* Vol. 9. New York: International Universities Press, 1954.
21. Piaget, J. *Play, Dreams and Imitation in Childhood.* Translated by C. Gattengo and F. M. Hodgson. New York: Norton, 1962.
22. Piers, M. W., and Landau, G. M. *The Gift of Play: And Why Young Children Cannot Thrive Without It.* New York: Walker, 1980.
23. Pines, M. A child's mind is shaped before age 2. *Life* 71:63, Dec. 17, 1971.
24. Schaefer, E. S., and Bayley, N. Maternal behavior, child behavior and their intercorrelations from infancy through adolescence. *Soc. Res. Child Dev.* 28(3):9, 1963.
25. Sears, R. R., Maccoby, E. E., and Levin, H. *Patterns of Child Rearing.* Stanford, CA: Stanford University Press, 1976.
26. Smilansky, S. *The Effects of Sociodramatic Play on Disadvantaged Preschool Children.* New York: Wiley, 1968.
27. Sutton-Smith, B. Children at play. *Natural History* 80(10):54, 1971.
28. Sutton-Smith, B. The useless made useful: Play as variability training. *School Review* 83:196, 1975.
29. Toffler, A. *Future Shock.* New York: Random House, 1970.
30. Udwin, O., and Shmukler, D. The influence of sociocultural, economic, and home background factors on children's ability to engage in imaginative play. *Dev. Psychol.* 17:66, 1981.
31. Vandenberg, B. Play: Dormant issues and new perspectives. *Human Dev.* 24:357, 1981.
32. Weikart, D. P., et al. *The Cognitively Oriented Curriculum: A Framework for Preschool Teachers* (an ERIC-NAEYC publication in early childhood education). Washington, D.C.: National Association for the Education of Young Children, 1971.
33. White, B. L. *The First 3 Years of Life.* Englewood Cliffs, NJ: Prentice-Hall, 1975.
34. Wolff, P. H. Operational Thought and Social Adaptation. In M. W. Piers (Ed.), *Play and Development; A Symposium.* New York: Norton, 1972.
35. Wolfgang, C. H. *Helping Aggressive and Passive Preschoolers Through Play.* Columbus, OH: Merrill, 1977.

16
Development of a Concept of Sexuality

Clara S. Schuster

Today's sin is the sin of ignorance where knowledge is available, of failing to seek for more knowledge now that we have the means of seeking it, of failing to believe that the truth will make us free.

—Margaret Mead

Sexuality is a critical aspect of each of our lives. Regardless of how egalitarian or nonsexist a person or family may try to be, subtle influences from our earliest years and the cultural or personal biases of other persons still tend to make an impact on our behavior, dress, and self-image.

Each culture establishes its own criteria for gender roles, and the persons within that culture tend to transmit the male or female scripts to the younger generation. From the moment of an infant's birth, people tend to respond to the infant based on their perceptions of gender-appropriate behaviors. As children grow and develop, these gender scripts become a part of their core identity, self-esteem, and personality and thus influence their relationships with other persons at all levels of contact.

PERSPECTIVES ON SEXUALITY

Sexuality has many different definitions. The narrowest definitions incorporate the concept that sexuality involves those physical characteristics and behaviors of an individual that lead to, or can lead to, copulatory behaviors. Slightly broader definitions indicate that sexuality includes all those behaviors and tendencies that are associated with sexual-social interactions. Both of these definitions appear to be too narrow, since sexuality is a macroconcept, pervading all four major domains. It is a very complex and personal construct comprised of many subcomponents.

Sexuality is the totality of an individual's attitudes, values, goals, and behaviors (both internal and external) based on, or determined by, perception of gender. This definition indicates that a person's concept of sexuality influences many aspects of life, including priorities, aspirations, preferences, social contacts, interpersonal relationships, self-evaluation, expression (or even acknowledgment) of emotions, career, and expressions of friendship. This is not meant to sound like a potpourri, but it must be recognized that one's concept of sexuality is so pervasive that it touches nearly every aspect of self-knowledge, self-expression, and self-ideal. The development or expression of one's concept of sexuality is also closely related to physical, cognitive, and moral development. The total significance of sexuality can be understood only in relation to one's adjustment to life, family, and society and not just in relation to activities engaged in for sensual pleasure or procreation [52]. It is essential to break down the concept of sexuality before synthesizing and applying the concept.

Components of Sexuality

One's concept of sexuality generally becomes more abstract, refined, and stable with age. The individual's gender-expression and gender-preference are usually compatible with a core gender-identity.

1. Core gender-identity. The identification of oneself as male or female. This cognitive categorization occurs early in life and is the foundation on which all other aspects of sexuality are based. It is the basic category a child assigns to her- or himself, and the only one that remains fixed throughout life [30].
2. Gender-role. The clusters of behaviors or characteristics that are associated with one gender more frequently than the other; an organized set of prescriptions and prohibitions on activities established by the culture [22]. The individual may choose among those behaviors deemed gender-appropriate to foster a unique identity acceptable within the cultural age and historical confines.
3. Gender-identity. The conviction that the individual has about his or her gender and its associated role. A subjectively determined concept of one's degree

of masculinity or femininity [31]; the private experience of one's gender-role [47].
4. Gender-typing. The developmental process by which culturally assigned behavior patterns that are deemed appropriate to each gender are taught and reinforced [49].
5. Gender-orientation. A stable, subjective sense of comfort with, and liking for one gender rather than the other for social/sexual relationships.
6. Gender-expression. The behaviors emitted by an individual that reflect his or her concept of gender-appropriate roles. These behaviors are usually compatible with gender-identity but are more likely to be compatible with cultural expectations.
7. Gender-preference. The gender-role an individual finds most desirable regardless of compatibility with a personal core gender-identity.
8. Masculinity/femininity. The very complex, abstract qualities of personality that are assigned individually and collectively by the culture on the basis of gender. Boundaries are imprecise. It is very difficult to construct operational definitions of masculinity and femininity, as will be seen in the next section.

Gender-Role Stereotypes

In earlier and more primitive cultures, roles were assigned on the basis of physical characteristics that were necessary to carry out tasks essential to the survival of the family or the culture. The childbearing and nursing abilities of the female relegated her to the raising of children, a task that kept her close to home and frequently involved in the more agrarian activities. The greater muscular and skeletal strength of the male was essential to hunting, warfare, and protection of the family.

Over time, many gender-related activities and occupational choices developed out of the woman's need to breast-feed the young and to stay near the children. Today, however, when alternative methods are available for infant feeding and contraceptive methods are readily available, many people are beginning to question the value of roles based on gender, and a renewed interest is being directed toward the detection of real versus imposed gender differences (see Chap. 29).

Gender-role stereotypes are culturally assigned clusters of behaviors or attributes covering everything from play activities and personal traits to physical appearance, dress, and vocational activities. Stereotypical personality characteristics popularly associated with gender in Western cultures include the following:

Male	Female
Aggressive	Passive
Controlling	Submissive
Independent	Dependent
Problem-solving	Nurturant
Exhibitionary	Self-abasive
Stoical	Expressive
Self-confident	Deferential
Dominant	Succoring
Instrumental	Affiliative

There is mounting evidence that core gender-identity and gender-appropriate roles are learned early in life. Gender-related differences in play behaviors are evidenced as early as 13 months [19]. Males are generally more aggressive in their play and problem-solving activities, whereas females exhibit more "refueling" behaviors. These early behaviors are apparently so critical to one's core gender-identity that children who experience gender reassignment after the age of 2 years are high-risk candidates for psychotic disorders [42].

Brown [7] devised a test for evaluating a young child's perception of gender-roles. The child is asked to choose an activity or an object depicted on cards for a stick doll called an "It." The "It" doll test evidences conflicting results, but the trend indicates that 3- to 4-year-old children make gender-appropriate choices according to Western stereotypes [13]. Three- to 5-year-old males appear to be more concerned about gender-appropriate play activities than are females [48], and by age 6 years, males exhibit extremely stereotyped behaviors [30]. Adolescent males also appear to be more conscious of gender-roles than females [3]. A cross-sectional study of seventh grade, twelfth grade, and adult males and females identified a positive correlation between chronological age and endorsement of gender-desirable traits. Adolescents were particularly rigid [56]. One would need to ask, however, if this positive correlation were due to chronological age, experience, or cultural-historical changes.

Because of culturally imposed roles, many myths have grown up regarding gender-related differences, mainly to justify role stereotyping. In actuality, only four gender-related differences have been identified through research [33, 55]:

1. Females have greater verbal ability.
2. Males have better visual-spatial skills.

3. Males excel in mathematical skills.
4. Males are more aggressive.

Even the physiological responses to sensual stimulation have been discovered to parallel each other in the two sexes, with four clearly identifiable phases that incorporate nearly identical somatic and genital responses [38] (see Chap. 27).

Nevertheless, gender-role stereotypes persist. Individuals frequently govern or check their own behavior and judge or react to the behaviors of others based on these stereotypes. Males and females experience differential pressure to conform to gender-role stereotypes [36]. Both males and females object to a gender-role that forces them into roles they deem undesirable, forces them to deny or relinquish a valued or desired aspect of self, or prevents them from expressing their perceived attitudes, values, and potentials. Males may object to restrictions on expressing tenderness or nurturant behaviors; females frequently object to restrictions of social and occupational aspirations. Both object to the stigmatization that frequently accompanies violation of cultural stereotypes. Fortunately, recognition of the universality of human characteristics and of the nonequation of physical and cognitive strength has fostered a more egalitarian approach to gender-roles. Research indicates that individuals with a dynamic, flexible orientation toward life have the most positive adjustment to life [37]. This androgynous identity enables the individual to tap both masculine and feminine elements as needed.

In spite of potential shortcomings associated with rigid gender-roles, these stereotypes also have some positive benefits for both the young child and the adolescent. Stereotypes are a very helpful mechanism for coding, categorizing, organizing, and remembering data; they reduce the number of schemata one has to deal with [40]. This aspect is particularly helpful to the young child with limited categorizing ability. Segal indicates that stereotypes facilitate personality organization by "allowing the ego to emerge out of chaos and to order its experience" [50]. Stereotyping may also help to reduce anxiety arising from gender differences and may aid in the process of psychic separation from one's parents. Stereotypes provide an external guide to behaviors until the child's gender-identity is sufficiently consolidated to provide internal guidance cohesive with other identities (e.g., body image, moral identity, cognitive skill identity). Stereotypes, then, can provide structure and facilitate development as well as potentially restrict development if they are too rigid or incompatible with a child's potentials.

THEORIES ON THE ORIGIN OF ONE'S CONCEPT OF SEXUALITY

It is very difficult to identify and document etiological factors in gender-role differences, even though the existence of such differences is broadly acknowledged [5]. The question is whether these differences are real or imagined or whether they are innate or environmentally induced. Major personality theorists place different emphases on the role of the sensual aspects of sexuality in personality development. To Freud, sexual-sensual pleasure was the focal point, or organizer, for the developing personality; to Maslow, it became an expendable primary need. We find the same divergence of attitudes in individual lives. Some make sensual pleasure the primary goal of their lives, whereas others all but deny its existence. These attitudes can be explained in part, but not entirely, by the different theories on child development. There are four major theories on the origin of gender-role differences.

Psychoanalytical View

Sigmund Freud postulated that one's sexual drive is biologically based and mandated. The psychosexual energy or libido becomes the energizer and organizer of one's perception of life experiences. He postulated a direct link between libido or sexual energies and emergent behaviors and motives for behaviors. He felt that all contact with or stimulus of a critical organ has protosexual meaning or influence (i.e., early sensual behaviors influence later behaviors). Since an individual is basically a sensual, sexual, pleasure-seeking being, culture (in the form of parents) must channel and control these primitive behaviors to prevent outbreaks of abnormal sexual activity [17]. Freud felt that the first 5 years of life were particularly critical to psychosexual adequacy.

PSYCHOSEXUAL PHASES

Freud postulated that individuals experience sexual-sensual pleasure from earliest infancy. Rather than seeing sensuality as being synonymous with sinfulness, Freud recognized that sensuality helps the child to become aware of the concreteness of the body and to grow to appreciate the everyday experiences life has to offer. In infancy the individual can learn some of the body's capacities for pleasure and comfort. Freud believed it was only when culture denied the reality

and beauty of sensuous experiences that neurotic behaviors emerged. He identified three erogenous zones, which, when manipulated, would afford sensual pleasure much as scratching relieves an itch [21]. Recent research on the vertical and horizontal organizations of the human brain and the response to sensual stimuli indicates that Freud's theory may be supportable [53]. However, the process is extremely complex and as yet is not clearly understood.

The Oral Phase. During early infancy, activity centers around the mouth for eating activity, play, vocalization, and exploration. Neurological development renders it one of the most mature and sensitive experience receptors of the body. Freud felt that the extent of satisfaction or dissatisfaction with the feeding experience would help to establish early attitudes about dependence and aggression [21]; Erikson later expanded this concept to one of learning to trust or to distrust events or persons in the environment. Pleasure is derived both from tactile stimulation and from incorporating into the mouth objects that satisfy sucking and hunger needs. The mouth has four major modes of relating to objects in addition to incorporating them: (1) holding on to, (2) biting, (3) spitting out, or (4) shutting out. Freud indicated that the need to overuse any one mode can lead to personality problems later on. The normally developing infant will incorporate or embrace objects and experiences not only with the mouth but also with the eyes, the attention, and as much of the body as the infant is able to involve. Later the individual may incorporate love, money, power, knowledge, or material possessions [21].

The Anal Phase. During the second year of life, myelinization of the central nervous system allows the child greater awareness and control of the lower parts of the body. Consequently, the child begins to be aware of pressure created by fecal matter on the lower rectal wall and the anal sphincter. This pressure may be perceived as pleasant or painful, depending on the degree of tension caused by tissue stretching and spasms. Parental coercion is usually exerted to encourage the child to control the location of evacuation. Evacuation usually brings relief of tension and increased pleasure. Many authorities, including Freud, feel that the attitude of the parents toward evacuation, feces, and toilet training influences later personality characteristics. Freud felt that the child's desire to please the mother though the gift of a bowel movement exhibits itself later in life through generosity and philanthropic activities.

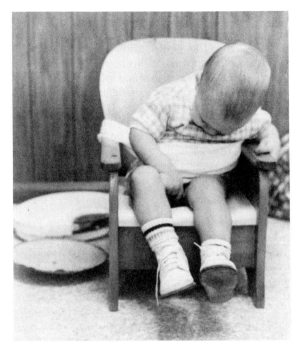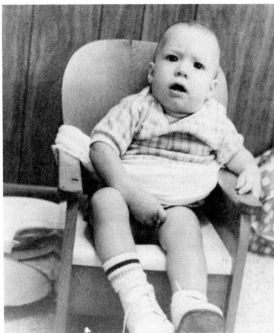

Figure 16–1. Discovery of one's anatomical structures may evoke many different reactions from the young child. It is only one step in the development of gender identity.

On the other hand, if the child feels forced to give up something valued, he or she may subsequently become very frugal, even possessive or stingy. The child also may have an aversion to dirty disorder or messiness if the mother indicates excessive distress at soiling.

The Phallic Phase. During the preschool years, the child becomes aware of genital differences. The child also finds that stroking and manipulation of the genitalia (penis or vagina) produces sensual pleasure and consequently may engage in masturbatory activities. This tendency can be augmented partly by curiosity and also by boredom. Masturbatory activities have a very different meaning for the preschooler than they do for the adult; however, parents observing the activity frequently execute strong, immediate restrictions. Freud felt that negative parental attitudes could cause the child to believe that the genital area was dirty or sinful, leading to problems in sexual adjustment later in life. On the other hand, it is obvious that children who engage in masturbatory activity to the exclusion of other valuable experiences may be restricting their social and emotional growth.

Freud hypothesized that awareness of genital differ-

ences leads to castration anxiety by boys and to penis envy by girls. These phenomena will be discussed further in the section on identification and the Oedipal complex.

The Latency Phase. At approximately 6 years of age (after the resolution of the Oedipal complex), Freud felt that the child enters a fairly neutral period in the development of sexuality. The child gradually integrates previous sexual experiences and reactions. Most relationships are with peers of the same gender. According to Freud, the child suppresses or even denies sensual needs during this phase, yet through the identification process he or she gradually incorporates more gender-appropriate behaviors. "Latency represents a repression of infantile sexuality and is inspired by the child's fear of punishment for his erotic interest in his same-sexed parent" [28]. Anna Freud postulates that there is a "transfer of libido from the parental figures to contemporaries, community groups, teachers, leaders" [14]. More contemporary psychoanalysts hypothesize that libidinal energies may be redirected to the cognitive and social domains, thus, psychosexual behaviors **appear** to be latent.

The Genital Phase. With the onset of puberty, the child experiences new emotions and new sexual direction. The desire to derive pleasure from the erogenous zones is increased. Freud felt that the three earlier phases must be relived and resolved before adult genital sexuality can be attained. The pregenital period (birth through 5 years) was characterized by primary narcissism, a self-love arising from pleasurable, sensual self-stimulation (self-cathexes). During adolescence, the individual seeks other persons to love. Sensual stimulation is exchanged as part of the social and mating process. Freud felt that "the displacements, sublimations, and other transformations of the pregenital cathexes become a part of the permanent character structure" [21]. During adolescence, one must identify and consolidate previous sexual experiences, gender commitments, and the identities learned during the pregenital period. Research indicates that adolescent girls are more likely to experience a crisis in this area than boys because of greater cultural restrictions on expression of their full potentials [57]; this observation is consistent with Erikson's theory. Adoption of cross-gender roles is associated with low-peer acceptance. However, a balance of both male and female traits (androgyny) is associated with high-peer acceptance [37].

Freud's psychosexual stages attest to his belief that biological processes and impulses are the foundation for affective and social adjustment. A secondary process, identification, is responsible for refinement of the affective and social orientation.

IDENTIFICATION PROCESS

Freud felt that sexuality in its broad sense is learned along with other behaviors in the socialization process. The major process through which social learning occurs is the identification process. **Identification** is a complex process through which the individual emulates the behaviors, attitudes, and emotions of a second, valued person. Identification allows the child to enjoy vicariously the values, powers, and experiences of the other. Freud postulated that the child sequentially experiences two types of identification [40].

Anaclitic Identification. Mahler and Piaget both indicate that the young infant is unable to differentiate self from environment [34, 46]. All experiences, therefore, are interpreted in terms of effect on the self. According to psychoanalytical thought, the child gradually begins to differentiate between self and others and to become intensely attached to those who meet his or her needs. This attachment becomes more specific as the caretaker is differentiated from other persons and as the child recognizes the dependence on the caretaker (mother) for comfort, pleasure, or even survival. When the mother exhibits warmth and nurturance, the infant cathects his libido to her (anaclitic identification). When mother and infant are separated, anger and frustration are experienced by the infant. Brief separations can be tolerated, but Spitz's classic studies on anaclitic depression indicate that the child's physical survival may depend on this love relationship (see Chap. 9). Both male and female infants appear to develop along the same pattern during the first 3 years; the mother is their first love and object of identification.

Identification with the Parent of the Same Sex. Freud indicates that when the boy realizes he cannot recapture his mother because of the possession of, and sharing of, the penis, or when the girl realizes she cannot attain a penis through favors to the father, each comes to accept his or her own gender and to identify with the parent of the same sex in order to possess the strength and the attributes deemed valuable in "capturing" persons of the opposite gender. It is the control of impulses and the resolution of the Oedipal complex or the Electra complex that helps to develop the conscience or superego and that assure appropriate gender-role identification. Freud felt that inappropriate resolution of this crisis leads to homosexuality later in life. Other theorists disagree with Freud's theory of castration fear and penis envy, stating that it is only one aspect of the development of one's concept of sexuality and not the origin of it [54].

Identification with the parent of the same sex helps to establish an ego ideal. Some psychologists observe that males have a more difficult time consolidating a gender-identity because they must transfer their identification from the mother (during anaclitic identification) to the father at the resolution of the Oedipal complex. This may be a factor leading to a less emotional, more impersonal approach to interpersonal relationships on the part of males, since the transference may be difficult and traumatic [33].

Psychoanalytical theory, then, holds that the sexual impulses are the core energizer and organizer of life experiences, but that gender-role is culturally and socially mediated.

Cross-gender Parental Love. At about 3 years of age, the separation-individuation process is essentially complete [34]. The child realizes that the mother is beginning to move away, and attempts are made to recapture her. At the same time (according to psychoanalytical thought), the child becomes aware of genital differences and feels that the difference is critical in the relationship with the mother. At this time, the child develops both a love and an anger or a jealousy toward the parents.

One of the central postulates of Freud's theory is that the preschool-age boy falls in love with his mother. The sexual impulses of the young boy toward his mother become very strong; as a result, he becomes very possessive of her and and jealous of the father's relationship with her (Oedipal complex). The child feels that he is in competition with the father for the mother's love. Since the father is bigger and stronger, he fears that his father will cut off his genitalia in retaliation (castration anxiety); he wonders if this is what happened to little girls, since he cannot imagine anyone without his most prized possession [15]. Gradually the boy learns to repress his sensuous desires, and the possession of a penis becomes a central focus of the relationship.

Freud also hypothesized that the preschool-age girl falls in love with her father (Electra complex) and attempts to make herself desirable to him. The young girl blames her mother for the lack of a penis and rejects her in favor of the father, who possesses the coveted appendage (penis envy). She becomes jealous of her mother because of the mother's relationship with the father. Freud felt that young girls pass through a masculine stage before reidentifying with the mother. According to Freud, both boys and girls develop love, jealousy, and rivalry with the parent of the same sex because of the possession of, or the lack of possession of, a penis. They may even deny their own gender-roles as they attempt to emulate the parent of the opposite sex. Karen Horney, however, denies this aspect of psychoanalytical psychology, stating that girls exhibit distinctly feminine traits between 2 and 5 years of age [27].

Biogenetic-Hormonal View

In contrast to the psychoanalytical view, which holds that one's sexuality is neutral at birth and is subsequently imposed by experiences with the culture, there are some who believe that sexuality is genetically determined and thus is incapable of modification. Social and cognitive behavioral differences come from the physiological makeup. Some believe that the infant is biased at birth in a way that facilitates learning gender-appropriate behaviors and resisting gender-inappropriate behaviors. This view holds that prenatal genetic and hormonal influences predispose gender-orientation; behavior and role have an initial direction at birth,

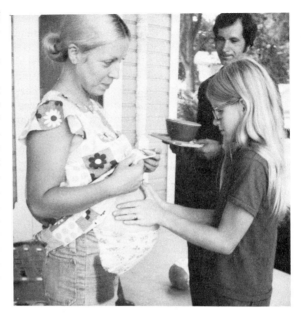

Figure 16–2. Identification with an adult of the same gender helps to establish an ego ideal. The best relationship is established with an adult who is comfortable with his or her own body and gender and their expressions.

which is only partially modified by experience. "Life experiences most likely act to differentiate and direct a flexible sexual disposition and to mold the prenatal organization until an environmentally (socially and culturally) acceptable gender-role is formulated and established" [8].

SUPPORTING EVIDENCE

The effects of early socialization make it very difficult to identify and to separate the effects of biological predispositions. Although female infants are about 4 to 6 weeks more mature neurologically at birth than male infants [4], this is hardly evidence of a foundation for gender-identity differences, and cross-cultural studies offer little support since they indicate wide variation in gender-related traits [39]. Most evidence supporting biogenetic predispositions comes from studies of primates. Harlow found a differentiation of nonsexual behaviors of rhesus monkeys raised by inanimate surrogate mothers. Males exhibited higher levels of gross-motor activity when engaged in free-play activities and more frequent and intense threat responses to intruders, whereas females exhibited more passivity and anxiety and more grooming behaviors [25]. He concluded that such differences were unlearned because no models were present.

In another study, Goy injected pregnant rhesus monkeys with testosterone. He postulated that prenatal hormones had a masculinizing effect on the developing brain, since genetically female offspring exhibited malelike behaviors [20]. Similar results have been found in genetically female human infants whose mothers had received large amounts of androgen during pregnancy. Even after corrective hormonal therapy, their psychosexual orientation remained essentially male [9, 10, 41]. One research study indicates that female homosexual adults tend to have higher plasma testosterone levels than heterosexual adult females, but the amount of overlap in subjects makes definitive conclusions impossible [18].

NEGATING EVIDENCE
John Hampson identifies seven significant variables that potentially influence gender-identity [24]:

1. Biophysical factors
   a. Chromosomal configuration (XX or XY)
   b. Gonad endowment (ovaries versus testes)
   c. Internal reproductive structures (uterus versus prostate)
   d. External genitalia (vagina versus penis)
   e. Hormonal balance (estrogen versus androgen)
2. Psychosocial factors
   a. Gender assigned at birth
   b. Response of the parent to the child's assigned gender

Hampson studied 113 individuals whose biophysical gender was not congruent with their assigned gender because of hermaphroditic incongruity. The results speak for themselves: of 19 individuals reared opposite their chromosomal configurations, all exhibited a gender identity for the gender assigned; of 30 individuals reared opposite their gonadal endowments, 27 fully accepted the assigned gender-role; of 25 individuals reared opposite their internal reproductive structures, 22 accepted the assigned gender-role; of 25 individuals reared opposite their external genitalia, 23 accepted the assigned gender-role; and of 31 individuals reared opposite their sex hormone balances and secondary sexual characteristics, 26 accepted the ambiguity and the assigned gender-role. Hampson indicates that those individuals who were ambivalent about gender-role either had parents who were ambivalent about the child's assigned gender or had experienced gender reassignment after 5 years of age [24].

A number of authors indicate that the period from birth to 3 years of age appears to be a critical period in the development of core gender-identity. Persons who experience assigned gender change after this point exhibit poor psychological adjustment [23, 24, 43].

Most evidence indicates that gender-role and gender-identity are not innate. The individual is psychosexually neutral at birth; sexuality and gender-orientation are shaped by experiences. Although hormones definitely influence primary and secondary physical characteristics, there is little evidence that they also influence social behaviors. This leads one to look at environmental factors that influence acquisition of gender-consistent behaviors.

Social Learning View
The social learning or behaviorist view of the acquisition of gender-consistent behaviors is based on the assumption that parents respond differentially to the assigned gender of the child and proceed to elicit and to reinforce what they assess to be gender-appropriate behaviors and traits while using various methods (e.g., punishment, withholding reinforcement, reinforcing incompatible behavior) to extinguish behaviors deemed gender-inappropriate. Although parents appear to treat children similarly across a wide variety of behaviors, they tend to expend more energy extinguishing feminine behaviors in boys [33]. The adoption of gender-roles appears to be influenced by two clusters of environmental variables: (1) the specific behaviors that the parents associate with the target gender, and (2) the effectiveness of the parent as a teacher [1].

EARLY LEARNING
Much of the parent's behavior toward the child is unconscious. However, gender-related differences are noted in the vigor of play, the frequency of parent-child interaction, and parental tolerance of aggression in very young children [17]. Whether these differences are governed by the parent's cognitive set based on gender-identity, subtle differences in the response of the infant and young child to interaction, or a combination of both factors is as yet unclear. Moss [45] did find that male neonates function less effectively and are more poorly organized than females, which may be due to the delay in neurological maturity in males. Males are more irritable, are more prone to physical distress, and appear to learn social cues less quickly than female infants. This could account for some of the differential behavior observed in mothers; for instance, they may hold, soothe, and attend to male neonates more than female neonates [55]. The cumulative effects of the mutual reinforcement patterns may lead to the measura-

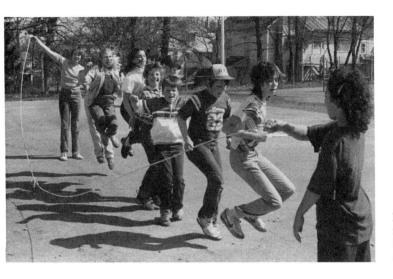

Figure 16–3. The nonsexist emphasis of today's culture allows children more freedom to enjoy joint activities without regard to gender-role stereotypes.

ble differences in attachment and play (touching and proximity) behaviors observed in females at the end of the first year [32].

Parents have different dreams, or goals, for their sons as opposed to their daughters (e.g., boys—tough, confident, protecting, career potentials; girls—soft, sweet, protectable, marriage potential). These feelings and attitudes may be directly or indirectly translated into differential behaviors [33]. Parents subtly give the children different messages. Toys may differ; the colors the child is exposed to may differ. The room and accoutrements of girls are more likely to be pink or yellow, whereas boys are exposed to blues and greens in our culture. Opposite-sex twins are usually dressed differently [32]—the female in dresses, the male in pants. The female's clothing is generally pink, red, or yellow, while the male twin is dressed in blue, brown, or green. These differences are subtle yet measurable. Many other differences have not yet been identified, or in some instances, measuring devices are not sufficiently refined to note differences.

Early learning is believed to occur on a stimulus-response model. Behavior that is compatible with the parent's conception of role-appropriate behavior is reinforced. Since children want approval, they emit those behaviors that are previously reinforced and omit those behaviors that are ignored or punished.

LATER LEARNING

Differential reinforcement must be combined with imitation in order to obtain the rate and breadth of gender-role acquisition observed. Such behavioral clusters are too broad for everything to be taught.

The social learning theorist believes that as children get older, they observe the behaviors of others, attend to details of behavioral differences, rehearse these behaviors mentally, and socially imitate what they see, independent of external reinforcements of behavior [40]. The elaborate attitudinal and behavioral characteristics and qualities associated with gender are absorbed early and become highly resistant to modification [33]. Parents are most likely to be imitated because of their availability. Children are also observed to imitate more readily those models who are nurturant or similar to themselves or who possess desirable characteristics, such as power or a particular skill [40, 49]. Children are influenced by siblings as well as the parents. As the child becomes older and is exposed to a wider range of potential models, he or she may choose a teacher, a popular hero, a historical character, or any other individual believed to possess desirable characteristics or skills. The process of imitation is similar to the process of identification presented by the psychoanalysts in that the child reproduces the actions, attitudes, and emotional responses of the adult. However, Freud believed that identification causes imitation; whereas the social learning theorists, such as Bandura, Sears, Bijou, and Baer, believe that imitation leads to identification [40]. The social learning theorists would interpret the sociodramatic play of the preschooler as preparatory for the assumption of appropriate gender-role behaviors in the adolescent and adult years. The psychoanalytical school would indicate that children engage in such activity to help them to cope with and to integrate roles already accepted as integral parts of their gender-identity.

Cognitive-Developmental View

According to the cognitive-developmental view, "The main difference among the theories does not reside in the specific manner in which the sex role behaviors are adopted or taught, but in the **motive** for modeling, adopting, or identifying with an adult figure" [2]. Lawrence Kohlberg presents us with still another motive: He feels that one adopts gender-consistent behaviors or roles in order to reduce cognitive dissonance and not to gain power or to capture a love object. As such, the emergence of behaviors and identifications is dependent on the cognitive organization of gender-identity and cultural stereotypes. Kohlberg states, "Sexuality constitutes the most significant area of interaction between biological givens and cultural values in human emotional life" [29]. He feels that children identify with the parent of the same sex because they recognize that parent as belonging to the same category. Children will identify with and imitate those whom they perceive to be similar to themselves.

During the first 2 to 3 years of life, the child is developing a core gender-identity, which becomes the bedrock of later sexual and gender-role attitudes. Kohlberg observes that gender conservation follows a developmental sequence and parallels object conservation in other areas as well as the emergence of concrete operational thought [30]. Prior to age 3, the child is able to label the self correctly and can identify the gender of others with partial accuracy. By 4 years of age, the child can label others correctly and becomes aware that one cannot change one's gender. At approximately 4½ years, the child begins to associate gender during childhood with adult gender-identity and roles. During the late preschool and early school years, curiosity about gender differences is at a peak. Nurse-doctor and "peeking" games are common during this period, before social taboos become internalized. Experimentation with changes of clothing in sociodramatic play helps the child to test the reality of a budding hypothesis regarding gender constancy. Around 6 to 7 years of age, the child becomes sure that gender is related to genital differences.

One's self-categorization begins to determine the value placed on objects and experiences. Since children want to like and to understand themselves, they seek out others like themselves (both adults and peers) to emulate. Children must see an objective basis for similarity between themselves and their models. This identification is usually made on the basis of gender, but it may take other criteria. Identification allows the child to exaggerate and concretize self-characteristics and to "structure and adapt oneself to physical-social

reality, and to preserve a stable and positive self-image" [29]. The child avoids what cannot be a part of the self. Consequently, we see increased association with peers of the same gender during the school years and increased antagonism or even hostility toward the opposite gender as a means for reducing cognitive dissonance and maintaining integrity. The child learns to control behavior in order to conform to the standards associated with his or her gender in the culture until such behaviors become well-established, internalized sets or patterns.

The child is concerned not only with gender-role, but also with his or her place in society and with moral aspects. There is a very complex interaction between cognitive development, social tendencies, and social experiences as one sorts out and organizes the attitudes toward self, love, work, and parenthood [30]. During the adolescent years, young persons develop a more unified construct of what they want to be, based on a "need for mutuality and equality of individuals in sexual relationships" [30].

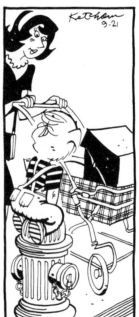
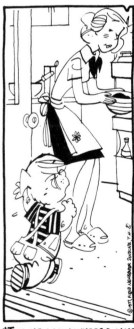

"NO KIDDIN'...UNDER A CABBAGE LEAF, HUH?"

"TELL ME AGAIN WHERE I CAME FROM. I BEEN HEARIN' SOME WEIRD STORIES."

Figure 16–4. Reprinted courtesy of *Dennis the Menace.* Copyright Field Newspaper Syndicate, T.M. ®

Masculinity or femininity, according to Kohlberg, is achieved by the child's desire to achieve cognitive consistency by adopting cultural behavioral standards associated with gender-identity. These behaviors include everything from the way a person positions the legs when sitting, to the holding of a teacup, the tilt of a head, the response to other people, the tone of voice, or even the colors worn. Kohlberg does not rule out the role of early reinforcement experiences, but he emphasizes the child's choice of a role because of its ability to reduce internal cognitive dissonance. The child learns the organized rules deducted from observation, experience, and guidance. These views may be oversimplified, exaggerated, stereotyped, or even distorted, but nevertheless they are adopted because they are deemed desirable by the child. Upon developing formal operational thought, the adolescent is able to generalize, abstract, and develop many personalized standards; however, for social and emotional reasons, he or she may remain rigid in some behaviors in order to retain peer group approval.

RELATIONSHIP OF SEXUALITY TO THE FOUR DOMAINS DURING ADOLESCENCE

From the foregoing discussion, it becomes obvious that one's sexual identity does not begin at puberty but develops concomitantly with other cognitive and social skills. However, the primary and secondary sexual changes that accompany puberty appear to highlight one's attention to gender differences, erotic sensations, peer relationships, and future adult role.

Biophysical Domain

The pubertal period—the period of maturation of the reproductive system—includes all the primary and secondary sexual developments that accompany the endocrine changes in an individual. These changes draw attention to the fact that one is no longer a child. The dramatic change in body configuration demands a change in one's body image, and hence in one's physical, sexual, and social identities. The individual usually becomes very interested in bodily development, is frequently confused by it, and is curious as to the final outcome. Variations in growth may cause concern over the normalcy of one's body, sexuality, ability to compete in athletics, and social and peer relationships. At a time when peer acceptance is so critical, variations in biophysical maturity can create major hurdles. In short, the physical changes of adolescence constitute a major developmental crisis for the individual. The

inability to control the changes may precipitate symptoms of the helplessness syndrome [51]. At no point in life is it more important to emphasize the concept of individuality than during the period of early adolescence, although if an emphasis on individuality has not been a priority throughout the earlier years, parental efforts during the pubertal period are unlikely to be convincing.

Those who mature early are frequently at a great advantage with their peers, since they appear to have left the world of childhood and to stand on the threshold of adulthood. The early-maturing male is at a particular advantage because he is usually able to compete in athletics more effectively. This advantage brings admiration and a concomitant elevation in value to both the self and others, which increases self-esteem. However, early-maturing females may find themselves in a social world of dating that they are not yet emotionally mature enough to handle, thus leading to increased stress and even to lowered self-esteem. Late-maturing individuals may become quite anxious about their eventual body configurations, their acceptability, and even their eventual ability to become parents.

It is not unusual for adolescents to tease one another about physical changes and to place a high sensual value on various attributes. The emphasis on "sex appeal" in television advertising and in books and magazines serves to accentuate the significance of possessing the right amount of a target physical characteristic. The adolescent, concerned about acceptance on a concrete, physical level, may experience great concern or great pride over his or her new body and appearance. In either case, much time may be spent at the gymnasium, at the clothing store, or in front of a mirror to make the most of what one has in order to fit the adolescent's concept of physical gender-identity.

Cognitive Domain

There is no evidence of real IQ differences between males and females, although there may be marked differences in performance because of motivational factors. Each culture places priorities on different characteristics for males and females. When a culture values physical strength over cognitive skills in males, a young male may feel that his sexuality is in jeopardy if he does well in school and exhibits superior cognitive skills. Consequently, adolescent females in such a culture may receive better grades in school because they are not exposed to the same pressure. On the other hand, if a female's concept of sexuality is to marry and to have children, she may not value educational pursuits either. One's concept of sexuality, then, will not affect the IQ but may prevent an individual from maximizing cognitive potentials if cognitive skills are seen as secondary to physical attributes. This observation is consistent with Kohlberg's cognitive dissonance theory: young persons choose to expand/repress those attributes that they view as consistent/inconsistent with their concept of sexuality.

Affective Domain

If the discrepancy between the gender-ideal and the real or recognized potential is too great, the adolescent may experience affective disequilibrium because of the inability to achieve cognitive consistency; he or she may achieve external conformity at the expense of internal conflict. Affective conflict may touch upon any aspect of life. The emergent young person may discover interests or skills that are seen as inappropriate for his or her gender. Since the adolescent is actively preparing for adult roles, this discovery may present a conflict. For example, a young man may find himself interested in women's hair styles or home decorating, or a girl may find herself skilled at auto mechanics or politics. If occupations utilizing these skills are incompatible with the individual's concept of gender-appropriate roles, he or she may experience considerable conflict in the consolidation of a cohesive self-concept. Discrepant interests or skills will have to be denied, repressed, or rechanneled into more gender-consistent outlets.

In other words, during adolescence the normally developing individual attempts to come to grips with various self-perceptions, ideals, and realities of life, to assess their compatibility, and to modify those perceptions or ideals that are incompatible with reality. Two major tasks are involved in this process. First, the adolescent is forced to review gender-identity, gender-role, gender-orientation, and gender-preference for consistency. In the process, he or she may evaluate his or her degree of masculinity/femininity. The adolescent may also question and decide on a homosexual versus a heterosexual expression of the sensual aspect of sexuality. Those who discover a homosexual orientation may experience alienation and a truncated development because of the repression of a significant part of their identity as well as peer rejection and the cultural sanctions on developing intimate homosexual relationships [35]. Self-repulsion and confusion may result if the gap between the ideal and the real cannot be bridged. Second, the adolescent may choose new models with whom to identify, models who possess

physical, cognitive, affective, or social characteristics that are deemed valuable. These characteristics may or may not be directly related to the adolescent's concept of sexuality but are generally compatible with it. The homosexual adolescent may have to wait until after his or her high school years to find acceptable role models. It is interesting to note the cumulative effect of parental influence during the adolescent years. As hard as the young person may try to deny parental standards or characteristics, the outside observer can usually note marked similarity of an adolescent's responses to stress and social situations with those of the parents.

It is during the period of adolescence that an individual is able to construct formally an ideal person or an ideal self, which can serve as a goal to stimulate and guide further affective and social growth. This ideal is usually a compilation of attributes extracted from qualities exhibited by parents, friends, teachers, cultural stereotypes, heroes, and other persons deemed to have valued characteristics by the adolescent. This "ideal" self is frequently at variance with the "real" or perceived self. This assumption automatically presents the adolescent with three major tasks:

1. Coming to grips with the discrepancy (or discrepancies) between the real self and the ideal self
2. Recognizing and integrating the many identities developed during earlier years (e.g., son, scholar, brother, musician, athlete) into a more cohesive view
3. Integrating the experiences or identities of the past into an identity of the present in order to achieve the ideal identity of the future (epigenetic principle)

In actuality, these tasks are not limited to adolescence. There is evidence much earlier of striving to reach ideals, and the process, it is hoped, continues throughout one's lifetime; however, adolescence appears to be a critical time for the integration of identities into a fairly cohesive, stable, heuristic model of self that allows maximization of self-potentials while minimizing energy expenditure to do so.

Maslow indicates that adolescence is a period of life when behaviors are motivated by the need for esteem and self-respect [36]. These needs are met as the individual bridges the gap between the real and the ideal by successfully mastering tasks imposed by the self or others. Self-esteem is heavily influenced by the feedback one receives from others. Incongruity between self-evaluation and evaluation from others can seriously undermine self-esteem. However, the individual who has developed a high degree of self-worth because of congruity of inner identities (or a small gap between ideal and real self) may be only minimally affected by external-internal incongruity. This is possible because such an individual is able to separate the projected identity from the inner self; the individual is able to look at the projected identity objectively without its reflecting on self-worth or self-value. If this individual has not reached the ideal self yet, he or she is able to see the self as a "person in progress." Many individuals are unable to differentiate between the two and consequently suffer identity diffusion, because their inner identities are not sufficiently identified and correlated to withstand incongruent feedback from peers, parents, or culture. The individual who has consolidated identities is able to be inner-directed, whereas the individual who is unable to identify and to coordinate identities is generally outer-directed and is much more dependent on feedback from others to maintain levels of self-esteem conducive to optimal or even adaptive functioning. These concepts are consistent with Witkin's theory of field-independent versus field-dependent persons [58]. Dependence on external feedback for identity formation or self-worth is normal in earlier stages of development, but continued reliance on the environment may indicate delayed development of identity consolidation.

Erikson notes that the individual who is unable to identify and to achieve compatibility among the various facets of his internal identities becomes "identity-diffuse." Witkin indicates such a person may remain field-dependent. Both indicate that the individual remains dependent on external input or circumstances for guidance or an identity for the moment, rather than developing an internally consistent identity that is independent of circumstances, events, feedback, or time. Events may modify external behaviors, but not internal identity or feelings of self-worth [28]. If the individual achieves compatibility among his or her concepts of self-potentials, gender-identity, gender-orientation, gender-preference, gender-role, and opportunities, this offers a feeling of security that may enable the pursuing of an occupation outside the culture-bound, stereotyped gender-roles without violating one's concept of gender-role or the concept of his or her degree of masculinity/femininity.

Robert Havighurst identifies critical tasks for the adolescent years [26] (see Appendix C). It is interesting to note that tasks 1, 2, 3, and 5 are intimately related to one's concept of sexuality. If a broad definition of sexuality is used, then all eight tasks are directly related to both the development and the expression of one's concept of sexuality.

Social Domain

During the school-age years and early adolescence, the individual generally spends much time with peers of the same sex (homosociality). This behavior appears to fit Kohlberg's theory that one attempts to spend time

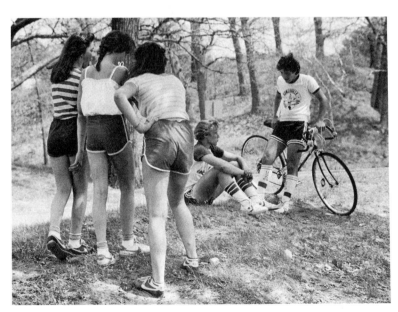

Figure 16–5. Gender-appropriate roles are heavily mediated by the environment and the culture.

with those perceived as being similar to the self. As mentioned earlier, there is much comparison during adolescence between self and others in the effort to assess one's normalcy within the peer group. Those who exhibit characteristics different from oneself (e.g., differences in race or gender, social or cognitive differences, or even differences in residential area or school) may be rejected, even declared to be enemies, in order to assure one's own integrity or superiority. Since these criteria are very arbitrary, they can be distressing to the "liberated" adult who is attempting to instill concepts of human dignity and equal value. However, intolerance for differences is an essential defense against identity diffusion during the school-age years and early adolescence [12].

Gender discrimination in relationships continues during the early adolescent years. With the advent of puberty, however, most adolescents begin to extend themselves toward heterosocial relationships [28]. Increased interest is shown in clothing, hair styles, scents, makeup, social behaviors, flirting skills, and physical attributes that are believed to encourage interest from the opposite sex.

Two issues become critical to gender expression during these years; the first is homosexuality. Evidence suggests that one homosexual experience during adolescence is not uncommon [44]. Perhaps this experience is part of the continued need to compare oneself with those deemed similar to self, or it may be seen as a "safe" environment for one's first extrafamilial attachment or love affair. However, the critical factor is whether or not the individual continues to maintain a homosexual orientation. According to the theories presented earlier, there is no evidence to support the hypothesis that homosexuality is biologically based. Freud believed homosexuality to be due to an overendowed anal zone or an incomplete resolution of the Oedipal complex. The behaviorist believes that homosexuality is due to environmental contingencies that lead the individual to find contact with persons of the same sex more reinforcing or less stressful than contact with the opposite sex. Kohlberg's theory would indicate either that the individual is unable to achieve cognitive consistency or that cognitive consistency is achieved but is not compatible with the norms for the culture. Even though one's gender orientation is established by adolescence, extensive research has not yet been able to identify the etiology of a homosexual versus a heterosexual orientation [5]. Individuals must be able to achieve a cohesiveness of gender-identity, gender-orientation, and gender-preference if they are to be truly secure and happy with their gender-expressions.

The second issue is one's role in the heterosexual erotic relationship. Premarital chastity has been the ideal for centuries, especially for women. The necessity was enforced by the possibility of pregnancy or venereal disease. As a result of advances in medical science, however, the threat of this outcome is reduced, although not eliminated. Many young people see adulthood as having more privileges than childhood, and sexual intimacy is seen as one of these privileges. Consequently, coitus may be engaged in as a symbol of one's emerging adulthood. For some it may represent an imitation of adulthood or even "avocational play," rather than "sex play" as it may be labeled by some adults [17]. Coitus may also be engaged in as a reassurance of one's gender-identity and sexual attractiveness, as an exchange commodity, or even as an opiate.

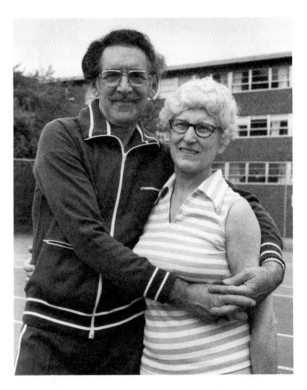

Figure 16–6. A person's concept of sexuality continues to influence his or her relationships for a lifetime. When coupled with intimate affective and social sharing, it can enhance one's enjoyment of life and can help problems to seem less oppressive.

The obvious danger is that an individual may use sexuality to achieve nonsexual goals and gratifications rather than concentrating on the internal state. Erikson's sixth developmental crisis is intimacy. However, physical intimacy is only one aspect of the task. Psychosocial intimacy, which builds from the ability to explore, to know, and then to share one's inner self with others, is the more critical component. When there is physical intimacy before internal identity is secure, it may increase the sense of identity-diffusion instead of helping to consolidate identity. Premature engagement in sexual intimacies, then, may create further cognitive dissonance and affective stress, rather than assuring one's sexuality. The externally controlled individual may experience a temporary reassurance regarding his or her sexuality and self-worth, but the internally controlled individual may experience a sense of disappointment, especially if a personal moral code is violated in the process.

The individual's concept of sexuality and its expression will continue to change over a lifetime. Mass media, cultural changes, the normal processes of maturation, and unique personal experiences all influence a person's value system, personality, and behaviors. Individuals who are comfortable with their personal concept of sexuality and who have found adequate outlets for its expression are more likely to actualize their potentials in other domains.

CONCLUSIONS

A survey of the literature indicates that environmental factors are more significant than biological factors in determining one's gender-identity, gender-orientation, and gender-preference. Gender-role stereotypes appear to be culturally produced and perpetuated. Advances in medicine and technology have reduced the need for gender-specific roles in the division of labor. Consequently, there exists today a greater concern for the unique needs of the individual than for the collective needs of society. The dichotomy of sexuality concepts implies inherent differences in the cognitive, affective, and social domains of individuals based on physiological composition, but this is not borne out in empirical research. Concerned scholars today are encouraging individuals to recognize both their strengths and their weaknesses realistically and to allow their human qualities to emerge regardless of gender so that both men and women can become more fully human and can actualize their potentials without ridicule or rejection [6].

Sears [49] recommends rearing children in a warm, accepting, nurturant, supportive home environment. Lerner [31] indicates that when parents are comfortable with their own gender-identity, gender-role stereotypes can be discarded without confusing the child. The Sex Information and Education Council of the United States (SIECUS) [52] suggests that sex education should include the following:

1. Knowledge about biophysical functioning
2. Information to decrease fears and anxieties associated with the rapid changes accompanying puberty
3. Assistance in developing an objective attitude toward one's body and its functions
4. Insight into relationships with others
5. Appreciation of the positive satisfactions emanating from a wholesome relationship
6. Guidance on the relationship of moral values and rational decision making
7. Prophylactic information on the misuses of erotic love experiences

Gagnon and Simon [17] observe that males are committed to erotic love expressions and are untrained in romantic love. Females, on the other hand, are committed to romantic love and are untrained in erotic love. They suggest that the dating and courtship periods are essential to train the peers of the opposite sex in the meaning and content of their respective commitments.

Child-rearing techniques should help the child to learn to appreciate all his or her potentials and identities without restrictions based on stereotyped, culture-bound gender-roles. Parents who have helped the child to appreciate the pleasures, comforts, and skills of the body during earlier developmental years should continue to be nurturant and supportive of the child's efforts to consolidate identity and other potentials. The body is the house of the spirit, the tool for its expression; it should not be a prison or a shackle. Only when the body is fully appreciated will sexuality become liberating and enjoyable.

REFERENCES

1. Anastasiow, N. J. *A Model for Predicting the Behavioral Aspects of Boys' Sex-Roles.* Bloomington, IN: Indiana University, Institute for Child Study, 1970.
2. Anastiasiow, N. J., and Homes, M. L. Identification and Sex Role. In J. J. Gallagher (Ed.), *The Application of Child*

Development Research to Exceptional Children. Reston, VA: Council for Exceptional Children, 1975.

3. Angrist, S. S., Mickelson, R., and Penna, A. N. Sex differences in sex-role conceptions and family orientation of high school students. *J. Youth and Adolescence* 6:179, 1977.

4. Argarian, M. Sex Differences in Early Development. In J. C. Westman (Ed.), *Individual Differences in Children*. New York: Wiley, 1973.

5. Bell, A. P., Weinberg, M. S., and Hammersmith, S. K. *Sexual Preference: Its Development in Men and Women*. Bloomington: Indiana University Press, 1981.

6. Boston Women's Health Book Collective. *Our Bodies, Ourselves* (2nd ed.). New York: Simon and Schuster, 1979.

7. Brown, D. G. Sex-Role Preference in Young Children. *Psychological Monographs* 70:14, 1956.

8. Diamond, M. A critical evaluation of the ontogeny of human sexual behavior. *Q. Rev. Biol.* 40:147, 1965.

9. Ehrhardt, A. A., and Baker, S. W. Fetal Androgens, Human Central Nervous System Differentiation, and Behavior Sex Differences. In R. C. Friedman et al. (Eds.), *Sex Differences in Behavior: A Conference*. New York: Wiley, 1974.

10. Ehrhardt, A. A., Epstein, R., and Money, J. Fetal androgens and female gender identity in the early treated adrenogenital syndrome. *Johns Hopkins Med. J.* 122:160, 1968.

11. Erikson, E. H. *Childhood and Society* (2nd ed.). New York: Norton, 1978.

12. Erikson, E. H. Identity vs. Identity Diffusion. In P. H. Mussen, J. J. Conger, and J. Kagen (Eds.), *Readings in Child Development and Personality* (2nd ed.). New York: Harper & Row, 1970.

13. Fling, S., and Manosevitz, M. Sex typing in nursery school children's play interests. *Dev. Psychol.* 7:146, 1972.

14. Freud, A. *Normality and Pathology in Childhood*. New York: International Universities Press, 1965.

15. Freud, S. *A General Introduction to Psychoanalysis*. Authorized English translation of the revised edition by J. Riviere. New York: Liveright, 1935.

16. Freud, S. *Three Essays on the Theory of Sexuality*. Translated by J. Strachey. New York: Basic Books. 1962.

17. Gagnon, J. H., and Simon, W. *Sexual Conduct: The Social Sources of Human Sexuality*. Chicago: Aldine, 1973.

18. Gartrell, N. K., Loriaux, D. L., and Chase, T. N. Plasma testosterone in homosexual and heterosexual women. *Am. J. Psychiatry* 134:1117, 1977.

19. Goldberg, S., and Lewis, M. Play behavior in the year-old infant; early sex differences. *Child Dev.* 40:21, 1969.

20. Goy, R. Organizing Effects of Androgen on the Behavior of the Rhesus Monkey. In R. P. Michael (Ed.), *Endocrinology and Human Behavior*. New York: Oxford University Press, 1968.

21. Hall, C. S. *Primer of Freudian Psychology*. New York: New American Library, 1979.

22. Hamburg, B. A. The Psychobiology of Sex Differences: An Evolutionary Perspective. In R. C. Friedman, R. M. Richart, and R. L. Vande Wiele (Eds.), *Sex Differences in Behavior: A Conference*. New York: Wiley, 1974.

23. Hamburg, D. A., and Lunde, D. T. Sex Hormones in the Development of Sex Differences in Human Behavior. In E. E. Maccoby (Ed.), *The Development of Sex Differences*. Stanford, CA: Stanford University Press, 1966.

24. Hampson, J. L. Determinants of Psychosexual Orientation. In F. A. Beach (Ed.), *Sex and Behavior*. New York: Wiley, 1965.

25. Harlow, H. Sexual Behavior of the Rhesus Monkey. In F. A. Beach (Ed.), *Sex and Behavior*. New York: Wiley, 1965.

26. Havighurst, R. J. *Developmental Tasks and Education* (3rd ed.). New York: David McKay, 1972.

27. Horney, K. The Denial of the Vagina. In H. M. Ruitenbeek (Ed.), *Psychoanalysis and Female Sexuality*. New Haven, CT: College and University Press, 1966.

28. Horrocks, J. E. *The Psychology of Adolescence* (4th ed.). Boston: Houghton Mifflin, 1976.

29. Kohlberg, L. A Cognitive-Developmental Analysis of Children's Sex-Role Concepts and Attitudes. In E. E. Maccoby (Ed.), *The Development of Sex Differences*. Stanford, CA: Stanford University Press, 1966.

30. Kohlberg, L., and Ullian, D. Z. Stages in the Development of Psychosexual Concepts and Attitudes. In R. C. Friedman, R. M. Richart, and R. L. Vande Wiele (Eds.), *Sex Differences in Behavior: A Conference*. New York: Wiley, 1974.

31. Lerner, H. E. Adaptive and pathogenic aspects of sex-role stereotypes: Implications for parenting and psychotherapy. *Am. J. Psychiatry* 135:48, 1978.

32. Lewis, M., and Weintraub, M. Sex of Parent and Sex of Child: Socioemotional Development. In R. C. Friedman, R. M. Richart, and R. L. Vande Wiele (Eds.), *Sex Differences in Behavior: A Conference*. New York: Wiley, 1974.

33. Maccoby, E. E., and Jacklin, C. N. *The Psychology of Sex Differences*. Stanford, CA: Stanford University Press, 1978.

34. Mahler, M. S., Pine, F., and Bergman, A. *The Psychological Birth of the Human Infant: Symbiosis and Individuation*. New York: Basis Books, 1975.

35. Malyon, A. K. The homosexual adolescent: Developmental issues and social bias. *Child Welfare* 60:321, 1981.

36. Maslow, A. H. *Motivation and Personality* (2nd ed.). New York: Harper & Row, 1970.

37. Massad, C. M. Sex role identity and adjustment during adolescence. *Child Dev.* 52:1290, 1981.

38. Masters, W. H., and Johnson, V. E. The Sexual Response Cycles of the Human Male and Female: Comparative Anatomy and Physiology. In F. A. Beach (Ed.), *Sex and Behavior*. New York: Wiley, 1965.

39. Mead, M. Cultural Determinants of Sexual Behavior. In W. C. Young (Ed.), *Sex and the Internal Secretions*, Vol. 3 (3rd ed.). Baltimore: Williams & Wilkins, 1961.

40. Mischel, W. Sex-Typing and Socialization. In P. H. Mussen (Ed.), *Carmichael's Manual of Child Psychology* (3rd ed.). Vol. 2. New York: Wiley, 1970.

41. Money, J. Sexual dimorphism and homosexual gender identity. *Psychol. Bull.* 74:425, 1970.

42. Money, J., and Ehrhardt, A. A.   *Man and Woman, Boy and Girl: Differentiation and Dimorphism of Gender Identity From Conception to Maturity.* Baltimore: Johns Hopkins University Press, 1972.

43. Money, J., and Hampson, J.   Imprinting and the establishment of gender role. *AMA Archives of Neurology and Psychology* 77:333, 1957.

44. Money, J. W., and Tucker, P.   *Sexual Signatures: On Being a Man or a Woman.* Boston: Little, Brown, 1975.

45. Moss, H. A.   Early Sex Differences and Mother-Infant Interaction. In R. C. Friedman, R. M. Richart, and R. L. Vande Wiele (Eds.), *Sex Differences in Behavior: A Conference.* New York: Wiley, 1974.

46. Piaget, J.   *Play, Dreams and Imitation in Childhood.* Translated by C. Gattengo and F. M. Hodgson. New York: Norton, 1962.

47. Rosen, A. C., and Rekers, G. A.   Toward a taxonomic framework for variables of sex and gender. *Genet. Psychol. Monogr.* 102:191, 1980.

48. Ross, S. A.   A test of generality of the effects of deviant pre-school models. *Dev. Psychol.* 4:262, 1971.

49. Sears, R. R.   Development of Gender Role. In F. A. Beach (Ed.), *Sex and Behavior.* New York: Wiley, 1965.

50. Segal, H.   *Introduction to the Work of Melanie Klein.* New York: Basic Books, 1964.

51. Seligman, M. E. P.   *Helplessness: On Depression, Development and Death.* San Francisco: Freeman, 1975.

52. SIECUS (Sex Information and Education Council of the U.S.).   *Discussion Guide #1.* New York: SIECUS, Oct, 1965.

53. Stephens, G. J.   Creative contraries: A theory of sexuality. *Am. J. Nurs.* 78:70, 1978.

54. Stoller, R. J.   *Sex and Gender: On the Development of Masculinity and Femininity.* New York: Aronson, 1974.

55. Thomas, J.   Adam and Eve revisited—The making of a myth or the reflection of reality? *Hum. Dev.* 20(6):326, 1977.

56. Urberg, K. A., and Labouvie-Vief, G.   Conceptualizations of sex roles: A life span developmental study. *Dev. Psychol.* 12:15, 1976.

57. Waterman, C. K., and Nevid, J. S.   Sex differences in the resolution of the identity crisis. *Journal of Youth and Adolescence* 6:337, 1977.

58. Witkin, H. A., et al.   *Psychological Differentiation: Studies of Development.* New York: Wiley, 1974.

17
The Effects of Ordinal Position

Clara S. Schuster

> The family is the child's "Rock of Gibraltar."
>
> —William C. Smith, *The Stepchild*

Introduction

Hierarchical Position
   The oldest child
   Only children
   The middle child
   The youngest child

Variations in Birth Order
   Twins
   Adoption
   Stepchildren
   Foster children

The Adult Years
   IQ and career choices
   Marital success

Summary

For generations, parents have been aware that, in spite of their best efforts, each child in the family develops a unique interactional pattern, even if two are identical twins. In a moment of either awe or frustration, the parents may ask, "How can two children be so different when they are raised in the same family?" Parents often try very hard to be fair and to treat each child equally. At Christmas or on other special occasions, each child may receive **exactly** the same gift (except a different color), but one child will still feel that the occasion is somehow unfair—and it probably is. One child may not have really wanted that particular gift, or the older child may resent the fact that the younger child is receiving a privilege at an earlier chronological age.

The truth is that **no two children are ever born into the same family,** even though they share the same parents and the same experiences. The simple fact that one child is born first may allow him or her the privileges of uncontested parental attention in the early years and may result in the development of higher level physical and cognitive skills than later-born children have at the same age. A child may be the oldest of five, the second of two, the last of six, or the fifth of nine; each child experiences an entirely different family milieu.

Although all the children within a family system may experience a significant event, such as the death of a grandparent, the arrival of a new family member, or the move to a new home, the difference in developmental level of each child at the time of the event changes the meaning of the experience for each child and thus the impact on their developing attitudes and behavior. Parents themselves continue to develop and to change over the years, modifying and altering their expectations for, and approaches to, each child. Consequently, even though two or more children may share the same parents, the family experience is different for each of them. As a result, two entirely different ways of thinking, reacting, and interacting can develop in two children with the same parents, the same IQ potential, and the same sociocultural advantages.

Each child has a unique position in the hierarchy of the family system. This position embodies and establishes particular rights, responsibilities, privileges, and roles. Each unique position influences both the quantity and the quality of relationships with others within the family. The oldest child is often given responsibility for caring for the younger children; seldom is the youngest put in charge of the others while the parents are away. Theories of ordinal position posit that the encouragement and reinforcement of differential interactions within the family cause the child to develop attitudes toward self and other people that can result in specific patterns of behavior. The behavior patterns learned in the family setting carry over into relationships outside the family system, with peers, and at school. Studies indicate that the patterns of interaction established during the early years of life can continue to influence social interactions during the adult years—both positively and negatively [24, 33, 61, 63].

When looking at the effects of birth order, or ordinal position, on personality development, one must be careful not to stereotype individuals. However, professionals can use the suggested characteristics associated with birth order as tools for understanding both themselves and others. Many factors (e.g., gender of the child, gender of siblings, family size and spacing, discipline, cultural factors, general emotional tone of the home, educational level and ordinal position of the parents) impinge on a person during the early developmental years, so that each person must be met as a unique individual—a product of a total life experience. The study of differences in interpersonal relationships as related to the perceived ordinal position of a child within the family offers a social theory of personality development [3]. In this view, personality is derived from the child's perception of his or her status and subsequent role within the family system. The differential reinforcement of behaviors based on the ordinal

position lends strong support to the behaviorist view of development.

HIERARCHICAL POSITION

The Oldest Child

In most families, no child is awaited more impatiently or greeted more eagerly than the first. The arrival of this baby is a new and unique experience for the couple; the birth may symbolically fulfill their obligation to society, proclaim their maturity, or assure their immortality [25]. This child makes them parents. The successful culmination of the pregnancy may be a symbol of adulthood to the parents as well as a confirmation of their sexuality. To many, the responsibility for perpetuation of the family bloodline or name is fulfilled. The child may also hold religious, legal, moral, or political meaning for the couple. They may see the neonate as an extension of themselves, as another way to fulfill their own hopes and dreams. Parents often vow to provide their child with the advantages they missed as children.

New parents usually feel that the arrival of their first child is the most fantastic event to ever occur—their baby is prettier, stronger, healthier, more alert, hungrier, or cries better than any other baby in the nursery. Each new accomplishment by the baby is eagerly anticipated, encouraged, noted, and cheered: holding the head up off the mattress, following with the eyes, grasping the parent's finger in the fist, eating solids, the first smile, the first tooth, the first word, the first step. Each milestone is eagerly shared with anyone who will listen.

RELATIONSHIP TO PARENTS

Although few parents admit it, the first child is usually their "guinea pig" for learning parenting skills (e.g., child care, discipline, child development information). Parents are usually tense about the first diapering, dressing, bath, or solid feeding. To the parents' amazement, the infant does survive!

Parents of first-born infants usually respond more quickly to the baby's signals, because there are no other children to compete for the parents' attention and because they are so fascinated by the novelty of their new offspring [55]. They spend more time comforting, playing with, and cooing and talking to the first baby. They encourage the baby to smile, to laugh, to talk, and to walk. As the child grows older, communication is channeled into reading and other "special sharing experiences." This early contact with adult language has a very positive effect in that it forces the oldest child to extract the rules of language in order to engage in meaningful dialogue with the parents. The oldest child becomes very sensitive to structure, meaning, and use of language [33]—a recognized asset in academic skills. Older children are usually better prepared for school than later-born children [20]; they also consistently score higher on National Merit Scholarship qualification tests because of better developed verbal skills [12] and attain higher academic levels than later-born children [23].

IDENTIFICATION PROCESS

Identification with a strong role model can inhibit feelings of inferiority or worthlessness. Most children feel that their parents have numerous desirable skills, characteristics, and privileges that they would like to have, such as physical strength, the ability to give and receive love and to command authority, special talents, and academic skills. The child's observation of the parents or an older sibling deriving power or pleasure from an activity functions as a stimulus to imitate the behavior in hopes of deriving similar power or pleasure. By emulating or imitating the attitudes, feelings, and behavioral characteristics of another person, the child learns to cope with life. Many examples of such imitation are seen in children's play (see Chap. 15).

The more common factors the child is able to identify between self and another person, the more likely the child is to choose that particular person as a role model. Gender is a powerful common denominator; younger children usually identify with the parent of the same sex. The child gradually incorporates the model's behavior patterns, attitudes, and characteristics. Individuals may identify with several different role models as they mature. Some may choose a teacher; teenagers often choose a movie star or an athlete. Children are most likely to identify with a warm, nurturing person—a source of love, acceptance, and security.

The first child, whether he or she is the oldest or an only child, is "adult-civilized" [33]; this means that the parents are actively involved in nurturing, civilizing, guiding, and grooming. As subsequent children are added to the family, the parents spend less and less time in direct care. Parental contact time is diluted as the oldest or older children assume more responsibility for caring for, and playing with, the younger children. These younger children, then, are more likely to be "peer-civilized" because of greater distance from the parents. The oldest, or adult-civilized, child identifies closely with the parents, absorbing their behaviors, prohibitions, values, and goals. Adult-civilized

children are recognized as holding more traditional views and being more conscientious than later-born children because of this close association with adult values. Since younger children more commonly identify with an older sibling, they more frequently identify with peer values rather than family values and goals.

Parents may try to use the first child to realize their own frustrated hopes and ambitions [33]; in other words, they try to force the child to identify with their own values and ideals. In the process, they fail to recognize the child's uniqueness or developmental level. Consequently, they may set unrealistic goals and expectations or may expect perfection. A child who is unable to meet these expectations may experience much anxiety, anger, or even guilt. This is especially true if the young person cannot please or gain the approval of the role models, even after valiant efforts. The only or oldest child may have to struggle harder to achieve the final step in the separation-individuation process from the parents.

Oldest children usually remain closer to the parents

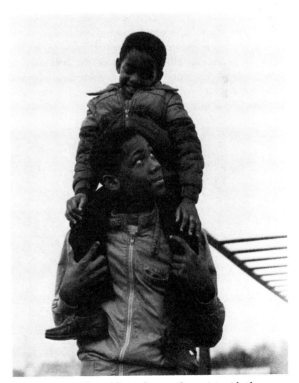

Figure 17-1. Older siblings frequently assist with the care and guidance of younger siblings—a factor that affects the development of both.

than later-born children [24] because of their close identification and communication with adults. They tend to exhibit higher standards of moral honesty and place higher value on "doing things the right way" [24].

RELATIONSHIP TO SIBLINGS AND PEERS

For the first year or two of life, the first-born child is the center of adult attention. As other children enter the family unit, the older child has to learn to share attention. When the second child is born, there is frequently a decrease in maternal attention (especially reinforcing responses), a decrease in mother-initiated games and activities [21], and a decrease in maternal warmth [62]. At the same time, the older child may show an increase in activity, in aimless wandering, temper tantrums, and sleep problems [65]. Consequently, there is generally a marked increase in negative confrontations and negotiations about control issues [21].

Alfred Adler suggests that the oldest child is rudely "dethroned" when the second child enters the family system [2]. The child may develop intense feelings of sibling rivalry and even hatred. A desire to overcome the situation by fighting can precipitate unattractive interactional behaviors, such as peevishness, clinging, or disobedience. The child may also become withdrawn or depressed or may even regress to an earlier stage of behavior—all symptoms of the helplessness syndrome. If the child is well prepared, is allowed maximal contact with the mother during her hospitalization, [65] is offered warm support, and is reassured

frequently of a secure position in the parents' affections, the crisis of transition from only to oldest child can pass with less trauma and without permanent ill effects (see Chap. 32).

The oldest child is usually given more responsibility in the home than are younger children; he or she is expected to "set an example" for the younger children and is often required to assume a parent-surrogate position. This responsibility usually fosters earlier social maturation and more serious work habits. Occasionally, however, the oldest child may be called on to assist with parenting to the point that it interferes with the development of the child's own potentials and realization of life plans [61].

Since the oldest child has greater access to the parents, he or she is more vulnerable to the effects of either outstanding or poor, weak parents. Consequently, first-born children have the highest rate of academic and career success, but they also have the highest rate of severe emotional problems [7]. They also have a significantly greater tendency to adopt the role of being sick when confronted with stressors [26].

Both parents and siblings may expect the oldest child to function as a communication liaison, forcing the child to bridge the gap between adult and peer goals and values. Rules are generally more lenient for later-born children; it is the oldest child who must "pave

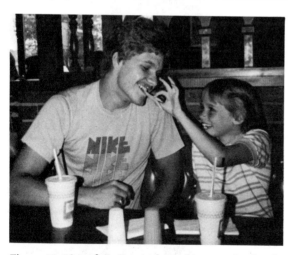
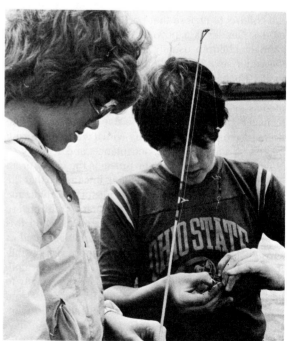

Figure 17–2A and B. Deep relationships can develop between siblings when they are able to share common interests and experiences, teach one another, or solve problems together.

the way" for new privileges, such as slumber parties, wearing makeup, dating, or driving the family car. The first-born must often fight for what he or she wants. These interactional patterns may carry over into the school situation, where the first-born may be too bossy or stubborn to be a congenial partner but becomes a good leader.

EFFECTS ON THE DEVELOPING PERSONALITY

Being the oldest child can be a source of both pride and strength. Through the childhood years, the oldest is someone special to the parents. Greater physical, cognitive, and social-emotional maturity lead to refined skills, greater strength, and special privileges. Oldest children recognize that they can perform many skills better than siblings. Problems can arise if the oldest child feels that this superior competence is due to factors other than greater maturity. They may continue to feel that they are more adequate than other persons during the adult years [24].

Severe identity crises can develop in oldest children when their younger siblings mature and the post–high-school society no longer endorses them as "superior" [33]. Ambitions may also outstrip ability and patience. Some oldest children may turn to any activity, either extremely good or extremely bad, just to recapture that recognition as a "special person"; this may be one reason why first born children participate more frequently in volunteer work. They exhibit a higher need for recognition and approval [39]. First-borns who are unable to achieve special status, may suffer depressive episodes of nonfunctioning self-doubt [33]. The oldest child needs to learn to balance goals with reality: "I cannot always **be the best,** but I can always **do my best.**"

Because oldest children generally are used to exercising leadership and authority, they have a greater respect for an autocratic structure rather than an egalitarian or democratic power structure within organizations [49]. However, they occasionally make more dangerous political leaders than younger siblings because they would "rather fight than switch" [61]. Oldest children learn to organize thoughts and people. They appear to be self-assertive, confident, and ambitious, and these skills prepare them for leadership positions in adult life. A higher percentage of first-born children become presidents or executives or occupy other positions requiring administrative skills.

Oldest children are most likely to experience conflict over dependent versus independent relationships in adult life [53]. They find it difficult to accept directions from peers and are quick to anger when rules are bro-

ken or their ideas are not accepted. Fortunately, they usually learn as children to react verbally rather than physically to such conflicts [39]. During adult life they are apt to become either very stubborn, choosing to forfeit their position rather than their principles, or they may seek to work out an agreement quickly in order to maintain peer acceptance [53]. Under stress, oldest children usually seek to affiliate more with respected peers [39]. This may be a way of testing the normalcy of their own emotional state by comparing their reactions to those of others [75], or it may represent a fear of repetition of the "dethronement" experience of earlier childhood. It may also be reflective of more positive experiences of affiliation with the parents [19].

Only Children

Five percent of the adult population are "only born" children [31]. The relationship of only children, or "singletons," to their parents is very similar to that of oldest children. They are closely exposed to the adult world, values, and pressures. Because of the lack of siblings with whom to associate, the only child may develop a very close, intense relationship with the parents. Singletons may develop behaviors and interactional patterns that are very similar to those of the parents yet may criticize them intensely [24]. During the adult years this adult-civilized child is more likely to seek advice from competent leaders or psychiatrists [55]. The parents may be extremely overprotective and overconcerned about the child's progress and health, since they do not have other children with whom to make comparisons or to absorb their attention. As a result, adult-civilized children tend to exhibit more fear and anxiety during the adolescent and adult years than later-born children when facing the same physical or emotional stressors [23, 55]. Other singletons may exhibit extreme self-confidence because of the support and security they felt during the developmental years.

RELATIONSHIP TO PARENTS

If the family is extremely child-oriented, the singleton may feel that the world revolves around him or her, and may use this role as "the child" to get his or her way with the parents. The parents need to find a healthy balance of recognizing and meeting the needs of each individual in the family. Overly demanding behavior is a reflection of the parents' overindulgent relationship rather than a characteristic inherent to only children [31]. The adult singleton may experience much difficulty when no longer the center of attention [3]. Only children may develop a fear of siblings who would upset the interactional patterns of the family; at the same time, the child may express loneliness and a need for peer companionship. The greater sociability and assertiveness [58] may reflect the singleton's efforts to recreate the milieu of earlier years.

RELATIONSHIP TO PEERS

Although only children exhibit less jealousy because they are not subject to competition within the family [24], the only child may experience immaturity or difficulty in peer relationships because of not having learned the normal give-and-take experiences of sibling life. Children need the experience of both losing and winning in order to learn how to face life successfully (table games are very helpful in this situation). Feelings of inferiority may also arise if singletons feel that they should be able to duplicate adult behaviors beyond their developmental levels. Close contact with large extended families, friends, and neighbors can help to simulate sibling relationships and thus mitigate some of these pressures.

EFFECT ON THE DEVELOPING PERSONALITY

Myth has it that the only child is selfish, lonely, and uncooperative. Granted, the family experiences of a singleton differ greatly from those of a child reared with five siblings. However, the only child has full access to the family's financial and social assets; thus, special talents are more likely to be fostered. The singleton also has more opportunity to learn to be comfortable with the self and to be self-entertaining. Much depends on the parents: Are they hovering and overprotective, or are they able to set developmentally realistic limits to guide the child's relationships? A balance must be found between exploitation and overindulgence of the child when family responsibilities are allocated for care of the home. It is the quality of interpersonal relationships and the opportunity to develop one's potentials in all domains that are most significant to personality development—not just ordinal position. The singleton can learn to share, to respect others, and to be a good team member if the parents provide the learning experiences.

A child who is the only child in a family for more than 6 to 7 years, will probably continue to act and think as an only child rather than as the oldest. The second or younger child will then also develop as an "only child" [24] due to the great amount of time each is able to spend with the parents during the early, formative years.

Only children are most secure with adult leadership. As adults, they often prefer to be leaders rather than

joiners [31]. Realizing that the parents will not always be available stimulates them to become independent and self-competent [24]. They are generally high achievers, strongly motivated, and trustful. If the parents have been developmentally oriented to the child's needs and have also asked the child to respect their needs as individuals, the only child can be very adaptable and cooperative.

The Middle Child

The second, third, or fourth (or more) child is usually not welcomed with as much joy and enthusiasm as the first. The couple has already passed the social and personal initiation into parenthood. The novelty of starting solid foods, toilet training, and the first word has worn off. The second child's accomplishments are not quite as spectacular, although they are still encouraged. With more experience, the parents begin to relax their expectations for both themselves and the child. Less time is spent with the child, and discipline is modified. This relaxation is reflected in research that reveals that older children view their parents as strict disciplinarians five times more frequently than later-born children [53].

RELATIONSHIP TO PARENTS

Later-born children seek more parental attention during the toddler years. When this behavior is associated with close spacing of siblings, it may be due to deprivation of adequate adult attention during early infancy when the mother was trying to meet the needs of two children in order to prevent sibling rivalry [45]. Later-born children are not afforded the same protection as the first-born; they must put up with the noises of the older sibling and the bangs, pinches, and bruises that usually accompany being the smaller of the two. They learn to fight back physically in self-protection. First-borns, who did not have to make a place for themselves are more cautious and may even fear to venture out to new experiences [53]. In adult life the middle child experiences less anxiety and fear of new or threatening situations [55, 72]. If the older child is too bossy or restrictive, the younger child may become very stubborn in order to be recognized as a unique person rather than as an extension of the older sibling.

RELATIONSHIP TO SIBLINGS AND PEERS

Because of the contact with the older sibling, younger children do not feel as much need to depend on the parents and are less likely to embody parental values and goals. Identification may occur with the older sibling rather than with the parents. The younger child knows he or she cannot match the parental skills but might be able to match the skills of an older sibling—especially if they are of the same sex. It can be very difficult for the second child to keep up with the academic or athletic record of an older sibling. Some will become very hard workers and strive to meet and surpass the elder child; others may develop inferiority feelings and give up without trying.

The dreams of children may reveal competitiveness based on ordinal position [3]. Oldest children frequently dream of flying just above the crowd but are not sure they can remain on top. Younger children more often dream of being unable to catch a train or to match the leader in a bicycle race. It is significant to note here that parents should help children to recognize their own individual talents and skills and should discourage destructive competition.

EFFECTS ON THE DEVELOPING PERSONALITY

Middle children are able to move gradually from childhood to adulthood; their experienced parents are more consistent and relaxed in their expectations. The guidance and discipline given by peers is more understanding, using child rather than adult standards. Middle children usually learn how to adjust to both younger and older siblings, those who are more competent and those who are less skilled. Consequently, the interpersonal skills developed by middle children within the home enable them to be more popular with peers at school [49]; they have greater sensitivity to the feelings and needs of other people [22].

The middle child is most likely to accept self and others at face value. He or she is able both to seek and to give help as needed [24]. Greater peer contact during the developmental years fosters greater self-confidence because the child is able to validate values, goals, and skills against those of comparable models. During adulthood, the middle child is able to draw upon inner resources and thus experiences lower affiliation needs [53]. The middle child has the fewest behavior problems [64], the best rate of adjustment to life, and the lowest need to seek counseling [7]. Less rigid and more relaxed about rules and goals than the oldest child, the middle child is thus able to take time to enjoy the pleasures, beauty, and wonder of the world.

Middle children are more concerned about peer norms than are older children [33]. Whereas the oldest child wants to be different (but not too far out of line), the middle child is content to be a part of the gang; he or she does not mind going along unnoticed. This may be because middle-born children and closely born children have lower self-esteem [38]. There has been nothing unique about their place in the family to give them special status or recognition. Middle children do not have the same need as oldest children to be recognized as a "special person." Volunteer work is more an outflow of their own joy and satisfaction with life. They will usually accept and use peer advice readily [33]. The middle child has less respect for autocratic approaches and prefers democratic decision making. Later-born children are also more concerned with practical "here and now" events rather than the theoretical or philosophical outlook on problem solving; their goals are more realistic. They do not have to live up to an exaggerated sense of self-worth, as the older child does.

The Youngest Child

The youngest child is received with a wide variety of emotions, depending on parental age and goals, ages of other children, and whether or not the pregnancy was planned. Because of the lack of empirical data, the author is forced to ignore those children who are "surprise" and "change-of-life" babies, and will concentrate on children who are no more than 6 years younger than the last child in the family.

RELATIONSHIP TO PARENTS

Parents generally have fewer opportunities to give concentrated attention to younger children. The youngest child can not enjoy the privilege of undivided parental attention until after the older children leave home. The older children (and parents) often treat the youngest as a "baby doll," encouraging "cute" behaviors and absorbing the child's stressors and responsibilities. In short, the youngest is frequently pampered. The parents may be lax in expectations and discipline; whatever the baby wants, the baby gets. Occasionally last-born children may attempt to keep parental attention by deliberately not learning self-care or self-sufficiency, which can be disastrous when they become adults and marry. The youngest child is usually very outgoing and optimistic as an adult, as a result of the indulgence experienced during the early years. However, because of greater parental age, the youngest child is most likely to lose the parents while still young, which can be a source of anxiety.

RELATIONSHIP TO SIBLINGS AND PEERS

The youngest child is the only one who is never "dethroned." On the other hand, he or she has many peers with which to identify and to compete. Many fairy tales, such as *The Three Little Pigs, Cinderella, The Seven-League Boots,* and *Beauty and the Beast,* relate how the youngest conquers the foe through patience, wit, or kindness. Even the biblical stories of Jacob and Esau, and Joseph and his brothers show the younger son gaining power over the elders.

The youngest child may feel that it is impossible to compete with older children. Rather than developing feelings of inferiority, "the later child generates and moves into relationships uniquely its own—the 'principle of unoccupied space'—specifically different from the role of the 'achieving child' which is already filled in the family" [29]. The later-born child is reinforced by novelty rather than the repetition of sibling behaviors. This quality can foster very spontaneous, creative individuals, especially in the social domain. They learn to give and take with great comfort.

The youngest child is frequently heard to complain that the older children will not let him or her win a game or that they are "picking on me." The mother's response is typically, "Come on, kids, how would you feel if you were the baby? Let her win, too." The baby of the family learns early to appeal to authority for help in solving problems rather than formulating viable alternative solutions.

The youngest child frequently feels less capable than other persons but feels secure that there will always be someone around to offer needed care and support [24]. Perhaps this explains in part why the youngest child as an adult is more likely than others to seek alcohol as a solution to life's problems [55]. Some youngest children do not learn how to identify priorities and options during childhood; they do not have to live with the consequences of their decisions, and their affective growth is stunted. Throughout childhood they are most likely to exhibit behavior problems [64].

The following lists summarize the personal characteristics that are frequently associated with the oldest child, the only child, the middle child, and the youngest child:

Oldest Child
Anxious and cautious
Conservative
Matures earlier
Serves others
Conceptual thinker
Rigid about principles
Prefers leadership position
Seeks signs of appreciation
Interested in heritage
Rules are important
Ambitious, high goals
Domineering

Protective of others
Quick-tempered
Honest
Extrovert
Serious
Conscientious
Critical
Self-assertive
Conformist
Competitive
Strong-willed
Self-important
High self-esteem
Internal laws of control

Only Child
Conceptual thinker
Interested in heritage
Difficulty in sharing
Loner
Anxious and fearful
Academically oriented
Independent
Honest, conscientious
Self-centered
Critical

Middle Child
Competitive
Good leader
Hard, steady worker
Sociable
Carefree, play-oriented
Friendly
Peer-oriented
Empathetic, sensitive to peers
Self-confident
Realistic self-acceptance
Most adaptable to others
Popular with peers
Analytical thinker
Practical
Realistic goals
Accepts advice readily

Youngest Child
Leisure-time oriented
Peer-oriented
Makes excuses
Dependent
May feel inferior
Affectionate
Lower academic achievement scores

Creative
Entertaining
External locus of control
Easygoing

VARIATIONS IN BIRTH ORDER

Many factors can significantly affect a child's perception of ordinal position. The oldest female child of a large family may assume the role of the oldest child even though she has one or even two older brothers; the same may happen to the oldest boy in a family that values male offspring. If the first-born child is developmentally delayed, the second child will assume the responsibilities of the older sibling. It is the perceived hierarchical status rather than the birth order per se that is significant to the development of interactional patterns.

First-born females tend to be more strong-willed [49] and are more likely to obtain college degrees [33]. Male children reared in families with all female siblings may feel different or isolated and may put great emphasis on their masculinity [3]. However, males with one or more older female siblings and no brothers may also have more gender-role conflicts; research indicates that they experience a greater tendency toward homosexuality. In one study, alcoholism was found to occur two and one-half times more frequently in men without brothers [6]. A female child with only brothers may develop very feminine or very masculine qualities [3]. In other situations, the gender uniqueness may elevate the person's self-esteem [38].

Twins

Twins have a unique scenario to enact because they simultaneously develop two early symbiotic ties—one with the mother, the other to the twin [54]. The early separation-individuation process must occur on two fronts rather than only one. Parents may inadvertently delay this process because they bond to the twin unit before they can bond to each twin separately [30]. During the first year, the twins tend to exchange dominance/passivity patterns several times, which makes intimate knowledge of each twin difficult, thus delaying the parent's ability to see them as separate, unique individuals.

Only 60 percent of twins are identified during the pregnancy [30]. Consequently, the mother, without the opportunity to fantasize and attach to two babies before the birth, may feel as if the second child is a "tag

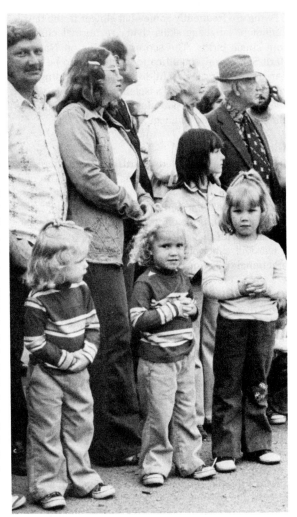

Figure 17-3. Even twins experience each event differently by their selective attention to different stimuli.

along." This normal response may create bonding difficulties that result in unconscious favoritism.

Twins, even when they are identical, tend to develop complementary interactional patterns, with one twin gradually assuming more dominance in the relationship [18]. Parents, without realizing it, may reinforce the outgoing behavior of one twin and the dependent behavior of the other one. One study shows that by the age of 2 years, the first-born twin is more eager, alert, social, and extroverted, whereas the second-born twin is more affectionate and placid. In school, the first-born twin is likely to be more successful both academically and socially [70].

Twins are frequently somewhat slower in the development of language skills than are normal children from single births. The scores of twins on National Merit Scholarship qualification tests tend to be lower than those of first-born children [11]. This finding may be a reflection of Breland's isolation hypothesis, which states that undivided parental attention is essential to get a good start in language skills.

Adoption

Children who are adopted at birth or shortly thereafter develop the interactional patterns of natural-born children. A child who is adopted after having an opportunity to develop a pattern of behavior based on a particular sibling role often continues to behave in accordance with that role. Any child more than 2 years of age will experience some carry-over of earlier interactional behavior patterns [24]. By the time a child is 3 years old, interactional patterns are well-established.

One research study indicates that the success of adult adjustment for individuals who were adopted depends on the age of the child at the time of placement [46]. The best adjustment was experienced by children who were less than 4 months of age at the time of placement, although good adjustments were achieved in placements as late as 18 months of age. However, children more than 2 years of age at the time of placement showed clear evidence of feelings of insecurity. Such feelings may be explained by the child's cognitive understanding of the loss; the separation from the original caretaker may be interpreted as the death of the caretaker by the child (see Chap. 20). Such an adoptee may continue to be vulnerable to experiences of loss, rejection, and abandonment [66]. The maturity and sensitivity of the adoptive parents to the child's experience of loss are critical to the child's long-range adjustment.

Many investigations reveal a much higher incidence of problems in emotional adjustment among adopted children than among nonadopted children [4, 8, 46, 48, 59, 60]. One of the reasons offered is the greater incidence of maternal deprivation and neglect the child may have experienced during the early months of life [8]. Some children may have to cope with multiple caretakers, caretaking styles, and interactional patterns before placement with a permanent adoptive family. Repeated fractionalization of relationships or the rupture of even one intense relationship with a caretaking figure can impede the development of the young child.

Even though a child may have experienced one or more emotionally traumatic events, children are amazingly resilient. They can withstand several major insults if they are provided with a good environment [44]. Many adoptive families are able to compensate for the emotional deprivation experienced by the child prior to placement [40]. Studies repeatedly indicate increased performance when children are placed in a better environment [17, 71].

The ultimate success of an adoption depends on the basic attitudes in the family toward all children whether adopted or not [46]. Prior to placement of a child, most adoption agencies undertake an extensive home study in order to ascertain the prospective parents' motives for adoption, their potentials as parents, and the best child match for the family. Parents must possess a spontaneous and real love for children—a love that accepts the child for his or her own potentials, **not** as an extension of the parents' ideals. One research study indicated that all the adoptees with poor or abnormal adult adjustment had come from homes in which the parents had questionable motives for adoption (e.g., to keep the mother company, or to care for the parents in old age) [46]. The parents must be able to accept the child emotionally as their own and yet view the child as a unique, independent person. Factors, such as parental age, the presence of natural children, and socioeconomic class, do not show high correlation with the success of the adoptive situation [42, 46]. Adopted children need to be treated as natural members of the family by parents, peers, and community members.

The attitudes of the community toward adoption can be very significant to the child's attitudes about self. For reasons known only to themselves, some parents do not allow their children to play with children known to be adopted. In some subcultural environments, comments about illegitimacy, adoption, or adoptees may be very derogatory; the child may feel hurt, embarrassed, angry, or depressed [4]. Adoptive parents or relatives may fear that the child has inherited a proclivity for sexually aggressive or deviant behavior and thus may become overly strict or protective. When the child misbehaves, they may blame "bad blood in the background." It is obvious that a child reared in such a milieu may develop feelings of insecurity and inferiority.

Some adoptive parents become emotionally labile and insecure because of the narcissistic hurt [42] or even guilt associated with the experience of infertility. The long waiting period associated with potential adoption is a further source of anxiety. The parents may exhibit insecurity or feelings of unworthiness through ambivalent, overprotective, or tense interrelationships with the child. Adoptive parents, then, need to be able to identify and work through their own attitudes toward infertility, illegitimacy, and adoption before assuming the responsibility of adoptive parenthood.

One of the critical questions facing every adoptive couple is whether or not to tell the child he or she is adopted. Each side has its advocates, with strong reasons as to when and why or why not to inform the child. Those who advocate not telling the child feel that the adoptee should be spared the adjustment to the community's stigmatizing attitude toward adoption. Joseph Ansfield feels that the option to tell or not to tell should be left up to the adoptive parents [4]. However, many experts, including Ansfield himself, recognize some critical problems inherent in not telling the child. First, it is very difficult to keep the secret. At some point, a clue will inevitably slip and the alert child will begin to suspect that all is not as represented. Most children will ask questions about their past, early months, birth, or even prenatal experiences. Children question their origins as a natural phenomenon of development. Between the ages of 8 and 12, almost all children, whether they are adopted or not, will question their parents at least once as to whether or not they were adopted. What will the parents say? They will have to correlate their stories early in the adoption to prepare themselves for these later experiences. The best response is, "Why do you ask?" However, the parents may eventually find that the stress of coping with the secret is more threatening than open sharing of the true relationship. As Ansfield says, "The feeling of having something one strongly believes in and not sharing it with others can be frustrating" [4].

To keep the secret successfully, the couple will have to prevent their relatives from knowing the details of the child's entry into the family system and will have to cut off social relationships by moving to a new community shortly after the child arrives. Otherwise, news of the child's adoptive status becomes public information. Eight, 10, 15, or 20 years later a relative, peer, or community member may accidentally or intentionally tell the child that he or she is adopted. The child who learns of adoption in a surreptitious manner may feel that the parents are ashamed of the relationship [66]. One study indicates that only about one-half of the children who learn of their adoption through others verify it with their parents [46]. The child's faith in the adoptive parent's honesty and the security of the relationship can also be greatly shaken. Adopted children, whether they were told of their adoption by their adoptive parents or by others, uniformly agree that the news should come directly from the adoptive parents [46, 66]. Adoptees generally feel that truth and openness in sharing enhance respect for the parents [66].

Most authorities on adoption and child development today feel that the child should be informed. Some advise telling the child before the fifth birthday [46]. Adoptive information can be shared with very young children in a natural, matter-of-fact, straightforward manner. However, parents should not expect the young child to understand the true meaning of the relationship. Many children will not really react until later when the meaning of the adoption has its impact [4]. At this time, some children may feel rejected by their natural mother and fear abandonment by the adoptive parents [10, 66]. Children should be helped to realize that their release for adoption was in no way related to their own behavior or desirability, but to the natural mother's choice. One option is to share the concept that "your natural mother loved you enough to realize she could not give you the kind of home she knew you needed to develop your potentials."

The strength of the love bond between the adoptive parents and the child before the adoptive relationship is understood will determine whether the discovery of the truth is a passing episode or a traumatic and isolating experience. A poor relationship will deteriorate even further after the knowledge of an adoption [46], whereas knowledge of the adoptive state can strengthen the child's ego-identity when a warm, supportive relationship exists [42]. It is obvious that the child should never be told during a time of anger, nor should the adoptive status ever be used as an explanation for maladaptive social behavior or a call for gratitude or loyalty to the adoptive parents for their benevolent spirit to an unfortunate waif! On the other hand, the adoptive parent must be careful that the child does not develop a superiority complex because of a "chosen" status.

The adoptive parents should not view the child's desire to learn more about the biological parents as a rejection of the adoptive state [13, 51]. Most individuals experience major identity conflicts during adolescent years, and interest in one's own "roots" is a normal phenomenon. Many adopted children will request detailed information about the adoption to help in the establishment of their identity. When one's ancestry is unknown, it is difficult to resolve completely Erikson's task of identity, which requires, in part, establishing continuity between past and future. Lack of adequate information about one's past can create a "genealogical bewilderment" [59]. An essential part of the self is

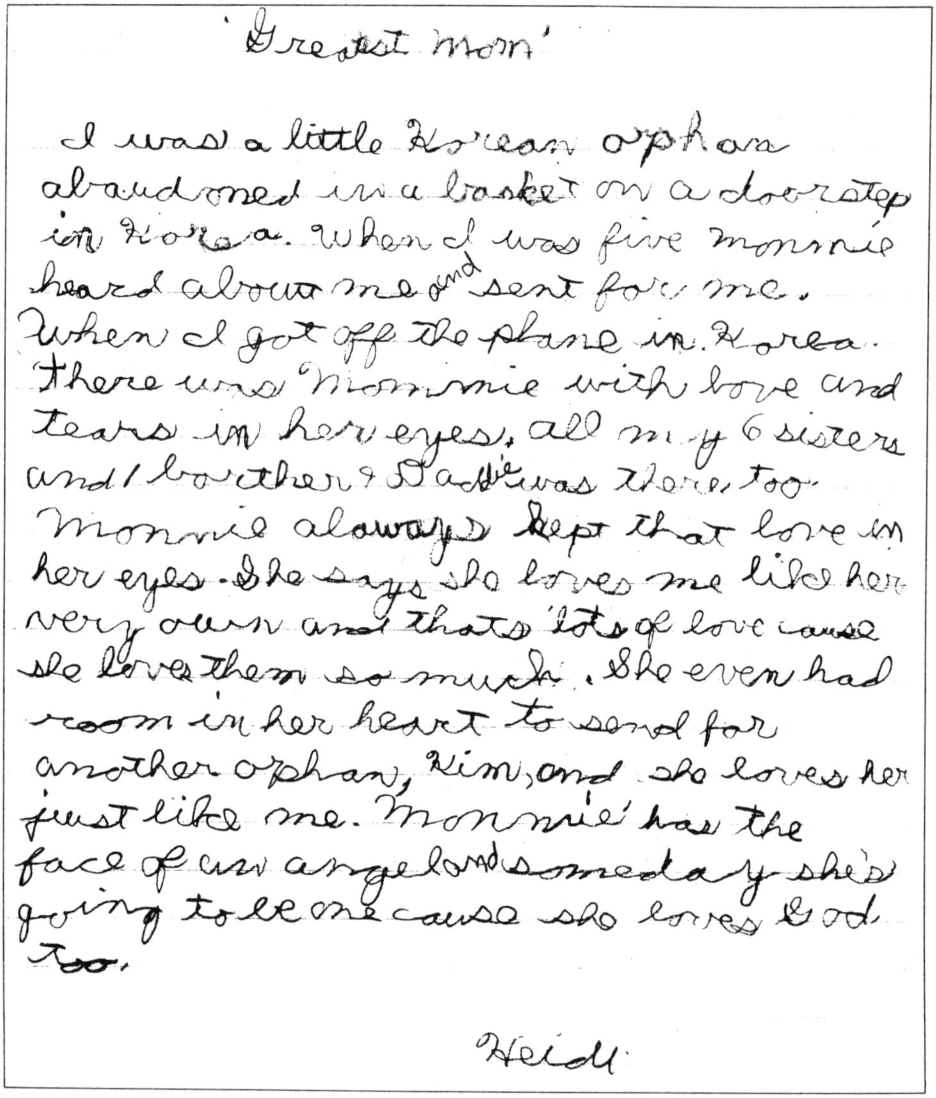

> 'Greatest mom'
>
> I was a little Korean orphan abandoned in a basket on a doorstep in Korea. When I was five mommie heard about me and sent for me. When I got off the plane in Korea. There was 'mommie' with love and tears in her eyes, all my 6 sisters and 1 brother & Daddy was there too. Mommie always kept that love in her eyes. She says she loves me like her very own and thats lots of love cause she loves them so much. She even had room in her heart to send for another orphan, Kim, and she loves her just like me. Mommie' has the face of an angel and someday she's going to see one cause she loves God. Too.
>
> Heidi.

Figure 17–4. Winning essay for a Mother's Day contest written by a 10-year-old girl.

cut off and can prevent the development of a healthy "genetic ego"; a "hereditary ghost" may take its place. For some adoptees, this block to the past may represent a block to the future as well [59].

The background information that adopted children commonly want to obtain includes why they were placed for adoption as well as the physical appearance, personality, age, and occupation of their biological parents. Possession of a picture of the biological mother can be very supportive. Other adopted children want to know about the health status of the biological parents (e.g., the existence of blood dyscrasias, diabetes, heart disease, cancer, and so on). Such knowledge is important when adoptees plan to marry or become pregnant, especially if they need or request genetic counseling.

It is normal for adopted children to threaten to seek their original parents or even to make attempts to do so [13, 59]. If the search is precipitated by the lack of satisfying relationships within the adoptive family, the actual meeting with the biological parents may create a further conflict with fantasy and a disillusionment with life [59, 66]. If the search is precipitated by a genuine desire to resolve the genealogical bewilderment and to strengthen identity, then increased self-confidence and serenity may result from the reunion [51, 59, 60]. So many variables are involved, however, that each case must be evaluated separately. Many adoption agencies today are willing to counsel and to assist with reunion efforts; but other agencies feel that such efforts may constitute a breach of privacy. It is recommended that adoptees wait until young adulthood to effect a reunion. Ninety percent of these introductions bring about new peace, self-integration, recognition, and understanding [59, 60]. One agency that facilitates reunions is Adoptees Liberty Movement Association (ALMA), P.O. Box 154, Washington Bridge Station, N.Y., N.Y. 10033.

The hazards for the adopted child are different and greater than those for the natural-born child. However, when adopted children experience unhappiness and disillusionment with life, it is not related to adoption per se but to (1) emotionally sterile early family life or (2) adverse life experiences [66]. Both of these situations can occur with nonadopted children as well. Given a warm, supportive family who accept the child on his or her own merits, naturally and lovingly, the adopted child will develop inherently in the same way as the biological children within a given family. Maximal development is more likely when all children are treated with respect and individuality by parents who love and respect each other.

Stepchildren

The family is the major source of affection and emotional security for the child as well as the provider of basic physiological needs. It is within the home that the child learns basic values, goals, interactional patterns, and behavior standards. The consistency of persons and interactional patterns helps the child to develop a well-integrated and well-balanced personality. When a stepparent enters the family, he or she brings new rules, values, standards, and interactional patterns into the child's life.

It is estimated that about one out of every six children in the United States has a stepparent [14]. Besides coping with grief over the loss of the biological parent, the stepchild is frequently forced into two new social roles, both of which can consume extensive amounts of emotional energy. First, the stepchild is frequently placed with a new parent who has different interactional patterns and behavioral standards. Behaviors previously learned or allowed might need to be exchanged for behaviors more in keeping with the stepparent's expectations.

The stepparent must help the child to resolve any guilt associated with loss of the biological parent. Memories of, or loyalty to, the biological parent may interfere with development of close bonds with the new parent [57]. The biological parent must help the children to expand their love relationships rather than shutting out the new family members. If the loss is by divorce, it is recommended in most situations that the child have free access to both biological parents. The majority of stepchildren appear to adjust to the stepparent situation, but permanent scars may be left if the process of learning to love and to be loved has been interrupted.

The second factor the stepchild may need to cope with is a change in ordinal position. This is particularly difficult if the change is from only child to oldest child [24]. As with adopted children, the younger the child, the easier is the transition to the new ordinal position. Stepparents frequently end up with two or even three sets of children—"hers," "his," and "ours." Rules must be consistent for all children. Severe sibling rivalries can evolve if the children do not feel that they are adequately represented, accepted, loved, and respected by both parents. The parents need to be careful that they do not get so wrapped up in each other that one or more children "get lost"—lose their individual identity—in the shuffle for new hierarchical positions within the family. Each child needs to feel valued and recognized for uniqueness.

Every child feels deprived, neglected, or mistreated at some point. The stepparent relationship makes a good scapegoat for these feelings—real or perceived. Adjustment is generally easier with a stepfather than a stepmother [24]. The fact that the mother usually spends more time with the child than does the father often makes the stepmother-stepchild adjustment more difficult. This may be a universal phenomenon, since more than 500 Cinderella stories (involving the wicked stepmother) have been identified around the world [56]. The two persons are forced into a close relationship, perhaps without really knowing or liking one another. Resistance may develop as each tries to modify the other's behavior into a more familiar, more acceptable pattern. The patient stepparent who recognizes the differences in values and behaviors, individualizes guidance, and tempers the tensions with humor will facilitate adjustment for everyone involved in the new family system. The new family can be a success if each member is willing to understand, give, and love.

The conscientious stepparent may find the normal criticism expressed by adolescents particularly difficult [57]. The young person may become resentful of the authority and the counsel the parent may offer when a desire for independence outruns the adolescent's experience and judgment, and he or she may attempt to blame the stepparent relationship and a lack of love for the strictness. In situations like this, the stepparent may find it difficult to be both fair and firm.

Foster Children

No one really knows how many foster children there are in the United States. Many of these children come from situations where they have been legally removed from a home because of neglect or abuse. Sometimes children are in foster placement because of parental illness or temporary inability to cope with an onslaught of stressors. Many children become permanent foster children because the mother, or parents, refuse to release the child for adoption, even though they do not feel they can support or care for the child.

In addition to the changes in ordinal position and other adjustment hurdles faced by adoptive children and stepchildren, foster children may need to adjust to multiple caretakers throughout their lives. The crisis that precipitated removal from the natural parents or foster family often results in unplanned placements and inadequate preparation for, or assistance with, the adjustment to a new family system with its subcultural values and interactional patterns. The child may develop justified feelings of insecurity. Although a child enters the foster care system through no fault of his or her own, the foster child, like the stepchild, may feel a sense of guilt over the fractionalization of the primary family unit.

During the school years, when being one of the group is so important, the foster child may move from place to place so frequently that the formation of close relationships is prevented. Other children may question why the foster child's name is different from that of the family with which he or she lives. These stigmatizing factors inherent in the foster child relationship may cause feelings of inferiority [52]. The child who feels that he or she does not really belong to a family may have reduced motivation to learn the family's rule system or to cooperate in family activities.

The foster child becomes extremely vulnerable to additional stressors and needs understanding, caring, nurturing, sensitive parental substitutes. Many families offer excellent, supportive foster homes; others may have questionable motives for caring for foster children [34]. Social workers need to choose homes carefully for their warmth and emotional support potentials. Siblings are usually kept together as much as possible in order to offer some stability and "genuine belongingness." The stability and availability of social workers are also significant to identification and security [34]. Foster children need the opportunity to "belong" to someone. They often feel that life has been unfair to them, that they have been cheated. Consequently, whether their grievances are real or not, they may interpret family rules as unreasonable and family relationships as noncaring or nonunderstanding. The best prophylaxis is an adult who listens with the heart—not just the ears.

The foster child's developing ego-identity is gravely threatened and can be permanently scarred by the multiple placements. Recognition of this has encouraged many agencies to develop more assertive programs to support the biological parents in concrete and constructive ways that enable a child to remain in the family unit [16, 67]. When this is not feasible, agencies are developing long-term placement agreements and earlier custody hearings in order to provide stable home environments and to free the children for adoption when rehabilitation of the original family seems unlikely within a reasonable period. More aggressive efforts are made to place hard-to-adopt children. Many successful adoptions now occur across racial lines. Studies indicate that black children adopted by white families have greater ego-strength than those left in foster placements [40]. Asian children show marked improvement in IQ scores [17].

When foster children or adoptive children move into a new home, they tend to go through four phases [15]:

1. Moving toward the family, the child is bewildered but cooperative and well behaved. He or she wants to be accepted and liked (honeymoon period).
2. Moving away from the family, the child feels depressed, distrustful. The reality of the situation and the child's helplessness to change things begins to sink in; solitude may be sought to think things out (withdrawal period).
3. Moving against the family, the child begins to express anger over the loss of the former situation. He or she becomes demanding and hostile (rebellion period).
4. Gradually the child is able to incorporate the loss and the new situation into a new lifestyle.

Warm, understanding supportive foster or adoptive parents can shorten the trauma of this time.

The child who feels misunderstood usually begins to display discontent through undesirable behaviors. The natural-born child, adopted child, stepchild, or foster child who feels that life in the family is unreasonable has eight behavioral options [57]: (1) withdraw from the situation by leaving home; (2) yield to the pressure and conform outwardly; (3) regress in behavior; (4) daydream and fantasize over the parent that "I could or should have"; (5) stubbornly refuse to obey; (6) become openly aggressive; (7) adopt a rational adjustment to the situation; or (8) develop a unique and creative adjustment to the situation. The parent can avoid much undue stress in the family system for the child (and others) by providing warm, secure, accepting attention that recognizes individual problems and potentials. Respect and love are the key concepts involved.

THE ADULT YEARS

Many characteristics associated with ordinal position have already been discussed. Attitudes toward self and others often carry through to the adult years. In adulthood, individuals tend to select friends, careers, and spouses that will allow them to perpetuate the relationships experienced during the developmental years. Success is more likely if the individual can invest energies in the task at hand rather than in coping with perceived hierarchical changes. If two oldest children want to remain friends, then one or both must be able to curb their tendency to want to dominate. If the stress

created by modifying one's approach outweighs the benefits of the relationship, the friendship will dissolve, often without either person's really understanding why, except to blame the failure on a "personality conflict." Adult interpersonal relationships are facilitated when the individual has had an opportunity to experience a variety of peer relationships during the developmental years [47]. The middle child obviously has the advantage here. However, participation in scouting and other community group activities can offer all children compensatory experiences.

IQ and Career Choices

First-born children who have learned organizational and leadership skills through family experiences are more likely to assume administrative positions in which they can continue to organize and give guidance to others. The identification with adult values, goals, and power structures during childhood gives them a tendency to perpetuate traditions and autocratic relationships. Responsibility for others during childhood fosters the development of nurturing skills, which frequently leads to a strong commitment to, and participation in, volunteer work, such as Red Cross, scouting, or church activities. Oldest children often choose careers, such as teaching or medicine, which

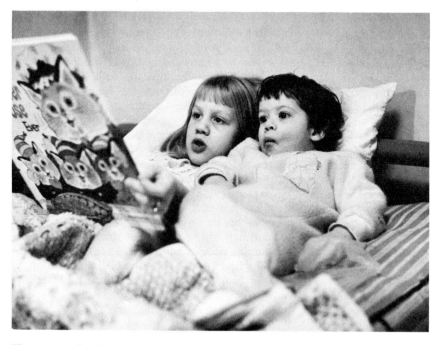

Figure 17–5. The older child experiences many opportunities to practice language skills with younger siblings.

allow both service and leadership. The oldest female in the family is more apt to choose nursing than are her sisters. Within the field of nursing, pediatric nursing is most popular with oldest sisters [24]. Very few youngest or only children are found in nursing [50].

Some scholars refer to the "intellectual primogeniture" of the first born [25], implying that first-born children are more intelligent. They cite evidence that first-born children are more likely to become eminent scientists, scholars, and potential leaders. This external evidence must be attributed to socialization patterns, since no relationship has yet been found between ordinal position and creative intelligence [33, 49]. However, Brian Sutton-Smith has identified a significant difference in thought patterns. His studies indicate that first-born children use a more synthesizing, conceptual approach to reality, whereas later-born children are more analytical [61]. This ability enables the first-born child to learn easily and to impress high school and college teachers. However, this same cognitive approach may be too general or speculative for upper division and graduate level courses, where there is a greater need to focus on details [33].

There appears to be a significant difference in learning style between first-born and later-born children [32]. Educational systems that encourage independent study favor the adult-civilized person who can think abstractly and synthesize data. The later-born child, who depends more on personal contact to aid in offering the connecting support for learning, may be handicapped by independent learning modules [33]. Educators should consider these factors when planning learning opportunities and should provide alternative methods for obtaining the desired goal.

Like older children, only children score well on the National Merit Scholarship qualification tests. However, their scores tend to fall below those of first-born children [12]. Hunter Breland feels that the close association with adult language and values during the early years is advantageous to academic achievement (isolation hypothesis); language skills are further stimulated when the first-born must act as a "go-between" for parents and younger siblings (interlocutor hypothesis). Again, verbal adeptness is reflected in higher IQ scores.

Robert Zajonc has compiled data from several sources, which indicate quite graphically that there is a drop in IQ scores that is related to both birth order and spacing of children in the family. Tested intelligence decreases with birth order. Zajonc's theory hypothesizes that the intelligence of the child is correlated with the "average" of the family's intellectual environment [73, 74]. In order to identify the total quantity of intelligence at the child's disposal, he arbitrarily assigns the parents an IQ of 100 each; this means that the parents have achieved 100 percent of their potential intelligence. When an infant enters the family, the average of the family's intellectual environment is $100 + 100 + 0 = 200 \div 3 = 67$.

If a second child is born when the first child is 4 years old, the average becomes $100 + 100 + 15 + 0 = 215 \div 4 = 54$. (Percent of adult IQ obtained by children is arbitrarily assigned by Zajonc.) Thus the average available for the second child's development is less than that available to the first. If the two children are only 2 years apart, then the older child would only have achieved 4 percent of adult intelligence. In this case, the family average would be $100 + 100 + 4 + 0 = 204 \div 4 = 51$. Consequently, the greater the spacing of children, the higher is the average. Results from several studies appear to bear out his theory. Twins, who would dramatically lower the average, tend to obtain lower scores.

Last-born children experience a greater drop in IQ scores than would be expected from birth order. Like Breland, Zajonc feels the opportunity to be a teacher of a younger child is significant in developing intellectual potentials. Zajonc's confluence theory has opened up much debate [5, 9, 27, 28, 74].

Marital Success

Both ordinal position and gender of siblings become important factors in understanding and living with a spouse. Children who grow up with siblings of the same sex may have difficulty accepting the opposite gender in a marital relationship [63]. Walter Toman has observed that marital relationships that match the individual's ordinal relationship have a greater chance of stability and success [63]. The ideal marriage, according to Toman, is one that joins the older male of a sister with the younger female of a brother. This combination offers the best chance of success because both partners are used to the male seniority position, which reduces conflict over seniority rights. Although there are currently strong outcries and movements against the male-dominated marriage relationship, many persons still find this to be the most comfortable relationship for couples in our culture. Since both partners have experienced living with the opposite gender during childhood, the sexual adjustment is also easier for them.

When the oldest female marries the oldest male, the couple frequently experience conflict over seniority rights, and each may attempt to place the other in a younger-sibling position. They may have many conflicts and arguments until children arrive, at which point interpersonal relationships become smoother [63]. On the other hand, the nurturing qualities learned by both of them during the developmental years may create a very warm, giving, nurturing atmosphere in which each cannot do enough to make life easier for the other. The difference between the two situations may lie in (1) how strongly the need to dominate accompanies the need to be nurturing, and (2) the ability of each partner to receive as well as to give attention.

Toman observes that a reversal of the culturally accepted dominance roles occurs when the younger male marries an older female of a sibling relationship; she is used to seniority rights and he to juniority rights. Actually such a marriage can be very successful if comments of parents and well-meaning friends are ignored. Constant reminders from others about the breach in cultural norms concerning "who wears the pants in the family" can undermine an otherwise successful match. The couple may need to take time to recognize, discuss, and accept their individual roles when societal pressures to change roles impinge on their marital comfort.

Conflict over juniority rights may occur when two youngest children marry [63]. Each wants the spouse to become the leader in the family, and both may avoid assuming responsibility. This couple frequently does not want children to care for. If they do have children, the parents may treat them as toys and then force them into the role of an older sibling as soon as possible [63]. The child may be asked to make decisions for the family, care for the home, or even to provide financial support.

The adult-civilized only child tends to look for a parent in a spouse [63], this match is most frequently found in a first-born child. Middle children, because of the variety of peer relationships, are most flexible in their personality and behavior patterns. They can make a successful marriage with a person representing any combination of ordinal position [69].

Research indicates that the order of combinations in terms of marital success is as follows [69]:

High Success
1. First-born male and later-born female
2. First-born female and later-born male
3. Middle-born (male or female) and any birth order

Medium success
4. Only child (male or female) with first-born

Low success
5. First-born male and first-born female
6. Youngest male and youngest female
7. Only child (male) and only child (female)

Obviously, birth order is only one of many factors involved in adjustment to adulthood and to marriage. The reader is referred to Chapters 28 and 29, and especially to Chapter 30 which discusses choosing a marital partner.

SUMMARY

Identification is a significant process in the formation of self-concept, work habits, gender-role behaviors, and social skills. Differences in the behaviors of children who fill different positions in the hierarchy of the family system appear to be related more to the affective and social domains than to innate cognitive differences. A child's birth order frequently determines the amount of time parents have available to nurture the child and hence whether the child will be adult- or peer-civilized. Each ordinal position is subject to different patterns of interaction, and as a result, children within the same family system have different social learning experiences. Differential reinforcement of behavior patterns by parents and siblings can foster leadership and independence in first-born children, dependence in later-born children.

Marital and career choices tend to be more successful if they allow the individual to continue interpersonal relationships similar to those experienced within the nuclear family. Adopted children, stepchildren, and foster children may experience special difficulty in establishing interactional frameworks when the new family hierarchy creates a change in the child's perceived ordinal position. Warm parental understanding and support, which includes helping each child to recognize and to realistically develop his or her unique skills and contributions to the family system, can enable each child to enjoy positive interpersonal relationships while maximizing individual potentials.

REFERENCES

1. Adams, B. Birth order: A critical review. *Sociometry* 35: 411, 1972.
2. Adler, A. Characteristics of the first, second, third child. *Children* 3(5):14, 1928.
3. Adler, A. *The Individual Psychology of Alfred Adler*, Ed-

ited and annotated by H. L. Ansbacher and R. R. Ansbacher. New York: Harper & Row, 1956.

4. Ansfield, J. G. *The Adopted Child.* Springfield, IL: Thomas, 1971.

5. Berbaum, M. L., Gregory, B. M., and Zajonc, R. B. A closer look at Galbraith's "Closer Look." *Dev. Psychol.* 18:174, 1982.

6. Blane, H. T., and Barry, H., III. Sex of siblings of male alcoholics. *Arch. Gen. Psychiatry* 32:1403, 1975.

7. Bossard, J. H. S., and Boll, E. S. Adjustment of siblings in large families. *Am. J. Psychiatry* 112:889, 1956.

8. Bourgeois, M. Psychiatric aspects of adoption. *Ann. Med. Psychol.* (Paris) 2(1):73, 1975.

9. Brackbill, Y., and Nichols, P. L. A test of the confluence model of intellectual development. *Dev. Psychol.* 18:192, 1982.

10. Braff, A. E. Telling children about their adoption: New alternatives for parents. *Am. J. Maternal Child Nursing* 2:254, 1977.

11. Breland, H. M. Birth order and intelligence. *Dissertation Abstracts International* 33-A:1536, 1972.

12. Breland, H. M. Birth order, family configuration, and verbal achievement. *Child Dev.* 45:1011, 1974.

13. Bright, R. I found my father. *Good Housekeeping* 188(6):129, 1979.

14. Byrne, S. Nobody home: The erosion of the American family, a conversation with Urie Bronfenbrenner. *Psychology Today* 10(12):41, 1977.

15. Child Welfare League of America, Inc. *Parenting Plus* (2nd ed.). New York: Child Welfare League of America, Inc., 1976.

16. Christensen, M. L. Schommer, B. L., and Velasquez, J. An Interdisciplinary approach to preventing child abuse *Am. J. Matern.-Child Nurs.* 9:108, 1984.

17. Clark, E. A., and Hanisee, J. Intellectual and adaptive performance of Asian children in adoptive American settings. *Dev. Psychol.* 18:595, 1982.

18. Collier, H. L. *The Psychology of Twins* (3rd ed.). Phoenix, AZ: Collier, 1980.

19. Conners, C. K. Birth order and needs for affiliation. *J. Pers.* 31:408, 1963.

20. Doreen, M. P. Evaluation of studies on birth order and sibling position. *Dissertation Abstracts International* 33-A:5548, 1973.

21. Dunn, J., and Kendrick, C. The arrival of a sibling: Changes in patterns of interaction between mother and first-born child. *J. Child Psychol. Psychiatry* 21:119, 1980.

22. Falbo, T. Relationships between birth category, achievement, and interpersonal orientation. *J. Pers. Soc. Psychol.* 41:121, 1981.

23. Farley, F. H., Smart, K. L., and Brittain, C. V. Implications of birth order for motivational and achievement-related characteristics of adults enrolled in nontraditional instruction. *J. Exp. Educ.* 42(3):21, 1974.

24. Forer, L. K. *Birth Order and Life Roles.* Springfield, IL: Thomas, 1969.

25. Fortes, M. The first born. *J. Child Psychol. Psychiatry* 15(2):81, 1974.

26. Franklin, B. J. Birth order and tendency to adopt the sick role. *Psychol. Rep.* 33:437, 1973.

27. Galbraith, R. C. Just one look was all it took: Reply to Bernbaum, Markus and Zajonc. *Dev. Psychol.* 18:181, 1982.

28. Galbraith, R. C. Sibling spacing and intellectual development: A closer look at the confluence model. *Dev. Psychol.* 18:151, 1982.

29. Glass, D. C., Neulinger, J., and Brim, O. G., Jr. Birth order, verbal intelligence, and educational aspiration. *Child Dev.* 45:807, 1974.

30. Gromada, K. Maternal-infant attachment: The first step toward individualizing twins. *Am. J. Maternal Child Nursing* 6:129, 1981.

31. Grosswirth, M. The myth of the only child. *Parents' Magazine* 52(1):42, 1977.

32. Harris, I. D. *The Promised Seed, A Comparative Study of Eminent First and Later Sons.* London: Free Press of Glencoe, 1964.

33. Harris, I. D. Differences in Cognitive Style and Birth Order. In J. C. Westman (Ed.), *Individual Differences in Children.* New York: Wiley, 1973.

34. Jacobson, E., and Cockerum, J. As foster children see it: Former foster children talk about foster family care. *Child. Today* 5(6):32, 1976.

35. Jenkins, S. Children of divorce. *Child. Today* 7(2):16, 1978.

36. Jenkins, S., and Norman, E. *Filial Deprivation and Foster Care.* New York: Columbia University Press, 1972.

37. Kammeyer, K. Birth order as a research variable. *Soc. Forces* 46(1):71, 1967.

38. Kidwell, J. S. The neglected birth order: Middleborns. *J. Marr. and Fam.* 44:225, 1982.

39. Knight, G. P. Cooperative-competitive social orientation: Introduction of birth order with sex and economic class. *Child Dev.* 53:664, 1982.

40. Ladner, J. A. *Mixed Families: Adopting Across Racial Boundaries.* Garden City, NY: Anchor Press/Doubleday, 1977.

41. Lawder, E. A., et al. *A Followup Study of Adoptions: Post-Placement Functioning of Adoption Families,* Vol. 1. New York: Child Welfare League of America, 1969.

42. Lawder, E. A., et al. *A Followup Study of Adoptions: Post-Placement Functioning of Adopted Children,* Vol. 2. New York: Child Welfare League of America, 1969.

43. Littner, N. The importance of the natural parents to the child in placement. *Child Welfare* 54:175, 1975.

44. McCall, R. B. Nature-nurture and the two realms of development: A proposed integration with respect to mental development. *Child Dev.* 52(1):1, 1981.

45. McGurk, H., and Lewis, M. Birth order: A phenomenon in search of an explanation. *Dev. Psychol.* 7:366, 1972.

46. McWhinnie, A. M. *Adopted Children, How They Grow Up; A Study of Their Adjustment as Adults.* New York: Humanities Press, 1967.

47. Mendelsohn, M. B. Successful heterosexual pairing, sib-

ling configuration, and social expectancy. *Dissertation Abstracts International* 33-B:4521, 1973.

48. Mikawa, J. K., and Boston, J. A.   Psychological characteristics of adopted children. *Psychiatr. Q. Suppl.* 42 (Part 2): 274, 1968.

49. Miller, N., and Marieyama, G.   Ordinal position and peer popularity. *J. Pers. Soc. Psychol.* 33:123, 1976.

50. Muhlenkamp, A. F., and Parsons, J. L.   Characteristics of nurses: An overview of recent research published in a nursing research periodical. *J. Vocational Behavior* 2:261, 1972.

51. My adopted daughter wanted to find her natural mother. *Good Housekeeping* 188(3):30, 1979.

52. Prosser, H.   *Perspectives on Foster Care*. Atlantic Highlands, NJ: Humanities Press, 1978.

53. Sampson, E. E.   The study of Ordinal Position: Antecedents and Outcomes. In B. A. Maher (Ed.), *Progress in Experimental Personality Research*. New York: Academic Press, 1965.

54. Sater, J.   Appraising and promoting a sense of self in twins. *Am. J. Maternal Child Nursing* 4:218, 1979.

55. Schacter, S.   *The Psychology of Affiliation*. Stanford, CA: Standord University Press, 1965.

56. Simon, A. W.   *Stepchild In the Family: A View of Children in Remarriage*. New York: Odyssey Press, 1964.

57. Smith, W. C.   *The Stepchild*. Chicago: University of Chicago Press, 1953.

58. Snow, M. E., Jacklin, C. N., and Maccoby, E. E.   Birth-order differences in peer sociability at thirty-three months. *Child Dev.* 52:589, 1981.

59. Sorosky, A. D., Baran, A., and Pannoc, R.   Identity conflicts in adoptees. *Am. J. Orthopsychiatry* 45:18, 1975.

60. Sorosky, A. D., Baran, A., and Pannor, R.   *The Adoption Triangle: The Effects of the Sealed Record on Adoptees, Birth Parents, and Adoptive Parents*. Garden City: Anchor Press/Doubleday, 1979.

61. Sutton-Smith, B., and Rosenberg, B. G.   *The Sibling*. New York: Holt, Rinehart and Winston, 1970.

62. Taylor, M. K., and Kagan, K. L.   Effects of birth of sibling on mother-child interaction. *Child Psychiatry Hum. Dev.* 4:53, 1973.

63. Toman, W.   *Family Constellation; Its Effects on Personality and Social Behavior* (3rd ed.). New York: Springer, 1976.

64. Touliatos, J., and Lindholm, B. W.   Birth order, family size, and children's mental health. *Psychol. Rep.* 46:1097, 1980.

65. Trause, M. A.   Separation for childbirth: The effect on the sibling. *Child Psychiatry Hum. Dev.* 21:32, 1981.

66. Triseliotis, J. P.   *In Search of Origins: The Experiences of Adopted People*. Boston: Beacon Press, 1975.

67. Velasquez, J. Christensen, M. L., and Schommer, B. L.   Intensive services help prevent child abuse. *Am. J. Matern.-Child Nurs.* 9:113, 1984.

68. Watson, K. W.   Adoptive and Foster Parents. In L. E. Arnold (Ed.), *Helping Parents Help Their Children*. New York: Brunner/Mazel, 1978.

69. Weller, L., Natan, O., and Hazi, O.   Birth order and marital bliss in Israel. *J. Marr. Fam.* 36:794, 1974.

70. Werner, E. E.   From birth to latency: Behavioral differences in a multiracial group of twins. *Child Dev.* 44:438, 1973.

71. Yarrow, L. J., and Klein, R. P.   Environmental discontinuity associated with transition from foster to adoptive homes. *Int. J. Behav. Devel.* 3:311, 1980.

72. Yiannakis, A.   Birth order and preference for dangerous sports among males. *Res. Q.* 47(1):62, 1976.

73. Zajonc, R. B.   Dumber by the dozen. *Psychology Today* 8(8):37, 1975.

74. Zajonc, R. B.   Family configuration and intelligence. *Science* 192:227, 1976.

75. Zimbardo, P., and Formica, R.   Emotional comparison and self-esteem as déterminants of affiliation. *J. Pers.* 31:141, 1963.

76. Zimmerman, B. M.   The exceptional stresses of adoptive parenthood. *Am. J. Maternal Child Nursing* 2:191, 1977.

18

Development of Self-Discipline

F. Franklyn Wise

If a man does not keep pace with his companions, perhaps it is because he hears a different drummer. Let him step to the music which he hears, however measured or far away.

—Henry David Thoreau, *Walden*

Two major characteristics of the mature individual are the abilities to exercise self-sufficiency and to maintain self-direction. Both are essential components of self-discipline. Self-sufficiency means that an individual can exercise initiative and take the appropriate steps to meet physiological, psychological, and social needs. These skills are learned gradually within the context of the family and the culture.

Self-direction is the ability to direct one's behavior in a way relatively free from the coercion of outer social pressures and inner impulses. Whenever the demands of society are consistent with an inner value system, one's behavior can be directed with ease. However, if external demands, societal pressures, and the perceived expectations of others conflict with one's conceptual and operational value systems, temptation and conflict will be experienced. The sharper the conflict, the greater the degree of temptation will be, and the more self-direction must be exercised.

The development of self-discipline is shaped by the individual's irresistible drive toward self-consistency [37], which is manifested in the conflict between the idealized self (what one wants and thinks one is) and the real self (what one really is). The individual cannot tolerate too much discrepancy between the conceptual and operational value systems. **Conceptual values** are those objects and activities that the individual considers important. **Operational values** are those the individual uses to direct everyday choices, behavior, and appearance. To reduce inconsistencies, the individual will resort to various ego-defense mechanisms or will make important adjustments in behavior.

The factors important for the development of self-discipline are both internal and external. All individuals have needs and goals that they wish to fulfill (internal factors). However, the individual must exercise the right to need-fulfillment within the multifaceted context of the rights of others to fulfill their needs. That is, in order for the various groups within a society to function smoothly, society formulates rules along with certain expectations and delegates authority and power to persons and institutions to enforce its rules (external factors).

A very important inner aspect of the development of self-discipline is the conscience. It is the inner cybernetic system that normally provides continuous feedback to the individual about the degree of behavioral consistency that exists between one's deeds and value system. Also important are the capacities of ego-control and self-discipline that the individual has learned as a result of external factors influencing internal ones. The family has the most significant influence on self-discipline: the method of child-rearing used by the parents, the characteristics of various emotional interactions, and the type of models observed in the family context. Families that are characterized by authoritative discipline, love between the members, and consistent models of moral behavior will be more likely to rear autonomous children who will cooperate with society's rules and values. Authoritarian or permissive disciplinary practices and cold, indifferent, uncooperative parents are more likely to raise children who rebel or disregard societal expectations and who are impulsive and self-centered.

Moral behavior is the operational description of the responses individuals make throughout life to societal demands. If these responses are consistent with societal expectations, they are regarded as moral; if they contradict expectations, they are considered immoral. While the behavior is observable and can be evaluated in terms of society's code, the dynamics of the behavior must be inferred as well as the level of development of the basic cognitive skills. One's intellectual development, the content of one's value system, and the characteristics of the self-concept (with its contingent self-esteem) are additional significant factors influencing moral behavior.

The development of self-discipline, which is contingent on conscience and moral development, is a life-long process. The basic foundations are laid in childhood. During adolescence, individuals begin to probe their own value systems seriously. Some aspects of the value system learned in childhood will be discarded, and some will be permanently adopted and internalized. Adulthood brings new evaluations, new adaptations, and new internalizations. Moral behavior and the wider applications of self-discipline (or self-indulgence) will fluctuate with the individual's degree of commitment to a set of values. This commitment is subject to ego-control and intellectual evaluation. Any consideration of the development of the capacity to make moral decisions will inevitably involve the role of the conscience in self-direction.

DEVELOPMENT OF CONSCIENCE

Definition of Conscience

By derivation, **conscience** means **together** (con) and **to know** (scire), that is, an idea held in common with others. However, most theorists concentrate on the personal aspects of the concept.

Menninger [44] described conscience as, "The function of approving or disapproving what the instincts and the occasion impel one to do. . . . " Jourard [30] states that "Conscience is made up of ideals and taboos for a person's behavior. Each socialized person internalizes the social value-system and acquires a personal value-system. . . . Conscience refers only to the values and ideals which pertain to the self."

Conn [14] enlarges this concept somewhat: "Conscience, then, involves all the subject's conscious and intentional operations insofar as they are practical, heading toward decision and action."

Eby and Arrowood [17] point out that "Conscience is a standard of life, an ideal of conduct that the individual implicitly agrees with others to maintain and chooses himself to observe."

Theories of Development of Conscience

Many researchers have been concerned with how the conscience develops. Several theories have resulted from their work.

PSYCHOANALYTIC THEORY

Personality. Freud [20, 21, 22] postulated personality as being comprised of three systems: the id, the ego, and the superego. The id includes the basic inherited drives of the individual, including the instincts, the reflexes, and the survival needs as well as the self, sex, and social urges. The id operates on the pleasure principle.

The ego includes the processes of learning, perception, memory, and rationality. It functions as a problem-solver and an ongoing repository of the individual's self-perceptions. The ego responds to the expectations and realities of the physical and social environment. It operates on the reality principle. Conflicts between the id and ego systems often develop.

The superego continually monitors the individual's behaviors and motives because it is shaped by the primary socializing agents in the environment whose values and social expectations have become an integral part of the perceptual-emotional-volitional processes of the personality. To the degree these expectations are internalized, the superego regulates and provides feedback to the individual regarding how closely one's behavior conforms to the personal value system. The sense of personal responsibility for actions is also proportionate to the degree of internalization.

There are two separate parts of the superego: the conscience, which discourages the expression of undesirable behavior, and the ego-ideal, which encourages approved behavior. The punishment of the child by significant adults, the threat of withdrawal of their love, or the adult's expressions of pointed disdain for particular behaviors sensitize the child's superego, hence the conscience. Some writers have characterized the conscience as the "no-saying" voice of the parents [20]. Its chief function is to restrain unacceptable behavior and to engender feelings of guilt and shame when the behaviors run counter to internalized values or societal expectations.

On the other hand, the ego-ideal is shaped by positive rewards and feedback from significant adults in the child's environment. Praise for accomplishments, expressions of approval for particular behaviors, and rewards earned in the form of privileges shape the ego-ideal. It is hoped that the child who receives a preponderance of positive rewards will develop an ego-ideal that will be the predominate, internalized, motivating force for positive and appropriate moral action. Of course, both ego-ideal and conscience are needed as counterbalances in development [20].

Pattison [50] suggests that the source of moral behavior is neither the conscience nor the ego-ideal per se but is the result of ego-strength. Morality is " . . . an evaluating and coordinating function of the ego which is part of its autonomous function, concerned with defining and directing one's life in accord with

values one has chosen." If this is true, then, the ability to be self-directing is directly affected by one's self-concept. A strong self-concept is characterized by high levels of autonomy.

Identification and internalization. Children incorporate parental values and a moral code through identification and internalization. Generally children want to become like their parents. This desire has a two-fold basis. Since parents dispense rewards and punishments, they appear to the children to be powerful. Children want to receive the rewards that parents have to give and to escape the punishments that parents can inflict. Children adopt parental values to receive praise and to avoid punishment.

Identification is " . . . a process whereby one individual takes on the behavior of another individual and behaves as if he were that individual" [28]. Children observe that the adults in their lives appear to exert control over events and to receive approval from others. Consequently, children want to emulate the behaviors of parents and other significant adults whom they admire and respect, so that they might obtain this same strength.

Parental values are internalized as children use them to guide behavior. This internalization is unquestioned in childhood and results in a conforming behavior. As they grow into adolescence, children will struggle with any conflicts between parental values and peer group values. As they face the conflict between identity and role confusion described by Erikson [18], adolescents will decide which values to adopt or to drop in order to forge their own personal behavioral codes.

SOCIAL LEARNING THEORY

Closely aligned with the psychoanalytic theory is the social learning theory [3, 23, 30]. Both theories focus on the key role of identification in conscience development. The social learning theory, however, stresses the component of modeling and imitation to a greater degree. Kagan [31] defines identification as an "acquired, cognitive response" in which one assumes attributes, motives, characteristics, and affective behaviors of a model into the psychological organization.

As children begin to imitate adult behavior, they do so to please the parents and to avoid their disapproval and punishment for misconduct. Later they realize that good conduct is rewarding in itself, and they find obedience is pleasant for its own sake. Thus children will act morally, with conscience serving as a self-regulatory function. Their consciences reward them with high self-esteem for good conduct and with shame and guilt for bad conduct.

In addition to the parents, children see other persons in their environment who provide models for them. They hold these models in high esteem and want to be like them. These persons may be television characters, athletes, teachers, or older siblings. Children identify with the models and the models' behavior influences the behavior of the children. It might be asked, "Why does the child choose a particular person as a model?" Identification is more likely to occur when the subject (S) and the model (M) have frequent contact, and the model has the power to reward S for behaving in approved ways. The more direct the contact between M and S, the stronger will be the identification [31]. The home and family situation provide the most direct contact between M and S. Thus parents are very influential models [27], and the critical role of the parents in developing conscience as well as in the moral development of children is strongly substantiated.

COGNITIVE THEORY

Jean Piaget [52] also studied the development of the moral capacities of children. He emphasizes the development of the cognitive powers of children, but little emphasis is placed on moral teachings or parent-child interactions. Piaget stresses the fact that parents make the rules and children react to them on the basis of their own level of cognitive development.

Moral development. There are specific stages in the development of the child's attitudes toward rules, justice, morality, and punishment, which parallel the child's mental development. Two broad stages of moral development are identified by Piaget: a respect for rules and a sense of justice. The stage of respect for rules (approximately 3 to 11 years of age) is called by Piaget a "morality of restraint." At this stage, rules are sacred to the child, probably because they are handed down by dominant and omnipotent adults. During this stage of practice of the rules, the child progresses from the imitation of older children to cooperation and completion. The ego develops from the impulsive through the self-protective to the conforming stages. The rules are sacred; morality is heteronomous (defined as an inflexible code of rules and punishments imposed by outside forces). In the judgment of the child, the punishment for breaking the rules should be either vengeful or fair compensation. The child has little recognition of the contingencies in a situation that may influence an offender's behavior and little comprehension of the intentions that may prompt it.

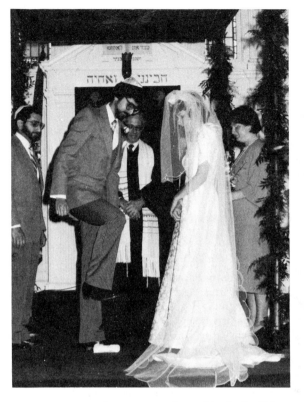

Figure 18-1. Social events are often a blend of religious beliefs and cultural traditions.

A "morality of reciprocity" characterizes the older child (12 years of age or more) for Piaget. An advancement to the level of abstract thought and operation enables the young person to develop a new conscientious, internally sensitive, and changing codification of the rules. Intentionality and abstract concepts of justice emerge. Along with these, a sense of autonomous operation (primarily an internally monitored value response) develops in the cause of mutually advantageous rule-making and operation. Thus two adolescents may consent mutually to change the rules of a game they are playing as an aid to adventure and new experience [24].

Concept of justice. In the earlier stages, intentionality has no bearing on the punishment deemed proper by a child. The child judges any behavior in terms of physical consequences rather than motivation or intention. The child is an "eye-for-an-eye" judge; retribution is the mode of moral perceptivity. In later stages, the child may develop the ability to be more forgiving or at least may take extenuating factors into consideration before rendering a verdict; reconciliation becomes a goal of justice. Interaction with peers is the vital element from which rational morality and a mature concept of justice emerge from the earlier egocentricity and moral realism.

Recent research [26, 38, 39] has questioned the applicability of these concepts of moral development to females. Researchers have built a strong case to support the idea that males are more concerned with maintaining rules and legal codes. Females are more willing to allow exceptions to the rules because they look at the issues of responsibility for the well-being of others.

Moral judgment. For Piaget, the dynamic interaction between the developing child and the rules creates new facets of personality and a higher creation functioning [52]. While Piaget's theory has found wide support, it has raised some questions. Bandura [3] found from his research that the vast majority of young children are capable of exercising autonomous subjective judgments and most older children display varying degrees of objective morality. However, other research appears to indicate that

> . . . the relationship between moral action and moral judgment depends on the moral stage an individual already has attained. A child at a lower stage is affected much more by the actions and opinions of others—that is, by the principles of social learning. At more advanced stages of moral development a child is more likely to follow his own cognitive understanding of the situation and be less easily influenced [55].

PECK'S STAGES OF CONSCIENCE
Based on their research, Peck and his associates [51] identified four stages in conscience development: (1) a conscience that is a crude, harsh, punitive collection of "don't's"; (2) a conforming conscience that is not really internalized but is ready to do what society expects and wants (a passive morality); (3) a conscience composed of moral rules that are deeply internalized and adhered to with unvarying, stereotyped behavior; (4) a conscience composed firmly of internalized moral principles that are constantly reexamined to be sure that they reflect a genuine moral purpose.

From these studies of the evolvement of conscience, several conclusions may be drawn. First, conscience is not fully shaped at birth, although the capacity for a conscience is present at birth. Second, conscience is inferred because humans experience feelings of guilt and shame if they violate its expectations. Third, con-

science develops through discernible, describable stages. Fourth, different moral structures operate at each level of development. Fifth, each stage is influenced differently by environmental events. In babyhood and early childhood, environmental contingencies determine one's principles; identification with the parental model is crucial to early internalization of moral structures. In early childhood, children expand their rule-awareness by observing adult models. In late childhood, cognitive development begins to interpret and to mediate moral behavior beyond particular environmental factors.

Critical Factors in the Development of Conscience
While many factors impinge on conscience development, only two will be discussed—(1) empathy and role-taking and (2) the effects of guilt and shame.

EMPATHY AND ROLE-TAKING
Role-taking is derived from the empathetic ability to understand the motives involved or expressed in another's behavior in a social situation. This skill requires that individuals be able to put themselves in another's place, to understand the motives involved in or expressed by that person's behavior, and to assess the responsibility of the other person on that basis. Because of their egocentrism, young children project their own motives and understandings when making moral judgments about another's actions. Role-taking results from the decentering factor that is so essential in helping the child to make the transition from the lower, self-centered level of moral and conscience functioning to the higher level of consciousness of others. Empathy and role-taking [29] enable one to deal with the questions, "What should I do?" "What is fair, just, and equitable for all concerned?" Self-directed decisions then become more attainable.

Differential opportunities for role-taking among cultures or among individuals within a given culture can have a significant impact on the rate of development of conscience. The fewer opportunities the individual has to participate in peer groups and egalitarian family structures, the slower will be the rate of moral reasoning and conscience development [58].

GUILT AND SHAME
The intrapersonal communication system of the conscience is guilt and shame along with self-approval. It is the cybernetic feeling system. When one violates accepted moral principles, guilt is felt. When one acts in ways that are not socially approved, shame is felt. If

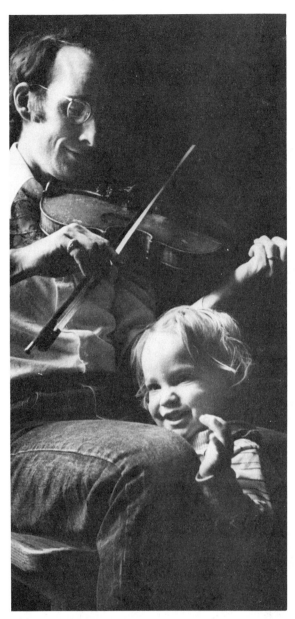

Figure 18–2. Values and aesthetic appreciation are formed by the experiences of early childhood as well as by the influences of the culture and the era.

ered, and self-disapproval will be felt. To avoid these feelings, the individual will attempt either to withstand temptation or to perform his or her duty. The inner positive self-approval that is felt reinforces the function of the conscience and enhances self-direction.

MORAL DEVELOPMENT

The term **moral development** refers to the gradual emergence of the capacity to incorporate more dimensions and higher level structures when making decisions regarding right and wrong. Since "moral" implies the quality of motivation as well as the knowledge of rules and the ability to make decisions, this term suggests that morality follows developmental principles. The type and level of moral development is reflected in behavior. In turn, the individual's behavior provides a consistent index to the degree of self-direction the individual has achieved thus far in the developmental process.

Aspects
Moral behavior involves the ability to make judgments in complex situations. Clearly, infants and very young children are incapable of these kinds of actions and decisions. They are too egocentric, too impulsive, too uninformed. A moral decision necessitates the ability to envision alternatives, and to anticipate the possible consequences of alternative choices. It requires positive, assertive action in some situations and self-restraining efforts in others (resisting temptations). At times moral behavior requires one to "go with the crowd," to engage in some assertive actions that advance the well-being, the happiness, and the good of self and others. At other times, one feels the evils in society must be protested, and moral behavior will dictate, for example, the participation in public demonstrations that support human rights issues, women's equality, or the opposition to the nuclear arms race.

Stages of Moral Development
Moral behavior depends on the cognitive development of the individual. Progressive moral maturation unfolds with intellectual development as well as with purposeful training. This unfolding has been described as the stages of moral development. The degree to which purposeful training by significant adults can accelerate the movement from lower to higher levels of moral functioning has not been clearly established by research. However, the various levels have been quite clearly articulated by Peck [51] and Kohlberg [35, 36].

an individual's behavior is consistent with a self-concept and a value system, the individual will feel self-approval. On the other hand, if an individual's behavior contradicts a personal value system, the conscience will register shame and guilt. Self-esteem will be low-

PECK'S FIVE LEVELS

Peck found a strong correlation between cognitive developmental periods and the predominant characteristics of the various levels of moral behavior [51].

Amoral. The amoral level is typical of infancy. At this early stage, the infant has neither the knowledge nor the self-direction to respond to any motivation but that of meeting immediate personal needs and desires. Behavior is impulsive and insensitive and is expressed without regard for its effect on others or its degree of conformity to societal expectations. The individuals who become arrested at this level are called sociopathic, that is, they have no internalized moral principles. They are egocentric in their interpersonal relationships and have no sense of remorse or guilt when they behave in ways that violate societal expectations. These individuals are blind to the moral implications of their behavior and its impact on others.

Expedient. The expedient level of moral behavior is most characteristic of early childhood. At this stage, children behave in ways that are mostly self-serving, which will gain for them perceived advantages. These advantages may be in the punishments avoided by being obedient or the rewards distributed for compliance to an authority figure's demands. In fact, these children are still very ego-centered but are willing to forgo short-term self-indulgence in order to obtain longer-term advantages. They see other persons as primarily the means by which they can satisfy their present, pressing wants and needs. These children behave in subtle ways that manipulate others for their own selfish ends. In the absence of external authority, they do what they want to do. Their behavior is characterized by an overall self-centeredness.

As adults, expedient persons have no internalized set of moral behavior codes. They manipulate their interpersonal relationships and give as little of themselves to others as possible. They see other persons only as objects to be used to satisfy their impulsive wants and not as persons of intrinsic worth.

Conforming. The conforming level of moral development is most characteristic of late childhood. Children conform to the group's demands on them. They take their behavioral cues from other persons and groups. When the peer group expects specific social or religious behaviors, the individual will behave consistently with these expectations. When the peer group rewards immoral or socially nonconforming behavior,

the individual will do what the crowd expects, even if such behavior violates earlier training. The basic rule is, "When in Rome, do as the Romans do." Ethics are based on the situation rather than a core set of principles. Behavior is externally mediated. As adults, such individuals may be faithful to their marriage commitments and church vows when at home. When they attend a convention in a distant city, they may forget those commitments. The attitude is that a behavior is OK if you don't get caught.

Conforming individuals have internalized few principles of moral responsibility on which to build their characters. They feel little guilt whenever they break a rule. They may experience shame in some cases because they are quite concerned about what others think of them but will feel no guilt for violating principles of honesty, loyalty, or truthfulness.

Irrational-Conscientious. The irrational-conscientious level of moral development may characterize individuals in later childhood and/or early adolescence. They are at the opposite end of the obedience-to-rules spectrum from conforming persons. These individuals have an internalized code of moral behavior to which they rigidly adhere, applying this code to themselves and to others almost without exception. The rules must be upheld and enforced; the penalty must be imposed without mercy or amelioration, and there is no consideration of extenuating circumstances or motives. They are as demanding of themselves as they are of others.

Because of such high personal expectations and their intolerance of individual failure, these individuals are often besieged with deep feelings of guilt and shame when failing to act in a morally acceptable manner. In severe instances, such persons may need psychotherapy to help free them from the bonds of irrational guilt.

On the positive side, irrational-conscientious persons try very hard to behave morally and to uphold the moral expectations of their religious faith and society. They become deeply involved in social issues. Perhaps because of many of them, the quality of life in their communities is significantly better.

Rational-Altruistic. The rational-altruistic level of moral development includes adolescents and adults who have moved beyond merely fulfilling legal rules to implementing internalized principles. They have not abandoned articulated rules altogether, but they use them as guides for moral behaviors. They have adopted the "good-of-others" principle as their operational

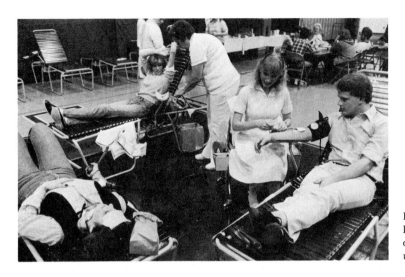

Figure 18–3. The American Red Cross Bloodmobile offers young people the opportunity to translate their inner values into active concern for others.

value system. They constantly seek to direct their behavior in all societal interactions and relationships in ways that implement their basic principles. Thus they choose courses of action based on reason rather than impulse as much as possible. They seek to enhance the welfare of others as much as their own, even if they must curtail the satisfaction of their own needs to do so.

At this level, persons seek to work with others in constructive ways. They enjoy life; they are not afraid to express their emotional reactions in appropriate ways. They are authentic persons because their conceptual and operational values are closely correlated. They are well-adjusted and quite undefensive about their actions. They admit their errors; they feel guilt and shame at times, but seek earnestly to rectify their mistakes, make amends, and restore the damaged egos of others. In short, they are fully developed moral persons, who try to behave conscientiously and morally because it is the right thing to do, and not merely to escape a guilty conscience or societal censure.

Summary. As adults, few individuals will fit into any one particular stage all the time. Different social situations and complex moral dilemmas may evoke different behaviors. Thus some persons may adopt the expedient response in one situation and the rational-altruistic in another. The businessman who gives generously of his time and money in community activities may be afraid to protest female discrimination at his company because it is an unpopular cause. Or, when

dealing with their children, some parents may be irrational-conscientious but may be rational-altruistic when interacting with other adults.

KOHLBERG'S THEORY
The interest in moral development has been greatly stimulated by the work of Lawrence Kohlberg [35, 36] who classified moral development into three levels with each level further divided into stages. The levels and stages move gradually from the extreme egocentrism of the neonate to the adults who are willing to die for their faith.

Preconventional Level. Moral behavior at the preconventional level is egocentric. The moral quality of an activity is determined by what the action will do for the individual. Whatever brings pleasure and helps the person to escape pain is morally right.

This level is divided into three stages. Stage 0 is characterized by the feeling that whatever is wanted and liked is morally acceptable. If children obtain what they want, they will show love to the adult; if they receive pain or are frustrated in their selfish pursuits, they will react with anger and rejection.

By the end of the second year, children are moving into stage 1. They will obey and perform as expected because they fear the power of an authority figure. All actions are grounded on the basis of fear and the avoidance of punishment. At this stage, might makes right. The potential physical consequence of an act is the major reason the child obeys.

At approximately 4 years of age, children move into stage 2. They try to "do good" because the consequences are personally advantageous. Children see others as the principal source for meeting needs, so that their approach to others is principally with the attitude, "I'll do this for you, if you'll do that for me;" and "On the other hand, if you hurt me, I'll hurt you." Thus their moral code is that of an "eye-for-an-eye."

Conventional Level. At this level, children begin to appreciate other people's feelings and the desire to please other people increases. Children have also begun to internalize the expectations of others and sincerely want the high regard of these important persons. They begin to judge the moral quality of their own and others' actions on the basis of partially internalized social codes.

During the early school years (7 to 8 years of age), children progress to stage 3. By now, children have become aware of the moral values of others. Their basic premise for deciding how to act is the kind of behavior they think parents or peer group would approve. Children are very anxious to please and to help others as well as to perpetuate the stereotypical images of what is appropriate. They are aware of their own and others' intentions, thus they temper judgments and decisions. Expediency takes precedence over integrity.

Stage 4 begins to develop at about 10 years of age. This stage is called the law-and-order stage. Moral decisions are made on the basis of established authority. Authorities establish the rules for the good of society. Morality is demonstrated by "doing your duty," or "obeying the law," because it **is** the law. The authority source may be a teacher, a parent, or a scout leader. For adults functioning at this level, the authority source may be the employer, a social or religious group, the legal system, or the conventions of the culture. In any case, the rules must be obeyed if society is to be stable.

Postconventional Level. The postconventional level is the highest level of moral development, and according to Kohlberg, is attained by only a few. At this level, principles are the basis of moral decisions. These principles, thoughtfully deduced by the individual, reflect a concern for the welfare and dignity of living beings and are capable of universal application.

The emergence of stage 5 depends on the cognitive skills associated with formal operational thinking (see Chap. 26). Rules are not arbitrarily imposed but are social contracts with specific purposes. The good of

the majority is more important than the rule itself. Moral decisions are influenced by reason, the rights of others, or the welfare of the whole group. Sometimes exceptions to the rules must be made; for example, "the end does not justify the means."

The person achieving stage 6 is characterized as mature, moral, self-motivated, and self-evaluating. The individual has a fully internalized set of ethical principles that are accepted as the individual's guidelines for behavior. At times a person's principles may demand disobedience to the rules of civil authority if actions stemming from the rules violate personal principles. A person may see his or her ethical value system as universal, extending beyond mere laws or guidelines that are written. This person does what is considered to be right, regardless of legal restrictions or the opinion of others (e.g., a strong stance on the abortion issue). An individual functioning at this level could not undertake an action that would purposely harm the self or another person. People who reach stage 6 act in accordance with internalized standards knowing they would condemn themselves if their basic principles were violated. Integrity takes precedence over expediency. Few people achieve this level of moral development or the proposed next level.

Recently Kohlberg [36] has suggested a seventh stage. This stage involves an infinite, cosmic orientation that includes an awareness of the "reason for existence" for the individual. The individual internalizes principles that go beyond the teachings of an organized religion to a consideration of the self as a part of the cosmic order [58]. Persons in stage 6 may be willing to **die** for their principles, but persons in stage 7 are willing to **live** for their beliefs—a much more difficult task.

Table 18–1. Kohlberg's Level of Moral Development

Level	Stage	Age	Underlying Principles
Preconventional	0	0–2	Do what pleases me
	1	2–3	Avoid punishment
	2	4–7	Do what benefits me
Conventional	3	7–10	Avoid disapproval
	4	10–12	Do duty, obey laws
Postconventional	5	13–	Maintain respect of others
	6	15–	Implement personal principles
	7	18–	Live by eternal, universal principles

Only the rare individual achieves this level. Socrates, Joan of Arc, Martin Luther King, Jr., and Mother Teresa of Calcutta represent a few such individuals.

GILLIGAN'S THEORY

Carol Gilligan [26], working with Kohlberg at Harvard, has challenged the rigid stage theory of Kohlberg. She observes that most research and writing on moral development has been done by males with a heavy component of male subjects to form the basis for their conclusions. Gilligan contends that the female's pronounced orientation toward empathy and caring tends to place her at a less advanced stage of moral reasoning when Kohlberg's model is used.

Gilligan's research involved 29 women who came to a research center after being referred to it by various abortion and pregnancy-counseling centers. The women were of diverse ages, ethnic backgrounds, socioeconomic levels, and marital statuses. They were interviewed in the first trimester of pregnancy while they were making a decision about having an abortion. During the interview, the women were asked about the decision they faced, how they felt their decision would affect their relationship with others, and how they felt about themselves. They were also asked to respond to Kohlberg's classic presentation of a moral dilemma: Heinz, whose wife was sick and facing certain death, was unable to secure the curative drug. The local druggist was unwilling to make a cure he had discovered available to Heinz except for an exorbitant price. Kohlberg asked his subjects what they would do and why if they were in the same situation.

Gilligan concludes that because men and women experience attachment and separation in different ways, each sex perceives a danger that the other does not see—men in connection, women in separation. Thus, women construct the moral problem as an issue of "care and responsibilities in relationships rather than as one of rights and rules" [26]. Moral thinking is tied to the development of changes in their understanding of responsibilities and relationships. Their conception of morality as justice ties development to the logic of equality and reciprocity [26].

Gilligan feels that the different parameters used by men and women for making moral decisions should not be regarded as the basis for judging one moral development system superior to another, but must be seen as a true difference. While this statement is not denied, when comparative studies of moral development are made of males and females, no statistically significant differences are found [25, 64].

INFLUENCES AFFECTING THE CONSCIENCE AND MORAL DEVELOPMENT

The influences that are basic to the development of self-discipline are factors such as self-concept, patterns of discipline used by families, and the emotional-social interaction systems that characterize the families in which children are reared.

Self-Concept

One's self-concept plays a critical role in determining interpersonal relationships [48]. Those with poor self-concepts see themselves as inferior and may become withdrawn and/or may refrain from taking a stand on a moral issue until they know what the crowd wants. They find it difficult to relate to others in a give-and-take situation. Or, they may adopt a compensatory reaction pattern that seeks to draw attention to themselves by engaging in bizarre behavior or to gain peer acceptance by performing immoral or antisocial acts as proof of their "self-confidence."

Individuals with realistic self-concepts who have learned to know and to accept themselves are released from the constraints of overconformity and undue submission to authority. They are self-directing, autonomous and self-reliant, and free from overdependence on the approval of others. Thus the conscience and moral decisions are under their own control [19].

Patterns of Discipline

Research has shown some correlation between the patterns of discipline used by the family and the development of personality patterns in children [7, 33, 53, 54, 59]. Discipline has many meanings. To some, it means guiding children to self-actualization and self-discipline; to others, it means harsh, punitive control of another person's behavior. In the context of this discussion, the purpose of discipline is to teach children acceptable societal behavior patterns and prepare them for successful adulthood. On the part of adults, discipline is a conscious and continuous effort to assist children to develop all their capacities and potentials.

PARAMETERS

In spite of the difficulty of assessment, parental behaviors and disciplinary practices generally fall within the discernible axes of love versus hostility and autonomy versus control (see Fig. 18–5).

Love versus Hostility. Loving parents are described as trying to see life through their children's eyes; accept-

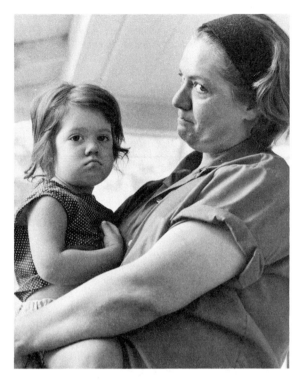

Figure 18–4. Discipline is difficult for both the adult and the child because the goals of each appear to be temporarily thwarted. However, when respect for the individual is maintained, even difficult situations can prove to be growth-producing for both.

ing their uniqueness; respecting their freedoms and rights; affirming their intrinsic worth frequently; explaining the basis for rules to them; and shaping their behavior by frequent, positive rewards rather than physical punishment or other harsh restraints. Parents characterized as hostile would be inclined to treat their children in an exactly opposite manner.

Autonomy versus Control. Parents who allow their children an increasing amount of freedom to make decisions as they develop would be placed on the autonomy extreme of the axis. They would make few demands on their children and would impose their personal expectations on them only when the children's developmental stage did not provide the necessary physical, social, or intellectual skills for the children to cope successfully with the specific environmental demands they were facing. The imposed parental expectations would be prompted by the par-

ents' concern for the children's needs and development toward self-direction and self-actualization and not by the need for convenience and comfort on the part of the parents. Freedom would be increased as the children gained the required skills.

Such parents would be more tolerant and accepting of children's behaviors, such as sexual exploration, immodesty in very young children, a noisy atmosphere, and verbal and physical aggression toward others, since these parents have fewer restrictions on, and lower expectations about, these behaviors. Controlling, restrictive parents would be much less tolerant and would structure their expectations for their children to be more consistent with adult behaviors.

Other Factors. The axes of love versus hostility and autonomy versus control provide the identifiable parameters of Figure 18–5. However, their implementation by parents involves other factors that strongly affect child-rearing practices and disciplinary concepts. For example, one set of parents may allow their children a high degree of autonomy and freedom, but they do so in a calm and detached manner. Their disciplinary pattern would be described as democratic. Another set of parents may allow the same degree of freedom, but they are motivated by anxiety and emotional involvement. These parents would be described as indulgent.

Another factor is the parent-centered versus child-centered orientation on the dimensions that describe the love-hostility axis. Generally parents who are rigid, demanding, and dictatorial are more concerned with their own comfort, rights, freedoms, and pleasure than those of their children. At the opposite pole are those parents who respect their children's rights and seek to guide them. They regard discipline as something done **for** and **with** children, not **to** them [2]. When all the factors are considered in their possible combinations, several probable outcomes of these variables can be plotted on the model shown in Figure 18–5.

EFFECTS ON PERSONALITY DEVELOPMENT
The various combinations of parental disciplinary practices used in rearing children have differing short-term and long-term effects on the children's personality development. The greater the component of freedom and love tempered by calm detachment on the part of the parents, the greater the degree of self-discipline and the happier and better adjusted socially are the children. Even restrictive practices administered with love and acceptance have beneficial results [5, 6].

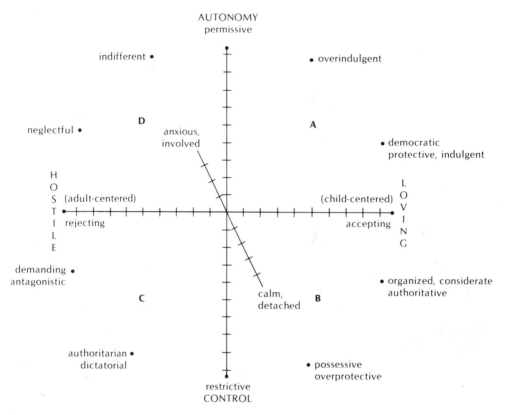

Figure 18–5. Three-dimensional hypothetical model of parental behaviors and attitudes toward the child (anxious-involved versus calm-detached is the arm of the third dimension).

Children of hostile, rejecting parents generally have poor self-discipline and make poor social adjustments, regardless of whether or not the parents are effective in their control.

Permissive-Accepting (Quadrant A). Parents who are permissive and accepting are regarded by some psychologists as being ideal parents. They allow their children the freedom to make choices and to be themselves and accept their behaviors, even undesirable ones, in a calm and detached manner. This does not mean they do not try to shape their children's behavior, but they do so by using positive reinforcement rather than punishment. They let children suffer the logical consequences of their behavior. As the children mature, freedom is increased. Rules are established by cooperation and the consent of the family members. In short, they are democratic parents.

Such parents tend to have children who are more likely to adopt adult roles [39] and who are low in hostility toward others as well as extroverted, active, au-

tonomous, and creative [7, 33, 42]. Outsiders, however, may see such children as being disrespectful toward adults, dominating and aggressive toward their peers, and at times disobedient at home.

If the parents tend to be more anxious and emotionally involved than detached, they are more likely to be overly indulgent. Their children are more likely to behave on the basis of their feelings rather than being self-directing. Nevertheless, even though these children may appear spoiled to outsiders, they are likely to become sociable, achieving, highly motivated individuals.

Restrictive-Accepting (Quadrant B). Authoritative parents have high expectations for their children and exercise considerable control over them [6]. Their child-rearing practices reflect what they themselves are; they are models of what they expect their children to become. Even though these parents are restrictive, they are loving and accepting. They consciously seek to earn the right to exercise authority over their children and do not impose authority because of their inherent right as parents to do so. They tend to be calm and detached in their dealings with their children.

Children raised by such parents have a positive self-concept [15] and are highly motivated, self-actualizing, and self-directing individuals. However, they tend to be less creative and more introverted, dependent, and conforming than children of permissive-accepting parents.

The effect of restrictiveness varies with the age of the child [33]. Prior to 3 years of age, restrictiveness has more long-term inhibitory effects than it does when it is imposed between 4 and 10 years of age. Early restrictiveness produces greater dependence, whereas in older children it results in more hostility and aggressiveness toward the parents, especially the mother.

On the other hand, overly protective parents are more anxious and emotionally involved with their children. They impose strict controls because they want to shield their children from the harsh realities of life, not to help them to develop their social skills. Children of such parents are frequently immature, dependent, and introverted; they resent controls and the smothering, solicitous attitudes of their parents. They may not become the autonomous, self-actualized individuals they should be because they were denied the opportunities to set their own goals, to solve their own problems, and to experience the success or the failure of their own decisions.

Restrictive-Rejecting (Quadrant C). Parents described as being restrictive-rejecting are either authoritarian and dictatorial or demanding and antagonistic. Authoritarian parents are classic examples of all that child-rearing experts deplore. They exercise rigid control and impose arbitrary rules on their children. Punishment is frequently used to shape the child's behavior. Because these parents are adult-centered, they cannot empathize with the problems the child faces in the world as he or she perceives it. The difference between the authoritarian and the demanding parent is the degree of emotional involvement. Authoritarian, dictatorial parents are calm and detached as well as rejecting; demanding, antagonistic parents are anxious and emotionally involved.

Children of restrictive-rejecting parents tend to be more neurotic than other children [34, 53, 54]. Since they cannot express their hostility outwardly and openly, they repress and internalize it [7]. Consequently, they feel a strong need to punish themselves even for minor misdeeds, have more suicidal tendencies, and are more accident-prone than other children. They are also more introverted, more socially inept and unresponsive, less motivated, shyer, and more immature than other children [33].

Authoritarian parents may have different effects on the personalities of their children when they become adolescents [51]. As young children, they conformed to their parents' demands as long as they could reasonably expect to be punished for their misbehavior. When the parents were out of sight and the children felt they could break rules and not be punished, they were more likely to do so. As adolescents, such individuals merely conform to what is expected of them

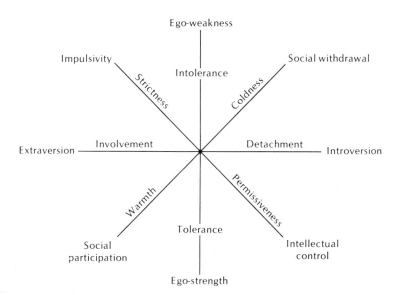

Figure 18–6. Relationship between personality and perceived parental behavior. (From P. E. Slater, Parental behavior and personality of the child. *J. Genet. Psychol.* 101:65, 1962. With permission.)

by the immediate social group. If they are in a situation where the pressure to conform is absent, they will disregard the rules. For example, a young person goes away to college and is arrested for shoplifting or becomes involved in an activity that is extremely atypical of his or her life-style at home. Why? In the past, this person had merely conformed to parental and peer pressure without internalizing his or her own value or self-discipline system.

The alternative possibility is that children will internalize authoritarian models as a part of their personalities. In this instance, they develop into strict, legalistic adults, who strongly enforce the rules regardless of their appropriateness or their effect on another's physical or psychological well-being. Often such individuals find their place in society as policemen or prison guards when they become adults. Milgrim's research [46] provides a chilling profile of the behaviors this extremely authoritarian personality is capable of carrying out—the ultimate of the "irrational-conscientious" person [51].

Permissive-Rejecting (Quadrant D). Parents in the permissive-rejecting category are either indifferent or neglectful; both are equally detrimental in their effects on children's behaviors. The parents are neither involved nor controlling. Children reared in this environment are confused about their own intrinsic worth as a result of this lack of love and structure; they equate such detachment with their own worthlessness and inadequacy. They have a poor self-concept [15] and are hostile toward their parents. They are also more likely to be impulsive and aggressive toward their environment and other persons [7]. To alleviate their repressed hostility, they are more likely to "act out" their anger and to engage in delinquent behavior as adolescents to achieve peer acceptance, which they feel powerless to gain in socially acceptable activities [33, 45].

Implications. From the preceding discussion, it appears that democratic and authoritative parents are more likely to rear children who have higher levels of self-direction, a more positive, healthy self-concept, more motivation, and a greater degree of self-actualization [15]. These children are more likely to move into the principled level of Kohlberg's moral development model. It is highly probable that they will become rational and altruistic adults who have internalized their own moral principles and implement them in such a way as to promote the well-being of others [51]. They tend to be self-reliant, happy children and adults. On the other hand, parents who are hostile, rejecting, and

self-centered tend to produce children who are immature, shy, and outer-controlled. Homes in which hostile, rejecting parents impose strict discipline inconsistently or are highly permissive produce children who are more likely to act out their aggression and, as juveniles, to become antisocial and to engage in delinquent behavior.

Thus far the discussion has imposed all the responsibility on the parents for how their children turn out. However, not all who have studied theories of discipline agree totally with this concept. One writer points out, " . . . a study finding a correlation between severe punishment and children's aggressiveness is often taken to show that harsh discipline produces aggressive children, yet it could show instead that aggressive children evoke harsh child-rearing methods in their parents" [58]. The question is a valid one. Do aggressive, self-assertive children tend to view their parents as being harsh, punitive, and authoritarian more than do compliant children? Or do such "difficult" children stimulate harsh, punitive, authoritarian reactions in their parents? Further research is needed to establish the causative factors in children's personality development [59].

IMPLEMENTATION OF DISCIPLINE

Although research indicates that the most desirable patterns of applying parental discipline are the authoritative and democratic ones, not all parents use them. Each set of parents implements the methods and processes of discipline in their own manner. While the specific reasons for variations in implementation of discipline are complex and multifaceted, some generalizations are valid.

Variables. Why do certain parents discipline their children the way they do? A part of the answer is supplied by the personality of the child and another part by the specific situation involved. Probably the past experiences and the personalities of the parents themselves provide the most important variables. Parents with high self-esteem are more likely to rear children who have high self-esteem [47].

Parental Perceptions of Themselves. Parents who have a healthy, positive self-concept feel more confident in their parental role. They are more likely to perceive their children as unique individuals who are the objects of, and partners in, the teaching-learning enterprise of family living. Parents with a poor self-concept tend to view their children as extensions of themselves and try to force their children to achieve their own previously unfulfilled goals rather than allowing the children to strive for goals of their own choosing. By imposing their own goals on their children, parents generate hostility in the children, ensure lowered achievement, and increase parent-child hostility and friction.

Previous Experiences. Parents tend to adopt the disciplinary patterns they themselves experienced from their parents. To the extent that parental discipline affects personality development, as discussed above, discipline becomes self-perpetuating. If the model was harsh and punitive, it is likely to be imitated [3]. Since spanking frequently involves more emotion and less reason on the part of parents than other types of discipline, it is easily perpetuated in succeeding generations. Many parents who batter their children were themselves the victims of abuse as children.

This fact may explain the increasing number of children in contemporary Western society who are abused, battered, or killed by their parents. When the parent's adult-centered need for rigid restrictiveness is motivated by repressed hostility and displaced onto the child under the guise of "making him behave," the parent is prone to lose control and the child becomes another statistic of child battering. Or, if the parent feels lonely and isolated, with no one to share problems, he or she vents the anger onto the child.

Temperaments of Children and Parents. Neonates generally fall into three categories: "easy," "difficult," and "slow to warm up" [12, 63]. Easy infants are warm, cuddly, and regular in their biological rhythms. They adjust to new situations with a minimum of frustration. Difficult infants react to new stimuli by withdrawing or becoming irritable. They are often negative in their responses and do not adjust quickly to novel situations. On the other hand, slow-to-warm-up babies will respond to new stimuli if allowed to do so gradually. They tend to retreat from close contact with other persons.

These different temperaments affect discipline in two ways. Since these patterns of responses tend to persist into adulthood, parents have their own peculiar way of interacting with their children. To the extent that the child's temperament evokes a particular response from the adult and that this response is involved in patterns of discipline, the child influences the type of discipline received. Thus if the parent was a difficult child, he or she is more likely to be punitive toward a difficult child; an easy-tempered parent is inclined to be more accepting of a difficult child.

If parents are disappointed with their child's temperament and either openly or subtly hold the easy pattern as their preference, they may fail to reinforce the difficult or slow-to-warm-up responses. Indirectly, they will communicate to the child his or her inadequacy. Since the child cannot understand the reason the parents are displeased and cannot change the parents' feelings, he or she may become anxious and develop low self-esteem.

PROCESS OF DISCIPLINE

Discipline may be implemented in positive, punitive, or counterproductive ways. Positive methods depend on rewarding acceptable behavior. Punitive processes involve the withholding of rewards or the infliction of painful consequences on the child for unacceptable behavior. Some of the ways in which parents discipline their children are counterproductive, defeating the purposes of discipline.

Positive Processes. Effective discipline results when adults and parents consciously plan strategies of behavior management. Parents and other adults who believe that discipline basically involves teaching children to be autonomous, socialized individuals can learn to apply these principles to guide children's behavior [6]. First, the parents must decide and agree on the type of behavior they want their children to learn or which behaviors they want to change. They then discuss with the children and agree on the expectations and the rewards to be given for successful accomplishment of a specific task. Parents are responsible for observing the children's behavior and for consistently rewarding their successes. A chart of the desired behavior and progress toward reaching it must be kept. Older children find that self-monitoring and recording of successes provides motivation for them to maintain the desired behavior. Obviously, parental expectations must be compatible with the developmental level of the child.

Rewards must be chosen carefully; they are effective only when they are what the child wants. Often children will express a strong desire for something (e.g., a new bicycle or going to a baseball game). Or, parents can use television viewing, allowing an overnight guest, or even chewing gum or serving a favorite dessert as rewards. Tokens may be earned and saved toward a more significant reinforcer. In any case, the parents must have total control of the reward. The children must not be able to circumvent the requirements and still receive the reward; otherwise the behavior management system breaks down and the children learn how to manage the system rather than their own behavior. Therefore, persons who plan to implement a behavior management program should be sure of the goals and contingencies as well as the behavior-modification principles before starting.

In addition to extrinsic rewards, parents find social rewards to be effective. Children want to be loved and appreciated by their parents and other adults; they are rewarded by compliments and verbal approval just as adults are. Statements such as "I'm glad you remembered" or "I appreciate your help with the dishes" are very rewarding to the other person. Verbal approval should always accompany extrinsic rewards.

Rewards may be either unexpected or contracted. After the child has done something the parent appreciates, the child can be thanked: "Thank you, Susie, for being so quiet while your baby brother was asleep." Or, the parent may give the child a cool drink and say, "Because you were so quiet while your baby brother was sleeping, here is a glass of orange juice."

Several results evolve from the use of such techniques. Because children are treated as individuals, and not as objects to be manipulated through love or adult power, they become inner-directed persons. They learn that they are involved in what happens to them and assume the responsibility for their own behavior; this is the best insurance against the helplessness syndrome and the "copping out" complex. They also learn to respect the individuality, rights, and freedoms of other children and adults. In short, positive methods of behavior-shaping help children to attain the goal of discipline—self-discipline.

Children learn to trust others through this process, since parents involved in bargaining are careful not to agree to give a reward that is impossible for them to fulfill. They must also be extremely careful to keep their end of the bargain when the children have fulfilled theirs. Once the reward has been promised it must be given. To be trusted as a parent by an adolescent, one must have built a foundation of trust throughout the child's earlier years.

Punitive Measures. Unfortunately too many parents equate discipline with punishment. Punishment may take either of two forms. The parent may actively inflict pain on the child by spanking. Or, the parent may withhold a positive reward or curtail temporarily the child's freedom because of the misbehavior. Of the two forms, the second is the most desirable and effective. If the child disobeys by going outside after being told to stay in, the parent may require the child to sit on a chair for a brief period of time.

Spanking is not as effective. Usually the result is that the child will obey as long as the parent is around to observe and to enforce the rule. Should the child think a behavior will not be noticed, the child will disregard the parental admonition.

Perhaps a more serious consequence of spanking is the possibility of escalating its severity. When persons give vent to strong emotions, they often experience an increasing intensity of it. Thus, when the parent is angry with the child and begins to spank the child, the parent's level of anger may increase uncontrollably. As a result the child may suffer injuries or even death.

Because of the increasing incidents of child abuse, several groups are strongly proposing that spanking be prohibited in this country as it is in Sweden. In most public schools, spanking has been banned because of its ineffectiveness as well as its dangers. The goals of discipline can usually be accomplished by the positive methods.

DENNIS the MENACE

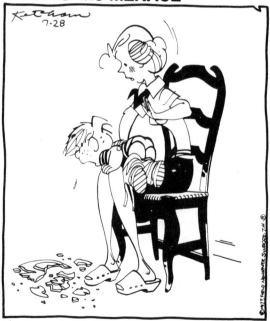

"AM I HAVIN' A UNHAPPY CHILDHOOD?"

Figure 18–7. Reprinted courtesy of *Dennis the Menace.* Copyright Field Newspaper Syndicate, T.M.®

Counterproductive Measures. Whenever parents or caretakers fail to carry through with the threatened consequences of disobedience, make unreasonable demands on children, or use punitive measures too harshly or too frequently, the disciplinary measures become counterproductive in developing self-discipline. Conformity (compliance) or rebellion are generated and passivity or self-assertiveness (aggression) may become the dominant behavioral pattern. In adulthood, the person may become antisocial.

PRINCIPLES OF DISCIPLINE

Effective discipline involves the proper use of some basic principles that apply in all situations to all children (Table 18–2). If properly used, these principles help children to achieve the goals of discipline—guiding them to become self-actualized, self-directed, socialized adolescents and adults.

Consistency. Parental expectations must be uniformly maintained for the children. Behavior that is acceptable today must be required tomorrow; tomorrow's code must reflect the same principles and values as yesterday's. In such a dependable climate, children are less likely to become delinquents [45]. Consistent parental expectations and consequences of behavior result in children who are more highly motivated to control their own behavior, who have better self-concepts [15], and who are happier and better adjusted.

Follow-through. The principles of follow-through entails parental attention to the child's responses to discipline. If the parent tells the child to sit on a chair for 3 minutes as a punishment, the parent must see that the child does so. The length of the sitting must be reasonable and definite. To say, "Sit there until I tell you

to get up" is unfair. It is better to specify the time and to make sure that the child sits there all the time. Most children will attempt to get up earlier. A good response is, "Every such attempt adds 1 more minute to your time."

Pacing. As was discussed earlier, freedom must keep pace with the maturational level of the child. Adolescents need more freedom than do babies; preschoolers require closer supervision than do children in junior high school. Physical intervention may be more appropriate for young children who cannot reason than it is for adolescents. Sometimes older children complain to their parents that they treat the younger siblings differently from the way in which they were treated when they were younger. Usually an explanation to the effect that parents have to learn to parent and that their experiences over the years has given them the confidence they lacked as younger parents will ease the tensions. If siblings understand the principle of individual differences, they can accept the differences in parental disciplinary practices used with older and younger children.

Modeling. Children learn a great deal about behavior by observing and imitating adults' responses [3, 4, 43]. Parents are usually the most influential models. "If you want your child to accept your values when he reaches his teen years, then you must be worthy of his respect during his younger days. . . . This factor is important for . . . parents who wish to sell their concept of God to their children. They must first sell themselves. If they are not worthy of respect, then neither is their religion,

Table 18–2. Basic Principles of Discipline

Principle	Description
Consistency	Rules are applied as uniformly as possible
Follow-through	Reasonable consequences are carried out; no escape for the child
Pacing	Expectations are consistently based on justice and freedom, but adapted to the child's developmental level
Modeling	Adults and parents monitor their own behavior so children learn approved behavior by imitating and identifying with them
Immediate feedback	Consequences of behavior are felt as soon as possible after it occurs, or just before it takes place
Truthfulness	Parents are truthful about their reasons for their expectations
Trust	Adults verbally express trust in, and act trustingly toward, their children until such trust is broken by the children
Logical outcomes	Consequences of behavior are logical results of the behavior
Self-disclosure	Parents are not afraid to disclose their own feelings and mistakes to children
Genuine love	The key to all effective discipline is genuine, unearned love

or their morals, or their government, or their country, or any of their values" [16]. The following remarks are in the same vein: "If they want their children to value honesty, parents must daily demonstrate their own honesty. If they want their children to value generosity, they must behave generously. If they want their children to adopt Christian values, they must behave like Christians themselves. This is the best way, perhaps the **only** way, for parents to 'teach' children their values" [27].

Immediate Feedback. The quicker the consequences of an action are experienced, the more learning takes place. Delayed consequences are ineffective in changing behavior. Although much of the research in this area was conducted on organisms lower than humans, this principle applies to all. Some research [66] found that children who were punished just before they were to engage in a forbidden play activity, or just afterward, had more resistance to engaging in it later than did those whose punishment was delayed. However, because human beings have better memories and verbal skills, delayed punishment is better than none at all. Delayed punishment can be effective with older children if the total situation and the forbidden activity are described and reenacted as fully as possible for the child at the time of punishment [1].

Truthfulness. Adults must be truthful with children at all times. For a parent to tell a child that he or she cannot have a piece of candy because the store is not selling any will make it difficult for the parent to establish credibility when another child is seen to be buying some. Why not tell the child, "When you eat candy you drool all over the front of your clothes. I want you to look neat when we go to your grandmother's house as soon as we leave here." Instead of instructing a child to tell the man at the door that Mommy is not home, why not be honest and tell the child to say, "Mother is not interested in buying anything today."

Trust. Effective child-rearing practices involve trust on the part of both adults and their children. Since parents have the children from birth, they are primarily responsible for establishing a trusting relationship. If parents genuinely trust their children, their offspring will be more likely to hold that trust sacred and inviolate. Adolescents are very sensitive about whether or not their parents trust them [32]. Teenagers are likely to perceive any inquiries from their parents about where they are going after the basketball game as a sign of mistrust and an invasion of privacy. A valid rationale for all such inquiries helps to allay the adolescent's fears about mistrust.

Logical Outcomes. Discipline is effective when the outcomes of behavior are logical consequences of that behavior. If a child disobeys the rule against batting the ball in the back yard and breaks a window, he or she learns more by having to pay for it out of an allowance than by being spanked. If a teenager comes in later than the time agreed upon to be home, he or she may learn more by losing driving privileges than by being denied the television.

Self-Disclosure. Children need to feel that their parents are human and fallible just as they are. They need to know that parents often can and do make mistakes. A parental apology for overreacting in anger when disciplining thereby assures the child that adults are also human. Adolescents take guidance better from parents who can acknowledge that they also made mistakes when they were younger. Does self-disclosure destroy parental authority? On the contrary, it helps to establish it. Self-disclosure helps to bridge the generation gap because parents forsake the citadel of perfection and join the human race as believable persons.

Love. Finally, the most important principle of discipline is love. Adults and parents who really love children rarely fail in raising autonomous, socialized, and self-actualized children. Whatever other mistakes parents may make, they can be overcome when an abundance of love tempered with calmly enforced high expectations characterizes the parent-child relationship.

Love is not an accident; it must be learned and pursued. Some children are easy to love, whereas others are very difficult. A son arrested for dealing in drugs may bring about feelings of anger in his family. An unmarried daughter who is pregnant may bring deep sorrow to a religious family with strong traditional values. Children of all ages, like adults, need love most when others may feel they deserve it least. Love is redemptive, whereas hostility and rejection destroy.

Love cannot be won, earned, bought, or feigned. It is given and deserved because one is human. A boy in nursery school was overheard to say to another child, "Mrs. S. likes me; Mrs. W. loves me."

MAXIMIZING SELF-DIRECTION SKILLS

The need for the ability to direct one's behavior is a lifetime need. The foundations for this ability are laid in childhood but profoundly affect the person through adolescence and adulthood. Some attention needs to be given to this aspect of self-direction.

Childhood

Just as moral development and conscience are profoundly affected by childhood experiences, especially because of the impact of parents and teachers [60], so can significant adults affect self-direction in childhood. They can maximize this by giving specific directions in the development of basic skills essential to self-direction. They can provide opportunities for children to experience self-direction.

SKILLS

Research [47, 48] has shown that children can learn self-control by using self-instructional and self-monitoring techniques. Self-instructional techniques involved preschoolers in telling themselves they were not going to look at a distracting talking "clown box" while they were doing an assigned task [48]. Self-monitoring involved children in recording the instances when they did not pay attention to their assignment in an individualized math curriculum. They were to return to their task whenever they noted these lapses. Sixth graders who used this technique did better and worked longer than did the control group [56]. "Self-monitoring and self-instruction are important means by which children learn to control and regulate their behavior" [48]. The same techniques are useful throughout life.

PARENTAL INITIATIVES IN MORAL DILEMMAS

Biehler [9] urges parents to encourage their children to talk about real moral dilemmas rather than hypothetical ones, especially those dilemmas in which they most likely will be required to make moral choices. Parents can help children feel how immoral behavior hurts another individual [29]. For example, a child whose bike is stolen may react in a "get-even" manner. Parents should help the child realize that unpleasant feelings of hurt and anger provoked by the theft would simply be passed on to another child through any tactics of getting even. The person so affected might then attempt to get even by finding someone else to victimize, and a vicious cycle of hurt and anger would thus be perpetuated. To the extent such empathetic encounters are used, children will be assisted in internalizing their own codes for appropriate behavior.

Parents should be careful not to scold children for failing to act morally in a certain situation but should try to help them understand the specific dynamics of the situation to which they responded.

The story of a child named John illustrates this point. One day John, 6½ years old, came home with a frog

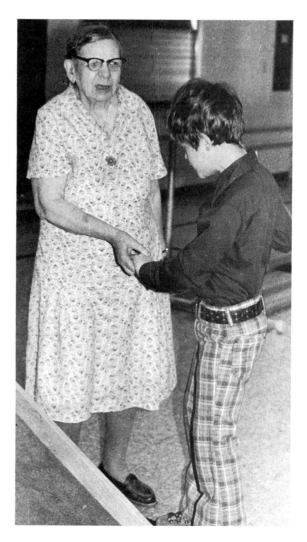

Figure 18–8. Adults can foster an allocentric orientation by offering opportunities for young people to become involved in the needs of other persons.

in a cottage cheese carton. Showing it to his father, he exclaimed, "Isn't this a neat frog, Dad?" Dad agreed it was indeed. About that time, John's sister, 7½ years old, reported to her father that John's friend was crying. "Why is he crying?" Dad asked. "Because John took his frog." Immediately, Dad had several impulses in response to the situation: power-assertion, nonintervention-permissiveness, love-withdrawal, frustration, and moral superiority—"God doesn't love a thief."

However, John's father resisted all such temptations and decided, after ascertaining the facts of the case, to use the incident as training in self-direction. Dad asked John if he would want the results reversed if the facts were reversed (role reversal); that is, would he want his friend Danny to take the frog to his house if it was found in John's yard. John answered quickly, "No way!" Endeavoring to secure empathy, Dad talked to him about Danny's hurt feelings, which did not seem to make much of an impression. An effort to place responsibility by asking "Who is responsible for Danny's hurt?" received only a noncommittal reply: "Man, how should I know?" Only two things were left to do at this point, offer some value education and extend autonomy. Dad endeavored to accomplish the first by saying something like this: "John, your Dad has lived six times as long as you have and may be at least twice as smart as you are at your present level of cognitive development. And there's one thing I've noticed in my lifetime. It's simply this: It has always been easier to find frogs than it is to make friends."

The second objective was attempted by this verbalization: "Now, John, it's time to decide what to do about that frog and that friend. It will be completely your decision. I will never question you about what you do about it or why you do it. There will be no punishment, no matter what you do. You will also, however, be totally responsible for the results of both your decision and your action. The consequences will be yours to live with. It's decision time!" Dad stood up and went into the house, and 20 years later, neither Dad nor John has mentioned that frog to the other. His sister had a tattletale spirit, though, so it was less than 10 minutes before she came and told Dad that John took the frog and gave it back to Danny. Dad still believes that the moral development resulting from the "episode of the frog" was well worth the time and the effort [24].

Hoffman [29] points out that parents can enhance moral development and self-discipline by showing love to their children when they fail. He also suggests that parents can assist the child in developing self-directed moral behavior to the degree that they are willing to admit their own failures to the child. Should the cashier at the supermarket give the parent 50 cents too much in change, the adult should take it back and discuss the reasons for doing so with the child. Or, an adult or a parent who goes through a stop sign should confess the error to the child. A child who sees the human frailties of parents will be better able to understand and to accept his or her own shortcomings.

Parents can also assist children to develop self-direction by assigning certain tasks to them [57]. The family has the responsibility for encouraging and facilitating children's mastery of tasks as they strive toward independence. The major way in which the parents foster mastery of Erikson's task of industry is by gradually increasing children's responsibilities. They can be responsible for setting the table before meals, picking up the clutter in their rooms, or making their beds. Parents will increase the complexity and the amount of the children's responsibility in proportion to their ages, as well as pacing them to the unique needs and opportunities available within the family. Assigned chores contribute to the sense of well-being of children by making them feel important, contributing members of their family systems. The mastery of relatively simple tasks lays the foundation for mastery of the more complex tasks and the responsibilities to be assumed during the adolescent and adult years. Parents rob children of essential opportunities to learn responsibility, perseverance, and self-control when they absorb all the household tasks or are too lenient in standards of task performance. Families, irrespective of socioeconomic level, can provide children with these opportunities.

Adolescence

The transition from childhood to adolescence increases the need for self-direction. Teenagers increasingly move from the close scrutiny of their behavior by their parents into the world of the peer group with its opportunities for greater freedom of choice. Unresolved conflicts of self-concept are intensified as they try to establish an identity. The sexual drive creates new temptations and the peer group exerts increasing social pressures through either acceptance or rejection.

A basic conflict must be faced: The resolution of the ego identity versus role confusion which Erikson proposed [18]. Adolescents ask, "Who am I?" The appeal and the power of a peer group to many youths is its offer of help in resolving this conflict. Adolescents will be able to exercise a balance between self-direction and compliance to the degree they have acquired a realistic self-concept.

Another conflict is the decision adolescents have to make in regard to the value system they will internalize. Will they accept as their own the system they learned from their parents, or will they reject it and find another system? Whichever the outcome, adolescents need the skill to see the alternatives and to weigh the possible outcomes of each. Sometimes this process involves them in a period of trying out other lifestyles, such as joining a cult or experimenting with drugs. In any case, their behavior is an exercise in deciding for themselves and carrying out their decisions. To the degree adolescents escape bearing the brunt of the consequences for their choices, they fail to learn self-discipline.

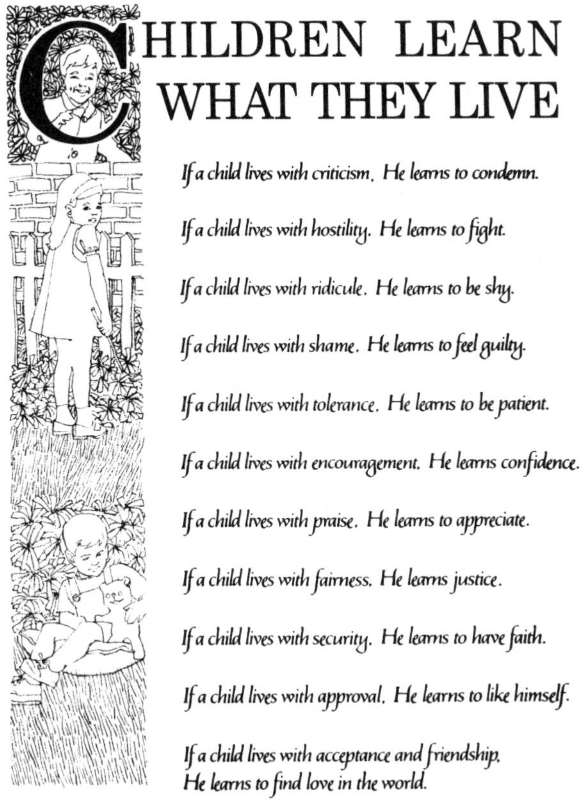

CHILDREN LEARN WHAT THEY LIVE

If a child lives with criticism, He learns to condemn.

If a child lives with hostility, He learns to fight.

If a child lives with ridicule, He learns to be shy.

If a child lives with shame, He learns to feel guilty.

If a child lives with tolerance, He learns to be patient.

If a child lives with encouragement, He learns confidence.

If a child lives with praise, He learns to appreciate.

If a child lives with fairness, He learns justice.

If a child lives with security, He learns to have faith.

If a child lives with approval, He learns to like himself.

If a child lives with acceptance and friendship, He learns to find love in the world.

Figure 18–9. Children learn what they live. Reprinted courtesy of Dorothy Law Nolte and Ross Laboratories.

Implicit in adolescent decision making, of course, is the necessity for adults and parents to discuss clearly the alternatives open to adolescents that will help them envision the consequences. But in the last analysis, parents must allow youth to make their own choices and to accept the consequences, even though the decision seems to be the wrong one to the adults.

Parents should continue to assign some responsibilities to adolescents for household tasks. Failure to fulfill the tasks should incur the denial of freedoms and privileges. Faithful cooperation will bring rewards. Self-direction will be learned as the youths learn to assume and to fulfill responsibilities appropriate for them.

Adulthood

Perhaps the ultimate test of self-direction is faced in adulthood when individuals achieve relative independence and freedom. They make commitments to mar-

riage partners, careers, jobs, and families. If individuals have achieved a satisfactory development of conscience and morality, and have acquired the skills of self-monitoring and self-instruction along with a healthy self-concept, they will be able to assume and fulfill their commitments and responsibilities with little outside coercion. These individuals will reinforce self-direction as they realize the inner satisfaction and peace that its exercise brings to them.

CONCLUSION

Parenting is an awesome but exciting challenge. The parents who can balance the five L's (love, limits, learning, liberty, liability) [23] discover that they themselves continue to grow and to develop as individuals because discipline's goals of self-direction, self-actualization, and socialization are accomplished by the parents as well as the children.

1. Every child has the right to be **loved** unconditionally. Not loved "if" or loved "when," rather, each child should be accepted with a positive regard, which includes care, concern, contact, communication, cuddling, caring, caressing (so many words begin with "care"). The child's total environment should be love; the child should never have to worry or wonder if he or she is loved.
2. Every child needs **limits**, physically, emotionally, mentally, socially, morally, and spiritually. Limits

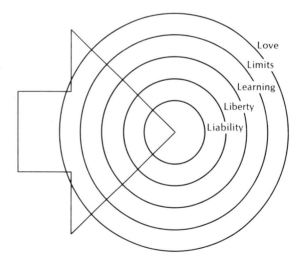

Figure 18–10. Child-rearing on target. (Adapted and expanded by Jarrell W. Garsee from a model proposed by Jerome Folkman.)

must not be provided for the convenience of the parent but always for the safety of the child and his or her proper development. Limits must be realistic, flexible, capable of being changed at different need levels, and consistent.

3. Every child needs examples and an environment conducive to appropriate **learning,** a process that includes good modeling and:
   a. Telling a child what is expected
   b. Explaining why it is expected
   c. Defining the consequences if something is not done
   d. Showing a child how to do what is expected
   e. Sharing the task with the child; doing it together
   f. Watching the child perform the task
   g. Evaluating the results
   h. Rewarding positively the appropriate response
   i. Rewarding negatively the inappropriate response
      As can be seen, discipline (disciplining) is a vital part of learning (and teaching).
4. Every child needs **liberty** to develop the ability to make appropriate choices. Begin with small decisions; help the child to evaluate the differences between bad, good, better, and best decisions.
5. Every child needs to assume the **liability** for the consequences of behavioral choices.

These five factors must be kept in relative balance—not too much or too little of any one of them—if child development is to proceed optimally. The factors are like circles that must gradually expand outward to increase individual responsibility and function with each new level of increased ability and maturity on the part of the child. The cause for disruption in communication between parents and child can often be diagnosed by endeavoring to evaluate which of these factors is not in proper proportion to a child's particular level of development. When the five circles have expanded outward to the point where an individual bears all liability, has optimal liberty, imposes the environment for self-learning, sets limits for the self, and is capable of unselfish, reciprocal love, that individual is ready to begin a new generation and to build a marriage, a home, and an independent life [23].

Self-discipline emerges gradually over a lifetime as the individual considers alternatives, establishes goals, commits the self to action, delays immediate gratification, and considers the effects of behavior on others besides the self. Satisfaction and self-esteem emerge from the ability to operationalize the conceptual value system with available skills.

REFERENCES

1. Aronfreed, J. The Concept of Internalization. In D. A. Goslin (Ed.), *Handbook of Socialization Theory and Research.* Chicago: Rand, McNally, 1969.
2. Auerback, A. B. *The Why and How of Discipline* (rev. ed.). New York: Child Study Association of America, 1974.
3. Bandura, A. M. The Role of the Modeling Processes in Personality Development. In A. M. Snadowsky (Ed.), *Child and Adolescent Development.* New York: Free Press, 1973.
4. Bandura, A. M., and Walters, R. H. *Adolescent Aggression.* New York: Ronald Press, 1959.
5. Baumrind, D. Current Patterns of Parental Authority. In R. F. Biehler, *Developmental Psychology: An Introduction* (2nd ed.). Boston: Houghton Mifflin, 1981.
6. Baumrind, D. Authoritarian *vs.* Authoritative Parental Control. In J. F. Rosenbith, et al. (Eds.). *Readings in Child Development.* Boston: Allyn and Bacon, 1973.
7. Becker, W. C. Consequences of Different Kinds of Parental Discipline. In M. L. Hoffman and L. W. Hoffman (Eds.), *Review of Child Development Research.* Vol. I, New York: Russell Sage Foundation, 1964.
8. Berne, P. H., and Savary, L. M. *Building Self-esteem in Children.* New York: Continuum, 1981.
9. Biehler, R. F. *Developmental Psychology: An Introduction* (2nd Ed.). Boston: Houghton Mifflin, 1981.
10. Boverman, I., et al. Sex-role stereotypes: A current appraisal. *Journal of Social Issues* 28:59–78. 1972.
11. Bull, N. J. *Moral Judgment from Childhood to Adolescence.* Beverly Hills: Sage Publications, 1969.
12. Chess, S. Temperament in the Normal Infant. In J. Hullmuth (Ed.), *The Exceptional Infant.* Vol. I. Seattle: Special Child Publication, 1967.
13. Chodorow, N. Family Structure and Feminine Personality. In M. Z. Rosaldo and L. Lamphere, (Eds.). *Women, Culture and Society.* Stanford: Stanford University Press, 1974.
14. Conn, W. E. *Conscience: Development and Self-Transcendence.* Birmingham: Religious Education Press, 1981.
15. Coopersmith, S. *The Antecedents of Self-Esteem.* Palo Alto, CA: Consulting Psychologists Press, 1981.
16. Dobson, J. C. *Dare to Discipline.* Wheaton, IL: Tyndale House, 1981.
17. Eby, F., and Arrowood, C. L. *The History and Philosophy of Education: Ancient and Medieval.* Englewood Cliffs: Prentice Hall, 1940.
18. Erikson, E. H. *Childhood and Society* (2nd ed.). New York: Norton, 1963.
19. Felker, D. W. *Building Positive Self-concepts.* Minneapolis: Burgess, 1974.
20. Freud, S. *The Basic Writings of Sigmund Freud.* Translated and edited by A. A. Brill. New York: Random House, 1938.
21. Freud, S. *Beyond the Pleasure Principle.* Translated and edited by J. Strachey. New York: Liveright, 1950.
22. Freud, S. *The Ego and the Id.* Translated by Joan Reviere, revised and newly edited by J. Strachey. New York: W. W. Norton, 1960.

23. Garsee, J.   Unpublished material, 1977.
24. Garsee, J.   The Development of an Idealogy. In C. S. Schuster and S. S. Ashburn, *The Process of Human Development: A Holistic Approach*. Boston: Little, Brown, 1980.
25. Gibbs, J. C., Arnold, K. D., and Burkhart, J. E.   Sex differences in the expression of moral judgment. *Child Dev.* 55:1040, 1984.
26. Gilligan, C.   *In a Different Voice*. Cambridge, MA: Harvard University Press, 1982.
27. Gordon, T.   *Parent Effectiveness Training*. New York: New American Library, 1975.
28. Hamachek, D. E.   *Encounters with the Self* (2nd ed.). New York: Holt, Rinehart and Winston, 1978.
29. Hoffman, M. L.   Empathy, Role-taking, Guilt and Development of Altruistic Motives. In T. Lickonona (Ed.). *Moral Development and Behavior*. New York: Holt, Rinehart and Winston, 1976.
30. Jourard, S. M.   *Personal Adjustment* (2nd ed.). New York: Macmillan, 1967.
31. Kagan, J.   The Concept of Identification. In P. H. Mussen, et al. (Eds.). *Readings in Child Development and Personality* (2nd ed.). New York: Harper & Row, 1970.
32. Kagan, J.   A Conception of Early Adolescence. In J. Kagan and R. Coles (Eds.). *Twelve to Sixteen: Early Adolescence*. New York: Norton, 1972.
33. Kagan, J., and Moss, H. A.   *Birth to Maturity: A Study in Psychological Development* (2nd ed.). New Haven: Yale University Press, 1983.
34. Kessler, J. W.   *Psychopathology of Childhood*. Englewood Cliffs: Prentice-Hall, 1966.
35. Kohlberg, L.   The development of children's orientations toward a moral order: I. Sequence in the development of moral thought. *Vita Humana* 6:11, 1963.
36. Kohlberg, L.   *The Philosophy of Moral Development*. San Francisco: Harper & Row, 1981.
37. Lecky, P.   *Self-consistency: A Theory of Personality*. Fort Myers Beach, FL: Island Press, 1982.
38. Lever, J.   Sex differences in the games children play. *Social Problems* 23:478–487, 1976.
39. Lever, J.   Sex differences in the complexity of children's play and games. *American Sociological Review* 43:471–83, 1978.
40. Levin, H.   Permissive Child Rearing and Adult Role Behavior. In D. E. Dulaney et al. (Eds.), *Contributions to Modern Psychology*. New York: Oxford University Press, 1958.
41. Lickona, T.   Research on Piaget's Theory of Moral Development. In T. Lickona (Ed.). *Moral Development: Current Theory and Research*. New York: Holt, Rinehart and Winston, 1976.
42. McCord, W., McCord, J., and Howard, A.   Familial correlates of aggression in non-delinquent male children. *J. Abnorm. Soc. Psychol.* 62:72, 1961.
43. McLaughlin, B.   *Learning and Social Behavior*. New York: Free Press, 1971.
44. Menninger, K.   *Whatever Became of Sin?* New York: Hawthorn Books, 1973.
45. Meyers, C. E.   The effects of conflicting authority on the child. University of Iowa Study. *Child Welfare* No. 409, 1944.
46. Milgrim, S.   *Obedience to Authority: An Experimental View*. New York: Harper & Row, 1974.
47. Mussen, P. H., et al.   *Child Development and Personality* (4th ed.). New York: Harper & Row, 1974.
48. Mussen, P. H., et al.   *Child Development and Personality* (6th ed.). New York: Harper & Row, 1984.
49. Patterson, C. J.   Self-control and Self-regulation in Childhood. In T. Field et al. (Eds.), *Review of Human Development*. New York: Wiley, 1982.
50. Pattison, E. M.   The Development of Moral Values in Children. In C. E. Nelson, *Conscience*. New York: Newman Press, 1973.
51. Peck, R. F., et al.   *The Psychology of Character Development*. New York: Wiley, 1960.
52. Piaget, J.   *The Moral Judgment of the Child*. New York: Free Press, 1965.
53. Rosenthal, J. J., et al.   A study of mother-child relationships in the emotional disorders of children. *Genet. Psychol. Monogr.* 60:65, 1959.
54. Rosenthal, J. J. et al.   Father-child relationships and children's problems. *Arch. Gen. Psychiatry* 7:360, 1962.
55. Rothman, C. R.   An Experiment Analysis of the Relationships Between Levels of Moral Judgment and Behavior Choice. In B. Sutton-Smith, *Child Psychology*. New York: Appleton-Century-Crofts, 1973.
56. Sagotsky, G., Patterson, C. J., and Lepper, M. R.   Training Children's Self-control: A Field Experiment in Self-monitoring and Goal Setting in the Classroom. In Mussen, P. H. et al., *Child Development and Personality* (6th ed.). New York: Harper & Row, 1984.
57. Schell, R. E.   *Developmental Psychology Today* (4th ed.). New York: Random House, 1983.
58. Skolnick, A.   The myth of the vulnerable child. *Psychology Today* 11(9):56, 1978.
59. Slater, P. E.   Parental behavior and the personality of the child. *J. Genet. Psychol.* 101:53, 1962.
60. Stengel, S. R.   Moral education for young children. *Young Children* 37(6):22, 1982.
61. Sutton-Smith, B.   *Child Psychology*. New York: Appleton-Century-Crofts, 1973.
62. Symonds, P. M.   *The Ego and The Self*. New York: Greenwood Press, 1968.
63. Thomas, A., Chess, S., and Birch, H. G.   The origins of personality. *Sc. Am.* 223(2):102, 1970.
64. Walker, L. J.   Sex differences in the development of a moral reasoning: A critical review. *Child Dev.* 55:677, 1984.
65. Walsh, K., and Cowles, M.   *Developmental Discipline*. Birmingham, AL: Religious Education Press, 1982.
66. Walters, R. H., et al.   Timing of punishment and the observation of consequences to others as determinants of response inhibition. *J. Exp. Child. Psychol.* 2(1):10, 1965.
67. Zimbardo, P. C.   *Psychology and Life* (10th ed.). Glenview, IL: Scott, Foresman, 1979.

19
Adaptation to Uniqueness

Clara S. Schuster

The encouraging thing is that every time you meet a situation, though you may think at the time it is an impossibility and you go through tortures of the damned, once you have met it you find that forever after you are freer than you were before. If you can live through that you can live through anything. You gain strength, courage and confidence by every experience in which you really stop to look fear in the face.

—Eleanor Roosevelt, *You Learn by Living*

Introduction

Each one of us is a member of a minority group in some way. Perhaps it is because one wears glasses, or because one is the only girl in the family, or on the block. Skin color, extremes of body height, or unusual hair color (or naturally curly hair) may also identify one as different from the majority of one's peers. Other individuals may achieve minority status because of high IQ, ethnic affiliation, physical disability, or religious beliefs. Readily identifiable interindividual differences, especially those based on physical characteristics, frequently become an index by which others label or categorize people (e.g., redheads have bad tempers, blind people are withdrawn, fat people are jolly, people with cerebral palsy are retarded, people of Spanish descent are emotional, gifted people are snobbish).

Information about interindividual differences can be valuable when used objectively for guiding our interactions. For example, we may avoid arranging a business transaction on a day that we recognize as the Sabbath or a high holy day for the individual with a known religious affiliation. We also might assume that blind persons cannot see well enough to identify us by visual cues and consequently, identify ourselves verbally when we greet them. Some may label as unfriendly a blind person who does not respond to a greeting on the street, when in fact the visually impaired person did not hear or recognize the speaker.

Stereotypes derived from misunderstandings of the behaviors of others can deprive us of many rich relationships and experiences, since they fail to identify the factors mediating the behaviors and do not allow recognition of interindividual similarities.

From a holistic viewpoint, even with our interindividual differences, most of us are more like our peers than different from them. Each of us wants to think that we are average, that we belong to the group, that we **are** like the others. The sense of belonging and affiliation appears to be critical in the formation of an individual's identity and ego strength. A person's affiliations reflect his or her developmental level. There is a gradual broadening and then refining of one's identity through association with others. The infant affiliates with the caretaker, the preschooler with the family. The peer group, or gang, becomes significant to school-agers as they absorb the values, the goals, and the behaviors of the subculture; peers are also important to adolescents as they begin to identify their uniqueness within the subculture (28). Refinement of one's identity continues in both subtle and not so subtle ways throughout the adult years as individuals seek out others who have similar interests, characteristics, problems, or goals.

Some individuals seek a total affiliation with others similar to themselves. Consequently, many American cities have a Chinatown or Cuban, Polish, or Italian districts. Some persons will establish a communal lifestyle, whereas others seek more casual, yet equally significant, affiliations with social, recreational, or religious groups. At other times, the need for similar peer association is exhibited through the choice of friends who share common social values or educational levels. We are more comfortable with persons whom we feel are sympathetic to or in agreement with our own values and lifestyle.

We speak of America as the "melting pot of the nations." It is true that many customs, goals, and values of our forefathers have been moderated by the influences of contact with other ethnic groups and by the mass media. However, we also find areas in our cities and throughout the country where individuals with common ethnic backgrounds or interests have established a minicommunity within the larger populace. These individuals have effectively retained their lifestyle and cultural individuality by associating with others of similar background. Just as the beauty of an artistic masterpiece is achieved through the subtle blending as well as the contrasting of colors and textures, the blending and contrasting of different subcultures within our country has given it a unique beauty.

As we go through life, we find that we are not a carbon copy of our peers. An an early age, we begin to be aware of our interindividual differences; they become even more obvious as we grow older. How we accept these differences is very significant to our ego-identity. If we are able to accept these differences objectively or positively, then affective energy is available to invest in social relationships and cognitive development. However, if these differences are translated into a negative self-identity, then affective energies may need to be used to protect the developing self, thus limiting the amount of energy available for creative activities.

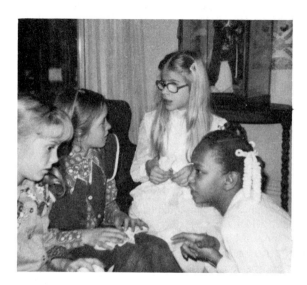

Figure 19–1. Two of these girls are legally blind and another represents a racial minority group, yet they are finding that their interindividual similarities are stronger than their differences and offer a basis for rich interpersonal exchanges.

PSYCHOLOGY OF EXCEPTIONALITY

The need to be an accepted part of the subcultural group is so strong during the school-age years that children often go to extremes to maintain their homogeneity. Clothing and hairstyles frequently become critical issues for confrontation between parents and children as the child tries to seek group identity through conformity to its values. Clubs or gangs are formed with arbitrarily designated criteria (e.g., gender, residence, grade) established to bring some children into, and to force others out of, the group [6]. The child who is different is often teased and rejected by peers; names such as "four eyes," "carrot top," and "honky" may be used to stigmatize the offender of the norm. The child may come to hate a part of self because of this ridicule. Children who belong to a religious sect that has explicit behavioral codes or religious observances may find themselves caught between parental and peer expectations. Clothing styles, participation in school social activities, or observance of religious rituals (such as Ash Wednesday by the Catholic child) may precipitate embarrassment or internal conflict.

Reaction of the Child to Exceptionality

When the child becomes aware of deviation from the norm of the community (his or her exceptionality), the child may respond in one of three ways:

1. Intense pride ("I am superior"). The difference makes the child feel better than others. This is especially true if the deviation is an excess of a desirable characteristic, such as money, physical skill, or beauty. As a person changes peer-group affiliation, status may change. Although the individual remains unchanged, the same characteristic that gave high status in one group may be an insufficient criterion in another. A young person may be the star football player in high school, but is unable to make the team in college. Another person may breeze through high school courses, but sweat through courses during the first years of college.

   The possession of a prized characteristic may be equated with personal worth, even though the trait is one that was acquired through heredity rather than achieved through personal efforts. The person who takes pride in a difference may be tempted to cheat or to lie in order to maintain a perceived superiority. When people use these superficial status symbols for group affiliation, scapegoating frequently occurs in order to main-

tain superiority by keeping others "where they belong." Human dignity is lost in such a situation. Individuals who are members of a culturally designated minority group may become very angry about the devaluation of their difference and may fight for equal rights and privileges.

2. Intense shame ("I am inferior"). Too often one's concept of "normality" is actually an ideal that few can ever reach [39]. Individuals who react in this way may feel that the difference makes them unworthy, unacceptable, or bad. They may accept the limitations imposed by others or reject themselves for their imperfections and become passive or even dependent or subservient in relationships with others. A person may find that a characteristic valued by one group is subjected to ridicule in a second. For instance, teachers may value a student's academic achievements while peers may value popularity, group solidarity, conformity, or physical prowess. Young people caught between conflicting value systems may consciously repress maximizing their own cognitive potentials in order to remain acceptable to the peer group.

3. Realistic acceptance ("I am me"). The development of this attitude requires a great deal of personal maturity and support from significant others. These individuals view their "imperfections" as but one aspect of a total life. They are comfortable with themselves and can see both assets and liabilities realistically, without stigmatizing value: They can proceed to identify their own limits rather than accepting those posed by sociocultural stereotypes. To identify limits means setting one's own goals and establishing a role based on personal interests and potentials. It also implies equal opportunity for, and evaluation of, each person for **who** they are, not for **what** they are; it is not based on what a person does or owns.

Disability versus Handicap

An impairment, a disability, and a handicap are not synonymous. It is generally assumed that an impairment causes a disability, which in turn causes a handicap. An **impairment** is an identifiable organic flaw, a defect in the biophysical domain. A **disability,** on the other hand, is an inability to execute a certain skill or to perform a function. A disability can be objectively identified, and the degree of the disability can be measured [61]. A **handicap** is more difficult to identify objectively because it involves a defect in the social and affective domains [41].

Impairment and disability are arbitrary concepts,

which are defined by the values and goals of the culture. Not all impairments are disabling. A large nose does not prevent one from smelling, nor does a birthmark hamper ambulation or the ability to smile. On the other hand, a disability is not necessarily the result of an impairment; it can result from the helplessness syndrome (see Chap. 14) or from the absence of a desired physical ability [61]. For instance, only a few individuals can run a 4-minute mile, span 10 notes on the piano with one hand, or hit high F when vocalizing. Thus a person may be normal but may be unable to perform a culturally desirable skill. A person's inability to execute a particular skill may be perceived by self or others as a disability because it prevents the individual from achieving a desired goal.

Handicaps, like beauty, are in the eye of the beholder. They are socially defined criteria that are neither universal nor permanent. Many factors can handicap one: disability, poverty, poor education, minority status, shyness, family encumbrances, and so on [62]. The Chinese once bound the feet of their female children to ensure what they considered a proper walking gait during adulthood. In their culture, our large feet would have been clumsy and unacceptable, a handicap, just as their shuffling gait would be a handicap in ours. In countries where Islam is practiced, blind men are honored because their prayers are believed to be more welcome to God than the prayers of the sighted. They are considered to bear a divine stamp. European women imitated the halting limp of Princess Alexandra, wife of Edward VI [41]. When a deviation from normal is socially valued, the self-esteem of the individual is enhanced. When a deviation is socially undesirable, the resultant social disapproval or rejection may lead to maladjusted behavior or an emotional handicap in the individual.

Sociocultural Handicaps versus Emotional Handicaps

A **sociocultural handicap** is any factor that is deemed undesirable by the social group or culture to which an individual belongs, and that consequently affects the quantity or quality of interpersonal relationships. Examples may include an Italian in a Polish community, a hearing person in a deaf community, a light-skinned Afro-American in a black community, or a woman in the political and/or business world. An **emotional handicap** is the psychological disequilibrium or behavioral maladjustment expressed by the person who perceives the self to be "different" or stigmatized. The altered affective state can inhibit realistic, positive ego-identity as well as learning and social growth.

There is a very close relationship between sociocultural handicap (impairment, disability, or deviance) and emotional handicap, but again, they are not synonymous. The following sequence of events can lead to an emotional handicap [41]:

1. The person lacks a tool or characteristic required for social acceptance or behavior within the culture and knows it is lacking.
2. Other people perceive this lack of an important characteristic or tool, and devalue the individual for the lack.
3. This person accepts the judgment of others (or self-judgment) that he or she is less worthy, and devalues him- or herself.

This sequence of events is a unit. If 1 or 2 does not occur, then 3 does not occur. If 3 does not occur, there is no emotional handicap. This concept is perhaps the central focus of the entire chapter. Deviance is an arbitrary, socially defined phenomenon that has no valid correlation with an individual's worth as a person. **It is the acceptance of these arbitrary values and subsequent devaluation of self that leads to the development of emotional handicaps and social maladjustment.** Interruption of the chain can prevent maladjustment and facilitate maximization of potentials in all domains. Children who think they can't—won't; children who think they can—will, somehow!

Prevention or Amelioration of Emotional Handicaps

Emotional handicaps can be prevented or ameliorated by reducing the stress load (liabilities) and increasing the powers (assets) of the individual. When a person is presented with a new situation, the response can be fairly readily predicted [41]. In order to achieve mastery or control, the individual will engage in trial-and-error behaviors in order to identify a potential solution. This behavior requires high amounts of emotional energy to cope with the accompanying anxiety. The rate of error is also high, which leads to frustration and emotionality. The person is placed in conflict. ("Should I attempt to reach this new goal or should I retreat to the safety of what I know?") Each new adventure brings a new challenge and the potential threat of failure; this is the source of the emotional disequilibrium.

For most people the number of new elements in novel situations is reduced by gradual assumption of new roles and experiences. An example of a novel situation is a person's first week at college. Although separation from family, introduction to new friends, and assumption of intensive studies are difficult, most people have had adequate preliminary experiences to help them make a successful adjustment. However, when a person's repertoire of experiences has been limited because of life-style, socioeconomic opportunities, ethnic affiliation, or physical disability, the adjustment becomes even more difficult.

ACCEPTANCE OF ONE'S DIFFERENCE

The most critical factor in adjustment to new challenges is realistic acceptance of one's difference or disability. Incorporated into this concept is the ability to establish realistic goals; this includes the ability to tolerate frustration when the goal is not immediately achieved, and the ability to stick to a task until it is mastered (Erikson's concept of industry). Realistic establishment of goals also includes the ability to set priorities. For example, a severely disabled person, because of time limitations versus ultimate goals, may need to choose between dressing and feeding self. Putting too much time and energy into nonessential activities may reduce one's ability to deal with essentials [35]. Thus the physically disabled person in any category may need to balance the stress of need for independence against the stress of need for dependence in order to ensure both psychological and physiological safety. Stress must be adequate enough to challenge but not to overwhelm the individual.

MASTERY OF SKILLS

The second factor that can facilitate adaptation to new situations is the learning of specific skills and behaviors that will facilitate structuring of new situations and permit goal achievement. This concept includes the skills essential for independence in the activities of daily living and culturally defined etiquette. When a person does not possess the physical tool for achieving a certain task, an alternative method must be learned. Consequently, deaf individuals can learn sign language and lip reading; blind individuals learn braille or use talking books; and some physically disabled individuals use animals for guidance or retrieval of objects. Parents who absorb all frustrations, pressures, and problems only serve to stifle the child's achievement of competence. Mastery of smaller tasks lays the foundation for handling more complex tasks later in life. Disabled individuals repeatedly state that a challenging parent, a sibling, or a teacher was the best preparation they could have had for adulthood [45].

The most important skill for a person to learn is how to solve problems or to make decisions—to think independently. The physically disabled child in particular needs assistance with generating viable alternatives in order to master tasks. A child can be taught when caught in a novel situation to observe the behavior of other persons and then follow suit. This method engenders lower levels of anxiety than the trial-and-error method.

EXPOSURE TO THE CULTURE

Young people, regardless of ethnic background or disabling condition, need to be exposed to new experiences as they develop. A person does not suddenly know how to live independently upon graduating from high school or upon marrying; growth-facilitating experiences must be offered during the developmental years. Children need to learn how to handle money through an allowance, a job, and self-planned shop-

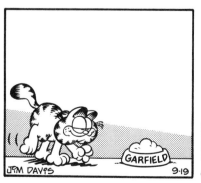
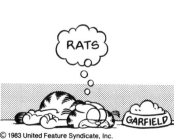
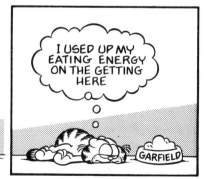

Figure 19–2. Disabled persons need to weigh the effort of accomplishing a task against the benefits received and request assistance as necessary so that available energies can be focused toward maximal goal achievement. (Reprinted courtesy of *Garfield.* Copyright 1983 United Feature Syndicate, Inc.)

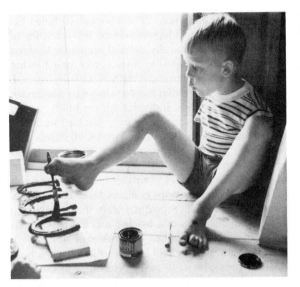

Figure 19–3. This young boy obviously has an impairment; he lost his arms in a farm accident at the age of 2. However, he is not necessarily disabled, since he has learned to do many things with his feet—including holding a pencil or a paintbrush between his toes. Here he is painting horseshoes for a family game. (Photograph by Carl Subitch.)

ping. Children need wide exposure to the elements of their culture (see Chap. 14). The wider the exposure to other lifestyles, cultures, environments, and ideas, the more understanding and flexible an individual can be when dealing with others or when solving problems. Individuals who have been deprived of the challenges leading to competence may develop the helplessness syndrome during the adult years because they have not learned how to control the environment [54]. Permissive, indulgent, child-rearing practices create insecurity in children. They must always rely on someone else rather than on their own talents and abilities; therefore, they are never secure in their own competencies and identity [67]. The overprotected child, whether normal or disabled, learns to be helpless.

NURTURING SUPPORT
One of the greatest challenges of parenting is to balance children's loads against their powers in such a way as to gradually guide children toward more independent functioning. This task requires a sensitivity to the individual child's developmental level in order to balance the stress of a situation against the challenge. The first criterion is that parents know their own values and goals well enough to offer stability and consistency in role modeling; the second is that parents

share experiences with their children. Sharing experiences means that parents do not do something **for** children, but **with** them, allowing the children to do as much for themselves as possible even if it takes a little longer. Thus the parent allows the 13-month-old child to walk, rather than be carried, to the car; he or she places the hands over those of the toddler or preschooler who is attempting to snap together some pop beads or to crack open an egg. When a problem arises at school, it may be more helpful if the parent, rather than handling the situation, allows the child to participate in the conference with the teacher. The parent may also engage in role playing with the child in the home setting, practicing teacher-pupil conferences or child-peer interactions. This method can have incredible short- and long-range results by increasing problem-solving skills, interpersonal relationship skills, and self-confidence.

AVOIDANCE OF SITUATIONS
Another way to reduce stress is to avoid situations that are potentially too traumatic; this is perhaps part of the realistic acceptance of one's limitations. A child who stutters may be able to communicate adequately in the classroom, but giving a speech in an assembly might represent a marked threat to self-confidence and self-esteem. This concept does not imply avoidance of growth-producing experiences, but avoidance of growth-threatening experiences (a thin line at times). To remove all challenge because of potential failure may signify to the child a lack of worthiness or confidence in him or her that can be more devastating than the public exposure [45].

EDUCATION OF THE PUBLIC
Individuals need to see themselves as whole and good persons. Since a person's attitude toward self is frequently a reflection of the attitude of others, major cultural attitudes toward ethnic and disability minority groups need to be changed. School textbooks are already reflecting such changes, and the mass media are beginning to give wider exposure to minorities. However, stigmatization is still a very individual matter. Each of us must reevaluate our own values and attitudes toward those who are different from ourselves. It is hoped that in so doing, we will begin to accept people for who they really are, not according to preconceived, stereotyped prejudices or a superficial value system. Minority representatives or physically disabled persons themselves can frequently help to change stereotyped public opinions by their own attitudes and unique approach to meeting life's responsibilites. Mi-

nority or disabled children should be prepared to handle the embarrassment or discomfort of others, and to hold up their own end of an interaction [3]. Role-playing experiences in church, scout, and social groups are potent sensitizers.

INDIVIDUALIZING RESPONSES
TO DISABLED CHILDREN

We need to be careful not to impose a handicap on top of a disability or a difference because of our own attitudes. Frequently experiences offered the disabled child create secondary disabilities or handicaps greater than the primary disability imposes [61]. Individuals can become who we think they are, especially if we are a significant person to them (the Rosenthal effect). In order to maximize potentials, we must accentuate the positive assets or powers of the individual. **Every child's performance should be considered in terms of assessed loads and powers, not in terms of norms.** This principle is also critical to the development of the gifted child. If the professional person or parent keeps good records of the child's progress, judicious sharing of these notes or charts can serve to spur more growth, since the child is competing against his or her own successes. Emotional disequilibrium does not accompany earned success. The rest of the chapter will focus on the physically impaired person.

STRESSORS AFFECTING THE DEVELOPMENT OF THE PHYSICALLY IMPAIRED CHILD

Persons with obvious deviations from culturally desired norms, whether these deviations are due to ethnic background or physical differences, share many common psychological experiences. The physically impaired child, however, faces even greater barriers to positive ego-identity and healthy adaptation to the deviation. The physically impaired child is always different, even in the earliest social affiliations with the mother and the family. Ethnic characteristics, on the other hand, usually do not pose difficulties until the child leaves the home for increased peer association during the school-age years [61]. The physically disabled child faces a number of potential sources of devaluation from the first day of life, the most critical of which are the parents. In light of all the barriers to high level mental health, it is amazing that so many disabled persons adjust as well as they do to life in the larger society. Most see themselves as "ordinary persons," not as "disabled persons" [45].

Role of the Parents

The parents are probably the single most critical source of stress or support to the impaired child. The impairment does not belong to the child alone—the whole family is impaired. All the reactions and problems discussed in the previous section can also be applied to the family as a unit. Since the parents provide the child with the earliest and most persistent relationships throughout life, their reaction to the impairment will affect the child's response to the deviance and the child's attitude toward self. The child frequently becomes what the parents think the child is.

The parents need to differentiate clearly between the superficial factors comprising sociocultural handicaps and emotional handicaps. They need to realize that

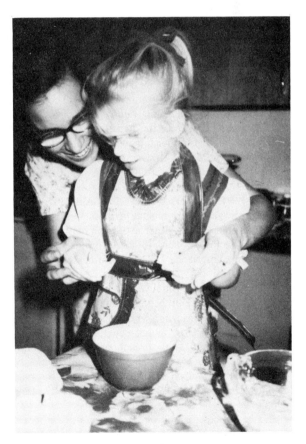

Figure 19–4. When a child has an impairment (blindness in this case) it is important that the parents start early to help the child to gain the appropriate skills for the culture. Lack of these tools for effective functioning constitutes a disability, which in turn becomes a handicap.

one's body is merely a tool for expression of the self; the body is not the self. When the requirements of the environment are matched with the skills of the child, frustration can be reduced and the self-esteem of both the child and the parents is increased. Having or being a disabled individual must never be equated with self-worth. Emotional maladjustment can be avoided or reduced if the child is afforded human dignity and acceptance for who he or she is and not for the ability to function according to the norms of peers. This is true for the gifted as well as for the impaired child. There is no need for a child to be ashamed of self when others offer respect, especially those most significant to the child—the parents. Most parents need some outside support to help them gain a healthy perspective. Parental reactions to a disabled child are covered in more depth in Chapter 35.

The Disabling Condition

Many stressors are specific to the type of impairment or disability a person has. Both the quantity and quality of interpersonal relationships can be altered. When these experiences are perceived as negative, the child becomes aware of deviance and may feel unacceptable or unworthy. The child may build a wall around the self as a protection from the pain of perceived rejection by others. (It is easier to cope with the pain if one has rejected the others first, or if one maintains only superficial involvement.)

IMPAIRMENT WITH OR WITHOUT DISABILITY
The person with a large facial birthmark or scar may find that other people either avoid eye contact (a sign of social rejection) or stare in horror or curiosity (a dehumanizing experience). In our culture, sustained eye contact (longer than 30 seconds) is reserved for objects, infants, the one you love, or someone with whom you are very angry [59]. A person may attempt to gain psychological superiority over another through sustained eye contact. In which category does the disabled person classify this breach of social etiquette? The person may feel caught between the extremes of social isolation and an intrusion of privacy because of the socially abnormal use of eye contact by other people.

The facial expressions of the viewers serve to remind the person of the undesirability of the impairment. Other people may actually be repulsed to the point of nausea by a deformity. Unless the person is assisted in separating the impaired physical self from the psychic self, he or she may feel that the self is undesirable. Since few young children are able to make such an abstract distinction, the parents may need to limit the child's exposure to others if public reactions are too traumatic to the child. The other alternative is to use cosmetic preparations or to dress the person in such a way as to minimize the visibility of the impairment. Some impairments can be improved or removed by surgery, which should be considered when the impairment constitutes a sociocultural handicap.

BLINDNESS
Vision is one of the most critical tools in social interaction. Mothers of blind infants indicate great difficulty in maintaining a natural, spontaneous interaction with their child because of the absence of eye contact [17]. The mother finds it difficult to learn to read the infant's behavioral cues, to respond contingently, and to establish the reciprocity of interaction so critical to the infant's early learning of self-other differentiation and cause-effect relationships [18]. This can lead to critical delays in ego development, passivity, cognitive delays, and learned helplessness. The mother of a blind infant needs to learn to be more responsive to postural cues, to expression of affect through the hand movements, and to changes in breathing patterns [8].

Brazelton finds that blind infants cry more than sighted infants, which can be an annoyance to the mother. He states that the sighted infant is able to orient the self to the environment and can use visual stimuli to organize and to control the state of consciousness (see Chap. 5). Vision is the coordinator of sensory experiences from the earliest days of life. Blind children exhibit marked delays in the mastery of early developmental milestones, even though cognitive potentials may be normal [18]. The blind person finds the constant assessment of the environment through auditory, olfactory, and haptic cues to be tiring; consequently, the blind infant or child is often observed to withdraw (a pause to refresh the self). Unfortunately, once withdrawn (i.e., head down, in state 3), the child may not return to an alert state unless stimulated to activity by another person. Thus these pauses are essential to organize environmental stimuli and to regain equilibrium, but if continued too long, they may interfere with a child's meaningful interactions with the environment, and thus delay development.

As the blind child continues to develop, he or she is unable to imitate many of the socially accepted behaviors unless given specific assistance. These behaviors may involve diverse aspects, such as how to sit in public, how to use the body for walking, maintaining an attractive hair style, or flirting behaviors during the adolescent years. It is obvious how significant vision is in learning the social use of facial muscles. Many congenitally blind individuals fail to adopt these nonverbal interactional cues. The failure to maintain eye contact with a speaker or even to face a person when speaking may seriously interfere with the other person's ability to feel comfortable during the interaction. Delays in, or absence of, spontaneous facial expressions during interactions may also be interpreted by the sighted person as signs of disinterest or rejection.

Because of these violations of culturally determined communication behaviors, the sighted person may feel very uncomfortable with blind individuals and consequently may avoid them. The sighted person may also interpret the lack of these behaviors as an indication of lowered cognitive functioning and thus may infantalize blind persons (treat them as being younger than their developmental level warrants).

The blind person may try very hard to minimize differences with sighted peers. He or she may become very quiet so that differences are not so obvious, or very loquacious in order to maintain control over what is happening. Some blind people may develop an extensive "visual" vocabulary as a means for decreasing differences [12]. Objects are described in terms of color, beauty, and grandeur rather than textures, sounds, and odors.

Gross- and fine-motor skills may also be altered in the blind person. Inability to observe the movements of others frequently makes learning to use one's own body more difficult. Inability to assess visually the topography of the environment may delay object-hand coordination, independent walking, running, and participation in group activities or sports involving rapidly moving objects and body contact.

Inadequate reception of meaningful stimuli by the blind person coupled with inadequate knowledge of culturally appropriate behaviors may also lead to the emergence of autostimulatory behaviors, such as body rocking and putting pressure against the eyeballs.

The absence of vision, then, can lead to alterations in ego development, socialization skills, communication patterns, and motor development. Difficulty in assessing environmental cues without vision can lead to higher levels of anxiety in the blind person than in sighted peers. This anxiety can limit the amount of energy that is available to invest in new experiences or learning unless steps are taken to reduce the stressors.

DEAFNESS

Because the earliest interactions with the environment are auditory as well as visual, the inability to receive auditory stimuli may be as disastrous as visual impairment for the young child. Although the child may possess normal cognitive potential, difficulty in learning the language code can seriously impede cognitive organizational processes because the tool of language may not be sufficiently developed to facilitate differentiation and clarification of relationships essential to effective categorization and development of schemata.

The person needs a means to communicate inner thoughts systematically. By 4 years of age, the deaf child should be able to master the major components of communication, either by the auditory-oral mode or the visual-sign mode [60]. Difficulty with communication skills may limit the attempts of others to communicate with the child, thus further decreasing opportunities to learn language and social relationships. Inappropriate, delayed, or nonexistent responses to communication efforts may cause the other person to infer that the deaf or hard-of-hearing person is cognitively delayed or noncompliant; this in turn may evoke infantalizing, avoidance, or hostile behaviors toward the deaf individual.

The deaf person may experience further frustration when a need, a problem, a thought, or an excitement cannot be adequately communicated to a significant other person. Any of these experiences can elicit high anxiety in the deaf individual. Limited social experiences, frustration with communication efforts, and the stigmatizing behaviors of others can prevent normal social development. Deafness, then, can lead to alterations in the development of communication skills, cognitive skills, social skills, and affective maturity.

ORTHOPEDIC AND NEUROLOGICAL DISABILITIES

The neurologically impaired child may also experience multidimensional alterations in development because of limitations in ability to experience the environment and because of insensitive responses of other persons to the child's repertoire of skills. Deficiencies in motor development or control may limit the child's mobility, secondarily limiting the child's quest for autonomy or independence. The child may experience great deprivation in the areas of general knowledge because of inadequate interaction with the culture. The parents may find it requires too much effort to take such a child shopping, camping, to the theater, to the zoo, to church, or even to a parade; thus the child may need to rely on the secondary sources of the mass media and the relation of experiences by parents and peers.

Lack of mobility, like sensory defects, may also interfere with adequate contact with peers. Since the child cannot participate in many of the gross-motor

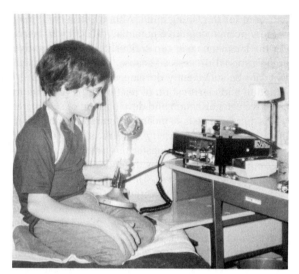

Figure 19–5. This home-bound adolescent has found great enjoyment and increased social contacts through use of a CB radio.

activities dominating the socialization experiences of normal counterparts, he or she may feel in the way or unwanted. Limited peer contact can lead to delayed development of social skills.

OTHER DISABILITIES

Many children who appear to be normal still may experience impairments or disabilities that can interfere with social relationships. The child with phenylketonuria (PKU), diabetes, or allergies may not be able to eat some of the food served at a party. The child with juvenile arthritis, osteoporosis (brittle bones), or cardiac problems may be unable to join in some of the physical activities of a peer group.

The impaired or physically disabled child offers an excellent example of the interdependence of the four major domains. When working with physically impaired children, one **must** use a holistic approach to habilitation and appreciate the mediating effect of the impairment on other areas of development.

Medical and Habilitation Therapy

Impaired or disabled children may experience hospitalization more often than the normal child, which may mean separation from family and parents as well as interruption of daily routines and activities. Surgery may evoke fear of castration, mutilation, abuse, or even death [68]. The child may see other children wrapped in bandages or wearing casts or may hear screams from the treatment room and envision torture or anticipate excruciating pain. Even a hypodermic needle may be interpreted as a lethal weapon. The whir of the electric cast cutter can frighten a child, even though no pain is involved.

Some children, especially during the preschool years, may feel that the hospitalization, separation, and treatment—or even the disability itself—represent a punishment for misdemeanors [68]. Children need a very careful, honest explanation of what is happening and why. This explanation should include preparation for the pain involved, the projected time schedules, and the anticipated outcome. Even the older infant's or young toddler's cooperation can be effectively elicited and trauma reduced when the explanation is geared to the level of comprehension. For example, after she had been given an explanation of what was happening, the author's 10-month-old daughter remained flat in bed without crying or attempting to get up for over 48 hours following eye surgery. (Although this child had exceptional language skills, the basic principle is still applicable to all children.)

A child can be so stressed during physical therapy sessions that he or she is unable to benefit from them [47]. It is important, then, in any therapy situation that the therapist make friends with the child, be honest with the child, and if possible, make a game out of the therapy in order to encourage the child's positive, active participation.

Limitations on Independence and Socialization

Disabled children are generally less mature for their age; experience more problems with social relationships; exhibit greater feelings of anxiety, conflict, and defensiveness; have a higher suicide rate; a higher incidence of psychiatric disorders; more somatic complaints; and less flexibility [22, 39, 52]. An intense therapy program or the need for assistance with the activities of daily living may effectively preclude the efforts of disabled adolescents toward emotional and physical independence from the parents. They may need to ask for or to accept assistance with tasks as simple as brushing their teeth or knowing when it is safe to cross the street. As the child matures, alternative methods for accomplishing the tasks can be learned, but only if the parents and teachers encourage it.

Difficulty with mobility and communication may severely hamper peer relationships. Other children may avoid initiating a relationship with a "different" child

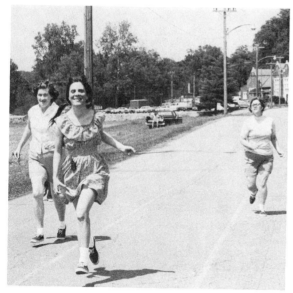

Figure 19–6. These mentally retarded girls are enjoying competition with peers in preparation for the Special Olympics. Such experiences facilitate affective and social growth in spite of disabilities in other domains.

because they do not understand the nature of the disability, may fear transfer of the impairment to their own body, are too wrapped up in their own interests to see the needs of another, fear the ridicule of peers for associating with someone who is "abnormal," or may not know alternative ways of relating to the exceptional child or how to overcome the communication barriers. Children are involved in the concrete here and now, in what they can see. Children often need help to relate to the **person** who has a disability, rather than to the **disabled** person. The same principle applies to any variation from the norm.

The exceptional child may increasingly feel left out of activities because of inability or lack of invitations to participate in events. Limited peer association and awareness of physical unattractiveness may also be associated with difficulties in expressing one's sexuality during the adolescent and adult years—another potential source of frustration. Children with "hidden impairments," such as diabetes or epilepsy, may carry a double burden of the condition itself and the stress of keeping it a secret from peers [7]. Parents are encouraged to invite other children to the disabled child's home for a party or special event to facilitate peer relationships; teachers are encouraged to teach all children about the difference between physical adeptness

and personal worth. Experiences simulating a disabling condition can help to foster an appreciation for the needs and problems of a disabled person [30].

Educational Arrangements

Although more details will be discussed in the next section, it is significant to recognize that disabled children face unique stressors in terms of receiving an education. The disabled child who attends a regular public school may find it very difficult to participate in all the activities. The child prone to exercise-induced asthmatic attacks may need alternative experiences during recess or physical education classes. The deaf child may miss much of what the teacher says; the blind child must carry around bulky books and have access to a typewriter for written assignments. The deaf child may not hear the fire alarm, whereas the blind child may hear but may not know where to go. Disabled children who attend school outside of their community may require long hours for transportation daily, further reducing the energy available for concentrating on studies. Other children attending residential schools may experience separation from the family for the academic week or month. These separations are especially difficult for the very young child who still looks to the parents for emotional support and guidance. The child may also feel rejected, punished, or deserted, which further reduces the energy available for learning. It is not unusual for a child in a residential setting to experience symptoms of grief and loss—mourning over the perceived loss of parents, home, and lifestyle (see Chap. 21).

Acceptance of One's Own Exceptionality

Very little research has been done in the area of how impaired children accept their exceptionality. It is frequently assumed that because these children have never experienced a "normal" life, they will not miss it and will automatically adjust to living with their disabilities. This simply is not so. As observational and cognitive processes develop, the child begins to realize that he or she is different. Even the blind child may become aware of difference shortly after the first birthday. During this first stage, the child usually does not interpret the difference as being abnormal and accepts the disability as a normal part of the developing self. During the second stage of awareness, the child begins to recognize that the disability is unusual but assumes that it will be outgrown. During the third stage, the child accepts the abnormality of the disability but maintains a fantasy of being cured someday. The child

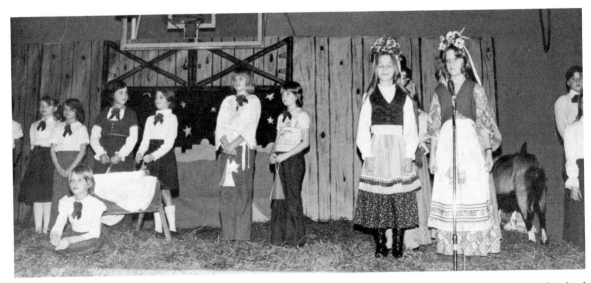

Figure 19–7. Appreciation rather than criticism of different cultural backgrounds and values can be fostered through school and scouting activities.

frequently sees the disability as a nuisance [36]. Unfortunately, many disabled persons may remain in this or the next stage, neither of which is conducive to successful habilitation. In the fourth stage, the child realizes that the disability is permanent and may respond in anger, feeling that the world is unfair, or with helplessness because he or she feels no control over fate. Fifty percent of chronically ill and disabled children can experience acute distress and depression by 10 years of age, as they mourn the loss of normalcy, unattainable skills and goals, or anticipated failures and death [42, 50, 53]. These feelings are especially prominent during the school-age and adolescent years and frequently interfere with activities, such as wearing a hearing aid, learning Braille, following a special diet, or practicing therapeutic exercises. Each of these activities is a reminder to the child of disability, a symbol of deviation from the normal. Twenty to 25 percent of physically disabled children have behavior-affective problems serious enough to be diagnosed as emotionally disturbed [43, 51].

Parents may feel very frustrated as they try to help the child adjust to a world limited in peer contacts at a time when peers are so critical; or as they try to maximize the child's potentials when the child is too full of hopelessness or anger to care or think rationally. The immaturity of cognitive skills prevents long-range perspectives or abstract thought processes; consequently, the disability may assume paramount importance in the child's life. The disability may be blamed for all

problems and failures; it may also be used as a weapon to elicit sympathy (attention getting) or to get one's own way (controlling the environment). Although these are common responses, they are unhealthy. The parents must exhibit great love, patience, restraint, and openness to help the child through this period to a realistic acceptance and healthy adaptation to living with a disability (the fifth stage). This degree of acceptance implies that the child is able to distinguish between the physical self and the psychic self; he or she uses the body as a tool, but maintains confidence in his or her value as a person.

Thus far we have spoken of the congenitally disabled child (one who is born with the impairment). The adventitiously impaired individual (one in whom the impairment occurs after birth) also experiences difficulty in adjustment to the change in body image. The individual has developed as a "whole" person and must now adjust to an impaired image of the self. Some people with newly diagnosed visual alterations will resist wearing glasses because they feel it makes them ugly. Other disabilities cannot be avoided as easily. A person who experiences a serious injury, such as extensive burns, an amputation because of bone cancer, or a spinal injury from an auto accident, is forced to face the reality of the body change. Such a person may experience marked grief over loss of the known physical self and may also feel that the events represent a punishment. Various factors contribute to the ability of these individuals to cope with the disability and a new body image: how they are treated by medical personnel, the support given them through the grief process, the previous self-image, and former relationships with family, siblings, and peers [68]. The type of disability, the age of onset, the individual's basic personality and coping strategies, and the parents' adjustment are also critical to the adaptation [39]. The individual needs to talk out fears, fantasies, and misconceptions in a loving, accepting environment that provides facts, comfort, and reassurance. An inability to resolve grief may delay the ability to accept the situation realistically and to adapt constructively to it.

As an exceptional adult, the support of peers and family members facilitates adjustment, but the ability to maintain independence through career, self-care, and leisure activities becomes even more critical. When parents make life easy for the developing child, they only make life harder for the individual as an adult. Disabled children must learn self-care and how to assume responsibilities within the home [45]. Some adults find they have not developed their self-care, travel, self-discipline, or interpersonal skills sufficiently to secure or retain employment.

The greatest burden to the disabled adult is the limitations imposed by society. Employment opportunities are limited because of accessibility and travel barriers and the biases of potential employers [65]. Many severely disabled individuals are unable to support themselves on the salary they receive when they have to pay others to help them dress and go to the bathroom, clean house, or cook a meal. Consequently they are forced to accept placement in a nursing home at a high cost to the welfare system instead of remaining employed, utilizing the skills they do have, and contributing to the welfare of others. A subsidized income, and/or accessible, independent-living homes would enable the individual to remain employed and independent [45]. Unemployment and underemployment have devastating effects on the individual's self-esteem. Bitterness, depression, and helplessness are common outcomes.

Some adults, because of the nature of their disability, experience career goal changes and actually maximize their potentials to a higher level than if they had not experienced the disabling condition [45]. A disabling condition does not have to be handicapping if the individual can work with it realistically and set appropriate goals. However, advocates are still needed to assure that disabled persons are granted their rights as full citizens [9].

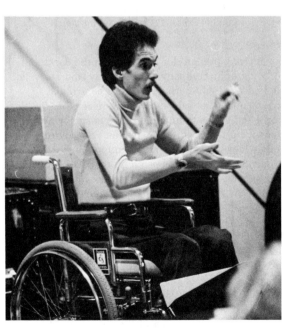

Figure 19-8. Physically disabled persons have talents and abilities that can enrich community life. Many obtain superior educations to compensate for motor disabilities and thus make outstanding employees.

LIVING IN TWO WORLDS

When we speak of handicaps, we are speaking of process and of interrelationships—not a hard fact or a static phenomenon. We are dealing with disabled individuals, the attitude of others toward them, and their response to the cultural attitude. When normal persons avoid contact with a disabled person, they are frequently aware that the avoidance behavior is unethical and that the disability is an unavoidable condition that is neither good nor bad, but they may rationalize their behavior by saying that the feeling "can't be helped" [41, 61]. By relating to the disability rather than to the person, the nondisabled individual prevents normal opportunities for the disabled person and forces him or her to adopt a "disabled" role. Everything stated here about the disabled person is equally applicable to individuals who are ethnically or linguistically different from the mainstream.

Disabled persons are often an object of curiosity when entering a new situation. They may be alternately or simultaneously pitied, sympathized with, helped, patronized, or exhibited. When a disabled person "makes it" in spite of disability, he or she is praised for spunk. In other words, the disabled person is seen not as an individual with potentials, but as an individ-

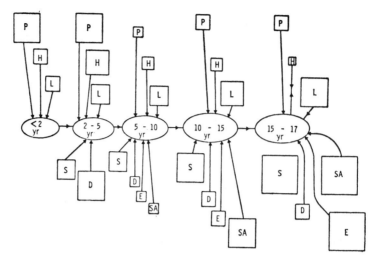

P . . . Stress arising from parents' reaction to child's handicap.

H . . . Stress arising from hospital visits, hospitalization physiotherapy, and operation.

L . . . Stress arising from limitations of activity.

S . . . Stress arising from social limitations and difficulties in social relationships.

D . . . Stress arising from dependence on others.

E . . . Stress arising from educational or employment demands.

SA . . . Stress arising from self-awareness. Realization of own handicap.

Figure 19–9. Hypothetical model of stressors for children with disabilities. The pattern and the intensity of stress in a child's life vary with age as well as with the type of disabling condition. (From J. Reynell, Children with Physical Handicaps. In V. P. Varma (Ed.), *Stresses in Children.* London: University of London Press, 1973. With permission.)

ual with limitations. Such an environment is stressful and stigmatizing.

When the disabled person is with similarly disabled peers, individual abilities, interests, beliefs, values, and goals receive more attention; he or she is more likely to be accepted for the real self. This situation provides a safe, comfortable environment. The disabled person, then, has two worlds to choose from when establishing adjustment patterns [41] for the achievement of life goals.

First, the individual may choose the world of the disabled because of its security and acceptance. When experiences with the larger culture and general knowledge are weak, many normal daily events are novel experiences for disabled persons. Things unknown are feared; therefore, they avoid what they fear [11]. The disabled world offers a small, restricted, but safe lifespace. Depending on the disability, the disabled person may join a social club for the deaf or live in a special community for disabled individuals, seeking minimal overlap with the normal world. Goals are confined to those situations in which the individual can function with equal or superior advantage; for instance, a blind

person may prepare for a position in the darkroom of a photography company or in an x-ray laboratory. Psychological disequilibrium can thus be avoided.

A second disabled person may reject the disabled world and aspire to function in the normal world as if there were no disability. A person who stutters may prepare for a career in radio announcing, or a neurologically handicapped person for a career in acting. Occasionally these persons are successful, but they encounter many problems. The gains may take more effort than they are really worth. These individuals are living in an unreal world—always pretending that their disabilities do not exist, and fearing that someone will challenge them. This feeling increases tension levels and precipitates much status-anxiety [61].

The third type of disabled person values the commonalities of the disabled and normal worlds [41]. These individuals do not deny or disregard their deviation or disabilities, but at the same time, they are not overwhelmed by them [61]. They see disability as only one aspect of life, and participate in the normal world as much as they can realistically, learning adaptive and alternative skills for achieving goals. The in-

However, the disabled individual does not achieve this realistic approach to life without help. He or she needs at least one other significant person who believes in and will challenge his or her potentials. This teacher of how to live and to enjoy life is usually a parent or a teacher at school. The disabled child will not achieve this high level affective and social wellness without an education that will support the maximization of potentials.

EDUCATION OF THE EDUCATIONALLY HANDICAPPED CHILD

The Bureau of Education for the Handicapped (BEH) estimates that there are approximately 8 million educationally handicapped children in the United States [46], or 10 to 12 percent of the school population. If gifted children are included in this group, it would add another 3 percent [26].

Educationally handicapped children are those who deviate from the norm in one or more domains to such an extent that they require specialized or modified techniques, equipment, or services in order to develop their potentials to maximal capacity and to function adaptively within the milieu. By law, this group includes children who are "mentally retarded, hard of hearing, deaf, orthopedically impaired, other health impaired, speech impaired, visually handicapped, seriously emotionally disturbed, or children with specific learning disabilities" [46]. Some cities and states also include gifted children in their special education program.

Relationship of Disabilities to Developmental Tasks

It is generally recognized and accepted that disabling conditions can interfere with normal growth and development. When children are under too much stress, the anxiety they feel may attenuate attention to the environment; if they feel unable to control events, motivation is decreased to learn cause-effect relationships. In short, the mediating factors of stress can decrease learning. Because parents and peers frequently treat disabled children differently, learning experiences are also altered, creating a different milieu for development.

ERIKSON'S TASKS

Erik Erikson's theory of personality development is based on sequential mastering of affective tasks. If the child does not have a positive feeling about the self, he

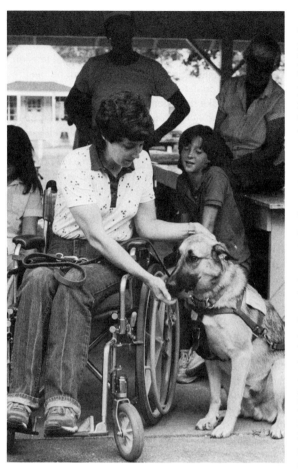

Figure 19–10. Many disabled persons are able to use animals to assist with orientation to the environment or for hearing, fetching, protection, and mobility. Although a close relationship develops between the disabled person and the dog, it is considered a working animal and not a pet. Thus friendly overtures toward the dog from strangers are not encouraged.

dividual views the self as "physically challenged" rather than "physically handicapped" and is able to participate with groups of disabled peers as well as normal persons and to enjoy both. These individuals do not accept the stereotyped role established by others in the culture; they establish their own roles, know their own strengths and weaknesses and work cooperatively with them to find challenge and joy in life. They see and feel the stigma that others associate with their disabilities but do not dwell on it. These individuals educate others through their own joy of living, their ease with their own limitations and potentials.

or she may develop the negative counterpart (see Appendixes B and C). Physically impaired children are known to have a higher emotional maladjustment rate than "normal" peers [39]. Since at least partial mastery of each stage is essential for progression to the next stage, altered experiences can impede affective growth. Some emotional handicaps can be directly related to incomplete resolution of Erikson's stages; examples are given in the following sections. If sensitive adults, are available to help impaired children, most of them should be able to master Erikson's tasks.

Trust versus Mistrust. If the infant's parents have not yet resolved their own shock and grief over their child's impairment, they may be very inconsistent in their responses. Their response to either cries or smiles may be delayed or inappropriate. If the infant is hospitalized, this may further increase the child's stress level and delay the establishment of trusting, affectionate bonds with the parent. The blind child's inability to predict when he or she will be picked up can lead to crying when the child is startled; consequently he or she should be warned by voice before being touched. The deaf child likewise may be startled when touched unexpectedly. In this instance, visual contact should be made before tactile contact.

Autonomy versus Shame and Doubt. During the toddler stage, children normally learn to get things for themselves, to control bowels and bladder, to walk, to run, and so on. Children with neurological disorders or cerebral palsy may have a particular conflict if they are unable to learn to control their bowels. They may still need to wear diapers at age 6, even though their cognitive functioning levels are normal. Although enuresis (bed-wetting) can be a sign of emotional tension, for neurologically impaired children it can be the creator of emotional tension. The inability of disabled children to make their bodies do what they want them to do can be an acute source of frustration, requiring sensitive parental assistance. Disabled adults also often experience considerable dismay and shame about lack of control in these areas. Understanding friends who have a sense of humor can be invaluable sources of support.

Initiative versus Guilt. It is very difficult for some children with specific health problems (for example, asthma, epilepsy, cerebral palsy, diabetes, or cardiac anomaly) to exert initiative in selecting activities because their choice may result in adverse physical effects. When cognitive processes have not yet sufficiently developed to allow the child to understand the reasons for, or the mechanics of, physical limitations, confusion and guilt may ensue when a diabetic crisis, a seizure, or a respiratory difficulty follows the child's attempts to set personal limits. It is difficult for the child to achieve independence from the parents and set personal goals or limits when so many limits have already been set by the physical disability. Parents need to balance sensitively the opportunity to make choices (offering two or three safe alternatives) and provide the necessary teaching, with protective restrictions, until the child is able to govern behaviors within safe limits.

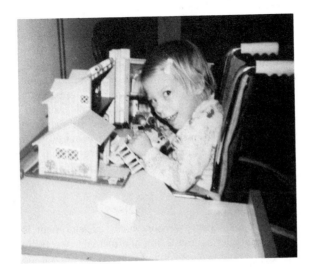

Figure 19–11. Even the toddler with severe cerebral palsy can be provided with meaningful, independent play activities by a creative parent.

The blind adult who must ask for assistance in locating landmarks or objects and the neurologically impaired adult who needs assistance with mobility may experience guilt feelings about the forced dependence on others, which can lead to lowered self-esteem.

Industry versus Inferiority. The school-ager develops the precursors for self-identity through the mastery of valued skills. If school-age children are disabled, the disability may prevent them from reaching goals. They may feel frustrated and cheated. It is rather common for them to give up efforts to be successful. The child of this age needs support in setting appropriate goals and learning alternative approaches leading to mastery (children of poverty may also experience frustration in goal achievement because of inadequate money for activities such as music lessons, bicycling, hobbies, or pet care). Helplessness and depression are common in this developmental stage. The disabled adult who is unable to secure compatible, challenging employment may develop feelings of inferiority.

Identity versus Role Confusion. The disabled adolescent may experience great conflict in attempts to blend the past, present, and future into a positive role identity. Questions about career and marriage may remain nebulous. Anxiety may increase as graduation from the semiprotected educational environment draws closer. ("Will I be able to get a job?" "Can I compete with nondisabled people?" "Is there a niche for me?") Career counseling is critical. If the disabled person's tools are carefully weighed against the skills needed to perform a job, success can be anticipated. It must be noted, however, that even if the tools and skills are matched well, the job may not be retained if interpersonal relationship skills have not been adequately refined.

Intimacy versus Isolation. Disabled adults may feel inferior or unworthy if they have not been given adequate support during earlier years. As a result, they may prefer to marry other disabled persons because they are "equals." In some situations this works out very well; however, a couple may withdraw further into the disabled world if they find that frustration in coping with their disability is the focus of their relationship rather than mutual respect and love. Many disabled persons, because of unresolved pain stemming from earlier interpersonal relationships and experiences, prefer to isolate themselves rather than face the risk of repeated social rejection. Others will accept any quality relationship in an effort to avoid loneliness.

Generativity versus Stagnation. Any adult who has not developed a positive concept of self and respect for personal skills will experience difficulty with the task of sharing this part of self with other persons. A limited physical skill repertoire may restrict the options available to expand a career or to enjoy hobbies. Consequently, the individual may become bored with life unless aggressive assistance is offered to expand professional and social horizons. Even the most severely disabled person, however, has the potential ability to offer ideas, encouragement, and a philosophy of life that can foster the development of other persons, providing he or she has a positive concept of self.

Ego Integrity versus Despair. Those persons who have been unable to integrate their inabilities, impairments, or cultural differences within a positive framework will experience difficulty in achieving a sense of satisfaction or personal value in their later years. They may feel that the negative aspects outweigh the positive experiences and draw the conclusion that life is "not worth the trip." Conversely, those impaired persons who have met and resolved each challenge as it emerged develop a sense of confidence in themselves and others. They recognize that everyone must face challenges during a lifetime and that their challenges are merely more obvious, not necessarily more difficult.

HAVIGHURST'S TASKS

Robert Havighurst, as the reader will recall, identifies specific skills to be mastered at each level of development. These skills, which are sequentially arranged, cover the cognitive, biophysical, and social domains as well as the affective domain. The practitioner can find these tasks to be a very helpful general guide for developing a habilitation program. The specific skills may need to be translated into conceptual tasks before they are applied to the disabled child. If the child cannot learn to perform a skill in the normal way, the practitioner can usually substitute an alternative skill to accomplish the concept that the task embodies. For example, a task for the toddler is to learn to talk. The deaf child may experience considerable difficulty talking. However, when one identifies the concept as learning to communicate, alternative methods become apparent; the child may learn sign language. In fact, deaf children who learn sign language during preschool years usually exhibit better command of language concepts and achieve higher academic skills than deaf children who are confined to lip-reading during preschool years [64].

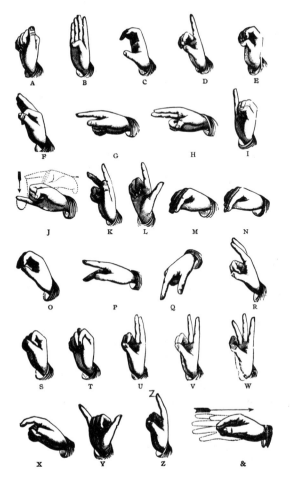

Figure 19–12. Manual alphabet for the deaf. Deaf persons also have a manual language with its own codes for words and syntactic structure for sentences. Some individuals are now using cued speech, a system of 32 hand signals that represent phonemes and that accompany lip reading. (Courtesy Ohio School for the Deaf.)

The school-ager is expected to develop fundamental skills in reading, writing, and calculating; the blind child can learn to use Braille, a typewriter, and the abacus or Taylor slate as alternative skills. A task of the adolescent is to achieve new and more mature relationships with agemates of both sexes. If orthopedically handicapped children cannot participate in all the activities, they may choose to develop expertise in one socially desirable skill that allows them to take part in an activity or brings others to them; for instance, an individual may become the timekeeper at the basketball games or the typist for the school newspaper.

Disabilities may pose barriers to the accomplishment of developmental tasks but need not prevent their accomplishment if a creative teacher is available to help the child assess and develop potentials.

Public Law 94-142

In 1974, BEH discovered that 50 percent of our nation's educationally handicapped children had inadequate educational programs and that more than 1 million children between the ages of 6 and 16 had no educational program at all [46]. This situation was felt to be a gross violation of the civil rights of these children. The United States Constitution states that all men are created equal; this does not mean that they all have equal potential, but that they all have the right to equal opportunity under the law [36, 61]. Each child has the right to receive an education geared to helping him or her to learn and to maximize potentials in order to live life to the fullest capacity.

In 1975, the 94th Congress passed Public Law (PL) 94-142. The Education for All Handicapped Children Act of 1975. It mandates that **all** children 5 to 21 years of age, regardless of type or degree of disability, **must** be offered a free, appropriate public education. (Most states include ages 3 to 21.) This law embodies a holistic approach to education, which can include adaptive functioning and self-help skills as well as academic skills. The goal is to help each child to achieve maximal developmental level [25]. Section 10 of the Education Act of 1974 provides similar safeguards in England [62].

MAJOR PROVISIONS OF PUBLIC LAW 94-142
PL 94-142 is very specific in its requirements in order to protect the educational rights of the disabled child.

Least Restrictive Alternative. The law stipulates that to the maximum extent possible, educationally handicapped children are to be educated with children who are not handicapped. Removal is to occur "only when the nature or severity of the handicap is such that education in regular classes with the use of supplementary aids and services cannot be achieved satisfactorily" [46]. Practitioners may interpret this statement to mean that all children must be "mainstreamed" or fully integrated, but this is not true. The law requires that each child be individually evaluated and placed in the program that is most advantageous to his total development. A hierarchy of educational programs is available to meet the unique needs of the child (see Fig. 19–14). One starts with the assumption of nor-

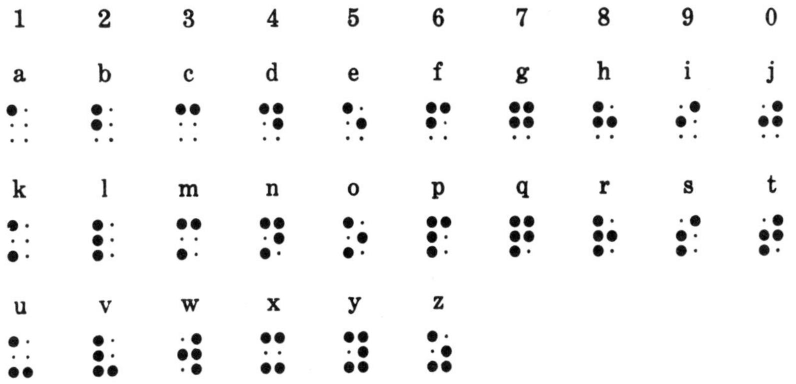

1	2	3	4	5	6	7	8	9	0
a	b	c	d	e	f	g	h	i	j

k	l	m	n	o	p	q	r	s	t

u	v	w	x	y	z

Figure 19–13. The Braille alphabet is developed around the six positions of a cell. The position of the raised dot indicates to the reader the letter represented. Variations of raised dots on this same six-position cell will indicate punctuation, letter combinations, or whole words. Even mathematics and music have been translated into this six-position cell code. (From M. B. Dorf and E. R. Scharry, *Instruction Manual for Braille Transcribing.* Washington, D.C.: Library of Congress, 1973. With permission.)

malcy and alters the environment only as necessary— to meet the needs of the **child,** not the needs of the school system.

Placement Team. No **one** person can decide on appropriate placement or program for a handicapped child. The team must include (1) a representative of the administration of the local educational agency (LEA), (2) the child's actual or potential teacher, (3) the parent or parents, and when appropriate, (4) the child. This team is to develop the IEP jointly. Whatever all agree upon is considered to be appropriate [66].

Individualized Educational Program (IEP). The real value of PL 94-142 centers around the fact that each child must be provided with a written statement that includes the following:

1. Present performance level
2. Annual goals (according to the child's needs, this is to include areas such as social adaptation, emotional maturity, prevocational and vocational skills, psychomotor skills, physical education, self-help skills, activities of daily living, and academic skills)
3. Short-term instructional objectives
4. Specific special services (e.g., physical therapy, transportation, special equipment) as needed
5. Extent of participation in the regular program
6. Objective criteria for evaluation
7. Date for initiation and duration of services

This written plan must be evaluated annually. It might be noted that special education may be a very small part of the child's total educational package [66].

This individualized approach has five very valuable assets. First, it prevents segregating and educating the child according to a labeled category. Second, it prevents relegating the child to a "back ward" once the child has been identified and labeled. Third, this approach recognizes the intraindividual differences of children and individualizes educational approaches according to the child's unique developmental level. Fourth, the IEP capitalizes on the child's assets. Fifth, it looks at the **total** child, not just the disabling condition. When unique, alternative approaches are used to meet the needs of the individual child, frustration can be lowered, successes earned, self-esteem elevated, and social-emotional adaptation problems prevented.

Due Process. Occasionally the team cannot agree on appropriate placement or program. In this case, the family is entitled to examine all records and to request an impartial hearing; they may even go to court if necessary. However, the law was developed to open up communication, not to create adversaries. Suits usually come about because of inadequate communication and poor IEP planning [66].

Multifactored, Nondiscriminatory Evaluation. For the white middle-class child, school is frequently seen as an extension of the family for continued enculturation and socialization. For children of other socioeco-

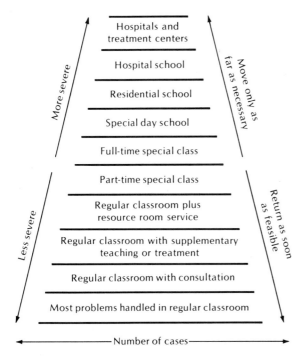

Move only as far as necessary

Return as soon as feasible

More severe

Less severe

Hospitals and treatment centers

Hospital school

Residential school

Special day school

Full-time special class

Part-time special class

Regular classroom plus resource room service

Regular classroom with supplementary teaching or treatment

Regular classroom with consultation

Most problems handled in regular classroom

◄──── Number of cases ────►

Figure 19–14. Hierarchy of services for special education programs. (From M. C. Reynolds, A framework for considering some issues in special education. *Except. Child.* 28:368, 1962. With permission.)

nomic levels and ethnic groups, however, there may be a marked discontinuity between school, subculture, and home values and norms [31]. As a result, children of different subcultural and ethnic backgrounds may fail to do well in school because they have had different life experiences, they do not understand the demands of the school, or they have a different value system [20]. As a result of these differences in experiences, a child may enter school with a different complex of general knowledge and repertoire of competencies. Unfortunately, although potentials for success may be high, many of these children have been labeled "slow learners" or "retarded" because of these cultural discrepancies. With PL 94-142, the school system must meet the child's needs rather than fitting the child into an existing program. Some schools are now offering classes in the child's native language (especially Spanish and the Indian languages); some school systems are providing portable schools for children of migrant farm workers; many schools are making more concerted efforts to honor and to extend value to sub-

cultures by including study of native arts and crafts or courses designed to meet the value systems of specific ethnic groups. Persons interested in the childhood experiences of ethnic groups within the United States may wish to read excerpts from David Gottlieb [23] or some of Lois Lenski's books.

A single IQ test can no longer be used as the basis for educational placement. The LEA must evaluate the needs of the **total** child. The testing must be given in the child's native language or mode of communication if necessary. The testing may be used to identify functional skills but cannot be used to discriminate against the child. This law, then, is affecting the education of not only individual children but also groups of children because of its stipulations.

Full Services. PL 94-142 also requires early identification of handicapped children. Recognizing that early intervention can frequently prevent later problems, it encourages states to provide programs for children 3 to 5 years of age. The law stipulates that all education and supportive services be given at no cost to the parents; this includes room and board if the child is placed in a residential setting at the recommendation of the placement team.

Now that the handicapped child's right to education is assured it is the responsibility of the educators to provide quality. Some educators find it difficult to include the parents as part of the team, but personal experience indicates that when parents are respectfully involved, their ability to work with the child is increased and the child's learning process is accelerated.

Resources

A truly holistic approach to the education of exceptional children is not limited to the home or the school. Children need experiences with community social agencies that expand or offer an outlet for their interests and provide for peer contact. The local American Red Cross and YMCA frequently have programs designed specifically for disabled children. Scouts, 4-H, and other clubs for children are frequently able to provide very sensitive, individualized peer and adult interactions. The local public library is also a rich source of resources and services.

Depending on the type and degree of disability, the child may attend a summer camp with nondisabled peers or may choose one that specializes in serving children with special needs [34] Porter-Sargent Publishers in Boston publishes several books of value in this area, including *Guide to Summer Camps and Summer Schools* and *Directory for Exceptional Children: A Listing of Educational and Training Facilities.*

Other sources of information or referral are given in the following list:

American Association for the Education of the
  Severely/Profoundly Handicapped
  Box 15287
  Seattle, WA 98115
American Foundation for the Blind, Inc.
  15 W. 16th St.
  New York, NY 10011
Association for Children with Learning Disabilities
  4156 Library Rd.
  Pittsburgh, PA 15234
American Association of Mental Deficiency
  5101 Wisconsin Ave., N.W.
  Washington, DC 20016
American Brittle Bone Society (Osteogenesis
  Imperfecta)
  1415 E. Marlton Pike
  Cherry Hill, NJ 08077
Association for Children with Down's Syndrome
  589 Patterson St.
  East Meadow, NY 11554
Association for Education of the Visually
  Handicapped
  919 Walnut St. Fourth Floor
  Philadelphia, PA 19107
Epilepsy Foundation of America, Suite 406
  1828 L St., N. W.
  Washington, DC 20036
Little People of America, Inc.
  P.O. Box 126
  Owatonna, MN 55060
National Association for Gifted Children
  8080 Springvalley Dr.
  Cincinnati, OH 45236
National Association for Retarded Children
  420 Lexington Ave.
  New York, NY 10017
National Association of the Deaf
  814 Thayer Ave.
  Silver Spring, MD 20910
National Camps for Blind Children
  4444 S. 52nd St.
  Lincoln, NE 68506

National Committee for Multi-Handicapped Children
  239 14th St.
  Niagara Falls, NY 14303
National Easter Seal Society for Crippled Children
  and Adults
  2023 W. Ogden Ave.
  Chicago, IL 60612
National Federation of the Blind
  1800 Johnson St.
  Baltimore, MD 21230
National Society for Autistic Children
  169 Tampa Ave.
  Albany, NY 12208
Spina Bifida Association of America
  343 S Dearborn St.
  Chicago, IL 60604
United Cerebral Palsy Association, Inc.
  66 E. 34th St.
  New York, NY 10016

The physically disabled child needs to be provided with as many normal extracurricular activities as are appropriate and comfortable. Experience with peers and brief separations from parents for experiences with independence are just as significant to the development of the disabled child as they are for the non-disabled child. The last section of Chapter 35 gives further sources of information or referral. The unique needs and problems of disabled adults are discussed further in Chapters 27 and 28.

CONCLUSIONS

Each person is a member of a minority group in some way. Unless an individual is able to accept his or her uniqueness in a realistic perspective, it may adversely affect the ability to maximize potentials and to adjust to the life-style and demands of the larger culture. The parents are critical in the establishment of trust in the environment and faith in one's ability to control events. Interactional patterns, attitudes, or "sets" formed during the developmental years can affect self-esteem and ego-identity for the rest of one's life.

The school-age years are spent in expanding beyond the family and learning skills that will initiate and introduce the child to society; this includes the explicit, or the formal learning that occurs in school as well as the implicit, or the informal, learning that is picked up from contact with family, peers, and society. The atti-

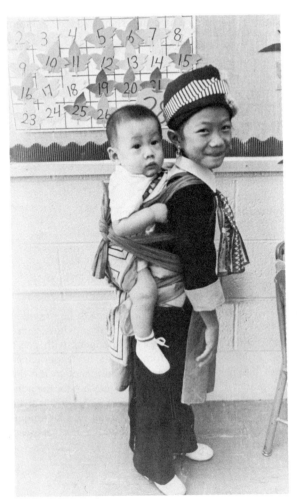

Figure 19–15. Pride in one's cultural heritage can be fostered by giving the child an opportunity to share native costumes and customs with teacher and peers.

tudes, values, and general knowledge gained through implicit learning usually have longer-lasting results than the specific facts learned through explicit methods. Consequently, the reactions of other persons to a child's deviation become critical to the budding self-esteem and ego-identity.

During the school years the child attempts to identify with the significant values and characteristics of the subculture. During adolescence one attempts to identify personal uniqueness within the society, while consolidating and synthesizing childhood identifications. The minority child (whether as a result of racial, cultural, or physical variation from the majority) is forced

to identify differences before identifying sufficient similarities and thus may feel alienated from the culture. Sensitive guidance from a significant adult can help to prevent the development of a socioemotional handicap; supportive guidance can facilitate the maximization of potentials.

Isolation from the mainstream of life can aid or hinder the child's ability to adjust to adolescent and adult living. If one plans to remain within the confines of a subculture, the isolation serves to perpetuate select cultural standards and goals (e.g., religious or ethnic values) [32, 56]. However, if the child must, or wants to, eventually blend into the mainstream of the culture, isolation during the developmental years because of factors, such as overprotective parents, a residential school, or inadequate opportunities, can present sufficient barriers to continue the alienation throughout one's life cycle. Since physically disabled children are most likely to be placed in these situations, it behooves all practitioners to become advocates for the child to assure adequate educational opportunities in order to be prepared to enter the adult world successfully.

Each of us should reexamine our attitudes toward persons of minority status and make conscious efforts

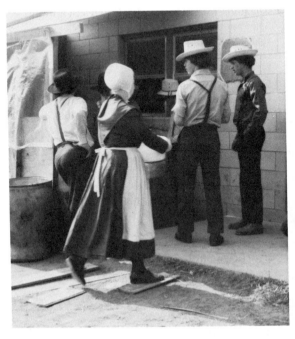

Figure 19–16. For subcultures that want to perpetuate their values and goals, isolation from the mainstream of the culture serves to prevent dilution of their lifestyle.

to get to know the **person** with whom we have contact, rather than responding to the external indexes. Inter-actions based on stereotyped concepts of individuals limit the potentials of everyone involved. Although it may take more effort to include a disabled or culturally different person in an educational program, place of employment, or social group, the benefits can far out-weigh any inconveniences.

REFERENCES

1. Abeson, A., and Zettel, J. The end of the quiet revolution: The Education for All Handicapped Children Act of 1975. *Except. Child.* 44(2):114, 1977.
2. American Association for Health, Physical Education, and Recreation and Bureau for Education for the Handi-capped, U. S. Department of Health Education and Wel-fare. Operational definitions for the mentally handicapped. *J. Sp. Educ. Men. Retard.* 12(2):129, 1976.
3. Ayrault, E. W. *Helping the Handicapped Teenager Ma-ture.* New York: Public Affairs Committee, 1974.
4. Ballard, J., and Zettel, J. Public Law 94-142 and Section 504: What they say about rights and protections. *Except. Child.* 44(3):177, 1977.
5. Barnes, B. Cued speech keeps deaf pupils ahead. *Child. Today* 7(4):28, 1978.
6. Bartel, N. R., and Guskin, S. L. A Handicap as a Social Phenomenon. In W. M. Cruickshank (Ed.), *Psychology of Exceptional Children and Youth* (3rd ed.). Englewood Cliffs, NJ: Prentice-Hall, 1971.
7. Bingham, D. M., and Guay, P. L. More special than dif-ferent. *Am. J. Nurs.* 81:2031, 1981.
8. Brazelton, T. B. "The Remarkable Talents of the New-born." Papers presented at symposium, *Parent to Infant Attachment.* Cleveland, Nov. 6, 1977.
9. Burgdorf, R. L. *The Legal Rights of Handicapped Persons.* Baltimore: P. H. Brookes, 1980.
10. Coopersmith, S. *The Antecedents of Self-Esteem.* Palo Alto, CA: Consulting Psychologists Press, 1981.
11. Cruickshank, W. M., and Johnson, G. O. (Eds.). *Education of Exceptional Children and Youth* (3rd ed.). Englewood Cliffs, NJ: Prentice-Hall, 1975.
12. Cutsforth, T. D. *The Blind in School and Society.* New York: American Foundation for the Blind, 1951.
13. *Directory for Exceptional Children: A Listing of Educational and Training Facilities* (9th ed.). Boston: Porter-Sargent, 1981.
14. *Due Process and the Exceptional Child, a Guide for Parents.* Philadelphia: Education Law Center, 1976.
15. Erikson, E. H. *Childhood and Society* (rev. ed.). St. Al-bans: Triad/Paladin, 1978.
16. *Federal Register,* Vol. 42, No. 163 (Aug. 23, 1977). Educa-tion of Handicapped Children, Implementation of Part B of the Education of the Handicapped Act, 1977.
17. Fraiberg, S. Blind Infants and Their Mothers: An Ex-amination of the Sign System. In M. Lewis and L. A. Ro-senblum (Eds.), *The Effect of the Infant on Its Caregiver.* New York: Wiley, 1974.
18. Fraiberg, S. *Insights From the Blind: Comparative Studies of Blind and Sighted Infants.* New York: Basic Books, 1977.
19. *Getting Your Baby Ready to Talk: A Home Study Plan for Infant Language Development.* Los Angeles: John Tracy Clinic, 1968.
20. Gitter, L. L. The underachieving child, Part 1. *J. Sp. Educ. Men. Retard.* 12(2):139, 1976.
21. Goffman, E. *Stigma: Notes on the Management of Spoiled Identity.* New York: J. Aronson, 1974.
22. Gordon, M., et al. Psychosocial aspects of constitutional short stature: Social competence, behavior problems, self-esteem, and family functioning. *J. Pediatr.* 101:477, 1982.
23. Gottlieb, D., and Heinsohn, A. L. *America's Other Youth: Growing Up Poor.* Englewood Cliffs, NJ: Prentice-Hall, 1971.
24. Harasymiw, S., and Horne, M. Integration of handi-capped children: Its effect on teacher attitudes. *Education* 96:153, 1975.
25. Haring, N. G. (Ed.) *Behavior of Exceptional Children: An Introduction to Special Education* (2nd ed.). Columbus, OH: Merrill, 1978.
26. Haring, N. G. *Exceptional Children and Youth: An Intro-duction to Special Education* (3rd ed.). Columbus, OH: C. E. Merrill, 1982.
27. Harrison-Ross, P., and Wyden, B. *The Black Child, A Par-ents' Guide.* New York: Wyden, 1973.
28. Hauser, S. T., and Kasendorf, E. *Black and White Identity Formation* (2nd ed.). Malabar, FL: Krieger, 1983.
29. Havighurst, R. J. *Developmental Tasks and Education* (3rd ed.). New York: David McKay, 1972.
30. Hedahl, K. J. Helping children establish positive attitudes towards disabled persons. *Pediatr. Nurs.* 7(6):11, 1981.
31. Hirata, L. C. Youth, Parents and Teachers in Chinatown. *Urban Educ.* 10(3):279, 1975.
32. Huntington, G. E. Children of the Hutterites. *Natural History* 90(2):34, 1981.
33. Irvin, T. Implementation of Public Law 94-142. *Except. Child.* 43:135, 1976.
34. Kawasaki, M. A. Summer camp and the disabled child. *Pediatr. Nurs.* 7(4):9, 1981.
35. Kershaw, J. D. Handicapped Children in the Ordinary School. In V. P. Varma (Ed.), *Stresses in Children.* London: University of London Press, 1973.
36. Kirk, S. A., and Gallagher, J. J. *Educating Exceptional Children* (4th ed.). Boston: Houghton Mifflin, 1983.
37. Klein, G. S. Blindness and isolation. *Psychoanal. Stud. Child* 17:82, 1962.
38. Kowalsky, E. L. Grief: A lost life-style. *Am. J. Nurs.* 78:418, 1978.
39. Lombana, J. H. *Guidance for Handicapped Students.* Springfield, OH: Thomas, 1982.
40. Lydon, W. T., and McGraw, M. L. *Concept Development*

for Visually Handicapped Children (Rev. ed.). New York: American Foundation for the Blind, 1973.

41. Meyerson, L. Somatopsychology of Physical Disability. In W. M. Cruickshank (Ed.), Psychology of Exceptional Children and Youth (3rd ed.). Englewood Cliffs, NJ: Prentice-Hall, 1971.

42. Minde, K., et al. How they grow up: Forty-one physically handicapped children and their families. Am. J. Psychiatry 128:1554, 1972.

43. Minde, K. "Coping styles of 34 cerebral palsied adolescents." Paper presented at the American Psychiatric Association, 1977.

44. National Advisory Committee on the Handicapped. "Education of the Handicapped Today" (excerpt from Annual Report 1976). Reprinted in American Education, June 1976.

45. Orlansky, M. D., and Heward, Wm. L. Voices: Interviews With Handicapped People. Columbus: OH: C. E. Merrill, 1981.

46. Public Law 94-142, Education for all Handicapped Children Act of 1975. Washington, D.C.: U.S. Congress, 94th, S. 6, Nov. 29, 1975.

47. Reynell, J. Children With Physical Handicaps. In V. P. Varma (Ed.), Stresses in Children. London: University of London Press, 1973.

48. Reynolds, M. C. A framework for considering some issues in special education. Except. Child. 28:367, 1962.

49. Reynolds, M. C., and Birch, J. W. Teaching Exceptional Children in All America's Schools (Rev. ed.). Reston, VA: Council for Exceptional Children, 1982.

50. Rodgers, B. M., et al. Depression in the chronically ill or handicapped school-aged child. MCN 6:266, 1981.

51. Rutter, M. A children's questionnaire for completion by teachers, preliminary findings. J. Child. Psychol. Psychiatry 8:1, 1967.

52. Rutter, M., Tizard, J., and Whitmore, K. Education, Health, and Behavior. Huntington, NY: Krieger, 1981.

53. Schowalter, J. E. The Chronically Ill Child. In J. D. Noshpitz (Ed.), Basic Handbook of Child Psychiatry. New York: Basic Books, 1979.

54. Seligman, M. E. P. Helplessness: On Depression, Development, and Death. San Francisco: Freeman, 1975.

55. Shea, T. M. Camping for Special Children. St. Louis: Mosby, 1977.

56. Shigaki, I. S. Child care practices in Japan and The United States: How do they reflect cultural values in young children? Young Child. 38(4):13, 1983.

57. Spock, B. M., and Lerrigo, M. O. Caring for Your Disabled Child. New York: Macmillan, 1965.

58. Steinhausen, H. Chronically ill and handicapped children and adolescents. J. Abnorm. Child Psychol. 9:291, 1981.

59. Stern, D. N. Mother and Infant at Play: The Dyadic Interaction Involving Facial, Vocal, and Gaze Behaviors. In M. Lewis and L. A. Rosenblum (Eds.), The Effect of the Infant on Its Caregiver. New York: Wiley, 1974.

60. Stokoe, W. C. Seeing and signing language. Hearing and Speech News, 42:32, 1974.

61. Telford, C. W., and Sawrey, J. M. The Exceptional Individual (4th ed.). Englewood Cliffs, NJ: Prentice-Hall, 1981.

62. Topliss, E. Social Responses to Handicap. New York: Longman, 1982.

63. Torres, S. (Ed.) A Primer on Individualized Education Programs for Handicapped Children. Reston, VA: The Foundation for Exceptional Children, 1977.

64. Vernon, M., and Koh, S. D. Early manual communication and deaf children's achievement. Am. Ann. Deaf. 116:527, 1970.

65. Wehman, P. Competitive Employment: New Horizons for Severely Disabled Individuals. Baltimore: Brookes, 1981.

66. Weintraub, F. "Federal Mandates for Handicapped Children." Paper presented at the Ohio Federation for Exceptional Children, Cleveland, Nov. 13, 1976.

67. Weller, J. Yesterday's People. In D. Gottlieb and A. L. Heinsohn (Eds.), America's Other Youth: Growing Up Poor. Englewood Cliffs, NJ: Prentice-Hall, 1971.

68. Zeligs, R. Children's Experience with Death. Springfield, IL: Thomas, 1974.

20

Development of a Concept of Death

Clara S. Schuster

He who does not know how to live is also not capable of dying; and he who fears death is really terrified of life.

—Maria Nagy

An individual's concept of death is the major organizer of the personality. No other concept has the integrating force embodied in this single macroconcept. Into this one complex concept are integrated personal concepts of past, present, and future—the affective, social, cognitive, physical, and spiritual domains. The uniqueness of humanity, human dignity, and, in fact, the value and meaning of life itself are all bound up in one's concept of death.

The development of a concept of death is never complete. A concept of death continues to be modified until death itself ends temporal life. The most dramatic changes in one's concept of death occur during the first decade of life, paralleling changes in cognitive functioning and ego development. The words, "I will die," have a different meaning to the child than to the adult because of the child's inability to think abstractly as well as the still weak ego-strength of the child. A mature understanding of "I will die" presupposes an understanding of the following subconcepts [27]:

1. I am a separate individual.
2. There is a difference between living and nonliving objects—I am alive.
3. Death is universal—this includes me.
4. Death is inevitable—I cannot evade all causes.
5. There is time present and time future—death is a future event.

6. The time left to live is unknown.
7. Death is permanent—an end to temporal life.
8. Death is separation from the known world.

Thus a mature understanding of "I will die" requires "self-awareness, logical thought operations, conceptions of probability, necessity, and causation, of personal and physical time, of finality and separation" [27]. Individuals must develop a concept of life before they can develop a concept of death. A concept of life also closely parallels the development of a concept of self [24]. Young children lack the mental operations to integrate all these concepts into a single concept of personal mortality.

Although the development of a concept of death is unique and personal to each individual, it has some universal qualities. It is also heavily influenced both by individual experiences and by the values and beliefs of the subculture milieu of which the person is a member. In order to appreciate the qualitative changes that occur in the development of one's concept of death, we must examine the role of culture and personal experiences as well as that of cognitive development. All three factors must be carefully evaluated in time of loss in order to aid the grieving person to use the crisis as a maturational rather than a destructive experience. This chapter will concentrate on the developmental aspects of a concept of death. How one's concept of death affects coping with imminent personal death will be discussed in Chapter 21.

EFFECTS OF WESTERN CULTURE THAT INHIBIT POSITIVE CONCEPT FORMATION

In past eras, death was an integral part of family life [1]. Several generations often lived in the same house. Death was an obvious part of the life cycle. Children were exposed to the process of dying—not just to death itself. When a loved one died, all the family members participated in the viewing, memorial, and burying events. Although the children might be too young to comprehend the significance of all the events, they were introduced to the fact of permanent separation and grief. The common sharing of grief supported the value of human life, allowed a therapeutic milieu for the expression of sorrow and frustration, and offered experience for further integration and growth of the psyche.

Death is no longer seen as a natural event in our culture [53]. Today families are smaller, and older persons usually live in their own homes, in a housing complex for the elderly, or in a nursing home. The child's emotional bond with grandparents is frequently weak because of distance or infrequency of contacts.

Advances in medical care have extended both the quantity and the quality of life. Death during childhood is rare. No longer does a family expect to lose at least one child before his or her tenth birthday. Whereas death was seen as an inevitable part of family life in the nineteenth century, now it is often seen as the result of personal negligence or a tragic accident. Consequently, it is approached as an avoidable illness or a physical stigma [1, 17].

Denial and ritual are frequently used to distort or to disguise death as a meaningful fact in our country [1, 39]. Health, youth, and vitality are valued; they are given visibility both within the home and through the mass media. Discussion of death is a taboo subject in many homes—just as discussions of sex and pregnancy were avoided in the Victorian era. When questions are asked, the parent frequently evades the issue or will admonish the child, "Oh, don't talk about that. It's too awful to think about!" Euphemisms such as "sleep," "pass away," or "rest" are often used to soften the reality of the finality of death; other euphemisms such as "shuffle off" or "croak" attempt to add humor as a form of denial of the reality.

When a death does occur in a family, it is usually in a hospital, not in the home. The wake and the memorial service are at the funeral parlor—no longer in the home. Death is removed as far as possible from the family setting. When a family member dies, the parents frequently attempt to hide the fact from young children. However, the child does not remain blissfully ignorant; subtle changes in parental attitude, affect, and approach indicate to the child that something is wrong. Lack of information tends to increase rather than to decrease the child's anxiety. The child may even suspect that he or she is somehow responsible for the event. Total exclusion from the event may have a damaging effect on the child's personality by depriving the child of a sense of belonging, of sharing, and of personal respect [22]. Participation in family grief with explanations appropriate to the child's comprehension level can help to avoid potential long-range negative effects [51].

No child is protected from the discovery of death. It is all around us. Leaves change color, die, and fall in the autumn; an animal is seen dead beside the highway; a fly is swatted; a pet dies. Each of these events provides experience with loss and offers an opportunity for the discussion of death. Television programs, including cartoons, "cops and robbers" programs, and the news, also offer examples of death and destruction. Most television programs portray death as being violent, accidental, or resulting from an infraction of society's rules. The National Congress of Parents and Teachers estimates that the average child views 11,000 television murders by 14 years of age [61]. A number of court cases in the past decade have centered around the effect of the mass media on murders committed by minors.

DISCOVERY AND ACCEPTANCE OF DEATH AS A PART OF LIFE

Throughout life, children are engaged in a series of death-discovering experiences. A child's concept of reality is constantly striving for definitions, direction, limits, reversibility, finality, and separation—all death-related concepts. The discovery of death by a child becomes a "private, individual experience of great magnitude," often because of the avoidance and denial tactics used by significant adults [49].

The child's understanding of death is closely related to developmental stage. Cognitively, the child cannot possess a well-developed concept of death without the basic tools for understanding life (i.e., animate versus inanimate objects). The child must also be able to comprehend cause-effect relationships in order to put his or her awareness of death into a more meaningful framework and to decrease the anxiety or fear that may accompany such awareness. Since a mature concept of death deals with philosophical issues, the future, and the unknown, young children must learn to deal with the concrete factors of death before they can deal with the more abstract issues.

Affectively, the child must develop sufficient ego-strength to face the concept of nonbeing. This is a difficult task when one is just beginning to recognize and to appreciate one's own separateness and uniqueness. The ego of the young child is very vulnerable. Being forced to face this reality before adequate ego-strength and coping skills have been developed can have serious long-range effects, which will be discussed later in the chapter.

Stages in the Development of a Concept of Death

The cognitive and affective domains are intimately related, but not synchronous, in the development of a concept of death. Each domain appears to go through a gradual progression of four phases: naiveté, awareness, rebellion, and acceptance. The cognitive domain appears to precede the affective domain as the two at-tempt to come to grips with the concept of death. It must be kept in mind that the ages given with each stage are arbitrary and are heavily influenced by experiences, intelligence, family communication patterns, religious orientation, and cultural mores. Affective changes are not as easy to assess as cognitive changes. Thoughts about death are most frequent and have the greatest affective impact during the times when the ego is least stable: between 5 and 8 years of age, when the superego is emerging and logical/causality thinking is being established; and between 13 and 16 years, when society demands that the individual be more adult and when there is a search for identity and ideology with a reorganizing of self-concept. Thoughts about death may be intensified at any point in the life cycle when the individual is experiencing radical personal changes (e.g., marriage, birth of a child, illness, job change, menopause, retirement, old age) [2].

COGNITIVE AND AFFECTIVE NAIVETÉ
(Birth to 2 Years)

Although there are many who disagree with him, Otto Rank, a psychoanalyst, states that the child's first experience with death is birth itself [45]. One would not deny the presence of an instinct for physical survival as exhibited by the frantic gasping for air by the neonate suffering temporary oxygen deprivation; however, this and other protective reflexive behaviors hardly fit into the complex integration of concepts discussed earlier as comprising a mature concept of death.

A concept of death presupposes a concept of life; a concept of life presupposes a concept of animism. According to Piaget, the child starts life with a primary assumption of universal life. The more refined concept of animism that appears with maturation is not a product of structure but rather of differentiation [43]. Piaget believes that the infant begins life with the concept of a continuum between the self and the environment [42] and is aware only of need gratification, not of separateness. Awareness of separateness is a gradual process of differentiation in the biological, social, and affective realms [32, 44]. The infant must begin to develop a concept of self before comprehending me–not me [11].

Although the infant cannot conceive of death, the child is aware of a lack of completeness, or discomfort. The earliest precursors to a cognitive awareness of death are awareness of object loss and separation anxiety, which are usually first evident between 5 and 10 months of age. The infant exhibits distress when a toy disappears and becomes aware that the parent can come and go at will. Losing sight of the parent is responded to as if it were a threat to the child's own survival.

Infants gradually learn to control the anxiety associated with separation and gain primitive skills for dealing with separation through games, such as peek-a-boo. An infant engaged in this game with a parent alternately experiences panic and delight; the body tenses, extremities flail, eyes widen, breath quickens, and, finally, the infant will begin to cry if the parent disappears behind the cloth or hand too long. Immediate joy is exhibited when the parent reappears. Peek-a-boo is an old English term meaning "life or death." Another activity facilitating acceptance of finality or loss is the concept of "all gone," which may be experienced by the infant while eating food or blowing away dandelion seeds.

As the child's cognitive skills mature, there is an increasing awareness of threats to survival, consequently, for the infant, separation is synonymous with death; it is a form of deprivation—a loss of possession, of affection, of nurturing and nurturance. The primary caretaker is the source of tension reduction and pleasure gratification and as such is life-sustaining. When one is learning to trust the environment, to predict events, and to invest oneself in others, loss of a significant adult may have permanent residual effects on attachment formation. It is important when the child is in the process of learning to love and to be loved that the process continue uninterrupted. If interruption does occur, a warm, affectionate, permanent substitute should be located as soon as possible [7] (see Chaps. 9 and 17 for discussions of separation, adoption, and foster children).

COGNITIVE AWARENESS, AFFECTIVE NAIVETÉ (2 to 4 Years)

The toddler gradually becomes aware that some things have an end, and sadness may be felt at the separation from a desired object. He or she continues to learn to cope with the concept of "all gone" as a final separation. The earliest dependable record of cognitive awareness of a finality to life, or a death discovery, is reported by Kastenbaum, who tells of a 16-month-old boy who said "No more" with a depressed, resigned manner after seeing an adult step on a caterpillar [28]. Janssen relates the processes of assimilation and accommodation of the concept of "dead" by a child between 21 and 36 months of age [25]. To the astute observer, attempts to accommodate this concept could be found in all levels of the child's relationship with self and environment. Janssen indicates that an anxiety related to the potty chair and the feces may be due

to the newly acquired concept of death rather than to castration anxiety or anxiety over the loss of a body part as postulated by Freud. Although young children are cognizant that some things have an end to their existence, toddlers are ignorant of the fact that they too will die. Yet, apprehensions about swimming, safety precautions, or even sleep indicate that toddlers have begun to develop a vague awareness that what has been seen to happen to animals or people could also happen to them.

According to Piaget, the young child's universe is governed by the idea of purpose; consequently, children endow all things with consciousness (ability to know, to think, to plan) and categorize anything that is active or useful in any way as both conscious and alive [43]. Egocentric thought leads children to believe that all things think, feel, plan, and experience as they do. (The bed sheet wrapped itself around a foot on purpose; the oven or poisons are alive because they can hurt.) By 3 years of age, concepts of life and living begin to be restricted to those things that move or make sounds. A radio or television, a swing, a mirror, a pendant necklace, or a bicycle may all be responded to as if they embodied purposeful actions directed specifically toward the child. Animal death is usually identified before plant death. The 3- to 4-year-old thinks that a toy feels pain when it is broken or that it hurts to sew the ear back onto a stuffed dog. Children of this age see parents as a source of strength and power. When parents cannot "fix" or "make all better" something that has broken, it can make the child very insecure [52]. When children become ill, they may rationalize that their parents failed to take care of them adequately or are punishing them. They may interpret the illness as a form of parental rejection and respond with separation anxiety (realized dependence) and aggression (anger at the parents).

Although toddlers may begin to have an awareness that others die, they are ignorant of the meaning of death. For toddlers, death is merely another phase of life, not a separate state [34]. "Dead" to them means "less alive." To them, the dead continue to grow, to get hungry, to walk about, and to continue vital functions [25, 49].

Since the child's concepts of time are vague, separation is difficult for the toddler to cope with. The toddler fears being left alone and being separated from the love object; consequently, death, divorce, and hospitalization can be synonymous for the young child. Absence is equated with loss of love. The loss of a toy or a security blanket may be as significant to the toddler as the death of a friend is to an adult. To the toddler it is the loss of a love object—something the child has invested with a part of self.

When loss of a loved person or object does occur, the grief reaction takes much longer for the toddler to resolve than for the adult, partly because the child needs to mature in order to understand what has happened. Lack of understanding can lead to distortion of reality, which can have long-range effects on personality development. Inadequate coping skills can prevent substitution of supportive alternatives for the loss. Transfer of affectional ties may be difficult, and thus deep depression may continue over time [7]. The child may express grief through misbehavior.

James Robertson, a British physician, studied the emotional responses of toddlers to hospitalization and separation [48]. He felt that separation from parents was more traumatic than the hospital procedures themselves. At that time the parents were only allowed to visit the children briefly once a day. On being hospitalized, the children experienced loss of love, fear of the unknown, and fear of punishment. Robertson felt that toddlers were too young to understand and to reason with the separation and lacked sufficient internal resources to cope with it. He noted three specific phases in response to prolonged separation from the parents:

1. Protest. The children become grief-stricken and panicky, calling for a parent and rejecting other people who offer assistance or comfort. They are hostile, uncooperative, and very active. All energies are extended to "recapture" the parent. Sleep comes only from sheer exhaustion.
2. Despair. The children become withdrawn, apathetic, and anorexic. They attempt to "mother" themselves through self-comfort measures, such as thumb-sucking, body rocking, attachment to a "security blanket," or assuming a fetal position. Toddlers continue to watch anxiously for the mother. The mourning can become so great that they may become even more upset when the mother does visit because the visit does not offer enough contact to satisfy them, or it reactivates the pain of loss. It also increases their sense of helplessness, since they have no control over the retrieval or the disappearance of the mother. Some children are noted to reject the mother when she comes to visit; it is felt that this behavior is used as a way to retaliate and to punish the mother in an attempt to retain some control over the situation. There is frequently a marked regression to earlier behaviors of soiling and infantile speech; this may be a way of letting others know that

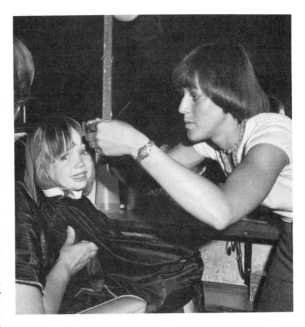

Figure 20–1. Loss of body integrity and fear of physical mutilation are major fears during the toddler and preschool years.

the child still feels helpless and in need of care, or it may be that inadequate energies are available to meet the needs of both the affective and social domains. The care of a mother substitute is no longer rejected, but passively accepted.

3. Denial and detachment. The children no longer act depressed. They begin to show interest in the environment and to accept attention in a detached way from anyone who gives it. Feelings for the mother are repressed. Parents may be ignored when they arrive for a visit, and no distress is shown when they leave. No attempts are made to control them or to make them stay. The children feel a loss of ability to control the environment; the helplessness syndrome appears.

It is significant to note at this point that these three stages can be prevented or attenuated if the hospital offers liberalized visiting policies or rooming-in. When parents cannot be present, attentive personnel can help to reduce the child's emotional trauma by encouraging trusting attachment to one or two staff members.

After separation and return to the home, children may become very "clingy" and may want to go everywhere with the mother. They do not want to lose sight of her again; the abandonment was too terrifying.

Other behaviors, such as sleep problems, crying, and continued infantile behaviors, indicate that a child fears a second separation.

Although Robertson's studies specifically involved a hospital setting, many similar behaviors are exhibited by children of this age in any setting when they are separated from their parents. Separation is a form of death, and death represents separation—a phenomenon the child is not yet ready to face as a reality. "Refueling" activities with the parents are still essential to autonomy [32]; loss of this source of strength can be devastating unless adequate substitutes are provided.

COGNITIVE REBELLION, AFFECTIVE AWARENESS
(5 to 6 Years)
Piaget states that the next level of differentiation of animate objects includes all things that move [44]. The table or a sheet is no longer seen as alive and conscious; however, the sun, the wind, or a clock is endowed with life and consciousness as are animals and people. Many children can identify characteristics of life, but few can identify characteristics of death. Thirty-two percent of children under 7 years of age are able to give adequate criteria for "animate," but only 6 percent are able to give an adequate criterion for "dead" [15].

The child in this phase accepts the fact of death as a cessation of movement but fantasizes that the dead person continues to experience emotion and biological functioning in the grave, even though the person does not move. Maria Nagy notes that many primitive people continue to conceptualize death on this level, as evidenced by the custom of putting food, drink, artifacts, and even servants and wives in the tomb with the deceased [41]. The child frequently feels that death is a gradual or a reversible process—if one is good. One's own death is not seen as a natural end of life. It is easier to conceive of death resulting from violence than death occurring through disease or natural processes [54]. One study [9] revealed that only 11 percent of 4-year-olds, 20 percent of 5-year-olds, and 22 percent of 6-year-olds admit to the universality of death. Even though one-third of the 4-year-olds acknowledged the irreversibility of death, not one of the 5-, 6-, or 7-year-olds was able to admit this belief—their emerging egos were still too fragile to acknowledge the probability of a personal nonexistence or a permanent cessation of being.

Children of this age frequently associate death with retaliation or punishment [3]; consequently, they may greatly fear the anger or the aggression of others, especially adults. This feeling may also cause the child

to try to please adults—a common characteristic of this age—as a way to avoid death [49]. The child begins to suspect that his or her own death is possible—but not probable in a loving environment. Play behaviors indicate that the children know that death is permanent [42], but affective factors protect them against acceptance of their own deaths. The ego, which is just beginning to recognize the self as a separate entity, is overwhelmed by the idea of nonbeing [49]. When loss does occur, the young child's delicate character structure finds an active acknowledgment of grief too strenuous on the fragile ego, frequently forcing the child to distance the self by denying the feelings or even the experience in order to assure personal psychological survival [20].

According to Kastenbaum, 75 percent of adults think that children never or seldom think about death. However, one study indicates that 80 percent of the young child's fears are associated with death, dying, being killed, or the death of a family member [46]. Sylvia Anthony reports that 50 to 60 percent of children 5 to 12 years of age refer to, or speak of, death in some form when completing stories [3]. Much spontaneous death-related talk and activity can be observed in play experiences: "Bang, bang! There, I killed you," or "I die, but you fix me and make me alive again," or "You can't move, you're dead." Play activities indicate that children know death is inevitable but they try to deny the idea through magical thought processes. As with many other anxiety-arousing events, the child tries to master the concept through play activities involving events, such as being frightened, lost, killed, or in the hospital. Cartoons involving violence, death, and revitalization may serve to perpetuate the child's confusion, since many children of this age have difficulty distinguishing between fact and fantasy. For others, the cartoons may offer a vehicle for working through their developing concept and dealing with loss in small doses.

The greatest fear of preschoolers is still separation and loss of love and security. They may worry about the death of a parent, since they still recognize their dependence on parents for support and guidance. If a parent does die during this phase, children may feel resentful, angry, and abandoned. They may believe the parent chose to die, since they still perceive parents as being all-powerful and all-wise. In turn, a child may also feel guilty or ambivalent regarding a parent's death because he or she had once wished that the parent were dead (as most preschoolers do at some time or another) [52]. The child, who believes the parent can read thoughts may feel that the death—permanent abandonment—is punishment for a bad thought or behavior [63].

The loss of a parent through divorce may precipitate analogous responses. Losing one parent heightens the child's awareness of the possibility of losing two parents. Children will often worry in silence with an imagination that works overtime. Knowing that there are many people who love them and who will take care of them "just in case" can be very supportive.

The death of a pet may be almost as significant to the preschooler as the death of a parent. To replace the pet too quickly is to teach the child not to invest self in others—that things are expendable [60]. Research with adults indicates that they cannot mourn the loss of a significant other and simultaneously form an attachment to a new family member [13]. The child is placed in an analogous situation when the pet is replaced too soon; one of the processes will be submerged. To deny the child the opportunity to mourn is to deny love and attachment. The prevention of mourning may prevent or hinder the growth of love [15]. The child's expression of grief should be encouraged and facilitated through the ceremony of burying, flowers, or whatever is deemed appropriate or meaningful. Discussion with the child of concepts of memory, love, sharing, and significant others can facilitate the grieving process while fostering personal integrity and maintenance of psychosocial security. Explanations must be very concrete and should be in terms of personal experiences because the child of this age finds it difficult to draw from the experience of others.

When loss does occur during this age, it is very difficult for the child to sustain grief for long periods of time. The child must forget, or rather repress, thoughts of the event for periods of time in order to survive psychologically [63]. The child may be frightened by his or her feelings and thus inhibit their expression. Frequently the child's mood may revert to the opposite emotion—that of laughing or acting excited. This response is a form of denial and coping, but it is very confusing to the adult who is dealing with the grieving child. Acceptance is gradual; reality is dealt with in small doses. True grief behavior may be shown much later as the child's concept of death matures.

COGNITIVE ACCEPTANCE, AFFECTIVE REBELLION
(7 to 9 Years)
According to Piaget's observations, during this phase of life any object that moves spontaneously is categorized as being alive [43]; this would include the sun and the wind but would exclude a bicycle or a tree. The child knows and accepts the fact that death is a

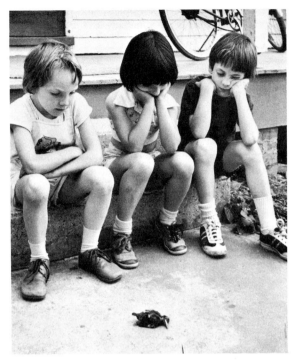

Figure 20–2. The preschooler uses sociodramatic play to cope with a growing awareness of death. Death concepts can be handled in small doses, at their own pace, and with a happy outcome. A funeral and burial for an animal facilitate respect for life as well as an emerging concept of death.

final state but may believe that the dead continue to see, hear, and feel [34]. The child no longer feels responsibility for the death of others—an idea that characterized the last phase—and gives up ideas of magical thought to logic and reason. The school-age child begins to realize the inevitability of death for all living things, but still finds it difficult either to accept or to deny personal death. Sixty-one percent of 7-year-olds, 75 percent of 8-year-olds, and 100 percent of 9-year-olds were able to acknowledge the universality of death in one study [9]. Twenty-five percent of 8-year-olds, 30 percent of 9-year-olds, and 63 percent of 10-year-olds admitted the irreversibility aspect of death [9]. The school-ager frequently takes a compromise stand that death is real, but it is external to the self. This position enables the child to assert that death can be avoided [41]. Efforts are extended toward achieving a biological understanding of death in the hope of learning how to control and to prevent the inevitable. In order to learn specific ways of controlling the event, children ask many questions, draw on the experiences of others, and discuss the matter openly and freely [30]. In short, school-agers are fascinated with the idea of death as a part of living, but they do not want to stop existing—not while they feel the richness of life and living [12].

Children in this phase begin to recognize the human fallibility of their parents and the need for other sources of strength. It is during this period that they frequently ask if they were adopted and also exhibit concern over who would care for them if the parents were to die. They begin to reach out to other adults and peers, extending their attachments and meaningful relationships. Realizing that death can occur in the young as well as in the old can have a disquieting effect. Children begin to realize that significant others can die without warning, and that the future offers many uncertainties. They may devise elaborate procedures that distort or deny the fact of universal death: sidewalk cracks are avoided, one's breath is held while passing a cemetery, and contact with dead people and funeral homes is avoided whenever possible.

Maria Nagy has indicated that many children of this age think of death in terms of personification. "Mr. Death" is an invisible bad spirit who can think, plan, and stalk a victim. He comes at night to take one's soul away. Mr. Death may be personified as a skeleton, ghost, black cat, bogeyman, goblin, or other form. If one is smart and quick enough, one can outwit or outrun Mr. Death. Doors are locked, dark rooms are avoided, heads are hidden under the covers; children run extra fast through a particular alley, vacant lot, or wooded area. Death is still seen as an event external to the self that is contingent on the aggression of others; therefore, it can be avoided. It **must** be avoided, especially if it is perceived as prolonged torture.

Television violence may serve to perpetuate this concept by showing how to outwit death; or, especially in the younger child, it may serve as a medium for "working through" concepts of death in small doses and at a safe distance. Peer associations also facilitate working through one's death concept. Games such as "tag," "king of the castle," and "cops and robbers" allow expression of mastery over danger, fear, or an "enemy." Unfortunately, peer approval may be so important in proving who is bravest that children of this age frequently disregard real dangers in games of "I dare you." Fantasy and daydreams also allow the child to try on roles and to gain emotional and intellectual mastery [12].

When the death of a significant other does occur, cognitive-affective dissonance in accepting reality may inhibit emotional response and grief expression. Many deep feelings are not shown on the surface [12]. The child is generally more upset than the parents realize [26]. The child may respond with jokes, crassness, or indifference in order to ward off the impact of grief. Some children may not appear to mourn at all but may mourn very heavily at a later time. Grief in this period is exhibited in short spans—the ego is still too weak to grieve for long periods. The child frequently finds it easier to mourn at a distance, for example, in writing rather than in person.

My Big Brother

My big brother:
  21 years old,
  Broad shoulders,
  Brown eyes,
  Freckles,
  Marines,
  Married,
  Strong.
Yet—
  You're the best brother
  I've ever had.
  In less than a month,
  You will have been dead for a year.

Grace Ellison, age 15

The school-age child may experience a great emptiness after mourning because release of sadness may be equated with release of the love object [63]. The death of a parent may permanently scar a child's development. Much sensitive support is needed to allow children to express their feelings—at their own pace. A wholesome, sensitive short story about death written for children of this age group is *A Taste of Blackberries* by Doris Smith [58]. It is a first-person narrative of a young boy's thoughts about his best friend and his inner response to the friend's death. This story is highly recommended both for developing a greater sensitivity to the emotions of children in this phase and for helping children to understand themselves and to cope constructively with death.

COGNITIVE AND AFFECTIVE ACCEPTANCE
(10 to 12 Years)

Piaget's observations indicate that the child of 10 recognizes that life is a quality possessed by, and restricted to, members of the plant and animal kingdom. As the individual enters the period of formal operations, he or she possesses the cognitive tools to comprehend time, space, causality, and quantity; therefore, the young person is able to form a concept of death similar to that possessed by adults. Death is understood in relation to natural laws [44]; it is no longer seen as merely the result of aggression or trauma. Illness and age, as well as accidents, are recognized as causative agents. Death is acknowledged as originating from within us rather than being external to us. The individual now accepts the biological finality of death; no longer does the dead person continue to live and feel in the grave. Death is accepted cognitively and affectively as being universal, inevitable, and irreversible.

With the recognition of physical death, most adolescents and adults believe in psychic immortality. This belief may be a protective coping mechanism perpetuated by the culture because the concept of nonexistence is difficult to accept even for the person capable of abstract thought, or it may be a truth discovered and shared with us through generations by persons who are more sensitive to out-of-body experiences, those who have had deep religious experiences, or those who have had near-death experiences.

Young people during this phase and the years that follow expend much energy in abstract thought, reviewing their experiences to integrate past, present, and future into a philosophy of life (see Chap. 26). The adolescent must come to terms with death as a prerequisite for building a philosophy of life [23]. Adolescents begin to realize that growth comes with caring deeply about others [12], and that death stops that growth. As they become more aware of the life-producing potentials of their own bodies and lives, they begin to recognize death as an enemy—a thief that can deprive them of life's plans, dreams, and goals. They think it unfair to have invested so much in the process of growing up only to have the threat of a life ended before one has achieved some sense of fulfillment or has tasted some of the adult pleasures and privileges. This is one reason why some young people resist and object to involvement in war; they do not want to die without the opportunity to live as an adult. Others may accept the challenge of war as a way to tempt fate and prove their ability to outsmart "Mr. Death." Other young people enjoy the mastery achieved over fear, or the "high" received when adrenalin levels are elevated during and after a fast ride in a car, on a roller coaster, or on water skis. The adolescent fears death and yet is fascinated by it.

Adolescents who are coming to grips with life may devote much thought to death as they explore options and alternatives in life. The more completely they resolve the issue of their own mortality, the stronger their own identities become. As adolescents become more secure in their ideologies, they experience greater resilience and coping skills when facing a life-threatening crisis. Kastenbaum indicates that "brighter" adolescents and more "psychologically alive" adults devote much thought to the issue and continue to modify their orientation toward death throughout life [27]. Many adults may continue to deny their mortality by giving little thought to death throughout much of their lives [59].

The death of a parent during adolescence is very traumatic socially as well as affectively. The process of grieving may be similar to that experienced by adults (see Chap. 21). However, the adolescent may feel stigmatized by the situation. At a time when peer support and companionship are so important, who is there to share this event with as a common experience? The bereaved adolescent feels different, singled out. The adolescent may also feel the need to replace a lost family member by assuming their responsibilities or even their mannerisms. If financial burdens are intensified by the death, the young person may have to change educational and career goals. Resentment and a sense of having been cheated are not uncommon feelings. Reintegration of past, present, and future, one's concept of God, and one's philosophy of life and death may be a very difficult task following the death of a loved one during adolescence. One's own mortality cannot be denied, and the search for a meaning in death may be painful.

Search for the Meaning of Death

A major task of each individual, especially during late adolescence and early adulthood, is to find meaning in life—to establish values, goals, and priorities, to find something to live for (see Chap. 18). This task requires a recognition and an integration of a concept of death [64]. "Death asks us for our identity" [18]. Edgar Jackson feels that the high suicide rates among adolescents and college students are partially explained by the anxiety felt by these individuals in acknowledging the fact of death and trying to find a meaning in life; the attempt to integrate the two and to bring this new concept into focus is sought at the price of self-destruction [23]. The value or meaning of life may be very difficult to identify when one is living under extemely adverse circumstances. The helplessness syndrome may prevail and prevent thoughts on this abstract, philosophical issue.

Edgar Jackson observes that when individuals tend to lose sight of the spiritual meaning of life, they become overwhelmed with a materialistic attitude [23]. Viktor Frankl in his autobiography of life in a Nazi concentration camp, *Man's Search for Meaning* [16], explains that meaning can be found to life under any circumstance. It is our attitude, not circumstances, that give life its meaning. He concludes that parents need to assist children to find meaning in life. This book is highly recommended for both its historical and personal value.

Edgar Jackson and many religious leaders believe that a deep religious experience can give life and circumstances meaning by bringing the two into focus, and giving a person the motivation to live. Such an experience can give an individual a realistic confirmation of the value of life and living [23]. In this context, the meaning of life is answered within the framework of a sacred doctrine. Death is seen as a personal matter between God and self [18]. The self is seen as a spiritual person living in a physical body.

LIFE AFTER DEATH

This view of life, the union of the physical with a spiritual self (soul or psyche), has been given more concrete support in the last few years by the research of Elisabeth Kübler-Ross and Raymond Moody. Kübler-Ross, a psychiatrist, became convinced that there is psychic life after death during conversations with critically ill and dying clients whom she interviewed to try to determine how they could be assisted with the process of dying [31]. Moody, a philosopher and physician, began a systematic investigation of reports of out-of-body experiences related by individuals who had had "near-death experiences" or who had been "clinically dead" and then revived [38]. After collecting data from approximately 150 cases, he noted striking similarities in the relation of the experiences, which included psychic disengagement from the physical body, a heightened awareness of environmental activities, an ability to move through space and to think, hear, and see, and the meeting with spirits of previously deceased friends and relatives. Almost every individual reported an encounter with a very bright light, which was identified as a spiritual being with a definite personality. They indicated that this "Being of Light" flooded them with warmth, acceptance, and love beyond description while asking one question, variously translated as "Are you ready to die?" or "What have you done with your life that is sufficient?" A very rapid, detailed, yet vivid review of their lives occurred. This "Being of Light" appeared to stress two factors in each life: (1) learning to love other people, and (2) acquiring knowledge.

After this encounter, almost all the individuals reported that they did not want to return to life. Most were very hesitant to reveal their experiences to others after their return but were frequently profoundly changed by the experience. Obviously, the data collected offer no proof of life after temporal life. However, the continual compilation of data from similar experiences makes the possibility impossible to deny. Moody's research also indicates that his observations are almost identical to the experiences of death or dying reported in diverse civilizations, cultures, and eras [38].

THE ROLE OF RELIGION

Sylvia Anthony observes that religious beliefs, doctrine, and rituals socialize an individual's attitude toward death [3]. Fulton feels that the rites and ceremonies for the dead are an expression of both subcultural influences and theological beliefs. As such, they reinforce social bonds and values by linking humanity, a supreme being, and society [18]. Theological positions are an attempt to help people to cope with all there is of reality [23].

There is a wide continuum of beliefs regarding the purpose of life, the nature of the human being, and the existence of God or a supreme being. One must come to terms with all three of these concepts both in the development of a concept of life and death and in the expression of that belief in a formal religion. At one end of the continuum are those who believe only in the concrete reality of the **now** experience. Adherents to this position see no ultimate purpose to life, describe the human as a biological being able to think and master part of the environment, and believe that there is no God. The idea that the human being may be an integration of physical and spiritual components is untenable to them; the concept of the existence of God is too abstract and metaphysical even to entertain. At the other end of the continuum are those who believe that the individual's ultimate purpose in life is to worship God; that the physical component of existence is secondary to the spiritual component and is merely a vehicle or tool through which the spirit can express itself; and that God is the supreme ruler of the universe, directly or indirectly orchestrating the activities within it.

Most cultures and religions believe that death and decay of the body are not synonymous with dissolution of the personality. They also presuppose the existence of God as a basic tenet of their beliefs. Most believe in the dual nature of the human. Some propose that the spirit or the soul enters another physical life when the present body dies (reincarnation). Other religions—particularly the Catholic and Protestant theological positions—believe that the soul has only one chance to live in the world we know as the planet Earth. They feel that if death is indeed the end of man, then life is empty and without meaning. To them, life on earth is a preparatory process for another life after death. Human dignity is the "consequence of the union in each man of his material body with an immaterial, immortal soul" [47]. To them, the concept of God gives meaning to both current life and eternal life. Concepts of heaven and hell assure continuity of self and also serve as a guide or check on temporal behavior as a contingency for future reward or punishment—the ultimate cause-effect relationship; the ultimate modifier of behavior.

Religious training does have a marked effect on the development of a concept of death, especially on the concepts of heaven versus hell, good versus bad, and temporal versus spiritual life. Some researchers note that "children from religiously oriented homes have more specific concepts of death than those who come from homes where religion plays a minor role" [5].

One 6-year-old child from a deeply religious home shared her feelings with the author [35]:

> People get sad when someone in their family dies. It is good for them to die, but people don't want them to die. But they have to, it is a part of life. When you die, you will not come back to Earth anymore. You will be with Jesus all the time. There will be no sickness, fights, stealing; no hurt. It will be a wonderful place. I think I will die—when I get to be old. Sometimes people die when they are young by a car accident, fall, or crack their head open. I think there will be happiness when I die. I don't think about it much. I just wonder how old I will be and what it will be like. I would feel sad if I thought I was going to die now. I would miss everybody.

This child's religious background (and cognitive functioning level) has obviously advanced her concept of death beyond that expected for her chronological age. She indicates that she has accepted death, both cognitively and affectively. She has realistically worked this feeling into a concept of life, about which she can talk easily and freely.

A 10-year-old girl from a similar religious background, who has been blind since birth, presents an interesting view on fulfilling one's purpose in life—even after death [55]:

> Death is not scary because I know I will go to Heaven. That's all I really care about death, and I'm ready to die. I don't want to now. I have too much to do and fulfill. My ghost would come back by its own choice to fulfill my task,

and then return to Heaven. In death your spirit merely goes on to another life—an eternal life. The meaning of life is to fulfill the purpose God made us for. You find out that purpose through prayer. In a subtle way, I look forward to death, because I'll be able to see again, be perfect.

The striking point in both of these girls' discussions of death is their attitude of acceptance. Death was a reality with which they lived, were prepared for, and did not fear. Life was an interlude in existence—a preparation for another existence. Death represented both an end and a beginning. They had learned to trust this life. The quality of this life for which they were already assuming responsibility would determine their future, and they were at peace with that idea. Thus, fear of death is not universal. Furth observes that persons can die in peace if the soma and the psyche are in harmony, regardless of age [17].

PREPARING THE CHILD TO COPE WITH DEATH AND LOSS

Preparation for coping with death begins in infancy by learning to cope with separation. The simple game of peek-a-boo was mentioned earlier as a significant activity for learning to cope with the temporary loss of contact with a significant other. The father's participation in child care helps the infant to accommodate to more than one approach of interaction. Gradual introduction of other caretakers and brief separations help the infant to learn gradually that existence can continue without direct maternal contact. Inadequate contact or overt rejection of the child can increase anxiety levels, however. A healthy balance between contact and separation must be based on the individual child's developmental level and tolerance of separation (see Chap. 9).

During the toddler years, a parent can begin to use flowers, insects, and pets to help the child develop a concept of death as a part of the life cycle. When death does occur, the child needs a trusted adult to fill the void and share the grief. Mourning should be encouraged in this and all later stages of the life cycle. Crying is not an infantile regression nor an effeminate behavior; it is a normal, natural expression of human sorrow that has no boundaries of age or gender. Stifling grief at any age will prolong the grief process, cause intensification of feelings, and lead to internalization with distortion of conceptualizations [7]. It is especially important not to equate death with sleep, since children may begin to fear sleep and going to bed and may exhibit marked disturbance of sleep patterns and night-mares [52].

The preschooler is ready for a simple, direct discussion of death. Death should be discussed openly during nonstressful times in a matter-of-fact, honest, but sensitive manner. As with other stressful subjects, the information needs to be presented in many ways, using different experiences as examples, so that children can begin to remember and to integrate the information into their repertoire of knowledge [26]. Many books are available that can offer a common experience for adults and children to share the emotions of love and sorrow, and to explore feelings about death [36]. Natural events and phenomena can continue to serve as examples to explain the life cycle—fallen leaves in autumn, butterflies, a bird found dead in the yard, or the animal at the side of the road. The child may find it difficult to incorporate the conventional metaphysical and religious explanations of death [54]; however, religious beliefs may help the child to accept the fact of death. Salk warns that these beliefs should only be expressed if they are a **real** part of the parents' life—otherwise they will tend to increase anxiety. The child is able to sense when parents are not honest or sincere and may believe the religious interpretation to be another fairy tale [52]. The love relationship should be stressed. When a loss does occur, the child should be assured that it was not his or her fault; that the deceased did not die on purpose; that no one will replace the deceased's unique relationship, but that new relationships are developed throughout life; and that the child will never forget the loved one—their memory can keep them with us whenever we want.

Even a young child should be told about the death of a person who is significant to the child. When a loved one just "disappears" it is very traumatic—more traumatic than the truth. One explanation that can be given the young child is that the body is the house where the "me" lives while on earth. Death is when the "me" has left a body that no longer works right. The body is worn out or cannot be fixed [46]. Children may have a great deal of difficulty with the development of a positive concept of God if they are told that God "wanted" the person who died.

School-agers often ask if the parents will die. They need to be told honestly, "Yes, I will die. But I don't expect to die for a long time." The underlying concern is generally, "Who will take care of me if my parents die?" Parents should assure children of the arrangements for child care in case of untimely illness or death [4].

One question that parents face is whether or not to allow the child to attend the wake (viewing) and the funeral. Observing the child's response to the death of a pet or other separation experience can give some clues as to readiness. The child should be included as much as possible; exclusion from all activities gives a sense of unreality and detachment to the event. Moderate sharing of grief by other mourners can help the child to feel less alone in the crisis and may help in the personal expression of grief. Most authorities recommend that children less than 7 years of age not be taken to the funeral, but this is a very individual matter. Some children in the 7- to 9-year-old age group are terrified by the prospect of a funeral. The author's daughter still remembers with great tenderness saying "good-bye" to her grandmother at her funeral, even though she was only 3½ years old at the time.

Religious beliefs may or may not offer support at this time, especially to the adolescent. Such support depends on the unique blending of the three major subconcepts (the purpose of life, the nature of human beings, and the existence of God), as well as the degree to which the individual has resolved his or her own mortality into a concept of life, and the depth to which this belief or concept of life has been translated into values, goals, and actions.

SUMMARY

Concern is expressed that in our modern, throw-away society, children may be desensitized in the art of becoming attached—the investing of oneself in another. The rapid replacement of pets and toys interferes with normal grieving and the development of the concept that death is inevitable, universal, and irreversible. The violence portrayed in the mass media may undermine the valuing of human life and perpetuate the myth that death is the result of external aggression and, therefore, avoidable.

The cognitive and affective domains are interdependent in the development of a concept of death. To the infant, who has relatively no concept of time or the meaning of death, separation from a significant caretaker may represent a death experience, as do games of peek-a-boo or toss and retrieval games. To the egocentric toddler, death is separation from a love object seen as essential to his or her existence. The preschooler acknowledges death as a cessation of movement but believes that revival is possible through the power of magical thought. The young school-ager feels

Table 20–1. Major Concerns of Each Age Related to a Concept of Death

Age	Concerns
Infant and toddler	Separation and deprivation
Preschooler	Biological integrity
School-ager	Psychological integrity
Pubescent	Social integrity
Adolescent	Philosophical and theological integrity
Adult	Life role and goals

that death is a form of punishment that can be avoided by "being good." The scary tales of school-agers and the interest they show in Halloween, ghost stories, exhibitions of omnipotence, and strivings for physical prowess may all be partially explained by the concept that death can be outwitted if one is wise enough, brave enough, or strong enough. Table 20–1 summarizes the major concerns of each of these age groups in relation to a concept of death.

When the fact of personal mortality is accepted, both cognitively and affectively, this acceptance must be worked into a philosophy of life that includes defining a purpose for life, a concept of God, and the potential for existence of the spiritual self beyond the life of the physical self. Many adults repress thoughts of personal death until times of critical life-change events [59]. Incomplete resolution of the issue prior to the crisis can increase anxiety levels and interfere with the implementation of constructive coping skills.

Parents who are sure of their own feelings toward life and death are the best resources in facilitating the development of a positive, integrating concept of life and death by the developing child. Parents who feel that they do not have the strength or the security to explain death to their children should seek professional assistance from the clergy, their pediatrician, or a child psychologist.

One's concept of death continues to be modified throughout the adult years as the quality of life changes and as a result of religious experiences. Readers who would like more knowledge in this area are encouraged to take a college course or to attend a seminar (frequently sponsored by church groups) that offers an opportunity to explore one's own concept of death and how to cope with the reality of death. Information on coping with one's own imminent death is given in Chapter 21.

REFERENCES

1. Ariès, P. *The Hour of Our Death.* Translated by H. Weaver. New York: Alfred A. Knopf, 1981.
2. Alexander, E. I., and Adlerstein, A. M. Affective Responses to the Concept of Death in a Population of Children and Early Adolescents. In R. L. Fulton (Ed.), *Death and Identity.* New York: Wiley, 1965.
3. Anthony, S. *The Child's Discovery of Death: A Study in Child Psychology.* New York: Harcourt, Brace, 1940.
4. Backer, B. A., Hannon, N., and Russell, N. A. *Death and Dying: Individuals and Institutions.* New York: Wiley, 1982.
5. Barclay, D. Questions of life and death. *New York Times,* July 15, 1962.
6. Becker, E. *The Denial of Death.* New York: Free Press, 1975.
7. Bowlby, J., and Parkes, C. M. Separation and Loss Within The Family. In E. J. Anthony and C. Koupernick (Eds.), *The Child in His Family,* Vol. 1. New York: Wiley-Interscience, 1970.
8. Bowlby, J. *Attachment and Loss,* Vol. 2, *Separation, Anxiety and Anger.* New York: Basic Books, 1973.
9. Childers, P. and Wimmer, M. The concept of death in early childhood. *Child Dev.* 42:1299, 1971.
10. Cook, S. S. *Children and Dying.* New York: Health Sciences, 1973.
11. Crase, D. R., and Crase, D. Death and the young child. *Clin. Pediatr.* 14:747, 1975.
12. Easson, W. M. *The Dying Child* (2d ed.). Springfield, IL: Thomas, 1981.
13. Evans, S., Reinhart, J., and Succop, P. Failure to thrive, a study of 45 children and their families. *J. Am. Acad. Child Psychiatry* 11:440, 1972.
14. Feifel, H. Psychology and the death-awareness movement. *J. Clin. Child Psychol.* 3(2):6, 1974.
15. Formanek, R. When children ask about death. *El. Sch. J.* 75(2):92, 1974.
16. Frankl, V. E. *Man's Search for Meaning.* Translated by I. Lasch. Boston: Beacon Press, 1962.
17. Fulton, R. On the Dying of Death. In E. A. Grollman (Ed.), *Explaining Death to Children.* Boston: Beacon Press, 1967.
18. Fulton, R. L., and Bendiksen, R. *Death and Identity* (rev. ed.). Bowie, MD: Charles Press, 1976.
19. Furth, G. M. The Use of Drawings Made at Significant Times in One's Life. In E. Kübler-Ross (Ed.), *Living With Death and Dying.* New York: Macmillan, 1981.
20. Glasberg, R., and Aboud, F. Keeping one's distance from sadness: Children's self-report of emotional experience. *Dev. Psychol.* 18:287, 1982.
21. Grollman, E. A. (Ed.). *Explaining Death to Children.* Boston: Beacon Press, 1967.
22. Grollman, E. A. "Explaining Death to Children." Paper presented at the Annual Meeting of the National Council of Family Relations, Salt Lake City, Utah, August 1975 (ERIC Document Reproduction Service No. ED 117 628).
23. Jackson, E. N. The Theological, Psychological, and Phil-

osophical Dimensions of Death in Protestantism. In E. A. Grollman (Ed.), *Explaining Death to Children*. Boston: Beacon Press, 1967.

24. Jackson, P. L.   The child's developing concept of death *Nurs. Forum* 14:204, 1975.
25. Janssen, Y. G.   Early awareness of death in normal child development. *Infant Mental Health J.* 4:95, 1983.
26. Johnson, P. A.   After a child's parent has died. *Child Psychiatry Hum. Dev.* 12(3):160, 1982.
27. Kastenbaum, R.   The Child's Understanding of Death: How Does it Develop? In E. A. Grollman (Ed.), *Explaining Death to Children*. Boston: Beacon Press, 1967.
28. Kastenbaum, R.   Childhood: The kingdom where creatures die. *J. Clin. Child Psychol.* 3(2):11, 1974.
29. Kliman, G., et al.   *Facilitation of Mourning During Childhood*. White Plains, NY: Center for Preventive Psychiatry (ERIC Document Reproduction Service No. ED 084 011).
30. Koocher, G. P.   Childhood, death, and cognitive development. *Dev. Psychol.* 9:369, 1973.
31. Kübler-Ross, E.   *Questions and Answers on Death and Dying*. New York: Macmillan, 1976.
32. Mahler, M. S., Pine, F., and Bergman, A.   *The Psychological Birth of the Human Infant: Symbiosis and Individuation*. New York: Basic Books, 1975.
33. McLure, J. W.   Death education. *Phi Delta Kappan* 55:483, 1974.
34. Melear, J. D.   Children's conceptions of death. *J. Genet. Psychol.* 123 (2nd half):359, 1973.
35. Miller, A.   Personal communication, 1977.
36. Mills, G. C.   Books to Help Children Understand Death. *Am. J. Nurs.* 79:291, 1979.
37. Mitchell, M.   Bereaved Children. In V. Varma (Ed.), *Stresses in Children*. London: University of London Press, 1973.
38. Moody, R. A.   *Life After Life*. Harrisburg, PA.: Stackpole Books, 1976.
39. Morrisey, J. R.   Death Anxiety in Children With a Fatal Illness. In H. J. Parad (Ed.), *Crisis Intervention: Selected Readings*. New York: Family Service Association of America, 1965.
40. Moseley, P. A.   "Developing Curriculum for Death Education: How Do Children Learn About Death?" Paper Presented at the Annual Meeting of the American Educational Research Association, San Francisco, April 1976 (ERIC Document Reproduction Service No. ED 123 191).
41. Nagy, M.   The child's theories concerning death. *J. Genet. Psychol.* 73:3, 1948.
42. Parness, E.   Effects of experiences with loss and death among preschool children. *Child. Today* 4(6):2, 1975.
43. Piaget, J.   *The Child's Concept of Physical Causality*. Translated by M. Gabain. Totowa, NJ: Littlefield, Adams, 1972.

44. Piaget, J.   *The Child's Conception of the World*. Translated by J. Tomlinson and A. Tomlinson. Totowa, NJ: Littlefield, Adams, 1972.
45. Rank, O.   *The Trauma of Birth*. New York: Harper & Row, 1973.
46. Reed, E. L.   *Helping Children With the Mystery of Death*. Nashville: Abingdon Press, 1970.
47. Riley, T. J.   Catholic Teachings, the Child, and a Philosophy for Life and Death. In E. A. Grollman (Ed.), *Explaining Death to Children*. Boston: Beacon Press, 1967.
48. Robertson, J.   *Young Children In Hospital* (2nd ed.). London: Tavistock Publications, 1970.
49. Rochlin, G.   How Younger Children View Death and Themselves. In E. A. Grollman (Ed.), *Explaining Death to Children*. Boston: Beacon Press, 1967.
50. Romero, C. E.   "The Treatment of Death in Contemporary Children's Literature." Master's Thesis, Long Island University, 1974 (ERIC Document Reproduction Service No. ED 101 664).
51. Rubenstein, J. S.   Preparing a child for a good-bye visit to a dying loved one. *J. Am. Med. Assoc.* 247:2571, 1982.
52. Salk, L.   *What Every Child Would Like His Parents to Know*. New York: David McKay, 1972.
53. Sardello, R. J.   Death and the imagination. *Humanitas* 10(1):61, 1974.
54. Schilder, P., and Wechsler, D.   Children's Attitude Toward Death. In L. Bender (Ed.), *Aggression, Hostility and Anxiety in Children*. Springfield, IL: Thomas, 1953.
55. Schuster, E.   Personal communication, 1976.
56. Siggins, L. D.   Mourning: A critical survey of the literature. *Int. J. Psychoanal.* 47:14, 1966.
57. Singher, L. J.   The slowly dying child. *Clin. Pediatr.* 13:861, 1974.
58. Smith, D. B.   *A Taste of Blackberries*. New York: Crowell, 1973.
59. Smith, D. W.   Survivors of serious illness. *Am. J. Nurs.* 79:441, 1979.
60. Toffler, A.   *Future Shock*. New York: Random House, 1970.
61. T. V. violence a threat to children's health. *American Nurse* 9(3):3, 1977.
62. Wolf, A. W. M.   *Helping Your Child to Understand Death* (Rev. ed.). New York: Child Study Association of America, 1973.
63. Wolfenstein, M., and Kliman, G. (Eds.).   *Children and the Death of a President*. Gloucester, MA: Peter Smith, 1965.
64. Woods, B. W.   *Christians in Pain: Perspectives on Suffering*. Grand Rapids, MI: Baker Book House, 1982.
65. Zeligs, R.   "Children's Experience with Death." (ERIC Document Reproduction Service No. ED 076 237), 1973.
66. Zeligs, R.   *Children's Experience with Death*. Springfield, IL: Thomas, 1974.

21
Concepts of Loss and Grieving

Darlene E. McCown

To everything there is a season . . . a time to be born, and a time to die.

Ecclesiastes 3:1–2a

During the past 50 years, the interest in loss and grieving has moved beyond the realms of poetry, philosophy, and religion and into the areas of scientific investigation and popular discussion. Scholars have been able to describe the grief experience and have identified stages commonly found in the bereaved [20, 39, 42, 73]. These stages and attendant behaviors formulate the basis for an understanding of the typical grief response. Manifestations of grief that differ significantly from the pattern are considered abnormal and become a matter for concern.

An insight into the processes of loss and grief can enlarge one's understanding of the responses to death as well as to other losses, such as graduation, divorce, surgery, and leaving home. Losses occur in every stage of life and in all four domains. Although every loss is unique, each one has features in common. This chapter will focus primarily on loss during the adult years. (See Chap. 20 for earlier coping patterns.)

ISSUES OF LOSS AND GRIEF

Definitions of Loss and Grief
Grief, bereavement, and mourning are the terms used to refer to the reaction to a significant loss in life. Grief and mourning signify the painful cultural, emotional, and physical processes that follow loss.

LOSS

Loss is experienced whenever one is separated from a significant object, person, goal, or event. It can be sudden or prolonged. It can be complete, partial, or seemingly unending, such as fire-induced facial scars, the birth of a mentally retarded child, or a family member who is missing in action. Loss poses a threat to the individual's lifestyle, values, and self-esteem [79]. Failure to achieve a desired grade on a paper, denial of entrance into the school of one's choice, menopause, misplacement of a special ring, or inability to attend a special event all represent significant loss experiences.

BEREAVEMENT

Bereavement designates the entire process of accommodating to a significant loss, usually of a loved one. After the loss of a significant other, a psychological process follows that brings mental images of that person into harmony with the reality of the situation. Bereavement has two primary components—grief and mourning [3]. Bereavement activities can accompany *any* significant loss, not just the loss of another person.

GRIEF

Grief refers to the intense emotional and physical feelings aroused by a loss. It is characterized by intense emotional suffering, distress, sorrow, and regret. It is accompanied by weeping, despair, and bewilderment. The suffering is a stimulus to which friends and relatives respond by offering help, companionship, and other forms of concern. Grief responses help maintain bonds and affection between people. "Anticipatory grief" can be experienced when one expects a significant loss to occur even though the person or object is still accessible.

MOURNING

Mourning is defined as the cultural response to loss [3]. It represents conventional behavior as determined by cultural mores and sanctions. For example, after a death there are the social expectations of a funeral, subdued clothing, expressions of sadness, and a family gathering. Usually mourning and grief are found together. However, grief may occur independently in situations that lack cultural mourning rituals, such as the loss of a job, the removal of a breast, a child entering school, or the death of a pet. In these cases, the mourning aspect is difficult because society lacks rituals that can enhance adjustment to these losses. Similarly, the mourning component may merely follow social ritual and incorporate little or no true feelings of grief.

Systems Theory and Loss

When loss occurs, particularly of a loved one, the whole family is affected. Following a death in the family, boundaries become less defined as the roles and the functions are reallocated to surviving members. A redefinition of family structure and the roles within the structure must occur.

The alignment of subsystems is also disrupted after a death. Support, trust, and assistance from other family members may be insufficient as each affected individual experiences a disruptive grief response. Leadership in the family system may be altered. For instance, the death of a powerful father will require a new member to assume the role of decision-maker. A diffusion of power may inhibit the family's resolution of grief and its reorientation to life without the deceased member.

A death in the family impacts the whole system, even succeeding generations [69]. Survivors of Hiroshima and the Nazi concentration camps experienced "death immersion," which can lead to death anxiety and guilt over survival. Research on the survivors of the concentration camps shows that many children and grandchildren of survivors manifest anxiety, depression, nightmares, guilt, feelings of isolation, estrangement and emptiness, generalized family insecurity, and high parental overprotectiveness.

Theories of Grief

Although grief is generally discussed in relation to the loss of a significant person, the reader should understand that the same affective responses may be experienced regardless of the type of loss experienced.

PSYCHOANALYTIC VIEW

Each theory of grief helps to explain the human response to loss. The psychoanalytic view emphasizes the human instinct toward life. Even the physiological struggle of the neonate to breathe and to balance physiological processes is viewed as an example of the drive for life [59]. Psychoanalysts indicate that individuals fear death and consequently develop grief as a symptom in response to the fear of death. Grief is seen as a departure from normal psychological functioning and thus is identified as a pathological condition. The psychoanalytic view of death can be diagrammed as follows: [85]

$$\text{Danger} \rightarrow \text{Anxiety} \rightarrow \text{Symptoms}$$
$$\text{(loss)} \qquad\qquad \text{(grief)}$$

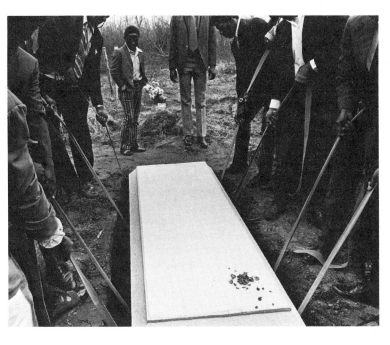

Figure 21–1. Death, like birth and marriage, is a social event surrounded by cultural traditions that help significant others to make the transition to the new relationships.

Freud identified four major characteristics of mourning: (1) dejection, (2) lack of interest in the world, (3) loss of capacity to love, and (4) inhibition of activity. He saw the adult grief response as a struggle to understand the reality of the loss. The bereaved person desires to keep the former attachment to the deceased, but gradually, an awareness of the reality of the loss develops. This awareness develops slowly, at the expense of time and energy. The lost object is gradually decathected (devested of emotional attachment) by a process of remembering, reality testing, and the separation of memory from hope [88].

LINDEMANN

Lindemann developed the concept of "acute grief." His grief theory resulted from work with 101 bereaved persons, including survivors of the classical and now famous Coconut Grove fire in Boston, which occurred in 1942.

Lindemann carefully observed and recorded the reactions of survivors. Gradually, a pattern of grief symptoms and responses became apparent. Common responses included [48]:

1. **Sensations of somatic distress,** which last from 20 minutes to 1 hour and include tightness, choking, sighing, shortness of breath, and energy loss. (Other practitioners find that somatic distress symptoms may continue for several weeks or until the person begins to decathect from the loss and invest in the future.)
2. **Preoccupation with the image of the deceased,** which results in sensory alteration (such as conversations with the deceased, sensing the presence of the deceased) and feelings of distance from others.
3. **Feelings of guilt** manifested by questioning how one's personal involvement might have affected or prevented the circumstances surrounding the death.
4. **Hostile reactions,** including loss of warmth in relationships with others.
5. **Loss of patterns of conduct** indicated by changes in social relationships, an increase in speech and restlessness, and an inability to initiate and organize activity.
6. **Assuming behaviors of the deceased** is common in survivors, which could include assuming the deceased's responsibilities as well as the mannerisms, the sayings, and the habits of the deceased.

Lindemann viewed grief as a normal response to the cessation of a social interaction. Grief work entails emancipation from emotional bondage to the deceased, readjustment to life without the deceased, and formation of new relationships. To accomplish "grief work," one must face as well as allow the emotional expression of pain.

ENGEL

George Engel described four distinct phases in the grief process following a death [17]. The initial reaction is **shock** and **disbelief,** which is accompanied by a sense of numbness and immobility. This phase is characterized by efforts to protect oneself against the event by raising the threshold against its recognition and the painful sequelae.

As the reality of the death and the meaning of the loss penetrate the consciousness, there are acute periods of anguish and pain that flood the bereaved [17]. This **awareness** of loss is often coupled with physical pain, emptiness, and anger. Crying characterizes this period and appears to function as an aid to the bereaved in acknowledging the loss, allowing a temporary dependent state, and expressing the need for help. Engel indicated that the inability to cry interferes with the normal grief process.

Restitution signifies the third stage of grief. Cultural rituals and shared moments with friends and family clarify the reality of the loss as well as provide comfort, activity, and support. However, even when the social-cultural mourning activities are finished, grief lingers.

With time, as the reality of death is accepted, the **resolution** of the loss occurs. This phase takes place in stages. The bereaved experiences a painful emptiness and frequently a lessening of self-esteem coupled with a difficulty in forming new relationships. For a time, physical ailments similar to those experienced by the deceased may develop as a means of suffering and maintaining a bond with the deceased. A preoccupation with thoughts of the dead loved one will range from a focus on the personal effects of the loss to the physical aspects of the deceased. Gradually, a generally positive mental image of the deceased person develops and an identification with his or her ideals, values, and aspirations occurs. When the mourner's interest in everyday life and new relationships returns, the grief process is completed. "The clearest evidence of successful healing is the ability to remember comfortably and realistically both the pleasures and disappointments of the lost relationship" [17].

KÜBLER-ROSS

Elizabeth Kübler-Ross pioneered the current interest in death and dying by interviewing terminally ill patients about their feelings and experiences [42]. A major contribution of her work has been the realization that dying people are not only able to share their thoughts about death but also want to do so. Five stages in the response to one's imminent death have been recognized from her interviews.

The first stage is **denial and isolation.** This is manifest by the response "No, not me." Denial serves to lessen the dreadful news and allows time to adjust and to mobilize defenses. Denial is usually temporary and gives way to a growing awareness of reality. **Anger** occurs in the second stage, when denial can no longer be maintained. The person demands to know, "Why me?" Anger is displaced in all directions. It is often directed at health professionals and other healthy people who represent the very aspects of life the dying person is losing. Gradually the dying person enters a period called **bargaining.** Most bargains are with God, whom many assume to be the ultimate giver of life. The person engages in an agreement in an attempt to postpone death, often setting a specific time extension related to a particular event, such as a wedding, a birthday, or an anniversary. Bargaining sets a deadline and includes a promise that one will not ask for more if the one favor is granted.

As the process of dying demands more and more of the person, the individual comes to a deep sense of loss and **depression.** Multiple losses accompany this process, for example, loss of health, loss of activity, loss of job, loss of social contacts, loss of future, all of which provide legitimate reasons for depression. Kübler-Ross distinguishes between two kinds of depression that occur in those who are dying. One is a **reactive** depression to the multiple losses and the other is a **preparatory** depression that results from a sense of impending loss. When depression stems from an impending loss, then encouragement and reassurances lack substance.

The final stage of dying is **acceptance.** Given adequate time, the dying person reaches a state that is free from denial, anger, and depression and is able to face death. This state is accompanied by an increasing need for sleep and a distancing of the self from life. It is not a happy state, but it is one that is relatively free from anguish. Kübler-Ross called it "the final rest before the long journey." Not all dying people reach acceptance, but those who do will progress through the stages in various orders and at different paces. These stages represent variable but commonly observed patterns.

Anticipatory Grief

Grief may occur prior to loss when the probability of loss is realized. In expectation of the death of a loved one, family members may experience the symptoms of grief identified by Lindemann, Engel, and Kübler-Ross. Anticipatory grief differs from conventional grief in that anticipatory grief has a definite end point—the time of actual death [2]. A grief that continues after this

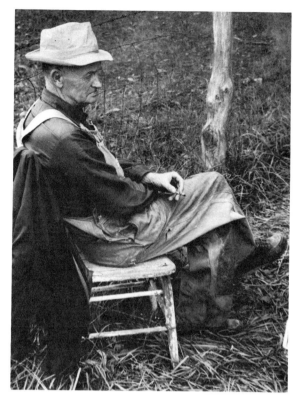

Figure 21–2. The older adult may spend much time in reflection. Erikson feels that satisfaction with one's past life and acceptance of death lead to a sense of dignity and ego-integrity during old age.

point is no longer anticipatory. Conventional grief lessens with time whereas anticipatory grief deepens.

Anticipatory grief involves a period of socialization in the bereaved role [28]. The anticipation of loss gives individuals an opportunity for preparation, but it also allows the expression of ambivalent and hostile feelings toward the dying person. A "death watch" may take place while waiting for the expected end [28]. Life without the loved one is envisioned and mourned. In some instances family members begin to distance themselves from the dying one. This grieving process can progress to the point where the bereaved has little emotional attachment to the dying person by the time of the actual death. Family members may need assistance to understand their feelings and reactions during the period of anticipatory grief and following the death. An acceptance of the fact that grief may take place before death and that little sadness may be felt at the actual point of death will help the bereaved resolve their loss and may allow them more energy to cope. There

has been time to say goodbye, to mend relationships, to reestablish communication and lines of responsibility, and to rehearse new roles while the loved one was still available.

Response to Loss

The response to loss varies from person to person. A variety of factors influences individual reactions [68, 83]:

1. Whether or not the loss was anticipated
2. The relationship between the bereaved and the lost object or person
3. The emotional makeup of the mourner
4. The cause of the loss or the death
5. The amount of real change that results from the loss
6. The importance of the object to the person
7. The typical coping pattern of the bereaved
8. Cultural and social standards
9. Attitudes toward loss and death
10. Special resources and liabilities of the survivor

The loss of a loved one may reactivate previous experiences of loss, such as separation. This factor highlights the importance of providing children with experiences of loss as a basis for gaining maturity in handling loss and grief experiences. The intense anguish and sorrow gradually give way to acceptance and a return to the activities of a happy, normal life, even though spontaneous, painful thoughts of the loss, and daydreaming about what might have been may arise.

Occasionally grief becomes pathological. "The most immediate and evident characteristic of pathological grief is its excessive and disproportionate nature and its protracted course" [83]. Grief may be considered abnormal if 6 months or more after a death the bereaved:

1. Intellectually acknowledges the death but demonstrates emotional denial
2. Frequently has unresolved dreams of the deceased
3. Is preoccupied with the dead
4. Speaks of the dead person in present terms
5. Uses highly emotional objects to keep a link with the deceased

Grief may follow the typical course described earlier or develop atypical forms. Unresolved grief requires professional intervention. Atypical forms include [30]:

1. **delayed grief,** in which the loss may be denied for months or years and erupts later in life, often related to an anniversary occasion:
2. **inhibited grief,** which is observed in people who exhibit a subdued, long-lasting mourning associated with disturbed physical symptoms; and
3. **chronic grief,** which is demonstrated by a prolonged and intensified grief reaction.

LOSSES THROUGHOUT THE LIFE CYCLE

Loss of Significant Persons
Many kinds of loss occur in a lifetime and each contains an element of grief.

DEATH OF A GRANDPARENT
The death of a grandparent frequently is the first death of a significant person that is experienced by the individual. Very little formal research and theory is available in this area. Children's literature, however, abounds with stories on the subject (e.g., *My Grandson, Lew,* Charlotte Zolotov; *My Grandpa Died Today,* Joan Fassler; *Annie and the Old One,* Miska Miles). Parents are encouraged to read stories with their children to aid in the development of an understanding of death and expressing grief. Although keenly felt, the death of a grandparent is less traumatic because death is associated with, and expected of, old age. Unless the surviving grandchildren are physically or financially dependent on grandparents, major disruptions do not occur. However, readjustments that involve supportive care and the role of the surviving grandparent arise as new issues to be resolved in the family system.

DEATH OF A PARENT
The death of a parent is a significant loss for a child of any age. Adult children experience readjustment in generational position following the death of a parent, accompanied by the realization of being the "oldest generation." The death of an older parent is felt deeply and painfully because of the break in a primary, lifelong relationship. Grief is experienced in its acute forms. However, several factors often combine to make the loss of a parent bearable for the adult:

1. Lack of physical and material dependence of the adult on the deceased parent
2. Increased expectation of death associated with advancing age of the parent
3. Responsibilities of adult children to their own succeeding generation
4. Increased physical distance between parents and children, which limits face to face involvement

5. Ongoing social and work obligations typical of the adult children's peak productive years (40 to 60-year-old age range)
6. Distribution of parental estate and family momentos
7. Burdensome activities associated with caring for aging parents
8. Suffering and pain associated with illness and aging

The more harmful repercussions of parental loss are generally felt by younger children [6, 15, 61]. They may demonstrate behavior problems reflecting anger, guilt, or apathy [35]. (See Chap. 20 for a more detailed description of childhood grief.) Long-term responses to early parental death, such as delinquency, acting out, adult depression, and psychiatric disorders, also have been identified [6, 10, 55]. A grief that reappears in adulthood, following the loss of a parent in childhood, may be maturational rather than pathological [37]. **Maturational grief** is an extension of normal grief that reflects a freshly discovered sense of loss associated with a new stage in life (e.g., with the birth of a baby, the previously bereaved daughter realizes anew the loss of her parent as a grandparent for the infant).

LOSS OF A SPOUSE

Death. The death of a spouse is a severe loss. Multiple additional losses attend the loss of a mate, such as the losses of income, companionship, a sexual partner, a provider or homemaker complement, or social status. The death of a spouse has been associated with an increase in physical (particularly for younger women) and emotional problems in the survivor [52]. Widows and widowers run a higher risk of dying than married people of the same age [51]. One study [66] showed that widows have specific immediate reactions, such as numbness, denial of the death, and extreme behavior outbursts. The widows experienced a sense of searching for the dead husband. They were preoccupied with thoughts of the deceased and the things associated with him. More than one-half of the widows were able to clearly visualize their husband at 1 month and even at the end of 1 year. The characteristics of grief gradually decreased over the first year, particularly crying, but were occasionally experienced by some widows even after 1 year. Anger, guilt, and restlessness accompanied the grief. One-half of the widows dreamed about their husbands. Severe sleep problems gradually decreased over the first year. Only 15 to 20 percent of the women who were widowed for 1 year exhibited a higher level of emotional health than they experienced before the death. Clearly, the death of a spouse is a critical event that alters the physical, social, and emotional patterns of the survivors.

Divorce. Marital conflict that results in the loss of a spouse can precipitate grieving behaviors similar to those experienced with death. Divorce involves the loss of an ideal marriage and a couple-relationship. It may include a sense of social failure—a loss of success and self-esteem. Guilt abounds regarding each partner's role in the conflict and often blame is placed on a particular party. The reaction to divorce includes shock, disbelief, anger, hostility, guilt, periods of reconstructive activity, and resolution [34]. A difficult part of the process of resolution involves formulating both a new image and a new role with the ex-partner with whom a relationship still exists, especially when children are involved. The grief experience related to divorce is complicated because society does not offer social rites or rituals, for example, as it does with a funeral, to acknowledge formally the lost relationship.

DEATH OF A SIBLING

The death of a sibling has profound meaning for surviving children. These youngsters frequently exhibit behavior problems [5, 12, 49]. In one study [49], more than one-third of the children showed behavior problems, such as school difficulties, somatic complaints, enuresis, nightmares, depression, clinging, crying, antisocial behavior, and jealousy. Children also are sensitive to parental sadness and grief and may feel the loss of parent-child intimacy and nurturance. Some children may assume responsibility for the loss, feel unworthy to have survived, or wonder when their turn will come. The guilt and anxiety accompanying these reactions exhibit themselves in affective disturbances and behavior problems.

Adults also experience the loss of a sibling. They, too, may feel unworthy to have survived. Surviving siblings may experience fears and anxieties related to health and may often experience symptoms similar to those of the deceased [18]. It appears that as bereaved adults experience grief for a deceased sibling, they become more acutely aware of their own vulnerability and future death.

LOSS OF A CHILD

Death.* The loss of a child in the latter part of the twentieth century has become a relatively uncommon event. Before the advent of modern drugs and advanced technology, parents might expect to lose half of their children in infancy or early childhood (see Chap. 1). At the present time, the loss of a child appears to have become the most distressing and long-lasting grief. Several factors may have contributed to this change of attitude: (1) The structure of the family is changing, with parents having fewer children; (2) the fact that childhood deaths are relatively uncommon leaves parents unprepared for such losses; (3) society, in general, is youth-oriented. It is difficult to explain the death of a child who has not had time to really enjoy life or to add significantly to society's welfare and who has not performed a deed that should result in such dire consequences.

In the presence of a prolonged illness followed by the death of a child, the emotional strain on the family is enormous. Throughout the course of the illness, the family faces continual challenges to identity, goals, standard of living, and values. The family may go through the same five stages faced by a dying adult—denial, anger, bargaining, depression, and acceptance. Parental behavior may be characterized by shock, disbelief, hostility, outbursts of grief, guilt, and anger. Each parent may react differently because of the differences in their pre-illness relationships with the child. Mothers, realizing a dramatic role loss, may experience the "empty-mother syndrome" [89], which can create a disquieting estrangement from the family for a prolonged period of time. Less-involved fathers tend to be more accepting of the crisis than mothers [44, 82].

Although, as in any crisis, there is opportunity for personal and family growth, the terminal illness of a child appears to be particularly lethal to the family system. One study [14] estimated that 80 percent of parents of leukemic children were divorced or were seriously considering the action during the first year after the child's death.

It is apparent that unless parents are helped in their expressions of grief, serious consequences may result not only to themselves but to the family as a whole. Regardless of how stable the marital relationship was before the diagnosis, it will be tested to the limit in the course of the illness and during the postdeath period. Unfortunately, few support systems, if any, are available to them in their time of greatest need. Even grandparents are frequently unable to offer emotional or practical support [65] and may be less accepting of the diagnosis than the parents themselves [26].

It is generally assumed that each of the parents can support the other. This is indeed a fallacy, because the parents may not even be able to communicate with each other; each parent may be experiencing a different stage of the grieving process, may blame the other

*This section was written by M. Patricia Donahue, Ph.D., R.N.

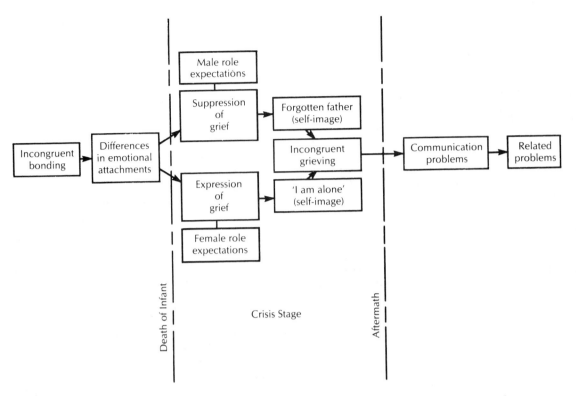

Figure 21-3. A model of husband-wife conflict. (From L. Peppers, *Motherhood and Mourning*. New York: Praeger, 1980. With permission.)

for the death of the child, or may be guilt-ridden about the fate of the child [62, 81]. Since men have frequently been socialized to hide or to deny their negative feelings, the father may become quiet or withdrawn and refuse to discuss the situation. Consequently, the mother may experience the "isolated wife syndrome" [25]. Neither is able to support the other in their grief processes.

In other families, the illness may become the focal point of all interaction. A bereaved mother commented, "When our son died, there was nothing left for us to talk about. Our entire family had revolved around our ill child for 7½ years, and there was nothing left to hold us together. It was as though each of us had died, along with our marriage, and were buried with our son." Although other children may be left, a great void is still present. Many parents wish to have another child soon after the death. However, it is very difficult to bond to a new child while grieving the loss of another. Each parent must be encouraged to complete the grief process in his or her own way and needs to be supported emotionally during that period.

Many deaths in childhood are sudden, the result of violent accidents, on the highway or elsewhere. These deaths are sharp and sudden tragedies for which the

parents are totally unprepared; thus available resources have not been mobilized, and a more acute and prolonged grief reaction may be experienced. No time is allowed for anticipatory grief or preparatory mourning. This situation may also occur with an acute, short-term illness. It is important to understand the difference that may exist between parental reactions to sudden death and reactions to a lengthy terminal illness. A fatal illness with a prolonged course provides a period in which anticipatory grief may be experienced before the ultimate death. The symptoms of grief are weakened over time and vary in intensity during the course of the illness. Some persons cannot face the stress of the perpetual mourning that accompanies chronic illness associated with a terminal process; consequently, they may withdraw emotionally from the dying child or person in an attempt to escape the mounting pressure and to renew their coping strategies [33]. The process of anticipatory grief is a healthy adaptation to a person's illness, which allows the continuation of more normal functioning and attention to other responsibilities during the illness, and serves to cushion the bereaved against the massive and disorganizing impact of a loved one's death. However, apparent abandonment may leave the terminally ill person without adequate support systems and bring social criticism, implying lack of love or of concern on the part of the parent (or spouse). It is very difficult to watch a loved one die. It is easier to have it done with. Often, after a lingering illness, the parents may feel only relief. They may have mourned for months or even years; no more tears are left.

Guilt feelings are the normal reactions of parents who are searching for an answer or for a cause of the illness. Guilt may simply be related to the fact that if the child had not been conceived, no death could have occurred. Other parents may feel guilt because of a previously ambivalent relationship with the child, a previous desire for the death of the child, a wish that more time had been spent with the child during periods of wellness, or even because of feelings of anger toward the child for "daring to die" and causing such intense emotional pain in the parent [29]. Guilt may also be related to feelings of incompetence, punishment, inadequate care and preventive measures, or transmission of the malady. It is much easier to deal with a specific cause for death than continually to face the unknown. One father expressed this idea quite clearly: "If they could only tell us what caused his illness and death, I could handle it." It is difficult to resolve a loss when no specific answers are available. In addition, parents may become overprotective or overindulgent to alleviate their guilt feelings [53]; they may be unable to treat the extremely ill child in a "normal" manner for the time remaining to him or her because of their self-blame.

Several behaviors characterize parents' relationships with dying children. Fatigue is a key factor. The increased work load of caring for ill children at home or in the hospital is energy-demanding. A fear of separation is evidenced by clinging to the child [62, 65]. Guilt and anxiety may eclipse the mother's ability to perceive the child's needs for inclusion and affection [72]. Some parents attempt to shield the child from the knowledge of the outcome of the terminal illness. However, research indicates that dying children are aware of the finality of their illness [80, 84]. The dying child's reaction to the illness is influenced by the developmental stage of the child. For some children and their families, the fear of separation, traumatic procedures, and death can be decreased by the practice of home care for dying children [57, 58].

The maturity level and the coping skills of the individual parents will affect their response to the dying child and to one another. In some cases, a strained marital relationship may be strengthened by a shared response to terminal illness; however, the chronic illness is more likely to provide merely a temporary mor-

atorium to an already fractionalized relationship. The quality of the parent-child relationship may also influence the experience and the resolution of grief. One thing remains clear: The parents must be able to feel that they did everything possible for their child, that no stone was left unturned. Then, and only then, can complete resolution occur.

Sudden Infant Death Syndrome. The sudden infant death syndrome (SIDS) precipitates reactions of intense loss. The majority of infants diagnosed as SIDS have no specific disease process or pathology to explain the death [8]. Because of the unexpected nature of SIDS, parents are particularly vulnerable to social blame and guilt for the death. If the parents are young and at the lower socioeconomic level associated with youth, these factors add to their vulnerability.

The consequences of SIDS on the family include the overprotectiveness of succeeding children, marital disharmony, and blaming one another. Parents experience the typical grief responses. In addition, many fear their own parental abilities and feel helpless and incompetent [63]. Social support groups are available for SIDS families. Technical advances in monitoring for apnea (absence of breathing) provide support for parents to use at home with succeeding infants.

Loss of a normal child. If a child is born dead or handicapped, a major loss occurs, yet there are no recognized mourning rituals. The parent of a handicapped child often feels a longing for the desired child, resentment of the reality of the situation, and guilt related to the child (see Chap. 35).

Parents of handicapped children experience a series of losses with each discovery of a new inadequacy in their child. Their mourning extends for years and may become what has been labelled "chronic sorrow," or unresolved grief [64].

Loss of Self

LOSS OF BODY PARTS AND FUNCTION
Because of the emphasis on physical beauty and prowess in our culture, a strong, healthy body can be a source of pride and esteem. The loss of a body part and/or ability is cause for grief [74]. Special meaning is often attached to particular body parts. The heart has great importance as the central organ of life. The breast, prostate, and testes are highly emotional organs, and their losses impact the individual's sexuality. The loss of body function following a stroke influences

the person's ability to perform his or her usual roles in life. Grief from the loss of a body part or function is accompanied by depression and anxiety.

The response to the loss of a body part varies with the importance of the part to the individual [74]. A male usually reacts more strongly to the loss of a body part that is associated with his work and his role as a provider [74]. Women respond more strongly to cosmetic losses. The individual's ability to adapt to losses of body parts depends on personality and body image. Sudden losses are more anxiety-producing than gradual chronic losses [74]. The sense of loss can be diminished by preparing the person for removal of the part and by a discussion of the importance of the part and life without it.

A concern for the effects of the disease process is predominant with internal organ losses, whereas concern for the surgical procedure is predominant with external losses [7]. The loss of the **function** of the part may predominate over the part itself. For instance, after removal of the colon, the person may be more concerned over the alteration in bowel elimination than the loss of the colon. Internal losses are easier to deny than the more obvious external losses. In both instances, however, a sense of incompleteness results.

The reaction to chronic conditions depends on multiple factors, including age, the nature of the illness, the type of disability, and the resources available to relieve the problems. The individual with a long-term condition must come to terms with the issues of resocialization, deviance, and grief. The newly disabled person not only has a personal burden of grief but also feels the impact of others' grieving for, and because of, him or her [85]. Resocialization, new role identifications, and redefinition of self, require indepth evaluation of family roles, sex roles, social roles, and work roles. One cannot run away from or leave behind a physical disability. It is always there [85]. Finding value in selfhood despite changes in one's repertoire of skills is integral to grief work.

BIRTH, ABORTION, STILLBIRTH
The birth of a child may also represent a partial loss of self. The mother loses the fullness of her body. She loses the center stage of attention, which must now be shared with the infant. The mother may mourn her empty body and the loss of freedom and uninterrupted sleep. Postpartum blues, or a sense of grief, may set in.

The interruption of a pregnancy before the delivery of a viable child may result in feelings of guilt and failure with a loss of self-esteem. Feelings of guilt and loss are as intense for these mothers as for those whose newborn infant dies [67]. It is a lonelier grief, however, because except for the parents, few other persons had formed relationships with the fetus [47]. Also, couples who experience infertility problems may experience recurrent grief each time the woman starts her menstrual period.

The grief experienced by a couple at the loss of a fetus is related to the degree of bonding already established with the unborn child. Because of the physical reality of the growing child within her, the mother bonds earlier than the father. A spontaneous abortion in the early months is felt more keenly by the mother than the father because he has less involvement. At the time, the male will usually remain calm and fulfill the social role of "protector" [67].

In the case of elective abortion, an early decision to terminate the pregnancy is apt to decrease a sense of bonding between the parent and the fetus. Fantasies and dreams of the expected child are actively discouraged and thus may lessen the sense of direct loss and grief. However, there is frequently a loss of self-esteem and sexual fulfillment along with feelings of guilt [87]. Anger may be directed toward those responsible for the pregnancy or its interruption. Delayed or postponed grief may be felt at the time the fetus would have been born and even for several months or sporadically for several years thereafter.

Developmental Losses

SEPARATION EXPERIENCES
Loss scenarios begin early in life with separation experiences. Separating from mother is an important milestone for the child in learning to cope with loss. Entering school, spending the night with a friend, and attending a week-long camp, are the means by which the child's ability to undergo a loss of the familiar environment is tested, and self-sufficiency is encouraged. These experiences should be encouraged for each child because they enhance the social-emotional maturation that is essential for a healthy personality. For example, the grief process as applied to high-school graduation can be analyzed in the following manner [22]. During the senior year, denial may take the form of failing to prepare for final tests and delaying completion of term papers. Anger is displayed in fighting over commencement speakers and proper dress. Anger may also be directed at teachers for not providing adequate preparation. The anger then gives way to depression: Students lack energy and zest; they miss classes and fail to get involved in activities ("Senioritis"). An acceptance of loss begins when students can

evaluate their educational program and see both the good and the bad. When they begin to make plans for the future, acceptance has been reached.

Social Losses

Moving to a new home; changing jobs; breaking habits, such as smoking, drugs, or alcohol; and the losses of aging represent social losses because they require the adoption of new coping behaviors.

STOPPING SMOKING

Loss theory can be applied to the personal experiences of giving up smoking [70]. Denial is a strong motivation to **not** stop smoking. Anger is apparent in irritability and overreactions. Bargaining allows one to identify with the circumstances under which one would smoke again. Depression, sadness, and longing for a cigarette accompany cessation of smoking. The acceptance of a nonsmoking life-style does not occur until 6 to 12 months after stopping smoking.

LOSS OF A JOB

The loss of a job requires that the individual grieve and feel anger and sadness related to the old job. Until the individual grieves, the plans and the adjustments essential for gaining a new position cannot be made. Three major factors influence the grief over a job or a career loss [38]: (1) the person's understanding of why the job loss occurred, (2) the effectiveness of the support systems available, and (3) the person's ability to cope effectively with stress. The management of the loss involves facing the reality of the situation; breaking ties with the lost job; and developing new interests, activities, and job opportunities [77].

LOSSES OF AGING

Aging subjects people to multiple losses. Health may be lost; cultural hallmarks of beauty may have faded; lifetime goals may be unreached; important jobs and sources of self-esteem may be gone. Some aging people follow a pattern of inhibited or chronic grief [30]. This is manifested through somatic pain and distress because the grieving is unexpressed.

The losses of aging are unique because there is limited opportunity for a reinstatement of the loss or to regain lost gratification in other ways [1]. Grief intensifies the fears of increased loneliness. The older person may also face repeated forms of anticipatory grief in relation to expected losses in the near future. Old age requires a process of reintegration, where losses are accepted and essential purposes are retrieved, re-

formulated, and reincorporated in a new way in the life of the individual [56].

CONFRONTATION WITH LOSS

Death Education

The goal of death education is to facilitate a realistic and positive attitude toward death and to aid people in understanding the grief process and the expression of emotions. Death education is available through formal courses in colleges and universities and as part of health education in the family-living courses of primary and secondary schools [60]. Death education content should be presented at a level consistent with the emotional-social-spiritual level of students as well as their cognitive development. However, the ideal death education for young children is one that takes advantage of the "teachable moment" and includes experiences with life processes—plants, animals, and people. It originates from the children's questions and experiences and is shared lovingly within the framework of the parents' beliefs. Healthy death education should assist in the development of accurate and positive death concepts.

Death education for adults is often directed toward professionals who work with dying persons and the bereaved. The focus is on affect, knowledge, and acceptance of death. Some community agencies also offer support groups and general content courses that focus on understanding death as a part of life. Many excellent resources are available for community death education courses [21, 27, 31, 32, 36, 37, 42, 44]. The death education teacher needs to evidence personal maturity and sensitivity to the topic as well as to the feelings of students.

Development of Faith

Several perspectives on the development of faith have been postulated [16, 23, 24, 25, 78]. These views generally follow the cognitive-developmental and psychosocial stages set forth by Piaget [9], Erikson [19], and Kohlberg [41]. James Fowler sets forth the most recent and thorough theory of the stages of faith [4, 23, 24, 25]. "Faith" for Fowler does not refer to a specific set of beliefs or religious dogmas. It is a dynamic, human activity by which one constructs the meaning of life. This faith, or "master story" provides an explanation for one's values, and offers a rationale for behavior and the direction of life. The individual's faith frame can be centered on career, family, religion, financial success, personal recognition, institutions, or even self-actualization. The content is insignificant, according to Fowler, because from a structural-developmental frame, the stages are universal. When confronted with the loss or death, people will struggle to understand the event in the light of a personally defined meaning of the purpose of life. Based on hundreds of personal faith interviews with people from 4 to 80 years of age, Fowler has identified six discrete and hierarchical stages of faith. The age ranges for the stages are arbitrary designations that reflect a general pattern. Faith can be arrested at any stage. Environmental stimulation, crises, and family/cultural role models significantly influence the timing and the movement through the following stages of faith.

UNDIFFERENTIATED FAITH

The first 2 years of life are critical in establishing the foundation on which the edifice of faith is built. During these years, a trust in the parents helps to offset the anxiety of separations. Children build trust in concrete, life-sustaining, soul-enhancing experiences. Gradually children discover, however, that life is transient, and living things die.

INTUITIVE PROJECTIVE FAITH: STAGE 1

In the intuitive projective stage, children combine their limited, often distorted perception of events with their feelings to create an image of the protective-threaten-

Table 21–1. Psychological, Cognitive, and Faith Stages: Optimal Parallels [24]

Psychosocial (Erikson)	Cognitive (Piaget)	Faith (Fowler)
Trust vs. mistrust	Sensorimotor	Undifferentiated (infancy)
Autonomy vs. shame and doubt	Preoperational	Intuitive-projective (early childhood)
Initiative vs. guilt		
Industry vs. inferiority	Concrete operational	Mythic-literal (school years)
Identity vs. role confusion	Early formal operations	Synthetic-conventional (adolescence)
Intimacy vs. isolation	Formal operations (dichotomizing)	Individuative-reflexive (young adulthood)
Generativity vs. stagnation	Formal operations (dialectical)	Conjunctive (midlife and beyond)
Integrity vs. despair	Formal operations (synthetic)	Universalizing

ing powers surrounding their lives. Children in these early childhood years (2 to 7 years of age) allow their imaginations to run wild and unchecked by logic, so that a meaning can be extracted from life.

Religious doctrine offers a representation of the transcendent through sacred writings [16]. Preschool and elementary children enjoy the simple religious stories. The true meaning of religious acts and symbols is vague, but the ritual aspects provide concrete acts and meaningful consistency. During these early years, the child imitates the behaviors observed in parents, siblings, and significant others. Children of this age may participate by imitation in social mourning rituals, such as crying or attending a funeral, without experiencing any value or meaning from the activity. Role models help young children establish early concepts of deity and life values.

MYTHICAL LITERAL FAITH: STAGE 2

The faith of school-agers, 7 to 12 years of age, is described by Fowler as mythical literal. For them the world is literally understood. The ability to think in concrete terms gives rise to a sense of causality and a diminishing of imaginative explanation. Children are able to use the perceptions of others (authority figures, such as parents, teachers, and clergy) to develop a logical meaning to life. Their sense of moral judgment is based on reciprocal fairness and imminent justice [41]—a legalistic concept of rigid reward-punishment rules. Children begin to extract the moral from stories and narrative accounts. Religious doctrine may then assist children in building a more mature faith and an acceptance of death.

SYNTHETIC CONVENTIONAL FAITH: STAGE 3

A synthetic-conventional faith emerges during adolescence (12 years of age and more). As adolescents struggle to understand themselves, the values and the beliefs of earlier years coalesce to support the emerging identity. The acceptance of a dogma tends to emotionally unite the person with others who hold similar explanations on the meaning of life—a factor that further supports the developing ego. Role models, whether peers, religious figures in writings, or a mentor, are crucial in translating the adolescent's values into behavioral patterns and in facing crises, including significant losses.

INDIVIDUATIVE REFLECTIVE FAITH: STAGE 4

An individuative reflective faith does not usually emerge until the individual's identity is firmly established (20 years of age or more). This stage reflects a movement away from a group (conformist) faith to a personally held perspective. Although the individual still recognizes the larger social system, a critical evaluation of values reveals that the locus of authority for the meaning of life resides in one's own judgment. The primary task of this stage is to take on the personal responsibility for one's own beliefs, commitments, and life-style. The young adult constructs personalized values and goals in response to philosophical questions, such as "Who am I?" and "Where am I going in life?" [24]. A death or significant loss may be a critical event, leading to a reflection on current beliefs about the meaning of life and death. Community-held beliefs about mourning rituals and social norms may be shunned or openly scorned.

CONJUNCTIVE FAITH: STAGE 5

As people awaken to the realization that truth is more multifaceted and complex than previously recognized, they enter the stage of conjunctive faith (35 years of age or more). The individual searches for new truths and meanings as the paradoxes and polarities of life's events and religious dogma are confronted. In this stage, the individual may willingly choose to follow the doctrine of a specific denomination or may create a philosophy more consistent with a personal concept of the meaning of life. There is often a reclaiming and reintegration of past faith into present circumstances. People at midlife know the realities of life and the pain of defeat, consequently they appreciate the depth of reality to which symbols, myths, and rituals refer.

UNIVERSAL FAITH: STAGE 6

The final stage of faith is not realized by all individuals. In the stage of universal faith, individuals become aware of a oneness with the source of power or being. They become devoted to the cause for which they have found meaning in life. Life is, paradoxically, both loved and held too loosely [24]. Individuals are willing to spend and to be spent for the cause and for the possibility of others receiving meaning and identity in their own lives. These persons are "contagious" in creating faith communities. There is a commitment to justice and a selfless passion for a transformed world. Two overriding characteristics of this stage are universal love and inclusiveness. Death is not feared by these individuals; it is incorporated into their living experience.

In summary, faith, by its very nature is an evolving philosophy of life, incorporating concepts of both life and death. Since faith, according to Fowler, is the structure on which people build their lives [25], it will influence how they respond to loss and their approach to resolving grief.

Resolving Grief

SOCIAL SUPPORT

Time is a great healer of grief. However, time alone is not enough; it is the help and the support received in the days and months following loss that facilitate recovery from, and resolution of, the loss. Social support systems are both formal and informal. Friends, neighbors, and family surround the bereaved with informal support in the form of companionship; material assistance, such as food; and aid in decision making. Their empathic understanding allows them to comprehend and to support the state of the bereaved. Empathy must be distinguished from sympathy. Sympathy focuses on one's own feelings and projects those feelings onto another. Empathy centers on the feelings and experiences of the bereaved other. It involves a loss of self-consciousness and an objective concern and an appreciation for the experience of the other [40]. Because of differences in early training and cultural expectations, empathy appears to be more developed in women and increases with age [11]. Empathy is a response that develops as a person learns to experience vicariously and to understand the feelings of another.

The formal expression of support comes from organized groups. These groups preserve the cultural responses to death and thereby facilitate and encourage the mourning process. Community support groups that are available to offer support are listed in Table 21–2.

HOSPICE CARE

A growing source of support for terminally ill persons is hospice care. The hospice concept encompasses a philosophy of care that allows the client and the family members to face death with dignity. Hospice programs offer an environment that gives relief from the distressing symptoms of disease, a caring milieu, expert medical and nursing care, a sense of security, and family-centered care [13]. These programs allow the dying person and family members to maintain control over a most critical life experience—the passage through dying. The process can be the peak of personal growth and development for the dying person and the supporting family members.

FUNERALS

Funerals and final rituals are the cultural, social expressions of grief. By participating in the prescribed mourning rituals, the bereaved are supplied with a pattern of activity in the early days of shock and numb-

Table 21–2. Community Support Groups for People Experiencing Loss

Group	Focus
Candlelighters Suite 1011 2025 Eye Street, N.W. Washington, D.C. 20006	Families of children with cancer
Compassionate Friends P.O. Box 1347 Oak Brook, IL 60421	Parents who have lost children of all ages
Parents without partners 7910 Woodmont Avenue, #1000 Bethesda, MD 20814	Single parents
Alcoholics Anonymous Association Box 549 Grand Central Station New York, NY 10017	Those in the process of loss of alcohol habits
Narcotics Anonymous P.O. Box 622 Sun Valley, CA 91352	People with drug habits
SIDS Support Groups National SIDS Institute 275 Carpenter Drive Atlanta, GA 30328	Families who have lost an infant through sudden infant death syndrome
Weight Watchers 800 Community Drive Manhasset, NY 11038	Overweight people

ness following a death. The funeral offers an opportunity for community support and sharing emotional expressions.

Questions arise concerning the value of funerals for children. The limited available literature is contradictory. Grollman suggested that funeral experiences al-low the child to view firsthand the reality of death and to receive comfort [31]. Others think children should be permitted to attend funerals because their fantasies regarding the event are worse than the experience (76). Some believe funeral rituals offer a sense of closure for the child just as they do for the adult [75]. Other studies show that children may have behavior problems related to funeral attendance [50, 75, 86]. Specifically, children under 7 years of age and female children may be particularly affected by funeral attendance [50]. However, each child is different, and the individual maturity, sensitivity, and preparation of the child must be considered when making the decision to attend a funeral. The experience can be a positive growth opportunity for the well-prepared child.

The trend toward cremation also has implications. Mourning rites and rituals that assist the bereaved need to be developed for cremation.

SIGNS OF RECOVERY

The recovery from loss takes time. Each individualized aspect of the grief process must be experienced in its intensity before grief can be resolved. Emotional energy must be released from the deceased and invested in daily living. Facing loss can be a maturing experience, but if it is denied or avoided, the individual may lose the opportunity to grow and may actually regress. Grief must be resolved before replacement of the loss, otherwise, it will interfere with an effective investment in new relationships. The course of grief depends on the ability of the bereaved to do the work needed to separate the self from the lost object and reinvest in new interests. Recovery from grief begins at the point when the bereaved returns to normal activities with a full capacity for life and pleasure. Even the normally recovering person, however, will reexperience periods

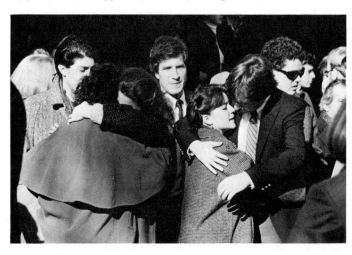

Figure 21–4. Losses are experienced in many forms throughout the life cycle. The presence of a caring, supportive person helps one to regain composure and control, so that a sense of overwhelming helplessness does not immobilize the individual.

of acute pain and loss awareness periodically, especially at holidays or anniversaries. Three months and one year after the loss appear to be particularly painful times as the person confronts the reality of loss and loneliness.

SUMMARY

Loss, grief, and mourning are a part of life. Grief is a period of acute sorrow and anguish, which can follow any kind of loss. The loss may be of a significant person, pet, object, event, anticipated experience, or goal. The normal duration of grief is time-limited and influenced by multiple factors. The resolution of grief occurs over time through religious or philosophical faith, social support, and cultural rituals. Adjusting to loss is part of the human experience. Successful adjustment leads to higher levels of personal maturity.

REFERENCES

1. Agee, J.   Grief and the Process of Aging. In J. Werner-Beland, *Grief Responses to Long-Term Illness and Disability.* Reston, VA: Reston, 1980.
2. Aldrich, C. K.   Some Dynamics of Anticipatory Grief. In B. Schoenberg, et al. (Eds.), *Anticipatory Grief.* New York: Columbia University Press, 1974.
3. Averill, J.   Grief: Its nature and significance. *Psychol. Bull.* 70:721, 1968
4. Betz.   Faith development in children. *Pediatr. Nurs.* 7(2):22, 1981.
5. Binger, C., et al.   Childhood leukemia: Emotional impact on patient and family. *N. Eng. J. Med.* 280:414, 1969.
6. Birtchnell, J.   Recent parent death and mental illness. *Br. J. Psychiatry* 116:289, 1970.
7. Blacher, R.   Loss of Internal Organs. In B. Schoenberg, et al. (Eds.), *Loss and Grief: Psychological Management in Medical Practice.* New York: Columbia Press, 1970.
8. Blugass, K.   Psychosocial aspects of the Sudden Infant Death Syndrome. *J. Child Psychol. Psychiatry* 22:411, 1981.
9. Brainerd, C.   *Piaget's Theory of Intelligence.* Englewood Cliffs, NJ: Prentice-Hall, 1978.
10. Brown, F.   Childhood bereavement and subsequent psychiatric disorder. *Br. J. Psychiatry* 112:1027, 1966.
11. Bryant, B.   An index of empathy for children and adolescents. *Child Dev.* 53:413, 1982.
12. Cain, A., Fast, I., and Erickson, M.   Children's disturbed reactions to the death of a sibling. *Am. J. Orthopsychiatry* 34:741, 1964.
13. Craven, J., and Wald, F.   Hospice care for dying patients. *Am. J. Nurs.* 75:1816, 1975.
14. Dempsey, D. K.   *The Way We Die.* New York: McGraw-Hill, 1975.
15. Dennehy, C. M.   Childhood bereavement and psychiatric illness. *Br. J. Psychiatry* 112:1049, 1966.
16. Elkind, D.   The origins of religion in the child. *Review of Religious Research* 12(1):35, 1970.
17. Engel, G.   Grief and grieving. *Am. J. Nurs.* 64:93, 1964.
18. Engel, G.   Death of a twin: Mourning and anniversary reactions. *Int. J. Psychoanal.,* 50(23):21, 1975.
19. Erikson, E.   *Childhood and Society* (2nd ed.). New York: Norton, 1963.
20. Feifel, H. (Ed.)   *The Meaning of Death.* New York: McGraw-Hill, 1965.
21. Feifel, H. (Ed.)   *New Meanings of Death.* New York: McGraw-Hill, 1977.
22. Fishel, A.   Graduation/Termination. *Am. J. Nurs.* 81:1156, 1981.
23. Fowler, J.   Towards a developmental perspective on faith. *Religious Education* 69:205, 1974.
24. Fowler, J. W.   *Stages of Faith: The Psychology of Human Development and the Quest for Meaning.* San Francisco: Harper & Row, 1981.
25. Fowler, J.   Moral Stages and the Development of Faith. In B. Munsey (Ed.), *Moral Development, Moral Education, and Kohlberg.* Alabama: Religious Education Press, 1980.
26. Friedman, S., Chodoff, P., Mason, J., and Hamburg, D.   Behavioral observation on parents anticipating the death of a child. *Pediatrics* 32:610, 1963.
27. Fulton, R. L. (Ed.)   *Death and Identity* (Rev. ed.). Bowie, MD: Charles Press, 1976.
28. Gerber, I.   Anticipatory Bereavement. In B. Schoenberg, et al. (Eds.), *Anticipatory Grief.* New York: Columbia University Press, 1974.
29. Goldberg, S.   Family tasks and reactions in the crisis upon death. *Soc. Work* 54:398, 1973.
30. Gramich, E.   Recognition and Management of Grief in Elderly Patients. In Ellard, J., Volkan, V., and Paul, N., et al. *Normal and Pathological Responses to Bereavement.* New York: MSS Information Corp., 1974.
31. Grollman, E. A. (Ed.)   *Explaining Death to Children.* Boston: Beacon Press, 1969.
32. Grollman, E.   Children and Death. In E. A. Grollman (Ed.) *Concerning Death: A Practical Guide for the Living.* Boston: Beacon Press, 1974.
33. Gyulay, J. E.   *The Dying Child.* New York: McGraw-Hill, 1978.
34. Hafer, W. K.   *Coping with Bereavement from Death or Divorce.* Englewood Cliffs, NJ: Prentice-Hall, 1981.
35. Hutton, L.   Annie is alone: The bereaved child. *Am. J. of Matern. Child Nurs.* 6:274, 1981.
36. Jackson, E. N.   *Understanding Grief: Its Roots, Dynamics, and Treatment.* New York: Abingdon Press, 1957.
37. Johnson, P., and Rosenblatt, P.   Grief following childhood loss of a parent. *Am. J. Psychother.* 35:419, 1981.
38. Jones, W.   Grief and involuntary career change: Its implications for counseling. *Voc. Guid. Q.* 27(3):196, 1979.
39. Kastenbaum, R., and Aisenberg, R.   *The Psychology of Death.* New York: Springer, 1976.
40. Katz, R. L.   *Empathy, Its Nature and Uses.* London: Collier-Macmillan, 1963.
41. Kohlberg, L.   *The Philosophy of Moral Development,* Vol. I. San Francisco: Harper & Row, 1981.

42. Kübler-Ross, E. *On Death and Dying.* New York: Macmillan, 1973.

43. Kutscher, A. H. and Kutscher, L. G. (Eds.) *Religion and Bereavement: Counsel for the Physician, Advice for the Bereaved, Thoughts for the Clergyman.* New York: Health Sciences, 1972.

44. Lascari, A. The dying child and the family. *J. Fam. Pract.* 6:1279, 1978.

45. Levinson, D. J., et al. *Season of a Man's Life.* New York: Knopf, 1978.

46. Leviton, D. J. Death Education. In Feifel, H. (Ed.), *New Meanings of Death.* New York: McGraw-Hill, 1977.

47. Lewis, E. Mourning by the family after a stillbirth or neonated death. *Arch. Dis. Child.* 54:303, 1979.

48. Lindemann, E. Symptomatology and the management of acute grief. *Am. J. Psychiatry* 101:1, 1944.

49. McCown, D. *"Selected Factors Related to Children's Adjustment Following Sibling Death."* Doctoral Dissertation, Oregon State University, 1982.

50. McCown, D. Funeral attendance, cremation and young siblings. *J. of Death Education,* 8:349, 1984.

51. Maddison, D. The Consequences of Conjugal Bereavement. In J. Ellard, et al. (Eds.), *Normal and Pathological Responses to Bereavement.* New York: MSS Information Corp., 1974.

52. Maddison, D., and Walker, W. Factors Affecting the Outcome of Conjugal Bereavement. In J. Ellard, et al. (Eds.), *Normal and Pathological Responses to Bereavement.* New York: MSS Information Corp., 1974.

53. Mann, S. Coping with a child's fatal illness. *Nurs. Clin. North Am.* 2:81, 1974.

54. Markel, W., and Sinon, V. *The Hospice Concept.* New York: American Cancer Society, 1978.

55. Markusen, E., and Fulton, R. Childhood bereavement and behavior disorders: A critical review. *Omega* 2:107, 1971.

56. Marris, P. Conservatism, innovation and old age. *Int. J. Aging Hum. Dev.* 9(2):127, 1978–79.

57. Martinson, I. M., et al. Home care for children dying of cancer. *Pediatrics* 62:106, 1978.

58. Martinson, I. M. (Principal Investigator). *Home Care for the Child with Cancer Final Report* (National Cancer Institute. Grant CA 19490). Minneapolis, Minnesota: University of Minnesota, 1980.

59. Maurer, A. Maturation of concepts of death. *Br. J. Med. Psychol.* 39:35, 1966.

60. Middleton, K. Strategies for teaching about death and loss. *Health Educ.* 10(1):36, 1979.

61. Munro, A., and Griffiths, A. Some psychiatric non-sequelae of childhood bereavement. *Br. J. Psychiatry* 115:305, 1969.

62. Natterson, J. M., and Knudson, A. G. Observations concerning fear of death in fatally ill children and their mothers. *Psychosom. Med.* 22:456, 1960.

63. Nikolaisen, S. The impact of sudden infant death on the family: Nursing Intervention. *Top. Clin. Nurs.* 3(13):45, 1981.

64. Olshansky, S. Chronic sorrow: A response to having a mentally defective child. *Soc. Casework* 43:190, 1962.

65. Orbach, C., et al. Psychological impact of cancer and its treatment: III. The adaptation of mothers to the threatened loss of their children through leukemia: II. *Cancer* 8:20, 1955.

66. Parkes, C. The first year of bereavement. *Psychiatry* 33:444, 1970.

67. Peppers, L. G., and Knapp, R. J. *Motherhood and Mourning: Perinatal Death.* New York: Praeger, 1980.

68. Peretz, D. Development, Object-Relationships, and Loss. In B. Schoenberg, et al. (Eds.) *Loss and Grief: Psychological Management in Medical Practice.* New York: Columbia Press, 1970.

69. Reilly, D. Death propensity, dying, and bereavement: A family systems perspective. *Family Therapy* 5:35, 1978.

70. Richard, E., and Shepard, A Giving up smoking: A lesson in loss theory. *Am. J. Nurs.* 81:755, 1981.

71. Salladay, S. A., and Royal, M. E. Children and death: Guidelines for grief work. *Child Psychiatry Hum. Dev.* 11:203, 1981.

72. Samaniego, L., et al. The physically ill child's self-perceptions and the mother's perceptions of her child's needs: Insights gained from the FIRO-BC—a behavior test for use with children. *Clin. Pediatr.* (Phila.) 16:154, 1977.

73. Schoenberg, B., et al. (Eds.) *Loss and Grief: Psychological Management in Medical Practice.* New York: Columbia University Press, 1970.

74. Schoenberg, B., and Carr, A. Loss of External Organs: Limb, Amputation, Mastectomy and Disfiguration. In B. Schoenberg, et al. (Eds.), *Loss and Grief: Psychological Management in Medical Practice.* New York: Columbia University Press, 1970.

75. Showalter, J. How do children and funerals mix? *Pediatr.* 89:139, 1976.

76. Schultz, C. Grieving children. *J. Emerg. Nurs.* 6(1):30, 1980.

77. Sheehy, G. *Pathfinders.* New York: William Morrow, 1981.

78. Shelly, J. *The Spiritual Needs of Children.* Illinois: Inter-Varsity Press, 1982.

79. Simos, B. G. *A Time to Grieve: Loss as a Universal Human Experience.* New York: Family Service Association of America, 1979.

80. Spinetta, J. J., Rigler, D., and Karon, M. Personal space as a measure of a dying child's sense of isolation. *J. Consult. Clin. Psychol.* 42:751, 1974.

81. Stebbens, J. and Lascari, A. Psychological follow-up of families with childhood leukemia, *J. Clin. Psychol.* 30:394, 1974.

82. Townes, B., Wold, D., and Holmes, T. Parental adjustment to childhood leukemia. *J. Psychosom. Res.* 18:9, 1974.

83. Volkan, V. The Recognition and Prevention of Pathological Grief. In J. Ellard, et al. (Eds.), *Normal and Pathological Responses to Bereavement.* New York: MSS Information Corp., 1974.

84. Waechter, E. Children's awareness of fatal illness. *Am. J. Nurs.* 71:1167, 1971.

85. Werner-Beland, J. *Grief Responses to Long-Term Illness and Disability: Manifestations and Nursing Interventions.* Reston, VA: Reston, 1980.

86. Wessels, M. The grieving child. *Clin. Pediatr.* 17:559, 1978.

87. Whitlock, G. E. *Understanding and Coping with Real-life Crises.* Monterey, CA: Brooks/Cole, 1978.

88. Wolfenstein, M. How is mourning possible? *Psychoanal. Study Child* 21:93, 1966.

89. Wong, D. Bereavement: The empty mother syndrome. *Am. J. of Matern.-Child Nurs.* 5:385, 1980.

VII
The School-Ager

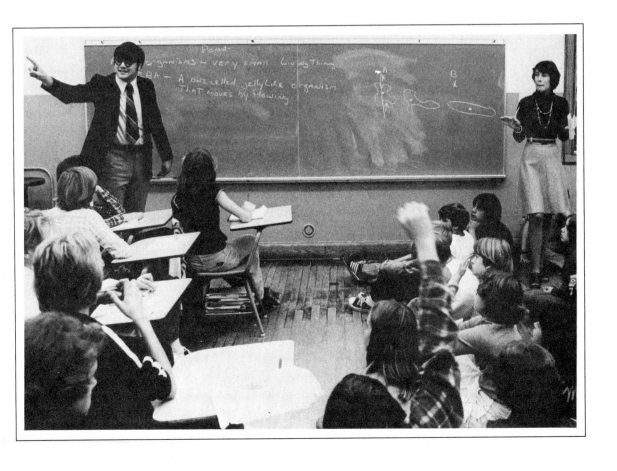

22

Biophysical Development of the School-Ager and the Pubescent

Clara S. Schuster

A little bit is better than nothing. Do something, begin in a small way.

—Anonymous

Introduction

Somatic Development

Maintaining Health

Allergies in Children

Summary

The biophysical growth and the development of the child in the early school-age years are singularly unremarkable. During the years from 6 to 10, most children experience a relative plateau in growth—a lull between the rapid growth of early childhood and that which they will once more experience during the prepubertal years (ages 10 to 13 years in females, 12 to 16 years in males). The changes that do occur are gradual and relatively subtle. The body appears to be undergoing a period of refinement, of hypertrophic development, rather than the hyperplastic growth that predominated in the earlier years.

There are minimal differences in body contour between males and females until the late school years. However, the individuality of children as influenced by both heredity and environment becomes more obvious. It is this individuality that makes it very difficult to establish norms for the school-age years. Although growth from child to child has many similarities, each child has his or her own growth pattern and timetable. Great variations in height and weight may still be considered normal when all the contributing factors are considered. Growth patterns are more significant than single measurements, therefore, growth and development charts should be used as reference points only— as tools to reinforce and improve clinical judgment (see Appendixes D and E). The periodic measurements of height and weight are imperative for evaluating growth patterns and identifying potential deviation. Accurate height and weight measurements are especially important with hospital admissions because body surface area is calculated from these two measurements. Many dosages of medications and fluid replacements are calculated on the basis of body surface area rather than by chronological age, height, or body weight alone.

By the time a child is 6 years old, evidences of future adult body proportions are already present. An individual's general relationship to norms usually does not change after the school years. One can begin to estimate, therefore, whether a child is going to be tall, petite, or stocky. Height can be predicted from the average height of the parents (Fig. 22–1). Although measurements can give an indication of the child's health status, it is the pattern of progress that becomes the critical factor. Unfortunately, deviations in growth will accompany or follow, not herald, a disorder.

The body proportions of the school-ager are quite different from those of the preschooler or the adolescent. At birth the head comprises one-fourth of the body length because of the rapid growth of the central nervous system during fetal life. During the toddler and early preschool years, there is a rapid increase in body length, giving the child a top-heavy appearance. During the late preschool years, the extremities grow rapidly, and the child appears to "thin out." By 6 years of age, the child is able to put an arm **over** the head and touch the opposite ear. By 7 years of age, parents often describe the child as being gangly and awkward and begin to complain about the expense of keeping the child in shoes and clothes that fit. During the pubertal years, trunk growth begins to accelerate again.

For many individuals, the school years represent one of the healthiest periods of life. Children of this age are able to fight off infections easily and tend to recover quickly when ill. The increase in organ maturity and in general body size enables the child to respond physiologically in a more adult manner to illness. In the school-age child, for example, there is a greatly reduced danger of occlusion of the airway during an infection of the respiratory tract, a reduced incidence of seizures accompanying high temperatures, and a greatly reduced chance of dehydration during an illness involving vomiting or diarrhea. As the body size increases, there is less body surface in proportion to the body mass; this fact combined with maturation of the skin decreases insensible water loss [5].

Figure 22–1. (A) These girls (8, 11, and 18 years of age) are all the same height. (B) The influence of genetics is readily apparent 6 years later when they are again seen standing with their fathers.

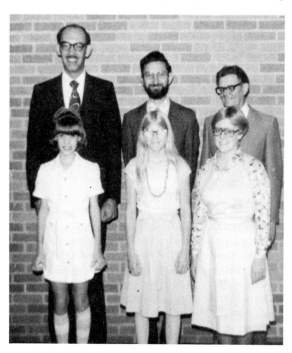
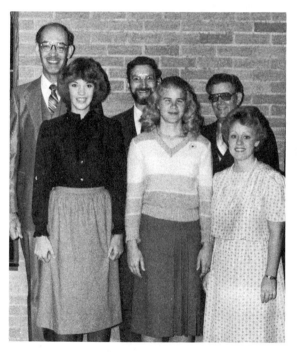

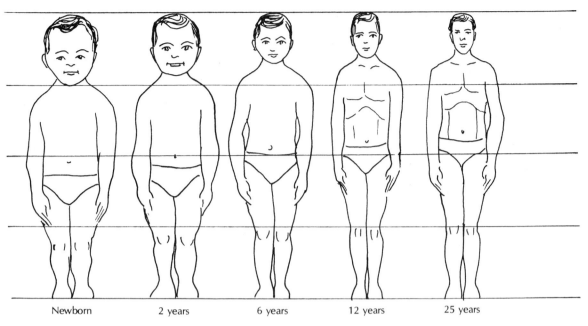

| Newborn | 2 years | 6 years | 12 years | 25 years |

Figure 22-2. Body proportions and form will change as individuals progress through the early years of the life cycle.

SOMATIC DEVELOPMENT

Skeletal System

The most rapid hyperplastic growth during the school-age years is experienced by the skeletal system. This growth is particularly obvious in the long bones of the extremities and in the development of the facial bones. The rapid growth of the preschool years now slows to a height gain of 2 to 2½ inches per year [3, 19] if nutrition is optimal and no disease processes interfere. Growth is most rapid in the spring and the fall. Females begin to surpass males in height and weight, and they will frequently remain taller until males enter the adolescent growth spurt that accompanies puberty.

Even with this slower rate of growth, however, the long bones are growing faster than the adjacent muscles. As a result, many children experience "growing pains," or muscle and ligament aches, due to stretching of these softer tissues [36]. Children are most likely to complain of pain when lying down at night. Although such pain is thought to be a normal phenomenon by some people, persistent complaints of pain should be checked by a physician because bone cancer, childhood arthritis, rheumatic fever, and other disease processes may exhibit similar symptoms in their early stages [36]. Taut, stretched muscles also have a tendency to respond with quick, jerky movements [37].

POSTURE

The curvature of the spine reflects the body's health state and balance. It changes throughout childhood as the center of gravity moves down the body and as muscle strength increases (see Fig. 22-3). Until there is adequate increase in the strength of adjacent muscles and

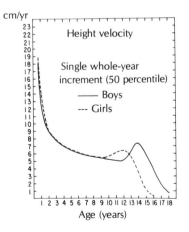

Figure 22-3. Average height gained each year from birth through 18 years of age. (From G. H. Lowrey, *Growth and Development of Children* [7th ed.]. Chicago: Year Book, 1978. With permission.)

ligaments, the child may appear to be loose-jointed, gangly, and swaybacked [36]. During the early school-age years, the child gradually loses the pot-bellied, swaybacked appearance of the early childhood years (lordosis). The child's posture becomes straighter as the pelvis tips backward and the abdominal muscles become stronger [3]. A convex curvature begins to appear in the thoracic spine area [16]. The shoulders continue to have a rounded appearance [19]. Although the neck appears to elongate and the chest becomes broader and flatter, a "military posture" (head erect, shoulders back, stomach in, chest out) does not appear until further growth of the trunk during the adolescent years [16].

Adequate exercise is needed to help maintain strength and flexibility and to encourage muscular development during the school-age years. However, exercise has minimal influence on posture because the vertebral curves are not fully under voluntary control. According to Lowrey, "Posture, to a degree, reflects strength and health, and these factors are the more basic conditions which should receive our consideration. The old idea of admonishing school children to 'stand straight' or 'sit straight' in the interest of better posture often confuses cause and effect. A child typically adopts the posture which keeps the parts of his body in proper balance. Frequent action and change of activity in school are excellent preventives of faulty posture" [19].

Poor posture can reflect fatigue as well as a major or minor skeletal defect. School-age children, especially females during the late school years and early adolescence, should have periodic spine checks for evenness of hips (pelvic tilt) and shoulders and for abnormal curvatures of the spine in standing or bending positions. Erect posture may be considered satisfactory if one is able to draw a straight line from the ear through the shoulders and then through the greater trochanter (hip) to the anterior part of the long arch of the foot [19]. Although parents and teachers may encourage this positioning, it should not be forced on the child. One should keep in mind that the posture assumed is usually reflective of body growth.

The toddler normally assumes a wide base or stance when standing. The toes point outward because of an outward rotation of the legs at the hip. As the lower extremities gradually rotate inward, flexibility for voluntary rotation increases. By the school years, the child is usually able to rotate the foot 30 degrees inward and 60 degrees outward [16]—valuable assets for ballet. If the leg rotates too far, the child may exhibit pigeon-toed walking (toes pointing inward). Although this phenomenon is occasionally due to a pathological problem, most cases are developmental and disappear spontaneously without treatment, especially if they are due to the normal "grip phenomenon" of utilizing the big toe for balance and for pushing off during walking. Both corrective shoes and poorly fitted regular shoes may increase stress points on the growing skeleton; thus the former alter skeletal development therapeutically and the latter negatively. Rapid growth of the foot in the late school years is one of the first indications of the onset of the adolescent growth spurt. The feet will reach their final growth 1 to 2 years before the long bones of the legs [29].

OSSIFICATION

Ossification, the formation of bone, continues at a rather steady pace throughout the school years. Fractures usually heal quickly because the body is already metabolizing the necessary constituents of bone tissue [5]. All the primary ossification centers of the long, tubular bones appeared during fetal life [4]. The body lays down a transverse disc along the cartilaginous tissues that are precursors to bone development. These discs serve as foundation structures for calcification, or bone formation, during the next two decades of life. The

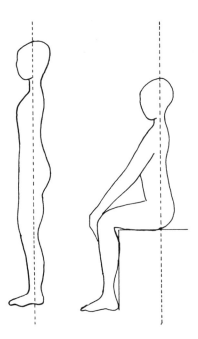

Figure 22–4. Correct standing and sitting positions for adolescents and adults. Good body alignment, whether standing, or sitting, should allow a straight line to be drawn through ear, shoulder, and hip.

discs gradually increase in length. The constant addition of cartilage at the ends of the ossification points allows continued extension of bone length.

Secondary ossification points appear after birth at the ends of bones. These oval discs grow outward and downward very slowly toward the epiphysis—the final point of ossification of the long bones [4]. The shaft of the long bone and the cap will fuse at, or near, the onset of true puberty. In fact, the maturation of the skeletal system and that of the reproductive system are synchronized. Menarche (the first menstrual period) usually occurs slightly before final epiphyseal fusion. The maximum increment in growth of the long bones occurs in the year prior to the onset of menarche. All linear growth of the long bones ceases within 2 years after menarche. Those individuals who mature early usually experience an earlier growth spurt and end up shorter than their peers in adult life.

Successive x-ray films of the hand reveal a definite schedule in the appearance and the union of the wrist bones. These x-rays can be used to assess biological age. However, by 10 years of age, it is common to have as much as a two-year discrepancy between bone age (skeletal maturity) and chronological age [19]. The determination of bone age can be very valuable in estimating biological age in predicting the onset of puberty. Children who are experiencing either delayed or premature maturation can be identified by comparing the maturity of the bone development with that of their somatic development as shown through x-ray. Both gender and race affect bone maturation. Females generally mature 2 years sooner than males, and Blacks mature more rapidly than Caucasians [19]. Bone age can also be altered (usually delayed) by disease, nutrition, or metabolic factors.

FACIAL DEVELOPMENT

Since the head attains 95 percent of its adult size by 8 to 9 years of age [6], only a minimal increase in the size of the circumference of the skull occurs during the school-age years. However, between 6 and 11 years of age, the head appears to enlarge greatly, and facial features exhibit marked changes because of the growth of the facial bones—in particular, the sinuses, the maxilla (upper jaw), and the mandible (lower jaw). The face literally grows away or out from the skull.

Many children experience a marked increase in upper respiratory infections during the early school years as a result of the increase in exposure to communicable diseases after entering school as well as the development of the sinal cavities. Between 5 and 7 years of age, the frontal sinuses become well-developed. Sinal growth continues rapidly over the next 5 to 6 years; by 12 years of age, adult size is nearly attained [4]. Although the sinuses strengthen the architectural structure of the face, reduce the weight of the head, and assist in providing resonance to the voice, they also offer potential foci for infection, since they provide a warm, dark, moist area that is conducive to bacterial growth.

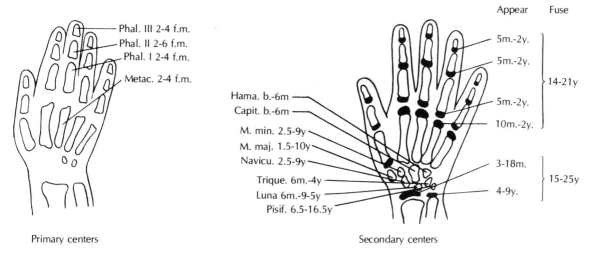

Primary centers | Secondary centers

Figure 22–5. Time schedule for the appearance of primary and secondary ossification centers and the fusion of secondary centers with the shafts in the hands. Key: f.m. = fetal month; b = birth. (From J. Caffey et al., *Pediatric X-Ray Diagnosis* [7th ed.]. Chicago: Year Book, 1978. [Modified from Scammon in Morris' *Human Anatomy*.] With permission.)

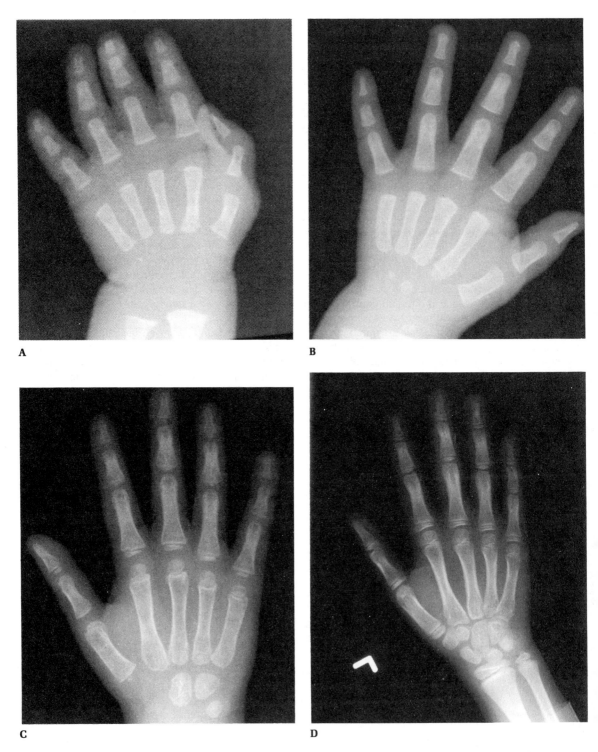

Figure 22–6. X-rays of the hand, showing ossification of the wrist bones. (A) 5 weeks; (B) 1 year; (C) 4 years; (D) 8 years. (Courtesy Department of Radiology, The Children's Hospital, Columbus, Ohio.)

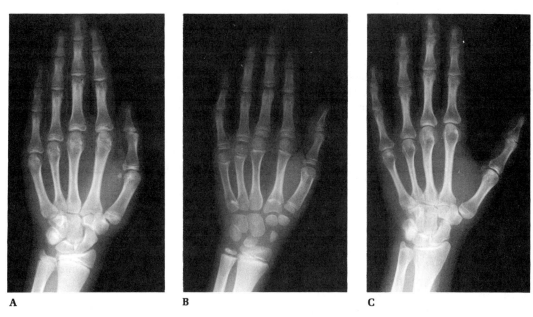

Figure 22–7. X-rays of the hand, showing ossification of the wrist bones. (A) 10-year-old female; (B) 10-year-old male; (C) 20-year-old. (Courtesy Department of Radiology, The Children's Hospital, Columbus, Ohio.)

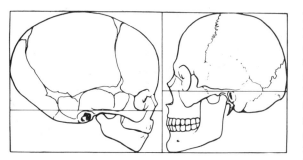

Figure 22–8. Facial growth. The skull of a neonate (left) and that of an adult (right) drawn to the same scale. Changes due to the differences in growth are apparent in the relatively large cranial vault of the infant and the greater increase in size of the facial bones in the adult. The horizontal lines cross the same bony landmarks in each illustration. (From G. H. Lowrey, *Growth and Development of Children* [7th ed.]. Chicago: Year Book, 1978. With permission.)

The mandible grows downward, forward, and away from the cranial vault. Concomitant growth of the maxilla and the nasal passageways allows for greater exchange of air to meet the needs of the growing, active body. Room is also made for the permanent molars and other secondary teeth. About 90 percent of facial growth is attained by age 12 [19]. Temporary disproportions in the shape of the face frequently lead schoolagers to consider themselves "ugly ducklings."

Muscular System

During the middle childhood years, the child gains about 3 to 3.5 kg (5 to 7 pounds) per year. A formula sometimes used for predicting weight (in pounds) for children 8 to 12 years of age is to multiply the age by 7 and then add 5 ([age $\times$ 7] + 5) [19]. This weight increase is due mainly to increases in the size of the skeletal and muscular systems as well as increases in the size of some body organs. There is a gradual increase in muscle mass and strength, and the body takes on a leaner appearance as "baby fat" decreases. The loose movements, "knock knees," and lordosis of early childhood disappear as muscle tone increases. At all ages, males have a greater number of muscle cells than females, apparently as a result of the higher levels of androgens (male hormone) [29]. Although females generally have more adipose (fat) tissue, the balance between muscular and adipose tissue in a child seems to be more closely related to the amount of exercise and activity than to gender [5]. The increase in muscular strength results from both genetic factors, which cause hyperplastic growth, and exercise, which facilitates hypertrophic growth. Children double their strength and physical capabilities during these years [37]. Because of their greater number of muscle cells, males, at all ages, are usually stronger than females [3].

Athletic prowess in a child is more closely related to biological age than to chronological age; this factor should be considered before children are allowed to participate in competitive, strength, and endurance sports. Muscles are still immature and are easily injured. In other words, athletic activities should be chosen according to the physical abilities of the child, not by peer, parental, or community pressures. This factor also needs to be weighed when a child is considering participation in coeducational sports.

Central Nervous System

The continuing sequential maturation of the central nervous system allows for the performance of increasingly complex gross- and fine-motor skills. Although the brain has reached 90 percent of its adult size by 7 years of age [19], the sulci (fissures or grooves) of the cortex of the brain continue to develop as intellectual function expands [5]. The growth rate of the brain is greatly slowed, with 95 percent of brain growth achieved by age 9 [6] and full growth achieved during adolescence. Improvement in diet cannot make up for nutritional deficits that have affected hypoplastic growth of the brain during the late fetal or early infancy periods of life (see Chap. 4). Since head circumference correlates well with the deoxyribonucleic acid (DNA) content of the brain, heads measuring more than two standard deviations below the expected norm are indicative of potential cellular deficiency. In general, the smaller the size of the head, the lower is the intelligence [29]. Children with superior intelligence quotients (IQ) often have larger-than-average head circumferences [19].

MYELINIZATION

Myelinization—the development of the myelin sheath around the axons (arms) of nerve cells—continues during the school years. The percentage of attainment of final development appears to be synchronized with growth of the brain. The increase in the thickness of the sheath appears to serve as an insulator to improve conduction of nerve impulses. The transformation of the clumsy 6-year-old into the coordinated 12-year-old is due in part to the maturation of the central nervous system and the improved transmission of nerve impulses to the muscles involved as well as to experience in using the motor pathways.

Gross-motor activity. The gross motor (large-muscle) skills of the 6- to 7-year-old far outstrip fine-motor (small-muscle) coordination. The child of this age is full of energy, enjoys gross-motor activity, and is enthralled with a new world. The sky is the limit. Control of impulses is limited; anything and everything must

be tried—hopping, roller skating, bike riding, running, climbing, wrestling, and so on. Even when the 6-year-old is sitting in a chair or lying on the beach (or in bed), the child seems to be in perpetual motion. The 6-year-old becomes so engrossed in activities that he or she often does not recognize tiredness when it occurs. Fatigue may be exhibited later in quarrelsomeness, crying, or a lack of interest in eating. The emotional roller coaster of the 6-year-old may be due in part to this sustained activity followed by the physical exhaustion of overactivity.

Seven- and 8-year-old children exhibit less restlessness. Although the energy level of these older children is just as high, their activities are more subdued and directed. Increased attention span and cognitive skills enhance their enjoyment of sit-down games. Bicycles can now be used for errands and transportation—not just for something to do. Increased myelinization im-

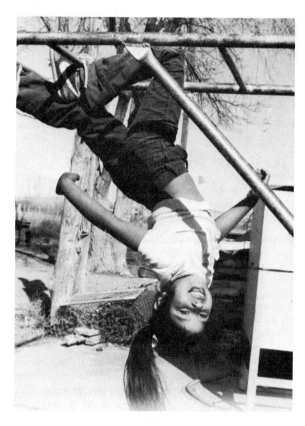

Figure 22–9. The young school-ager may not exhibit extraordinary skill, but loves to show off. Such early efforts need to be reinforced as a foundation for attempting more complex feats later.

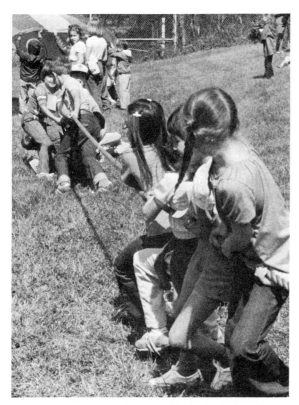

Figure 22–10. Six- and 7-year-olds possess excessive amounts of energy, which are frequently directed into gross-motor activities that may allow competition and cooperation with peers.

proves reaction time, which makes participation in group sports easier. The 6-year-old can throw and catch a ball with a fair amount of control; the 7-year-old begins to make connections between the bat and the ball. Running is directed toward races or to getting somewhere in a hurry—not just running for the sake of running. Swimming movements become more coordinated. In general, the 7-year-old uses a more cautious (and a more serious) approach to activities. Gross-motor activities seem to come under the control of both conscious will and cognitive skills.

Children between 8 and 10 years of age gradually exhibit greater rhythm, smoothness, and gracefulness of muscular movements. They consciously work to coordinate and perfect physical skills. Strength and endurance increase. These children engage in physical activities that require longer and more concentrated attention and effort, such as baseball and hiking. Hours are spent practicing new gymnastic stunts, ballet positions, batting and pitching skills, or judo and wrestling maneuvers. They compete individually in races on foot or on a bicycle to test their strength; they try to outdo one another in complexity or bravery on the skate board or in climbing trees. Group games in school or in the community give the older school-ager additional opportunity to develop and to test skills. Greater individuality is also exhibited during these years. As restlessness decreases, many children begin to prefer quieter activities, such as reading. Children begin to appreciate their individuality and seek opportunities to show off a newly acquired skill—whether a "Tarzan

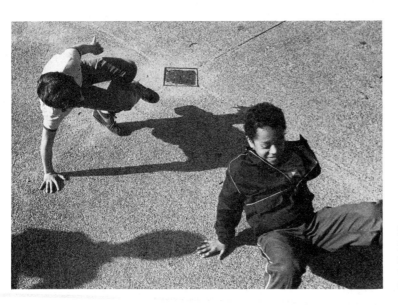

Figure 22–11. During the late school years, children participate in controlled gross-motor activities that allow them to refine movements and to increase strength. (Photo by Ed Slaman.)

swing" or the recitation of a poem. Admiration of the skill by an adult or peers enhances the child's self-esteem. Since the metabolic rate of children is higher per mass unit and their sweating capacity is still limited, they have more difficulty adjusting to extremes of temperature when exercising [1]. Dehydration and overheating create genuine threats to the child's health and life. Full hydration, frequent rests, and light clothing are essential.

Between 10 and 12 years of age (the pubescent years for girls), energy levels remain high but are well directed and controlled. The child now possesses physical skills almost equal to those of the adult—all that is required is practice. The body will do what the brain tells it to do. Further growth and development of the muscular and skeletal systems during adolescence will increase strength and endurance but will not necessarily improve the execution of a skill. Greater self-mastery is reflected in repetitious practice, increased self-confidence, and interest in self-development through physical activities. Although the pubescent child can sit still for prolonged periods of time, discharge of excess energy frequently occurs through foot tapping, finger drumming, and leg swinging—much to the distraction of parents and teachers.

Fine-motor activity. Increased myelinization of the central nervous system is reflected in the improvement of fine-motor or manipulative skills even more than in gross-motor activities. Balance and eye-hand coordination gradually improve. The hands are used more adroitly as tools. The 6-year-old is able to hammer, to paste, to tie shoes, and to fasten clothes. (The neurologically immature child may continue to have difficulty with tying anything for several years.) Handedness should be firmly established by age 6.

By 7 years of age, the child's hands become steadier. The child of this age prefers a pencil to a crayon for printing, and reversal of letters during writing is less common. Printing becomes smaller. Many children exhibit sufficient finger coordination to begin music lessons on the piano or another instrument. The 7-year-old is usually completely self-sufficient in dressing.

Between 8 and 10 years of age, the hands can be used independently with more ease and precision. Sufficient coordination develops to enable the child to write rather than print words. Letter size continues to become smaller and more even. Special abilities become more obvious and differentiated; that is, children begin to use fine-motor skills to express cognitive and cultural interests through activities, such as sewing, model building, or playing woodwind, brass, or stringed instruments. Parents are grateful to see improved eating skills at the table. Children should become completely self-sufficient in self-care during these years, including complete bathing and hair washing.

The child between 10 and 12 years of age, begins to exhibit manipulative skills comparable to the precision exhibited by adults. The complex, intricate, and rapid movements essential for producing fine-quality handcrafts or executing a difficult number on a musical instrument may be mastered. Recitals or exhibitions of their work help to foster positive self-regard in children with such accomplishments. Physical maturation and the social environment work together to help the child achieve Erikson's task of industry. During these years, children learn not only what they can do but also what they are interested in doing, and what activities have intrinsic and extrinsic value. A foundation is being laid for the emerging sense of identity—the central task of the adolescent years.

PERCEPTUAL SKILLS

Intact perceptual skills are critical to learning and performing in school. Five modalities are recognized that may be used in learning: (1) visual (discussed in the next section), (2) auditory, (3) haptic (touch), (4) olfactory (smell), and (5) gustatory (taste). The senses of taste and smell are fully developed before the school-age years. These senses are more commonly used as modes of learning in the preschool years, but they continue to offer valuable sources of information about objects throughout life. The young school-ager should be able to feel, to identify, and to locate points of cold, heat, skin touch, and pinprick on every body surface. The young school-ager should also be able to identify common unseen objects by touch (stereognosis). This skill provides the basis for many "feel" games in kindergarten through second grade.

Auditory perception is normally acute during both the preschool and the school-age years. The child should be able to discriminate fine differences in articulated sounds and voice pitch. Because of the ability to duplicate phonetic utterances and to comprehend translations, the school years are an optimal time to learn a foreign language. Children who are introduced to a second language during the preschool or school-age years frequently learn to speak the language as fluently and easily as a native. The ability to duplicate foreign sounds exactly may be lost after about age 12. Children who move to a foreign country or who learn a second language during adolescence frequently retain an accent, especially when under stress, even if

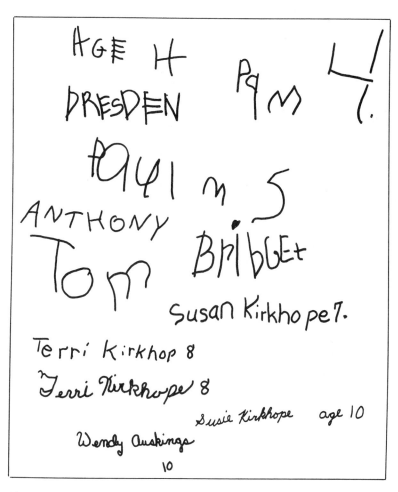

Figure 22–12. Improvement of fine-motor control is evidenced by changes in handwriting. These children were asked to write their names on a blank piece of paper. With increasing age, the size of their writing becomes smaller, and the evenness and the uniformity of letter configurations improve. Females generally exhibit more highly developed fine-motor skills during these years because of advanced neurological development. Note the immaturity in discrimination as well as coordination of the 4-year-olds; the reversal of letters of a 6-year-old (Bridget); the mixture of upper- and lower-case letters of the 6-year-olds; and the letter dropping of the 8-year-old. All are common phenomena for the ages of the children.

the new language becomes their primary form of verbal communication [23]. Evidence strongly suggests that foreign languages should be introduced during the primary school years.

DEVELOPMENT OF THE EYE

During infancy and toddlerhood, the eye is normally hyperopic. Because of the shortness of the eye from front to back, the image of an object focuses behind the retina, a situation that leads to farsightedness. However, the extreme malleability of the lens during early childhood allows the eye to refocus the image rapidly on the retina. In fact, during infancy the ability of children to accommodate for distance allows them to see objects held only a few inches from the nose [16]. During the preschool years, the eye becomes emme-

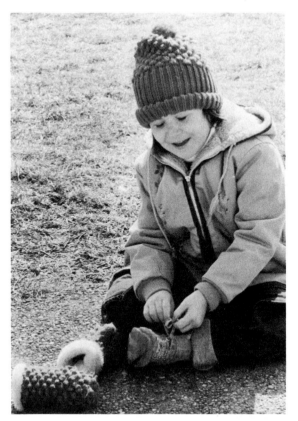

Figure 22–13. Some late preschoolers are able to tie their shoes. However, most children do not master this feat until the early school years because of the complex cognitive skills as well as the fine-motor skills involved.

other persons can see clearly at 40 feet (this is the estimated visual acuity of the 2-year-old). Visual acuity of 20/200 indicates that an individual can only identify an object from a distance of 20 feet that other people can identify at 200 feet (this is the estimated acuity of the 1-year-old child [29]; it is also the definition of legal blindness). Improvements in vision during the toddler and preschool years appear to be due more to increased discrimination skills and learning than to changes in the eye per se [16].

Depth perception (visual stereognosis) requires the coordinated use of both eyes. The optic center of the brain must fuse the two images. This ability is not present at birth; consequently, strabismus (crossed eyes)

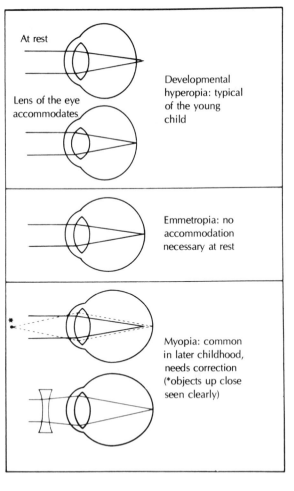

Figure 22–14. Changes in the eye during childhood. (From D. W. Smith, E. L. Bierman and N. M. Robinson, *The Biologic Ages of Man: From Conception Through Old Age.* Philadelphia: Saunders, 1978. With permission.)

tropic; the image of an object focuses on the retina without any accommodative effort from the lens. If the eye continues to grow, the image will focus in front of the retina, producing myopia (nearsightedness). Any time the image is not focused directly on the retina, vision will be blurred. The length of the eyeball appears to be genetically controlled; therefore, nearsightedness (myopia) and farsightedness (hyperopia) frequently appear in several generations of a family. The eye may have a slight growth spurt again during early adolescence, which may be responsible for an increased frequency of myopia during the pubertal period [33].

Most children with normal vision achieve 20/20 visual acuity by age 5; this means that the child (and those with normal vision) is able to see a particular object clearly at 20 feet. Visual acuity of 20/40 means that an individual can see an object clearly only at 20 feet that

is common during infancy and early childhood. As visual acuity and control of eye movements by the ocular muscles improve, the brain learns to fuse the images. Stability of depth perception usually occurs between the fourth and sixth years [19]. Strabismus that continues during the early school years can be due to an inability of the brain to fuse the images or to a decreased acuity in the deviating eye [19]. Children should be asked to indicate if they see a single image when looking at objects.

Visual maturity is usually reached between 6 and 7 years of age. Peripheral vision is fully developed, and the child is able to discriminate very fine differences in color [5]. Large-print books are not essential to aid in visualization. However, since differences in shapes and positions of letters are more obvious, large print helps the child who is just learning to read to discriminate letters and words more easily. Although visual screening tests (by professional or paraprofessional persons) are recommended during the preschool years, all children should have a visual examination by an ophthalmologist on entering school. Only one-third of the children who need visual correction are identified during the preschool years [17]. The child with a vision problem usually does not complain of poor vision because he or she has known nothing else. Although adults see things like leaves on trees, letters on signs, and features on faces, the child seems to assume that such powers of discrimination are yet to come. When peers exhibit discrimination competencies, the visually impaired child may accept such skills as another sign of individual differences. Many visual problems can be easily corrected with eyeglasses.

Cardiovascular and Respiratory Systems

By 5 years of age, the heart has quadrupled its birth size. At 9 years it is six times the birth weight, and by puberty it is almost ten times the birth weight [19]. Obviously, much cardiac growth takes place during the school years. However, the size of the heart is smaller, proportionately, to body size than at any other period of life. This accounts in part for the easy tiring [37]. Increased cardiac function is essential to meet the oxygen and circulatory needs of the growing, active body. As the heart grows, it assumes a more vertical position within the thoracic cavity. The diaphragm descends, allowing more room for both cardiac action and respiratory expansion.

Pulse and respiratory rates are affected by size, gender, and activity of the child (see Appendix E). As the rhythm of the heartbeat gradually comes under the influence of the vagus nerve, there is a slowing of the cardiac rate [19]. "Functional" or "innocent" heart murmurs are present in as many as 50 percent of children during the school years. These soft, "blowing" heart sounds are caused by the blood passing through normal heart valves [16]. These sounds, which have no particular significance, occasionally persist into the adolescent or adult years. Blood pressure increases as the left ventricle of the heart develops.

The respiratory tissues achieve adult maturity, with lung capacity being proportional to body size. The respiratory rate slows as the lungs' tidal volume (the amount of air exchanged with each breath) doubles between ages 5 and 10 [19], thus increasing tolerance and resilience for gross-motor activities.

Minimal changes are experienced in the constituents of the blood from infancy through 12 years of age. The hemoglobin and hematocrit are increased slightly, and the white blood cell count is reduced slightly from preschool levels.

Gastrointestinal System

The gastrointestinal system achieves adult functional maturity during the school years [16]. There are fewer upset stomachs. The toddler's "cow's–horn-shaped" stomach assumes a "fish-hook" shape between 7 and 9 years of age. The adult "bagpipe" shape appears during pubescence (10 to 12 years). The stomach is able to tolerate all foods, but dietary intake needs to be geared to the growth and metabolic needs of the child (see the section on maintaining health, following). The increased capacity allows children to go longer between meals. Abdominal pain is a common childhood complaint. Since this can be a symptom of either psychogenic or physical pathology, medical consultation should be sought for recurring complaints.

Genitourinary System

The urinary system is functionally mature during the school years. The renal system is able to conserve water adequately to maintain stable fluid and electrolyte balances [5]. The kidneys double in size between the fifth and tenth years to keep up with the increased metabolic wastes of the body. The constituents and specific gravity of the urine are similar to those of the adult. Five to 20 percent of school-age children have small amounts of albuminuria (protein in the urine); it is found most commonly in children with marked lordosis. The reason is unknown, but it appears to be related to the impaired venous blood circulation experienced by the kidney when the child is standing. This phenomenon normally disappears by puberty [19].

Five to 17 percent of children between 5 and 18 years

of age continue to have nocturnal enuresis (wet the bed involuntarily during sleep) [37]. Most cases of nocturnal enuresis show no organic cause, and the etiology is unknown. Evidence indicates that these children may have delayed neurological development, small bladder capacity, and a genetic predisposition [27]. The behavior creates intrafamily tensions that can lead to social and emotional problems for the child. Most cases are self-limited, and the child experiences a spontaneous "cure." Several treatments are available. The bed-alarm conditioning device appears to show the most promise [27].

Immunological System

The immunological system becomes functionally mature during the early school years. The body is able to localize infections well, but the school-ager still experiences 3.5 significant infections per year. Colds, gastrointestinal system infections, allergic disorders, communicable diseases, and pneumonia account for more than 70 percent of school absenteeism [16].

Lymphoid tissues, the producer of antibodies, reach a peak in size between 6 and 7 years of age. Once an individual has produced an antibody against a particular antigen (foreign material), the template is retained. The body can resynthesize antibodies against the same antigen at a later date very rapidly and in large quantities. Consequently, the number of major infections usually decreases with age, because the body can fight the antigen at an earlier stage.

Enlargement of the adenoidal and tonsillar lymphoid tissues is normal in the late preschool and early school years. These tissues often appear to be hypertrophied by adult standards, but they are normal for the child 5 to 7 years of age. The maximal development of these tissues coincides with the time when acute infections of the respiratory and alimentary tract are most common. Tonsillectomies and adenoidectomies are frequently incorrectly recommended because of the relative enlargement of these organs [2]. They do not need to be removed unless they are precipitating serious middle-ear infections, are obstructing swallowing or breathing, or are the foci for frequent, persistent infections. Growth of these tissues ceases after 7 years of age. Normal involution makes them appear small by puberty.

MAINTAINING HEALTH

A major task of the school-age years is to prepare oneself for adulthood. In fact, one-third of our lives is spent in preparation for the other two-thirds. During the school years, the child is rapidly learning how to use the strengths and to compensate for the limitations of his or her own body. Maximal development of the cognitive, social, and emotional domains is highly dependent on adequate functioning of the biophysical domain. The child who is ill, who has a low energy level, or who is physically incapable of learning a particular skill is limited in the ability to take full advantage of educational and social opportunities (see Chap. 19). An understanding of basic health needs can help to prevent many health problems. Regular health checkups can identify minor problems early, before they become more serious.

Metabolic Needs

Physical development is more significant than chronological age in determining the basal (resting) metabolic rate. The basal metabolic rate is highest during periods of most rapid growth. Since males have more muscle mass than females, they generally have a higher basal metabolic rate. Total metabolic needs (resting and energy) are affected by the energy expenditure of the individual child. The quiet, sedentary child who prefers fine-motor activity requires fewer calories than the athletically oriented child who utilizes every opportunity to express or exhibit gross-motor prowess.

NUTRITIONAL NEEDS

As children grow, they gradually require less food per unit of body weight; however, the total amount of food consumed increases until after the pubertal period (see Appendix E). Adequate nutrition is needed for five reasons during this period of life:

1. To meet the basal metabolic needs of the body. A certain amount of energy is needed just to keep the body functioning optimally.
2. To meet the body's energy needs. Great variation is seen among children in this area.
3. To meet cellular growth needs. Some hyperplastic growth is continuing, but much hypertrophic growth occurs during the school years.
4. To meet cellular replacement needs. Some cells are already beginning to exhibit signs of aging and must be replaced, if possible, to maintain optimal functioning of the system.
5. To meet cellular repair needs. Injuries—minor and major—are common during the school years. Even a hangnail requires extra calories for repair.

A formula sometimes used for predicting caloric needs of children of this age is 1000 plus 100 times the

Table 22-1. Recommended Daily Intake for School-Agers*

Type of Food	Amount
Milk	2–3 cups
Meat	2–3 servings
Fruit and vegetables	4–5 servings
Bread and cereal	4–5 servings

* Extra foods may be added in each group to ensure adequate caloric intake.

child's age (1000 + [100 × age]) [36]. The protein, calcium, vitamin, and mineral requirements are particularly high during these years to ensure adequate materials for growth of the muscular and skeletal systems. Although vitamins may not be essential if the child eats a well-balanced diet, many health-care practitioners recommend daily vitamins to ensure adequate vitamin and mineral intake. Table 22–1 gives the recommended daily amounts of different types of food for the school-age child. If the child is involved in sports and exercise programs, then very special consideration should be given to an adequate intake of not only calories and fluids but also to the right proportion of fat, carbohydrates, and protein ingested [22].

Since obesity in childhood is closely correlated with obesity during the adult years, parents are advised to maintain their child's weight within normal limits. Good eating habits are a critical factor. Food preferences and dislikes become strongly established during the school years; dietary habits are the result of cultural influences, family attitudes toward food, parental example, and individual tastes. Education and guidance offered to the child by the parents regarding nutritional intake will strongly influence intake. Some children will eat foods mainly composed of high amounts of sugar and starches and will avoid vegetable and protein foods because of inadequate guidance. Other children may begin to use food as an emotional weapon against the parents. As in every other aspect of the parent-child relationship, the parents must know themselves well and be secure in their goals in order to prevent and to remedy mealtime problems.

School-agers frequently become so involved in their activities that they neglect or forget to eat. Parents must establish a fairly regular schedule to ensure that the child obtains adequate intake to prevent undue fatigue and illness. Breakfast is critical for providing adequate calories to start the day. The child who attends school without breakfast exhibits fatigue and poor attention, and learning will obviously be affected. Many schools have established breakfast or lunch programs, or both,

to assist with this problem when a large number of their children come from homes where breakfast is not offered or encouraged. Children also need after-school and between-meal snacks. Energy expenditure and growth needs are so high during childhood and adolescence that the fasting period between meals is too long. Low-energy levels can precipitate irritability, headache, and lassitude—factors that can lead to family dissension. Illness, fatigue, excitement, and temporary emotional disturbances can all cause temporary decreases in food intake. Changes in food habits can be a sign of disequilibrium.

Table manners show interesting changes with age. The 6-year-old who is going through a brief growth spurt, who has a high energy level, and who is experiencing an expanding world generally has a good appetite. However, since there are so many more interesting things to do besides eat, the 6-year-old's table manners consist of grabbing the food, stuffing it in the mouth, and then talking with the mouth full of food; spills are frequent. Life seems too exciting to waste much time eating. The 7-year-old, as in other areas of life, becomes less expansive. Talking at mealtime decreases, but food continues to be bolted in order to rejoin the gang outside. The 8- to 9-year-old child begins to slow down. Manners generally improve (in those homes where they are encouraged), and the meal can become a time of brief socialization. The pubescent child may once again begin to eat rapidly in order to join (or rejoin) friends, but improved coordination improves manners and prevents the spills of earlier years. A better perspective of time and parental guidance can help make the dinner hour a very pleasant social activity.

Illness or dietary deficiencies can cause temporary setbacks in growth during this period. However, since the majority of growth is hypertrophic in nature, catch-up growth can occur if an adequate diet is provided. Replacement of the missing factor (nutritional or hormonal) frequently results in dramatic acceleration of growth [29]. Adequate growth following an illness or a deficiency depends on the age of the child, the severity and duration of the problem, and the actual tissue (or tissues) involved. The humoral negative feedback system (the cells secrete a particular protein that has an antimitotic effect when a certain level is reached) allows the cells to grow until the expected levels for the child's development are reached, and then growth continues at a more normal pace [19, 29].

As mentioned earlier, not all tissues develop at the same time; each has its own critical growth period. Deficiencies that extend beyond this critical hyperplastic growth period usually cannot be compensated for (e.g., brain growth during early infancy).

SLEEP NEEDS

Inadequate sleep can lead to daytime irritability, fatigue, lack of endurance, inattention, and poor learning. The 6-year-old needs about 12 hours of sleep per night; some children also continue to need an afternoon quiet time or nap to allow them to restore their energy levels. The 12-year-old needs about 10 hours of sleep at night [20]. Evening television programs often compete for sleep time.

Children of this age may continue to have nightmares. There are many different theories concerning the occurrence of nightmares: some postulate that they occur because of the maturation of the child's concept of death; some feel that they are related to indiscriminate watching of violence on television; others feel that they are related to energy expenditure and the continued search for one's own strengths and skills; still others feel that nightmares are a warning or indicator of excessive stressors in the child's life. Parents are urged to evaluate the child's environment in terms of his or her coping level. Bedtime is an excellent time to foster parent-child confidences. The activities of the day can be shared, and conflicts can be discussed and resolved. Ways to help the child relax prior to sleep include storytime, religious readings and prayers, physical ministrations, and exchange of loving assurances. Quiet music is also relaxing.

HEALTH CARE

Continued health care surveillance is essential to maintain a high level of physical health. Younger school-agers are too busy with the world to take time out for bathing or for washing faces, hands, or ears; many would wear the same clothes all week if the parents did not intervene. Fortunately, school-agers gradually begin to assume more interest in self-care. They also become more sensitive to exposure of the body and express interest in their own physical changes. By approximately 11 years of age, they begin to become more concerned about personal hygiene and will dress for social reasons.

Irritations and minor infections of the genitalia are relatively common, especially in females. Even though the child may experience vaginal itchiness or odor and even some discharge, she may not tell an adult [5]. Education in hygiene, health, and sexual functioning are essential, both by the family and at school, especially as puberty approaches. Of particular importance is teaching the young female child to wipe from front to back (toward the rectum) after urination and defecation, to decrease the possibility of introducing bacteria into the vagina or urethra. Other health maintenance measures include the provision of adequate nonglare lighting for reading and the avoidance of sudden loud noises or blaring music, which can damage the inner ear and cause hearing loss.

Health Supervision

School-age children should have one complete physical examination per year to assess growth patterns and to detect early signs of illness. Most visit their physicians several additional times each year for minor illnesses, infections, or injuries. It should be mentioned at this point that accidents are the leading cause of death in this age group. Curiosity, incomplete control over motor activities, delayed responses, impulsivity, inadequate knowledge, and poor planning or problem-solving skills are all interrelated. Education by example and discipline are both needed to help avoid accidents. Although the child may vehemently resist parental guidance, parents are wise to establish guidelines governing the activities and whereabouts of the younger school-ager. Public concern has encouraged laws requiring fireproof nightclothes, fences around swimming pools, and helmets for motorbike riding in order to help protect younger children. The child will gradually internalize parental rules and can then be allowed increased freedom with safety (see Chap. 18).

The "accident-prone" child, or the child who is involved in many minor accidents, needs to be evaluated. Neurological deficits may be a causative factor. Psychological and social factors also may be major precipitants of physically traumatizing events. (Is the child a daredevil? Why? Does the child lack self-discipline? Why?) An accident-prone child may consciously or unconsciously be seeking more adult attention. Depression may also prevent the child from foreseeing the results of an activity. Other children may be exhibiting an inability to correlate adequately the cause and effect relationships of their behaviors—a mild form of the helplessness syndrome (see Chap. 14).

Dentition

The child's face and permanent teeth are developing so rapidly during the school years that dental checkups are recommended every 6 months. Eighty percent of school-age children develop caries (dental cavities) at one time or another [16]; in fact, tooth decay is the leading "disease" in the United States. Research indicates that adequate fluoridation of water or a fluoride supplement can reduce the percentage of caries

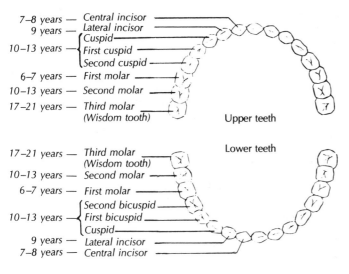

7–8 years — Central incisor
9 years — Lateral incisor
{ Cuspid
10–13 years — { First cuspid
{ Second cuspid
6–7 years — First molar
10–13 years — Second molar
17–21 years — Third molar
(Wisdom tooth)   Upper teeth

Lower teeth

17–21 years — Third molar
(Wisdom tooth)
10–13 years — Second molar
6–7 years — First molar
{ Second bicuspid
10–13 years —{ First bicuspid
{ Cuspid
9 years — Lateral incisor
7–8 years — Central incisor

Figure 22–15. Eruption of the permanent teeth. (From D. R. Marlow, *Textbook of Pediatric Nursing* [5th ed.]. Philadelphia: Saunders, 1977. With permission.)

by one-half [16]. (There is some evidence that adequate fluoride intake may also strengthen the bone structure and reduce fractures in the elderly [10].) The average 7-year-old is capable of assuming responsibility for dental hygiene, including the use of dental floss. It is particularly important that individuals of all ages brush adequately before bedtime. Prolonged contact of food particles with tooth enamel can cause rapid tooth erosion at the point of contact. Baking soda or salt may be effectively substituted for toothpaste.

Caries should receive prompt attention. They can become the foci of infection and send toxins (poisons) throughout the body system if untreated. Raw sugars and candies are common contributors to the development of caries. Primary teeth should not be pulled unless absolutely necessary because they affect the alignment of the other teeth; this in turn can cause alignment problems when the permanent teeth emerge.

Young children and adolescents frequently experience tooth pain or sensitivity, even though no pathology is present. A response to highly concentrated sugars or to temperature differences occurs because the large nerve of the young tooth puts it closer to the surface of the tooth. As the tooth ages, the nerve not only becomes less excitable, but the nerve also begins to shrink, putting more distance between it and the tooth surface, thus rendering it less sensitive to environmental influences.

The loss of the first tooth can be very frightening to the child who is unprepared for the event. To the child who is prepared, it is one of the first tangible signs of growing up, and the event is greeted with much enthusiasm. Children soon learn how squeamish many

adults are about loose teeth and blood and take great delight in wiggling the loose tooth for parents or relatives. When the first permanent central incisors

DENNIS the MENACE

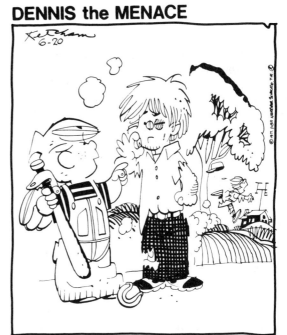

"NAW...THE TOOTH FAIRY WON'T CARE IF IT GOT KNOCKED OUT IN A FIGHT. IT ALL PAYS THE SAME."

Figure 22–16. Reprinted courtesy of *Dennis the Menace.* Copyright Field Newspaper Syndicate, T.M.®

emerge, they appear much too large for the mouth and face—another factor contributing to the "ugly duckling syndrome." Generally, the teeth of males are larger than those of females [19].

MALOCCLUSION

More than 75 percent of children have some form or degree of occlusional disharmony; at least 15 percent of them need treatment [32]. Normally the cusps (prominent structures) interdigitate with the fossae (depressions in teeth) to create a comfortable, tight, chewing surface. When cusps meet and prevent the close interdigitation essential for chewing or interfere with the relaxation of facial muscles or an attractive appearance, treatment is indicated. Malocclusions may be either skeletal or dental in origin. Disharmonies of bone growth frequently result from a mixed racial background [19]. The malposition of teeth may be due to: (1) prolonged sucking, which causes open bite and tongue thrust; (2) the early loss of primary teeth because of improper care, which allows permanent teeth to drift into abnormal positions; or (3) a disproportionate relationship between jaw length and tooth size, which causes either wide spacing or overcrowding [18] (see Fig. 15–5a).

BRUXISM

Some children grind their teeth while they are sleeping. This sometimes creates enough noise to be heard in the next room. Over a period of time, the child can grind away some of the enamel and dentin. Some people think that bruxism is a sign of severe tension in the child's life. However, this behavior can help with the positioning of teeth and can facilitate a good occlusion of permanent teeth. When teeth are malpositioned, bruxism is an attempt at self-righting. A dental evaluation should be obtained.

Health Screening

Many schools require or provide health and dental screening prior to entrance to school and periodically during the school years. Poor health status or deficient functioning of the senses can reduce the child's ability to learn at school. School systems require adequate immunization as a prerequisite for admission to, or staying in, school. If a child has completed all immunizations prior to school, none may be needed during the school years except on special occasions, such as when influenza shots may be recommended to prevent epidemics.

VISION

Twenty-five percent of children need eyeglasses at some point during their school years [16] to correct for accommodation problems, strabismus, or an astigmatism. An astigmatism, or uneven refraction of an object on the retina, can cause distortion and blurring of letters and numbers. All visual problems should be corrected as soon as possible. Visual screening should be continued throughout one's lifetime.

HEARING

Significant hearing loss is the most commonly overlooked serious handicap in young children [16]. The child may exhibit a mild to marked speech defect secondary to the hearing loss. The parents often feel that the child "is just not paying attention," "doesn't understand," or "forgets easily." Recurrent or chronic ear infections, fluid in the middle ear, frequent exposure to sudden loud noises, and illnesses, such as measles or mumps, can lead to decreases in auditory acuity. Five percent of children do not pass auditory screening tests [16]. Many hearing losses are temporary due to mild infections or allergies. Loss of hearing in one ear may create difficulty in picking up sounds and in determining directions for location of the source of a sound.

URINALYSIS

Urine tests can detect diabetes and silent or chronic urinary tract infection. One percent of females may have infections without symptoms [16]. Many adult urinary tract problems had their beginning in untreated childhood infections.

HEMATOLOGY

Blood tests may reveal an iron-deficiency anemia, a problem usually associated with inadequate nutrition. Increased susceptibility to infections, irritability, easy fatigability, and inadequate attention span are frequently associated with anemia. Once identified, anemia can be easily treated with an iron supplement and the addition of iron-rich foods to the diet (e.g., raisins, spinach, liver, egg yolk).

TUBERCULOSIS TESTING

Many schools require that children have periodic tuberculosis screening. If a child is discovered to respond positively to a test, the local public health officials attempt to identify every potential contact in order to locate the source of the bacteria in the family members or in contacts in the community. Follow-up

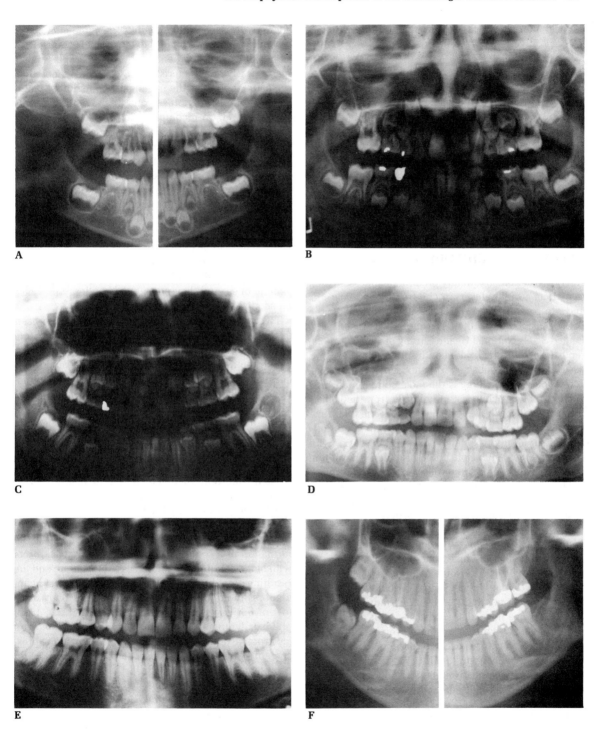

Figure 22–17. X-rays of the deciduous and permanent teeth. (A) 3 years; (B) 6 years; (C) 8 years; (D) 10 years; (E) 14 years; (F) 23 years.

medical intervention is essential for the child who has had a positive reaction to the test.

BLOOD PRESSURE

Blood pressure screening of children has been receiving more attention in the last few years. During childhood, in almost all cases, a cause for elevated blood pressure can be identified and treated. There is increasing awareness that elevated blood pressure in adults may be detected during childhood [25].

Adequate surveillance of health status during childhood can not only help to maintain high level wellness during the school years but can also help to prevent some chronic, residual problems of the adult years.

ALLERGIES IN CHILDREN*

Allergic reactions frequently precipitate illnesses (such as asthma and hay fever) in children and adolescents and are responsible for more health problems in the pediatric population than is generally realized. The United States National Health Survey of 1959–1961 [28] reported on chronic health conditions in children, and based on the data collected from household interviews, it was found that allergy is the most common chronic health problem occurring in children from newborns through age 17. The report showed that the total time lost from school due to chronic health conditions amounted to approximately 33 million days, with asthma being responsible for more than 7.5 million days and hay fever or other allergic illnesses accounting for 1.5 million days. Thus more than one-fourth of the days lost from school because of chronic health problems were due to allergic disorders.

The frequency of allergic conditions occurring in the total population is generally thought to be 10 percent or more [15], and the incidence of major allergies in children is reported to range as high as 28.5 percent [14]. However, the United States National Health Survey reports that nearly 33 percent of children less than 17 years of age have allergic diseases [28].

The frequency with which hay fever or asthma occurs in children whose parent (or parents) also had hay fever or asthma is approximately 58 percent [34]. In contrast, the incidence in a similar group of individuals whose parents did not have hay fever or asthma averages 6.4 percent [34]. These data strongly suggest that allergic conditions are transmitted by hereditary factors. It is the general opinion that it is a predisposition for allergy that is inherited rather than a specific

*This section was written by James Abel, M.D.

allergic disease. There is some disagreement as to whether the inherited allergic tendency is transmitted as a Mendelian dominant trait or as a simple autosomal recessive characteristic. However, evidence now seems to show that the genetically transmitted factor is an incomplete dominant one that is determined by two genes: H, an incomplete dominant gene for nonallergic individuals, and h, a recessive allergic gene. People who have HH genetic compositions are not allergic; those with hh genetic material are allergic. An individual with Hh may or may not be allergic, but even if the person is nonallergic, the h factor could be passed to an offspring and thereby account for the appearance of an allergic individual in a family with a negative history for allergy. In fact, a large number of allergic individuals are found in nonallergic families. On the other hand, there are some persons who believe that it is difficult to dissociate acquired factors from genetic ones, and they postulate that allergy may also be acquired.

Two general types of allergic responses have been described. One is the immediate reaction, which occurs quite suddenly after exposure to an antigen for which the host is sensitized. This type of reaction occurs as a result of antigen-antibody complex formation. The other type of response is the delayed reaction; in this case, the observed reaction is postponed a number of hours or days, and there are no demonstrable circulating antibodies. Common examples of the immediate type of reaction include urticaria, allergic rhinitis, eczema, and asthma (the major allergic diseases in children). Included among the delayed forms are fungus allergy, allergic contact dermatitis, and bacterial allergy (especially the tuberculin type).

The usual type I allergic reaction features the unification of an antigen with an antibody, resulting in the formation of a soluble complex. This synthesis reacts with blood components known as complement, and the resulting combination then releases or removes the inhibitors (found in serum or tissues) that normally serve to prevent special sensitized cells (mast cells, basophils, or lymphocytes) from undergoing a proteolytic (destructive breakdown) mechanism. Thus, in the presence of the antigen-antibody complex combined with complement, the sensitized cells in the shock organ(s) and tissue(s) undergo a proteolytic reaction that results in the release of chemical mediators found within these cells. These mediators are responsible for the ensuing allergic reaction(s) either entirely or in part, depending on the site of the reaction(s). The chemical mediators produce the symptoms of allergy primarily by their influence on smooth muscle, capillary blood vessels, collagen, and mucous glands with the usual results of constriction of smooth muscles, dilation of blood vessels with increased capillary permeability, inflammatory reactions in collagen tissues, and increased mucus secretion.

The responses produced in the delayed hypersensitivity reaction are mediated by the interaction of locally deposited antigen with antibody that was produced by, and bound to, a sensitized lymphocyte. This reaction can only be induced by special routes of antigen administration (subcutaneous or intracutaneous), after prolonged antigen contact with the skin (e.g., poison ivy dermatitis), with antigens that are living agents (e.g., the tubercle bacillus), or through certain chemical agents called adjuvants that enhance the development and the production of hypersensitiveness. No serum antibodies are demonstrable in the delayed hypersensitivity reaction, and no special shock tissue(s) or organ(s) are present. However, many of the body's tissue cells are susceptible to injury from these delayed reactions because such reactions can be elicited in nonvascular tissue(s).

After reviewing the preceding material, it becomes easier to understand allergic reactions: If one knows the nature of the antigen; the location of the antibody-containing cells or shock tissue(s) or organ(s); and the character, concentration, and route of entry (introduction) of the specific antigen, then one can predict the type of allergic response to be expected. Various kinds of predictable reactions are outlined in Table 22–2. In addition, a comparison of the actions of the different chemical mediators can serve to explain the various clinical manifestations of allergic reactions that occur, depending on the mediator (or mediators) involved. Table 22–3 gives an analogy of two chemical mediators and the clinical symptomatology evoked by them.

After studying these two tables, it becomes evident that different allergic reactions are similar in many respects except for the location of the shock (target) organ(s) and tissue(s) or sensitized cells. It also becomes apparent how the diagnosis, essential characteristics, and treatment of many of the different allergic ailments can be very similar (e.g., avoidance of the antigen). In addition, it is evident that more than one shock organ or tissue may be provoked by a single antigen to produce a combination of symptoms, or several different antigens may induce the same reaction in a given target organ or tissue. Finally, clinical examples of immediate and delayed forms of hypersensitivity may exist either together or at different times, and these reactions may occur as a result of exposure to the same antigen. Thus any organ, tissue, or system

may be affected, and there are no strict limits as to the combination of manifestations that may result. In addition, there are no restrictions as to the types of agents that can act as antigens to produce or to enhance the manifestations of allergy.

Lucretius stated in his *De Rerum Natura,* published in 65 B.C., "What is food to one man may be fierce poison to others." What has been said of antigenic inhalants, drugs, contactants, injectants, and infectants applies with equal force to foods and agents intentionally or unintentionally added to foods. It should be realized that one of the more troublesome problems of infant and child care is that of food allergy. Unfortunately, knowledge about this condition is far from complete, and many differences of opinion exist about food allergy disorders.

There are two principal kinds of food allergies: an immediate reaction that manifests itself within a few seconds or minutes after the offending agent is eaten, and a delayed reaction that appears several hours or days after the food has been eaten. With the immediate type of reaction, it is more likely that the antigen is a whole food or food additive, whereas in the delayed reaction, the antagonizing agent(s) may be some breakdown product(s) produced during the process of digestion; in either case, the insulting factor may also serve as an antigen. It must be realized that the development of so many varieties of processed foods and chemical additives* has produced a vast number of substances that can be antigenic in themselves or can act as antigens to cause a variety of allergic reactions† [24]. In each case of food intolerance, an attempt must be made to determine whether or not the reaction is a true allergy. This can be an arduous task, but there are differences between intolerance for food(s) secondary to a number of specific or nonspecific causes, and a true

---

*An inventory of food additives compiled by the Food Protection Committee of the National Research Council lists more than 2700 substances that are being added to American foods. These additives include preservatives, nutritive supplements, nonnutritive sweeteners, antioxidants, surface acting agents, emulsifiers, stabilizers, bleaches, food coloring and dyeing agents, buffers, texturizers, firming agents, anticaking agents, binders, enzymes, and natural or artificial flavorings. The largest group of additives are food flavorings, with more than 2100 different chemical agents (more than 1600 are artificial), and there are more than 30 food-coloring and dyeing agents. Nearly 80 percent of all food additives are coloring or flavoring agents that have no caloric or nutritive value; their only purpose is cosmetic—yet they have the potential to act as antigens.

†The scope of this text cannot include a listing of myriad unintentional food additives and their potentially harmful effects.

Table 22-2. Variable Allergic Responses to Different Antigens

Nature of Antigen	Specific Antigen affecting →	Shock (Target) to produce Organ or Tissue →	Clinical Manifestation
Inhalants	Pollens (trees, grasses, flowers)	Eye	Lacrimation, visual disturbances, conjunctivitis, iritis, uveitis, blepharitis
	House dust	Nose	Seasonal and/or perennial rhinitis, nasal polyposis
	Mold		
	Spores	Ear	Partial or complete hearing loss, serous otitis media
	Any animal dander (cat, dog, horse, gerbil, guinea pig, etc.)	Throat	Itching of mouth or tongue, sore throat, croup, edema of glottis and epiglottis, enlarged tonsils and adenoids, cough, salivation, swollen lips, mouth, or tongue
		Bronchi and lungs	Asthma, bronchitis, asthmatic bronchitis, Löffler's syndrome, pneumonitis, pleural effusion, pleurisy
Ingestants	Any food	Gastrointestinal system	Aphthous stomatitis or canker sores, cheilitis, geographic tongue, gastritis, duodenitis, jejunitis, ileitis, colitis, inflammatory bowel disease, diarrhea, constipation, vomiting, colic, abdominal pain, bloating, melena, proctalgia, pruritus ani, cyclic vomiting
	Any drug		
	Any swallowed inhalant		
	Any food additive (intentional or unintentional)		
		Musculoskeletal system	Arthritis, arthralgia, palindromic rheumatism, intermittent hydroarthrosis, myalgia, "leg pains"
		Skin	Angioedema, eczema, urticarias, purpuras, erythema multiforme, drug rashes, contact dermatitis, Arthus reactions
		Blood	Thrombocytopenic purpura, hemolytic anemia, leukopenia, agranulocytosis, eosinophilia
		Genitourinary system	Dysuria, frequency of urine, enuresis, vulvovaginitis, urethritis, pruritus vulvae, orthostatic and idiopathic albuminuria, idiopathic renal bleeding
		Nervous system	Headache (including migraine), convulsions, tremors, tension, fatigue, hyperactivity, lethargy, mental apathy and dullness, confusion, poor attention span, vertigo, mood changes, narcolepsy, insomnia, Meniere's disease, neuralgia
		Miscellaneous	Anaphylactic shock, Henoch-Schönlein purpura, fever, enlarged lymph nodes, flushing, pallor
Contactants	Plant oils (poison ivy)	Skin	Contact dermatitis
	Cosmetics		
	Clothing		
Injectants	Drugs	All tissues	Serum sickness or drug allergy
	Foreign serum		
Infectants	Viruses	All tissues	"Bacterial" allergy
	Bacteria		
	Bacterialike organisms		

Table 22-3. Comparison of Some of the Actions of Histamine and Acetylcholine to Produce Clinical Allergy Manifestations

Target Organ(s) or Tissue(s)	Histamine	Acetylcholine	Clinical Allergy Manifestation
Nervous system	Headache	Headache Excitement Depression	Headache Tension Fatigue
Respiratory	Bronchospasm Increased mucus secretion	Bronchospasm Cough Increased mucus secretion	Asthma Bronchitis Asthmatic bronchitis
Gastrointestinal system	Stimulates acid production Stimulates other gastrointestinal glands	Stimulation of gastrointestinal glands	Gastritis Pylorospasm Esophagitis Duodenitis Ileitis Colitis
Genitourinary system		Increased bladder tone	Frequency Enuresis
Cardiovascular system	Vasodilation Hypotension Whealing	Vasodilation Hypotension	Flushing Shocklike lowering of blood pressure Hives
Salivary glands	Salivation	Salivation	Salivation Drooling
Sweat glands		Increased stimulation	Increased sweating
Lacrimal glands		Increased lacrimation	Tearing
Skeletal muscle		Asynchronous fasciculation	Tremors

food allergy generated by an antigen-antibody mechanism. In the former instance, symptoms induced by the ingestion of the food are caused by either a deficiency in the digestive mechanism or a disturbance in digestive physiology.

Allergy to foods can be responsible for many clinical manifestations (see Table 22-2). Of interest are the neurological, neurotic, and psychoneurotic manifestations included in the food allergy-mediated disorder of "allergic toxemia" (or tension-fatigue syndrome [30, 31]). This disorder is characterized by symptoms, such as lethargy, fatigue, irritability, restlessness, mental confusion and dullness, headache, various gastrointestinal symptoms, tiredness, and body aches or pains [7, 8, 9, 11, 12, 13, 21, 24, 26, 31, 35, 38, 39]. When such symptoms accompany other allergic manifestations, such as hay fever or asthma, and if they improve or disappear when these other symptoms abate, it is not difficult to attribute the symptoms to allergy. However, when such diverse symptoms arise in the absence of a definite associated allergic reaction, many doubt that they occur secondary to an allergy and prefer to attribute their etiology to other causes—mainly psychoneurosis.

It is unfortunate that children who have the more diffuse constitutional allergic traits (e.g., tension, fatigue, hyperactivity, excessive sweating, salivation, pallor, lacrimation, or vague aches and pains) are usually considered to be either neurotic, hypochondriacal, or structurally inferior. When other reasons for such symptoms cannot be ascertained, the possibility of a syndrome due to food allergy should be investigated. If symptoms such as nervousness, irritability, hyperactivity, mental or physical fatigue, and sluggishness appear in children who have allergic disorders, the possibility that these symptoms are due to an allergic intolerance for one or more foods or food additives may be readily substantiated if the symptoms improve or disappear after elimination of the suspected food(s) from the child's diet and reappear with introduction of the food(s) back into the diet [13, 26, 31]. The allergic child deserves to be approached with an open mind and a willingness to consider the possibility that almost any symptom(s) may be of allergic origin.

Allergy is one of the greatest medical masqueraders for disease(s) and behavioral disorders in childhood. A typical sequence of ailments in an allergic child in the preadult years might be as follows: First, the infant may experience feeding problems due to a reaction to cow's milk, with symptoms of colic, vomiting, diarrhea, or constipation. Later, eczema may appear, and the child may begin to develop frequent "colds" characterized by rhinitis, cough, and congestion. Perhaps numerous bouts of ear infections begin, and recurring or persistent fluid in the middle-ear space(s) becomes a problem. Intermittent episodes of bronchiolitis, croup, bronchitis, or pneumonia may then appear. Concurrently or subsequently, the child may develop hay fever or asthma and all of its complications. It is possible that sinusitis, migraine headaches, abdominal pain, or colitis will also become an issue. Interspersed with this succession of events may be problems, such as bed wetting, leg pains, hyperactivity, urethritis or vaginitis, fatigue, learning disabilities, a seizure disorder, bouts of unexplained fevers, and behavioral disorders at home or school. The child may also suffer from canker sores, menstrual irregularity, dysuria, nasal polyps, arthritis, vertigo, sleep disorders, or hives. All the aforementioned ailments, and many more, could be due to one or more allergies. The potential combination of disorders, diseases, or disabilities is nearly uncountable.

SUMMARY

Growth is slower and more uniform during the early school years than during the preschool and adolescent years. Norms are valuable to indicate growth trends, but individual variance as affected by hereditary factors, gender, and environmental conditions must be kept in mind when growth tables are used. Measurements taken only one time may give one undue cause for alarm or a false sense of security; measurements need to be taken several times in order to identify the child's pattern of growth. Individual differences increase with age in all domains, including the biophysical. No child fits the norms in all aspects.

A poor state of health can affect the learning process. Good nutrition, careful hygiene, regular physical and dental checkups, and routine screening tests can help to maintain high level wellness in order to maximize potentials in all four domains.

Allergy can precipitate a plethora of diverse ailments. When faced with a child who manifests an unusual disparity or strange profusion of symptoms, the practitioner should consider the possibility of an underlying allergic provocation and refer the child for an allergy evaluation by a physician.

REFERENCES

1. American Academy of Pediatrics, Committee on Sports Medicine. Climatic heat stress and the exercising child. *Pediatrics* 69:808, 1982.
2. Behrman, R. E., Vaughan, V. C., and Nelson, W. E. (Eds.). *Nelson Textbook of Pediatrics* (12th ed.). Philadelphia: Saunders, 1983.
3. Brower, E. W., and Nash, C. L., Jr. Evaluating growth and posture in school-age children. *Nursing 79* 9(4):58, 1979.
4. Caffey, J. P. *Pediatric X-Ray Diagnosis: A Textbook for Students and Practitioners of Pediatrics, Surgery, and Radiology* (7th ed.). Chicago: Year Book, 1978.
5. Chinn, P. L. *Child Health Maintenance: Concepts in Family-Centered Care* (2nd ed.). St. Louis: Mosby, 1979.
6. Cooke, R. E. (Ed.). *The Biological Basis of Pediatric Practice.* New York: McGraw-Hill, 1968.
7. Crook, W. G. *Your Allergic Child: A Pediatrician's Guide to Normal Living for Allergic Adults and Children.* New York: Medcom Press, 1974.
8. Crook, W. G. *Can Your Child Read? Is He Hyperactive?* (Rev. Ed.). Jackson, TN: Professional Books, 1977.
9. Ellis, E. F. (Ed.). Symposium on Pediatric Allergy. *Pediatr. Clin. North Am.* 22(1), 1975.
10. Emmert, W. Personal communication, 1978.
11. Feingold, B. F. *Introduction to Clinical Allergy.* Springfield, IL: Thomas, 1973.
12. Feingold, B. F. *Why Your Child is Hyperactive.* New York: Random House, 1975.
13. Frazier, C. A. *Coping With Food Allergy.* New York: Quadrangle, 1977.
14. Freeman, G. L., and Johnson, S. Allergic diseases in adolescents. *Am. J. Dis. Child.* 107:549, 1969.
15. Gerrard, J. W. *Understanding Allergies.* Springfield, IL: Thomas, 1973.
16. Holm, V. A., and Wiltz, N. A. Childhood. In D. W. Smith and E. L. Bierman (Eds.), *The Biologic Ages of Man From Conception Through Old Age.* Philadelphia: Saunders, 1973.
17. Ismail, H., and Lall, P. Visual acuity of school entrants. *Child: Care, Health and Dev.* 7:127, 1981.
18. Kilman, C., and Helpin, M. L. Recognizing dental malocclusion in children. *Pediatr. Nurs.* 9:204, 1983.
19. Lowrey, G. H. *Growth and Development of Children* (7th ed.). Chicago: Year Book, 1978.
20. Marlow, D. R. *Textbook of Pediatric Nursing* (6th ed.). Philadelphia: Saunders, 1985.
21. Miller, J. B. *Food Allergy: Provocative Testing and Injection Therapy.* Springfield, IL: Thomas, 1972.
22. Narins, D. M., Belkengren, R. P., and Sapala, S. Nutrition and the growing child. *Pediatr. Nurs.* 9:163, 1983.
23. Oyama, S. A sensitive period for the acquisition of a nonnative phonological system. *J. Psycholinguist. Res.* 5(3):261, 1976.
24. Randolph, T. G. *Human Ecology and Susceptibility to the Chemical Environment.* Springfield, IL: Thomas, 1978.
25. Report to the Task Force on Blood Pressure Control in

Children. Prepared by the National Heart, Lung, and Blood Institute's Task Force on Blood Pressure Control in Children. *Pediatrics* (Suppl.), 59(5), May 1977.

26. Rowe, A. H. *Food Allergy: Its Manifestations and Control and the Elimination Diets, A Compendium.* Springfield, IL: Thomas, 1972.

27. Ruble, J. A. Childhood nocturnal enuresis. *Am. J. of Matern. Child Nurs.* (Jaunary–February 1981). 6:26.

28. Schiffer, C. G., and Hunt, E. P. *Illness Among Children.* U.S. Children's Bureau Publication, No. 405. Washington, D.C.: U.S. Government Printing Office, 1963.

29. Smith, D. W., and Bierman, E. L. *The Biologic Ages of Man: From Conception Through Old Age* (2nd ed.). Philadelphia: Saunders, 1978.

30. Speer, F. (Ed.). *The Allergic Child.* New York: Hoeber Medical Division, Harper & Row, 1966.

31. Speer, F. (Ed.). *Allergy of the Nervous System.* Springfield, IL: Thomas, 1970.

32. Stewart, R. E., et al. (Eds.). *Pediatric Dentistry: Scientific and Clinical Practice.* St. Louis: Mosby, 1982.

33. Tanner, J. M. *Foetus into Man: Physical Growth from Conception to Maturity.* London: Open Books, 1978.

34. Tuft, L., and Mueller, H. L. *Allergy in Children.* Philadelphia: Saunders, 1970.

35. Von Hilsheimer, G. *Allergy, Toxins, and the Learning-Disabled Child.* San Rafael, CA: Academic Therapy Publications, 1974.

36. Waechter, E. H., Phillips, J., and Holaday, B. *Nursing Care of Children* (10th ed.). Philadelphia: Lippincott, 1985.

37. Whaley, L. F., and Wong, D. L. *Essentials of Pediatric Nursing.* St. Louis: Mosby, 1982.

38. Wunderlich, R. C. *Kids, Brains, and Learning: What Goes Wrong—Prevention and Treatment.* St. Petersburg, FL: Johnny Reads, 1970.

39. Wunderlich, R. C. *Allergy, Brains and Children Coping: Allergy and Child Behavior, The Neuro-Allergic Syndrome.* St. Petersburg, FL: Johnny Reads, 1973.

Cognitive Development of the School-Ager

Thomas Clifford

"Oh, yes, once you know, you know forever!"

The remark quoted in the epigraph is attributed to a Swiss schoolchild by Inhelder and Piaget. Something like this has probably been said by nearly every school-age child—it is typical of the age. It is during the school years that children discover themselves as knowers, doers, thinkers, planners, adventurers, contrivers, and as individuals apart from their parents and, indeed, from anyone else. There is a break away from the magical, mysterious world of 4, 5, and 6 years old, as one finds oneself a discoverer of rules and order, of reasoned understandings and of secrets.

For some children, this transformation happens so gradually that nothing seems noteworthy or memorable; for others, it is dramatic. A school-age child whose parents are going through a divorce, for example, may awake one morning to realize that no amount of daydreaming is going to bring the parents back together. On a more sanguine note, some people remember the day they first discovered that printed words do not themselves contain stories but are, rather, the devices used by others to tell stories if one would learn to read. Many first and second grade teachers are sensitive to this critical developmental turning point and can facilitate their students' discoveries.

Such an event was reported by Anne Sullivan, the teacher of Helen Keller. Miss Keller became blind and deaf as a result of illness at the end of her second year of life. Miss Sullivan, who had herself experienced blindness as a child, arrived at the Keller home in Alabama when Helen was 6 years and 8 months old, in March of 1887. A month later, Miss Sullivan wrote in a letter, "She has learned that *everything has a name, and that the manual alphabet is the key to everything she wants to know*" [73]. Helen Keller related the event in her autobiography [39]:

> Earlier in the day we had had a tussle over the words m-u-g and w-a-t-e-r. Miss Sullivan had tried to impress it upon me that m-u-g is *mug* and that w-a-t-e-r is *water*, but I persisted in confounding the two. . . .
> We walked down the path to the well-house, attracted by the fragrance of the honeysuckle with which it was covered. Someone was drawing water and my teacher placed my hand under the spout. As the cool stream gushed over one hand she spelled into the other the word *water*, first slowly, then rapidly. I stood still, my whole attention fixed upon the motions of her fingers. Suddenly I felt a misty consciousness as of something forgotten—a thrill of returning thought; and somehow the mystery of language was revealed to me. I knew then that w-a-t-e-r meant the wonderful cool something that was flowing over my hand. That living word awakened my soul, gave it light, hope, joy, set it free!
> . . .
> I left the well-house eager to learn. Everything had a name, and each name gave birth to a new thought. As we returned to the house every object which I touched seemed to quiver with life. That was because I saw everything with the strange, new sight that had come to me. . . .
> It would have been difficult to find a happier child than I was as I lay in my crib at the close of that eventful day and lived over the joys it had brought me, and for the first time longed for a new day to come.

What Helen Keller had discovered was that language "is the key to everything she wants to know." She had captured that knowledge forever. It happened just short of 3 months before her seventh birthday.

CONCRETE OPERATIONAL THOUGHT

The period of concrete operational thought, which lasts from about 7 until 11 years of age, marks a transition from intuitive thought to objective thought, from egocentrism to relativism, and from dependence on reproductive imagery to anticipatory imagery. Hallmarks of the period are decentering, seriation, multiple classification, and conservation. Underlying these phenomena is a new capacity for reversal transformations, the foundation for concrete operational thinking.

Anticipatory Images

Piaget marks the emergence of anticipatory images, as distinguished from reproductive images, as occurring between 7 and 8 years of age [59]. Imagine a stick falling from a vertical position. The preoperational child can imagine the initial and final positions of the stick but has difficulty with the intermediate positions; this is reproductive imagery. The child capable of anticipatory imagery knows the intermediate positions even though they are not literally seen. It is as though the younger child has mental photographs of only the beginning and end states, whereas the older child has a mental movie camera that is capable of reverse, forward, and stop action at any point. The younger child can anticipate where the stick will fall, but the imagery is restricted to what has actually been seen, that is, to a reproduction of what is known from past experience. The older child can anticipate a change of state not immediately seen or experienced, although, because of the concrete nature of thought during this period, it could be experienced. Later on, when formal operational thought breaks away from the bonds of the concrete, analogous mental operations can be performed on abstractions without a physical referent.

Decentering and Relativism

Piaget asserts that anticipatory images "seem to be necessary for the representation of any transformation" [59]. The process of decentering, or decentration, that underlies the transition from egocentrism to relativism also exemplifies this concept. Place an apple, an orange, and a banana on a table, and photograph the arrangement from different points around the table. Seat a child at the table and place a teddy bear across the table from the child. Now ask the child to choose the photograph that shows how the fruit would appear from the opposite side of the table where the bear is sitting. The egocentrism characteristic of preoperational thought is reflected in the child's unquestioned assumption that everyone's experiences are from the same vantage point. In this case, the photograph taken from the child's seat is chosen. The older child picks the photograph taken from the bear's side with certainty, as if the mental movie camera had run around the table and stopped behind the bear's eyes to confirm the selection. One child shows egocentrism, the other relativism. This new capacity of the 7- to 8-year-old to see the world as others see it is particularly important in terms of moral development, as discussed in Chapter 18.

Reversal Transformations

The capacity to operate one's imagery as a movie camera with forward, reverse, and stop action illustrates the reversal transformations underlying the phenomena of this period. Just as egocentric thought melts into relativism, the mental transformations of the tangible world shape absolute concepts into more subtle relational concepts. Preoperational children comprehend the world as a series of discrete states connected by temporal proximity but not by logical necessity. They use and respond to relational concepts, such as "smaller," "faster," "heavier," and "longer," as being expressive of absolutes. Preoperational children are unimpressed by magic; if a rabbit comes out of a previously empty hat, they find it amusing but not incredible. After all, if they believe that they are followed by the moon and that the sun shines so they can play, why shouldn't a rabbit appear out of a hat? In dramatic contrast, the mind's eye of the concrete operational child differentiates all the small states required to change from one condition to another and comprehends them as being necessarily connected in an integral series, even though the intermediate states cannot be directly seen. The connection becomes essential, sensible, and logical. For the preoperational child, magic is the order of the day. For the concrete operational child, the world becomes inhabited by reasoned, sensible, essential relations; the tricks of a magician become, as they are to adults, incredible.

Relational Concepts and Seriation

Exercise of the newly emergent capacity for reversal transformations takes time. Initially applied to individual, isolated events, or centrations, comprehension of how objects undergo change gradually becomes coordinated across events. Something that is "small" in one circumstance is "big" in another, and the object is seen as maintaining its integrity while going through the relational transformation. As similar comprehensions occur, "smallness" and "bigness" become decentered from isolated events and become points on a transformational continuum; "same," "smaller," "small," "bigger," and "big" become related conceptually as relational concepts, and these concepts become decentered from their identities with insular events to become applicable across many events so that events can be compared. The concrete operational child knows that an event can stay the same while the name changes. Daddy is my daddy, but Granddad's son; I am bigger than the baby, but smaller than Mommy. Preschoolers with one sibling are inclined to assert that they have a brother or a sister but that their brother or their sister does not, as if "brother" were part of him or her and not part of "me." The concrete operational child is capable of understanding these multiple relations.

Children who are capable of concrete operational thought can place sticks and stones in order from small to large and from light to heavy. This activity is known as seriation—putting things in serial order. The intervals between integers become equal to permit addition, subtraction, multiplication, and division into fractions. Numbers become systems that are useful for counting and measuring. A row of seven pennies is separated from a large pile. "Now, will you make a row with the same number of pennies?" A 6-year-old picks pennies from the pile one by one and places them in one-to-one correspondence with the pennies in the row until the places are filled. The child agrees that both rows have the same number. Now the first row is collapsed to form a cluster. "Which has more, the row or the bunch?" The child says the row has more. The same sequence is followed with an 8-year-old. To the first question, the 8-year-old counts the pennies in the row, then picks seven from the pile and arranges them in a second row. To the second question, the child asserts that both the cluster and the row have the same number. If pressed, the child may express puzzlement, not about the correct answer but about the intelligence of the questioner; the 8-year-old is not in the least puzzled about the answer. Number has been conserved in spite of the transformation from a row to a cluster; whether the pennies are stacked, put in one's pocket, or used as buttons, there will still be the same number.

Multiple Classification

Concrete operational children are fascinated with multiple classifications. Take a handful of marbles, some red and some blue, and ask, "Of which are there more, red marbles or marbles?" The six-year-old will answer "Red marbles"; the 8-year-old will answer "Marbles." Inhelder and Piaget formed an L on a display with a row of pictures of leaves varying in color and a column of pictures of various green objects [31]. The intersect was left blank to be filled by the child from among a group of pictures. Children 9 to 10 years old quickly recognized the appropriateness of a green leaf. Younger children filled the space with a picture of anything green or with a leaf of any color; they did not understand the double classification. This is the age—at 9 or

10 years—when children become collectors: stamps, match covers, figurines, bubble gum cards, comic books, bottle caps, and dolls. These new acquisitive impulses express the meticulous orders of multiple classification; they facilitate the development of concrete operational thought.

The Conservations

The conservations appear in order, depending on their complexity. Conservation of quantity emerges at about 7 years of age. Apple cider is poured into two identical drinking glasses so that the levels are equal and the child observing is sure there is an equal amount in both. The cider is then poured from one of the glasses into a tall glass cylinder or alternatively, into a wide, shallow dish. "Which one has more?" the child is asked. The typical 6-year-old will choose either the glass or the new vessel; the 7-year-old will assert with certainty that the amounts of cider are still equal.

Conservation of quantity can also be tested with two balls of clay, one of which is then rolled into a cylinder. If the cylinder is squashed flat and the child is asked which one weighs more, one finds that conservation of weight normally appears at about age 9. Conservation of volume is the last to appear, just prior to the emergence of formal operational thought. The two balls of clay are immersed in water to demonstrate their equal volumes, and then removed. One ball is then broken up or otherwise distorted and the child is asked "Will the levels be the same when the clay is put back in the water?" [59].

Concept of Time

If one saw a hare move from point **a** to point **d** in the same time that the tortoise moved one-fourth the distance, from **a** to **b,** one could ask the following questions: "Who was fastest?" "Who went farthest?" and "Who took the most time?" The concrete operational child would answer all three questions correctly; the preoperational child would probably get the first two correct and the last one wrong. Piaget refers to this preoperational impression that time is peculiar to the event as "localized time" [61]. There is confusion of the distance moved, the velocity at which the movement took place, and the time elapsed. The concrete operational child, however, comes to conserve these different dimensions, although as yet unable to understand their interrelations on an abstract level.

Time is a tricky concept even for adults; it tends to be quite subjective and closely tied to circumstance. Each of us indulges in preoperational time and per-

haps, in some moments of abandon, in sensorimotor time. On the other side, many adults seem to be rather irrational about clock time and about time zones, and few probably clearly understand concepts, such as biological time or astronomical time. Thus, the understanding of time on which many adults operate emerges during the period of concrete operations, with seconds and minutes classified under hours and days, with speed and distance conserved apart from time, and with speed and distance forming dimensions along which time can be transformed.

VARIATIONS IN COGNITIVE FUNCTIONING

Intelligence Testing

A clear and precise definition of intelligence has not been agreed upon. However, it is assumed that intelligent people will attain high scores on intelligence tests and will do well in school. This assumption was the point of departure for Alfred Binet's work around the turn of the century when he was engaged by the Paris school system to devise a test that would detect children who would not do well in regular classes.

THE INTELLIGENCE QUOTIENT

The concept of intelligence quotient (IQ) derived from this early work. Modifications of Binet's test ultimately yielded a mental age (MA) in months. The outcome of dividing MA by chronological age (CA) was the intelligence quotient (IQ = $100 \times$ MA/CA). Contemporary tests usually use deviation IQs based on the statistical distribution of scores for a standard sample of people. IQs from 84 to 116 are considered to be in the average range.

INDIVIDUAL AND GROUP TESTS

A test frequently used today to assess intelligence, the Stanford-Binet test [76], takes its name from this early researcher. It measures intelligence through a range from 2 years to "superior adult." Like the Wechsler Intelligence Scale for Children-Revised (WISC-R) [83], the Stanford-Binet is an individual test, administered to one person at a time. Individual tests are more sensitive than group tests and are especially useful for diagnosing disabilities of exceptional children, but they require special training to administer and interpret. The summary sheet for an individual test records observations of the social, emotional, and behavioral characteristics of the person as well as notes on test performance. Group tests record less information and are less sensitive to the conditions of the individual child, but they are much more efficient in terms of administration.

Because the individual test is given by a skilled examiner in a one-to-one situation, characteristics of the child that might affect the validity of the score are easier to detect. A valid test score is based on the assumption that the child understood the instructions, felt physically and emotionally prepared for the test, and wanted to do well. Furthermore, it assumes that the child is a member of the group from which the standard statistical norms for the test were derived. If the child is different from that group, perhaps because of prevailing physical or cultural differences or because of a momentary condition, such as illness or emotional distraction, the score will reflect neither that person's intellectual achievement nor his intellectual potential; it will be invalid.

INTERPRETATION AND ERROR

But how is one to know? The fact that one cannot know all the factors influencing the validity of a test score and the fact that factors qualifying the validity of a test score are often ignored are two serious criticisms that have been leveled against intelligence testing in the past few years. Most intelligence tests were standardized on middle-class American children, and under these circumstances, the tests have high validity coefficients; that is, they correlate highly with school achievement and with other tests of intelligence. Even under optimal conditions, however, a test score is better interpreted as an approximation than as an accurately drawn point on a scale. For example, in recording a score from the Stanford-Binet test, rather than saying that Henry Uno has a score of 96, it would be more accurate to say that the chances are 19 in 20 that Henry Uno's IQ is between 90 and 102. We are assuming that Henry is representative of the standardization sample and that he understood the directions, felt well, was not bothered by problems at home, and wanted to do well. Extending the same assumptions to a class of, say, 100 sixth-graders, if we estimated each child's IQ as falling within 6 points of the child's point score, we would be wrong for five children out of the 100. If there were children in the group who were not familiar with the culture represented by the test, or who were otherwise handicapped, we would be wrong for more than five children. In fact, it is not hard to imagine situations in which we would be wrong for most of the children—and our errors might very well have enduring consequences for them.

Numbers have a way of commanding respect, and an IQ score can seem to be a secure guide for the assignment and treatment of a child. Indeed, the detection of children in need of special attention is the most valuable function of intelligence tests. When tests are not used well, however, children's education may suffer. This danger exists in any case, but it has special significance for children from cultural groups not representative of middle America, for example, for many blacks, Chicanos, and native Americans. The claim that many intelligence tests are biased against children from culturally different groups is convincing, and the latest edition of the manual for the WISC-R includes norms for other groups [83].

Children are treated differently according to their presumed intelligence both at an institutional level, by being placed on different educational "tracks," and by teachers and peers according to their attitudes and values. Teachers, being human, tend to favor winners, and the favoritism itself lends further advantage. Rosenthal and Jacobson call this phenomenon the "Pygmalion effect" or the "self-fulfilling prophecy" [68]. These researchers measured the IQs of a number of children, divided them into two equal groups according to their scores, and then gave their teachers erroneous information about their scores, some children being described as higher than measured and some as lower. At the end of the school year, a retest showed that the children's IQs had changed significantly toward the given scores; the deceptions had become prophecies. Could the distortions be corrected? Yes. But the Rosenthal and Jacobson study dramatically illustrates what may be the fate of many children.

A QUESTION OF RACE

Some researchers have interpreted the small but persistent difference between the average IQs of black children and those of white children to reflect a genetic difference. General comparisons between blacks and whites in the United States reveal that whites are advantaged; the list of items on which they average more than blacks includes income, education, and IQ. In an article that attracted nationwide attention 17 years ago, Jensen claimed that he controlled for these other factors with statistical adjustments and still found a difference in IQ, indicating a genetic distinction [33]. Others have examined this claim and found it wanting [37].

Quite possibly the question will never be settled, but

research in this area continues. In a recent study of children between ages 5 and 16 years in the rural South, the IQs of black children but not of white children were found to drop substantially as they grew older [35]. This contrast between blacks and whites might mean that the decrement was genetically determined or that it was a cumulative effect of chronic environmental deprivation. An earlier study of children in California, where educational conditions were more favorable and more equitable, showed no decrement for either blacks or whites [34]. From a comparison of these two studies, Jensen suggested that cumulative environmental deprivation better explained the drop [35].

COGNITIVE TALENT: GENERAL OR SPECIFIC?

The question of whether intelligence is unitary or multifaceted is an important one, particularly for educational policy. If intelligence were unitary, the design of educational programs and the selection of children for those programs would be greatly simplified. But the question turns on itself, since intelligence in children is defined in terms of success in school. Let us look at the factors that are related to scholastic achievement. Is there a single factor, or are there several?

During the preschool years, to the extent that later school performance can be predicted at all, the factors of attention and persistence seem to do the job most succinctly. During the school years and beyond, verbal facility, or ease in reading, writing, and comprehending language, is most highly related to school achievement. The fact that nonverbal factors correlate with both school achievement and with verbal measures of intelligence suggests a general factor underlying school achievement. The most sensitive tests of intelligence include a variety of subscales under the verbal and performance scales. The WISC-R, for example, includes general information, general comprehension, arithmetic, similarities, vocabulary, and digit span on the verbal scale; and picture completion, picture arrangement, block design, object assembly, coding, and mazes on the performance scale. That these factors are intercorrelated speaks to a general intelligence factor; that the different scales make distinctive contributions to the overall assessment of intelligence speaks to the diversity of intelligence.

GUILFORD'S MODEL

An approach to intelligence that is more directed to the diversity of mental facility is the structure-of-intellect model developed by Guilford and his colleagues

[24, 25, 26]. Guilford used a statistical approach, called factor analysis, to distinguish the diversity of intellectual abilities. This approach allows a mathematical assessment of degrees of interdependence and of independence in numerous tests. The structure-of-intellect model includes 120 distinctive intellectual factors, abilities, or categories.

Guilford has organized the model in a compellingly simple form. First, he asserts that intelligence can be analyzed in terms of contents, operations, and products—that is, in terms of basic ingredients, what might be done to them, and how they might turn out. These three parameters, as they are called, are the three dimensions of the model. This concept is analogous to a "shopping model" one might use to select building blocks in a toy store: one might order blocks by size, color, and form—a big red square, or a medium green triangle. Just as the size of blocks might be small, medium, or large, Guilford offers four categories of contents: figural, symbolic, semantic, and behavioral. Just as color might be red, orange, yellow, and so on, there are five distinctive categories of operations: evaluation, convergent production, divergent production, memory, and cognition. For products there are six categories: units, classes, relations, systems, transformations, and implications. Just as the number of possible kinds of blocks would be the number of sizes times the number of colors times the number of forms, the num-

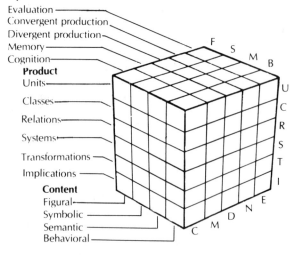

Figure 23–1. Guilford's three-dimensional model of the structure of intellect. (From J. P. Guilford, *The Nature of Human Intelligence*. New York: McGraw-Hill, 1967. With permission.)

ber of distinctive kinds of intellectual abilities in the structure-of-intellect model is $4 \times 5 \times 6 = 120$.

This introduction to Guilford's model is not as important for the particular kinds of intelligence delineated as for how eloquently the model speaks to two points alluded to earlier: that intellectual abilities are diverse and that standard intelligence tests tap a limited sample of these abilities.

Mental Retardation

DEFINITIONS
According to the American Association of Mental Deficiency (AAMD), "Mental retardation refers to significantly subaverage general intellectual functioning existing concurrently with deficits in adaptive behavior, and manifested during the developmental period" [23]. General intellectual functioning is assumed to be reflected by performance on individually administered IQ tests. The latest edition of the *Diagnostic and Statistical Manual of Mental Disorders* [2] identifies several levels of intellectual functioning below the average range of IQ scores: borderline intellectual functioning, 71–84; mild mental retardation, 50–70; moderate mental retardation, 35–49; severe mental retardation, 20–34; and profound mental retardation, below 20. It is noteworthy that the label of "borderline mentally retarded" is absent from the latest manual of the AAMD [23].

The term **adaptive behavior** refers to "the effectiveness or the degree with which the individual meets the standards of personal independence and social responsibility expected of his age and cultural group" [23]. The AAMD's 1973 revision of the Adaptive Behavior Scale includes two parts, one concerned with traditional adaptive behavior, such as independent functioning, physical development, economic activity, language development, numbers and time, self-direction, responsibility, and socialization; and a second concerned with idiosyncratic behavioral adjustments that would interfere with socialization and education, such as destructive behavior, nonconformance, untrustworthiness, withdrawal, odd mannerisms, unacceptable vocal habits, hyperactive tendencies, and use of medication. Norms for this scale have been established from a large multiethnic sample of California school children [45].

The term **educable mentally retarded** (EMR) is the legal designation used in the public schools for mildly retarded children who are capable of learning academic skills, such as reading and arithmetic; this term

is not included in the AAMD manual. The designation **trainable mentally retarded** (TMR) is used in public schools for children benefitting from special training in simple job skills and in caring for themselves. This designation is comparable to the "moderate" and "severe" AAMD classifications.

Although the definitions in the last two AAMD manuals [23, 28] place new emphasis on adaptive behavior in addition to IQ, the lack of a readily available standardized measure of adaptive behavior for the assessment of retardation has, in practice, left emphasis on individual measures of IQ. The reader will recall that tests of intelligence were first devised by Binet for the purpose of determining which children would better benefit from special instruction. Compared with achievement test scores and teachers' assessments, individual intelligence test scores remain the best predictors of a child's progress in school, at least for 1 or 2 years after testing. Given the essential cautions mentioned in the discussion of IQ testing and the qualifiers that scores do not necessarily indicate innate capacity and may change significantly over time, IQ scores can be helpful, but not definitive, in anticipating the need for special educational programs to meet the needs of individual children.

A COGNITIVE-DEVELOPMENTAL APPROACH
While intelligence is generally conceived of as an ability or as the content of one's thoughts, Piaget conceives of it as an adaptation that reflects the interaction between the individual and the environment [60]. Using the Piagetian cognitive-developmental perspective, Inhelder suggested four classifications of mental retardation: the slow learner, arriving late at formal operational thought (normally 11+ years); the retardate, capable of some level of concrete operational thought (normally 7 to 11 years) but never of formal operational thought; the imbecile, capable of intuitive thought (normally 2 to 7 years); and the idiot, with an ultimate potential limited to the sensorimotor period (normally birth to 2 years) [30].

In her discussion of mental retardation, Inhelder notes that the retarded child typically evidences oscillations or fluctuations between cognitive levels. In a normal child, such oscillations are most evident during transitional periods, when the child can easily be convinced of errors in thinking. The retarded child is not so easily apprised of errors, and whereas the oscillations of the normal transitional child are temporary and soon show resolution to the next phase of cognitive development, those of the retarded child are not. Inhelder also points out that the retarded child's attention is not as strong as that of a normal child. A review of research and theory on mental retardation from the Piagetian perspective has recently been compiled [41].

COMPLICATING FACTORS

School psychologists need be especially sensitive to other factors in addition to IQ in the determination and assessment of exceptional children with learning problems, particularly in instances of possible EMR children [45]. Inhelder's discussion of the retarded child's generally lower interest or attention level includes the qualifier that interest levels can range widely among children with high intelligence as well as among those with low intelligence [30]. This factor—interest, or attention—has broad significance for intellectual performance and learning facility [63]. For example, reading problems are significantly related to deficits in attention, especially in auditory attention [77]. A study of 16 different cognitive measures found that one for "listening," a test for aural comprehension, was distinguished for its prediction of intellectual development [3]. Retarded individuals with identical IQ scores may vary widely in learning abilities [6, 13]. It seems likely that differences in attention underlie some of this variation.

To complicate the picture still further, the achievements of the retarded are also affected by factors, such as high expectation of personal failure, tendencies to distrust personal attempts at solving problems, and negative reactions to adults who expect too much [48]. In sum, these observations speak to the necessity of thorough and sensitive assessment during the school years and to the need for continuing attention to children with mental or academic retardation.

Impediments and Impairments

The cerebral cortex of the brain is divided into two hemispheres. One of the more intriguing findings of recent brain-mind research is that these cortical hemispheres (left and right) process information differently [72]. The left hemisphere in most people processes information in a linear, sequential, and analytic manner and is associated with language, analysis, and planning. Perhaps, gratuitously, this hemisphere is also referred to as the dominant cerebral hemisphere. The right hemisphere interprets input in a spatial, intuitive, and holistic manner and is associated with pattern recognition, synthesis, and evaluation.

Traditional education systems and IQ tests tend to emphasize the analytical processing skills associated more with the left side of the brain. The highly creative individual who may perceive more globally, or holis-

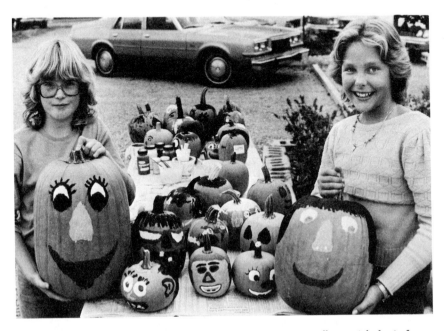

Figure 23–2. Creativity comes in many forms. Art projects supposedly tap right-brain functioning and offer the opportunity to develop all four domains.

tically, and who may be more comfortable with artistic expression is afforded little opportunity to express these traits in the traditional classroom or on an IQ test. Only within the last decade has the educational literature begun to attach equal importance to affective learning modes and creative learning styles. Research on learning styles has shown that individuals vary greatly in their dominant modes of learning. Much of this literature has emphasized the differences in hemispheric functioning of the brain as a simile for the emphasis and neglect of traditional education and IQ testing. Tradition emphasizes contents and outcomes, but these do not occur without synthesis and the creative process. Educators are now speaking to a need to nurture the creative process, and they are using the simile from recent research on the brain to strengthen their point. Separated, the cerebral hemispheres function, but with a loss to each and both. To best benefit a nation, education must foster creativity as well as transmit and preserve the past [54].

Learning disabilities are not synonymous with mental retardation. A learning disability can be understood as a disposition to process information through touch, hearing, kinesthetic experience, or sight in a way that does not fit into the expectations of present educational systems. Millions of people have learning disabilities from the slight to the severe in degree. Although information may not be processed in the conventional way nor in the allowed time, very complex problems can be analyzed. Thomas Edison and Nelson Rockefeller were learning-disabled. Problems arise when the educator tries to force the child to learn and to be assessed by traditional methods. For example, a 9-year-old boy was having severe problems in the third grade after having been at the top of his class in earlier grades. One of his problems was a strong disposition to process visual information from right to left. With English, this runs counter to convention. In earlier grades, one-syllable words and simple sentences had permitted a phonetic emphasis and the problem had been ignored. With more two-syllable words and the increasing importance of eidetic analysis of printed language (as happens in the third grade), the problem emerged as an impairment in learning, or, as we say, a learning disability.

The fragile ego of the child succumbs quickly to pressures to conform or to confrontation with the difference. Many of these children suffer from low self-esteem and helplessness syndrome, factors which may lead to general academic failure and social dysfunctions.

It is easy to understand that an injury or a disease that involves the brain can affect learning and thinking. It is not easy to understand how this happens. Neurologists and neurosurgeons are inclined to consider their work finished when a disease process is interrupted or a wound is healed. Neuropsychologists and behavioral neurologists are more sensitized to the behavioral and psychological consequences, which may last for years, even a lifetime, and significantly affect the individual's social and personal life. As a rule, the younger a person is when brain injury or disease occurs, the more readily compensations are made for any deficits in functioning whether in language, behavior, or thinking. Yet the author has seen many cases where the effects of a high fever or an injury in infancy or early childhood do not emerge until years later, in the middle-school years or in early adolescence when more abstract and complex thought is typically required in school and in social life.

Gifted Children

Shortly after sunrise one spring morning many years ago there was a ruckus in the front yard. High among the leafless branches of a large maple tree were a young orange cat and two blue jays. The jays were calling and flitting about, teasing the cat; they could have flown away. The cat was doing catlike things, stalking and climbing after the birds and making leaps across branches thirty feet off the ground. Propelled in its leaps as though shot from a cannon, the grace and the tension exhibited by the young cat as it split the air in the morning sunlight would have shamed the dreams of a ballet dancer. One became acutely aware of witnessing an ordinary event, punctuated by extraordinary skill. It was a cat possessed by a gift, a cat among cats, a supercat.

Most individuals are not gifted, but some of us are, and it is a rare person indeed who believes he or she cannot discern an extraordinary performance or achievement and who does not thrill to the sharing of that feat. It is also true that some individuals are gifted but do not know it. Furthermore, in spite of how expert we may feel about our judgments of who is gifted and who is not, these judgments are often wrong.

The catch phrase "genius is next to madness" is dispelled by a classic study begun in 1921 of 1500 school children with Stanford-Binet IQs of 140 or higher [74]. These people were evaluated at intervals over the years. Early tests revealed them as superior in a wide variety of factors other than IQ: physique, physical health, social adjustment, moral attitudes, and mastery of school subjects. Follow-up studies showed them as superior in social and personal adjustment later in life as well as in productivity and longevity. As Terman, who initiated these studies, put it, " 'Early ripe, early rot' simply does not hold for these subjects" [75].

The subjects of Terman's study may have been as lucky as they were gifted: They knew they were gifted by virtue of their participation in the study. We know little about those people who are gifted and who either are told they are not or are unable to practice their gift because of circumstances beyond their control.

The detection of talent is not an easy matter. Athletic teams go to great lengths to find young men and women with exceptional promise, but even with the benefit of in situ observation, the young people who are discovered often do not achieve prominence as professional athletes. Selection of intellectual talent is even more difficult. Comparisons of different ways of detecting intellectually gifted children and adolescents, such as teachers' nominations, IQ scores, grades,

and other test measures, show a striking failure of correspondence across the alternatives [17]. One study of junior high school students found that teachers identified only 27 percent of those designated as being gifted by IQ scores of 136 or above. In the same study, gifted students selected on the basis of IQ scores included only 45 percent of those identified as gifted by teachers [57].

The global embarrassment suffered by the United States upon the Soviet Union's launching of the first orbital satellite on October 4, 1957, inspired a search for scholastic talent unparalleled in American history. Since then, the United States has had serious debates in high levels of government about detecting and encouraging talent, and it has gone through cycles of a varying supply of, and demand for, scientists and engineers. What is gifted or what is extraordinary talent is largely defined in terms of the contemporary values of society. While it is true that gifted people are capable of achievement in many areas, and that people's achievements seldom if ever reflect their true range of potential, it is also true that much of the world's resources of human potential are wasted for lack of op-

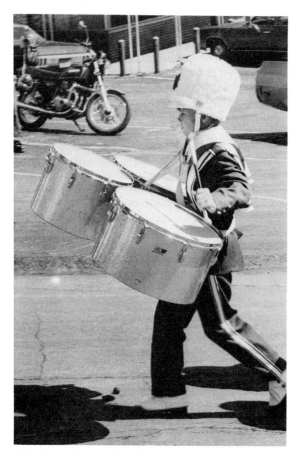

Figure 23–3. Each child has some special talent. It is a challenge to parents and educators to help the child discover and develop his or her special "gift."

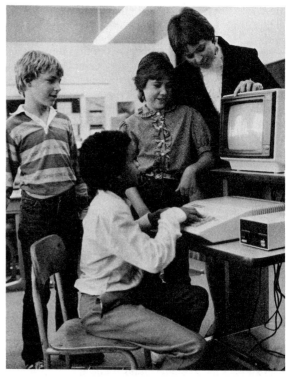

Figure 23–4. Computers are taking their place beside the basic "three R's" in classrooms today.

portunity or competitive disadvantage. Gifted people benefit from special opportunities [49]. While any child, including the prodigy, tends to be handicapped by the injunction or the requirement that they live in terms of someone else's ambitions, any child also benefits from a wealth of opportunities from which to choose. The issue of dealing with gifted children, in light of the difficulties in detecting giftedness and in light of changing societal values, directs attention more appropriately to how society can afford a wider range of opportunities for more children, how children can be encouraged to address these opportunities, and how children can be guided in attention to, and attraction toward, quality and value.

Problem Solving and Creative Production

A problem begins with a felt difficulty. If one ventures beyond this feeling, several steps follow: the difficulty is located and defined, various solutions are produced, the consequences are considered, and one of the solutions is accepted. These are the five steps of problem solving as described by John Dewey in 1910 [15]. Creative production was analyzed in terms of four steps by Wallas in 1926: preparation, incubation, illumination, and verification [82]. Guilford asserts that problem solving and creative production are basically the same phenomenon [25].

It can be argued that children have neither the store of information nor the command of their talents required for true creativity, where a creative idea is one that illuminates a problem, is unique, and is useful. However, research on problem solving in children typically uses problems requiring the generation of ideas that are familiar to the adult testers but not to the subjects. Thus the processes that children go through can be assumed to parallel the creative processes of adults. Furthermore, we might expect that the circumstances most conducive to the development and encouragement of creative talent in adults would be those most conducive to parallel processes in children.

CHARACTERISTICS OF CREATIVE PROBLEM SOLVERS
Barron studied adults who were judged to be especially creative by their colleagues in the professions of architecture, mathematics, science, and writing. Several characteristics were common to the creative individuals in these groups. Some of his descriptions are as follows [7]:

Appears to have a high degree of intellectual capacity
Genuinely values intellectual and cognitive matters
Values own independence and autonomy

Is verbally fluent; can express ideas well
Enjoys aesthetic impressions; is aesthetically reactive
Is productive; gets things done
Is concerned with philosophical problems; for example, religion, values, the meaning of life, and so forth
Has high aspiration level for self
Has a wide range of interests
Thinks and associates to ideas in unusual ways; has unconventional thought processes
Is an interesting, arresting person
Appears straightforward, forthright, candid in dealings with others
Behaves in an ethically consistent manner; is consistent with own personal standards

This is a diverse array of characteristics that appear to beg for opportunities to express themselves in order to maintain self confidence and sustain hope. Many questions could be asked about the potential hazards of extending these opportunities. If too much emphasis is placed on providing abundant opportunities, is there a danger of discouraging exploration and personal initiative? If hopes for a child's success are high, might not efforts to support those hopes exaggerate fears of failure? Might not efforts to supply an abundance of opportunities present instead an array that bewilders rather than enlightens?

CREATIVITY AND INTELLIGENCE
Answers to some of these questions are suggested by the results of a study of the relation of creativity and intelligence in fifth-grade boys and girls [81]. In this study, intelligence was measured with standard tests, and creativity was measured with items, such as, "Name as many things as you can that are sharp" and "Tell all the different ways to use a newspaper." One important finding of the study was that intelligence and creativity can be independent. Although there appears to be a certain level of intelligence that is necessary before an individual can be creative, a low or a high intelligence would not determine whether one is low or high in creativity. Furthermore, the social behavior of the girls, but not of the boys, was related to the combination of intelligence and creativity. If the difference between boys and girls reflects a difference in emphasis on factors underlying intelligence and creativity during the school years, the findings for the fifth-grade girls are of general interest. The girls who were high in both intelligence and creativity were self-confident and popular, whereas those high in intelligence but low in creativity were very popular but seemed more aloof and cautious in social initiatives. The girls low in both intelligence and creativity were also somewhat cau-

tious and hesitant socially, but they were still quite popular and outgoing. Most socially handicapped were the girls who were high in creativity but low in intelligence; they evidenced low self-confidence, were cautious and hesitant in their social relations, and tended to be unpopular. The major lesson to be learned here is from this last group. These girls had many unusual ideas; but they had difficulty making their ideas credible, understandable, or interesting, and evidently this interfered with their social adjustment. One imagines their peers as being impatient with their attempts to express a headful of seemingly farfetched ideas, and one would hope that these children would learn at some time to be more patient with their ideas, to take sufficient time for careful examination and exposition of their ideas, to tolerate the skepticism and resistance that often greets new ideas, and to value themselves and to find friends for support. Unfortunately, that is not always the case.

HANDICAPS TO CREATIVE PROBLEM SOLVING

The greatest handicap to creative problem solving in adults is fixedness of thinking—an inflexibility of assumptions or beliefs that is inconsistent with finding solutions. Adults are also handicapped by fears of failure or of being wrong. Preschool children typically fail in problem solving for different reasons: failing to understand the problem, forgetting the elements of the problem, or a lack of sufficient information. The school-age child shares the handicaps of the preschooler, but with the growing sensitivity to social judgment characteristic of this age, he or she is also handicapped by fear of failure [51]. Indeed, these factors may be combined. A child may be so distressed at the prospect of being wrong that the question or problem is not even heard or the task is not even attempted.

Evaluation is also an important component of problem solving, and it is a skill that develops over the school years. Marked increases in response times to problems occur across the years from 5 through 12, and marked decreases in errors occur across the same years. This finding suggests an increasing concern for errors, perhaps partly from a greater fear of being wrong, but also because of increasing care about being correct and, perhaps, because of increasing satisfaction or pleasure attendant upon a good solution [36].

FACILITATING PROBLEM SOLVING

How might problem solving be facilitated? Torrance offers five principles for teachers to follow in encour-

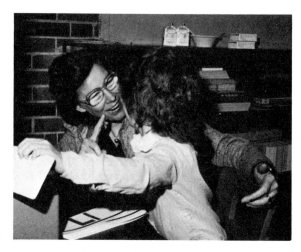

Figure 23–5. The focused, synchronized attention of a caring adult can facilitate learning. The enthusiastic response of an adult can give wings to the child's efforts.

aging their students; they might also serve as a guide for parents. The teacher should [79]:

1. Be respectful of unusual questions
2. Be respectful of imaginative, creative ideas
3. Show pupils that their ideas have value
4. Occasionally have pupils do something "for practice" without the threat of evaluation
5. Tie in evaluation with causes and consequences

Finally, Klausmeier offers some important suggestions toward fostering creative personalities [40]. He observes that creative individuals tend to be described as impulsive, sensitive, self-confident, independent, and unconventional rather than conforming, conventional, and dependent. A parent or teacher who would foster the creative personality must be prepared to encourage a wide variety of behaviors and ideas. The setting of clear boundary conditions is important, but so are wide tolerances for independence, autonomy, the unconventional, and the nonconforming.

MEMORY

Research on memory and its development has recently been accelerating. The many new ideas generated by this research present great promise for new understandings, just as they leave many new questions unanswered for the present. Several theories or models exist, each of which is especially useful for representing particular phenomena of memory and for organizing a body of research.

Information Processing

An information-processing model distinguishes three separate kinds of memory: sensory register, short-term memory, and long-term memory [4, 5]. This model presents a computer analogy of three common phenomena of memory. A variant of this approach, the depth-of-processing model, refers to a hierarchy of operations that control storage, or input processes, and retrieval, or output processes [14, 55]. The depth-of-processing model avoids the problems of distinguishing among the three kinds of memory, which is often difficult. It is potentially more useful for developmental research because ontogenetic changes in storage capacity have not been demonstrated and because changes in storage duration are assessed in terms of depth of processing within the hierarchy [64, 65]. However, this model represents more of a look forward than an assessment of the present state of the area. The precedence and didactic clarity of the three-stage model establish it as an important point of departure for any discussion of memory.

SENSORY REGISTER

The term **sensory register** refers to the impression left on the sensory end organ immediately following stimulation. This phenomenon was first studied by presenting subjects with information in the form of brief flashs of light; sensory register follows the initial pattern exactly and dissipates within one-half-second [71]. A study comparing people of different ages concluded that sensory register memory is the same across all ages studied: 5 years, 8 years, 11 years, and adulthood [69]. Memory failed with longer intervals up to 1 second in the younger children, possibly because of less effective processing of the impressions beyond initial registration.

As it has been studied in the visual mode, sensory register is similar in its photographic quality to eidetic images, although much shorter in duration. A person with eidetic imagery can recall, in amazing detail, parts of a display after a brief exposure, for instance, the spelling of a foreign word or the number of rungs in the back of a chair. One study found strong eidetic imagery in 8 percent of 8- and 12-year-olds [27]. A few people retain this talent into adulthood. It seems similar in quality to sensory register memory, but how the two phenomena may be related is not known.

SHORT-TERM MEMORY

Every person has had the experience of looking up a number in the telephone book and trying to carry it in the head across a room without losing it. Short-term memory is more impressionistic than sensory register, and it decays in a few seconds. Some kind of representational processing is assumed to be required in order to transfer information from sensory register to short-term storage [55]. The distinction is similar to that beween sensation and perception, the one being literal, the other interpretative and shaped by context and experience. The capacity of short-term storage is estimated at from five units [70] to nine units [50] of information, and items are susceptible to being "bumped" out of storage by additional information. Material in short-term memory can be retained longer with mnemonic, or memory, strategies, such as rehearsal (i.e., by repeating the information over and over). The use of such strategies becomes more effective with age, particularly during the school years.

Increasingly effective use of rehearsal over the school years has been indicated by recent research. When a series of words, for example, or a song is repeated over and over and tested for memory with each repetition, the typical result is that the first and the last parts are learned, or remembered, most readily, and the part in the middle is the most difficult. Remembering the first part well as opposed to the middle part is called the **primacy effect,** and remembering the last part well as opposed to the middle part is called the **recency effect.** A study of the serial learning of 18 unrelated words found the same recency effects for 8-, 11-, and 13-year-olds, but increasing primacy effects across these three ages. The primacy effects were greatest for the oldest children; that is, the older children had better memories for the first part of the list—but not the last part—than the younger children. These results were interpreted as indicating that there are no differences across ages in short-term memory (the recency effect) but increasingly effective mnemonic strategies with increases in age from 8 years to 13 years (the primacy effect) [52]; for example, older children rehearse larger numbers of words together than do younger children [53].

Short-term memory span is commonly included as one of the components of individual tests of intelligence. The number of digits that a child can recall after a single recitation increases with age and is correlated with intelligence at any age level. A 4-year-old can remember from three to four digits; a 12-year-old can remember six or seven.

Incidentally, children with reading disabilities frequently have poorer short-term memories than normal readers with the same IQ scores [77]. They are also less likely to use efficient rehearsal strategies [78].

LONG-TERM MEMORY

Long-term memory is the relatively permanent storehouse of what we know—the record of our lives and how we understand that record. The line separating short-term from long-term memory is not sharp, but the contents of long-term memory represent what one would generally refer to as memories or remembrances. Four conceptual categories suggested by Flavell and Wellman serve well to organize the relevant research; these categories are basic processes, knowledge, strategies, and metamemory [20].

Basic Processes

The most recent speculation theorizes that the basic "hardware" of memory systems, such as the elementary requisites for recognition and recall, is laid down by the end of the sensorimotor period, or by the second year after birth [21]. Habituation of the orienting response to a repeated sound, which indicates a primitive form of recognition, occurs as early as 4 weeks after birth [9], and Piaget's "deferred imitation," or the mimicking of a model not present, appears at the end of the sensorimotor period and indicates recall [58]. Thus, what little is known about the basic processes of memory (recognition and recall) concerns development during the first 2 years after birth.

Knowledge

Piaget and Inhelder distinguish between memory in the strict sense and memory in the wider sense [62]. The first category refers to a memory of a particular event, along with the feeling of certainty that the event really happened and that one was there when it did happen. The latter category includes what we generally refer to as knowledge, or our storehouse of understandings and cognitive schemes. A similar distinction is made between episodic memory and semantic memory [80].

One important point to be made here is that knowledge (or memory in the wider sense, or semantic memory) shapes perception; it shapes the storage of information as a constructive process; and it shapes information retrieval as a reconstructive process. A second important point is that one's knowledge changes dramatically over the period of concrete operations with the emergence of seriation, multiple classifications, the conservations, and relational concepts. Consequently, qualitative changes in memory may occur with the emergence of concrete operative processes. For example, an array of sticks increasing in height will be remembered differently according to whether or not a child is capable of seriation [62]. Furthermore, Piaget and Inhelder assert that memory may actually improve with a longer delay if this delay allows for further maturation of an important cognitive operation [62]. For instance, a serial array of sticks might be reconstructed by an 8-year-old as a random array at one point and as a serial array several months later without intervening exposure to the original array, presumably because of the further development of seriation, which is important in this context. This assertion has been supported by others [22, 46], and the phenomenon has been shown to be facilitated by training in seriation [47]. However, this particular example may illustrate changing reconstructive distortion rather than reconstructive correction; in one study a child was shown a disorderly array that was reconstructed several weeks later as an orderly series [1]. In any case, what is remembered changes dramatically during the school years according to systematic changes in cognitive operations.

Most of what we remember is not a literal depiction of an event but rather an inference or judgement based on our frame of reference and how we responded at the time. Research on memory as a reconstructive process has waxed and waned over many years [8]; interest in this process has recently been renewed [10]. Developmental research in this area has just begun, but early returns from research on school-age children indicate that the ability to apply inferential processes to develop a more meaningful memory from fragmented or partial information improves with age during the school years [56].

Strategies

There is a difference between knowing (semantic memory, or memory in the wider sense) and knowing how to know (what one does, actively and willfully, to enhance one's memory) [11]. Memory enhancers are known as **strategies** [20]. The strategies for improving memory and the storage of information include increasing study time, rehearsal, organization, and elaboration; strategies for improving memory upon retrieval include persisting in a search beyond the first failures, cross-referencing remote associations, and making a systematic search [21]. It is important to note that external strategies for improving memory exist as well as the internal strategies just mentioned. Taking notes, tying a string around one's finger, and asking someone for a reminder are examples of external strategies.

Definite changes in the use of strategies for improving memory occur across the school years. An illustration of such changes is the use of rehearsal by schoolchildren. The spontaneous use of rehearsal as a strategy was studied in 5-, 7-, and 10-year-olds by lipreading the subvocal, verbal rehearsals during a 15-second delay period before recall. With 20 children in each group, spontaneous rehearsal was detected in two 5-year-olds, in twelve 7-year-olds, and in seventeen 10-year-olds [18]. A subsequent study involved first-graders, some of whom rehearsed spontaneously and others of whom did not. The spontaneous rehearsers showed better memory than those who did not rehearse, but the latter group did just as well as the others when they were shown how to rehearse and did so. More than one-half of these same children, however, subsequently gave up rehearsing as testing continued [38]. The first-grade children who did not rehearse are said to be "production-deficient"; that is, they were able to rehearse, and when they did rehearse it improved their memory, but they did not produce this strategy spontaneously, without prompting [19]. Some children with reading disabilities are thought to be production-deficient with respect to rehearsal [78].

As children grow older, they tend more and more to produce the strategy of rehearsal spontaneously; thus the early school years compose a transitional period marking the emergence of rehearsal as a memory strategy. This development is paralleled by other simple strategies. When children were told that the waiting period between learning and testing would be longer than before, 8-year-olds spontaneously increased their study time, whereas 4- and 6-year-olds did not [66].

As one might imagine from an understanding of changes in children's abilities to classify during the concrete operational period, grouping items by categories also emerges as an effective mnemonic strategy during the school years, and it, too, goes through a transitional period of production deficiency, as did rehearsal [67]. The same may be true of elaboration, although the question remains undecided at this time. Flavell illustrates the strategy of elaboration in relating two disparate words, "elephant" and "pin," by suggesting that one "create an image of an elephant delicately balanced on the head of a pin, modestly acknowledging the applause of the audience" [21]. Then he challenges the reader to try forgetting the association! Although children may recognize the benefit of such elaboration for enhancing memory, it is unlikely that elaborations are spontaneously produced for this purpose until adolescence [67].

The little research currently available on develop-

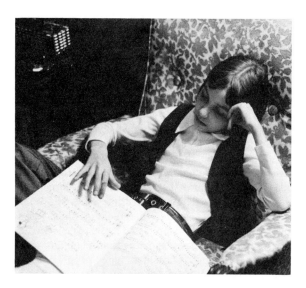

Figure 23-6. This girl is using sensorimotor memory skills to assist her with the memorization of highly abstract representational symbols (musical notes in this case).

mental changes in the use of retrieval strategies suggests a course similar to that of storage strategies: gradual and halting emergence through a transitional period, with production deficiency during the early and middle-school years and with spontaneous production and effective use toward the end of the concrete operational period [42, 43]. All the relevant research points to the elementary school years as being crucial for the development of knowing how to know.

It is worth noting that most research on memory concerns internal storage and retrieval processes. In the real world, however, we commonly benefit from many kinds of external assistance. When a teacher wants to send a message home, the child takes a note. Adults use external assists every day: leaving an envelope to be mailed in a prominent place, taking a grocery list to the store, or asking someone to remind one to pick up some stamps at the post office. There has been no systematic research on when these external devices develop in the individual, but children do use them and know that they help in remembering.

Metamemory

Children as young as 3 years of age know that when they are asked to remember where a toy is hidden, they will be expected to reveal its hiding place at a later time; they know what "remember" means [85]. Kindergarten and first-grade children know a lot more:

They know that they forget, and that events long past are harder to remember than recent events. They know that material may have certain aspects, such as meanings or relationships, that make it easier to remember, and that material learned once is easier to relearn. And they know that a lot is harder to learn and remember than a little. But compared with the third- or fifth-grader, the younger child's knowledge about memory, or metamemory, is diffuse and imprecise [44].

Although some first-graders know that older children remember better, third- and fifth-graders are more likely to understand that children of different ages study differently. Third- and fifth-graders know that distant events are harder to remember than recent ones, and that this is complicated by what goes on during the interval. They also know that the ability to remember varies over occasions, types of information, and individuals, and that these factors interact. For example, a long story requires more time to learn than a short story, and more still if retention is expected over a long interval, but less if recall is to be approximate but not verbatim, or less if only recognition will be required instead of recall [44].

Like strategies of memory, the development of metamemory undoubtedly varies with several factors. It has been suggested that one such factor is whether a problem is external or internal. An illustration of an external problem is as follows: "Suppose you lost your jacket while you were at school. How could you go about finding it?" [44]. Here is an internal problem: "Suppose you had a great idea about a present to buy your mother for her birthday and then forgot what it was. How could you find out what that present was?" [89]. When children 8 to 14 years of age were asked such questions, the number of solutions for external problems increased slightly from ages 8 to 10 years and leveled off thereafter; in contrast, the number of solutions for internal problems increased from ages 8 to 10 years and again from 10 to 12 years. This development parallels the transition from concrete operations to formal operations, with the shift away from necessary reliance on external events toward a greater facility with abstract thought.

Another dimension of metamemory, or knowing about knowing [11], is the knowledge of one's own memory capacity. Several studies indicate distinct changes in the middle-school years. In one study, children estimated how many pictures in a series they could remember completely after a brief look, the longest series consisting of 10 pictures. Twenty-four of 48 4-year-olds but only 5 of 48 8-year-olds said "all 10" [88]. In another study, the task was to inspect pictures for as long as necessary to memorize in anticipation of future recall. Second- and fourth-graders could do this fairly well, whereas kindergarten and nursery school children could not [19]. A third study examined the particular phenomenon referred to as "feeling of knowing": if you cannot recall the name of a thing seen, do you know whether or not you could select the name from the list? Third-graders were distinctly more accurate in their feeling of knowing judgments than kindergarteners or first-graders [84]. This finding was paralleled in a study of educable retarded children; accurate feeling of knowing judgments were made by children of mental ages 8 through 10 years but not by children with a mental age of 6 years [12].

The evidence on personal monitoring of memory capacity fits nicely with changes in ability during the school years. Apparently, children's sense of whether or not they hold something within themselves, such as a memory or an understanding, flowers during the middle-school years. This understanding emerges along with facilities for active and skilled learning. Children become executives over their cognitive processes during these years [51]. Increasing self-consciousness accompanies increasing self-awareness and a sense of effectiveness [86, 87]. Clearly, the school years bring dramatic changes in knowing about oneself and what one can do.

IMPLICATIONS

Safety
Pedestrian traffic accidents and drownings are leading causes of death for school-age children. Children sometimes know how to take care, but often they do not do so spontaneously and have to be reminded. The phenomenon of production deficiency referred to in the discussion of strategies for memory surely has a parallel in this area. As the school years proceed and as capacities for classification and analysis become more facile, the rules acquired here and there may become generalized and qualified to form constellations, including rules of safety or "how to take care of oneself."

Whether or not these rules are learned depends partly on the circumstances the children pass through and partly on the guidance of peers and elders. In part, coming to understand personal safety is a matter of survival; it is also a matter of growing to care for oneself as a valuable person who may eventually keep others safe with the same consideration as was received from parents and other adults.

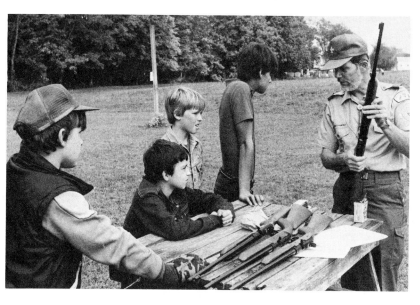

Figure 23–7. It is critical that children receive adequate instruction and develop a healthy sense of safety precautions before using new equipment.

Misdemeanors

Breaking out of the house, or home, sometimes coincides with breaking the law. Sometimes such an act (e.g., stealing) is rationalized within the new literalism of concrete operational thought: "I didn't steal that. All I did was take it from Rat. He gave it to me. How was I to know that it wasn't his?" And Rat says, "I just picked this thing off the counter and showed it to Bones. How did I know he would walk out of the store with it?"

Breaking rules, like lying, stealing, and cheating, can be a dramatic, desperate attempt to obtain recognition, as if the child were saying, "Look at me; pay attention to me. I can break your rules. Pay attention or I shall do worse!" Children who break rules often believe that their punishment is a necessary consequence of their misdemeanor. They know they have broken a rule, and they will not find relief until they are punished. Yet when they are punished, the adult who punishes them is demeaned by the act, as though the child's hypothesis of a vulnerable and fallible adult was denied by being caught but confirmed by being punished, to restore a lost balance. "You are worse than I for punishing one smaller than you. I am only a kid." Children in this situation are trapped in two ways: since they are not contained by adults, they break the rules of adults to capture their attention; when they are caught and punished, the adults who punish them are diminished in value. The result is a spiral of diminishing re-

turns. "If nobody cares about me except for punishing me, why should I care about anybody except for hurting them? They don't care about me. I don't care about them, or me, either!" As children try to measure their personal worth, some quickly learn that material goods and property are valued more than they. As long as they have the energy and the will, however, they can deny the lessons imposed by adults' punishment. They can lie, steal, cheat, and commit vandalism to get even, to confirm their knowledge that adults can be fooled, to bring attention to themselves, and to confirm their belief that they can reduce something more valuable than they to something no more valuable than they, to something of no value. They might wish for a different world, but they continually struggle to come to grips with the world that they think fate has dealt them.

Lying

Lying is sometimes done just to see if one can pull it off, to test one's ability to tell a tall story. Becoming acquainted with oneself as a distinct person includes understanding that one's knowledge, or what is in one's thoughts, is not obvious to others. Late in the intuitive stage and early in the concrete operational period, children are often very disturbed by people looking at them, especially parents or older siblings. "Don't look at me!" they shout. They are beginning to understand that they can have private thoughts, but they still are not sure as to whether the parental omniscience is really gone. Sometimes it seems as if parents can see right through them. After all, children's lies are often, as we say, transparent. The school-ager who resorts to lies may do so to avoid punishment or criticism for actions. Sometimes the child may lie to impress others, especially peers. Whatever motivates him or her, the school-ager is cognitively aware that the lies are untrue.

An 8-year-old was told by his parents not to go to play computer games with his buddy, as they had done before. A little after noon he and the friend left the house. The temperature was far below freezing, and a howling blizzard threatened to continue for the rest of the day. It did. "Where are you going?" "To ride bikes." Four hours later they returned. "Where have you been?" "Out riding bikes." There were no winners in that exchange. When "caught in a lie," the school-ager can be helped by an adult to better understand feelings if the adult guides the child in analyzing what he or she said and why it was said. A helpful approach such as this should aid children in self-evaluation without causing them to feel guilty.

Fears

The fears of school-age children become magnified with their imaginations and as they enter unfamiliar worlds. Five-year-olds fear the dark, bodily injury, and the parent's absence; six-year-olds are more afraid of strange noises, ghosts, and imagined phantoms in the closet or under the bed. Their intuition provokes more questions about what might be present behind facades or in dark corners. They also tend to fear the elements: fire, drowning, thunder and lightning, cyclones, and tornadoes. These fears continue into the next year, when a greater sensitivity to visual fears is added to the rest. (Do you remember trying to figure out how to turn out the light and get into bed safely before the mice [or whatever] jumped out and bit your toes? Hit the switch, one step, leap, and—zip—into bed and under the covers.) Seven-year-olds also worry about being late for school and about not being liked. Children of 8 and 9 years have fewer fears. Those that are mentioned tend to be reasonable, or more concrete—about personal failure or inadequacy, including not being able to understand the homework or to get it done in time. These fears usually diminish by 10 years of age.

In sum, children's fears change over the years. Some may persist for 1 year or more and be thoroughly resistant to explanation or assurance; others may appear abruptly and dissipate just as fast. A few fears are clearly tied to traumatic experiences, but these are the exceptions. More often, the fears of the school years are concrete representations of premonitions varying in vagueness. Whatever their origins, confrontation is to be avoided; assurance or refuge and security may help, and, if appropriate, so may opportunities for talking around an issue. The school-age child is capable of understanding explanations in concrete terms, and these explanations may sometimes afford encouragement. Most importantly, children's fears beg for respect. They may be "kid stuff" to older siblings and grownups, but to children going through them, they are real [29].

Beliefs

Doubts and questions about what lies beyond appearances begin to emerge around the fourth birthday. They increase exponentially for the next several years, throughout the intuitive stage. By approximately 7 years of age, a qualitative change has been accomplished: The child's knowledge of the world has changed. It is not that the 7-year-old knows more; rather, the 7-year-old has begun to know the world differently. Six and 7-year-olds hang their stockings at Christmas "just in case"; the 8-year-old does the same with the certain knowledge that Santa Claus is a myth promulgated by parents who are, occasionally, childlike. The stage of concrete operations has begun.

ASSUMPTIVE REALITIES

The emergent abilities of concrete operational children outstrip the egocentrism of preschoolers, that is, the inability to assume perspectives other than their own and the confusion of words and their referents. Because the operations of school-age children are emergent and not primarily shaped by experience, the revelations that reflect new mental facilities are treated as eternal verities newly discovered. These discoveries make their impression on the global, diffuse ideation that is typical of preoperational thought. The consequence is that the halo, or complex, of ideas surrounding a focus undergoes abrupt transformation on the basis of changes in an isolated idea. With respect to physical events, these new understandings typically coincide with those of others; with respect to interpersonal and social events, they often do not. Elkind calls these exaggerated and unqualified beliefs "assumptive realities" and explains them in terms of a characteristic tendency to confuse hypothesis or suggestion with reality [16]. This tendency to overgeneralize, to leap from a specific instance to a general conclusion, or for the intemperate exercise of induction, is a kind of egocentrism—a kind of confusion of subject and object. As Elkind puts it, "It is this lack of differentiation between assumption and fact that constitutes the egocentrism of the concrete operational period" [16].

COGNITIVE CONCEIT

A prominent manifestation of assumptive realities is "cognitive conceit" [16]. As the child's new concrete operational vision penetrates the aura of omniscience and omnipotence surrounding adults, particularly parents and teachers, the discovery that adults make mistakes is readily extrapolated to the conviction that all adults are clumsy, inept fools. The school-age child is not inclined to shout this discovery to the rooftops, but it is a delightful working theory that is sustained in spite of evidence to the contrary and that the child often goes to some lengths to support by contrivance. ("I *did* wash my hands. You didn't tell me to use soap!")

Evidence of cognitive conceit permeates children's stories and movies. The heroes of swashbuckling dramas often have preadolescent pals to demonstrate that their primary loyalties are really to kids. The other adult characters in these sagas are either well-intentioned folks who need a lot of help or villains who are either outwitted or bettered by skill and daring. There are also the extraordinary tales, such as *The Dana Girls* and *The Hardy Boys* mysteries.

In contrast to the imagined stupidity and ineptitude of adults, children imagine themselves to be adroit. This superiority is also presumed for close associates and perhaps a favorite adviser or teacher. Parents are sometimes baffled or frustrated in attempting to make what they believe to be a simple and obvious point when their child stands loyal to conflicting testimony related from a respected associate.

THE FOUNDLING FANTASY

An apparent by-product of cognitive conceit is the foundling fantasy that often appears in late childhood. Like the hero in *The Man in the Iron Mask* and Arthur in *The Sword in the Stone*, children imagine themselves to be foundlings born of aristocratic parents who will someday recognize them and elevate them to their true stations as heirs to power and wealth.

Continuities

It is important to recognize that cognitive conceit is practiced beyond the years of childhood and is, in fact, typical of the behavior of adults in many situations, individually as well as in groups. The exaggerated superiority of the in-group, the exaggerated inferiority and baseness of the out-group, and the leap to total acceptance or rejection on the most fragile evidence unfortunately characterize much of adult behavior as well as that of school-age children. The phrases "Love is blind" and "Don't throw the baby out with the bath water" illustrate the point. Analyses of calamitous errors of judgment made by high government officials—Pearl Harbor, the Bay of Pigs invasion, escalation of the Vietnam War, Watergate, and many other incidents—reveal many elements in common with the assumptive realities typical of childhood [32].

On the other hand, the same parallel might be drawn for some of the most heroic events in history—Masada, the Alamo, Stalingrad. Assumptive realities may exaggerate reality and denigrate other people, but they also provide the inspiration for exploration and taking chances beyond the given. An important task of childhood is the testing of assumptive realities. As they inspire children to venture beyond the present, these adventures further develop the storehouse of effective ways of dealing with the world. The next chapter will elaborate further on these tensions of childhood, where the major psychosocial crisis is portrayed as being between industry and inferiority.

Assumptive realities are treated as truths by children, but their salience as truths crests and ebbs above a sustaining ballast, partly afforded by previously formed senses of personal worth and continuity and partly afforded by trust in, and understanding of, guidelines set by parents. Cognitive conceit is an expression of hope for one's own competence; it is also an inspiration to adventure and a way to cope with one's foibles and failures. It results in many errors, but it also propels development forward. The process is facilitated by a basic confidence in personal continuity and that of the parents. Sometimes neither the parents nor the conceit offer much hope or security; such circumstances often provoke children to seek support outside of the home. Fortunate are those children whose parents can absorb the mental extravagances of school-agers and temper assumptive realities and cognitive conceit with the understanding that children's errors and foibles, as well as those of adults, may be treated with tolerance, resolution, and occasionally good humor.

SUMMARY

The cognitive development of the school-age child spans the intuitive thought of the 5- and 6-year-old through the concrete operational thought of the middle-school years to the threshold of formal operational thought in early adolescence. The ages of 7 and 8 years herald critical changes in cognitive functioning in the midst of increasing spheres of social interaction outside the home. Emergent modes of thinking leap from specific encounters to broadly applied generalizations about people and society as well as physical transformations and relations.

The new understandings of the physical universe approximate those of adulthood and receive a broad consensus of support from both peers and adults. The generalizations about people and society include significant peer groups outside the family and, far from receiving broad consensus, tend to separate people into various groups of "us" and "them." Furthermore, the affiliations with peers inevitably present to each child measures of competence against people who are comparable, as siblings and parents never were. These social interactions and their consequences for the school-age child are the subject of the next chapter.

REFERENCES

1. Altemeyer, R. A., Fulton, D., and Berney, K. M. Long-term memory improvement: Confirmation of a finding by Piaget. *Child Dev.* 40:845, 1969.
2. American Psychiatric Association. *Diagnostic and Statistical Manual of Mental Disorders, Edition 3.* Washington, DC: American Psychiatric Association, 1980.
3. Atkin, R., et al. Cross-lagged panel analysis of sixteen cognitive measures at four grade levels. *Child Dev.* 48:944, 1977.
4. Atkinson, R. C., and Shiffrin, R. M. Human Memory: A Proposed System and Its Control Process. In K. W. Spence and J. T. Spence (Eds.), *The Psychology of Learning and Motivation.* Vol. 2. New York: Academic, 1968.
5. Atkinson, R. C., and Shiffrin, R. M. The control of short-term memory. *Sci. Am.* 225:82, 1971.
6. Babad, E. Y., and Budoff, M. Sensitivity and validity of learning potential measurement in three levels of ability. *J. Educ. Psychol.* 66:439, 1974.
7. Barron, F. X. *Creative Person and Creative Process.* New York: Holt, Rinehart, and Winston, 1969.
8. Bartlett, F. C. *Remembering: A Study in Experimental and Social Psychology.* London: Cambridge University Press, 1964.
9. Brackbill, Y. The role of the cortex in orienting: Orienting reflex in an anencephalic human infant. *Dev. Psychol.* 5:195, 1971.
10. Bransford, J. D., and Franks, J. J. The abstraction of linguistic ideas. *Cognitive Psychol.* 2:331, 1971.
11. Brown, A. L. The Development of Memory: Knowing, Knowing About Knowing, and Knowing How to Know. In H. S. Reese (Ed.), *Advances in Child Development and Behavior.* Vol. 10. New York: Academic, 1975.
12. Brown, A. L., and Lawton, S. C. The feeling of knowing

experience in educable retarded children. *Dev. Psychol.* 13:364, 1977.
13. Budoff, M. Learning potential among institutionalized young adult retardates. *Am. J. Ment. Defic.* 72:404, 1967.
14. Craik, F. I. M., and Lockhart, R. S. Levels of processing: A framework for memory research. *J. Verb. Learn.* 11:671, 1972.
15. Dewey, J. *How We Think.* Chicago: Regnery, 1971.
16. Elkind, D. *Children and Adolescents: Interpretative Essays of Jean Piaget* (3rd ed.). New York: Oxford University Press, 1981.
17. Feldman, D. H., and Bratton, J. C. Relativity and giftedness: Implications for equality of educational opportunity. *Except. Child.* 38:491, 1972.
18. Flavell, J. H., Beach, D. H., and Chinsky, J. M. Spontaneous verbal rehearsal in a memory task as a function of age. *Child Dev.* 37:283, 1966.
19. Flavell, J. H., Friedrichs, A. G., and Hoyt, J. D. Developmental changes in memorization processes. *Cognitive Psychol.* 1:324, 1970.
20. Flavell, J. H., and Wellman, H. M. Metamemory. In R. V. Kail and J. W. Hagen (Eds.), *Memory in Cognitive Development.* Hillsdale, NJ: Erlbaum, 1976.
21. Flavell, J. H. *Cognitive Development* (4th ed.). New York: Wiley, 1983.
22. Furth, H., Ross, B., and Youniss, J. Operative understanding in children's immediate and long-term reproductions of drawings. *Child Dev.* 45:63, 1974.
23. Grossman, H. J. (Ed.). *Manual on Terminology and Classification in Mental Retardation.* Washington, DC: American Association of Mental Deficiency, 1977.
24. Guilford, J. P. Intelligence: 1965 model. *Am. Psychol.* 21:20, 1966.
25. Guilford, J. P. *The Nature of Human Intelligence.* New York: McGraw-Hill, 1967.
26. Guilford, J. P., and Hoepfner, R. *The Analysis of Intelligence.* New York: McGraw-Hill, 1971.
27. Haber, R. N., and Haber, R. B. Eidetic imagery: I. Frequency. *Percept. Mot. Skills* 19:131, 1964.
28. Heber, R. A manual on terminology and classification in mental retardation. *Am. J. Ment. Defic.* (Monograph Suppl.), 1961.
29. Ilg, F. L., Ames, L. B., and Baker, S. M. *Child Behavior* (Rev. ed.). New York: Barnes and Noble, 1982.
30. Inhelder, B. *The Diagnosis of Reasoning in the Mentally Retarded.* Translated by W. B. Stephens et al. New York: John Day, 1968.
31. Inhelder, B., and Piaget, J. *The Early Growth of Logic in the Child.* New York: Humanities Press, 1970.
32. Janis, I. L. *Victims of Groupthink: A Psychological Study of Foreign-Policy Decisions and Fiascoes.* Boston: Houghton Mifflin, 1972.
33. Jensen, A. R. How much can we boost IQ and scholastic achievement? *Harvard Educ. Review* 39:1, 1969.
34. Jensen, A. R. Cumulative deficit: A testable hypothesis? *Dev. Psychol.* 10:996, 1974.

35. Jensen, A. R. Cumulative deficit in IQ of Blacks in the rural South. *Dev. Psychol.* 13:184, 1977.

36. Kagan, J. Reflection impulsivity and reading ability in primary grade children. *Child Dev.* 36:609, 1965.

37. Kamin, L. J. *The Science and Politics of IQ.* New York: Wiley, 1974.

38. Keeney, T. J., Cannizzo, S. R., and Flavell, J. H. Spontaneous and induced verbal rehearsal in a recall task. *Child Dev.* 38:953, 1967.

39. Keller, H. A. *The Story of My Life.* New York: Grosset & Dunlap, 1903.

40. Klausmeier, H. J., and Goodwin, W. *Learning and Human Abilities: Educational Psychology* (4th ed.). New York: Harper & Row, 1975.

41. Klein, N. K., and Safford, P. L. Application of Piaget's theory to the study of thinking of the mentally retarded: A review of research. *J. Spec. Educ.* 11:201, 1977.

42. Kobasigawa, A. Utilization of retrieval cues by children in recall. *Child Dev.* 45:127, 1974.

43. Kobasigawa, A. Retrieval Strategies in the Development of Memory. In R. V. Kail and J. W. Hagen (Eds.), *Memory in Cognitive Development.* Hillsdale, NJ: Erlbaum, 1976.

44. Kreutzer, M. A., Leonard, C. A., and Flavell, J. H. An interview study of children's knowledge about memory. *Monogr. Soc. Res. Child Dev.* 40(1), Serial No. 159, 1975.

45. Lambert, N. M., Wilcox, M. R., and Gleason, W. P. *The Educationally Retarded Child: Comprehensive Assessment and Planning for Slow Learners and the Educable Mentally Retarded.* New York: Grune & Stratton, 1974.

46. Liben, L. S. Long-term memory for pictures related to seriation, horizontality, and verticality concepts. *Dev. Psychol.* 11:795, 1975.

47. Liben, L. S. The facilitation of long-term memory improvement and operative development. *Dev. Psychol.* 13:501, 1977.

48. MacMillan, D. The problem of motivation in the education of the mentally retarded. *Except. Child.* 37:579, 1971.

49. Martinson, R., Hermenson, D., and Banks, G. An independent study-seminar program for the gifted. *Except. Child.* 38:421, 1972.

50. Miller, G. A. The magical number seven plus or minus two: Some limits on our capacity for processing information. *Psychol. Rev.* 63:81, 1956.

51. Mussen, P. H., Conger, J. J., and Kagan, J. *Child Development and Personality* (6th ed.). New York: Harper & Row, 1984.

52. Ornstein, P. A., Naus, M. J., and Liberty, C. Rehearsal and organizational processes in children's memory. *Child Dev.* 46:818, 1975.

53. Ornstein, P. A., Naus, M. J., and Stone, B. P. Rehearsal training and development differences in memory. *Dev. Psychol.* 13:15, 1977.

54. Ostrander, S., et al. *Superlearning.* New York: Dell, 1979.

55. Paivio, A. *Imagery and Verbal Processes.* Hillsdale, NJ: Erlbaum, 1979.

56. Paris, S. G. Integration and Inference in Children's Comprehension and Memory. In F. Restle et al. (Eds.), *Cognitive Theory.* Vol. 1. Hillsdale, NJ: Erlbaum, 1975.

57. Pregnato, C., and Birch, J. W. Locating gifted children in junior high school: A comparison of methods. *Except. Child.* 25:300, 1959.

58. Piaget, J. *Play, Dreams, and Imitation in Childhood.* Translated by C. Gattengo and F. M. Hodgson. New York: Norton, 1951.

59. Piaget, J. Piaget's Theory. In P. H. Mussen (Ed.), *Carmichael's Manual of Child Psychology* (3rd ed.). New York: Wiley, 1970.

60. Piaget, J. *Science of Education and the Psychology of the Child.* Translated by D. Coltman. New York: Orion, 1970.

61. Piaget, J. *The Child's Conception of Time.* Translated by A. J. Pomerans. New York: Ballantine, 1971.

62. Piaget, J., and Inhelder, B. *Memory and Intelligence.* Translated by A. J. Pomerans. New York: Basic Books, 1973.

63. Pick, A. D., Frankel, D. G., and Hess, V. L. Children's Attention: The Development of Selectivity. In E. M. Hetherington, et al. (Ed.), *Review of Child Development Research.* Vol. 5. Chicago: University of Chicago Press, 1975.

64. Reese, H. W. Memory Development in Childhood: Life-Span Perspectives. In H. W. Rees, *Advances in Child Development and Behavior.* Vol. 11. New York: Academic, 1976.

65. Reese, H. W. Models of memory development. *Hum. Dev.* 19:291, 1976.

66. Rogoff, B., Newcomb, N., and Kagan, J. "Planfulness and Recognition Memory." Unpublished study, 1974 (cited in Kreutzer et al. [44]).

67. Rohwer, W. D. Elaboration and Learning in Childhood and Adolescence. In H. W. Rees (Ed.), *Advances in Child Development and Behavior.* Vol. 8. New York: Academic, 1973.

68. Rosenthal, R., and Jacobson, L. *Pygmalion in the Classroom: Teacher Expectation and Pupils' Intellectual Development* (Enlarged ed.). New York: Irvington Publishers, 1983.

69. Sheingold, K. Developmental differences in intake and storage of visual information. *J. Exp. Child Psychol.* 16:1, 1973.

70. Simon, H. A. How big is a chunk? *Science* 183:482, 1974.

71. Sperling, G. The information available in brief visual presentations. *Psychological Monographs* 74: Whole No. 498, 1960.

72. Springer, S. P., and Deutsch, G. *Left Brain, Right Brain.* San Francisco: Freeman, 1981.

73. Sullivan, A. Letters. In H. A. Keller, *The Story of My Life.* New York: Grosset & Dunlap, 1903.

74. Terman, L. M. Mental and Physical Traits of a Thousand Gifted Children. In L. M. Terman (Ed.), *Genetic Studies of Genius.* Stanford, CA: Stanford University Press, 1925.

75. Terman, L. M. The discovery and encouragement of exceptional talent. *Am. Psychol.* 9:221, 1954.

76. Terman, L. M., and Merrill, M. A. *Stanford-Binet Intelligence Scale*. Boston: Houghton Mifflin, 1973.

77. Torgesen, J. Problems and Prospects in the Study of Learning Disabilities. In E. M. Hetherington (Ed.), *Review of Child Development Research*. Vol. 5. Chicago: University of Chicago Press, 1975.

78. Torgesen, J., and Goldman, T. Verbal rehearsal and short-term memory in reading-disabled children. *Child Dev.* 48:56, 1977.

79. Torrance, E. P. *Rewarding Creative Behavior: Experiments in Classroom Creativity*. Englewood Cliffs, NJ: Prentice-Hall, 1965.

80. Tulving, E., and Donaldson, W. (Eds.). Episodic and Semantic Memory. In E. Tulving and W. Donaldson (Eds.), *Organization of Memory*. New York: Academic, 1972.

81. Wallach, M. A., and Kogan, N. *Modes of Thinking in Young Children: A Study of the Creativity-Intelligence Distinction*. Westport, CT: Greenwood Press, 1984.

82. Wallas, G. *The Art of Thought*. London: Watts, 1946.

83. Wechsler, D. *Wechsler Intelligence Scale for Children—Revised*. New York: Psychological Corporation, 1974.

84. Wellman, H. M. Tip of the tongue and feeling of knowing experiences: A development study of memory monitoring. *Child Dev.* 48:13, 1977.

85. Wellman, H. M., Ritter, K., and Flavell, J. H. Deliberate memory behavior in the delayed reactions of very young children. *Dev. Psychol.* 11:780, 1975.

86. White, R. W. Motivation reconsidered: The concept of competence. *Psychol. Rev.* 66:297, 1959.

87. White, R. W. Competence and the Psychosexual Stages of Development. In M. R. Jones (Ed.), *Nebraska Symposium on Motivation*. Vol. 8. Lincoln, NE: University of Nebraska Press, 1960.

88. Yussen, S. R., and Levy, V. M. Developmental changes in predicting one's own span of short-term memory. *J. Exp. Child Psychol.* 19:502, 1975.

89. Yussen, S. R., and Levy, V. M. Developmental changes in knowledge about different retrieval problems. *Dev. Psychol.* 13:114, 1977.

24

Psychosocial Development During the School-Age Years

Joseph Rapalje, Douglas Degelman, and Shirley S. Ashburn

> Childhood has its own way of seeing, thinking, and feeling, and nothing is more foolish than to try to substitute ours for theirs.
>
> —Rousseau

Introduction

Perspectives on Psychosocial Development
Psychodynamic views
Learning theories
Humanistic views

Widening the Social Environment
Family
School
Peers
Mass media

Developing a Positive Self-Image
Individualizing identity
Factors affecting the self-concept
Fostering positive self-esteem
Getting through the pubescent years

Developmental Concerns
Anxieties
School phobia
Illness and hospitalization
Incestuous assault

Summary

The school-age years are a time of new experiences, new challenges, and new adjustments. The excitement of entry into school is accompanied by new demands and pressures. Among the many developmental tasks confronting the school-age child are the following: (1) achieving personal independence, (2) forming friendships with peers, (3) developing fundamental skills of reading and writing, and (4) maintaining and further developing a healthy self-image [32].

Entry into school represents a major life event that is as radical for this age as the transitions to college, married status, and parenthood are later on in life. Each major life change embodies the potential for both growth and stress, since each of these transitions requires adaptation and orientation to a new environment [77].

PERSPECTIVES ON PSYCHOSOCIAL DEVELOPMENT

Each theorist provides a different perspective on the changes that occur during the school-age years. These perspectives generally are complementary rather than competing, and taken together, they provide a more balanced view of development.

Psychodynamic Views

FREUD

Although Freud (see Appendix B) paid relatively little attention to the school-age years (what he called the stage of latency), he highlighted several significant characteristics of children at this stage. First, there is an emphasis on same-sex relationships. Second, there is a rigid adherence to the rules of parents and society in general. Having resolved the Oedipal conflict of the phallic stage, the child has repressed the sexual urges of the first years of life. This repression of sexual urges not only leads to a preponderance of same-sex relationships but also to the control of thoughts that have a sexual focus.

The resolution of the Oedipal conflict also results in the child's adoption of the parental value system. This acceptance of the parental (and therefore society's) values leads to a rigid adherence to, and reliance on, "the rules of the game." This becomes a critical factor in the enculturation process.

Most neo-Freudians and most non-Freudians observe that school-agers exhibit strong rather than dormant feelings. School-agers channel these energies into their play, studies, and sports. Emotions are further mobilized in their avid interests in life, death, religion, politics, the arts, and social interactions. However, although an interest in sexual matters may continue, it is suppressed in conformity to social standards only to emerge again when the child reaches puberty.

ERIKSON

In Erikson's extension and refinement of Freud's theory, the school-age years are characterized by the psychosocial crisis of industry versus inferiority (see Appendix B). The emphasis is on meaningful effort or a desire to accomplish something of consequence [21]. The major theme of the phase reflects the child's de-

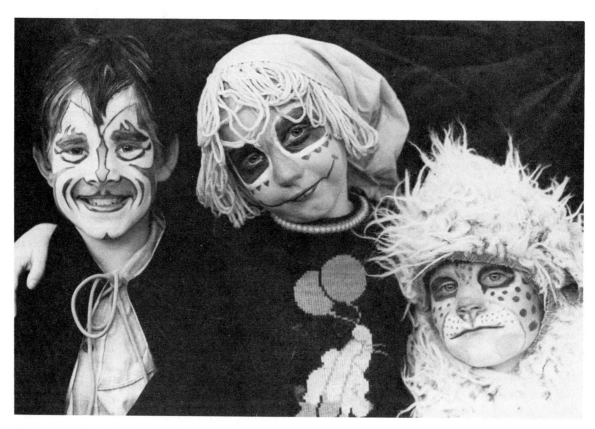

Figure 24–1. School-agers begin to recognize and to develop their uniqueness within the limits of peer boundaries and cultural opportunities.

termination to do something and to do it well. Children begin to extend efforts to learn tasks that are essential for successful adulthood in the culture. In American society, the focus is on formal education and competition. In other societies, the emphasis may be on farming, hunting, or survival. In American society, if a child has been adequately prepared for school and has been presented with appropriate tasks by parents, this period will foster feelings of competence and self-worth. On the other hand, if a child is ill-prepared for the tasks of school, feelings of incompetence, inferiority, worthlessness, and helplessness may result.

Children at this stage of development are usually eager to learn new tasks and skills. Success leads to increased eagerness to learn. Success functions as an immunization against the helplessness syndrome. Hobbies and collections are common among school-agers and play an important role in increasing the child's knowledge about a selected area (stamps, seashells, hub caps, types of dogs or cars, and so forth), giving the child some expertise, a source of respect from others, and pride in self. Some children may place so much importance on mastering technical skills (e.g., musical instrument, sewing, gymnastics, sports) that they may neglect their relationships with other people. Parents need to help them find a healthy balance between intraindividual and interindividual skills.

Learning Theories

Learning theorists present a different perspective on the years of middle childhood. Rather than emphasizing internal drives and repressed conflicts, the learning theorist looks to external factors in explaining the actions of children. In addition to emphasizing consequences of actions, learning theorists, such as Bandura, identify factors that are not unique to the school-age years but take on added significance during these years. Imitation may be the most important of these factors [4]. Observational learning is a complex process, but the basic ideas are clear—children learn by observing others in order to understand how they should act and how they may be responded to in the future. Many of the requisite skills involved in observational learning converge in children during the school-age years: the ability to attend to the relevant aspects of a model, the ability to assess and retain relevant information, and the ability to imitate appropriate behavior. Children concentrate on learning the skills they plan to use in later life, whether positive (such as piano playing, dancing, art, or swimming) or negative (such as shoplifting or cheating).

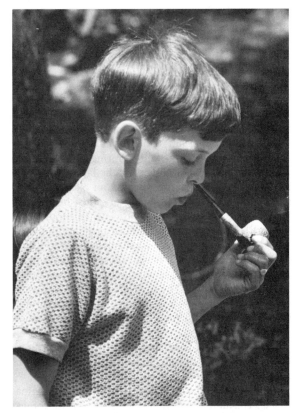

Figure 24–2. School-agers learn culturally approved roles by emulating the behaviors of adults. Unlike the preschooler, who imitates close family members, the school-ager may be influenced by others outside the immediate family.

Humanistic Views

Rather than emphasizing internal forces or external consequences, the humanistic perspective focuses on the distinctively human qualities of choice, freedom, self-actualization, dignity, and worth. Although not directly addressing significant characteristics of the school-age years, a few implications for these years can be extracted from the works of prominent theorists. The humanistic perspective does not pose stages of development; rather, it suggests a **process** of moving toward the actualization of potentials. As in Erikson's formulation of the psychosocial crisis of industry versus inferiority, the humanistic perspective emphasizes a desire to accomplish something worthwhile, a testing period in which individual efforts move the individual toward self-actualization. Many of the school-ager's efforts are directed toward unity with the culture (belongingness) and approval of the family and the peer group (love)—the third stage of Maslow's hierarchy (see Appendix B).

WIDENING THE SOCIAL ENVIRONMENT

Family

Two equally important conclusions can be drawn about the influence of the family during the school-age years: (1) The relative influence of the family is diminishing; and (2) the family remains an extremely important influence. Both conclusions must be kept in mind in order to have a balanced view. To support the first of these conclusions, we must examine the widening social environment—most obviously, the influence of the school. Teachers begin to serve as important adult models, and may, in some circumstances, serve as parent-substitutes. The time spent with peers is increasing, and the need to belong within the peer group becomes paramount. As a child becomes more competent socially, greater opportunities for peer contact emerge—trips with friends to school, church, or club. Necessarily, then, the proportion of time spent with family is diminished.

Nevertheless, the influence of parents remains strong. The family can provide a secure base for forays into the world while providing a haven for hasty retreats. The certainty of parental love remains a necessary anchor in the lives of school-age children. Further, parents serve as safe sounding boards for ideas and actions. At this age, even though children may verbalize less love and respect for their parents, they continue to look to parents as authoritative sources of information and sources of unconditional love. They use their parents as touchstones to evaluate their own abilities and goals. Parents of school-agers need reassurance that even the most critical children will not tolerate any outside criticism of their parents. Children's attitudes about their own abilities are influenced more by the parents' attitudes about the children's abilities than by the children's own past performances in those areas [58].

It is important for parents to retain a warm, accepting attitude, while gradually encouraging and supporting greater independence on the part of the child [6, 50]. The confident parent is able to assist the child in achieving greater independence (although probably not as much as the child says he or she wants), while still providing the necessary limits and authority without which the child would flounder.

When we think of a family unit, we typically think of the nuclear family with the father as the provider and the mother as the primary caretaker for the children. Marked variations in family constitution are present in every culture. Two increasingly important variations of familial relationships in the United States are the two-provider family and the single-parent family.

TWO-PROVIDER FAMILY

The two-provider family represents the most common variation of the traditional family. Nearly two-thirds of the mothers of school-age children in the United States are now employed either full- or part-time [85]. The reasons for this shift are varied, but economic necessity and the changing attitudes about the roles of women are cited. In 1979, over 25 million persons (11.6% of the population) lived below the official poverty line. Keniston has suggested that this figure presents too rosy a picture and estimates that between one-fourth and one-third of all children in the United States are born into families with "financial strains so great that their children will suffer basic deprivations" [43]. Since school-age children often develop sensitivities to externals, such as clothes and possessions, financial stress can impact significantly on the child's social as well as physical status during this period.

There is no clear pattern of evidence suggesting any adverse effects of two-provider families on the psychological development of school-age children. Most studies find no adverse effects, while a few studies have revealed some adjustment problems for the sons of lower and middle-class employed mothers [48]. This may result from the son's perception that the father has failed in his role as a provider. Child-rearing attitudes of employed mothers of school-age children differ little from those of comparable unemployed mothers [61]. Similarly, no differences in control or discipline are noted. The school-age child of an employed mother perceives the mother as no less loving or affectionate than children of unemployed mothers.

In some respects, children of two-provider homes may have an advantage. One clear result of recent research on two-provider families shows that both boys and girls have fewer sex-stereotyped attitudes when the mother is employed [27, 48, 55]. School-age daughters of employed mothers are likely to want to work when they grow up [37]. School-age children of employed mothers tend to have greater responsibilities in the home [36]. The mothers may encourage greater independence in the children, which may in turn tend to enhance feelings of self-esteem and competence in the children.

Interestingly, the movement of mothers into the work force has not been matched by a reciprocal move by fathers into a sharing of home responsibilities. This phenomenon in some cases may have to do with the site of the tasks rather than the nature of the tasks [7]. For example, cooking may be acceptable for a man on a camping trip, but not in the kitchen. Clearly, there are many factors that affect the willingness to share the division of labor in the home, such as the nature of each spouse's employment, whether the wife works full-time or less, the work schedule of each spouse, and the power division in the relationship [55]. Regardless of the reasons, the result has been an additional burden for many employed mothers who are expected to retain the bulk of work responsibilities in the home. Consequently, a child may still be exposed to traditional, stereotypic, culturally imposed gender roles even though he or she is verbally encouraged to assume a more egalitarian, nonsexist philosophy toward life.

LATCH-KEY CHILDREN

Because of the need for many parents to work outside the home, millions of children are left alone for prolonged periods before and after school and during vacations. These "latch-key" children are often given responsibilities beyond the usual age-appropriate norms and may be expected to perform in a manner beyond their developmental level. Some of these children are expected to come home after school, clean the house, do laundry, care for the younger children, and possibly even prepare the dinner. By giving children specific responsibilities, the parents not only lighten their own burden of housekeeping, but they believe that they keep the children's time sufficiently occupied to reduce the opportunities to "get into trouble." These children frequently are not permitted to waste time in activities considered unimportant by the parents. Consequently, latch-key children may not participate in school activities and may develop few peer friendships. Other latch-key children are left to "roam the streets" unsupervised, frequently feeling bored or lonely—factors that can lead to depression, restlessness, or mischief. It is important for all family members to share in homemaking responsibilities yet to allow children sufficient time to develop their own interests and skills.

Younger children need the security of access to a responsible adult (e.g., peer's mother, neighbor, grandmother). More mature preadolescents, if left alone for a period of time before and after school, should know how to reach help. A friendly note from Mom or Dad left on the refrigerator door combats the loneliness and helps to maintain family unity. Many communities are now providing appropriate and safe after-school programs, but the availability is not as great as the need.

SINGLE-PARENT FAMILY

The second common variation of family is the single-parent family. Although there are many reasons (e.g., choice, death of spouse, imprisonment of spouse, military service), most single-parent families are the result of divorce. The effects of the single-parent family on the psychological development of the children involved may have more to do with the child's perception of the causes of the absence rather than with the causes themselves. Over 90 percent of single-parent families are comprised of mothers and children. There are over ten million children in the United States in father-absent homes. It has been estimated that 20 percent of children today will spend at least part of their childhood in a single-parent home [47].

THE EFFECTS OF DIVORCE

The effects of divorce on children depend on factors, such as the age of the children at the time of separation, the number of children, the degree of financial stress, and the involvement and the relationship with the noncustodial parent following separation. Although divorce is usually a stressful time for both parents and children, there are some indications that the period immediately prior to divorce may be even more stressful because of the tensions between the parents [70].

Many studies examining the effects of divorce on children have focused on preschoolers. The conclusions emerging from these studies indicate that severe disruptions in play and social behaviors are evident for the first year following the divorce. For male children, these negative effects may endure for years, while for female children, most of the adverse effects have disappeared after 2 years [35].

There is "something very important about the ongoing, continuous relationship of a child with the same-sexed parent" [70]. One study examining the effects of divorce on school-age children compared intact families, father-custody families, and mother-custody families [70]. These investigators found that children with the same-sex custodial parent were more mature, more sociable, and more independent. Competent social behavior in these school-aged children was also positively correlated with authoritative parenting (in which there is a warm relationship and a clear setting of rules, but a willingness to discuss those rules).

A second study assessing the effects of divorce on school-age children examined families where the father had been present until the child was 6 years of age and then absent for the following 2 to 3 years [33]. Some important findings were that the negative effects of divorce were lessened when a positive relationship was maintained with both parents. The child's relationship with the noncustodial parent (the father) proved to be just as important as the continuing relationship with the mother.

Realistically, not all children are able to maintain a continuing relationship with the absent parent. One of the long-term consequences of divorce for both male and female children may be a less positive perception of their relationship with their fathers than the children from intact families [23]. Several factors may contribute to these differences, among them continued friction between mother and father, and court settlements that do not provide the noncustodial parent the opportunity to spend time with the children on a daily basis.

Richard Gardner, in *The Boys and Girls Book About Divorce*, speaks honestly and directly to children and adolescents about the feelings they may experience when their parents get divorced. For each problem he describes, he gives practical suggestions as to what these young people can do to make themselves feel better, and describes activities that will make life more pleasant for them and for their parents.

School

When a child begins school, dependence on the family diminishes as greater responsibility is assumed by the child. The child quickly learns that the criteria used in school to evaluate performance are different from those used in the home [20]. Until entry into school, children are judged on the basis of their past performances. In school, however, children quickly learn that they are being evaluated and compared with others. Elkind argues that the increasing assessment by testing has led to a "factory" model of education, where the emphasis is on accountability [18]. The result of this model, according to Elkind, is excessive pressure on the child and a shifting of focus from learning to the end result, grades. One result of this shift is a decrease in the amount of contact time between teacher and student. At least one researcher has argued that after taking into consideration the personal characteristics of teacher and student, the most important factor in the learning process may be the length of time the teacher and the student are together [11].

One crucial component of the educational process is the self-image of the child. School experiences are filtered through the self-image, while those same experiences may serve to modify the self-image. Thus, negative experiences early in the school career may change the child's view of self, which may in turn affect the actions in which the child chooses to engage. Clearly, the potential impact of schooling on self-image as well as self-image on schooling is great in both cases. As early as second grade, the level and the stability of self-esteem are positively correlated with academic achievement [45].

Children's attitudes about school are not formed exclusively at school. Parental support and encouragement of the child's involvement and participation in school activities are very important [57]. Parents can demonstrate this support by attending parent-teacher conferences, by spending time with the child talking about what is happening at school, and by involvement in the child's homework. What is common to all of these parental activities is a willingness to spend time on matters of importance to the child. The general level of family interest in intellectual pursuits also is a factor that contributes to the child's attitudes about school.

Although Rosenthal and Jacobsen's classic study of teacher expectations has generated considerable methodological criticism, the importance of teacher expectations on student achievement has been reaffirmed repeatedly [61, 68]. There are indications that the magnitude of these effects may be greatest during the first 3 years of school when children are aware that they are being evaluated but have a limited understanding of the bases of those judgments. Children want to be regarded as valuable human beings; consequently, they strive very hard to fulfill the teacher's expectations and to avoid disapproval. The teacher frequently becomes a surrogate parent during school hours and plays a very important role in molding a child's self-esteem.

Rosenthal has identified four factors which may account for the teacher expectation effect [68]. First, teachers may interact in a more friendly, concerned manner with students who are expected to do well. Second, teachers may provide more feedback, both positive and negative, to these students. Third, teachers may simply spend more time teaching the children of whom they have high expectations [51]. Fourth, teachers may require more responses from these students.

Peers

The peer group (classmates, playmates) provides many of the same opportunities for socialization that siblings do—how to deal with aggression, competition, inti-

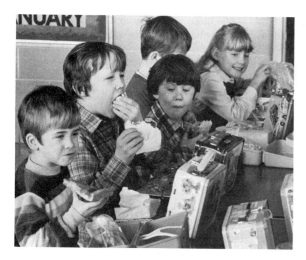

Figure 24–3. Lunch time provides opportunity for free social exchanges, which aid in the development of interpersonal relationships.

macy, and so forth. But peers also begin to introduce the child to the broader culture and to the differences between families and individuals. Companionship, broadened knowledge, and flexibility are valuable contributions of peer relationships.

FUNCTION OF PEERS

Peers provide the school-age child with the opportunities to develop social competence. They also serve as a measure for comparing the child's status in the group and as a sounding board for the child to obtain information about self. Children learn about the rules of behavior in a peer group and will experience various degrees of acceptance and rejection. Rejection tends to cause a downward spiral: Unpopular children are more likely to be low achievers in school [8, 13], to experience learning difficulties [1], and to drop out of school [84] than are their socially accepted peers. The consequences of low-peer acceptance, however, may go beyond academic problems [3]. Childhood unpopularity is highly correlated with behavior problems, such as juvenile delinquency [67], bad conduct discharges from military service [65], and the occurrence of emotional and mental health problems in adulthood [17] that include adult schizophrenia [80], neuroses [66], and psychoses [45, 65]. It is difficult to know whether peer rejection is based on deficiencies in the target child or itself creates the deficiencies.

A recent study of popular and unpopular children found that unpopular children were perceived by teachers as being more unpopular, depressed, and deviant than were popular children [86]. Classroom observations indicated that unpopular children spent significantly less time on-task than popular children and engaged in significantly more negative interactions. There was a tendency for popular children to perform at a higher academic level than unpopular children.

Unpopular children, when attempting to enter groups, tend to disrupt the ongoing activity and frequently attempt to call attention to themselves by physical contact, stating their feelings and opinions, talking about themselves, or asking redundant or irrelevant questions. These strategies frequently cause these children to be ignored or rejected by the group rather than accepted. Several interventions are suggested [63]. First, any intervention should involve teaching children ways to prevent situations that will lead to disagreements (for example, giving a general reason for a disagreement and suggesting an alternative action for the child). Second, any intervention should attempt to reduce children's use of behaviors that draw negative attention to themselves. They should be encouraged to determine the group's frame of reference, to find points of agreement, and to exchange information with group members. A third approach is to teach the child how to handle a difficult situation with confidence through role-taking.

Children develop social skills through these interactions with their environment. Through the active process of resolving social and cognitive conflicts, the child constructs his or her way of viewing the world. An important function of the peer group is to teach the child how to view the world through the eyes of other people. Jean Piaget has stated that the interactions that enhance role-taking allow a diminishing of egocentrism [60]. Such interactions are more effective when each participant modifies his or her intended behavior in anticipation of the other's reaction. Cooperative social interaction allows this modification to occur because children functioning in a group must recognize the difference between their own preoccupations and those of others. "It is cooperation that leads to the primacy of intentionality, by forcing the individual to be constantly occupied with the point of view of other people so as to compare it with his" [60].

Clubs and social groups introduce the child to the community, community needs, and community resources (e.g., church, scouts, Junior Red Cross, 4-H, YMCA). The time spent with nonneighborhood peers and community adults helps the child to learn more about the broader culture. The laws, the customs, and the relationships that operate outside the family system are learned. Clubs offer an arena to test one's emerging skills and to learn how to blend into the larger culture.

Classrooms using cooperative peer-initiated group learning have been compared with other more traditional teacher-centered methods [10]. Role-taking was found to be enhanced by cooperative interdependence. Support is found for Piaget's assumption that cooperative peer exchange promotes perspective taking. There is also a high positive correlation of cooperativeness and supportiveness with social preference [15]. Helping the child to see the view of another peer is clearly a valuable function of the peer group. The peer group also helps the child to interpret parental behavior as the group discusses rules and shares experiences.

When evaluating a child's behavior, an account must be taken not only of peer norms (approval or disapproval) for behavior but also of peer standards for parental behavior as well [40, 75]. While peer influences may take precedence in certain behaviors and fads ("*Everybody* wears blue on Monday"; "*Nobody* eats that kind of sandwich"), parental values are likely to have greater influence on more fundamental issues, such as life goals, especially those concerning education. In most middle- and upper-class groups, scholastic success is positively valued and explicitly rewarded not only by the teacher but also by the parents and the peers. Lower-class children are less likely to be encouraged by parents or peers to strive academically [56].

GROUP FORMATION

One of the tasks of middle childhood is to make attachments to age-mates. As children increase their interactions with peers, they form groups that possess common goals, aims, and rules of conduct. They learn the value that peers place on cooperation and competition as well as on the hierarchical organization or structure of a group.

Prior to the ninth birthday, children tend to mingle in informal groups composed of who is available and who is interested in the same activity. At about 8 or 9 years of age gender groupings begin to appear. At first they are small and unstable ("Yesterday April was my best friend; today it is Kim"). The intensity of relationships increases and will peak in the junior high-school years and will abate around pubescence. Affiliations gradually form around particular interests and activities (e.g., science club, swim team), and the number of affiliations increases.

As groups form, children begin to feel a cohesive-ness that binds them to the group. One study was designed to instill cohesiveness and solidarity within two separate groups of male children [74]. When these children were first divided into two groups, they expressed considerable resentment at being separated from their friends. The members of the first group stated that 65 percent of their friends were in the opposite group; the members of the second group likewise stated that 65 percent of their best friends were in the first group. The members of each group participated together in many enjoyable events, such as camping out, cooking meals, improving a swimming hole, clearing athletic fields, boating, and various games. Eventually, each group achieved its own identity and even selected its own name (tough-fighting names, such as Bull Dogs and Red Devils). Each group created flags and other identifying symbols. Within 5 days, the initial resentment had vanished, and new friendships became firmly established. Ninety-five percent of the Red Devils now chose fellow Red Devils for friends, and 88 percent of the Bull Dogs similarly chose friends from their own group. This study and others clearly show the importance of cooperation and common goals in the formation and cohesion of groups [74]. Moreover, even a grouping together of people that is entirely independent of any prior association or shared interest can make them discriminate against an outgroup [80].

Older children and dominant children tend to be highly influential in the formation of groups, especially in our highly competitive American society. Older children tend to base status structures on appearance, leadership skills, pubertal development, athletic prowess, and academic performance [71]. Dominant children tend to have less dominant children cluster around them and may play a particularly influential role in the formation of groups. A recent study of children in a free-play session found that dominant children were observed and imitated by the other children more than nondominant children [1].

Probably the most crucial factor in the formation of groups is the competition involved. Competition is an integral part of many of the activities that enable the child to gain desired goals. Sullivan uses the term **social accommodation** to indicate how the child learns the give and take in peer associations as well as flexibility in approaching situations [79]. The formation of clubs and gangs can help the child to find the balance between personal rights and group responsibility. The gang offers social protection while the individual sorts out personal values from those of the family, the culture, the school, or the gang.

CONFORMITY

With the formation of the peer group, a pressure is exerted to conform to the beliefs and norms of conduct that are viewed as desirable by the group. The need for peer conformity may become so strong that there is some rebellion against adult authority. Often schoolagers will make up their own rules and demand strict conformity to them. The child is caught between conforming enough to the group so as not to be rejected as odd by peers and being punished by others for peergroup conformity. The child eventually learns how to balance personal and group rights.

The degree of conformity of elementary school children varies with age and with the ambiguity of the task being performed. When tasks are easy or unambiguous, the agreement of the child with the responses of a peer decreases with age; the child learns to depend on his or her own skills. However, on hard or ambiguous tasks where children are uncertain about correct responses, there is an increasing tendency with age to agree with the response of a peer [38].

Another factor that influences conformity is the socialization of male and female children toward achievement. Females typically have been taught to be more conforming than males [39]; however, if the conformity task is presented as an "achievement" task, males (who are generally taught to be more achievement-oriented than females) are likely to show greater peer compliance [69]. In American society, males generally have been taught to be achievement-oriented in order to earn money and status later in life, in some high-paying professions that conform to more traditional gender stereotypes. Other factors in conformity include group size, the relationship among members, the degree of agreement with the group, and the importance of the issue to the group [59].

PREJUDICE

Even before kindergarten, many children acquire prejudices toward minority groups. Attitudes of tolerance and fairness must be specifically taught and practiced if they are to be learned [82]. If such teaching and practice are combined with the changes already taking place in the larger sociocultural milieu, it can be expected that American children will be less likely to develop the biases that are a handicap to a democratic society.

One study found that both white and black children are biased in favor of whites in the first four grades [88]. This bias is present even among preschoolers and remains fairly constant for black children through the early school years, while for white children it increases until second grade and then declines.

In nonracial situations, both black and white preschoolers tend to evaluate the color white more favorably than black. For example, they perceive a pictured white horse to be kinder than a black horse [9]. Children who strongly prefer white over black carry over this preference in their attitudes toward people and will demonstrate a more prowhite, antiblack bias there as well [9]. These studies support the view that racial attitudes begin to be formed very early in childhood. Three overlapping phases are identified: **awareness** of racial differences begins at about age 2½ years; **orientation** toward specific race-related words and concepts at about age 4 years; and true **attitude** toward various races, begins at about 7 years [28].

One of the major influences is the attitude of the parents. Children who are the most prejudiced tend to have authoritarian parents who use strict disciplinary techniques and are inflexible in their attitudes [88]. In contrast, children whose parents are more tolerant are able to respect themselves more and are better able to appreciate others.

Other people can help to reduce prejudice in children: open, warm, nonprejudiced teachers, camp counselors, school advisers, and so forth, can offer models of flexibility and show how to maintain positive relationships. One study compared four different techniques to counter the racially biased attitudes of white second and fifth-grade children who scored high on tests of prejudice. The techniques used were: (1) increased positive racial contact, in which children worked on interracial teams at an interesting puzzle and were all praised for their work; (2) vicarious interracial contact, in which children heard an interesting story about a sympathetic and resourceful black child; (3) reinforcement of the color black, in which children were given a marble every time they chose a picture of a black animal instead of a white one; and (4) perceptual differentiation, in which children were shown slides of a black woman whose appearance and name were varied and then were tested to see how well they remembered the names and different appearances. Two weeks after the experiment, the children's prejudice levels were measured again. Children who were exposed to any of the four techniques showed less prejudice than did children in control groups [41].

One method that schools have successfully used in attempting to alleviate racial prejudice has been the introduction of interethnic curricula [87]. The assumption that the mere acquisition of knowledge about other races and cultures reduces the level of prejudice toward racial minorities has been supported by research [71, 89]. Young children's prejudicial attitudes can be changed.

By the time children reach school age, their parents can no longer completely protect them from the prejudice of others that may exist because of a child's size, appearance, beliefs, color, ethnic background, family social class, or neighborhood. Parents can initiate measures, however, to help their children build self-confidence and the ability to relate tolerantly to those who are prejudiced. In working with a situation where there is prejudice against a child, parents, teachers, rabbis, priests, and other leaders can make use of the available literature and music that provides the child with a sense of belonging and reassurance about his or her difference. The child can thus deal with this byproduct of life in a diverse society without a severe loss of self-esteem or a detriment to psychosocial development [54]. When children question why they or someone else is different, they need direct, honest answers. They especially need consistent reassurance that difference does not mean they are "bad" or less worthy than their peers (see Chap. 19).

Mass Media

It has been estimated that by the age of 18 a child born today will have spent more time watching television than in any other single activity besides sleep [49]. What are and what will be the effects of this cumulative exposure?

Seventy-seven percent of 67 studies conducted between 1956 and 1976 reported a positive correlation between TV violence and aggressive behavior, 20 percent reported no association, and about 3 percent reported an inverse relationship (with TV violence associated with lower levels of aggression) [2].

The idea that certain factors may "predispose" a child to react to TV violence was first raised in the 1972 Surgeon General's Report on TV violence. A literature review [17] came to the following conclusions: (1) Televised violence seems to be capable of affecting viewers of varying ages, social classes, ethnicities, personality characteristics, and levels of aggressiveness; (2) Males and females are equally influenced by exposure, but within each gender, those who are more aggressive are more likely to be influenced. Children between 8 and 12 years of age are somewhat more likely to be affected than are either younger or older children; (3) In actual behavior, male children are more likely to be aggressive than female children; 4) Males are more likely to watch and to prefer televised violence than females; similarly, members of the working-

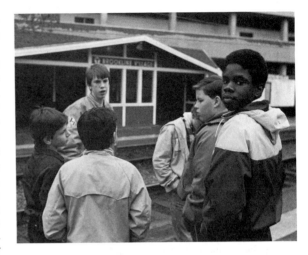

Figure 24–4. School-agers gradually assume more independence from parents as they exchange ideas with peers. (Photo by Ed Slaman).

class are more likely to watch and to prefer televised violence than members of the middle-class.

As male and female children develop, they are reinforced in sex-type behaviors by their parents. Females are typically reinforced in feminine activities and nonaggressiveness, while males receive encouragement to be aggressive and to participate in more physical activities. These outcomes are later perceived as norms. As a result of this socialization process, males are more likely than females to watch and to prefer televised violence.

Three of the specific effects of TV violence have been identified [49]. First, a high action content appears to arouse viewers. Arousal dissipates quickly, but for a period of time—varying between a few minutes and a few days after exposure—a child may act more aggressively, more vigorously, or more impulsively because he or she has been aroused by TV violence. Presumably, this is the price that is paid for being aroused, which seems to be a major element in successful entertainment [81].

Second, TV violence may be imitated either impulsively or when environmental circumstances invite acts that have been modeled in TV shows. Many children and adolescents thus gain the **potential** for acting in a more aggressive and antisocial manner as a result of exposure to TV violence. Whether or not these examples will be acted out depends on other factors, such as the consequences (positive or negative) received by the model and the opportunity to replicate the act.

Third, TV violence conveys attitudes and values

about violence, aggression, and antisocial behavior. It must be remembered that although older children and adolescents discount particular content as being "just a story," they describe the roles, role relationships, and interactions of characters as highly realistic. Admired characters are presumed to behave in appropriate or desirable ways, and their approval of aggression or antisocial behavior elevates it in the eyes of young viewers.

Television also has the potential to convey prosocial values. Although most studies suggest that prosocial television can have desired effects, the ability to magnify these effects and minimize undesired ones is in its infancy [49]. Moreover, it is evident that the entire process of socialization is highly complex. For example, there are a number of studies that indicate that the prosocial episodes of "Mister Rogers' Neighborhood" and "Sesame Street" can have prosocial effects but that the influence is limited to situations that are quite similar to those presented on the program [49]. In addition, while a single exposure to a prosocial segment of "Sesame Street" apparently produces immediate effects, these do not last even for a day [49]. No one knows if watching Laura painfully tell Pa the truth on "Little House on the Prairie" will instill similar values in school-age children. The First Lady, Nancy Reagan, believed so strongly in the influence of television on children that she appeared on "Diff'rent Strokes" to make a plea against the use of hard drugs.

There are indications that the rapid pace and generally unchallenging character of most television fare has affected the ways in which children process information and use their imagination [42]. It is thought that children who view increased amounts of fiction and fantasy are not inspired to actively use their minds to explore and to learn. Nevertheless, television is often an important part of a school-ager's life. With wise use, it can become an enriching tool to be used in opening doors to other worlds, cultures, and ideas. Excessive use, as with any activity, can prevent the school-ager from applying the energy to master the skills that are essential for successful development.

DEVELOPING A POSITIVE SELF-IMAGE

Individualizing Identity

During the school years, the child begins to identify and to develop his or her own special abilities, which leads to the development of a set of identities that the child can use to interpret and to code both the external environment and the internal self. This process occurs over a long period of time and never really ends during the life of an individual. During the late school-age years and early adolescence, the child begins to identify and to consolidate these identities and to compare or to relate them to those of peers or to those of individuals valued by the culture. These identities must be tested and modified, strengthened, or eliminated as reality proves them to be inappropriate or ill-conceived. In the early years, for example, a school-ager may feel the need to prove that he or she can walk a fence that is longer or higher than that attempted by anyone else on the block. Another may feel compelled to take music lessons "like everybody else" and will then attempt to win the weekly contest for practicing the longest. Gradually, as school-agers become adolescents, the well-adjusted individuals will possess the self-confidence to "try on" new identities, not necessarily those attempted by their closest friends. The individual's behaviors and self-identity are no longer as heavily influenced by peer behaviors and identities. One begins to appreciate one's own uniqueness, so that behavior becomes more inner-directed than outer-directed.

Factors Affecting the Self-Concept

Self-concept or self-identity is defined as the perception one holds of oneself as a total person [62, 73, 90]. The anchor points for a developed concept of self include the body, significant others, and the physical environment [22, 29]. Studies on the development of the self-concept in the preschool child suggest that in the early years, the prime components of self are recognition of physical qualities, motor skills, sex-type, and age [53]. There is a considerable expansion of self-concept in middle childhood. The breadth of self-description has increased from a few categories to as many as 25 possible categories, including ethnic awareness, ambition, ideal self, ordinal position, conscience development, and functioning aspects of self [22]. While very young children may represent themselves primarily as similar to other children ("I am a girl"; "I am 6 years old; "I go to school"), the self representations of upper grade school children are in terms of how different they are from their peers ("I am the tallest girl in the class"). The older child's responses become increasingly less global in their descriptions and evaluations of self. At approximately 6 years of age, there begins to emerge the distinction between self and ideal self: "I am plain Jane" (actual self) versus "I would like to have long curly hair and be thin" (ideal self).

The child whose surroundings permit him or her to

do things independently and successfully (because the tasks are suited to development) grows in self-confidence and self-respect. Havighurst states that along with developing and perfecting the tools of society and the skills of social interaction, the child wants to gain mastery over the body [31]. The child works for hours developing the dexterity and the control to improve competence in games. Tossing a ball, swimming in a pool, running—these tasks are important for the child to accomplish, and they help the child to grow in self-confidence. The self-concept is formed in the process of accomplishing or not accomplishing these tasks. The child may come to label the self as competent or not so competent. The major theme of Erikson's industry versus inferiority stage reflects this determination to master selected tasks. The young child eagerly embarks on the journey of learning the skills and the tools of society to carry out adult work eventually. As the child learns to use culture's tools, an understanding seems to develop that this type of learning will be helpful in becoming a more competent individual. As the child successfully builds the skills necessary to complete a grade in school, or to function successfully on the playground, the child also builds self-esteem and self-respect [21].

A clearer picture of developing self-conceptions might be possible if the content and the structure of self-perceptions are separated and their interaction evaluated. Harter has developed a model of the self-concept that is divided into four stages [30]. In the first stage, children who think they are good at one skill (drawing) will also anticipate being good at a variety of skills (e.g., puzzles, numbers, colors). Gradually, there is an integration of behaviors with umbrella-trait labels (for example, smart or dumb). When traits are opposites, the child feels that he or she can control only one trait label in the pair, and therefore thinks of the self as all "dumb" or all "smart" based on one or two key abilities or lack of abilities. In stage two, the traits become more differentiated. The child realizes that he or she can be "dumb" at one thing (math) and "smart" at another (art). Single abstractions based on an integration of the traits emerge in the third stage. When an adolescent recognizes differences in skill competency levels but finds that the skills balance one another, the adolescent may conclude that he or she is of average intelligence. Single abstractions also become more differentiated; for example, an adolescent who is a skilled writer and also a skilled painter may combine these perceptions into a single perception of an artistic, creative person. In the fourth stage, these single abstractions become further integrated so that there are no longer apparent contradictions and the self does not seem fragmented. For example, a young adult may have a nonconformist self-concept,—that is, as one who rejects conventional intellectual values of the society in favor of the pursuit of personal artistic endeavors.

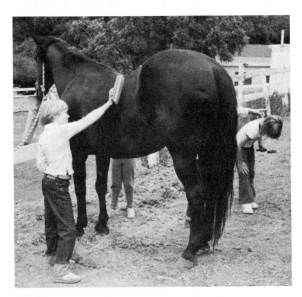 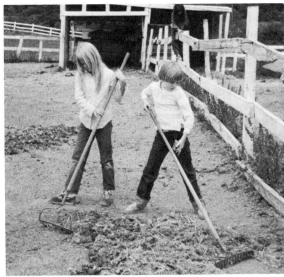

Figure 24–5. School-agers soon learn that caring for an animal has both its pleasant and unpleasant aspects. Such responsibility is excellent preparation for the adult years while offering many rewards along the way.

Coopersmith has examined self-esteem through extensive interviews with 10- to 12-year-old boys and their mothers. He concluded that an individual develops a self-concept in terms of four factors [16]:

1. Significance (how much he is loved and approved of by significant others)
2. Competence (how well he performs tasks that he considers to be important)
3. Virtue (to what extent he feels he has attained the expected moral standards of his culture)
4. Power (how much and how well he can control himself and influence others)

The higher a child feels he or she rates on these four factors, the higher will be the self-esteem.

Carol Gilligan [26] has explored the differences in the way males and females experience issues of dependency and relationship:

> For boys and men, separation and individuation are critically tied to gender identity since separation from the mother is essential for the development of masculinity. For girls and women, issues of femininity or feminine identity do not depend on the achievement of separation from the mother, but on the progress of individuation. Since masculinity is defined through separation while femininity is defined through attachment, male gender identity is threatened by intimacy while female gender identity is threatened by separation. Thus males tend to have difficulty with relationships, while females tend to have problems with individuation. [26]

Physical development and body image can affect the self-concept (for example, a child feels too short, too thin, has freckles, wears glasses or braces). A child's self-concept can be negatively affected if the child is teased excessively for prominent physical characteristics.

Another variable that can potentially affect self-concept is family income. Some studies have suggested that economically disadvantaged children have more positive self-concepts [76, 83]. It is possible that children in low-income families blame their environment for poor performance rather than themselves. Other researchers have found, on the other hand, that partly because their present status appears to be more dependent on factors over which they have no control (such as parents' employment or the characteristics of a landlord), lower-class children are more likely to believe they have little control over their future; therefore, they do not try as hard and accomplish less [5]. Children who do not feel they are in command of their

school performances are more likely to suffer a decrease in self-esteem and to think their teacher expects too much of them or blames them too much.

Fostering Positive Self-Esteem

Self-concept is the individual's picture of self and ideal self, whereas self-esteem is a measure of personal worth or value. Self-esteem reflects how important one feels the self to be in the world and will range from self-love to self-deprecation. Ironically, the child who appears to love the self to the point of conceit may actually hate the self to the point of disdain and use boastfulness to cover the true feelings of low self-esteem. Self-esteem, like self-concept, is a reflection of others' opinions and treatment of the child. Feelings of personal uselessness and unworthiness can be learned through continual criticism, failure, and punishment. Feelings of high esteem come from success, encouragement, and praise.

From an early age, without being deliberate about it, the child acquires ideas and attitudes about self and others. Many persons will acquire persisting feelings of inferiority or other unhealthy attitudes regarding their personal worth, which represent either an irrational estimate of themselves or a failure to accept themselves realistically as they are [39]. New learning experiences can raise or lower self-esteem. It seems that one of the central tasks for parents and teachers is to help children to accept themselves as a "person in process," and thus help to keep self-esteem high.

Concern, respect, and acceptance by the family will contribute to a child's developing self-esteem. The parents' interest and concern about companions, as well as their availability for interaction and discussion of problems, will facilitate the development of high self-esteem [16]. When Coopersmith interviewed a group of parents about their children's upbringing, he found that the parents of male children who had high self-esteem were likely to have positive self-concepts themselves. In addition, he found very different attitudes about childrearing. Young males who were high in self-esteem had parents who showed a great deal of interest in them. The parents knew all of their sons' friends and spent time with them discussing problems and engaging in joint activities. They set high standards for behavior, were consistent in enforcing the rules and relied on rewards rather than physical punishment as a means of discipline. These parents clearly indicated that they regarded their sons as significant persons worthy of their interest. As a result, the children came to regard themselves in a favorable light [16].

On the other hand, the parents of male children who

were low in self-esteem demonstrated less interest in their sons' welfare, were less likely to spend time with them, were less likely to know their friends or activities, and rarely considered their opinions in family decisions. These parents tended to be permissive, having no clear-cut rules for behavior. The young males who were low in self-esteem thus had neither daily feedback about their importance as persons nor a consistent set of standards for behavior. As a result, they came to have doubts about their own value and effectiveness. Coopersmith concluded that a child's opinion of the self is derived from the day-to-day personal relationships with parents, teachers, and peers [16].

Although the parents of high-esteem children encourage self-reliance and independent behavior, they also need to protect their children from tasks that might be too difficult and too frustrating. Parents need to be particularly aware of the pressure they may exert that may cause a child to form a self-ideal beyond his or her capabilities. This in turn could cause conflict and frustration between what the child is and what the child feels he or she must become. Poorly adjusted children may grossly overestimate what they should become, leading to feelings of inadequacy and rebellion. Parents and teachers can help children improve themselves, so that self-concept can approach the ideal self. The child can also be challenged concerning the realism of the ideal self. Can he or she truly hope to meet such high standards? If not, perhaps they are too high. Our "musts" and "shoulds" often guarantee that we shall make ourselves absolutely miserable by constantly shooting too high and failing to pat ourselves on the back for our actual accomplishments [19]. Adults can help children decide that the areas in which they do not do very well are not as important as the ones in which they succeed. For example, the less physically attractive individual may strive to become more entertaining or skilled in a peer-valued task. This accentuation of the positive, or compensation, is an excellent form of adjustment for children if it is in line with appropriate values. At other times, adults need to help children to work harder at achieving their standards of excellence or to compromise by accepting a good rather than a perfect performance. One can be proud of **doing one's best** even if it is not **the best** when compared to others.

The ability to compromise is an extremely important ability for children to learn. Children in our society are often encouraged to be "better than the others," but they may find that this conflicts with being "the most popular." Thus, along with learning to compete, the child must also learn to compromise. Compromise, ac-

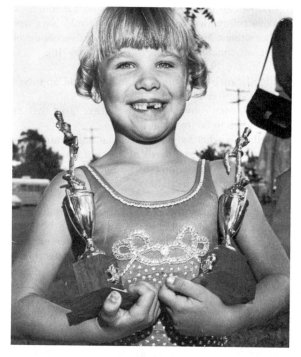

Figure 24–6. Our society encourages competition by promoting contests and awarding trophies. Many school-agers will practice diligently to become "number one."

cording to Sullivan, means learning to give and take. It is a high form of winning. "If you do this for me, I'll do that for you." The child eventually learns the rules of the game and, being realistic, understands that he or she will win sometimes and lose at other times. Adjusting and adapting to the wishes of others while maintaining one's own self-worth is an important interaction tool the school-ager must learn to implement. "If we do this together, we will both get what we want" [79]. Cooperation benefits everyone.

In conclusion, a child's self-concept is an internal construct by which the child views or describes the self—abilities, identity, weaknesses, perceptions, beliefs, feelings, attitudes, and values. Parents and peers serve as a mirror, reflecting back the type of person the child is.

Getting Through the Pubescent Years

American preadolescents usually spend time in gender-segregated groups. As adolescence approaches, they begin to participate in more heterosexual groups. To further facilitate social-emotional development, the preadolescent begins to move away from the parents toward a more intense relationship with peers. Peer groups are beginning to demand a higher level of conformity. The preadolescent observes older peers who pride themselves on their increasing independence and shun conformity to adult authority.

Not only are preadolescents caught in making a transition from the home to the peer group, but they also face the challenge of developing deeper, same-gender friendships. Sullivan finds that the surest predictor of trouble in adult relations is the absence of an intimate friendship in preadolescence [79]. Conversely, an effective relationship with a chum can go a long way. The formation of extra-familial intimacies provides a kind of affirmation by others; as one looks at oneself through a chum's eyes, the self-concept is expanded and self-esteem is enhanced. This provides courage and strength to begin thinking about pursuing the individualized interests and identities that are essential to successful adolescence and adulthood.

Preadolescence is a time of cognitive and social conflict as the child looks toward adolescent issues of sexuality, autonomy, and identity. To complicate this social

development even further are the changes in the body as well as in the body image. It is true that the most evident and rapid changes during puberty are physical; nevertheless, developments also occur in mental functioning, social interactions, and conceptions of the self. Fritz Redl offers some suggestions to parents and teachers to help the preadolescent through these trying times [64]:

1. Avoid counter-hysterics. Study the situation and decide when to ignore behaviors and when to intervene. Whatever the decision, intervention should be realistic and free from hysteric over-emotionalism.
2. Don't fight windmills. Some preadolescents will challenge parents around issues, such as hair style, dress style, TV program selections, and so on. Parents should interpret the cause of the behavior first (Is the child really asking the parent to set limits that she is having difficulty establishing for herself?), and then judge how much and in what way to intervene.
3. Provide a frame of life adequate for growth. Every preadolescent needs some space for personal

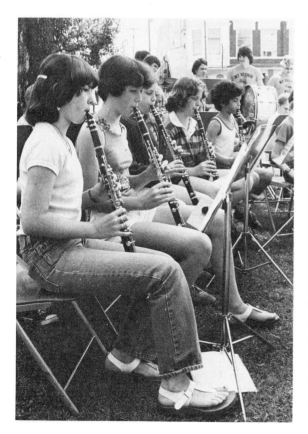

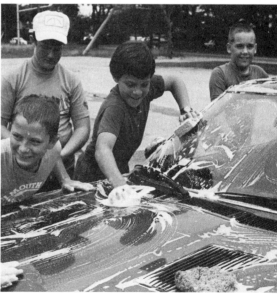

Figure 24–7. Determination and hard work focused toward mastery of a goal can contribute to a positive sense of self. Active participation in activities aids the school-ager in refining skills. Through collaborative efforts, the school-ager begins to find his or her identity within the group. With time, opportunity, and experience, the middle-schooler begins to identify his or her uniqueness and interests—which aid in the solidification of identity. (Right photo by Ed Slaman.)

growth. The adult should decide when behaviors are adaptive and growth-producing and when they are maladaptive, and should try to establish physical and social-emotional limits that are safe yet allow the child freedom to construct and test some of her own emerging skills and ideas.

4. Watch out for preadolescent "corns". There are many sensitive areas. Many preadolescents will reject what their parents want, not because they feel it is unreasonable or unjustified, but because of the way in which parents put the issue. The child needs to feel that he is assuming more of his own decision-making responsibility.

5. If in doubt, make a diagnostic check-up. The parents should obtain information from relevant books or seek the counsel of a professional.

DEVELOPMENTAL CONCERNS

Anxieties

Conflicts with parents, a change in a residence or a school, and a change in physical appearance are all factors that can create stress in children. High expectations from parents can also create stress and lead to feelings of anxiety. Some typical worries of school-agers are those, such as parental illness and death, poor school grades, getting into trouble, lack of peer acceptance, and accidental injury. Gradually, fears become more realistic and more closely tied to learned or experienced objects and situations, such as specific animals, fire, poison oak, and deep water [52]. Fear of the dark largely disappears after 7 years of age. Fears of nonexistent entities, such as monsters, the boogeyman, ghosts, witches, and animated skeletons, are typically abandoned around 10 years of age. Fears of people and their actions doubles from ages 5 to 12 years and includes divorce, people with guns, and child enticers.

Anxiety can manifest itself in a variety of ways, among them daydreaming, nightmares, bedwetting, insomnia, psychosomatic illness, withdrawal, overaggressiveness and rebelliousness. Anxiety and conflict are often the chief determinants of childhood headaches, stomach aches, lack of appetite, obesity, diarrhea, and tiredness [72]. Psychosomatic illnesses are genuine physical disorders, caused or aggravated by stress. Children with allergies, asthma, and diabetes are especially susceptible to exacerbation of their disorder by stress.

The child may express anxiety directly through symptoms, such as shyness, clinging, overdependence, or social isolation. There are a number of behaviors that children may develop that can handicap their social life, for example, stuttering. Tics may also be a symptom of anxiety. Emotionally caused tics may arise from stress in the child's past or current relationships. Some psychiatrists feel that children release emotional tension in this way. Tics are most common in tense children with fairly strict parents [43]. These children are only partially successful at bottling up their irritations and impulses.

School Phobia

When parents have extreme anxiety about letting go and freeing their child for the new experiences that school makes available, the child's response may result in school phobia. This intense fear arises out of an acute separation anxiety between the school-ager and the primary caretaker who has indulged in consistent overprotection. Most children are occasionally reluctant to go to school, but a persistent fear of leaving home and going to school is a symptom of underlying conflicts both with the child and the caretaker. Since severe physical symptoms from headaches to severe abdominal pain and vomiting may develop, counseling is frequently indicated for both the parent and the child.

Illness and Hospitalization

The individual school-ager's understanding of, reaction to, and method of coping with illness and hospitalization are related to how significant the child views the separation, the loss of control over events, and any bodily injury and pain associated with it.

SEPARATION

The stress imposed by illness or hospitalization may increase the school-ager's need for parental security and guidance. Young school-agers, who are still adjusting to school, may require the frequent presence of primary caretakers during illness or hospitalization.

Older school-agers also miss their parents but may verbalize more concern about being apart from peer activities. They might even admit to missing school—the academically oriented especially fear "getting behind" in classroom and homework studies.

School-agers, afraid of being called "baby," may not ask for the parental guidance and the adult support that they need during this time of crisis. The need to express negative feelings (hostility, anger, depression) often is transformed into irritability, withdrawal, or rejection of meaningful relationships.

LOSS OF CONTROL

The school-age child, in the endeavor to be independent and productive, is especially susceptible to feeling that he or she has lost control when ill or hospitalized, for example, having to stay in bed or not being able to choose certain favorite foods. When such children are allowed to exert some allotment of power, regardless of how limited it may appear (for example, deciding whether to have a bath before or after breakfast), they usually maintain some of their self-esteem.

BODILY INJURY AND PAIN

The school-ager may fear that pain will lead to prolonged illness, disability, or even death. Taking an active interest in bodily health, the child knows that there are certain parts of the body that must keep working if he or she is to continue living.

Although routine physical examinations are usually fairly well-tolerated by school-agers, their concern for privacy becomes increasingly evident. A 7-year-old female may be reluctant to remove her blouse in front of a male doctor; both male and female children prefer to pull down their pants and sit covered with a sheet or an examination gown while the doctor is out of the room.

By the age of 9 or 10 years, most school-agers overtly resist painful procedures. They may have developed their own coping skills to get them through—gritting their teeth or closing their eyes. A few try to bargain with "Let's wait 'til the clock says 5 minutes are up!" or a reasonable facsimile. Even painful procedures can be endured if the child is given some opportunity to decide when they will be done or the order of events.

Incestuous Assault

Incestuous assault has been defined as "any manual, oral or genital sexual contact or other explicit sexual behavior that an adult family member imposes on a child, who is unable to alter or understand the adult's behavior because of his or her powerlessness in the family and early stage of psychological development" [14]. Most incestuous relationships begin when the child is in the school-age years. The average age of onset is 9 years, with an average duration of 3 years [33] A recent review indicates that approximately 15 percent of white, middle-class women report having had a childhood sexual encounter that involved physical contact with an adult. Because of the nature of the sample, this figure may underestimate the actual rate of incidence [33]. Father-daughter incest is by far the most common type, accounting for approximately 97 percent of parent-child incest cases. A conservative estimate is that 1 million American women have been involved in incestuous relationships with their fathers [24]. Father-daughter incest is coercive, even if force is not employed. The father is in a position of power. The child is not in control and therefore cannot freely choose to take part in the relationship. Because children are in a dependent relationship, they will do "whatever they perceive to be necessary to preserve a relationship with their caretakers. If an adult insists upon a sexual relationship with a dependent child, the child will comply" [33].

Theories abound to explain why a father would engage in a sexual relationship with his daughter. Poor impulse control, maternal deprivation, paternal deprivation, unsatisfactory marital relationship, and excessive change are among the explanations [12]. There have been no studies of the family as a system that explore what causes incestuous behavior [12]. From the studies of incest that have centered on the individual, certain conditions appear to be associated with the development of father-daughter incest. First, members of incestuous families tend to be highly enmeshed with one another (see Chap. 30), even though strong feelings of hostility may exist between the parents. What may appear to be a stable relationship may actually involve high degrees of emotional dependence on the part of one or more members rather than a healthy interdependence. Second, families in which incest occurs are often characterized by borderline coping skills of one or more members [12]. This behavior is found at all socioeconomic levels and in all ethnic and religious groups.

The range of possible negative effects of incestuous assault on a child include poor self-esteem, guilt, depression, and shame [12, 33]. Some physical effects include infections, lacerated vaginas, rectal fissures, and perforated anal or vaginal walls. Victims of incestuous assault are also at greater risk for repeated victimization in adult life. Sexual contact with an adult, especially a trusted relative, is a significant emotional trauma when it occurs and may have long-lasting, deleterious effects on the victim during his or her young adult years [33] that prevent the assumption of a positive, trusting, heterosexual relationship. Counseling is essential both immediately and whenever anxiety reappears.

SUMMARY

Although children are inherently social, they do not come into the world equipped with the necessary traits and techniques for social living. As they enter school, they learn how to function in the social aspects of the culture. Children must learn the skills of cooperative give-and-take in the midst of a very competitive world. They learn more about themselves as they come to understand others. The more children learn about individuals who exhibit characteristics, values, and behaviors different from their own, the less they have to defend themselves from those individuals, and consequently, prejudicial behaviors are decreased.

As the child progresses through the school-age years, he or she develops and learns to use the skills of social subordination, accommodation, competition, compromise, and cooperation to achieve a sense of social competency and self-balance. The child's good opinion of self is highly affected by physical attractiveness, height, weight, social class, and skills in particular areas, such as school and play activities. Self-esteem and the psychosocial development of the school-age years are affected by the personal, day-to-day relations with parents, teachers, and peers.

REFERENCES

1. Amidon, E. J., and Hoffman, C. Can teachers help the socially rejected? *El. Sch. J.* 66:149, 1965.
2. Andison, F. S. TV violence and aggression: A cumulation of study results 1956–1976. *Pub. Opinion Q.* 41:314, 1977.
3. Asher, S. R., Oden, S. L., and Gottman, J. M. Children's Friendships in School Settings. In L. G. Katz (Ed.), *Current Topics in Early Childhood Education.* Vol. 1. Norwood, NJ: Ablex, 1977.
4. Bandura, A. *Social Learning Theory.* Englewood Cliffs, NJ: Prentice-Hall, 1977.
5. Bartel, N. R. Locus of control and achievement in middle- and lower-class children. *Child Dev.* 42:1099, 1971.
6. Baumrind, D. Childcare practices anteceding three patterns of preschool behavior. *Genet. Psychol. Monogr.* 75:43, 1967.
7. Bernard, J. The good-provider role: Its rise and fall. *Am. Psychol.* 36:1, 1981.
8. Bonney, M. E. Assessment of efforts to aid socially isolated elementary school pupils. *J. Educ. Res.* 64:345, 1971.
9. Boswell, D., and Best, D. The measurement of children's racial attitudes in the early school years. *Child Dev.* 46:494, 1975.
10. Bridgeman, D. L. Enhanced role taking through cooperative interdependence: A field study. *Child Dev.* 52:1231, 1981.
11. Brickell, H. M. How to change what matters. *Educ. Lead.* 38(3):202, 1980.
12. Brooks, B. Familial influences in father-daughter incest. *J. Psychiatr. Treat. and Eval.* 4:117, 1982.
13. Buswell, M. M. The relationship between social structure of the classroom and the academic success of the pupils. *J. Exper. Educ.* 22:37, 1953.
14. Butler, S. *Conspiracy of Silence: The Trauma of Incest.* San Francisco: Volcano Press, 1982.
15. Coie, J. D., Dodge, K. A., and Coppotelli, H. Dimensions and types of social status: A cross-age perspective. *Dev. Psychol.* 18:557, 1982.
16. Coopersmith, S. *The Antecedents of Self-Esteem.* San Francisco: Freeman, 1967.
17. Cowen, E. L., et al. Long-term follow-up of early detected vulnerable children. *J. Consult. Clin. Psychol.* 41:438, 1973.
18. Elkind, D. *The Hurried Child: Growing Up Too Fast Too Soon.* Reading, MA: Addison-Wesley, 1981.
19. Ellis, A. *Reason and Emotion in Psychotherapy.* New York: Lyle Stuart, 1962.
20. Entwisle, D. R., and Hyaduk, L. A. *Early Schooling: Cognitive and Affective Outcomes.* Baltimore: Johns Hopkins University Press, 1982.
21. Erikson, E. H. *Childhood and Society* (2nd ed.). New York: Norton, 1963.
22. Fahey, M., and Phillips, S. The self concept in middle childhood: Some baseline data. *Child Study J.* 11:155, 1981.
23. Fine, M. A., Moreland, J. R., and Schwebel, A. I. Long-term effects of divorce on parent-child relationships. *Dev. Psychol.* 19:703, 1983.
24. Finkelhor, D. *Sexually Victimized Children.* New York: Free Press, 1979.
25. Gardener, R. A. *The Boys and Girls Book About Divorce.* New York: Bantam Books, 1981.
26. Gilligan, C. *In a Different Voice.* Cambridge, MA: Harvard University Press, 1982.
27. Gold, D., and Andres, D. Developmental comparisons between ten-year-old children with employed and nonemployed mothers. *Child Dev.* 49:75, 1978.
28. Goodman, M. E. *Race Awareness in Young Children* (Rev. ed.). New York: Collier Books, 1964.
29. Gordon, I. J. *Human Development, From Birth Through Adolescence* (2nd ed.). New York: Harper and Row, 1969.
30. Harter, S. Developmental Perspectives on the Self-System. In P. H. Mussen, (Ed.), *Handbook of Child Psychology,* formerly *Carmichael's Manual of Child Psychology,* (4th ed.). New York: Wiley, 1983.
31. Havighurst, R. J. *Developmental Tasks and Education* (2nd ed.). New York: McKay, 1965.
32. Havighurst, R. J. *Developmental Tasks and Education* (3rd ed.). New York: McKay, 1972.
33. Herman, J. L. *Father-Daughter Incest.* Cambridge, MA: Harvard University Press, 1981.
34. Hess, R. D., and Camara, K. A. Post-divorce family relationships as mediating factors in the consequences of divorce for children. *J. Soc. Issues,* 35:79, 1979.
35. Hetherington, E. M., Cox, M., and Cox, R. Play and social interaction in children following divorce. *J. Soc. Issues* 35:26, 1979.
36. Hoffman, L. W. Changes in family roles, socialization, and sex differences. *Am. Psychol.* 32:644, 1977.
37. Hoffman, L. N. W., and Nye, F. I. *Working Mothers.* San Francisco: Jossey-Bass, 1974.

38. Hoving, K., Hamm, M., and Galvin, P. Social influence as a function of stimulus ambiguity at three age levels. *Dev. Psychol.* 1:631, 1969.

39. Jersild, A. T. Self-understanding in childhood and adolescence. *Am. Psychol.* 6:112, 1951.

40. Kandel, D. B., et al. *Adolescents in Two Societies: Peers, School and Family in the United States and Denmark.* Washington, D.C.: Department of Health, Education and Welfare, Office of Education, 1968.

41. Katz, P., and Zalk, S. Modification of children's racial attitudes. *Dev. Psychol.* 14:447, 1978.

42. Kelley, H., and Gardiner, H. Viewing children through television. *New Direct. Child Dev.* 13:100, 1981.

43. Keniston, K. *All Our Children: The American Family Under Pressure.* New York: Harcourt-Brace Jovanovich, 1978.

44. Kessler, J. W. *Psychopathology of Childhood.* Englewood Cliffs, NJ: Prentice-Hall, 1966.

45. Kohn, M., and Clausen, J. Social isolation and schizophrenia. *Am. Sociol. R.* 20:265, 1955.

46. Kugle, C. L., Clements, R. O., and Powell, P. M. Level and stability of self-esteem in relation to academic behavior of second graders. *J. Pers. Soc. Psychol.* 44:201, 1983.

47. Lamb, M. E. Parental Behavior and Child Development in Nontraditional Families. In M. E. Lamb (Ed.), *Nontraditional Families: Parenting and Child Development.* Hillsdale, NJ: Erlbaum, 1982.

48. Lamb, M. E. Maternal Employment and Child Development: A Review. In M. E. Lamb (Ed.), *Nontraditional Families: Parenting and Child Development.* Hillsdale, NJ: Erlbaum, 1982.

49. Liebert, R. M., Sprafkin, J. N., and Davidson, E. S. *The Early Window: Effects of Television on Children and Youth* (2nd ed.). New York: Pergamon Press, 1982.

50. Martin, B. Parent-child Relations. In F. D. Horowitz (Ed.), *Review of Child Development Reseach* (Vol. 4). Chicago: University of Chicago Press, 1975.

51. Martinek, T. J., and Johnson, S. B. Teacher expectations: Effects on dyadic interactions and self-concept in elementary age children. *Res. Q.* 50:60, 1979.

52. Maurer, A. What children fear. *J. Gen. Psychol.* 106:265, 1965.

53. McCandless, B. R., and Trotter, R. J. *Children: Behavior and Development* (3rd. ed.). New York: Holt, Rinehart and Winston, 1977.

54. McElroy, E., and Tackett, J. J. Potential stresses in Families with School-age Children. In J. J. Tackett and M. Hunsberger (Eds.), *Family-Centered Care of Children and Adolescents.* Philadelphia: Saunders, 1981.

55. Moen, P. The two-provider Family: Problems and Potentials. In M. E. Lamb (Ed.), *Nontraditional Families: Parenting and Child Development.* Hillsdale, NJ: Erlbaum, 1982.

56. Mussen, P. H., et al. *Psychological Development: A Life-Span Approach.* New York: Harper and Row, 1979.

57. Parkinson, C. E., et al. Research note: Rating the home environment of school-age children; A comparison with general cognitive index and school progress. *J. Child Psychol. Psychiatry* 23:329, 1982.

58. Parsons, J. E., Adler, T. F., and Kaczala, C. M. Socialization of achievement attitudes and beliefs: Parental influences. *Child Dev.* 53:310, 1982.

59. Patel, H. S., and Gordon, J. E. Some personal and situational determinants of yielding to influence. *J. Abnorm. Soc. Psychol.* 61:411, 1960.

60. Piaget, J. *Judgment and Reasoning in the Child.* Translated by M. Warden. Totowa, NJ: Littlefield, Adams, 1976.

61. Pilling, D., and Pringle, M. K. *Controversial Issues in Child Development.* New York: Schocken Books, 1978.

62. Purkey, W. W. *Self-concept and School Achievement.* Englewood Cliffs, NJ: Prentice-Hall, 1970.

63. Putallaz, M., and Gottmann, J. M. Social Skills and Group Acceptance. In S. R. Asher and J. M. Gottman (Eds.), *The Development of Children's Friendships.* Cambridge: Cambridge University Press, 1981.

64. Redl, F. *Pre-Adolescents—What Makes Them Tick?* New York: Child Study Association of America, 1974.

65. Roff, M. Childhood social interactions and young adult bad conduct. *J. Abnorm. Soc. Psychol.* 63:333, 1961.

66. Roff, M. Childhood social interaction and young adult psychosis. *J. Clin. Psychol.* 19:152, 1963.

67. Roff, M., Sells, S. B., and Golden, M. M. *Social Adjustment and Personality Development in Children.* Minneapolis: University of Minnesota Press, 1972.

68. Rosenthal, R., and Jacobsen, L. *Pygmalian in the Classroom.* (Enlarged ed.). New York: Irvington, 1983.

69. Sampson, E. E., and Hancock, T. An examination of the relationship between ordinal position, personality, and conformity: An extension, replication, and partial verification. *J. Pers. Soc. Psychol.* 5:398, 1967.

70. Santrock, J. W., and Warshak, R. A. Father custody and social development in boys and girls. *J. Soc. Issues* 35:112, 1979.

71. Schafer, S. A. An evaluation of the effectiveness of the green circle program in stimulating and reinforcing positive racial attitudes in children. *Dissertation Abstracts International* 32:2492, 1971.

72. Senn, M. J. E., and Solnit, A. J. *Problems in Child Behavior and Development.* Philadelphia: Lea and Febiger, 1970.

73. Shavelson, R. J., Hubner, J. J., and Stanton, G. C. Self-concept: Validation of construct interpretations. *R. Educ. Res.* 3:407, 1976.

74. Sherif, M., and Sherif, C. W. *Social Psychology.* New York: Harper and Row, 1969.

75. Siman, M. L. Application of a new model of peer group influence to naturally existing adolescent friendship groups. *Child Dev.* 48:270, 1977.

76. Soares, A. T., and Soares, L. M. Self-perceptions of culturally disadvantaged children. *Am. Educ. Res. J.* 6:31, 1969.

77. Stewart, A. J., et al. Adaptation to life changes in children and adults: Cross-sectional studies. *J. Pers. Soc. Psychol.* 43:1270, 1982.

78. Strain, P. S., Cooke, T. P., and Appolloni, T. *Teaching Exceptional Children: Assessing and Modifying Social Behavior.* New York: Academic Press, 1976.

79. Sullivan, H. S. *The Interpersonal Theory of Psychiatry.* New York: Norton, 1953.

80. Tajfel, H., and Billig, M. Familiarity and categorization in intergroup behavior. *J. Exp. Soc. Psychol.* 10:159, 1974.

81. Tannenbaum, P. H. Entertainment as Vicarious Emotional Experience. In P. H. Tannenbaum (Ed.), *The Entertainment Functions of Television.* Hillside, NJ: Erlbaum, 1980.

82. Trager, H. G., and Yarrow, M. R. *They Learn What They Live: Prejudice in Young Children.* New York: Harper, 1952.

83. Trowbridge, H., and Trowbridge, L. Self-concept and socio-economic status. *Child Study Journal,* 2:123, 1972.

84. Ullman, C. A. Teachers, peers and tests as predictors of adjustment. *J. Educ. Psychol.* 48:257, 1957.

85. United States Bureau of the Census. *Statistical Abstract of the United States: 1981* (102d edition). Washington, D. C., 1981.

86. Vosk, B., et al. A multimethod comparison of popular and unpopular children. *Dev. Psychol.* 18:571, 1982.

87. Westphal, R. C. *The Effects of a Primary-grade Level Interethnic Curriculum on Racial Prejudice.* San Francisco: R and E Research Associates, 1977.

88. Williams, J., Boswell, D., and Best, D. Evaluative responses of preschool children to the colors white and black. *Child Dev.* 46:501, 1975.

89. Wright, E. A. *Educating for Diversity.* New York: John Day, 1965.

90. Wylie, R. C. *The Self-concept* (Rev. ed.). Lincoln, NE: University of Nebraska Press, 1974.

VIII
Adolescence

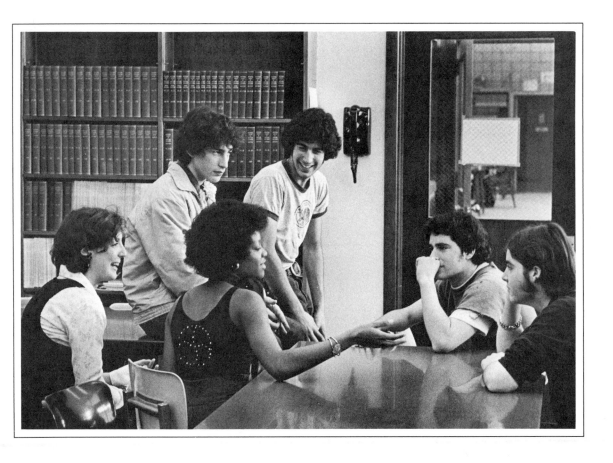

25

Biophysical Development of the Adolescent

Clara S. Schuster

I think what is happening to me is so wonderful, and not only what can be seen on my body, but all that is taking place inside. I never discuss myself or any of these things with anybody; that is why I have to talk to myself about them.

Each time I have a period—and that has only been three times—I have the feeling that in spite of all the pain, unpleasantness, and nastiness, I have a sweet secret, and that is why, although it is nothing but a nuisance to me in a way, I always long for the time that I shall feel that secret within me again.

—Anne Frank, *The Diary of a Young Girl*

Introduction

The Pubertal Period
Hormonal control
Somatic changes
The menstrual cycle

Somatic Development
Skeletal system
Muscular system
Central nervous system
Cardiovascular system
Respiratory system
Gastrointestinal system
Basal metabolic rate

Common Problems Associated with Adolescent Growth
Juvenile obesity
Weight loss
Acne
Poor posture
Dentition
Headache

Conclusions

One of the major milestones in the development of the individual is the period of transition from childhood to adulthood. Many cultures have dramatic rites to celebrate the young person's initiation into the adult world. Although Western societies do not have such clearly defined launching points into the rights and responsibilities of adulthood, each individual is expected to gradually assume more adult roles in all four domains. Even with the best foundation, however, this transition is frequently marked by disequilibrium and crises.

Definitions
Adolescence is the term used to identify the period of transition from childhood to adulthood. This term recognizes the marked changes occurring in all four major domains. Adolescence is conceptualized as the period of life during which the individual is forming a sense of personal identity and gaining emancipation from the family unit. As such, it is primarily a cognitive, sociological, and affective process, rather than a physical phenomenon. Adolescence has no clear-cut beginning or end. However, in order to establish more definitive parameters—at least for the discussion of the development of the biophysical domain—the authors

have arbitrarily chosen the years from 11 through 19 to represent the period of adolescence, with the specific understanding that the boundaries can be extended at either end to encompass the variations in development found in individuals. The authors agree with Horrocks, who notes that some persons continue to function as adolescents for many years beyond the twentieth birthday [23].

Puberty is restricted to physiological development, in particular, those phenomena associated with final maturation of the reproductive system. Many persons use the word **puberty** to refer to the entire transition period. However, a precise definition of puberty, or **true puberty,** is the point at which reproduction is first possible. Unfortunately, it is very difficult to identify that point precisely because both ovulation and spermatogenesis are internal phenomena. Consequently, most persons use external phenomena to identify the point of puberty rather than attempt to identify the point of true puberty. **Menarche** (the first menstrual period) is the identification point used to divide the prepubertal from the postpubertal female; the onset of **nocturnal emissions** (wet dreams or involuntary orgasm experience during sleep) is frequently used as an arbitrary division between prepubertal and postpubertal males. Some authorities use coarsening and curling of pubic hair as the point of puberty in males, since this phenomenon frequently coincides with spermatogenesis. However, none of these external phenomena indicates that the individual is biologically capable of reproduction, since gametogenesis is usually delayed 1 or 2 years after the external phenomena are exhibited. Adolescence and puberty, then, are interdependent, but independent developmental processes.

General Development

The early years of adolescence are characterized by very rapid growth. The individual is usually very interested in bodily development, is frequently confused by it, and is curious about the final outcome. The physiological changes require a change in one's body image and concept of self. Chronological age is an inadequate parameter for biophysical development; in a group of 14-year-olds, a 4-year spread in sexual and somatic development is not uncommon. These variations in growth may cause concern over the normalcy of one's body, sexuality, ability to compete in athletics, and social and peer relationships. At a time when blending with one's peers is so important psychosocially, variations in biophysical maturity can create major hurdles. In short, the physical changes of adolescence constitute a major developmental crisis for the individual.

Imbalances in biophysical growth as well as in the development of the four domains are common. The adolescent may be awkward in gross-motor activity—it takes time to get used to one's new body. Many adolescents experience temporary difficulty in adapting to the changes. A marked increase in modesty frequently accompanies sexual changes. Others may become sharply critical of their own features. One's hands, feet, or nose—all of which increase in size before the arms, legs, or the rest of the face "catch up"—are common sources of embarrassment to the adolescent. Some adolescents are embarrassed and fear ridicule because of excessive height or shortness, breast development, or a squeaky voice.

These changes, along with fluctuations in hormonal balance, frequently lead to heightened emotionality in the adolescent [24]. The inability to control the changes may precipitate symptoms of the helplessness syndrome. Peers and other social contacts frequently interact differently with an individual who appears to be physically mature. The new role expectations, combined with the essential psychological readjustments, can lead to symptoms of stress.

Adolescents need much supportive reassurance during the pubertal period, and they need to understand how and why changes occur. An understanding of the concept of variability of normal development is essential to facilitate adjustment. Comparisons can be devastating. At no point in a person's development should the concept of individuality be stressed as much as in early adolescence.

THE PUBERTAL PERIOD

The pubertal period—the period of maturation of the reproductive system—includes all the primary and secondary sexual developments precipitated by the endocrine changes in the individual. The pubertal period may last 8 to 10 years, although 3 to 5 years is more common [43]. **Primary sexual development** includes the maturational changes occurring in all those organs directly related to reproduction (e.g., ovaries, penis, breasts, uterus). **Secondary sexual development** includes the physiological changes that occur in other parts of the body as a direct result of changes in hormonal balance (e.g., development of facial and pubic hair, voice changes, fat deposits).

Hormonal Control

During early childhood, males and females have small amounts of both estrogen (female hormone) and androgen (male hormone) [32]. At about age 7 to 8 years, both of these hormones begin to increase gradually until **pubescence** (the first half of the pubertal period, which precedes the onset of external puberty). During pubescence, females experience a more rapid increase in the production of estrogen, whereas males have a rapid increase in the production of androgens.

The mechanics that initiate the pubertal process are as yet poorly understood. It appears that the hypothalamus initiates the process through secretion of neurohumoral releasing factors, which directly affect the activity of the anterior pituitary gland [26]. It is postulated that the hypothalamus is held in check during the childhood years by central nervous system immaturity [43]. The amygdala, a structure within the limbic system that forms a rim around the brainstem, appears to exert an inhibitory effect on the hypothalamus, which in turn prevents release of luteinizing hormone (LH) and follicle-stimulating hormone (FSH) by the anterior pituitary [7] (see Chap. 3).

Two other hormones secreted by the anterior pituitary are pituitary growth hormone (PGH) and thyroid-stimulating hormone (TSH). Growth hormone levels remain relatively constant throughout life [26]. The main function of PGH appears to be the stimulation of deoxyribonucleic acid (DNA) synthesis and hyperplastic cell growth, particularly of the bones and cartilage. Since the increased androgen levels that accompany puberty in both males and females are antagonistic to PGH, increased androgen levels are partially responsible for the decrease in rate of body growth.

During the pubertal period, there is a slight increase in thyroxin secretion by the thyroid under the influence of TSH [26]. Thyroxin levels directly increase total body metabolism. Adequate thyroxin levels are essential throughout life, for (1) hypertrophic and hyperplastic cell growth of all body systems—especially the brain and skeletal systems—and (2) primary and secondary sexual development. The increased metabolic rate leads to a higher body temperature, which frequently causes teenagers to complain of feeling too warm (thus explaining their rejection of an extra sweater offered by a concerned parent).

It is important to realize that the secretion of each of these hormones is interdependent with the levels of other hormones through a delicate feedback mechanism. During the pubertal process, imbalances in hormonal levels are common. Because of their intimate relationship to the hypothalamus, emotional states in an individual, such as fear or anxiety, can directly affect the efficiency of the total process. Normal maturation depends on a complicated and sensitive balance among the endocrine glands.

Somatic Changes

Although the point of onset of the pubertal process varies greatly from one individual to another, the sequence of events, once started, is fairly predictable. The maturational pattern of males parallels that of females. In discussing the sequence of these events, it is important to keep in mind that one phenomenon is not complete before another begins. Each characteristic may take 1 or 2 years to reach its adult maturity level.

FACTORS AFFECTING ONSET

The most critical factor controlling onset of the pubertal process is the gender of the individual: Females mature an average of 2 years earlier than males. It is postulated that this difference is due to the more rapid maturation of the central nervous system in females. Many factors appear to affect the onset of puberty: Hereditary factors and climate show significant correlation with the onset of menarche [1, 11], and chronic disease is known to delay the onset of puberty [26]. Black females tend to initiate the menstrual cycle a few months earlier than white females. However, when females from various racial backgrounds are exposed to similar environment and living conditions, differences in the onset of menarche disappear. Some research indicates that females have an earlier menarche if they have fewer siblings, are blind or obese, or live in lower altitudes or urban settings [1].

An improvement in the nutritional and health status of children in western cultures has been reflected by a gradual decrease in the age of onset of menarche from 17 years in Europe in 1850 to 14.5 years in the United States in 1900 [26]. The current average age of 12.5 to 12.8 years for onset of menarche has remained stable for the past 30 years, suggesting that, overall, adolescents appear to be approximating optimal nutritional and health levels.

Nutrition and health status have a marked influence on the maturational process. The evidence indicates that a minimal weight for height is essential for the initiation and maintenance of the menstrual cycle [16]. Although two females may vary widely in height, the percentage of body weight to fat is essentially identical at menarche. This is one of the explanations for delayed menarche in young female athletes—they have a very low body-fat ratio [38]. This "critical-fat theory" explains why females in poverty situations tend to have delayed onset of menarche as well as delayed resumption of the menses following childbirth and lactation. The critical-fat theory also explains why there has been a decrease in the age of menarche in advanced industrial nations.

Menarche that occurs any time between 9.5 and 15.5 years is considered to be within normal limits, although menarche before 11 years of age is considered early. Many males experience nocturnal emissons at about 14.5 years; 11.5 to 17.5 years is considered the normal range for regular onset of this phenomenon (Table 25–1). Although the neural pathways underlying orgasm are present much earlier, true ejaculations do not occur prior to external puberty [42].

SEQUENCE OF CHANGES
The earliest hormonal changes are so minute and gradual that external physical and emotional correlates are usually not recognizable. However, young females may

Table 25-1. External Phenomena Marking the Point of Puberty

Phenomenon	Normal Age Range (yr)
Menarche (female)	12.5 ± 3
Nocturnal emissions (male)	14.5 ± 3

have minor fluctuations in hormonal levels that can have corresponding physical and emotional manifestations that are discernible to the astute observer. When the author's daughter was about 8 years old, her mother began to notice temporary withdrawal behaviors and a single pimple on the side of her nose, occurring at about 6-week intervals. One day the daughter came to her mother, greatly disturbed because "I am so depressed and I don't know why." They mutually explored many potential sources of her depression, all of which proved to be unfounded. After exhausting the various avenues, her mother said, "Have you noticed that you have a pimple on the side of your nose?" The

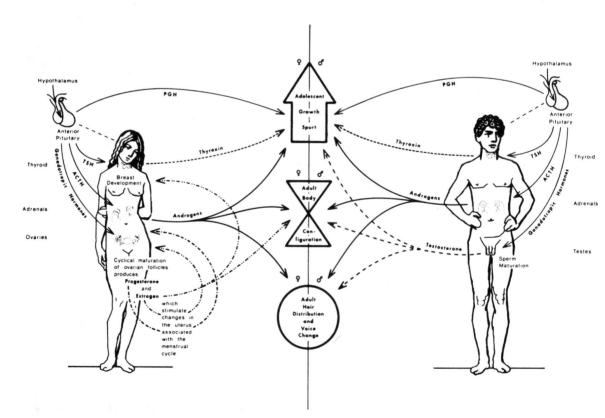

Figure 25–1. The endocrine system at puberty. (From I. Valadian and D. Porter, *Physical Growth and Development: From Conception to Maturity*. Boston: Little, Brown, 1977. With permission.)

daughter reached up to feel, wondering how a pimple could relate to her depression. Her mother then went on to explain briefly the cyclic effect of hormones in a woman's body, ending with the comment, "I don't think anything is wrong with you. I think your depression is just the result of your hormonal balance." Relief and a huge smile flooded her face. She hugged her mother and responded, "I'm so glad I talked to you about it. Now I am happy and excited about feeling depressed. I'm growing up!" So goes the paradox of maturation—one is happy about being depressed!

The first overt sign that the pubertal process is under way is usually the maturation of the eccrine and apocrine glands. The young person who typically hates to take time out to bathe must now wash and use deodorant regularly to protect both clothes and friendships.

The second physiological phenomenon experienced by males and females is pelvic enlargement. Males have a thickening and strengthening of the bone structure; in the female there is an increase in the diameter of the internal pelvis, which is preparatory for the birth process. These anatomical differences are clearly distinguishable by 10 years of age [26].

The third step in the somatic maturation of females is enlargement of the ovaries and uterus. The male experiences a corresponding increase in testicular and scrotal size. The testes become very sensitive to touch at this time. Most young men find an athletic support protective as well as comfortable for sports activities. Androgens may also cause the scrotum to begin to darken at this time. Some health care personnel workers are advocating that testicular examination on a regular basis is as critical to males for early detection of tumor growth as self-breast examination is to females [46].

The fourth developmental characteristic to appear is hyperplastic and hypertrophic growth of breast tissue. About 33 percent of males have some degree of unilateral or bilateral breast tissue enlargement [32], which may be a source of much embarrassment. It usually disappears after several months.

Female breast development occurs in five stages: (1) preadolescent breast bud; (2) increase in areolar diameter, slight breast mound; (3) breast and areola enlargement; (4) continual enlargement with secondary mound for areola; and (5) mature breast with projected nipple [2]. The breast continues to experience growth and contour changes for 3 to 5 years after the breast buds appear. The breasts are frequently tender during the early phases of growth. Slight differences in the size of the breasts are normal, since one breast may

respond more rapidly to circulating hormones than the other. Females should be encouraged to begin breast self-examination each month after the menstrual period; literature on this subject can be obtained free of charge through the local chapter of the American Cancer Society.

The fifth characteristic is darkening and coarsening of the pubic hair. However, it will be 1 to 2 years before it assumes adult color, texture, and curliness. Pubic hair may eventually spread to the thigh areas.

The sixth area to exhibit changes is the external genitalia. The penis now "catches up" to the growth experienced earlier in scrotal size. Young males need reassurance that the size of the nonerect penis has no relationship to the size of the erect penis or to the sexual satisfaction of either partner during sexual intercourse. Females experience growth in the labia and the size of the vagina. Many begin to secrete a thin, milky substance as early as 12 months before menarche. The amount secreted is often cyclic in pattern, reflecting changes in the hormonal levels. This secretion causes a yellow staining of the underpants, leading many mothers to question their daughters about "wetting their pants" or having poor hygiene habits.

Midway through the pubertal period, about the time the pubic hair begins to curl, females experience their first menses and males may begin to experience regular nocturnal emissions. However, the onset of menarche does not indicate sexual maturity. The early menses are often irregular, both in frequency of onset and in the duration and characteristic of flow. This irregularity is probably due to a lack of the modifying influence of progesterone, since progesterone is not produced until ovulation occurs. Early menstruation is caused by cyclic fluctuation of estrogen levels. Nocturnal emission, an involuntary release of semen from the penis during sleep, is also a poor indicator of the onset of true puberty in the male. Some males may experience nocturnal emissions fairly regularly during the late school-age years. The emissions, usually occurring every 1 to 2 weeks, are independent of sexual stimulation. Nocturnal emissions, like menarche, can create a developmental crisis if the young person is not prepared for the event. Young males may experience either deep shame and guilt or pride about the phenomenon, depending on family and peer attitudes and pressures. Others may fear or even receive punishment from their parents for "wetting the bed." Spontaneous erections and ejaculations can be puzzling, troublesome, and embarrassing to the adolescent male. However, nocturnal and spontaneous emissions are as normal for males as menstruation is for females. Both should be accepted as signs of healthy development of the reproductive system. Masturbation activities can relieve genital tensions and provide the adolescent with information on how the body works.

The eighth characteristic to appear is axillary hair. Hair holds odor, which makes good hygiene mandatory. Many girls prefer to shave the axillary hair for reasons of both hygiene and appearance. The appearance of axillary hair may occur much earlier in the sequence of events, even before the appearance of pubic hair.

Gametogenesis generally occurs 12 to 24 months after the external indicators of puberty appear. Occasionally, ovulation may precede menarche. Male gametogenesis can be confirmed by finding mature sperm in the urine or seminal fluid.

The last major physiological change is broadening of the body frame. Females have broadening of the hips and males experience broadening of the shoulders, giving each the mature body contours of the adult. However, the internal diameter of the pelvis continues to broaden for at least 3 years after menarche. The final growth is usually not complete until after the eighteenth birthday [28], which is a major reason why adolescent females have a higher incidence of difficult childbirth.

Both males and females experience vocal-pitch changes with laryngeal growth and thickening of the vocal chords. In just 12 months, the laryngeal membranes grow from 8 mm to 16 mm [45]. Males characteristically experience dramatic changes, with "cracking" of the voice. Females may also experience vocal cracking but to a lesser degree. These changes occur throughout the pubertal process. Like facial hair in the male, vocal changes in males and females usually begin to occur at the point of true puberty, although they may not occur until the end of the pubertal period.

Hormonal changes and rapid growth cause about one-third of all adolescents to develop striae (stretch marks) on gluteal areas, thighs, and lower abdomen. They are a deep reddish purple when they first appear but gradually fade to near invisibility [26]. The somatic changes of the pubertal period in males and females are summarized in Table 25–2.

The Menstrual Cycle

The anticipation and the onset of menarche raise many questions in a young female's mind. Foremost is the question, "Am I normal?" Inherent in this question are concerns over sexuality, health status, and child-bearing ability as well as curiosity about the unknown. A knowledge about normal physiology and characteristics of the menstrual cycle with its variations can greatly reassure the young woman who is learning to deal with her new body functions.

NORMAL CHARACTERISTICS
During the first year following menarche, the length of the menstrual cycle (onset of one menses until the onset of the next menses) is frequently very irregular. After the establishment of a regular pattern, a cycle may range from 21 to 35 days and still be within normal limits. Variations from month to month are also common; 60 percent of females frequently vary as much as 5 days from the expected date of onset [36].

There are three distinct phases of the menstrual flow: premenstrual discharge, major discharge, and postmenstrual discharge. Premenstrual discharge may be pink-mucoid to dark brown in color, lasting up to 1½

Table 25-2. Somatic Changes of the Pubertal Period

Step	Females	Both Genders	Males
1		Apocrine gland development	
2	Increased diameter of internal pelvis	Pelvic changes	Thickening and strengthening of bone structure
3	Growth of ovaries and uterus	Growth in gonad size	Growth of testes and scrotum
4		Breast enlargement	
5		Appearance of pubic hair	
6	Growth of labia and vagina	Growth of external genitalia	Growth of penis
7	Menarche	External puberty	Nocturnal emissions
8		Axillary hair	
9	Oogenesis, ovulation	True puberty	Spermatogenesis, sperm in urine and semen
10	Broadening of hips	Broadening of body frame	Broadening of shoulders
11		Vocal changes throughout	

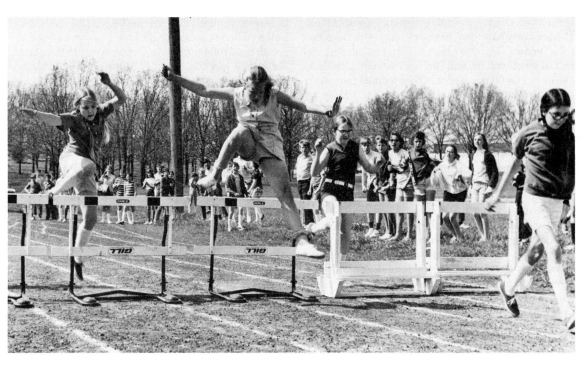

Figure 25–2. Increased activity of the apocrine glands during exercise requires greater attention to personal hygiene.

days. The major discharge, which is bright to deep red in color, lasts an average of 3 to 5 days. Many women experience a postmenstrual discharge, lasting up to 2 days. This last type takes several forms: pink-mucoid secretion, yellow-brown serous fluid, red watery fluid, or thick brown secretions. Some women may experience very little or no premenstrual or postmenstrual discharge. Women report that the total menstrual flow period lasts 4 to 8 days when the premenstrual and postmenstrual flows are included; the average is 5 to 6 days [39].

The major flow is a bloody, nonclotting, viscous fluid with occasional tissue particles and mucus. The average blood loss is about 44 ml (1½ ounces); young adolescents average about 34 ml (1 ounce) [20]. Small clots and pieces of the endometrial lining are not unusual during the first 24 hours. However, large clots or pus, or both, are indicators that medical attention is needed. The odor of the menstrual flow is a bloody, musty, "earthy" smell. An unpleasant odor develops when the flow comes in contact with air. Good hygiene is essential to prevent both odor and infections. Menstrual pads or tampons can be a reservoir of bacteria and potential infection if not changed frequently (three to four times daily, or every 3 to 4 hours during heavy flow).

PREMENSTRUAL SYNDROME

The drop in estrogen and progesterone levels prior to the onset of the menses is often accompanied by both physical and emotional symptoms. Approximately 40 percent of women experience some degree of distress prior to their menses [13]. The symptoms of premenstrual syndrome (PMS) are related to decreased hormonal levels that cause fluid retention. This factor is responsible for temporary weight gain (often as much as 5 pounds), sensitivity of the breasts, abdominal enlargement, irritability, and headache. Some women, especially those who sing, may note minor changes in vocal quality before or during the menses due to edema of the vocal chords. Women who use their eyes for fine details such as in needlework or for extensive reading, may become aware of visual acuity changes before and during the menses. The fluid is lost through increased urine production during the first 2 days after onset of the menses. Decreased blood flow to the uterus and uterine contractions appear to be responsible for pelvic discomfort, cramping, and backache. Some women may experience mild hypoglycemia (low blood sugar) as part of the premenstrual syndrome, which may be partially responsible for fatigue and dizziness as well as nausea, paleness, sweating, weakness, and a craving for sweets. Some women experience constipation, but others may have diarrhea symptoms with the onset of the menses. Many women experience varying degrees of emotional tension such as irritability, restlessness, or even mild depression. Older women frequently complain of increased facial hairs, which must be shaved or plucked out. Nonmedical treatment may include extra sleep and rest, small frequent meals, decreased fluid, sugar, and salt intake, increased physical exercise, and decreased caffeine and nicotine intake. Medical treatment may include biofeedback and hormonal therapy.

DYSMENORRHEA

Dysmenorrhea (painful menstruation) is experienced by about 33 percent of adolescent females after ovulation occurs [11] (nonovulatory cycles do not cause hypertrophy of the secretory endometrial lining and consequently are relatively painless [44]). Primary dysmenorrhea is experienced as spasmodic uterine or lower abdominal and back pain during the first 12 to 24 hours of the major menstrual flow [33]. The etiology and mechanisms of primary dysmenorrhea are unknown, but there appear to be several contributing factors. Recent research indicates that the secretory endometrium produces prostaglandin, which causes contraction of the smooth muscles (uterus and blood vessels) [2]. The pain may also be due to ischemia (lack of oxygen) of the uterine muscles. Because of the anatomical position of the blood vessels, the blood supply is decreased when the uterine muscles contract. This phenomenon is an essential asset during and following childbirth but is somewhat of a nuisance at other times. Contractions of the round ligaments that support the uterine body by attaching to the spinal column are responsible for the backache. Primary dysmenorrhea often disappears spontaneously at about 24 years of age when uterine maturation is complete [44] or after the birth of a baby as the result of dilation of the cervix. The small cervix of the nulliparous woman causes the uterus to work harder to rid itself of the menstrual contents.

Primary dysmenorrhea should be evaluated by a physician to rule out any organic problems and to offer emotional support to the young woman. The fact that only ovulating women experience primary dysmenorrhea can be reassuring to the young female.

The treatment of dysmenorrhea may include warmth (e.g., application of a heating pad) to increase the blood supply to the uterus and a mild analgesic, such as aspirin. Exercise throughout the month maintains good muscle tone and flexibility; exercise during the menses

is helpful in alleviating backache. Occasionally, physicians will recommend a diuretic to reduce symptoms due to fluid retention, an oral contraceptive to be taken for 3 to 6 months in order to produce anovulatory cycles, or a medication to relax the uterine musculature. If dysmenorrhea is associated with the first menstrual period, the young female should be seen by a physician [2].

Secondary dysmenorrhea is characterized by severe, constant, or radiating pain (pain that appears to "shoot" down the leg), which may begin 2 to 3 days before the onset of the menses or may extend beyond the first 24 hours. These are symptoms that should be evaluated by a physician.

AMENORRHEA

Amenorrhea, or absence of a menstrual period, is frequent during the first year after the onset of menarche. Once the cycle is clearly established, the most common cause of amenorrhea is pregnancy. Amenorrhea can be caused by emotional factors, such as unresolved stressors that lead to anxiety. Fear and fatigue can also cause amenorrhea. The apparent link to the endocrine system that governs the hormonal levels is through the hypothalamus. Oligomenorrhea (cycles of 35 to 90 days) and amenorrhea are more prevalent in college students than in the general population [4]. Several female college students have told the author that they never have a menstrual period during the academic quarter or semester; however, when their examinations are over and they return home for a well-deserved vacation, the menstrual period returns. Female inmates of penal institutions report similar menstrual behaviors. Cases of amenorrhea should be checked by a physician, however, since amenorrhea can also be a symptom of a pathological process or pregnancy.

SOMATIC DEVELOPMENT

About 2 to 4 years before the onset of external puberty, the child enters the pubescent period, which is characterized by a rapid acceleration in the rate of body growth. At the beginning of this period, most children have already attained 75 to 80 percent of their height and 50 percent of adult weight [11]. Although all body systems undergo rapid maturational changes, the growth is most easily observed in body height.

The prepubertal growth spurt is arbitrarily divided into two stages. The first stage, the adolescent growth spurt, is identified by an increase in the growth rate.

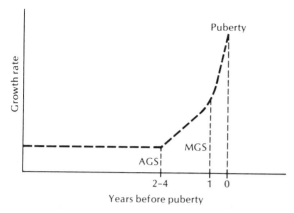

Figure 25-3. The prepubertal growth spurt. AGS = adolescent growth spurt; MGS = maximal growth spurt.

This growth spurt is basically the product of increased hormonal activity. The second stage of prepubertal growth, known as the maximal growth spurt, begins about a year before the onset of true puberty. The individual again experiences a marked acceleration in the rate of height increase. Growth continues at a rapid pace until it reaches a peak that generally coincides with the onset of external puberty, which is followed by a rapid decrease in the growth rate.

Another interesting change that occurs during the pubescent period is the change in hairline. During childhood, the hairline of both males and females circles evenly around the face at the temples. During pubescence and the early adolescent years, the hairline on males begins to recede at the temples, giving the face a more rectangular appearance.

Skeletal System

The correlation between the maturation of the skeletal system and that of the reproductive system is very high

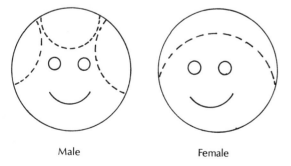

Figure 25-4. The hairline of females continues to encircle the face after puberty, whereas the male's hairline begins to recede at the temples.

[26], probably because they are both under the influence of the hypothalamus [11]. Activation of the hypothalamus appears to initiate the sequential growth changes in the young adolescent. The feet and hands are the first to experience rapid growth, followed by the long bones of the arms and legs. Before puberty, both males and females experience lengthening and broadening of the body frame. After onset of the external signs of puberty, the growth rate is greatly slowed. As ossification slows and the epiphyseal areas of the long bones mature under the influence of the sex hormones, long-bone growth stops. The African Black has longer legs and arms in proportion to sitting height, more muscle, and heavier bones per unit weight than Caucasian youths, giving many Blacks a marked advantage in racing and other sports [42].

Although the adolescent may experience a height increase of 2 to 3 more inches following the onset of menarche or nocturnal emissions, most of this growth is caused by an increase in length of the trunk rather than the long bones [11]. The longer prepubertal growth stages experienced by males allow for greater limb growth [40].

One-third of the females and one-half of the males of high-school age participate in some competitive sports [30]. Since androgen influences the density of skeletal structure, the bones of males are more dense than those of females. For example, the humerus of the male is one-third more dense than that of the female [11]. The implications for sports or activities requiring leverage are obvious. It should also be noted at this point that fractures of the long bones—especially in the epiphyseal area—during the prepubertal growth spurt can create a growth imbalance by arresting growth of the affected bone.

Not all fractures are easily recognized. Many adolescent athletes develop stress fractures from overuse or stress on the young bones. X-ray examination may show no bone changes, but the child can continue to complain of generalized pain in the leg or adjacent joints. Some may have focal tenderness, swelling, or decreased range of motion. Resting the bone is critical to healing and the prevention of a complete fracture. A switch to swimming will result in minimal disruption of training and loss of muscle tone [37].

Since growth in both height and weight is closely related to maturation of the reproductive system, the onset of which is genetically as well as environmentally determined, the establishment of norms for this age group is very difficult. One child might grow 6 to 7 inches in one year, while a peer may grow only 1 inch. The assessment of growth must be highly individualized, taking into account parental height, previous growth pattern, sexual maturity, and environmental conditions (see the grids in Appendixes D and E for growth trends). Males may continue to increase in height through their early twenties.

Muscular System

Prior to the pubertal period, males and females experience only minor differences in muscle mass [11]. The maximal growth of muscle mass correlates with the maximal growth of the skeletal system [26]. The peak period of growth in females is 1 year before menarche, and in males, about 6 months before puberty [11]. Androgen appears to be directly related to the marked increase in muscle mass experienced by males [7]. By 17 years of age, muscle mass is about two times greater in males than in females, causing the average male to be two to four times stronger than the average female [11].

Central Nervous System

The growth of the cerebrum, cerebellum, and brainstem is essentially complete by the end of the tenth year of life [26]. Consequently, in contrast to the other systems of the body, the central nervous system does not experience a sudden growth spurt during the pubertal period. However, the myelinization of the greater cerebral commissures and the reticular formation of the central nervous system continue until the middle adult years [7]. Brain tissue appears to reach quantitative and qualitative maturity with puberty. Gradual increases in fine-motor control and intellectual capacity are discernible during the adolescent years. However, it is difficult to determine whether this improvement is due to practice or to continued neurological development.

Cardiovascular System

The heart experiences a growth spurt during the prepubertal growth period. This growth enables the heart to pump the blood with increased strength, thereby elevating the blood pressure. Although the pulse rate may exhibit a transient increase during the peak periods of growth, the increased size allows the pulse rate to stabilize at a lower rate. Females generally maintain a pulse rate about 10 percent higher than males [7]. Blood volume, which is directly related to weight, increases more rapidly in the male. In late adolescence, males average 5000 ml and females 4200 ml of blood. By the sixteenth year of life, the heart has usually adopted the adult rhythm [26]. There is an increase in the length and the thickness of the blood vessel walls and in the size of the heart. The heart growth is relatively greater, however, than the growth in the diameter of the veins and the arteries. This delay in increase in the size of blood vessels, combined with the increased heart size, stroke strength, and blood volume, may cause the young adolescent to experience transient chest discomfort or fullness combined with "thumping," especially after periods of activity. Hormonal changes also create some differentiation of blood values (see Appendix E).

Respiratory System

The increase in vital capacity (the greatest volume of air that can be expressed from the lungs following a maximal intake of air) correlates with the structural frame; the greater the height of an individual, the larger is the vital capacity and the slower is the respiratory

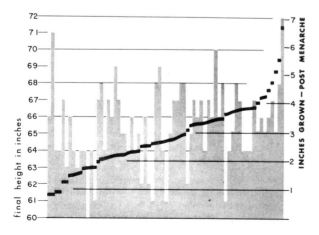

Figure 25–5. Growth following menarche in 68 normal American girls. The dark line indicates the final height; the shaded areas indicate the inches grown after menarche. There does not appear to be any correlation with final height. (From G. H. Lowrey, *Growth and Development of Children* [7th ed.]. Chicago: Year Book, 1978. With permission.)

rate, regardless of gender [7]. On the average, however, males breathe more slowly than females.

Gastrointestinal System

During adolescence, the organs function at widely varying levels of maturity—even within the same system (Table 25–3). These variances can and do lead to temporary metabolic, hormonal, and functional imbalances.

The adolescent growth spurt requires a corresponding increase in the size of the stomach to accommodate the increased need for the food required to implement growth. The stomach becomes both longer and wider and also experiences an increase in gastric acidity in order to facilitate digestion of the increased intake [40]. This increased acidity frequently causes abdominal pain and may occasionally lead to symptoms of gastric ulcers in adolescents. The stress of coping with the myriad of physiological changes may also increase gastric secretions and thus bring about ulcer symptoms.

Basal Metabolic Rate

The basal metabolic rate (BMR; the rate at which the body uses calories to maintain body function when at rest) correlates closely with the rate of body growth. It increases with periods of growth spurt, reaching a peak at external puberty, and declines gradually as the growth rate decelerates. At the end of adolescence, the BMR of males is about 10 percent higher than that of females [26]. One theory for the gender difference is the greater muscle mass in males; another is that increased BMR is a direct result of higher androgen levels [7].

Because of the very rapid growth, the pubescent child may not have sufficient energy left for strenuous activities. He or she tires easily and may frequently

Table 25-3. Average Weights of Organs at Different Ages (gm)

	Newborn	1 Yr	6 Yr	Puberty	Adult
Brain	350	910	1200	1300	1350
Heart	24	45	95	220	300
Thymus	12	20	24	30	0–15
Kidneys (both)	25	70	120	170	300
Liver	150	300	550	1500	1600
Lungs (both)	60	130	260	410	1200
Pancreas	3	9	20	40	90
Spleen	10	30	55	95	155
Stomach	8	30	60	80	135

Source: G. H. Lowrey, *Growth and Development of Children* (7th ed). Chicago: Year Book, 1978. With permission.

complain of needing to sit down. Gradually the child is able to increase both speed and stamina during exercise. An increase in muscular and skeletal strength, as well as the increased ability of the lungs and heart to provide adequate oxygen to the tissues, facilitates the maintenance of homeostasis and the rate of recovery after exercise. The body reaches its peak of physiological resilience during late adolescence and early adulthood [7]. Evidence of this peak is reflected in the age of many Olympic competitors. Both strength and the tolerance for strenuous activity can be increased by regular physical training and an individualized conditioning program.

NUTRITIONAL NEEDS

An increase in caloric needs parallels the rate of body growth and the increased metabolic rate. Teenagers frequently feel as if they can never get enough to eat. Meals are frequent and voluminous. Parents are awed and sometimes angered at the amount of food their adolescent consumes. At peak growth periods, females may consume as much as 2600 calories per day, and a male may take in 3600 calories or more [11] (see Appendix E for further details). Careful attention should be paid to fluid, protein, and calcium needs during this period of rapid growth.

Protein needs are closely related to the growth rate. During adolescence, proteins should comprise 12 to 16 percent of the total daily energy intake [34], with higher proportions during the earlier years, when growth is most rapid. Protein needs may not be met if the adolescent is on a severe reducing diet, is from a lower socioeconomic environment, or is on a diet that eliminates animal proteins. Strict vegetarian diets can also lead to deficiencies in vitamins and minerals.

Adequate calcium intake is essential for continued bone growth and formation of teeth. Adolescents, especially males, are at risk for suboptimal calcium intake during periods of rapid skeletal growth. The weight-conscious female may also unknowingly reduce her calcium intake dangerously. Milk and cheese are the richest sources of calcium. The female's iron needs vary according to the blood loss during her menses; a daily intake of 1.2 gm of iron is recommended for replacement and maintenance needs [31]. Periodic blood checks will indicate if additional intake is needed. Many physicians recommend a regular iron supplement even when dietary intake appears to be adequate. Inadequate vitamin C is another frequent nutritional problem, since fruit juices, fresh fruit, and vegetables may be overlooked.

Caloric needs are further increased if the adolescent

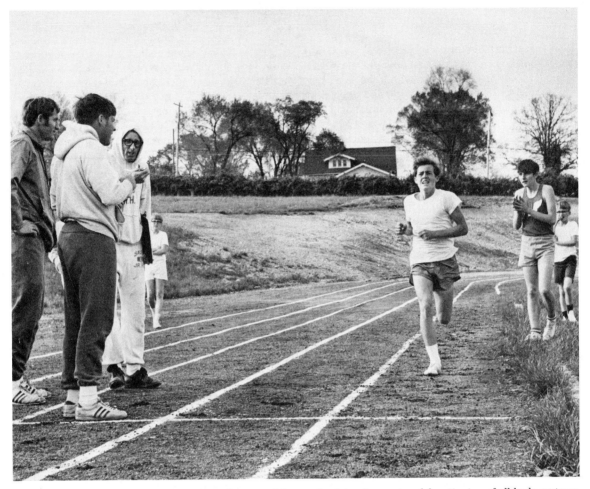

Figure 25-6. Adequate exercise continues to be critical for maximal development and functioning of all body systems.

is involved in sports. The amount and the frequency of food intake can affect the athlete's strength and endurance. Athletes may consume as much as 6000 calories per day. The recommended pattern of food intake is 15 percent protein, 30 percent fat, and 55 percent carbohydrate [30]. Fat and carbohydrate, but not protein, are converted to immediate energy. Paying attention to adequate hydration and salt intake is also important for athletes. There is no evidence that massive intake of vitamins increases physical prowess, but well-balanced meals and regular vitamin, mineral, and iron supplements are recommended to assure adequate nutrition. Muscle development also depends on regular, appropriate exercises.

The recommended daily intake for adolescents in the four basic food groups is given in Table 25–4.

Busy schedules and the need for frequent intake of

food lead many adolescents to skip breakfast and rely on quick-energy foods, such as carbonated beverages and snack chips. Inadequate nutritional intake is common even though calories may be adequate. A daily vitamin supplement can help to ensure the adequate intake of essential vitamins.

Table 25-4. Recommended Daily Intake for Adolescents*

Food Group	Amount
Milk	3–4 cups
Meat	3–4 servings
Fruit and vegetables	5–6 servings
Bread and cereals	4–5 servings

* Extra foods may be added in each group to ensure adequate caloric intake.

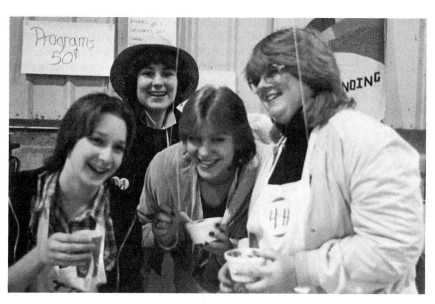

Figure 25-7. Many adolescent social activities center around or include food consumption.

FATIGUE

Easy fatigability was mentioned earlier as a side effect of the consumption of calories by the body for growth; fatigue may also be precipitated by overactivity. There is so much for the young adolescent to do and to become involved in that he or she may not set appropriate limits on activity or involvement. The adolescent needs to plan some quiet time every day to allow for both physiological and psychological rest. Many adolescents hate to go to bed—and hate to get up in the morning. All the interesting things happen at night (or so it seems). The lack of adequate sleep can also lead to a feeling of chronic fatigue. Adolescents need 8 to 9 hours of sleep at night.

Faulty nutrition is another major cause of fatigue. Poor eating habits established during the school-age years, combined with the typical quick-service, quick-energy food consumption patterns of adolescents, frequently lead to anemia. Females must be especially careful to obtain adequate iron intake because of the loss during each menses. Testosterone levels in males help to retain higher hemoglobin levels [40].

COMMON PROBLEMS ASSOCIATED WITH ADOLESCENT GROWTH

A number of common problems during adolescence present additional hurdles to the establishment of a positive self-concept and body image. Although these conditions are not unique to adolescence, they seem to occur more frequently during these years, creating more stress in a period that is already full of stressors and crises.

Juvenile Obesity

Obesity can be a serious health problem because it increases the incidence of some diseases, heightens surgical risks, and augments death rates [12]. Obesity is defined simply as excessive amounts of fat on the body. Many pubescents deposit extra fat during these years in preparation for the adolescent growth spurt. Those who consistently overeat and select nutritionally unbalanced foods may accumulate too much body fat. Once these additional cells are formed, they may predispose the individual to lifelong obesity. Ten to 16 percent of adolescent females are more than 20 percent overweight for their height [40]; 80 percent of these females will remain overweight as adults. Obesity may occasionally be caused by a malfunction in metabolism; calories may be converted into fat instead of heat energy [11]. However, the major cause of obesity is hyperphagia (overeating).

Food consumption patterns may facilitate storage rather than use of energy. Some teenagers have the "night eating syndrome." In the mornings they do not feel like eating, so breakfast is skipped. When they are unable to sleep at night, they eat. Eating before sleeping leads to storage of the calories, since they are not used for energy. Other teenagers face stress with the "eating binge syndrome." They consume great quantities of food in short periods of time and subsequently

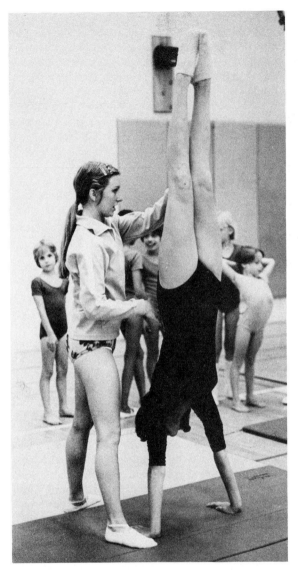

Figure 25–8. Adolescents tend to become involved in so many different activities that parents may need to help them set some limits to ensure adequate rest in order to prevent fatigue and the depression or the discouragement that will sometimes accompany it.

suffer severe discomfort and self-criticism. Their attempts at reduction diets are short-lived, since intermittent stress precipitates the eating binge again. The adolescent may develop negative feelings about the self because of being fat, yet he or she attempts to comfort the self with food. Thus a vicious cycle can be established. The teenager with the "eating without satiation

syndrome" finds it very difficult to stop once eating is started—the food just "feels so good going down." This type of hyperphagia usually has no correlation with stress, and the individual expresses little or no self-criticism after the spree [11].

Weight Loss

The treatment of juvenile obesity is very difficult during periods of rapid growth. Good nutrition—a diet that includes the basic four food groups—is essential. Caloric intake is usually reduced in the form of foods high in carbohydrates (sugars and starches). However, many health professionals try to assist the adolescent only to maintain, not to lose, weight until the growth spurt is completed. (This policy often results in an appearance of weight loss, since the adolescent gains in height what is lost in width.) Athletes who try to lose weight to fit into another weight category also lose muscle strength. They should limit weight loss to no more than 2 pounds per week [30].

Some young people may benefit from attending camps or "rap-session" groups for overweight children and adolescents. They are encouraged to lose weight by learning how to establish good eating and exercise habits. These programs include group discussion periods for the sharing of common problems and concerns. The "fat" adolescent rarely uses normal peer groups for support and physical activity [25]. Their embarrassment over their physical condition often sentences them to a life of loneliness, thus affecting social-emotional development. Group activities need to be provided that focus on constructive experiences that will assist the participants to recognize and to mobilize their potentials or assets. Obese adolescents need assistance in recognizing what they **can** do and what they **can** eat when out with the gang. Dieting and exercise are very difficult for the adolescent who developmentally needs instant results.

ANOREXIA NERVOSA

One to 3 percent of adolescents become so obsessed with the idea of losing weight that they restrict their intake and increase their activity level so severely that their very lives are threatened by the weight loss. Ninety percent of the anorexia nervosa population are female [3]. The etiology is unknown, but it is hypothesized that anorexia nervosa is a reactivation of the separation-individuation issue that is precipitated by events of puberty or independent living, since the peak periods of incidence are in the 12- to 13 and 19- to 20-year-old age groups. The adolescents are usually "ideal" children prior to the onset of symptoms. They have been rigidly obedient to parental and societal (external) expectations. The anorexia appears to be an attempt to extricate themselves from parental control by rigidly controlling what happens to their bodies (internal control). This control offers a sense of effectiveness in the face of developmental and maturational crises. Fifteen to 21 percent of anorexics die from the disorder [29].

Anorexia nervosa is not an attempt at suicide but at psychological self-preservation [8]. The irony is that the physical self is dying while the psychological self is emerging. The anorexia takes on a life of its own once it gets started. Physical changes include decreased weight, blood pressure, pulse rate, and temperature. The individual has dry flaky skin and may develop lanugo (fine downy body hair). Females experience amenorrhea as their weight falls below the critical-fat level. Perceptual changes include viewing the self as bloated, although the individual may have a 25 percent weight loss or more. There is a denial of hunger along with sensations of fatigue. The attempts to reason with anorexic individuals and to present facts and norms are useless. A distorted perception of personal appearance convinces the victims they are obese, although in reality, emaciation may threaten survival. They are proud of their strict, stoic, Spartan existence. Anorexics may also avoid school as a way to prevent control by teachers.

Many disciplines need to work together to help the anorexic adolescent to return to a safe weight and to gain a sense of self-control, pride, and independence. All of the members of the family must be involved in the therapy, since a careful assessment of the family dynamics may reveal inadequate individuation and gross overprotectiveness [6]. Anorexics who are cured tend to stabilize at 85 to 90 percent of ideal weight for their height [9].

BULEMIA

Some adolescents maintain or lose weight through self-induced vomiting, which may be used regularly or only after an eating binge. Nineteen percent of college-age females and 5 percent of college-age males use this method of weight control [21]. Bulemics may be obese, average, or underweight. Some bulemics may experience an erosion of tooth enamel because of the frequent vomiting (stomach acids eat the enamel away) [35]. Many bulemics have associated behavior problems, such as drug taking, promiscuity, and stealing [3] (all abnormal "taking in" activities). Laxatives and diuretics may be used by anorexics or bulemics to hasten weight loss. Most bulemics realize their behavior is ab-

normal and attempt to prevent discovery of their actions [35].

Since 23 percent of bulemics may attempt suicide [18], referral to counseling is strongly suggested when discovered. Both anorexics and bulemics should be referred for medical evaluation because of the threat to life. Additional information can be obtained through the National Association of Anorexia Nervosa and Associated Disorders, Box 271, Highland Park, IL 60035.

Acne

More than 80 percent of adolescents experience some degree of acne vulgaris between 9 to 20 years of age [41]. The increased androgen levels at puberty stimulate the production of sebum by the sebaceous glands of face, neck, shoulders, and upper chest. The small, immature ducts leading from the glands to the surface of the skin may be inadequate to transport the large amounts of material produced, forcing the sebum to occlude the ducts and to dilate the glands. The normal bacteria of the skin colonize the sebaceous follicle, releasing free fatty acid as a substance that irritates surrounding tissue. The closed comedo (whitehead) has two fates. It can continue to dilate until it becomes an open comedo (blackhead), or it can rupture below the skin surface, spreading its contents into surrounding tissue. The skin sets up a localized foreign-body response to the comedonal core and the acids from the ruptured comedos. Occasionally, two or three comedos may merge, creating nodules or cysts. When bacteria are involved, abscesses may form.

Most cases of acne disappear spontaneously sometime after the twentieth birthday. Although there appears to be a genetic predisposition toward acne vulgaris, it can be precipitated or aggravated by poor hygiene, working around greases, and the use of ordinary cosmetics. Forehead acne has been reported from the use of pomade on the hair, and perioral acne from the use of fluoridated toothpastes.

The general management of acne includes a well-balanced diet, good hygiene to remove surface pore blocks and to reduce bacteria count, the avoidance of known irritants, and the reduction of emotional tension and anxiety. Research does not document the need for dietary restrictions [41]. However, individuals may find that particular foods appear to be associated with increased comedo formation, and that adequate sleep and exposure to sunlight appear to help [31]. Pinching and squeezing may spread the contents into the adjacent tissues, thus increasing the chances of infection and scarring. Superficial pustules may resolve more quickly, however, if the contents are squeezed out to the surface, using gentle pressure and clean hands [41].

Several breakthroughs have been made in controlling the formation and the treatment of acne. For severe cases, antibiotics may be used. Synthetic oral Vitamin A preparations appear to decrease the formation of new comedos. Topical benzoyl peroxide and tretinoin are also helpful in reducing the severity of acne [15]. The adolescent may wish to obtain medical consultation for further advice or assistance in controlling the condition of the skin during this period of life.

Poor Posture

Poor posture is a common phenomenon of both male and female adolescents. One causative factor is the rapid skeletal growth. Since the long bones grow faster than the adjacent muscles, keeping the joints bent relieves tension on stretched muscles. Many young adolescents complain of muscle cramps or leg aches for the same reason. Some adolescents are uncomfortable with, or ashamed of, their height and will slump to achieve an appearance of being shorter. Some females who are embarrassed by an increase in breast size may round their shoulders and lean forward slightly to deemphasize their maturing figure. There is also speculation that some poor posture is due to inadequate exercise and too much sitting to watch television. Poor posture may also be caused by unequal leg length. A difference of one-half inch at maturity is still within the normal range [17]. Frequently a shoe lift is all that is necessary to achieve balance.

Medical evaluation may be appropriate to rule out the presence of a skeletal anomaly. Scoliosis, a lateral deviation of the spine, is often first diagnosed in early adolescence. Since it is progressive and can lead to complications, early intervention is warranted. Although evidence now suggests some genetic basis for scoliosis, the exact mechanisms and underlying causes are unknown [17]. Some physicians recommend routine screening for scoliosis during the junior high school years.

Dentition

Permanent dentition is usually completed during the late adolescent years. The third molar (wisdom tooth) usually erupts earlier in females. Many young adults need to have one or more wisdom teeth removed. The major reasons for removal of the wisdom teeth are as follows: (1) There may be inadequate room in the dental arch to support the extra tooth, and removal prevents overcrowding of teeth and resultant malocclusion; (2) since the third molar is the last tooth to develop, calcification may cease before the enamel is complete; eruption of the poorly calcified tooth leads to rapid decay, necessitating removal.

Adolescents are frequently in need of dental attention to prevent or to cure malocclusion, a significant deviation of the normal alignment of teeth that causes poor bite. Straightening of the teeth is usually done during adolescence when the supportive structures are still soft enough to allow gradual repositioning. Straightening of the teeth can decrease some speech defects due to tooth alignment; it can also decrease the occurrence of emotional trauma due to unattractive appearance.

Headache

Forty percent of children experience headache by 7 years of age, and 75 percent have headaches by age 15 [19]. Eighty to 90 percent of persons experience headache at some point in their lives [10], 90 percent of which are benign [5]. Headaches can be divided into three categories: symptomatic, psychogenic, and vascular (migraine). Symptomatic headaches are secondary to problems such as disease, trauma, sinusitis, metabolic imbalances, eye strain, head injury, fever, allergies, brain tumor, bruxosis, hunger, or encephalitis. Psychogenic headaches, or tension headaches, are the most frequent recurrent form of headache. Tension headaches are rare before adolescence [27]. The individual tenses the muscles—especially those of the neck and the scalp in response to stress. A headache ensues, which may last from several hours to several days. It is frequently a dull, persistent, band-like pain felt on both sides of the head.

Seventy percent of those experiencing vascular or migraine headaches have a family history of similar headaches [5]. These headaches may begin during the toddler years [27]; by 15 years of age, the incidence is about 5 percent [14]. Vascular headaches typically have three phases. In the preheadache phase, the individual may experience an aura that may consist of transient neurological signs and distorted perceptual processes and cognition. During the second phase, the scalp vessels become dilated and pulsatile, which produces a unilateral, pounding headache. In the third phase, edema of the vessel walls and tightening of the muscles leads to a steady, intractable, tension-type headache. The causes of vascular headaches are unknown, but stress, fatigue, loss of sleep, menstruation, bright lights, eye strain, alcohol, and foods with tyramine (milk products, chocolate, coffee, cola beverages) are known to trigger these headaches [27].

Recurring headaches in children should be evaluated by a physician. The child's total life-style and life-space need to be included in the assessment, such as school grades, peer relations, potential environmental toxins, and the parents' marital adjustment.

CONCLUSIONS

The pubertal period can be one of great happiness with the anticipation of adult characteristics or a period of intense anxiety and apprehension as the young person observes the unfolding of adult body configuration and functions. Although the total changes occur over a span of 8 to 10 years, the young person may be consciously aware only of those events that represent the most dramatic changes over a 2- to 3-year span of time. Menarche is the most clearly defined overt sign of female puberty, but true puberty does not usually occur until 1 to 2 years later when the ovaries begin to produce viable ova. Males have no clear demarcation for identifying the onset of true puberty.

Good hygiene and health practices as well as meaningful education about sexuality are essential to maintain high level physical and emotional wellness during, and following, the pubertal period. All females should be encouraged to have a pelvic examination and Pap smear annually after 18 years of age, or sooner if they are sexually active.

Energy and nutrition requirements during adolescence are directly related to the rate and the stage of growth, with the highest requirements at the peak rate of growth. Adolescents may need guidance to assist them to care for and to use their bodies appropriately in order to maximize their vast potentials. Dental visits should continue at 6-month intervals, and a complete physical examination should be obtained at least once a year. A diphtheria-tetanus "booster" immunization is recommended at approximately 14 to 15 years of age [1]. Health education classes can help adolescents to obtain the information that will help them to understand body functioning in order to become more independent in health maintenance.

At no time is individuality more critical than during adolescence. The young person needs to be assured of his or her normalcy while appreciating the individual variations contributing to uniqueness. Adolescents should be assessed in terms of individual health status and abilities. A carefully planned, individualized athletic program should be provided for each adolescent, including proper conditioning, competent coaching instruction, rigid regulations to protect the athlete's safety, and promotion of the enjoyment of the game.

Each individual needs to learn to appreciate, to use, and to care for the body properly during adolescence so that it can be used as a tool for self-expression in the years ahead.

REFERENCES

1. Adams, J. F.   Earlier menarche, greater height and weight: A stimulation-stress factor hypothesis. *Genet. Psychology Monographs* 104:3, 1981.
2. *Adolescent Gynecology.* Report of the 7th Ross Roundtable. Columbus, OH: Ross Laboratories, 1977.
3. Andersen, A.   Anorexia and bulimia. *J. Adol. Health Care* 4(1):15, 1983.
4. Bachmann, G. A., and Kemmann, E.   Prevalence of oligomenorrhea and amenorrhea in a college population. *Am. J. Obstet. and Gynecol.* 143:98, 1982.
5. Barrett-Griesemer, P., Meisel, S., and Rute, R.   A guide to headaches—and how to relieve their pain. *Am. J. Nurs.* 81:50, 1981.
6. Boyle, M. P., Koff, E., Gudas, L. J.   Assessment and management of anorexia nervosa. *Am. J. of Matern.-Child Nurs.* 6:412, 1981.
7. Chinn, P. L.   *Child Health Maintenance: Concepts in Family-centered Care* (2nd ed.). St. Louis: Mosby, 1979.
8. Ciseau, A.   Anorexia nervosa: A view from the mirror. *Am. J. Nurs.* 80:1468, 1980.
9. Collins, M., Hodas, G. R., and Lieberman, R.   Interdisciplinary model for inpatient treatment of adolescents with anorexia nervosa. *J. Adol. Health Care* 4:3, 1983.
10. Conway-Rutkowski, B.   Getting to the cause of headaches. *Am. J. Nurs.* 81:1846, 1981.
11. Cooke, R. E. (Ed)   *The Biologic Basis of Pediatric Practice.* New York: McGraw-Hill, 1968.
12. Craft, C. A.   Body image and obesity. *Nurs. Clin. North Am.* 7:677, 1972.
13. Dalton, K.   *The Premenstrual-Syndrome and Progesterone Therapy* (2nd ed.). Chicago: Year Book Publishers, 1984.
14. Debrun, S. R.   Headaches in adolescents. *Am. J. of Matern.-Child Nurs.* 6:407, 1981.
15. Domonkos, A. N., et al.   *Andrew's Diseases of the Skin* (7th ed.). Philadelphia: Saunders, 1982.
16. Frisch, R. E., and McArthur, J. W.   Menstrual cycles: Fatness as a determinant of minimum weight for height necessary for their maintenance or onset. *Science* 185:949, 1981.
17. Gallagher, J. R., Heald, F. P., and Garell, D. C.   *Medical Care of the Adolescent* (3rd ed.). New York: Appleton-Century-Crofts, 1976.
18. Garfinkel, P. E., et al.   The heterogeneity of anorexia nervosa: Bulimia as a distinct subgroup. *Arch. Gen. Psychiatry.* 37:1036, 1980.
19. Golden, G. S.   The child with headaches. *Dev. and Behav. Pediatrics* 3(2):114, 1982.
20. Hallberg, L., et al.   Menstrual blood loss: A population study. *Acta Obstet. Gynecol. Scand.* 45:320, 1966.

21. Halmi, K. A., Falk, J. R., and Schwartz, E.   Binge-eating and vomiting: A survey of a college population. *Psychol. Med.* 11:697, 1981.

22. Heim, K., et al.   Cervical cytology: The need for routine screening in the sexually active adolescent. *J. Pediatr.* 91(1):123, 1977.

23. Horrocks, J. E.   *The Psychology of Adolescence* (4th ed.). Boston: Houghton Mifflin, 1976.

24. Katchadourian, H. A.   *The Biology of Adolescence*. San Francisco: Freeman, 1977.

25. Langford, R. W.   Teenagers and Obesity. *Am. J. Nurs.* 81:556, 1981.

26. Lowrey, G. H.   *Growth and Development of Children* (7th ed.). Chicago: Year Book, 1978.

27. McCarthy, A. M.   Chronic headaches in children. *Pediatr. Nurs.* 8(2):88, 1982.

28. Moerman, M. L.   Growth of the birth canal in adolescent girls. *Am. J. Obstet. and Gynecol.* 142:528, 1982.

29. Moore, J. A., and Coulman, M. U.   Anorexia nervosa: The patient, her family and key family therapy interventions. *J. Psychiatr. Nurs.* 19(5):9, 1981.

30. Narins, D. M., Belkengren, R. P., and Sapala, S.   Nutrition and the growing athlete. *Pediatr. Nurs.* 9:163, 1983.

31. National Research Council. Committee on Dietary Allowances. *Recommended Dietary Allowances* (9th ed.). Washington, D.C.: National Academy of Sciences, 1980.

32. *Nelson Textbook of Pediatrics* (12th ed.). R. E. Behrman, V. C. Vaughan; senior editor W. E. Nelson. Philadelphia: Saunders, 1982.

33. Oriatti, M. D.   Dysmenorrhea. *Pediatric Annals* 4(1):60, 1975.

34. Pipes, P. L. (Ed.). *Nutrition in Infancy and Childhood* (2nd ed.). St. Louis: Mosby, 1981.

35. Potts, N. L.   Eating disorder: The secret pattern of binge/purge. *Am. J. Nurs.* 84:32, 1984.

36. Reeder, S. J., et al.   *Maternity Nursing* (15th ed.). Philadelphia: Lippincott, 1983.

37. Rosen, P. R., Micheli, L. J., and Treves, S.   Early scintigraphic diagnosis of bone stress and fractures in athletic adolescents. *Pediatrics* 70(1):11, 1982.

38. Sanborn, C. F., Martin, B. J., and Wagner, W. W.   Is athletic amenorrhea specific to runners? *Am. J. Obstet. and Gynecol.* 142:859, 1982.

39. Schuster, C. S.   "Characteristics of the Menstrual Period." Unpublished research, 1974.

40. Smith, D. W., Bierman, E. L., and Robinson, N. M. (Eds.). *The Biologic Ages of Man: From Conception Through Old Age* (2nd ed.). Philadelphia: Saunders, 1978.

41. Stone, A. C.   Facing up to acne. *Pediatr. Nursing* 8:229, 1982.

42. Tanner, J. M.   *Foetus Into Man: Physical Growth from Conception to Maturity*. London: Open Books, 1978.

43. *Textbook of Medicine* (16th ed.). J. B. Wyngaarden and L. H. Smith (Eds.). Philadelphia: Saunders, 1982.

44. Watson, J. E.   *Medical-Surgical Nursing and Related Physiology* (2nd ed.). Philadelphia: Saunders, 1979.

45. Weiczorek, R. R., and Natapoff, J. N.   *A Conceptual Approach to the Nursing of Children: Health Care From Birth Through Adolescence*. New York: Lippincott, 1981.

46. Williams, H. A.   Screening for testicular cancer. *Pediatr. Nurs.* 7(5):38, 1981.

26

Cognitive and Psychosocial Development During Adolescence

Gerald A. Winer

Although I'm only fourteen, I know quite well
what I want, I know who is right and who is
wrong, I have my opinions, my own ideas and
principles, and although it may sound pretty mad
from an adolescent, I feel more of a person than a
child, I feel quite independent of anyone.

—Anne Frank, *The Diary of a Young Girl*

"When I was a boy of fourteen, my father was so ignorant I could hardly stand to have the old man around. But when I got to be twenty-one, I was astonished at how much he had learned in seven years." So wrote the famous author Mark Twain [25].

Twain's quote, besides being humorous, tells us several things about the nature of the 14-year-old adolescent. To begin with, it suggests that adolescents are critical of their parents. The theme of adolescent censure and conflict with parents is central in the study of adolescence, although it is also widely disputed. Frank's quote also suggests why the adolescent is so critical of his or her parents. The criticism stems from the strong belief that youths' own thoughts are correct even in the face of contrary information from more experienced persons. To the adult, such an inflated belief in the rightness of one's own thoughts and ideas represents an arrogance and a form of egocentrism. To the adolescent, it represents a way to enforce recognition of individuality, to ensure worth, and to protect the still vulnerable concept of self.

COGNITIVE DEVELOPMENT

Piaget's Theory
Jean Piaget proposed that cognitive development consists of the gradual emergence of specific systems of

logic that underlie the child's behavior (see appendices B and C). The school-aged child develops a system of logic that allows understanding of number, space, time, classification, and ordering. But despite the fact that the child shows an ability to reason in these areas, the preadolescent's thought is narrow and essentially limited to dealing with problems that make reference to tangible or concrete objects. In short, the preadolescent, or the child in the concrete operational stage, cannot reason abstractly or on a symbolic level. During adolescence, we see the appearance of formal operational thinking or the emergence of a new level in the ability to employ abstract constructs for problem solving.

FORMAL OPERATIONAL THOUGHT

Piaget offers an example that helps to differentiate between the concrete thought of the preadolescent and the more abstract thought of the formal operational thinker. The example involves ordering. In one version of the problem, a child is shown two objects of different sizes, (e.g., a short red pencil and a slightly taller green pencil). The objects are placed side by side, and then the child is asked which is taller. There is no difficulty, of course, since the child can actually see that the green one is taller. Next the child is asked to compare the green pencil with an even taller one (e.g., yellow). Again the pencils are placed side by side, and again the child experiences no difficulty.

The challenge occurs when the experimenter asks the child to make a comparison between the objects that lie on the extremes (e.g., the shortest pencil [the red] and the tallest pencil [the yellow]). This time the experimenter does not line up the pencils side by side and thus does not permit the child to derive the correct answer by simple observation. Instead, the child must rely on reasoning about sets of relations to infer the correct choice. The reasoning might go something like this: The yellow one is taller than the green one and the green taller than the red, therefore, the yellow must be taller than the red.

This type of problem is termed one of **transitivity,** and it can be solved by children in the 7 to 11-year-old age range. But those children who are capable of reasoning about concrete objects will have difficulty if this same problem is posed in the abstract, with verbal terms substituted for the concrete objects, (e.g., If Joan is taller than Phyllis, and Phyllis taller than Mary, who is taller, Joan or Mary?). In brief, although the concrete operational child is capable of reasoning with respect to concrete objects, it is not until adolescence that the

ability to manipulate symbols and symbolic reasoning appears [47].

The preceding example only hints at the nature of Piaget's stage of formal operations. Actually Piaget and his followers have provided us with a number of characteristics of this stage. In describing some of these characteristics, it is important to recognize how Piaget plumbed the mind of the adolescent. Essentially, he and his followers presented a number of tasks that required solving of physical problems, that is, problems that depend on the discovery and understanding of physical principles. One such problem, for instance, required the child to reason about the variables that govern how fast a pendulum swings. From elementary physics, we know that the speed of a pendulum is determined by the length of the line holding the weight. With a shorter line the pendulum swings faster. But the actual weight of the object suspended by the line is irrelevant to the speed of the swing. In Piaget's problem, the adolescent has to discover this principle. The solution means eliminating the role of variables, such as the weight of the object or how high it is held before it is released [28].

PROPERTIES OF FORMAL THOUGHT

By analyzing performance on tasks of physical reasoning, Piaget and his followers discovered the properties of thought as revealed in behavior and a system of logic that underlies the thought of the adolescent. The details of the logical system will not be discussed here. Instead we will examine some of the manifestations of this thought and its implications for practical behavior.

Combinatorial reasoning. To begin with, we find the adolescent capable of what Piaget terms **combinatorial reasoning,** the ability to form combinations of events. Combinatorial reasoning was studied in a task in which the child was presented with five flasks containing colorless chemical solutions and told that when the fluid from one of four flasks was combined with that from the fifth, the liquid would change color. The task was to determine which combination of four flasks was critical for producing the colored precipitate. (Liquid from one of the four actually negated the reaction and prevented the child from simply mixing all the chemicals together). Young children approached this task haphazardly, missing many combinations. The adolescents, however, systematically combined liquids from each of the four containers with one another [28].

We might not suspect that the ability to form combinations is a very significant one, unless the adoles-

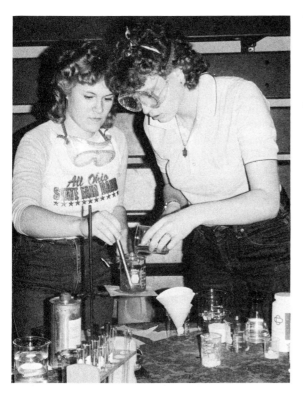

Figure 26–1. The adolescent is able to engage in systematic, hypothetical-deductive reasoning, which opens the door to scientific research and experimentation.

cent is confronted by a problem that requires systematic pairing of events, (like arranging playoff schedules for teams in a baseball league). However, combinatorial reasoning is significant in a more general way in that it represents the mobility and the activity of the adolescent's thought, a mobility that might be described as an increased capacity for generating possibilities. This type of flexibility is of importance in solving problems, since it underlies the capacity to derive multiple solutions to problems.

Hypothetico-deductive thought. Combinatorial thinking is closely related to another property of adolescent thinking: **hypothetico-deductive thought.** This form of thinking actually is the basis of most scientific reasoning, and at the most basic level, it can be thought of in terms of the formation of hypotheses and the use of "if-then" statements. When the car does not start in the morning, one might suspect that the battery is dead. The reasoning might then follow that if the battery is dead, other mechanisms, such as the lights and the

horn, might not work. It is obvious how this form of reasoning lies at the basis of problem solving, especially if one is engaged in science or research.

It is important to recognize that when adolescents employ hypothetico-deductive thought, they are often reasoning about, and with, a particular form of symbols, namely, verbal statements, or in Piaget's terms, verbal propositions. Moreover, they are exercising an ability to think logically, that is, to deduce consequences from various premises. The use of verbal propositions and logic in hypothetico-deductive thought becomes particularly meaningful, insofar as this type of thought and reasoning can be extended beyond the realm of the present and the actual to the realm of the possible. Thus we see adolescents engaged in theory building in which they formulate idealistic models, such as utopias and ideal forms of governments and societies. The adolescent, in short, becomes a theoretician and a thinker, or to put it in slightly different terms, a philosopher. Using newly developed skills, many adolescents spend time thinking about questions that concern the nature of God and reality.

A particularly significant by-product of the adolescent's theorizing concerns the adolescent's concept of self. Inhelder and Piaget [28] point out that adolescents have the ability to construct concepts of roles in society (e.g., gender roles, social-class roles, religious orientation roles). Such concepts play a major part in the adolescent's evaluation of the nature of the self and self-identity because to a large extent, the self can be thought of as a composite of roles.

Hypothetico-deductive and combinatorial thinking result in the construction of theories, which require reasoning with verbal propositions and consequently are signs of the adolescent's capacity to deal with symbols. There are other manifestations of the symbolic nature of adolescence. For instance, the ability to utilize symbolization might lead to a greater sense of creativity (the symbolic expression of thought or value system). Adolescents, also, sometimes engage in activities, such as writing of poetry or even the keeping of a diary. One can argue that this activity is one of giving new form to their inner feelings by using tools that were previously not as readily available.

Thinking about thought. Closely related to the aforementioned characteristics of adolescent thought is what Inhelder and Piaget [28] term thinking about thought. Adolescents, in contrast to younger children, can have their own thoughts and ideas serve as the object of thought. This feature of adolescent cognition is also closely related to another product of formal operations, namely egocentrism.

Egocentrism. Egocentrism, generally conceived as a reference to the self, takes many different forms throughout the life of the child. In infancy, egocentrism is shown by the fact that the infant discovers the body and the self before the external world. In childhood, egocentric thought is manifested by a variety of different confusions; however, it is commonly illustrated by difficulties in taking multiple perspectives, that is, in appreciating the viewpoint of different observers. Young children, for instance, often cannot imagine what a person can see who is standing in a different physical location from the one they are occupying. Inhelder and Piaget argue that adolescent egocentrism arises from the adolescent's preoccupation with one aspect of the self, namely the power of thinking. Adolescents, giving undue attention to their own intellectual processes, magnify and enhance the significance of their own ideas. Thus we find adolescents show a form of intellectual arrogance or aggrandizement in believing that their ideas are better than those of others and thus more likely to be correct. Recall in this connection Mark Twain's observation.

Like Piaget, Elkind [17] believes that the adolescent focuses on thinking but suggests that the adolescent also becomes concerned with the thinking of others. In other words the adolescent's thought becomes preoccupied with thinking about what other people are thinking. And what are these others thinking? Here Elkind assumes adolescents cannot differentiate the concern of their thought from the object of concern of the thoughts of others. Since the adolescent is concentrating on the self, other people must be doing the same. The adolescent thus walks around with a sense of self-consciousness, imagining that others are thinking about him or her. This type of thinking becomes so extreme that some adolescents will construct an "imaginary audience."

Another aspect of adolescent egocentrism is similar to the arrogance Piaget describes. Adolescents invest so much importance in their own thought processes, that they begin to believe their insights are special. Thus we frequently hear adolescents saying things, such as "You can't possibly know what I'm thinking and feeling, my feelings are so unique." This belief in the uniqueness of one's own thought is termed "personal fable." The research with tests constructed to measure imaginary audience and personal fables suggests that they decline as children progress from the

sixth through the twelfth grades [18] and egocentrism decreases.

Social Cognition. Also developing in adolescence is a broader type of thinking termed **social cognition.** Social cognition generally involves the extent to which an individual takes the perspective of another person (i.e., lack of egocentrism). It is an awareness of the way others are thinking and feeling, an appreciation of their perspectives. Social cognition begins with an inability to take the perspective of another person and progresses to taking first the perspective of others, and then, of others and the self. Finally, in adolescence the individual (1) views the interactions of the self with another from the standpoint of a third, external observer, and (2) believes in the necessity of social conventions to mediate discrepancies among perspectives [51].

In summary, from the Piagetian perspective, we see a number of changes in cognition that evolve from an increased capacity to symbolize. Thus we find gains in the ability to abstract and in flexibility and the capacity to construct and to test hypotheses. The resulting theories and constructs are used, in part, to assess and to guide the self but also to foster egocentrism. There is a gradual decline in egocentrism as adolescents develop skills in social cognition.

However, an increase in the ability to abstract does not solely account for the adolescent's idealization. Nor does it necessarily completely explain behaviors, such as keeping a diary and writing poetry. To be sure, symbolization is necessary for these to occur. But many adults have the capacity for advanced logical thought and are not compelled, as many suspect a number of adolescents are, to express themselves artistically or symbolically. For indeed, many of these artistic activities require a bedrock of emotionality, and this dimension of feeling most assuredly influences the quality of adolescent thought. It should be noted that Piaget did not stress the significance of emotion in affecting thought, although he did recognize that affect or emotion played a role. To the degree that we can say that certain feelings are driving the machinery of the mind, we have an interaction between different processes and thus evidence for a holistic system. Werner's theory would argue for an interaction between emotion and reasoning [61].

The Role of Experience and Education

Up to this point, the advances in thought have been stressed that supposedly accompany adolescence. In

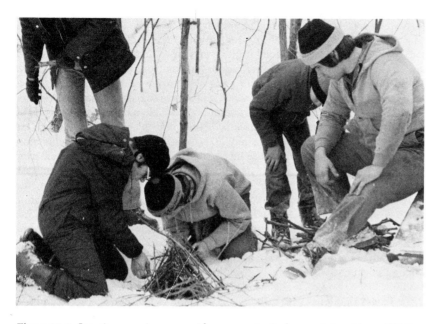

Figure 26–2. Scouting experiences provide an opportunity for scouts to achieve affiliation, to receive guidance, and to learn mastery of skills outside of their family setting.

discussing the role of experience and education, it might be rewarding to look at another aspect of adolescent thought, one of which every parent is well-aware: Namely, the advanced types of logical reasoning, which are presumably characteristic of adolescents, are not always shown by one's child, who often acts recklessly and impulsively. The parent's observation contains more than a grain of truth, for there are now studies that suggest many shortcomings in the adolescent's thought. These studies, which suggest that logical thought is not exercised along with evidence that adolescents do show high levels of reasoning in certain circumstances, can perhaps best be reconciled by stating that adolescents have the capacity for high-level cognizing, but that this capacity is not always demonstrated in performance. It is in the realization of these potentials in performance that the role of education and experience can be observed.

Before turning to an examination of the role of educational experiences in fostering adolescent thought, it should be emphasized that one of the major differences between the periods of preadolescent and adolescent thought lies precisely in the extent to which the individual spontaneously demonstrates the logic of his or her stage. In the period of concrete operations, most children who have mastered the logic of that stage can demonstrate appropriate reasoning without any special coaching or training.

Such is not the case in formal operations. The utilization of the logic of formal operations is not demonstrated by large numbers of adolescents. This capacity must be elicited by training of a formal sort or experiences of a more natural, ecological type. Numerous studies have demonstrated that educational experiences can facilitate the development of formal operations [32]. Moreover, research also suggests that merely exposing the student to problems that demand the discovery and employment of strategies can be effective in producing thought processes characteristic of the formal-operations period [34]. In other words, gains in thinking can be produced without training of a direct or a didactic sort in which the teacher demonstrates the correct solution.

Piaget also maintained that formal education is not necessary for the development of logical skills. He postulated that development occurs when one naturally adjusts to the environment. The precise mechanism of development is one of conflict resolution. The individual, in confronting a problem, experiences some internal conflict. The process of resolution stimulates cognitive development. This mechanism was termed **equilibration.**

In a recent addition to his theory, Piaget [48] explained why formal operations are not shown in all dimensions of life. He maintained that we only show formal operational thought in those areas in which we have aptitudes and receive specific training or apprenticeship. The physician, for instance, employs formal operations when serving as a doctor, but not necessarily when he or she attempts to work on a car. Note that Piaget is not arguing that occupational training formally teaches one logical skills. Nowhere in a physician's training is he or she directly taught formal operations. Rather, the needs and demands of the occupation force this mode of thinking on the individual. De we hold then that people only use formal operations in their occupations? Such a proposition would be absurd. The idea is that success in achieving certain goals requires the utilization of formal operations. These goals can be encountered in one's occupational life or indeed in one's avocational life.

There is some limited support for Piaget's notions. Thus in one study, researchers compared college science and nonscience majors on their solutions to Piaget's balance-beam problem [62]. Here subjects are presented with a see–saw-like apparatus and must decide how to achieve a balance through a combination of weight and the distance of the weight from the focal point. The science majors had more success with this problem, precisely as the theory predicts. However, it could be the case that science majors were specifically taught the solution to the problem, since the study of levers is common in high-school physics courses.

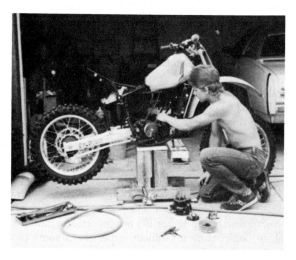

Figure 26–3. Working on complex problems, such as motor repair, requires hypothetical-deductive, problem-solving approaches.

Piagetian theory suggests the importance of experience in problem solving and also the significance of special training similar to that received in apprenticeship training for an occupation. But is this sufficient? Are more general experiences significant? There is now convincing evidence suggesting that the presence of formal operational thought must be accompanied by the accumulation of more general experiences. One clever study [37] presented students with a dilemma. The case involved an adolescent who was considering some facial surgery to remove a bump. Information was presented under various conditions. In one situation, two doctors provided contradictory information (one who receives pay for the operation and thus has a vested interest in advocating the surgery, and one who does not, who advises against the operation).

The results showed some interesting trends in comparing seventh- through twelfth-graders. The older students made more reference to the future, indicating that the decision might depend on the effect the surgery would have later on; younger students were more concerned with the immediate impact. Older students also wisely chose to obtain outside consultation from an expert. Finally, the older students were more aware of the problems of taking the advice of the doctor with the vested interest. Note that all of these adolescents are in the stage of formal operations, presumably, and yet the older students showed more mature judgments, reflecting no doubt their increased experience and sophistication, if not sheer insight.

A similar lack of conventional wisdom in younger adolescents is also seen in some of the older research on occupational choice. The results of a number of studies show that adolescents do not make judicious decisions early in their lives. Vocational preferences, for instance, often do not relate to the adolescent's abilities or interests [59]. Indeed, many adolescents seem downright unrealistic in assuming that they can enter occupations for which they have little ability or inclination. For example, one study showed that 40 to 65 percent of adolescents expect to enter professions, but only about 12 percent reach this goal [27]. Another study demonstrated that over 50 percent of sophomores in a poor rural school system expected to enter professional occupations and that the number of students showing unrealistic expectations increased as the students developed [13]!

Finally, although adolescents can often pick out the flaws in the reasoning or the information presented in advertising and, indeed, in many cases feel that advertisers are lying, a surprising number still tend to be influenced by the commercial and say that they will

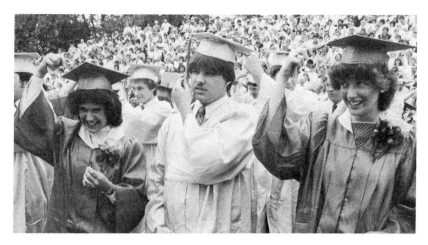

Figure 26–4. High-school graduation marks the culmination of formal education for some young people, but it is only the beginning for others.

purchase the product [38]. It appears that although adolescents have the ability to refute the advertisement, they do not utilize their skills. Such results again suggest the importance of experiences that lead to the use of an analytical attitude.

In summary, whether we examine performance on the traditional tasks used to measure the presence of formal operations or indeed more pragmatic aspects of behavior, there is much to lead us to believe that the adolescent is not an intellectually mature individual. Perhaps the potential for abstract reasoning exists, but the exercise and the application of this ability very much depends on additional experiences of a formal or informal sort.

Decision Making and Responsibility

The preceding characterization of adolescent thought leads to an interesting paradox when it comes to the critical decisions that adolescents frequently face in today's society (e.g., whether to continue education, to engage in sexual relations, to partake of drugs). The paradox consists of the fact that while the adolescent has the reasoning power and indeed the potential to make mature judgments, this ability is impeded by an absence of appropriate experience and self-discipline.

There are many nonrational factors that also militate against making reasoned judgments. Endocrine functioning precipitates a heightened drive state or emotionality that might lead the adolescent to override what his or her reasoning dictates. This often occurs when adolescents engage in sex without contraceptives. Peer pressure may also override good judgment. When the accident rate, drug abuse, or pregnancy sta-

tistics associated with adolescence are examined, it becomes obvious that the ability to engage in hypothetico-deductive thinking, (to identify appropriate alternative routes and to project probable consequences) is not sufficient to prevent adolescents from getting into difficulties. Cognitive processing is suppressed by emotional processing. The immediate goal outweighs future consequences.

What role, then, should adults play in the decision making of adolescents? It must be recognized that there is no absolutely correct or incorrect answer to this question. The position one takes is based on personal philosophy and inferences as to the import of various studies and theories in the area of adolescence. Some developmentalists stress the importance of free choice, an orientation that emphasizes the adolescent's ability to cognize at a high level [4, 7]. They advocate presenting adolescents with a series of choices (e.g., educational options versus no school) and then allowing the adolescent to make up his or her own mind. The adolescent presumably will have been trained to use reasoning in making decisions and also will have been given the appropriate information as to possible outcomes. Some decisions once made, however, can have lifelong import—usually of a negative nature—because of the adolescent's difficulty with priority setting based on long-term goals.

The principles advocated in this text are based on the notions of structure and guidance. Structure in the sense that certain choices are allowed and others disallowed based on the parents' assessment of the adolescent's maturity. Limits can and should be set as a way of protecting young persons from potentially traumatic decisions and to guide them toward greater independence. Limits are lifted gradually as the adolescent evidences increased skill at making decisions based on long-range results. The young adolescent might argue that to stay out all night for a party is not going to lead to ill effects nor will associating with a person of whom the parents disapprove. In fact, the adolescent might advance what appear to be rational and cogent arguments on his or her behalf. But the parent still has the right and indeed the responsibility to take an instrumental role in determining that these matters are not open to choice nor decided solely on the basis of egocentric adolescent logic and argumentation.

Two considerations are critical when dealing with the issues of adolescent decision making. One deals with how structure should be implemented. In other words, what style or manner should the parent adopt? The parent should not be heavy-handed and autocratic in dealing with the child but instead should employ a dialogue governed if possible by an appeal to logic. In other words, the parent should rely on the adolescent's reasoning capacity and ability to imagine consequences, by explaining why a particular course of action is liable to produce ill effects.

The parents should also provide guidance, especially through education, and timely consideration of issues. The time to discuss sex or drinking is not after the adolescent has begun to date or to party seriously, but beforehand, when an appeal to logic is removed from the emotionality of ongoing events. Guidance is offered in the sense of providing an appropriate role model. Such a model lives by the rules he or she proposes and behaves consistently with them in a number of ways. For instance, if parents do not want their children to drink or to smoke, they should behave consistently with this view, tempering or eliminating their own drinking or smoking. They should also be supportive of community and church efforts that are consistent with their value systems. Some communities, for instance, are now considering registering parties so that the parents can call in advance to find out who is chaperoning, or whether liquor will be served. Support of programs of this sort provides a model for the values conveyed to the adolescent.

A corollary consideration is how to provide the adolescent with adequate and appropriate practice and experience in making decisions. Which decisions should be left to the adolescent and under which conditions should the adolescent be given responsibility? Again, there are no absolute answers to issues of this

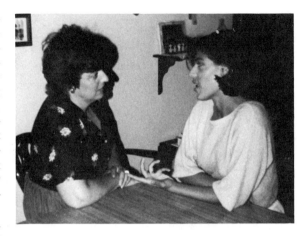

Figure 26–5. During adolescence, the parent begins to assume a mentor role, encouraging the adolescent to consider alternatives and outcomes when facing issues.

sort. To a large extent, the answer depends on the behavior of the adolescent and the extent to which he or she illustrates mature judgment. The responsibility for decision making is released gradually as both the parent and the adolescent build up a trust in the younger person's ability to assume responsibility for lower-level decisions.

Perhaps one way of describing such a strategy is to say that the amount of decision making the parent leaves to the adolescent should be somewhat above the adolescent's current level of decision making, but not at a level too far removed from the realm of experiences and judgment of the adolescent. This suggestion is similar to another notion in psychology that is described as a matching mechanism. According to this mechanism, providing stimulation that is slightly above the individual's capacity to process such input—thus creating a slight discrepancy between level of functioning and level of stimulation—is optimal for provoking maximum growth. The effective use of this process ultimately depends on a judgment about type and level of functioning, an assessment that is subjective and almost clinical in nature.

Finally, it should be noted that many critical decisions are made on a developmental timetable over which the parent has little influence or control. As the adolescent experiences emancipation from the parent by way of schooling, occupation, and friendships, the locus of decision making gradually shifts, and the matters we have discussed become irrelevant. It is hoped that the values, the guidance, and the processes have become internalized by this time. The adolescent in a sense begins to parent the self.

CONSOLIDATING ONE'S IDENTITY

One of the most significant tasks of adolescence is the formation of a sense of identity. The foremost theoretician in this area is the psychoanalyst, Erik Erikson. Erikson proposed that adolescence is a developmental stage defined by the crisis or the conflict between identity and identity diffusion [19, 20]. The task is one of establishing a consolidated, acceptable sense of who one is. In Erikson's framework, this involves an appreciation of the past, present, and future selves. That is, it involves an understanding of one's history or past, one's present, and an articulated idea of one's future self.

During adolescence, the individual develops either a clear sense of the uniqueness and separateness of self, or if one fails, an unclear, that is, diffuse, sense of self. One process that Erikson described in analyzing the development of self was the **moratorium period** [20]. Technically, the word *moratorium* means a delay, and the delay referred to is the accepting of adult roles and responsibilities. But this period is not to be conceived as a time of inactivity, for during this time the adolescent is actively experimenting with various persona, or senses of self, discovering thereby the real nature of his or her self. Notice how the Piagetian processes discussed earlier, those of hypothesis formation and of theorizing, can play a role in the construction of self.

Today, much of the work on development of identity from an Eriksonian perspective has followed the pioneering studies of James Marcia. Marcia conceptualized the process of identity formation as entailing four levels, or statuses, of identity [40, 41, 42]. The levels are best understood by referring to the manner in which Marcia measures them. Individuals are questioned on areas in which decisions are often reached. The significant factors center around the extent to which one finds crisis in an active process of decision making and the extent to which the crisis is resolved by achieving a sense of commitment or closure. The presence and the absense of crisis (active decision making) and commitment (closure) determines the level of identity.

Presumably, the most advanced level of identity is termed **identity achievement.** Here, individuals report having experienced a sense of crisis and having resolved the crisis by achieving a commitment. An illustration of this level would be the college student who experiments with different majors, thus demonstrating an active process of decision making that ends with a final choice and ultimate closure. This level represents an optimal state of affairs from the Eriksonian perspective: The individual has gone through an identity crisis, a normal stage of development, and has resolved the crisis.

The level that quite possibly represents the heart of the identity crisis of adolescence is termed the **moratorium status.** Individuals at this level are currently experiencing a crisis (i.e., engaged in decision making) and thus have no commitment. The third level is described by Marcia as **foreclosure.** Individuals have arrived at a sense of commitment, but in doing so, they have never experienced a crisis. Such individuals are often strongly influenced by their parents. They may indicate that they have always known what profession they were going to enter, perhaps because their father or mother held that occupation.

The remaining level is termed **identity diffuse.** Here, individuals have no sense of commitment, nor do they have a firm sense of crisis. They do not have a clear sense of their own uniqueness, and they have not yet identified a goal toward which their self-system can focus energies. One characterization of this level is to say that it describes the person who is directionless and aimless. This individual would represent the lack of differentiation Werner describes (see Chap. 2) and possibly Witkin's construct of "field dependence."

The levels of moratorium and identity achievement are seen as the most developmentally advanced and presumably also represent the healthiest individuals. These individuals are accorded this characterization because they reflect an attitude of exploration and discovery that is thought to be significant in the formation of self-identity [23]. Research with adolescents tends to support the idea that foreclosure and diffusion statuses are very common among students of high-school age [1, 2] and that as they progress through the college years to early adulthood, there is an increase in the percentage of individuals in the identity-achievement status [2, 44]. Thus for many individuals, Marcia's levels represent a normal developmental continuum during adolescence and not a static state. More specific analyses of students in college [60] suggest that as subjects progress through college, there is a shifting of moratorium or foreclosure levels into identity-achievement statuses. It should be noted, however, that there is a large number of adults who remain in the identity-diffusion category. Thus in one study

[44] 56 percent of 24-year-olds were in the identity-achievement category, but 24 percent were still at the identity-diffusion level.

The Influence of Family and Other Factors on Identity

One question that arises in connection with identity status concerns the relationship of identity status to the various experiences that an individual has. Varying experiences appear to have differing impact on identity level. Thus in one instance, a positive relationship was found between identity achievement, socioeconomic status, and parental education, leading the author to suggest that more highly educated parents foster a greater opportunity for choice [1]. There have also been some fairly extensive analyses of the types of familial relations and various levels of identity. The results suggest that high levels of exploration as represented in the moratorium and identity-achievement levels can be fostered by parents who encourage family members to express disagreement or separateness. These parents demonstrate similar traits [23]. In brief, the attitudes of the parents suggested an ability to negotiate conflict of opinion without a loss of integrity.

Connectedness, as demonstrated by cohesiveness and support among family members, was also shown to be a significant correlate of high levels of exploration [23]. But interestingly, only moderate levels of openness and connectedness were associated with the more exploratory levels. Parents who were highly accepting of disagreement and strongly inclined to stress independence often had children who were at the foreclosure and moratorium levels [23]. These results are consistent with the "matching hypothesis" presented earlier, which suggested that maximum growth occurs under conditions of a moderate discrepancy between the level of functioning and the input of stimulation from the environment.

Intrapersonal Sense of Identity

Marcia's work has provided an insight into some of the critical factors underlying Erikson's issue of identity formation, but another major component of Erikson's identity that is not addressed in his scheme concerns the sense of who one is, the self as perceived by the self. When children of different ages are asked who they are, they express qualitatively different responses as to the nature of the self.

One researcher asked children and adolescents what a person who knows them best would know about them that other people would not know [49]. In comparing the responses of children from 8 to more than 16 years of age, it was shown that the older the child, the greater the tendency to answer this question by referring to inner thoughts and feelings. The older adolescents tended specifically to answer by saying that a person who knows them best would know how they feel emotionally, would know when they are worried, sad, hurt, and so forth. Older subjects also showed more of a tendency to answer by referring to interpersonal attitudes (indicating that people who know them best would know how the individual felt about other people). Finally, older children were more likely to mention private or intimate aspects of the self, such as secrets or personal desires. Notice how all of these responses make reference to the inner self.

Younger children tended to answer the questions by referring to external behaviors that in certain respects are punishable. Thus, one child responded that her mother knew that she crossed Bradley Road. In short, the younger children conceived the self an an actor who engages in behaviors that are often evaluated in moral terms. They also made reference to physical features, such as height, and to traits or achievements, such as good in arithmetic. Note how the younger child is more concrete than the older, precisely what would be expected from the cognitively oriented theory of Piaget.

The older adolescent becomes increasingly aware of the dual nature of the self: an external self that others see and an internal one that only the self knows [11]. From the perspective of general systems theory and Werner's continuum, this development can be viewed as a form of differentiation. The growing awareness of the inner self and the theorizing and discovery that go along with this self account for the adolescent's penchant for loneliness, secrecy and privacy, and (it might be speculated as well) the adolescent's tendency toward introspection, that is, to look inward and examine the self. One interesting issue concerns the extent to which preoccupation with this private self reflects pathology or deviance, since some theorize it is precisely this sense of division that is at the heart of schizophrenia [11]. However, this sense of divided self and the preoccupation with the private are important and normal characteristics of adolescence [11].

The awareness and the exploration of the meaning of a divided self, that is, the differentiation of the exterior from the interior self, is normal and indeed beneficial. This understanding is pivotal to the process of coming to know who we are and of constructing a theory of how and what the self is. This process is also significant in helping the adolescent to adjust or to modify his or her behavior in order to adapt to the expectations of society. Many social situations call for external behaviors that may not be consistent with the needs and the structure of the inner self. When we understand this inner self and are aware of the limits of deviance from this self that we can tolerate, we are able to adjust and to adapt to the environment without violating our own needs and value systems.

The less mature individual who equates external behaviors and acceptance with inner reality, identity, or values will experience marked tension and disequilibrium when the environment calls for behaviors that

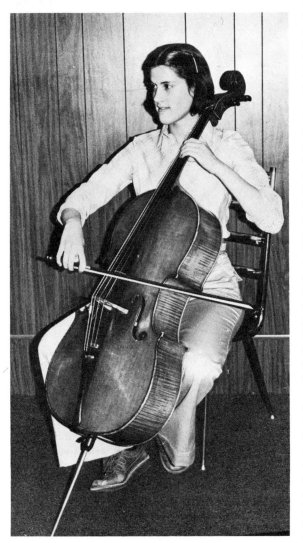

Figure 26–6. Skills mastered during the early years continue to be refined in order to achieve proficient levels of functioning.

threaten personal integrity. Consider an adolescent who finds him- or herself in a major institution, where limits are placed on behavior and modes of expression. Certain corporations have fairly rigid dress codes, allowing in some instances only white shirts, ties, and suits. It might be extremely difficult to function in this type of institution if the inner and private self finds adherence to these behaviors superficial or repugnant. One might find oneself a hypocrite, pretending to be what he or she is not, to secure social approval.

An understanding of the dual nature of the self is important in other respects as well. An understanding of the inner nature of the self allows one to look at the self as an outsider, setting the stage for self-criticism, self-guidance, and improvement. Over time, changes will occur, but positive development is based on evolution and planning. It is only through knowing our faults that we can improve.

On the opposite side of the coin, there is evidence that preoccupation with the inner self can be associated with pathological states. Kenneth Keniston [33] studied alienated students of the 1960s. These students attended a major prestigious university, but felt themselves to be separate from the formal aspects of the institution, such as clubs and student organizations, and also had extreme desires to be alone. Keniston discovered that alienated students were inclined to overly examine their lives and, in the process, evaluated themselves quite negatively. In fact, this preoccupation with self affected their relations with members of the opposite sex, since they used them in an exploitative fashion to gain additional insights into their own characters. Keniston's analysis of the causes of alienation stressed cultural factors and variables related to family background. But a necessary condition for the students' behavior was the ability to differentiate between different aspects of the self. Unfortunately, they seemed to become overly fixated on analysis of the inner self.

There are many adolescents similar to these alienated students, who become extremely concerned with their experiences and internal selves. Often they spend excessive amounts of time on introspection in the attempt to derive a more complete understanding of who they are. Although introspection is a significant part of adolescence, when it is carried to an extreme, it is detrimental to the continued development of the adolescent. It results in the withdrawal of the adolescent from the more active world where he or she can test the nature of the self against reality and experiment and determine the validity of the construction of the self. How many times, for instance, have we convinced ourselves through self-analysis that we are bright, cowardly, unacceptable, or whatever, only to have our beliefs dashed in the face of new evidence from the outer world.

In conclusion, during adolescence the individual becomes aware of a sense of a differentiated self, comprising inner thoughts and outer behavior. This differentiation is consistent with Werner's theory that development consists of increasing differentiation. It is also consistent with Piaget's theory, which stresses the adolescent's ability to think in symbols and to construct a symbolic system. In many respects each of us constructs a theory about the self. This theory can have positive or negative consequences on self-esteem and future development.

Differentiation of Self and Integration

The distinction between inner and outer aspects of self is only one type of differentiation that occurs in adolescence with respect to self. As the child matures, there is an increasing realization that there can be many self-concepts, depending on the particular situation in which one is involved and on the particular roles one adopts. Thus, there is self as student, as friend, as son or daughter, as musician or craftsman. During adolescence, individuals begin to consolidate these many identities into a central cohesive sense of self with a recognition of many modes of expression or interfaces. The concept of self as a compilation of multiple roles is replaced with a sense of core unity with multiple facets.

It might appear that the increased differentiation of discrete facets of self would lead to increasing fractionation and thus diffuseness, or a lack of coherence. However, results suggest that even contradictory facets of self become increasingly integrated into a more stable, flexible coordinated system [5,15] (just as Werner's theory would suggest). The adolescent, in short, develops a superordinate structure in which many parts of the whole dovetail and function together.

One distinction long-recognized as significant involves real versus ideal self. The real self is what a person feels or knows he or she is, the ideal self represents the end to which a person aspires. It serves as a goal toward which to work and monitor self-development. The ideal self may serve to bridge the gap between the external and internal self, or it may serve as a source of anxiety when there is too much discrepancy from the real self. Notice how the construction of the ideal self might depend on the logic of the formal operational period.

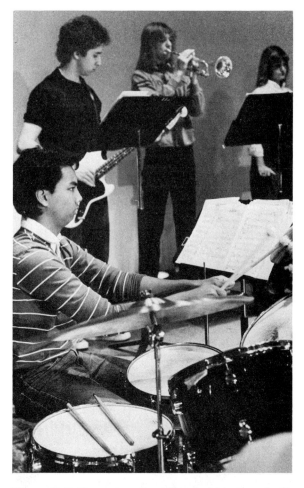

Figure 26–7. Possession of a skill prized by others facilitates social participation and acceptance.

Self-Esteem: A View in the Mirror

A final aspect to be considered in the discussion of self-concept is that of self-esteem, which is the feeling of worth or value we have about the self, a sense of pride or satisfaction. A high sense of self-esteem is viewed as an important component of identity, or self, for various reasons [14]. For one, self-esteem is frequently thought to be associated with mental health. Thus high levels of self-esteem are associated with increased life satisfaction and happiness, and low self-esteem is related to depression, anxiety, and maladjustment. Moreover, self-esteem is correlated with school performance: Those with low self-esteem perform more poorly in school than people with higher feelings of self-worth [14]. Given the importance of this construct, let us examine a few influences on the adolescent's self-esteem.

SELF-ESTEEM THROUGHOUT ADOLESCENCE

The early theorizing on the nature of adolescence led psychologists to believe that adolescents experience a disruption in feelings of self-worth. Thus in 1904 G. S. Hall, the father of the modern study of adolescence, characterized the years of adolescence as a period of storm and stress, that is, a period of extreme turmoil and conflict [24]. Such conflict would presumably be reflected in lowered or rapidly shifting levels of self-worth. This characterization has led to an interest in whether adolescents, as opposed to those in other age groups, experience a discontinuity in their levels of self-esteem. Such discontinuity might be revealed by rapidly changing levels of self-esteem over time or by general declines in self-esteem as the individual passes through adolescence. Interestingly enough, the results of research do not lend general support to the notion of changing levels of self-esteem throughout adolescence. In fact, a number of studies [16, 47, 49] generally show moderate to extremely stable levels of self-esteem, at least through later adolescence.

SELF-ESTEEM CHANGES IN EARLY ADOLESCENCE— IMPACT OF SCHOOLING

There is some impressive evidence that suggests there is a distinct lowering of self-esteem as the individual progresses through the early years of adolescence. Thus in comparing the percentages of students at different ages on measures of global or general self-esteem, one study found that there was a strikingly lower level of self-esteem among 12-year-olds as compared to 11-year-olds. This decline was most evident for females [49, 54].

Different types of analyses revealed that the critical variable in this study was not the age of the student but whether the student was entering junior high school. For instance, when 12-year-olds in the sixth grade were compared with 12-year-olds in the seventh grade of the junior high school, only the seventh-graders showed the lower self-esteem. The same finding was bolstered in an additional study that compared children in settings in which they went from kindergarten through grade 8 in one school, (in other words, a system in which there was no junior high school) with a system in which children changed schools as they entered a junior high school. The results supported the earlier findings. Female students who transferred to junior high school from the sixth grade

showed lower self-esteem compared to the students in the school with kindergarten to eighth grade [53]. In this investigation, incidentally, male students experienced no such decline. The lowest self-esteem was found among those females who had matured early and had started to date. The psychosocial changes and pressures associated with changing schools and assuming more mature heterosocial behavior were clearly threatening to these individuals. This threat took its toll on the feelings of self-worth.

While it is clear that physical maturation and the types of social interaction that are affected by maturation might contribute to a lowered self-esteem, there are other potential causes as well. As students shift from the classrooms of elementary school to those of junior high school, they are shifting from a setting which promotes close personal relationships to a setting, which by its very nature, is more formal and distant. The adolescent is thus in danger of losing the support that is gained through the presence of constant and caring others, such as a teacher who knows the individual's strengths and weaknesses and has time to address specific needs. In one instance, an elementary sixth-grade teacher told of being approached by a seventh-grade instructor who asked how to cope with a particular child. The child's former teacher replied that the child needed much personal attention (what is colloquially known as "strokes," or what psychologists might term *affectionate positive reinforcement*). The seventh-grade teacher lamented that the setting made it impossible to give the attention the child needed.

Another factor that may contribute to the decreased sense of self-worth associated with the transition to junior high school is the increased demand for organization and structuring. The young adolescent must contend with what might appear to be relatively complex schedules. These demands for scheduling and management of time alone can place a stress on the individual.

What is particularly interesting is that the change from junior to senior high schools is not associated with a similar drop in self-esteem [54]. In short, it is mainly in the years of early adolescence that the self appears vulnerable to conditions of change and presumably to a threat that is associated with what many consider to be normal transitions of youth. This is not to say that the early experiences in adolescence are short-lived or have only temporary effects. There is evidence that female students who experience lowered self-esteem after changing to a junior high school continue to have a lowered sense of self-worth throughout the early years of high school [10]. Moreover, during the years of both junior high school and high school, these students are active in fewer clubs and school activities.

THE EFFECT OF OTHER CHANGES

What do the aforementioned results suggest about other aspects of the adolescent experience? It seems reasonable to suppose that in early adolescence there is an increased vulnerability to a number of changes, especially those that might place demands for certain types of maturity upon the child (e.g., going away to camp or overnight sleeping away from home) or those that relate to physical changes the adolescent is experiencing.

Other transitions, such as being hospitalized for medical treatment, might also be particularly threatening to the adolescent. In fact, there is reason to speculate that any type of medical intervention is a potential threat to adolescents. An analysis of the anxieties that children experience in dental settings shows that as

preschoolers reach the elementary school years, they demonstrate fewer signs of fear. However, as children approach adolescence, their anxiety begins to increase [63]. In sum, a variety of transitions might be threatening to the adolescent's self-esteem, and some changes might be anxiety-provoking in general.

THE BODY AND SELF-ESTEEM

The adolescent is coping with major changes in the body's function and appearance. The adolescent's perception of body image has an impact on self-esteem and self-confidence. Physical attractiveness is positively associated with higher levels of self-esteem [52], although there is a stronger relation between physical attractiveness and self-worth for females than for males. For males the instrumental effectiveness of the body, that is, the extent to which the body is effective in achieving goals, is more important for self-esteem than physical attractiveness [35]. Moreover, instrumental effectiveness is more significant for males than it is for females. Imagine then, how especially damaging it is for males to suffer some physical handicap

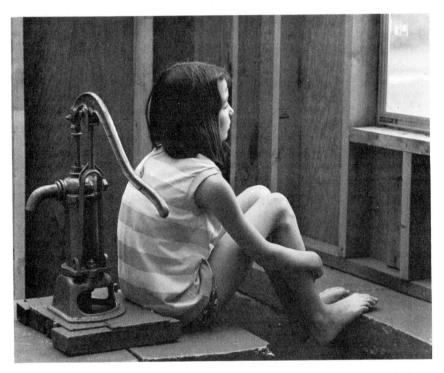

Figure 26–8. The imaginary friends of preschoolerhood give way to the fantasies of schoolagers. During pubescence, time is spent in daydreaming, and, during adolescence, in dream building.

that limits the effective use of their bodies. Weight is a preoccupation with many teenagers, and indeed many adults in our society. Adolescents, especially females, are very much concerned with weight [21], and being overweight is correlated with a more negative self-image, as measured by self-esteem, in early maturing girls [9].

RACIAL AND MINORITY STATUS AND SELF-ESTEEM
Racial and minority status might be thought to affect self-esteem, but the results are not that clear-cut and suggest complex relations. In the supreme court proceedings that culminated in the desegregation of schools, it was argued that black children suffered damage to their self-esteem because they were in segregated schools. Such decreased self-esteem was presumed to have a negative impact on scholastic performance [57]. More recent evidence shows that segregated black children do not have lower self-esteem than those in desegregated schools [12]. It appears that self-esteem is more closely related to the various traits that the adolescent ascribes to the self, such as brightness, good looks, and ease in getting along with others, than to pride in a religious or a racial group [49]. In fact, a large variety of studies suggests that belonging to a minority group per se does not have a negative impact on the value or worth the individual ascribes to the self. Even where there are studies that show that belonging to a minority group can be associated with lowered self-esteem, there are other studies that show no difference [49].

Minority-group affiliation may be secondary to more critical factors. Thus one study reported that those students who had negative views of their race or religion and who strongly depended on these factors for their identity had lower self-esteem. Another study found that when black children entered an integrated school, their grades were depressed compared to those of white children and their self-esteem also diminished [22]. Incidentally, the latter finding is not taken to mean that desegregation does not work; rather, the implication is that if desegregation leads to a lowering of grades and academic success, then self-esteem might also decline. When steps are taken to reduce competition, self-esteem rises [3].

In summary, self-esteem is inclined to decrease as children are presented with the stress of change and the demands for increased social interaction and maturity during the early years of adolescence. Self-esteem is less vulnerable to environmental variations in later adolescence.

EMOTIONAL SEPARATION FROM THE FAMILY AND DEVELOPING TIES TO OTHERS

Separation from the Family
The major features of the adolescent years are a decreased reliance on the family, an increased reliance on the self, and a turning toward other people and activities. Various names and characterizations have been used in reference to this process. Thus from the perspective of Werner's theory, one might characterize the increasing separation of the children from the parents as a form of increased differentiation, while from the standpoint of Witkin's theory, one might view the increasing separation as a form of field independence. Others have termed this phenomenon an "emancipation" [26], with the term emancipation connoting a liberation and an increased sense of freedom. However it is labeled, clearly one of the major tasks in this period is to develop an increasing sense of self-direction and responsibility that allows the individual to enter society and function as a productive adult.

Psychoanalysts have utilized the concept of **cathexis** to describe the changing allegiances of the adolescent. Cathexis is the emotional attachment, or bond, that one individual feels toward another individual. During childhood, the child is cathected to the parent; gradually starting in preadolescence, the strong cathexis to parents is loosened and broken and replaced first by a cathexis toward self (thus the egocentrism), then toward a close peer, and later directed toward another person who is seen as an intimate friend or as a sexual partner.

As part and parcel of this process of the separation from the parent and the attachment to others, the child branches out in terms of interests and commitments. That is, as the child breaks away from the parents and looks for other objects of attachment, he or she begins to form affiliations and commitments to a larger group of people or to other activities. Thus many adolescents turn toward external events, such as hobbies [8], clubs, and activities in school, which serve as a focus of attention and commitment. These new outlets ultimately will allow adolescents to come into contact with new ideas and thoughts [29] and to expand their personal "worlds" as they test self-concepts, value systems, and social identities.

Even with separation, the influence of the parent is not lost on the child. Despite the increasing independence, the child continues in certain respects to identity with, or to fashion him- or herself after the parent, albeit frequently at an unconscious level. One particularly pernicious manner in which the influence of the parent can be felt is through the formation of what is termed a **negative identity.**

Erikson [20] described negative identity as an identity based on the roles and the identifications of others that are presented as most undesirable. In other words, the adolescent becomes the opposite of what he or she should become. In describing the underlying dynamics for this type of identity, Erikson suggests that the child sees the parent emphasizing one negative trait or another. For instance, the parent might always harp on the dangers of stealing. The child thus comes to an understanding that by possessing such negative traits, he or she will attract the attention of the parent. In short, adoption of those values the parents oppose is likely to increase the involvement of the parent with the child.

But Erikson's description suggests an even more complex reason for the development of a negative identity. When individuals adopt negative traits, they often put themselves in a position to succeed, as in the statement of a woman who claimed, "at least in the gutter, I'm a genius" [20]. To put the matter in slightly different terms, by adopting negative roles and identities, the child lowers his or her level of aspiration and thus increases the chances of meeting with success. It is obvious that this process can account for the development of pathological personalities.

For some, forming an identity contrary to parental expectations allows them conscious control over their own life. To them, it is the final step in asserting their own identity. Their ego-identity is still too fragile to incorporate a parent's positive values or goals. To do so would make them an extension of the parent's self-system. They must forge their own unique identity and value frame even if it results in negative self-esteem and negative consequences.

There is some evidence that this view of negative identity is consistent with Erikson's concept of identify formation. Thus adolescents who engage in drug use and premarital sexual relations are found to score low on measures of conventional behavior [30, 31]. These adolescents will show lower levels of achievement in school and a decreased participation in formal activities, such as clubs, sports, and church. Most critically, they also show a tendency to adopt values that are discrepant from those of their parents.

In concluding the section on family, brief mention should be made of the storm-and-stress hypothesis postulated by Hall. One manifestation of storm and stress is conflict between the adolescent and the members of the family. It is controversial, however, whether adolescents do in fact have conflictual relations with parents. When adolescents and their parents are asked to characterize their interpersonal relations through questionnaires, children and parents usually state that relations with one another are generally harmonious.

However, there is evidence of storm and stress when we use other ways of defining and measuring such conflict. Thus in one interesting pair of studies [55, 56], it was shown that as adolescent males progressed through puberty, they tended to interrupt their parents more frequently and often did not bother to explain themselves. (Note how this finding supports Twain's anecdote.) Adolescents were not the only culprits; parents also showed similar tendencies to interrupt their sons and to explain themselves less. Also consistent with the storm-and-stress hypothesis is the fact that when the adolescent leaves home, parents often report an increase in their life satisfaction. In sum, then, there is at least limited support for the idea that parent-child relations are stressful during adolescence.

Adolescent Friendships

With the gaining of independence from the parents, adolescents become increasingly more reliant on peers and friends. Current theories and research give some insight as to why friendship is an important concern of adolescence. Sullivan [58] observed that preadolescents feel a need for friendships outside of the family and developed at least one close homosocial relationship with persons of the same gender (a chum). True friendship involves a concern for the other person or an ability to place the needs of the other person first. Later in adolescence, this need for friendship is generally transferred to a person of the opposite gender (heterosocial relationship).

One major component of friendship, according to Sullivan, is the ability to comprehend and to empathize with the needs of another person. Such an ability depends on the realization of a difference between the exterior and interior selves discussed earlier. It reflects the individual's ability to take the perspective of another person—the role-taking skill. Adolescence is a period in which one acquires the ability to take these perspectives.

Thus when adolescents are asked to describe what a friend is, there is an increasing tendency to refer to the sharing of thoughts and feelings with another person [5]. A close friendship sets the arena for affirmative intimacy as presented by Erikson. Intimacy and sharing contribute to a sense of positive self-regard when individuals can provide one another positive

others may feel a sense of unease and uncertainty and attribute these feelings to a personal defect or a short-coming. In discussing and sharing intimate views with others, the adolescent may come to realize that his or her friends share this same sense of being ill at ease.

In concluding the discussion of friendships, it is important to recognize that an increasing sense of intimacy involves more than an increasing ability to take perspectives or an increasing desire to receive validation and positive evaluation of certain aspects of the self. This section started with a discussion of cathexis and how in adolescence is found a further separation of the self from the parents. Such separations leave the adolescent in need of another "object" to love. To put the matter in slightly different terms, friends provide an opportunity to express love and affection and to avoid loneliness. Friends also help to move an adolescent out of "personal-fable" thinking by providing a mirror that reflects the nature of the individual's feelings, behaviors, and values.

Group Identity

Adolescents are influenced by their affiliations with groups as well as their interactions with specific people. Early adolescence can be characterized as involving the crisis of forming a sense of group identity versus a sense of alienation [45, 46]. The positive resolution of the conflict, the establishing of a sense of group identity, involves the affiliation with a specific group, which provides a sense of belonging and security. The negative pole, that of alienation, eventually leads to negativism and a sense of isolation.

The formation of an identity with a group has a variety of consequences. The group prescribes and proscribes specific behaviors, clothing styles, activities, and even attitudes and values. As such, group affiliation makes a strong contribution to the adolescent's goals and sense of self-identity and self-esteem. Individuals will characterize, construct, and evaluate a concept of self in light of the rules governing the behaviors of those with whom they are affiliated. The group also provides a context for learning various social skills and provides a network of friends and associates with whom the individual might continue to affiliate in adulthood [45, 46].

There are many different pressures toward the formation of a group by adolescents [45, 46]. Parents generally encourage their children to participate in groups that uphold parental values. The individual adolescent seeks group affiliation as a way to gain more independence from parents. Peers themselves encourage and reinforce affiliation behaviors. Teachers also provide

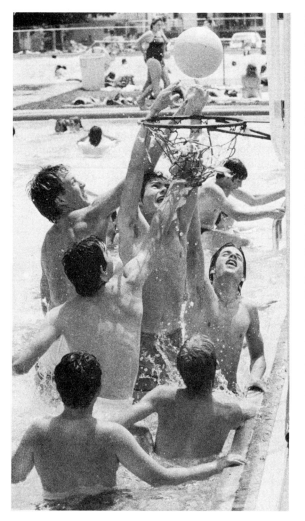

Figure 26–9. Adolescent friendships offer opportunities for competition as well as companionship. Same-gender companionship and activities are just as important to identity formation as cross-gender companionship and activities, since they foster the development of different aspects of the self-concept.

feedback and evaluations of innermost ideas and values. This becomes increasingly significant for adolescents, whose values and ideas might clash with those of the parents and who thus seek a validation of their ideas and values from peers. Whatever the interpretation, the results of studies show that adolescents with close friends generally have higher levels of self-esteem [5, 39].

Friendships can also correct fears and fantasies about the self [58]. A young person interacting with

an impetus for the formation of groups and actively assist in the creation of homogeneous groupings, such as segregating children who have similar academic skills. Passively, teachers foster group identification by doing little to discourage the spontaneous groups formed by children.

THE NORMAL ADOLESCENT

In this concluding section, we will try to form a composite picture of the nature of the normal or typical adolescent. This task, however, is easier said than done, for almost any of the classic characterizations are open to controversy and dispute. A simple case in point is the concept of adolescence as a period of storm and stress. Evidence can be marshalled both for and against this notion.

Perhaps one way of managing this cumbersome task is to admit that for many people, the period of adolescence does represent a time in which the number and the variety of major changes precipitate internal and external conflict. We have examined some of these profound changes in this chapter: the emergence of an advanced form of reasoning (yet to be tempered by experiences of life), the expansion of an understanding of self, the changing of one's social network. There are of course a host of other changes covered in other sections of this text, not the least of which are the biological transitions. The exact nature of the individual's turmoil depends on the complex blending of personality, cognition, circumstances, opportunities, support systems, and previous experiences.

To stress the transitional quality of adolescence might seem to be somewhat exaggerated, for surely, there are other phases of life that present even more dramatic instances of change: (1) Infancy emcompasses perhaps the most rapid and complete change; (2) adulthood brings its many changes, such as bearing and raising children along with midlife crises and other rough periods of transition, (3) in the elderly years, people are confronted with the transitions of retirement and facing death. But, despite these examples, adolescence still seems to be a period most heavily laden with physical and psychological change. The infant is not aware of the degree of change experienced, and adults experiencing change in one facet of their lives generally have years of experience to fall back on, an enduring network of friends, and a clear sense of identity.

The adolescent, however, is confronted with changes for which he or she may feel unprepared or may not desire. The very nature of our society and the biology and psychology of the human organism create a trajectory without a stop or a reverse button to slow the process to a rate with which the adolescent can be comfortable. There is the sense of self developing and an awareness of others, a change in the quality of the relationship with the parents, a change in the social support system, and the necessity to chart one's future. In today's world, there is no "normal adolescence." Each person must forge a unique blending of skills, knowledge, and experience to meet the demands of transition to adult independence.

SUMMARY

This chapter has dealt with four core areas of development and change for the adolescent: cognitive or mental growth, the development of self and identity, the relations with family, and the relations with friends.

The analysis of cognition shows many profound changes during adolescence. Thus in comparison to school-agers, we find among adolescents increased symbolic reasoning and abstraction, hypothesis testing, generation of possibilities, and an enhanced awareness of the process of thinking itself. Such changes are necessary for the advancement of the individual in society either by way of progress through formal social structures, such as schools, or merely in terms of adjusting to the adult world of problem solving. Although there are major gains in thinking and problem solving during this period, there is also much room for growth. The adolescent is often egocentric and, despite an ability to reason, in need of experience and guidance.

With respect to personality, the major change that occurs in adolescence involves a crystallization of the self and the ego. Erikson captured this idea in his characterization of adolescence as a period involving a conflict or crisis between the formation of a diffuse or unclear identity, versus a clear and sharp sense of identity. The research directly aimed at verifying Erikson's construct suggests that adolescents undergo different levels or statuses of ego identity. Such statuses reflect the presence or the absence of crises, or extended decision-making episodes, and the resolution of these episodes with a sense of closure or commitment. It is the facing and mastering of these challenges that enables the person to mature and assume a positive self-concept. Escape from facing life's crises through increased dependence on others, or the use of drugs or alcohol, effectively prevents healthy maturation. The sense of self and intrapersonal identity should expand in adolescence. Older adolescents become aware of a differentiated self, that is, an inner self known only by the individual as well as other selves that are available to others—a self that is comprised of different roles and ideals.

The more complex and multifaceted nature of self, however, does not represent a fractionated composite but rather a more integrated identity. Development, here, resembles the formation of a superordinate system, comprising integrated components, and is consistent with the theorizing of Werner and holistic-system theorists. Yet another aspect of self to undergo experimental scrutiny is self-esteem. This property of self is so central that it relates to one's achievement and mental status. Self-esteem is affected by many variables, including environmental transitions and bodily changes.

Socially, the period of adolescence can be characterized as involving a decreasing connectedness to parents, and an increasing connectedness to peers. Such changes reflect differentiation and integration: a differentiation of self from family and integration of self toward others. The process can be rocky at times, with adolescents and parents showing evidence of storm and stress. But there are new feelings and experiences arising, including an increased sense of intimacy and sharing.

In short, the period of adolescence is one of rapid growth and maturation on a number of levels that prepares the adolescent to approach the decisions, responsibilities, and social relationships of adulthood.

REFERENCES

1. Archer, S. L. The lower age boundaries of identity development. *Child Dev.* 53:1551, 1982.
2. Archer, S. L., and Waterman, A. S. Identity in early adolescence: A developmental perspective. *Journal of Early Adolescence,* 3:203, 1983.
3. Aronson, E., Blaney, N., Stephan, C., Sikes, J., and Snapp, M. *The Jigsaw Classroom.* Beverly Hills: Sage Publications, 1978.
4. Bereiter, C. *Must We Educate?* Englewood Cliffs, NJ: Prentice-Hall, 1973.
5. Berndt, T. J. The features and effects of friendship in early adolescence. *Child Dev.* 53:1447, 1982.
6. Bernstein, R. M. The development of the self-system during adolescence. *J. Gen. Psychol.* 136:231, 1980.
7. Berzonsky, M. D. *Adolescent Development.* New York: Macmillan, 1981.
8. Blos, P. *On Adolescence: A Psychoanalytic Interpretation.* New York: The Free Press, 1962.
9. Blyth, D. A., Bulcroft, R., and Simmons, R. G. "The Im-

pact of Puberty on Adolescents: A Longitudinal Study." Presented at the 1981 Meetings of the American Psychological Association.
10. Blyth, D. A., Simmons, R. G., and Carlton-Ford, S. The adjustment of early adolescents to school transitions. *Journal of Early Adolescence* 3:105, 1983.
11. Broughten, J. M. The divided self in adolescence. *Hum. Dev.* 24:13, 1981.
12. Cook, S. W. Social science and school desegregation: Did we mislead the Supreme Court? *Personality and Social Psychology Bulletin* 5:420, 1979.
13. Cosby, A. G. Occupational expectations and the hypothesis of increasing realism of choice. *Journal of Vocational Behavior* 5:53, 1974.
14. Damon, W. *Social and Personality Development: Infancy through Adolescence.* New York: Norton, 1983.
15. Damon, W., and Hart, D. The development of self-understanding from infancy through adolescence. *Child Dev.* 53:841, 1982.
16. Dusek, J. B., and Flaherty, J. F. The development of self-concept during the adolescent years. *Monographs of the Society for Research in Child Development* 46:No. 4, 1981.
17. Elkind, D. Egocentrism in adolescence. *Child Dev.* 38:1025, 1967.
18. Enright, R. D., Shulka, D. G., and Lapsley, D. K. Adolescent egocentrism-sociocentrism and self-consciousness. *Journal of Youth and Adolescence* 9:101, 1980.
19. Erikson, E. H. *Childhood and Society* (2nd Edition). New York: Norton, 1963.
20. Erikson, E. H. Identity and the life cycle: Selected papers. In *Psychological Issues.* Monograph 1, Vol 1, 1959.
21. Frazier, A., and Lisonbee, L. K. Adolescent concerns with physique. *School Review* 58:397, 1950.
22. Gerard, H. School desegregation: The social science role. *Am. Psychol.* 38:869, 1983.
23. Grotevant, H. D. The contribution of the family to the facilitation of identity formation in early adolescence. *Journal of Early Adolescence* 3:225, 1983.
24. Hall, G. S. *Adolescence.* 2 Vols. New York: Appleton-Century-Croft, 1904.
25. Harnsberger, C. T. (Ed.). *Mark Twain at Your Finger Tips.* New York: Beechhurst Press, 1948.
26. Horrocks, J. E. *The Psychology of Adolescence* (4th ed.). Boston: Houghton Mifflin, 1976.
27. Hutson, P. W. Vocational choices, 1930 and 1961. *Vocational Guidance Quarterly* 10:218, 1962.
28. Inhelder, B., and Piaget, J. *The Growth of Logical Thinking.* New York: Basic Books, 1958.
29. Jacobson, E. *The Self and the Object World.* New York: International Universities Press, 1964.
30. Jessor, R., Jessor, S. L., and Finney, J. A social psychology of marijuana use: Longitudinal studies of high school and college youth. *J Pers. Soc. Psychol.* 26:1, 1973.
31. Jessor, S. L., and Jessor, R. Transition from virginity to nonvirginity among youth: A social-psychological study over time. *Dev. Psychol.* 11:473, 1975.
32. Keating, D. P. Thinking Processes in Adolescence. In

J. Adelson (Ed.), *Handbook of Adolescent Psychology.* New York: Wiley, 1980.

33. Keniston, K.   *The Uncommitted: Alienated Youth in American Society.* New York: Dell, 1970.

34. Kuhn, D., and Angelev, J.   An experimental study of the development of formal operational thought. *Child Dev.* 47:697, 1976.

35. Lerner, Orlos, J. B., and Knapp, J. R.   Physical attractiveness, physical effectiveness and self-concept in late adolescence. *Adolescence* 11:313, 1976.

36. Lerner, R. M., and Karabenick, S. A.   Physical attractiveness, body attitudes and self-concept in late adolescence. *Journal of Youth and Adolescence* 13:307, 1974.

37. Lewis, C.   How adolescents approach decisions: Changes over grades seven to twelve and policy implications. *Child Dev.* 52:538, 1981.

38. Linn, M. C., de Benedictis, T., and Delucchi, K.   Adolescent reasoning about advertisements: Preliminary investigations. *Child Dev.* 53:1599, 1982.

39. Mannarino, A. P.   Friendship patterns and self-concept development in preadolescent males. *J. Gen. Psychol.* 133:105, 1978.

40. Marcia, J. E.   Identity in adolescence. In J. Adelson (Ed.), *Handbook of Adolescent Psychology.* New York: Wiley, 1980.

41. Marcia, J. E.   Development and validation of ego identity status. *J. Pers. Soc. Psychol.* 3:551, 1966.

42. Marcia, J. E.   Ego identity status: Relationship to change in self-esteem, "general maladjustment" and authoritarianism. *J. Pers.* 35:119, 1967.

43. McCarthy, J. D., and Hoge, D. R.   Analysis of age effects in longitudinal studies of adolescent self-esteem. *Dev. Psychol.* 18:372, 1982.

44. Meilman, P. W.   Cross-sectional age changes in ego identity during adolescence. *Dev. Psychol.* 15:230, 1979.

45. Newman, P. R., and Newman, B. M.   Early adolescence and its conflict: Group identity versus alienation. *Adolescence* 11:261, 1976.

46. Newman, B. M., and Newman, P. R.   *An Introduction to the Psychology of Adolescence.* Homewood IL: The Dorsey Press, 1979.

47. Piaget, J.   *The Psychology of Intelligence.* Totowa, NJ: Littlefield, Adams, 1981.

48. Piaget, J.   Intellectual evolution from adolescence to adulthood. *Hum. Dev.* 15:1, 1972.

49. Rosenberg, M.   *Conceiving the Self.* New York: Basic Books, 1979.

50. Savin-Williams, R. C., and Demo, D. H.   Conceiving or misconceiving the self. *Journal of Early Adolescence* 3:121, 1983.

51. Selman, R. L.   Social-cognition understanding: A guide to educational and clinical practice. In T. Likona (Ed.), *Moral Development and Behavior: Theory Research and Social Issues.* NY: Holt, Rinehart & Winston, 1976.

52. Simmons, R. G., and Rosenberg, F.   Sex, sex roles and self-image. *Journal of Youth and Adolescence,* 4:229, 1975.

53. Simmons, R. G., Blyth, D. A., Van Cleave, E. F., and Bush, D. M.   Entry into early adolescence: The impact of school structure, puberty, and early dating on self-esteem. *Am. Sociol. Rev.* 44:948, 1979.

54. Simmons, R. G., Rosenberg, F., and Rosenberg, M.   Disturbance in the self-image at adolescence. *Am. Sociol. Rev.* 38:553, 1973.

55. Steinberg, L., and Hill, J. P.   Patterns of family interaction as a function of age, the onset of puberty and formal thinking. *Dev. Psychol.* 14:683, 1978.

56. Steinberg, L. D.   Transformations in family relations at puberty. *Dev. Psychol.* 17:833, 1981.

57. Stephan, W. G.   School Desegregation: An evaluation of predictions made in Brown vs. Board of Education. *Psychol. Bull.* 85:217, 1978.

58. Sullivan, H. S.   *The Interpersonal Theory of Psychiatry.* New York: Norton, 1953.

59. Super, D. E., and Overstreet, P. L.   *The Vocational Maturity of Ninth-Grade Boys.* New York: Teachers College, Columbia University Press, 1960.

60. Waterman, A. S., Geary, P. S., and Waterman, C. K.   A longitudinal study of changes in ego identity status from the freshman to the senior year at college. *Dev. Psychol.* 10:387, 1974.

61. Werner, H.   *The Comparative Psychology of Mental Development.* Chicago: Follet, 1948.

62. White, K. M., and Ferstenberg, A.   Professional specialization and formal operations: The balance task. *J. Genet. Psychol.* 133:97, 1978.

63. Winer, G. A.   A review and analysis of children's fearful behavior in dental settings. *Child Dev.* 53:1111, 1982.

IX
Young Adulthood

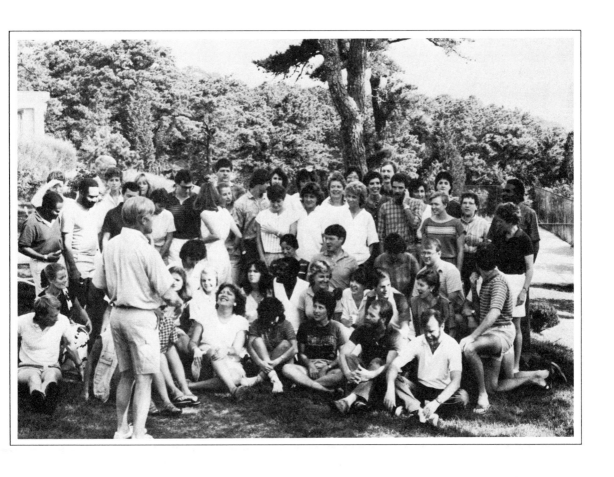

27

Biophysical and Cognitive Development in Young Adulthood

Shirley S. Ashburn

The secret is not to live less intensely, but more intelligently.

—Hans Selye, *The Stress of Life*

After spending 18 to 20 years undergoing rapid physical, cognitive, and social changes, the young adult often feels as if he or she has finally arrived, and that growth and development is complete. It is a surprise to the same person 15 to 20 years later, when approaching the end of the young adult period, to discover that developmental changes are still occurring. The early adult years are merely one more unique phase in the life cycle.

Age-related somatic changes continue to occur during these years. Optimal biophysical functioning is not a given. The maintenance of high-level functioning depends on understanding the body's unique needs and continuing to provide adequate care. Some people take better care of their cars than they do of their own bodies!

Hypothetically, it is during these young adult years that biophysical and cognitive skills reach their peak. Unfortunately, it is also a period of life when social and affective pressures tempt one to misuse and to abuse the newly acquired physical and cognitive skills. College students may spend night after night studying or socializing, thereby denying themselves the sleep they need to function optimally. Young mothers may skip meals in order to finish housework while their children nap. Aspiring, career-oriented young individuals may deny themselves proper nutrition and rest while they spend day after day pushing themselves toward success. Many young adults defer regular preventive medical attention. Statements such as "I'm too young to worry about overdoing it," or "I'll start thinking about my health after I'm 40," are attempts to justify these actions.

Optimal cognitive functioning depends on adequate physical functioning. Inadequate sleep, exercise, and nutrition will decrease intellectual acumen. Understanding how the cognitive system functions can help people to maximize their potentials and skills.

BIOPHYSICAL CHANGES

Young adults come in all shapes and sizes. Their differing heights and weights are influenced by many factors, including heredity, life-style, nutritional habits, and gender. For these reasons, it is more appropriate to decide the desirable weight for an individual by gender and body build rather than by an age-related norm. **Desirable** weights are not the same as **average** weights; instead, they are usually 15 to 25 pounds below average weights. Desirable weights are calculated in this way because they show positive correlation with the lowest mortality rates (see Appendix F). Even if an individual's weight remains constant throughout these years, the proportion of fatty tissue in the body may increase. "Overfat" is just as unhealthy as overweight. Although authorities disagree, it is probably safe to say that the maximum for fat in a healthy person is 15 percent of total body weight for males, and 22 percent of total body weight for females [2]. Fatness can be estimated by measuring the thickness of the fat folds of skin at selected body sites with special calipers. Other more refined tests also exist that more accurately calculate the percentage of body fat.

Skeletal System

The growth of the skeletal system is essentially completed around 25 years of age with the final fusion of the epiphyses of the long bones. However, since the vertebral column continues to grow until about age 30, another 3 to 5 mm may be added to one's height [51]. The smaller leg bones, sternum (breastbone), pelvic bones, and vertebrae (back bones) attain adult distribution of red marrow at about 25 years of age [28]. The red marrow is responsible for the production of blood cells and hemoglobin. Although the bone has achieved final growth, it does retain the ability to form new bone at any time, which is essential for the healing of fractures [53].

Neuromuscular System

Muscular efficiency is at its peak performance between 20 and 30 years of age [53]. Thereafter, muscular strength declines, but the rate of aging may vary according to the muscle group and the activity level of the individual. Reaction times generally peak just before the onset of young adulthood and remain constant until the late twenties. Since professional athletes must perform at optimal levels in order to compete successfully, the decline in muscular strength and reaction time may explain why many are considered too old to compete and retire between 30 and 35 years of age.

Integumentary System

After adolescence, the skin begins to lose moisture, gradually becoming more dry and wrinkled with age. "Smile lines" are usually noticeable in a person by the late twenties. Lines at the corners of the eyes ("crow's feet") may be upsetting to people in their early thirties, since they are interpreted as one of the first signs of the inevitable aging process. Many women approaching this age attempt both to increase the flow of facial circulation and to moisturize their drying skin by applying creams and lotions. Although these measures combined with adequate cleaning may aid in attaining a smoother, younger-looking skin, consuming adequate amounts of fluids and following a well-balanced diet are also helpful (see Table 27–1 and Appendix E for recommendations).

Unwanted hair growth, often the side effect of birth control pills, may be removed by tweezing, waxing, or electrolysis. Although gray hair and baldness are most often associated with old age, the first signs of these changes may appear in young adulthood. Both appear to be influenced by heredity (see Chap. 36).

Cardiovascular System

The cardiovascular system has established adult size and rhythm by 16 years of age. The total blood volume

Table 27–1. Dietary Recommendations for Adults

Food Group	Daily Amount
Milk group	2 cups or more equivalent[a]
Meat group	2 or more servings
Vegetable-fruit group	4 or more servings[b]
Bread-cereal group	4 or more servings

[a] Three cups or more for pregnant women; four cups or more equivalent for lactating women.
[b] One should be a citrus fruit to provide vitamin C; a dark green or deep yellow vegetable for vitamin A is needed every other day.

Although much research has been performed, there is no agreement as yet on the mechanisms by which diet affects serum cholesterol levels [1]. It has been demonstrated that modification of the dietary intake of fats (which includes cholesterol) can modify the elevated blood lipids (fats). Since cholesterol is a precursor of vitamin D and is closely related to some of the hormones in the body, it should not be considered an abnormal substance [1] or eliminated entirely from the diet. Wise young adults should use moderation in the amount and types of fat in the diet (see Chap. 36 for further discussion of cholesterol). They should also make sure that they remain physically active to keep muscle tone (especially the heart muscle) in a healthy state.

Race, gender, and weight influence blood pressure in young adults [24]. Black females tend to have the

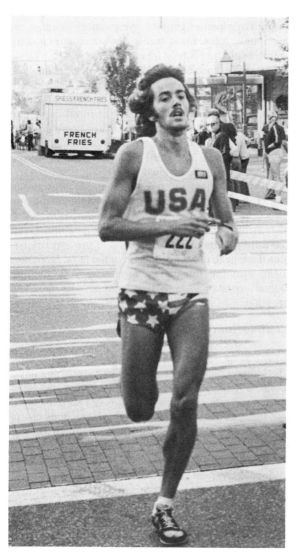

Figure 27–1. Young adulthood is the peak period for physical strength and endurance but must be carefully cultivated with long hours of exercise to achieve maximum performance.

in a young adult is 70 to 85 ml per kilogram of body weight [28]. Blood pressure rises slowly from early childhood (see Appendix E), and cholesterol levels increase from the age of 21 years. Cholesterol levels are of concern because high levels are correlated with fat deposits in blood vessels, which can lead to circulatory problems, especially in the heart muscle. Young males are more likely to have elevated cholesterol levels than are young females.

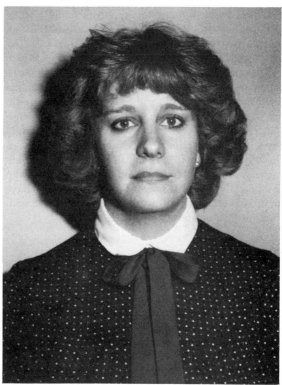

Figure 27–2. Many adults discover asymmetrical development of the face or body. Hyper- or hypoplagia of body tissues does not usually interfere with functioning. If one covers one half of this young woman's face, she will appear to be two different people. Note in particular the dissimilar shape of the nose, mouth, and jawline, as well as uneven eye height.

highest incidence of hypertension (high blood pressure), followed by black males, white males, and white females, in that order. Obesity was found to have the greatest influence on blood pressure because the heart must work harder to accommodate the accompanying increased blood volume.

Oral contraceptives, which are used by many women during the childbearing years, are suspected of increasing the risks of diseases of the cardiovascular system, including venous thromboembolism, high blood pressure, myocardial infarction (heart attack), and cerebrovascular diseases [37].

Respiratory System

Although most organs of the body thrive on work and increase their functioning mass (hypertrophy) when a chronic workload is necessary, the lungs possess a limited capacity to do so. The body's ability to use oxygen optimally is much more dependent on the efficiency of the cardiovascular system and the needs of the skeletal muscles than on the maturity of the lungs [32]. The greatest natural stress that human lungs endure is providing adequate oxygenation to the blood in high-altitude environments, since oxygen concentration in the air is decreased. Mobile and active young adults who are attracted to skiing, hang-gliding, piloting, or mountain climbing may feel short of breath or physically tired when attempting strenuous physical activity in these environments. The natives of high-altitude climates possess slightly larger lungs than do those who reside at sea level. The lungs of these natives also have an increased oxygen-diffusing capacity compared with those of their sea-level visitors [32].

Gastrointestinal System

The digestive tract displays a decrease in the amount of some digestive juices after 30 years of age. The amount of ptyalin (enzyme used to digest starches) in the saliva decreases after 20 years of age [53]; otherwise the digestive system remains fully functioning. Healthy young adults do not experience any noticeable changes in their patterns of digestion or elimination. The rate at which food travels through the gastrointestinal tract is still influenced by factors, such as the nature of the food (e.g., high fiber content or saturated fat) and the state of physical health. The previously established habits of elimination should continue to exist (i.e., frequency, consistency, and color of bowel movements). Most stools are brown in color due to the bile pigment they contain. Various foods and medications affect stool color. Stools that are externally coated with bright red blood might be a symptom of bleeding hemorrhoids, a condition that is not uncommon among young adults, especially females.

The appearance of "wisdom teeth," or third molars, is another age-related change in the alimentary canal. These third molars normally erupt between 20 and 21 years. Their roots are completely matured anywhere from age 18 to age 25 [28]. There are normally four third molars, although some individuals may not fully develop all four. The third molars frequently create problems for the individual. Their eruptions are unpredictable in time and presentation; it is not unusual for wisdom teeth to come in sideways, or facing any direction. They can also force the other teeth out of alignment, making chewing difficult and painful. Often the third molars must be removed to prevent irreparable damage to proper occlusion of the jaws. Even normally erupting third molars may be very painful. Dental assistance may be necessary to facilitate eruption.

Genitourinary System

RENAL FUNCTIONING
The kidneys play a dominant role in maintaining physiological homeostasis. They aid in excreting metabolic waste products and in regulating water content, salts, and the acid-base balance of the body. The body chemistry norms for adults reflect this combined work of the kidneys with other body organs. Total urinary output in a 24-hour period ranges between 1000 and 2000 ml for the average young adult.

Interestingly, some people are born with only one kidney. This single kidney is not uncommon and presents no difficulty if it functions properly.

GENITAL TRACT AND ORGANS
The uterus reaches its maximum weight at about 30 years of age. Although some women experience premenstrual syndrome (see Chap. 25) from the beginning of puberty, many develop it after a significant interruption of their cycle, such as pregnancy or use of the birth control pill. It is not uncommon for a healthy female to experience a minimal amount of menstrual bleeding ("spotting") either at the midpoint of the cycle or at the time when she would usually have a menstrual period. There are times when she may actually skip a menstrual period, even though she is not pregnant. Statistically, the optimal period for reproduction in females (in terms of the greatest frequency of successful pregnancies) is between 20 and 30 years of age [53].

The Leydig cells, which are a source of male hormones, begin to decline slowly in number when the individual is approximately 25 years of age [52]; this is accompanied by a gradual decline in androgen secretion. However, no significant weight loss occurs with age in the healthy human testes even in the elderly male. Since spermatogenesis continues throughout adulthood, the male's biophysical ability to father a child should not be affected by these somatic changes.

Biophysical Responses to Environmental Stimuli

SEXUAL RESPONSE

Many young adults are concerned about what is biophysically normal when they are engaged in sexual intimacies. Research by Masters and Johnson has advanced the knowledge of human sexual response patterns. From their studies, they found that the sexual response cycle in both men and women can be divided into four stages [30]. Phase 1, **excitation** (sometimes lasting hours), develops from any source of somatogenic or psychogenic stimulation and takes place more rapidly (perhaps in a few seconds) in men than in women. It is characterized by the erection of the penis and the secretion of lubricating fluids in the male; it is demonstrated by production of lubricating fluid, enlarged diameter of the clitoris, and increased blood congestion in both sets of vaginal labia (lips) in the female. Most women experience nipple erection during this phase, as do about one-third of men. If effective sexual stimulation is continued, the individual will progress to the next stage of the sexual cycle.

Phase 2, **plateau,** is characterized by an increase in blood congestion and sexual tension in the pelvic area for both men and women. Both experience a "sexual flush" on the chest, neck, and forehead. Women also experience a flush on the lower abdomen, thighs, and lower back more frequently than men. The duration of the plateau stage is dependent on the effectiveness of the stimuli employed and the individual drive for orgasm. It is from this second stage that the person may ultimately move to orgasm.

Phase 3, **the orgasmic stage,** consists of those few seconds when the climax of sexual tension is reached. This phase occurs in two substages for the male: First, he experiences contractions of his penis and the adjacent internal male reproductive structures; second, his contracting pelvic muscles produce the ejaculation (emission of seminal fluid). The female orgasm, occurring in one longer stage, is characterized by contractions of the uterus, vagina, and clitoris. In both men and women, there may be contractions of the rectal sphincter muscles as well as of other body muscles. Both may experience hyperventilation (rapid, shallow breathing) and tachycardia (rapid heart beats up to 180 beats per minute) [30]. Sometimes, the person perspires—men on the soles of the feet and palms of the hands; women over the back, thighs, and chest.

Both the man and the woman resolve from their orgasm into phase 4, **resolution.** This stage is an involuntary period of tension loss, when the congestion of many of the blood vessels involved in the sexual response cycle decreases. The purpose of resolution is to return the person through the plateau and excitement levels to an unstimulated state. Women have the response potential of returning to another orgasm from any point in the resolution phase, and they may experience multiple orgasms over a relatively short period of time. Men, after completing the orgasm, require a "refractory period" or a period of return to the plateau stage before another orgasm can be achieved. This period can be relatively short in men under the age of 30; men over 30 years of age usually require complete resolution and need to initiate a new response cycle [30].

Masters and Johnson emphasize that there is "wide individual variation in the duration and intensity of every specific physiologic response to sexual stimulation" [30]. For many reasons, most of which are psychogenic in origin, some women never achieve phase 3 during their lifetime, or at least during the younger years. Sensitive, synchronized attention from the woman's partner can facilitate and heighten the sexual tension, with excitement and enjoyment achieved by both. Many men fail to achieve phase 2 and/or 3 (impotence) on their first attempts, or when the need to perform is critical to self-esteem, such as on the honeymoon. Again, patience on the part of both partners and relaxation of one's attempts to impress or to succeed are usually all that is necessary to eventually achieve a satisfying orgasm.

Masters and Johnson do not believe that enough data have been collected to date to explain precisely all the mechanisms of the sexual response, but their research continues to pave the way for a greater understanding of human sexual adequacy and inadequacy.

PERCEPTUAL SKILLS

The major organ involved with cognition, the brain, reaches physical maturity before 20 years of age. Many 10-year-old children have a brain weight as great as that of an adult [28]. Final myelinization and differentiation in the central nervous system occurs at about

25 years of age [53]. The relative weight of the entire central nervous system at full maturation is about one-fiftieth of the total body weight. The brain is the organ with the highest metabolic rate, using 3.5 ml of oxygen for each 100 gm of tissue per minute [28].

The senses also experience age-related changes. The lens of the eye begins the aging process during infancy. Since it continues to grow without shedding older cells, it becomes thicker, less elastic, and more opaque with age [55]. The lens functions of accommodation and convergence are affected by this phenomenon. These changes are so gradual that the average young adult will not notice changes in visual acuity.

Hearing levels usually peak at age 20 years, and thereafter acuity gradually declines. The high tones are often lost first, then the low tones [55]. In most cases, the tones that are lost have no bearing on the activities of daily living, so behavior is not usually affected.

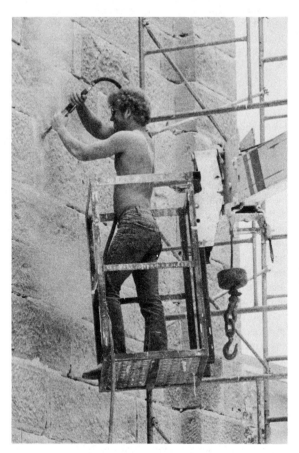

Figure 27–3. Many adults work in environments that may lead to hearing impairments or eye injuries.

Many factors, such as nutrition and heredity, affect how much and how fast hearing is lost. A substantial increase in noise levels can accelerate progression of hearing loss.

Taste, touch, and smell remain keen during young adulthood. No deterioration in these three senses is usually seen until middlescence.

SENSORY DEPRIVATION

Alterations in sensory input have been noted to cause serious behavioral changes. Phenomena, such as marked changes in the ability to think and reason, feelings of disorientation, anxiety, fear, depression, hallucinations, and delusions, have been described by individuals undergoing sensory deprivation [47]. Sensory deprivation is classified under three dimensions [9]: (1) decreased sensory input, or sensory underload; (2) decreased meaningful activity, or lack of stimulus relevance; and (3) alteration of the reticular activating system.

Sensory underload occurs when environmental stimuli are below the level needed to attract attention. This state can be caused by continuous repetition of a stimulus, stimuli of insufficient intensity to activate the receptors, inadequately functioning body receptors that fail to receive stimuli, or excess anxiety that decreases the ability of the body to attend to the normal stimuli being received by the receptors.

Relevance deprivation occurs when either an alteration in the stimuli or a blockage of the receptors restricts the reception of useful information. Stimuli can be altered in terms of size, intensity, or repetition. Introduction of a new communication code (such as during foreign travel or learning computer language) can constitute relevance deprivation. Relevance deprivation may also be experienced during periods of unemployment or when one's peer group or spouse is not "in tune" with one's needs or interests. Blockage of a receptor can occur through loss of its use, such as in deafness or blindness, or through interference by inattention, boredom, or anxiety.

The third type of sensory deprivation can occur when the reticular activating system is altered. This system is a mechanism located deep in the center of the brain through which an individual receives and organizes stimulation patterns to orient the self to the external environment. If a less than normal amount of stimuli is processed by the reticular activating system, the individual's normal potential for cognition and patterns of behavior are decreased in efficiency.

Too much stimulation can also affect the individual's interaction with the environment. When stimuli are at too high an arousal level (too intense or too great a volume), they interfere with the incoming and outgoing signals traversing the reticular activating center, causing the information it is carrying to lose meaning (sensory overload). Such excess information may overwhelm and interrupt the individual's normal range of behavior and cause him or her to function at a less effective level in a given situation. A balance must be found between the overall needs to accommodate and to assimilate new input. Thus it is not only the amount of stimulation but also the level of stimulus variation and the meaning of the stimulation that are related to human behavior. It is important for an individual to provide the self with changes in stimulation that present a meaningful interpretation of the world. Maintaining one's health in all four domains requires more than just keeping the body in shape.

COGNITIVE DEVELOPMENT

By young adulthood, one reaches the highest level of cognitive development and intellectual efficiency. In general, people exhibit their maximum levels of intellectual and creative effectiveness, perceptual clarity, and learning and memory capability during this period. With relatively few exceptions, the cognitive performances of young adults remains at a high plateau through the middle adult years. When adequate physical and psychic energies are available, and opportunities allow, cognitive prowess can create meaningful social and occupational achievements for young adults.

Intelligence
In general, young adults have reached a stable point in their achievement scores on intelligence tests.

CROSS-SECTIONAL DATA
The normative data on which intelligence quotient (IQ) scores are based are secured by ranking within age-group raw scores. Thus an individual 25-year-old's test achievements are compared to the test achievements of a sample of 25-year-olds. Cross-sectional norms show that a higher raw score level is achieved by 25-year-olds as a group than 15-year-olds or 60-year-olds.

The Wechsler Adult Intelligence Scale (WAIS) test is made up of two subtests: the performance subtests and the verbal subtests [57]. The WAIS performance subtests require reasoning, pattern perception, and problem solving. These raw score averages decline slightly toward the end of early adulthood. The WAIS verbal subtests emphasize general information, verbal rea-

soning, and vocabulary. These scores remain high throughout adulthood.

FLUID AND CRYSTALLIZED INTELLIGENCE
When a factor analysis of intelligence test items was made, two types of intelligence were identified [22]. **Fluid intelligence** is the capacity for dealing with spatial relations (geometric figures and matrixes), inductive reasoning, and nonsense memory (use of novel material requiring short-term memory). It is closely related to neurological and physiological function because it depends on spread of thinking, dexterity, and short-term memory.

The second entity, **crystallized intelligence,** is the scope of general understanding and knowledge. It is largely a product of socialization, education, and experience. Measures of crystallized intelligence include general reasoning (problems of everyday living) and verbal comprehension. WAIS performance scores are thought to be measures of fluid intelligence, while WAIS verbal scores reflect crystallized intelligence [21]. It is theorized that when aging processes produce declining neurological and physiological efficiency, then

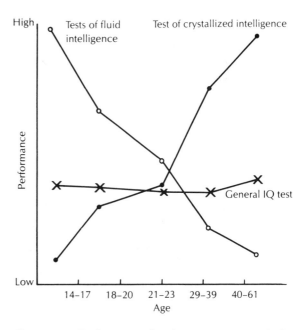

Figure 27–4. Performance of various age groups on tests used to define fluid, crystallized, and general intelligence. (From J. L. Horn, Organization of Data on Life-Span Development of Human Abilities. In Goulet and Baltes (Eds.), *Life-Span Developmental Psychology: Research and Theory.* New York: Academic Press, 1970. With permission.)

lower levels of fluid intelligence are reflected in lower WAIS performance scores.

Crystallized intelligence is said to be derived from environmental stimulation and cultural experience. Since the quality of these factors depends on the lifestyle of the subject, crystallized intelligence may or may not diminish with age. The average decline of WAIS verbal scores is less rapid. Both forms of intelligence are essential for effective processing of environmental stimuli, which the healthy person must continue to assimilate and to accommodate all through life if adaptation is to be successful.

LONGITUDINAL STUDIES

Evidence somewhat contrary to the theory of fluid and crystallized intelligence is found in longitudinal examinations of intelligence. Longitudinal studies of intelligence involve the retesting of the same individuals after a period of years.

As early as 1920, intelligence tests were administered to large numbers of college freshmen. Retests of these subjects when they were mature adults produce surprising results. The scores went up with age. Both performance and verbal test scores increased as these subjects progressed through their thirties, forties, and fifties [34]. Not until these subjects were in their sixties was a leveling trend evident. Some decline was found when they were in their seventies.

This finding of an increase in IQ with age is limited to a sample of the ex-college student population. Retests of adult populations with a full range of education and intelligence levels do not show that intelligence

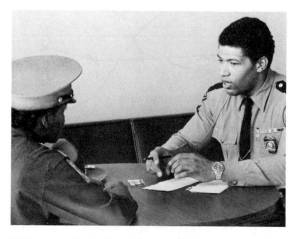

Figure 27–5. It is critical that one have access to individualized learning opportunities to maintain high performance levels in many careers.

test scores automatically increase with age, but neither do they show decreases [45].

There seems to be a pattern here. Individuals who exercise their intellectual skills during their adult years tend to enjoy some improvement in these skills, and this improvement is evident in their intelligence test scores. Individuals whose adult careers do not require an unusual exercise of mathematical and verbal efforts or abstract reasoning are likely to retain a steady state or capacity as measured by the tests. Declines in intelligence test scores are somewhat more likely in their performance tests than in the verbal tests.

Why is it that the longitudinal studies of intellectual skill indicate a good retention of skill, or even an improvement of skill during adulthood, while cross-sectional studies indicate a decline after 30 years of age? One possibility is that there is a "secular trend" of intelligence test scores. Just as there has been an improvement and increase in the height, weight, health, and physiological maturation rates over the last few generations, it may be that there has been a similar improvement in intellectual skills.

During the fifty years after the invention of intelligence tests in the first decade of this century, each generation of children earned higher raw scores on these tests than did the previous generation. This may well be due to the higher levels of education and literacy enjoyed by these generations [55]. Since cross-section studies sample different generations, the older, less advantaged subjects do less well on the intelligence tests. However, longitudinal studies follow the same sample of individuals over the years, so that these data are not influenced by cultural differences between generations.

It may be that this upward direction of intelligence test achievement is being reversed. During the 1960s, 1970s, and early 1980s, there has been a general decline in achievement test scores in secondary school and the performances on college entrance examinations [11]. If these lower scores truly reflect lower competence in recent graduates, then these individuals may score less well on intelligence tests during the middle and later years of the life cycle than individuals who finished school before 1960. However, if the lower scores are a reflection of the broader cross section of students taking the test (as opposed to just top, college-bound students of earlier years), then no differences should emerge.

Cognitive Performance

Young adults tend to do well in measures of learning and memory efficiency. The findings here closely parallel the findings on intelligence test performance. Young adults achieve a high level of performance and maintain this superiority throughout the span of young adulthood [55].

The efficiency of learning and memory, as with the other intellectual functions, appear to be closely related to the life activities of the individual. If an individual's daily experiences demand little in the way of intellectual effort, there is a tendency toward a gradual decline of intellectual performance during the adult years. On the other hand, if the individual's current activities require intellectual effort, and if these activities are interesting and rewarding, there is a tendency for intellectual capacity to grow. The relationship seems to be one of "use it or lose it" [55].

COGNITIVE PROCESSES

One approach to problem solving and creativity during young adulthood is to examine the organization of thought processes during this period.

Piaget's formal operations. For Piaget [17], young adulthood is a period when the individual refines the formal operations style of cognitive functioning. Formal operational thinking, begun during adolescence, involves the use of higher order abstractions. These processes are organized into systematic interrelationships, which Piaget called cognitive rules.

The young adult begins at the abstract level and compares the idea mentally or verbally with previous problems, memories, knowledge, and experience. The steps of a task are mentally combined or integrated instead of thinking about or doing each step as a separate unit. The alternatives to a situation are considered and ideas or information are synthesized and integrated into the individual's memory, beliefs, or solutions, so that the end result is his or her unique product. Adult thought is different from adolescent thought in that the adult, because of experience and education as well as inductive and deductive reasoning, can differentiate among many perspectives and outcomes in an objective, realistic, and less egocentric manner. The adult is able to entertain more options, to hypothesize the potential products or effects of an action and thus choose a solution with the "best fit," considering all current and long-range factors.

Mathematical calculus is an example of a cognitive skill that requires the use of formal operational thought. This process is one whereby new information that does not fit preconceived categories is used to innovate new concepts of organization. Piaget considered cognitive accommodation to be the essence of intellectual func-

tion. Flavell suggests that accommodation is the basis of the creative act [19].

Whether through lack of environmental opportunity or intellectual limitations, some adolescents and young adults fail to achieve the formal operations level of cognitive development. A few of these individuals may never possess the intellectual competence to perform at the formal operations level. Piaget states that individuals progress to each cognitive level of development at different speeds. Thus, some young people who appear to have come to an intellectual arrest may eventually attain formal operational thought. Such differences are due, he says, to the quality and frequency of intellectual stimulation. This stimulation is not only the result of social and environmental transmission, but the interdependence of the four domains is an integral factor in the development of one's cognitive competence and performance.

The achievement of formal operations may be limited or temporary, depending on the individual's response to environmental stressors. There are instances when even the most intellectually gifted individuals will resort to preoperational thought. Piaget [38] himself has noted " . . . I am, for example, at an operatory level for only a small part of the day . . . the rest of the time I am dealing with empirical trial and error." Without exercise, formal operations wither, so that some adults may become rigid in cognitive functions, losing the ability to be intellectually creative.

Quantitative versus qualitative changes. Piaget discusses intellectual development in terms of quantitative versus qualitative or structural changes. Quantitative intelligence refers to the amount of knowledge or information an individual has at his or her disposal at any given time; qualitative intelligence refers to the way information is organized for use. It involves the intellectual structuring or categorizing process and the rules used to manipulate the information for problem solving. While qualitative changes in cognitive structure cease after the individual has mastered the skill of formal operations (at approximately 15 years of age), quantitative changes in the content and the function of intelligence continue. Schemata are continually being modified throughout the life cycle.

Piaget states that a major change in the cognitive development of the young adult involves the loss of adolescent egocentrism. Egocentrism subsides when individuals learn to use logic effectively in relation to the realities of life, not just in relation to life as they think it should be [56]. Relative objectivity of thought with respect to conflicting issues is attained when adolescents assume adult roles in the real world and can differentiate the many possible points of view [56]. This is not to say, however, that all young adults are flexible in understanding the viewpoints of others.

Many adults do not attain the level of formal operations in all areas of intellectual growth [3]. Elkind, for example, found that 92 percent of college students conserve mass and weight, but only 58 percent conserve volume [17]. At this point it is important to recall that "intelligence" is a difficult entity to measure. The current battle over the validity of IQ testing exemplifies the controversy over the term and the interpretation of standards used to measure intelligence.

The vast number of uncontrollable variables (e.g., social class, culture, life experiences, religion) that go into formulating an individual's thought processes make it difficult to establish a comparative norm. The individual who may be considered an intelligent person in our society may be thought to be quite naive among people in a foreign culture requiring different adaptive skills. Although Piaget's framework for describing approaches to learning and problem solving appears to have universal applicability, the individual's data base, or schemata, is heavily influenced by his or her culture and life experiences.

Piaget notes striking differences in the levels of development attained by different individuals. He hypothesizes that up to the age when formal operations are mastered, certain behavior patterns of individuals characteristically form cognitive stages with general properties. Beginning at some time during formal operations, individual differences in aptitude become more important than the general characteristics that determine the individual's type of formal thinking [8]. Piaget feels that these individual differences influence a person's career choice. Thereafter, he says that the working environment contributes even more to the knowledge base and consequent thoughts that individuals possess [40]. Law students hope to build their career on their abilities to apply precise logic to abstract concepts; electricians take pride in their capabilities of "trouble shooting" and planning repairs of electrical equipment.

CREATIVE PRODUCTIVITY

A second approach to the study of creativity and the problem-solving patterns of young adults is to consider the nature and the frequency of the products of creativity. Several studies indicate that important discoveries and inventions occur with relatively high frequency during late adolescence and early adulthood [26]. Important creative works continue to be pro-

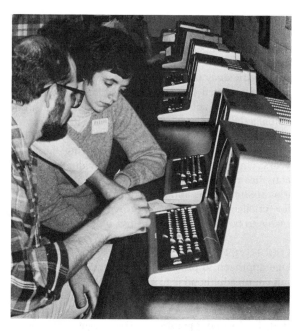

Figure 27-6. Continuing education may take the form of visiting other places of employment as well as formal workshops.

duced during middle and late adulthood as well as in old age [14]. Often the initial insight or discovery comes during early adulthood, and the contributions that come later emphasize elaborations and implications of the original study. Albert Einstein is supposed to have said that during his whole life, he had only two really good ideas, both of these as a very young man. He spent the whole of his life searching out the significance of these two ideas. This pattern is typical of some creative thinkers.

THINKING AND FLEXIBILITY

The capabilities needed for additional learning and for adjusting to new situations (i.e., analytical reasoning, comparison formations, creative imagination, information recall, and verbal skills) generally reach their peak when individuals are in their twenties [41]. Abstract thinking processes can be developed and facilitated through education and critical discussions with others. Students and faculty alike sharpen their understandings and clarify their own positions by engaging in dialogue about conflicting views or philosophies. A person's receptivity to new ideas partially depends on affective development, or the individual's outlook toward self and his or her world. The more affectively mature and secure individual is usually able to accept a broader range of differing opinions or viewpoints and is also usually able to concentrate more effectively on cognitive activities. The affectively secure person does not feel a need to defend his or her own view or ideas, and thus can utilize the modifying and expanding input from others.

In terms of thinking, young adulthood is likely to be the time when people have the maximum flexibility to form new concepts and can easily shift their thinking in order to solve problems. This ability to shift the thinking in an approach to a problem is usually displayed when the solution involves discovering the details of categories and using the information at hand. Again, however, age is not the only determinant; emotional maturity, intelligence, education, memory, opportunity, and motivation all contribute heavily to thinking and flexibility.

Interface of Intelligence and Socioemotional Skills

The individual's cognitive development rests on a complex of intellectual capacity and past experience that is played out against a unique, dynamic cultural environment. The interaction is a very personal one. In the ideal case, the individual's social life-space offers opportunities and challenges that may be mastered with reasonable intellectual effort. Social and financial recognition of competence facilitate continuous growth.

During adulthood, there are two themes that support the expression of cognitive maturity. These themes are

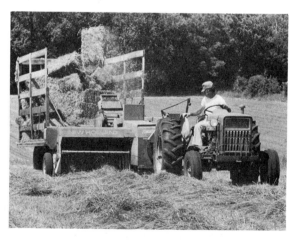

Figure 27–7. Traditional jobs, such as farming, require a higher knowledge of machinery and business as well as agricultural techniques in today's world.

found in the Freudian dynamic, which suggests that maturity is sought by sublimation in love and work [18]. The most successful (and happiest) individuals are those who feel in control of their lives and who evaluate their progress by their own standards, not those of others. At the same time, deep, significant, mutual relationships with others provide contexts for release of cognitive/affective energies where meaningful, productive, personal reality may be found. Employment that is challenging, rewarding, satisfying, and fun provides a framework for fostering cognitive creativity. The author agrees with Daniel Levinson's [27] concept that people need a dream (a realistic goal for commitment), a mentor (someone older and experienced as a guide), and another special person to serve as a source of affirmation in order to have sufficient affective energies to invest in strenuous cognitive pursuits.

EMPLOYMENT CHOICES

Tradition defines young adulthood as the time when individuals are expected to go to work full time. More and more women, as well as men, now work full time. Even more important than the economics or employment may be the social role and meaning that work provides. Employers who provide job opportunities, challenge, support, recognition, and reward in the work environment tend to have cognitively creative workers [36]. Morale is high and the companies prosper. The young adult who finds employment that contains these elements is challenged and supported. An individual's intellectual skills, especially his or her perception of them, are likely to affect self-esteem.

It is possible that how well young adults work with their peers and co-workers in certain job- or task-oriented situations is in part a determinant of how successful they are viewed by others. Flavell believes that adult cognitive changes focus far more sharply on interpersonal skills (conveying of judgments, attitudes, and beliefs), than on logical-mathematical procedures [19]. It is important to note that although job choice is affected by one's interests, motivations, and satisfaction in self, job success is largely determined by attitude, emotional maturity and interpersonal skills and not just ability and aptitude.

Young adulthood is usually when the first vocational choices are made. A person's job is a major aspect of self-identity. Many people answer, "Who are you?" with "I'm Nancy Jones, I'm a computer technologist."

In the past, one's first occupational choice decided the direction of one's life occupation. However, today, young adults think more in terms of a career, realizing that one may be employed at several different jobs before retirement. The individual's thoughts are therefore focused on a series of positions, which offer experience and personal satisfaction, that lead in a general direction toward an ultimate goal. The average person today can expect to hold six to seven different jobs during a lifetime [54].

Little research is available on how most young adults start to work in a particular field. Obviously, propinquity plays a major factor even in our mobile society. A person who grows up in a farming region is more likely to become a farmer than a scuba diver. One's choice of career may be an expression of personality ("I want to be a nurse because I want to help people").

An individual's pattern of interests—likes and dislikes—is one of the most thoroughly studied personality factors in vocational choice. Guidance counselors often advise young people to take vocational interest tests to determine what line of work they might enjoy. It is important to complement these interest tests with a realistic assessment of one's abilities and a willingness to secure an appropriate education to realize one's potentials.

Intelligence is related to job choice in a number of ways. Certain jobs require an above-average degree of intelligence for successful performance (e.g., lawyers, nurses, scientists), and thus are open only to people of relatively high intellect. In general, IQ scores correlate about 0.50 with "economic success," defined in terms of financial income and social prestige [6].

COLLEGE STUDENTS

Many people today are going to college or technical schools to prepare themselves for a specific career. Others attend college while they explore interest options with the hope that a career choice will eventually emerge. Many young adults of today prefer employment that places equal emphasis on challenge, the ability to express one's self, and free time for outside interests [60]. A good marriage between the individual's skills and the job's requirements are more significant than the money one can earn, the social status, or the chance to "get ahead." Young adults must be willing to sacrifice personal pleasures and economic security temporarily while they prepare themselves for more challenging and rewarding positions later in life.

NONCOLLEGE ADULTS

Many blue-collar young adults are becoming disinterested in their work, feeling that their jobs do not have a good future [60]. These young people also desire more self-fulfillment and individual expression in their work and in their lives. Theirs is a case of high expectations

but low opportunities or poor preparation/education. Their values clash with the built-in rigidities and limited responses of the traditional work place. Employers are encouraged to respect workers as individuals who bring to each position a desire for work that also will satisfy some of their deepest cravings—for community, fellowship, participation, challenge, self-fulfillment, freedom, and equality [60]. When the emotional-social needs of employees are met, they are more likely to fill the expectations and needs of the employer.

LEARNING PROBLEMS

The educational opportunities for each individual must be synchronized with the individual's needs, so that he or she can maximize the potential for growth in all domains.

Illiteracy. Twenty percent of adults in our society today are functionally illiterate: They do not possess the reading and writing skills that could help them to be self-confident, self-sufficient participants in their homes, communities, and society.

A few of these people have never been exposed to any type of formal learning or tutoring. Many of these individuals live in socioeconomically disadvantaged areas, and there are those who have not been encouraged to develop their cognitive talents. Some of these people may have been sheltered from the outside world, and only taught the survival skills (e.g., shooting game, gardening, cooking) of their introverted community. Another person may have been disabled and was sheltered from the community because the family thought he or she was "too different," thus creating a doubly handicapped adult.

An alarming number of these functionally illiterate individuals have attended elementary school, and many of them have been awarded high-school diplomas. The fact remains, however, that they cannot satisfactorily compose letters, fill out employment applications, write a check, read directions, or find a number in the telephone directory. In addition, many of these functionally illiterate individuals cannot perform simple arithmetic, so that they cannot add, subtract, multiply, or divide.

The functionally illiterate usually possess a low self-esteem, and feeling ignorant, are afraid others will discover their problem and make fun of them. Although their children come home from school learning the alphabet, and later, the difference between a subject and a predicate, many illiterate parents may make no attempt to learn from their children. Moreover, some parents may make fun of learning and instill a disrespect for education in their children—perhaps creating a bond of illiteracy between generations. Other illiterate parents try to hide their deficit from their children.

Most illiterate adults can learn to read and write by enrolling in, and completing, special classes offered by departments of adult education in community school districts. Those who wish to obtain a high school diploma or its equivalent can take courses that help them to attain this goal. Some community colleges accept adults who have not finished high school and make the necessary classes available to them that enable them to graduate from college with either certification in a special area of training or an associate degree in an occupation. Should an adult want to further academic or professional growth, he or she can pursue a degree elsewhere at the baccalaureate level.

Persons who possess vocational aptitudes that incline them toward specialized training can also take advantage of the services made available via continued education workshops, adult education classes, regional occupational programs, and high-school vocational courses. Some businesses and corporate organizations either contribute financially and/or offer such training. The military services provide other sources of educational opportunities.

Fear of Success. While some young people fear failure in their attempts to get ahead in the world, others may actually be afraid of the responsibility and the expectations of success. They may be fearful of making a change in their lives. Some of these individuals may need professional counseling to aid them in increasing their self-esteem. Others may benefit from special sessions and discussions geared expressly for young adults who in some way feel disadvantaged, for example, members of racial minorities, students who are also parents, working single parents, and those who have been out of school or work for a few years. There are also special services within most educational institutions to provide assistance and guidance to those students who have poor study habits or actual perceptual-learning problems.

Nurturing Cognitive Development during Young Adulthood

Relinquishing one of the major premises of our society, that working hard will always bring success, may be difficult for the young adult. They must realize that "trying" is not always enough and that making excuses for one's efforts or mistakes will not usually suf-

fice. Other young adults must disengage from the idea that there is only one right way to do things. One must redirect energies into cognitive pursuits that complement one's abilities, competence, interests, and individualized style of learning. One's satisfaction and morale are usually highest when both cognitive interests and performance meet society's expectations.

The same systems that provide services to those with learning problems also offer varied courses that serve as outlets for creativity. In addition, many social clubs, churches, community recreational departments, businesses, and local interest groups present lectures and seminars to impart knowledge and skills. Adult education classes cover both academic and leisure-time information, such as American literature, furniture refinishing, budgeting, assertiveness, and ceramics. Many professions mandate continuing education, and many institutions provide regular inservice programs for their employees.

AGE-RELATED VARIATIONS

Young adulthood is traditionally the time for searching for a place for oneself in society. Finding a mate, establishing a family, and initiating a career are major tasks during this period. Even the individual who possesses high level wellness in all domains may find these tasks difficult to master; obviously they can be much more difficult for the individual who is disabled in some way.

Accidents

Despite the general state of good health in this period of life, accidents are one of the leading causes of disability in the young adult. Disabling injuries may occur as a result of a number of situations, including work-related incidents, thrill-seeking pleasures, gunshot wounds, automobile accidents, and war injuries. The majority of disabling accidents occur before 35 years of age. Most of these accidental disabling injuries occur in the late teenage years or early twenties. Males are consistently involved in more accidents than females throughout the life cycle. This phenomenon has traditionally been explained by the more aggressive behavior exhibited by males in our society, and by the fact that males are exposed to more hazardous environments (e.g., combat, industrial work).

The four major types of accidents seen in the young adult generally result from motor vehicles, aggressive behavior (e.g., fighting), handling objects (e.g., power equipment, assembly line), and foreign bodies in the

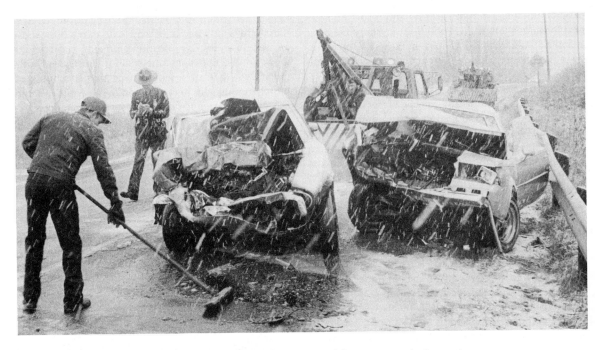

Figure 27–8. The leading cause of death and disability in young adults is motor-vehicle accidents.

eyes. Since accidents are most likely to occur when a person is under strain (emotional or physical) and many young adults are under duress either voluntarily or involuntarily, it follows that this is an age group that experiences accidents. The enthusiasm and spontaneity of youth are not always tempered by experience.

HEALING

Fortunately, many of the physical injuries resulting from accidents leave little or no residual impairment in the activities of daily living. The young adult's body mechanisms for restoration are impressive. Each system of the body heals in a different way. The healing of a simple skin wound can be divided into three phases [29]. The complexity of the healing process depends, of course, on the severity of the wound.

The first phase of the process, **traumatic inflammation,** is characterized by the sealing together of the wound edges (or traumatized area) by a fibrous clot. This seal is formed by the interaction of fibrinogen, a component of the hemorrhaging blood, with other body proteins; these two elements dry to form a seal that prevents fluid loss and bacterial invasion. The capillaries (small blood vessels) along the edge of the wound dilate, causing redness and swelling. At the same time

this process is occurring, the second phase of healing is under way.

During this **destructive phase,** white blood cells (leukocytes and macrophages) come to the scene and ingest dead and dying tissue. These two phases together take 4 to 6 days. The third phase is concerned with replacing and restoring the injured tissue; it is aptly called the **proliferation phase.** The existing capillaries sprout new offshoots, and collagen is laid down by fibroblasts to reinforce and to strengthen the bond between the wound edges. This whole process takes about 14 days.

Healing can be further categorized by first, second, or third intention. **First intention healing** refers to the simple closure of an uncomplicated wound (or one in which little tissue destruction has occurred). Healing by **second intention** takes longer and is necessary when the wound is complicated by infection or size. (Infection interrupts the simpler healing mechanisms.) Large or deep wounds require the body to produce granulation (scar) tissue to close the gap; healing is complete when new skin grows over the granulations. Often, if a wound is large, sutures (stitches) or skin grafting will be used to aid the healing process (healing by **third intention**). In addition to infection, conditions such as inadequate nutrition, body overactivity, poor circulation, and systemic diseases, such as diabetes, can delay or inhibit the healing process [7].

PAIN

In any discussion of injury or disease, one element often comes to mind—pain. Pain is a very individualized, purely subjective experience. For this discussion, however, an operational definition will be used: Pain is whatever the experiencing person says discomfort is, existing whenever he or she says it does [31]. The phenomenon of pain has four component parts: (1) reception of the pain stimulus by pain receptors, (2) conduction of the pain stimulus through impulses by the nerves, (3) perception of pain in the higher centers of the brain, and (4) interpretation and reaction to pain, which are both physical and affective in nature.

All pain is real, regardless of its cause. "Pure" psychogenic pain (caused by emotional events) probably is rare; "pure" organic pain (caused by physical stimuli) is, in all likelihood, also rare. Most bodily pain probably is a combination of both. An individual's attitude toward the self as well as the origin of the pain-producing stimulus affects the intensity of discomfort. An example of this phenomenon can be seen in the reactions of women of various cultures to childbirth. When the birth process is seen as a healthy, normal state that a woman has prepared for and looks forward to, discomfort is perceived to be much less intense than for a woman whose culture steeps childbearing in taboos and secretive fears.

The physical reaction to pain can be further divided into autonomic and skeletal muscle reactions. Autonomic reactions include elevated blood pressure and increased heart rate (measured by pulse), which serve to increase blood flow to the brain and muscles; rapid, irregular respirations, which increase the oxygen supply for the brain and muscles; dilation of the pupils, which allows for an increased amount of light entering the eye; and increased perspiration, which carries away body heat to regulate body temperature. The skeletal muscle response involves an increase in muscle tension, which results in increased neuromuscoloskeletal responsiveness. The totality of this physiological response prepares the body to "fight or flee" the painful stimulus [35] (see the discussion of stress in Chap. 36).

The discovery of endorphins has done much to add to the understanding of how the mind and body work together to produce natural analgesia [58]. Endorphins are compounds with opiatelike properties that include the potential to alter pain perception, mood, and breathing [59]. They are located in the synapses (places where nerve impulses are transmitted from one nerve cell to another) between nerve fibers. They probably transmit, modify, and inhibit noxious stimuli. Some people have higher endorphin levels than others. The release of these compounds is encouraged by physical stimuli, such as electrical nerve stimulation, pressure at acupuncture points, massage, and specific relaxation techniques (such as Lamaze breathing [see Chap. 30]). Psychological mechanisms, such as giving the individual anxiety-reducing information ("This ice pack should make the swelling go down") and distraction (using guided imagery to focus on pleasant thoughts), are believed to induce the flow of endorphins.

Pain can be further described by its duration (continuous or throbbing), its intensity (severe or mild), the nature of its feeling (dull or sharp), and its location (specific to one body area or generalized). In essence, pain is what an individual feels as a physical manifestation or response to a stimulus based on past experience, attitudes, culture, and nature of the stimulus.

STRESS

The perception of pain is a subjective response to a physical stimulus. Stress, on the other hand, involves a physical response to a subjective stimulus; it is the result of any consciously or unconsciously perceived threat to the integrity of an individual. The symptoms of stress as described by Selye [46] are presented in Chapter 36. Since stress is a universal experience, it is not specific to young adulthood. A big examination, a wedding (especially one's own), the first child, a new job, and a physical injury are all common precipitants of stress. Everyday life can also provide some chronic stress experiences, such as, driving in city traffic, rushing to meet deadlines, listening to screaming children or a barking dog, and waiting in cashier lines at the supermarket. The list could go on forever.

In the young adult, chronic low-intensity stress is experienced as a response to everyday pressures. Four years of graduate school can result in a Ph.D., but it can also produce an ulcer or a weight problem if the individual does not cope positively with frustrations. Insomnia is not uncommon during young adulthood, nor is excessive fatigue. Young adults need to learn to pace themselves and not to "burn the candle at both ends." Excessive physical activity or weight can be precipitating factors in the symptomatology associated with hemorrhoids and varicose veins, especially in the female.

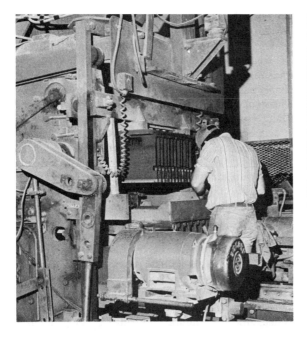

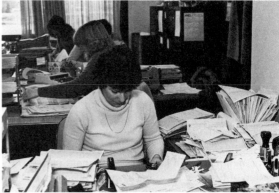

Figure 27–9. One reason men are consistently involved in more accidents than women is their more frequent choice of occupations using heavy machinery. However, more women than men choose secretarial positions—positions that several studies have concluded are among the most stressful. (Photograph on right by Marilee Caliendo.)

Emotional stress is known to weaken body defenses against physical illness. Upper respiratory infections and influenza occur more frequently in the young adult than any other acute illness. Young adults should take the time to take care of themselves. When they do develop an acute condition, they should seek medical attention before it becomes chronic. Young adulthood is a time when most people can maintain high level wellness with a minimum of effort.

The Disabled Young Adult

Nearly 5 million adults living in the community need assistance with everyday activities, such as bathing, feeding, and shopping. Some disabilities are severe enough to require special equipment or assistance in getting in and out of bed or using the toilet. Preparing meals, completing household chores, or driving a car may be impossible for some individuals unless extraordinary assistive devices are employed. Career potentials may be severely limited. Amputations, brain damage, or spinal cord injury, with resulting paralysis, or any alteration dramatically affect the individual's ability to carry out the routine activities of daily living independently.

This period in the life cycle is one in which much productivity is expected of young adults by the society they live in as well as by the individuals themselves.

A sudden interruption in the physical health of a young adult creates frustration beyond description when role expectations cannot be met. Aside from the psychosocial assault, which plays a crucial part in adjustment (see Chaps. 19 and 28), the disabled young adult has serious physical threats with which to contend.

The human is intended to be an ambulatory creature. When mobility is reduced, every body system is affected. There is a threat to life when a person is confined to a bed or a wheelchair from the impairment of the normal functions of various systems of the body. It takes the average healthy adult 6 weeks of mobility to reverse the cardiovascular changes that are acquired when immobilized for only 3 weeks [33]. Three physiological effects on the respiratory system may occur as a result of immobility: decreased respiratory movement, decreased movement of secretions, and disturbed oxygen-carbon dioxide balance. For many individuals, the effects of both physical and socioaffective immobility lead to problems with ingestion, digestion, and elimination. The neuromuscular and skeletal systems decrease motor function if immobility is prolonged. Metabolic homeostasis is threatened when a person cannot move about in an accustomed manner.

Perhaps the largest and most cumbersome barrier for physically disabled young adults is society's reaction to them. Social ignorance is the biggest offender; individuals in wheelchairs may be forced into dependent situations by well-meaning people when they are well able to handle certain tasks themselves. After an individual experiences a disabling accident, there is a long and often costly struggle ahead. The importance of strong support systems—especially family and friends—cannot be overemphasized during this struggle. The incidence of suicide and "loss of will" is too high to ignore the impact the mind has on the body. The disabled person's perceptions of the environment (e.g., time, people, what is said to him or her, body sensations) are also altered and may temporarily affect the ability or motivation to learn (see the helplessness syndrome in Chap. 14).

Many rehabilitation programs dedicated to aiding the disabled individual in the attainment and maintenance of optimal levels of functioning are available throughout the country. Many barriers can be overcome, but the process is not easy. Various self-help items (e.g., modified eating utensils, books recorded on cassettes, modified automobile controls) are available for those who need them as well as cosmetic and functional prostheses for amputees. Financial assistance and vocational training are also made possible through supportive systems at the local, state, and federal levels.

A most crucial facet of rehabilitation for the young adult is the resumption (or initiation) of a "normal" sexual relationship. Physical disability is **not** synonymous with sexual impotence [12]. Sexual partners should be included in counseling sessions, so that emotions and alternative means of gratification can be explored and worked through. Variation in positions for coitus can solve most difficulties presented by amputations of extremities. The major hurdle in sexual activity is the acceptance by both partners of the missing limbs, or stumps, since body image is an important part of a satisfying relationship. Spinal cord injury can be a more serious problem, depending on the location of the injury. In such situations, it is essential for the partners to keep an open mind and to remember that sexual intimacy can be reached in many ways.

An individual who is totally disabled by arthritis or other disabling conditions is also vulnerable to the complications resulting from immobility. Arthritics are often the victims of shams and quackery. Driven by pain and frustration, they may be tricked into trying copper bracelets, mineral baths, low-grade uranium exposure, ointments, and other "cure-alls" in an effort to find relief. These procedures can be costly and could lead to delay in seeking reliable medical treatment.

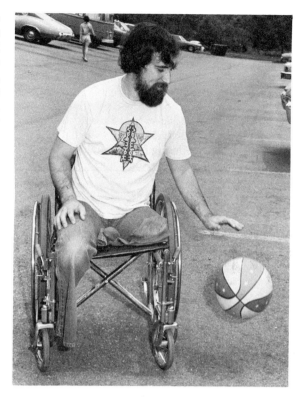

Figure 27–10. The disabled young adult faces many barriers to full participation in the work and leisure opportunities of the culture. However, with creativity and a willingness to be flexible, alternative methods can usually be found to accomplish a goal.

HEALTH MAINTENANCE

Nutritional Needs

As at any other age, good basic nutrition is essential during the young adult years to meet the metabolic requirements for maintaining body functioning. After the body stops growing, large numbers of calories are no longer necessary. The young adult needs only enough calories to maintain the development of new cells that are replacing old, worn-out cells in various systems. Poor adolescent eating habits are often carried into the young adult years; the result can be obesity or malnutrition. The traditional gauge of adequate caloric intake in an adult is to check one's weight regularly; caloric intake should be sufficient to maintain weight without gaining. Caloric needs are based on occupation, amount of physical activity, mental efforts, affective state, age, body size, climate, and metabolism. The adult male requires approximately 2700 calories per day after 22 years of age; an adult female needs approximately 2000 calories daily through young adulthood. A pregnant woman requires approximately 300 additional calories, and a nursing mother needs at least 500 more calories per day [44].

The model of the basic four food groups serves as a rough estimate that allows consumers and health professionals to check the intake of essential foods in order to plan a diet offering the basic nutrient requirements for optimal health. Adult nutritional requirements are given in Table 27–1. In using this model, it is important to consult nutrition resources to determine in which of the four groups a specific food belongs, to understand the types and amounts of foods that serve as substitutes for others, and to know how large the various servings are in each category. Overprocessing destroys the nutrients in many foods, and for this reason some foods may no longer represent the nutrient content of any given food group. Although other limitations exist in the model of the basic four food groups [23], it continues to be a good system for evaluation of an adequate diet.

Many individuals in our society (especially young adults) are becoming aware of the need to prevent diet-related diseases (e.g., coronary heart disease, obesity). Some propose that the future of our health now depends on the "adequate" diet becoming the "prudent" diet [23]. The prudent diet still contains foods from the basic four food groups, but emphasizes the use of more skim milk, poultry, fish, fiber-rich vegetables, fresh fruits, whole grain breads and cereals, and a maximum of three eggs a week. It also stresses judicious use of salt and sugar.

After 18 years of age, the young adult male needs more protein, vitamin C, riboflavin, and vitamins E and B_6. The female needs more vitamin C after age 18 [1], but her needs for protein and iron remain the same. The male requires fewer B vitamins (except riboflavin) and less iron; the female nutrient requirements of the B vitamins are also reduced. These reductions occur because the accelerated growth periods have ended, and prime physical maturation has been completed. The exceptions to these reductions include smokers and women taking certain birth control pills; both groups need to increase their intake of B vitamins, since their bodies metabolize these vitamins differently. Most adults (the young and the older) should consume an average of 2000 to 3000 ml of fluid in a 24-hour period to maintain electrolyte balance, to excrete kidney wastes, and to provide fecal softening.

Exercise

Regular exercise will help to control weight and to maintain a state of high level wellness. Muscle tone, strength, and circulation are enhanced by exercise, which affects the health status of the young adult by facilitating blood flow to the heart and thereby maintaining body functioning in all areas [55]. The amount of exercise each person needs is highly individualized. When most people think of exercise, deep knee bends, touching the toes, and push-ups come to mind. However, daily activities, such as walking, climbing stairs, and running for the bus also qualify as exercise. Problems arise especially when sedentary life-styles decrease the amount of exercise; therefore, extra effort must be made to assure adequate daily physical activity.

The increased involvement of people today with activities, such as jogging, cycling, aerobic dancing, and using a mini-trampoline, reflects a general concern with physical fitness. There are many health salons and exercise programs that are appealing to young adults; such programs usually produce results if the individual consistently practices good health habits (such as eating less "junk food") while carrying out an individually designed exercise program. These programs include monitoring the response of the heart to exercise, alternating different aerobic exercises, and usually exercising at least three times a week.

Sleep

Most scientists agree that sleep has a restorative function, and uninterrupted sleep is necessary for the well-being of the individual's body and mind. The exact physiologic mechanisms involved in sleep are not known [15]. A lack of sleep results in progressive sluggishness of both physical and cognitive functions. It is most common for young adults who are actively pursuing careers to sacrifice sleep in their efforts to get ahead.

Electroencephalograms (EEGs) have been used to compare brain-wave activity during awake and sleeping states. EEG recordings display rapid, irregular waves while we are awake and alert. As we begin to rest, these waves change to an **alpha** rhythm, a regular pattern of low voltage with frequencies of 8 to 12 cycles per second. While we are asleep, a **delta** rhythm occurs, which is a slow pattern of high voltage and 1 to 2 cycles per second. During certain stages of sleep, sleep spindles, or sudden, short bursts of sharply pointed alpha waves, occur with frequencies of 14 to 16 cycles per second. EEG tracings of sleeping babies demonstrate that they experience the same stages of sleep as adults. The difference between babies and adults lies in the amount of time spent in each stage [43].

Normal sleep consists of the cycling of four different stages. Stage 1 is a light state of sleep. Rapid eye movements (REM) appear during this stage. **REM sleep** refers to the periods during regular sleep that are characterized by mild involuntary muscle movement. Most, but not all, dreams occur during REM sleep. During stage 1 sleep, the adult heart rate decreases, the arterial blood pressure decreases 30 mm Hg below normal, and the basal metabolic rate decreases 10 to 20 percent [20]. A newborn baby spends about 50 percent of sleep time in REM sleep. REM sleep normally decreases from birth to the age of 5 years. Since these higher levels of REM sleep correspond to the time during which the brain is growing at its fastest rate, the question is raised as to whether or not the REM sleep may facilitate the vast amount of cognitive growth that occurs during this span of life [10, 43].

Under normal circumstances, 20 percent of the adult sleep cycle consists of REM sleep. It usually occurs three to four times during every sleep period at intervals of 80 to 120 minutes. Each segment of REM sleep lasts from 5 minutes to 1 hour. The exact physical reason is unknown, but the amount of REM sleep determines the amount of actual rest. When REM sleep is interrupted consistently, extreme tiredness and serious neurotic tendencies develop [20].

Stage 2 sleep is medium-depth sleep. Stage 3 sleep is even deeper and can be reached about 20 minutes after falling asleep. Stage 4 sleep is demonstrated by the person who is extremely hard to awaken. Sleepwalking, bedwetting, and nightmares occur during this stage. Although stage 4 sleep lasts only 10 to 20 minutes at a time, the person who is awakened during this stage may be confused. During adulthood, the total hours of sleep an individual needs and the amount of REM sleep remains fairly stable [55]. Deep sleep begins to be replaced with longer periods of lighter sleep after 30 years of age. Each person has a particular REM pattern, which changes throughout the life cycle.

Sleep patterns, as well as types of dreams, often change during pregnancy. The drowsiness of early pregnancy may be caused by increased estrogen levels, leading to increased sensitivity to serotonin, the brain's tranquilizer. By the third trimester, some women may have become desensitized to serotonin, leading to a withdrawal that includes insomnia.

Each person has an individual sleep cycle. Many young adults need approximately 7 to 9 hours of sleep, while others appear to do well with less. The evidence suggests that delta sleep is good, efficient sleep in terms of how a person feels after experiencing it. It remains to be seen whether the total time needed for sleep could be shortened if research could determine a healthy way to increase the time spent in delta sleep. Anyone who has more than occasional problems with obtaining refreshing sleep should assess his or her life-style and seek medical attention. Many young adults are vigorously exercising or eating too close to bedtime; these activities are stimulants that promote alertness and not sleep. Chronic insomnia is usually the result of a severe, long-term psychological disturbance, which suggests that pills will not cure the cause. Sleep is not the lack of activity [43]; rather, it is a complex physiological and psychological function that is essential to an individual's total well-being.

Measures for Maintaining Health

As with the care of any fine machine, preventive maintenance for the body can play a major role in assuring high level wellness for the young adult. Health maintenance is often neglected, since the young adult often feels immune to any kind of illness. Annual physical examinations are recommended, with more frequent visits if the individual has any particular problems. Most young women are encouraged to have annual Pap smears (checks for cervical cancer). This procedure, which also includes a pelvic exam, can aid in the detection of many other gynecologic problems. Monthly self-examination of the breasts should be practiced by all women during the week after the menstrual flow ceases. Dental examinations should be performed on a 6-month basis to avoid the possibility of teeth and gum disorders later in life. Routine eye examinations are encouraged every 2 years. For young adults who are on limited incomes, many clinics are available across the country that provide low-cost medical attention. Planned Parenthood, family health centers, and hospital clinics are only a few examples of these facilities.

Immunizations should be maintained during young adulthood; this is particularly important to women during the childbearing years. Most physicians and clinics keep records of immunizations and can guide the individual in the need for booster shots or renewal of protection (see Chap. 7 for immunization maintenance recommendations throughout the life cycle). Overseas travel also requires an update of immunizations. Since specific requirements vary from country to country, information should be obtained from a physician or the local health department.

PRESCRIPTION: HUMOR

A sense of humor can aid a person in attaining, maintaining, and regaining holistic health. Recent clinical evidence [13, 48] suggests that humor and laughter control pain, speed healing, and decrease the negative effects of stress. This may be accomplished by: (1) distracting attention, (2) reducing muscle tension, (3) encouraging a more positive outlook on life, and (4) increasing production of endorphins.

SUMMARY

Young adulthood is the period when peak physical fitness and superior intellectual performance can prove most complementary to the maximization of potentials. It is a time when much is expected and also the time when one is most capable of meeting these expectations. It can be a truly exciting period of life—sharing new relationships, enjoying a healthy body and its use, and continuing to learn much about oneself, others, and the world in general.

Maximization of cognitive potentials depends on the successful development and interface of the other three major domains. Skill in the use of hypothetical-deductive thinking increases with exposure to more experiences, knowledge, and opportunities to exercise abstract thinking skills. Personality and motivation impact heavily on career choice and success. Lack of opportunity to develop cognitive skills and knowledge base can negatively affect self-esteem and the ability to deal with the exigencies of life.

Since accidents and their consequences present a major threat to the health of young adults, this age group should be especially aware of the rules and regulations of the various activities they undertake (whether this involves driving a car, riding a bicycle, or enjoying a sport). Observing caution around machinery and thoroughly reading the instructions for new devices can help to prevent serious accidents.

The research on endorphins should continue to prove valuable by resulting in increased knowledge about how the brain and the central nervous system function in the perception of, and the response to, pain.

Disabled young adults face many problems when expectations cannot be met. Social values and the ability to establish relative independence play a major role in their struggle for self-fulfillment and physical homeostasis.

REFERENCES

1. Anderson, L., et al.   Nutrition in Health and Disease (17th ed.). Philadelphia: Lippincott, 1982.
2. Bailey, C.   Fit or Fat. Boston: Houghton Mifflin, 1978.
3. Beard, R. M.   An Outline of Piaget's Developmental Psychology for Students and Teachers. New York: Basic Books, 1969.
4. Bearison, D. J.   The construct of regression: A Piagetian approach. Merrill-Palmer Q. 20:21, 1974.
5. Botwinick, J.   Aging and Behavior (3rd ed.). New York: Springer, 1984.
6. Bowles, S., and Gintis, H.   I.Q. in the U.S. class structure. Social Policy 3(4):65, 1972.
7. Brunner, L. S., and Suddarth, D. S.   Textbook of Medical Surgical Nursing (5th ed.). Philadelphia: Lippincott, 1984.
8. Carrier, N. H. (Ed.).   Stages of cognitive development. Psychol. Digest 1(3):3, 1973.
9. Chodil, J., and Williams, B.   The concept of sensory deprivation. Nurs. Clin. North Am. 5:453, 1970.
10. Clark, M., et al.   The mystery of sleep. Newsweek, July 13, 1981; p. 48.
11. College Board scores change only slightly.   Chron. Higher Educ. 27(4):1, 1983.
12. Cornelius, D. A.   Who Cares? A Handbook on Sex Education and Counseling Services for Disabled People (2nd ed.). Baltimore: University Park, 1982.
13. Cousins, N.   Human Options: An Autobiographical Notebook. New York: Norton, 1981.
14. Dennis, W.   Age and creative productivity.   J. of Gerontol. 21:1, 1966.
15. Dinner, D. S.   Physiology of sleep. Am. J. EEG Tech. 22(2):85, 1982.
16. Elkind, D.   Quantity concepts in college students. J. Soc. Psychol. 57:459, 1962.
17. Elkind, D.   Children and Adolescents, Interpretative Essays on Jean Piaget (3rd ed.). New York: Oxford University Press, 1981.
18. Fenichel, O.   The Psychoanalytic Theory of Neurosis. New York: Norton, 1945.
19. Flavell, J. H.   Cognitive Changes in Adulthood. In L. R. Goulet and P. B. Bates, (Eds.), Life-Span Developmental Psychology: Research and Theory. New York: Academic Press, 1970.
20. Guyton, A. C.   Basic Human Physiology: Normal Function and Mechanisms of Disease (2nd ed.). Philadelphia: Saunders, 1977.
21. Horn, J. L.   Organization of Data of Life-span Development of Human Abilities. In L. R. Goulet and P. B. Bates (Eds.), Life-Span Developmental Psychology: Research and Theory. New York: Academic Press, 1970.
22. Horn, J. L., and Cattell, R. B.   Age differences in fluid and crystallized intelligence. Acta Psychol. (Amst). 26:107, 1967.
23. Howard, R. B., and Herbold, N. H. (Eds.).   Nutrition in Clinical Care (2nd ed.). New York: McGraw-Hill, 1982.
24. Johnson, A. L., et al.   Evans County, Georgia, cardiovascular study: Race, sex, and weight influences on the young adult. Am. J. Cardiol. 35:523, 1975.

25. Kuhn, D., et al.   The development of formal operations in logical and moral development. *Genet. Psychol. Monogr.* 95:97, 1977.

26. Lehman, H. C.   *Age and Achievement.* Princeton, NJ: Princeton University Press, 1953.

27. Levinson, D. J.   How men grow up: The necessary search for a dream, a mentor, and a special woman. *Psychology Today* 11(8):89, 1978.

28. Lowrey, G. H.   *Growth and Development of Children* (7th ed.). Chicago: Year Book, 1978.

29. Luckmann, J., and Sorensen, K. C.   *Medical-Surgical Nursing: A Psychophysiologic Approach.* Philadelphia: Saunders, 1974.

30. Masters, W. H., and Johnson, V. E.   *Human Sexual Response.* Boston: Little, Brown, 1966.

31. McCaffery, M.   Understanding your patient's pain. *Nursing '80* 10(9):26, 1980.

32. Murray, J. F.   *The Normal Lung: The Basis for Diagnosis and Treatment of Pulmonary Disease.* Philadelphia: Saunders, 1976.

33. Olson, E. V., et al.   The hazards of immobility. *Am. J. Nurs.* 67:779, 1967.

34. Owens, W. A.   Age and mental abilities: A second adult follow-up. *J. Educ. Psychol.* 57:311, 1966.

35. Pain, Part 1: Basic concepts and assessment, programmed instruction. *Am. J. Nurs.* 66:1085, 1966.

36. Peters, T. J., and Waterman, R. H.   *In Search of Excellence: Lessons from America's Best-run Companies.* New York: Warner Books, 1983.

37. *Physicians' Desk Reference: PDR.* Oradell, NJ: Medical Economics, 1984.

38. Piaget, J.   The Definition of Stages of Development. In J. Tanner and B. Inhelder (Eds.), *Discussions on Child Development.* Vol. 4. New York: International Universities Press, 1960.

39. Piaget, J.   Comments on Vygotsky's Critical Remarks Concerning *The Language and Thought of the Child,* and *Judgment and Reasoning in the Child.* Translated by A. Parsons. Attachment to L. S. Vygotsky, *Thought and Language.* Edited and translated by E. Hanfmann and G. Vakar. Cambridge, MA: M.I.T. Press, 1962.

40. Piaget, J.   Intellectual evolution from adolescence to adulthood. *Hum. Dev.* 15(1):1, 1972.

41. Pollak, O.   Some challenges to the American family. *Children* 11:19, 1964.

42. Riegel, K. F.   Dialectic operations: The final period of cognitive development. *Hum. Dev.* 16:346, 1973.

43. Riley, H. D., and Berney, J.   Infant sleep. *American Baby* 87:40, 1976.

44. Robinson, C. H.   *Basic Nutrition and Diet Therapy* (4th ed.). New York: Macmillan, 1980.

45. Schaie, K. W., and Geiwitz, J.   *Adult Development and Aging.* Boston: Little, Brown, 1982.

46. Selye, H.   *The Stress of Life* (Rev. ed.). New York: McGraw-Hill, 1978.

47. Shelby, J. P.   Sensory deprivation. *Sigma Theta Tau Image* 10:49, 1978.

48. Simonton, O. C., et al.   *Getting Well Again.* New York: Bantam Books, 1978.

49. Smith, D. W., Bierman, E. L., and Robinson, N. M. (Eds.).   *The Biologic Ages of Man; From Conception Through Old Age* (2nd ed.). Philadelphia: Saunders, 1978.

50. Smith, J., and Bullough, B.   Sexuality and the severely disabled person. *Am. J. Nurs.* 75:2194, 1975.

51. Tanner, J. M.   *Foetus Into Man: Physical Growth From Conception to Maturity.* London: Open Books, 1978.

52. Tillinger, K. G.   Testicular morphology: A histopathological study with special reference to biopsy findings in hypogonadism with mainly endocrine disorders and in gynecomastia. *Acta Endocrinol.* 30:1, 1957.

53. Timiras, P. S.   *Developmental Physiology and Aging.* New York: Macmillan, 1972.

54. Toffler, A.   *Future Shock.* New York: Random House, 1970.

55. Troll, L. E.   *Early and Middle Adulthood: The Best is Yet to be—Maybe* (2nd ed.). Monterey, CA: Brooks/Cole, 1984.

56. Wadsworth, B. J.   *Piaget's Theory of Cognitive Development* (2nd ed.). New York: Longman, 1979.

57. Wechsler, D.   *Wechsler's Measurement and Appraisal of Adult Intelligence* (5th ed.). Baltimore: Williams & Wilkins, 1972.

58. West, B. A.   Understanding endorphins: Our natural pain relief system. *Nursing '81* 11(2):50, 1981.

59. Wilson, R. W., and Elmassian, B. J.   Endorphins. *Am. J. Nurs.* 81:722, 1981.

60. Yankelovich, D.   *The New Morality: A Profile of American Youth in the 70s.* New York: McGraw-Hill, 1974.

28

Psychosocial Development of the Young Adult

Cecil R. Paul

> The unexamined life is not worth living.
>
> —Socrates

The hills have been climbed and the valleys traversed, and what one had assumed to be a peak is but another hill in the ongoing struggle to be and to become. Like those experiences one has in hiking of climbing up and down the approach hills to a slope, the adolescent period is at times a struggling experience, with high points of perspective and hope followed by low points of task diffusion and relational frustration. As the young adult years emerge, many of these small hills have been conquered and one feels that he or she has paid the price. There is a transitional sense that one is on that edge of readiness for a steady upward climb toward the pinnacle of what has begun to be perceived as the measure of success and fulfillment—adulthood.

However, as one approaches these young adult years, there may be an initial sense of letdown. There is often some sense of loneliness because the struggle to get there has left behind the familiar road-marks. There are initial demands for the assumption of responsibility through "plugging in" and settling down. It is a time for the experiences from that long struggle to be integrated into new adult objectives that connect one with society. The individual discovers that there are new hills and valleys with new risks and pressures. Those hazy hills of adulthood are not as clearly visible as one had anticipated; new tasks and crises await the weary traveler. There is the sense of a demand for the

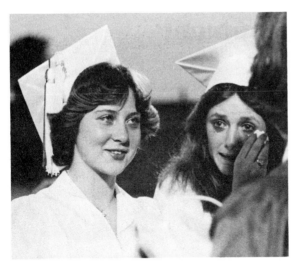

Figure 28–1. Graduation marks a point of mastery and launching; it is a time of joy and sadness, with mixed feelings of omnipotence and fear.

utilization of past experience and of a responsibility toward the surrounding society and environment. The new tasks involve the integration of previous experiences with dependence and independence into more complex levels of interdependence.

Robert Havighurst [9] observes that the young adult years constitute one of the most difficult periods in an individual's life. Prior to this time, many activities, responsibilities, and roles were determined by chronological age or grade in school. New privileges and responsibilities were regularly attained, earned, and bestowed when predetermined milestones or peaks had been reached. The pinnacle—perhaps the eighteenth birthday or graduation from high school—was seen as the ultimate goal or achievement, the signal for departure from the world of childhood, the launching point for adulthood. However, many young people discover when they have reached the end of the ladder that they are stepping off into a nebulous world devoid of preestablished goals, the achievement of which would bring acclaims of success. They discover that prestige and power are dependent on psychomotor skills, affective strength, and the ability to apply knowledge, rather than being automatically conferred with the passage of time or the move to a new class. In some situations, they discover that privileges and opportunities are based on family connections rather than on innate potentials or skills.

For 18 years (or more), the individual has been waiting to "grow up," to reach that point where he or she would "know," "understand," and "be in control." (Parents often tell the child, "When you grow up, you'll understand. . . .") That time has arrived, but the young person realizes that little has changed on the inside. Havighurst recognizes that the young adult has many decisions to make (see Appendix C), such as selecting a mate, getting started in an occupation, and managing a home, but minimal assistance is available. In the desire for independence, the young adult often breaks away from the family, which leaves the individual lonely and without guidance or support systems. Many young people find that they have had minimal educational preparation for making the critical decisions in life or executing the essential skills. At a time when they are most highly motivated to use help (from other than family), many realize that there are minimal resources available to help them establish appropriate goals (or they do not know how to make contact with sources that are available). As a result, it may take several years before the young adult is able to establish goals clearly. Many young adults need a moratorium, a period of delay in the pursuit of the tasks and goals of mature adulthood. Although it may take many behavioral forms, internally, the young adult is caught in the crosscurrents of the demands for task fulfillment while feeling the need for time and space to sort them out. The moratorium thus becomes a part of the process of focusing objectives and making appropriate choices.

The interim period—"youth"—can be one of intense searching for one's unique identity, goals, and affiliations. During this time, the individual begins to solidify identity and to define the adult role. Some may appear to make a very smooth transition to the new responsibilities, but on the inside they still do not quite feel "adult." Suddenly at age 30, they may say to themselves at a point of crisis, "My parents said I would know what to do when I'm an adult. I don't know what to do. Maybe I'm not an adult yet." This is a startling revelation and requires a redefinition of one's concept of adulthood and maturity.

When is one an **adult**? Legally, it may be at 16, 18, or 21 years of age; but is it a matter of age, as is so commonly expressed? This is how society cues and responds to the developing person. Whether the age is 16, 18 or 21 (and it is more likely to be viewed as 18 for more recent generations), our culture, like every other, establishes specific expectations for the young adult. In Chapters 25 and 26, adolescence was noted to end when "the individual consistently interacts constructively with the environment in all four domains in the role of an adult as defined by the culture in which he or she lives." Nevertheless, there are numerous practical problems for the young adult in being accepted as an adult. Is a 23-year-old college student an adult if he or she is still dependent on the parents for financial support? Is a 16-year-old married mother of twin sons an adult? The young adult who has experienced a delay or deviation in physical maturation may continue to be responded to as a younger person by society (infantilization); thus society may handicap an otherwise "normal" individual. How does one define adulthood for a 25-year-old retarded person? After entertaining questions such as these, one begins to realize that there is no one criterion, or even one simple grouping of criteria, that can be readily used to separate the adolescent from the adult. The transition is gradual. Physical development, chronological age, individual achievements, and responses to society all mesh to play a significant role in whether or not an individual is treated as a mature adult. The responses of society will continue to have an important influence on the psychosocial processes of the young adult years.

Definitions of **maturity** emphasize adjustment. The adjustments that an individual is expected to make in becoming mature involve three general dimensions of

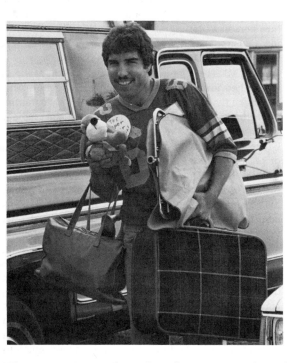

Figure 28–2. Leaving home for college or a new place of residence is one more step in the separation-individuation process.

life. First, there are the adjustment demands of the emerging self, which will be examined in terms of the pressures for differentiation and integration. The second dimension is interpersonal, in which one is learning how to deal with the reciprocal relationship between personal needs and the needs and expectations of others. The third area of adjustment is environmental, which has to do with managing the economic and physical needs of life. Thus maturity involves processes of differentiation, integration, relating, and coping.

THEORIES OF PSYCHOSOCIAL MATURATION

Perspectives on Maturity
There are many models for understanding personality that might be utilized in exploring the nature and process of maturity. Salvatore Maddi [13] has grouped these theories into three major models: conflict, consistency, and fulfillment.

CONFLICT
The conflict model views the human being as caught between two powerful opposing forces, which are never fully resolved. Consequently, life is a process of attempting to balance these forces in such a way that the individual is, relatively speaking, able to function with some degree of satisfaction without becoming the victim of paralyzing anxiety and guilt. Obviously, the most significant example of this approach is Sigmund Freud's psychoanalytical model.

Freud did not give attention to the adult years as involving stages and tasks beyond the genital psychosexual dynamics that begin at pubescence. The concept of defensiveness is essential to this view of personality and thus of adjustment and maturity. According to Freud, maturity is the process of adjusting to the demands and pressures of both the instincts and the outside society. At best, maturity is a maintenance of some balance between the two, but it is not without its price. The defensiveness posture protects the individual from an awareness of instincts while blocking out sensitivities to the guilt and the anxiety of nonconformity to society's expectations. The concept of degree is important in distinguishing adjustment from pathology. The degree of defensiveness may be such that one's awareness of reality is weakened, undermining the individual's potential to become both a productive member of society and a fulfilled person. Basically, the hypothesis is that there are forces in conflict that impinge upon the developing personality, either pushing the individual forward toward maturity or blocking that process, which leads to pathology.

The balance of maturity is between love and work. The maturity of love is expressed in sexual intimacy, friendships, and nurture; the maturity of work is expressed in productive social and cultural involvement. Erik Erikson, as a psychoanalytical conflict theorist, has enriched this theory with insights beyond adolescent genital psychosexuality into the psychosocial dynamics of the maturing adult. No one is better known for the phrase "psychosocial processes" than Erik Erikson. It would be difficult to write about the question of adult development and the nature of its tasks and crises without giving important attention to this internationally respected figure who has expanded the psychoanalytical understanding of the individual to include the long-neglected areas of adult development and cross-cultural variables in psychosocial development.

CONSISTENCY

Salvatore Maddi contrasts his own theory of consistency with the conflict theories, noting that "in the consistency model, there is little emphasis upon great forces, be they single or dual, in conflict or not. Rather, there is emphasis upon the formative influence of feedback from the external world" [13]. As in the general field of learning theories and behavioral models, the stress is on the stimulus-response relationship. Conflict is not viewed as inevitable, nor are there predetermined possibilities or ideals that serve as the indicators of meaningful living. This theory is basically a homeostatic view of the individual. Maddi's central emphasis is on the activation level of the personality. The personality is shaped in early childhood to expect a particular level of activation; thereafter, the person seeks to maintain the level of activation to which he is accustomed (that is characteristic of him). Behavior may serve the purpose of either increasing or decreasing the level of activity, depending on what is most familiar.

There is little evidence of a developmental theory in the consistency model. Once the formative years are behind, the developing person utilizes both differentiation and integration to manage the impact of the external world. It is important to stress that Maddi has a view of personality that is quite rich in its typology. Two general types are high-activation people and low-activation people. According to Maddi, "High-activation people will spend the major part of their time and effort pursuing stimulus impact in order to keep their

actual activation levels from falling too low, whereas low-activation people will spend the major part of their time and effort avoiding impact so as to keep their actual activation level from getting too high" [13]. The high-activation type has a need for intensity, variety, and meaningfulness in life. If a person is more external in his or her traits, this need is expressed in the external environment, both physical and social. If a person is more internal in his or her traits, these high needs are expressed in cognitive and emotional differentiation. The low-activation type avoids intensity, variety, and meaningfulness. If characterized by external traits, the individual is a conformist and a conservationist of what has been. If characterized by internal traits, the individual seeks the uncomplicated life, in which excess and indulgence are avoided. If maturity is defined in terms of adjustment, there are problems in defining the characteristics of the mature person according to this model. The definition of maturity would depend on an individual's activation type and whether he or she is an external or an internal type of personality. The consistency model does not provide us with a statement on the nature and the process of maturity, and there is no significant development of a stage theory with the tasks and adjustment demands of the adult years. Perhaps it could be said that in general, the mature person is coping most effectively with maintaining a customary level of activation.

FULFILLMENT

Other theories interpret personality as the natural unfolding of the potential of the individual. This potential might be in the form of a genetic blueprint, which, when expressed, blossoms without major conflict. Other slightly different theories emphasize the ideals of perfection the individual is capable of achieving. Conflict is neither necessary nor inevitable in these approaches. These theories focus on the processes of actualization and maturity that are neglected by both conflict and consistency theories. Gordon Allport, Carl Rogers, Arthur Combs, and Abraham Maslow are four of the more influential theorists of maturity as an actualization or "becoming" process. What is particularly valuable to us here is the degree to which these theorists develop their theories beyond the determinism of early childhood and adolescence into the adult years. Little attention has been given by others to the tasks, the needs, and the psychosocial dynamics of the early adult years, and thus these writers have much to say to us in our endeavor to understand maturity and the nature of the individual's being and becoming.

Conflict theorists identify maturity in terms of compromise and adjustment in the struggle between personal drives and the expectations of society. Consistency theorists emphasize the process of maintaining customary levels of activation in sorting out the feedback of the environment. For the fulfillment theorists, maturity is expressed as a natural unfolding of potential and the actualization of human ideals. Inasmuch as this is a highly optimistic view, it has a strong appeal to the young adult who is looking for goals and a sense of hope in confronting the tasks and crises of this phase of development. At no other point in life are individuals more keenly aware of their potentials and of the possibilities and pressures that confront them.

The Self-Actualizing Person

THE PROCESS OF SELF-ACTUALIZATION

Carl Rogers develops his theory of personality around the concept of self-actualization, as does Maslow. In describing his view of human development, Rogers writes: "The organism has one basic tendency and striving—to actualize, maintain, and enhance the experiencing organism" [19]. Rogers' view is highly optimistic: He sees the individual as being capable of growth toward self-reliance, autonomy, and self-government. This tendency toward self-actualization is present throughout development from the time of conception to maturity. Development is an ongoing process throughout adult life wherein the person is seen as a "fluid process, not a fixed and static entity; a flowing river of change, not a block of solid material; a continually changing constellation of potentialities, not a fixed quantity of traits" [20]. Rogers perceives maturity as an ongoing process that is both exciting and threatening; it is an ever-growing process of self-discovery.

The term **becoming** is highly expressive of how both Allport and Rogers view human development; less emphasis is placed on general norms for development and more emphasis on the uniqueness of becoming. There are many parallels between Maslow's theory and those of Rogers and Allport. They share highly optimistic views of the nature and potential of the individual to become. Like Rogers and Allport, Maslow places limited emphasis on a developmental stage theory and concentrates more on the themes of actualization and maturity. There are parallels of emphasis on the basic goodness of the individual; consequently these theorists are often grouped together under the "humanistic" category. There is an idealism that permeates their work to the extent that conflict is discussed only minimally as a barrier to the process of actualization. Although the importance of nurturing relationships is recognized by these "personologists," the thrust of their approach is on the resources within the individual, which is why the emphasis is placed on the individual's becoming and on the process of self-actualization.

Maslow's concept of a hierarchy of needs provides us with a model for identifying the different levels of need at which adults function. Consequently, there is a wide range of life-styles and values in adult life. While Maslow maintains his idealism throughout, the prepotency of lower-level needs brings the realities of the individual's circumstances into focus. Maslow establishes the primacy of physiological needs in his motivational theory. There is a homeostatic basis for this concept, since the human organism demonstrates "automatic efforts to maintain a constant, normal state of the blood stream" [16]. Most of Maslow's emphasis within the first level in the hierarchy has to do with food-seeking behavior, although he does note that there are other physiological needs such as coition and comfort [16]. An individual's perspective on life is significantly influenced by the level of need that dominates. If the adult is dominated by physiological needs, then these needs become reflected in the life-style and the focus of activities. In the extreme, the individual with significant food deprivation would evidence little of the higher level needs; he or she would be preoccupied in both thought and behavior with physiological need gratification.

The unemployed young adult male who is without family support will likely find himself preoccupied with meeting his basic physical needs. This situation makes it difficult for him to deal with the tasks of building a meaningful intimacy and establishing a family. If in fact he is married and has a family, his unemployment demands a concentration of thoughts on this lowest level of needs in the hierarchy. What are the possibilities for higher-level functioning for a pregnant young woman recently rejected by her boyfriend and family, or for an abandoned mother of four? They are going to be preoccupied with securing food and shelter for themselves and their children. The chronically ill individual is likely to be depressed by the dominance of illness over the capacity to rise to new levels of need fulfillment. When personal and family health problems are critical, the idealism of youth is easily lost. It is when these physiological needs are relatively ensured that the individual can move to higher levels of need experience. The new unsatisfied needs then dominate the individual's behavior, and when these needs have been satisfied, the next level of yet-to-be-satisfied needs emerges.

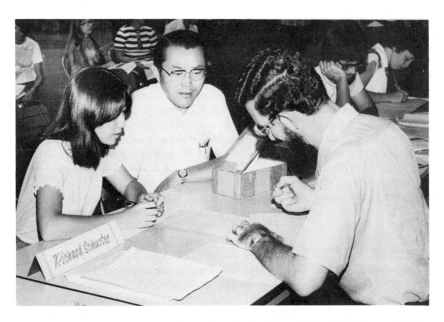

Figure 28–3. Entering college or applying for one's first job can be both exciting and frightening. Hopes for the future are mixed with fears of failure, yet it is only as one dares to expand that advances to higher levels of affective and social development are realized.

The needs of safety emerge and are evidenced in those patterns of behavior that are self-protective and cautious. There is a fear of helplessness and environmental crisis. These safety needs are more clearly revealed in the helpless child who has a high attachment need. Looking at the adult in our society, Maslow writes, "The healthy, normal, fortunate adult in our culture is largely satisfied in his safety needs. The peaceful, smoothly running, good society ordinarily makes its members feel safe enough from wild animals, extremes of temperature, criminal assault, murder, tyranny, etc. . . . Therefore, in a very real sense, he no longer has any safety needs as active motivators" [16]. This statement is helpful in understanding the impact of one's general cultural milieu and environment. When a community or country is torn by civil strife, social instability, or environmental extremes, the necessity of concentrating on this level of need stifles further development.

When physiological and safety needs are relatively satisfied, the need for "belongingness" and love becomes focused. This need for affection may become the dominant theme of the individual's thought and behavior. Mature and well-adjusted members of society have a sense of belonging and evidence reciprocity in the loving and caring dimensions of social life. The need for love is assumed by many theologians, philosophers, and psychologists to be the most central need of mankind and the highest expression of human values. There is a need to differentiate the different types or levels of love: infantile, dependent love is quite different from mature, responsible love and reveals important differences in self-awareness and insight.

Beyond the belonging needs, the developing personality reaches the level of esteem needs. Maslow sees the need to be valued and appreciated as a mixture of the need for achievement, competence, and recognition. The contrasting situation is that of being locked into a syndrome of low self-esteem, inferiority feelings, and blocked motivation due to feelings of inadequacy. An individual reaches relative satisfaction when he or she is moving away from these crippling feelings.

The satisfaction of the other levels of need in the hierarchy does not lead to a state of quiet reflection and satisfaction as though the final goal has been attained. Instead, individuals are pulled forward by the need to be what they are capable of being and begin to establish goals for the actualization of their potentials. The concept of "metaneeds" was developed by Maslow to identify the "being values" of the individual; it is the process of working at fulfilling one's destiny or calling in life. The goal of growth-motivated persons is to fulfill their vocation for purposes of ultimate satisfaction

[15]. This concept raises questions as to the basic characteristics of what Maslow refers to as the "self-actualizing" person or what Rogers refers to as the "fully functioning" person. Allport's concept of a "mature sentiment" and Combs' concept of the adequate personality add strength to these perspectives on the meaning and nature of maturity.

CHARACTERISTICS OF THE MATURE PERSONALITY
These four fulfillment theorists have given considerable attention to defining the specific characteristics of maturity. Their approaches are of particular value here, since there is fundamental agreement among them concerning the basic characteristics of maturity.

All these theorists give initial attention to the importance of being **open to experience.** Rogers sees the fully functioning person as being nondefensive, open to change, flexible, and able to tolerate ambiguity. The mature person is open to what is going on in his or her current life process. Allport characterizes the immature personality as one who is dominated by biological drives and immediate gratification; the mature personality would be one who has mastered impulse control and whose behavior reflects this. All these theorists see the absence of defensiveness as being characteristic of the self-actualizing or fully functioning mature adult; this concept implies being more open to reality and to others. The tasks on which Havighurst focuses are obviously more likely to be fulfilled by this type of person. To become intimate, to make a marriage work, and to relate responsibly to family and community requires the energy and investment of a relatively nondefensive personality.

A second area of agreement among these theorists in their emphasis on mature characteristics is the quality of **self-acceptance** or **self-objectification.** The mature person is "better able to permit his total organism, his conscious thought participating, to consider, weigh and balance each stimulus, need and demand, and its relative weight and intensity" [20]. Self-acceptance is the process of listening to oneself in order to let the inner self emerge. It might be added that a media-oriented culture leads to less of this process. Can individuals become psychosocially mature if they seldom meditate or listen to their inner needs and potential to become? Beyond self-acceptance is the capacity to be self-objective. This is the ability to look at one's self from another's perspective; to emotionally separate one's self from an interaction and to view the self as a third person. One has the advantage of seeing external behaviors as well as internal thoughts and motives. The individual who is able to do this is less likely to

become emotionally enmeshed in a scenario and is able to remain more objective and thus more sensitive to the needs of all involved—including the self. The mature personality has "the ability to objectify oneself, to be reflective and insightful about one's own life. The individual with insight sees himself as others see him, and at certain moments [seems] to glimpse himself in a kind of cosmic perspective" [1].

The apex of this process of self-objectification is what Maslow identifies as a "peak experience," which is most likely to occur when a person is facing a crisis with a full awareness of all the dimensions involved and a full utilization of capacities. It is the obverse of the acute helplessness syndrome. The capacity to view life with a combination of insight and humor is another way of expressing nondefensive living. Because the individual is able to think clearly, he or she is able to respond in synchrony to the needs of the immediate situation while keeping in mind the long-range effects. This is in contrast to the person who reacts when a person or an event touches a "trigger button."

The mature individual is free to enter into intimacies and responsibilities more completely and effectively. Events, such as selecting a mate, building a marriage, and creating a family life experience that is mutually enjoyable and fulfilling, are far more likely to occur in the life of such a person.

A related characteristic of the mature personality is that of **assuming responsibility** for one's own life in an honest manner. This also means that one expects and allows other persons to take responsibility for their own lives, actions, and values. The open and self-objective person will confront reality and the tasks of life in a responsible manner. In discussing the fully functioning person, Rogers identifies this quality as possessing an "internal locus of evaluation" [20]. Individuals are no longer driven by the dictates of a severe conscience or the traditions of the culture; rather, they have sorted out and integrated those values that are most important to their own becoming. They assume responsibility for their own lives and decisions. Maslow suggests that such individuals may have to be nonconformist and swim upstream against the currents of conformity. To put this in the language of a contemporary moral theorist, Lawrence Kohlberg, the individual has moved beyond the conventional law-and-order approach to morality to the postconventional level of principled living (see Chap. 18). This self-aware internalization is reflected in an individual's sensitivity to justice and **reciprocity in relationships** with others. Obviously, such a person is most capable of fulfilling the tasks of assuming civic responsibility and establishing reciprocal social care. (See Havig-hurst's tasks, Appendix C.)

The mature person views life as involving **ongoing change** and is willing to be a significant part of that process. The individual has the capacity to continue to differentiate and to integrate the experiences of life. Changes in culture and the institutions of society do not overwhelm the person. He or she is able to maintain integrity while expanding a sense of identity. This capacity is particularly important in the light of significant changes in gender-role and marital-role expectancy in our society. Rather than becoming overwhelmed, defensive, or isolated, the mature person participates in the process of differentiating and integrating roles that are mutually beneficial. Thus the mature man whose wife is seeking the fulfillment of her deferred educational and vocational objectives is capable of entering into that process in a contributing and mutually rewarding manner, which may be reflected in a cooperative endeavor to fulfill the ongoing tasks of rearing children and managing the home.

There is consensus among these theorists as to the critical importance of a **philosophy of life** that is both unifying and directing. Allport sees the attributes of humor and religion as complementary and balancing functions in the mature personality. This mature religious sentiment or philosophy of life is rich in its diversification due to a combination of discriminations and reorganizations. While it is shaped by formative childhood experiences, it is dynamic and fundamentally autonomous of its origins. This philosophy of life is unifying because it is "productive of a consistent morality." The mature outlook is one that endeavors to take into consideration all other perspectives and data. There is a quality of tolerance that saves the individual from a narrow dogmatism that would reject the views and opinions of others [1]. This philosophy is comprehensive inasmuch as it makes sense out of life for each person, which includes coming to grips with the major dilemmas of human suffering and death. The individual is able to function wholeheartedly even without absolute certainty.

In the face of life's complexities and humanity's sufferings, the mature person demonstrates the capacity to take risks for the good of our fellow man. "To the genuinely mature personality a full-faced view of reality in its grimmest aspects is not incompatible with an heuristic commitment that has the power to turn desperation into active purpose" [1]. People involved in the helping and healing professions are constantly confronted with these dilemmas. Providing both med-ical care and strength of character in the face of an individual's suffering and pain is a challenge that confronts the medical and psychiatric practitioner. This challenge may also confront a young couple facing the grim reality of a chronic disease process in their child, or a young man whose wife has just died, leaving him with the care of two young children. A comprehensive philosophy of life provides a sense of hope and purpose that enables the individual to continue to function even in the presence of sickness and death.

The experience of becoming fully functioning or self-actualizing is ongoing. However, it is attained to a relative extent in the development of those characteristics we have discussed. The fully functioning individual is actualizing potentials. Such self-actualization is possible only if lower-level needs are met; if they are not met, the individual has a pattern of deficiency motivation. The quality of the individual's life and that of others becomes negatively influenced. The growth motivation required to effectively establish intimate and mutually responsible relationships in marriage and family is missing, as is the growth motivation essential to building community. The growth-motivated person, on the other hand, is expressing self rather than simply adapting; relationships with others are spontaneous and natural rather than forced or defensive.

Maslow has an appreciation for the ongoing need for the renewal of the human spirit in its struggle to become self-actualized. This renewal is expressed in spiritual rather than in traditional religious ways. Maslow sees the need for persons periodically to achieve a peak experience that is somewhat mystical in nature. Although such an experience may be transient, it has a powerful influence on the ongoing process of actualization [15].

Gaps: Expectations and Realities

There are differences in the nature of developmental tasks and the timing of the psychosocial crises for each stage of development. These differences create gaps in time perspective and energy investment and may lead in turn to major differences in values and priorities in life-style. A "generation gap" may occur when two persons do not understand or appreciate their differences in values and priorities. However, the generation gap is not primarily chronological, any more than a chronological definition of either adolescence or maturity is adequate. A generation gap may also occur between two persons of the same age who have markedly differing developmental levels or primary value systems. There are gaps in approach, style, and values in dealing with the major areas of differentiation and integration of identity, establishing psychosocial reciprocity, and managing one's life.

One of the major gaps exists in the area of role definitions and expectations. The adolescent has to invest time and energy in sorting out strengths and capacities. This process of differentiation and integration often involves role playing or role experimentation, which is evidenced in everything from clothing styles to fluctuating interests in various activities. The adolescent is faced with the dilemma of finding a role in relation to a changing culture. It is somewhat like getting on a moving vehicle that you know you have to get on, but you have not had enough time to decide whether or not you want to go in the direction it is heading. Dealing with goals is secondary to finding a role. However, roles are constantly shifting as the culture and its institutions are shaped by technology and the media. The adult may have great difficulty understanding or relating to the adolescent who does not demonstrate a stability and a direction in goals.

Young adults in their thirties who have adolescent children often find themselves polarized around style, values, and choices. The young adult is generally much more goal-oriented than the adolescent. The heterosexual polarizations within the psychosocial experience of the adolescent are relatively resolved in the young adult, enabling the person to deal with issues of intimacy. The young adult has already dealt with the differentiation of personal drives, individual abilities, and the place of family and peer group in his or her values. Experimentation with the capacity to fulfill certain roles is generally behind the young adult, enabling a move toward consideration of direction or goal orientation for the expression of identity.

Gaps exist on intrapersonal as well as interpersonal levels. There are problems with time diffusion in the experience of the adolescent; the pressures are so great that time may go out of focus. Integrating the past into the present as well as responding to the demands of others to make future choices becomes an overwhelming task. A more stable sense of time enables the young adult to maintain a focus on tasks that involve both present commitments and future goals. The young adult is able to invest time and energy with less diffusion in accomplishing the tasks that society expects this individual to fulfill. Undertaking marital and family responsibilities in adolescence poses a much higher risk than in the young adult years.

There are gaps that exist within the experience of the young adult. Those who have not mastered prior tasks and psychosocial crises will experience gaps between current social expectations and their resources to respond. We will explore these unresolved psychosocial crises as factors that frustrate the transition into maturity. Other gaps exist that are due to combinations of environmental and decision-making problems; perhaps the attainments of an individual do not measure up to self-expectations. There may be a recurrence of old task demands due to failures or breakdowns in those tasks that were once thought to be completed.

One of the most common task-breakdown experiences is failure to make a marriage work. The experience of separation and divorce is on the increase in our society and leaves individuals with ego problems as well as problems with role and goal conflicts. The 30-year-old man who is now back in the single group, separated from his wife and family, has trouble sorting out roles and goals. He experiences a type of regressive episode in his psychosocial development; he is back climbing old hills and struggling through valleys of identity diffusion he thought he had conquered. At the same time, he feels the demands from self, children, and society to continue to function as a good father. How is he to put it all together? Feelings of failure, loss, hurt, and bitterness over a lost marriage may block the fulfillment of the task of finding a partner and making a second marriage work. The response of the surrounding community may compound the problem. The divorced woman who joins community organizations for the sake of her children may find herself forced into isolation; she may be viewed as a threat to the stability of other marriages and rejected by couples. One of the major problems in such situations is to find a congenial social group that will help the divorced young adult cope with the ongoing demands of social and family responsibilities.

The failure to make a marriage work generally includes the sense of failure in rearing children. There are gaps between what one had anticipated in parenting and the realities of separation. The breakdown in the time and space dimensions of the relationship involves a separation of shared growth experience. Failure in parenting adds to the feelings of defeat and loss that began with the disruption of the marriage. In addition, the task of vocational fulfillment may break down into the frustrations of job inadequacy to meet the economic pressures of marital and family separation. The loss of role often throws the sense of goals into a new state of diffusion.

The processes of differentiation and integration of identity are ongoing. The idealism of the fulfillment theorists focuses the possibilities for self-actualization and maturity. However, the existence of gaps between expectations and realities suggests that, whether or not conflict is inevitable, it is a significant factor in young adult experience. This tension is most evident as the young adult explores the psychosocial crises of intimacy and his or her relationship to the culture.

THE ISSUES OF INTIMACY AND CULTURAL CONTINUITY

Inasmuch as this chapter is concerned with the psychosocial dimensions of the young adult years, the germinal work of Erik Erikson warrants a central place in our explorations of this stage. Erikson has combined the strengths of the psychoanalytical intrapsychic understanding of personality development with a creative model for understanding psychosocial processes from birth to death. In his development of the psychosocial dynamics and polarizations for each stage, emphasis is given to specific behavioral evidences of how the different crises are dealt with in the life of the developing personality [5].

The epigenetic principle is an important point of departure in a discussion of Erikson's stage theory. He draws an analogy with the sequential physiological development of the embryo through the fetal period of development. If there is some developmental defect in one of the organ systems, a developmental arrest occurs that can have a significant influence on ongoing development. Postnatal maturation follows this same basic principle in the areas of biophysical, cognitive, and social development. In relating these events to psychosocial development, Erikson feels that in the sequence of significant experiences, the healthy child, if halfway guided, merely obeys and, on the whole, can be trusted to obey inner laws of development, which create a succession of potentialities for significant interaction with others. The expectations of the surrounding culture create pressures for adjustment to which the developing ego must respond.

The processes of psychosocial development carry demands for adaptation. The problem of time is critical for the developing personality. When the ego makes the necessary adaptations and meets the challenge of external society, the sequence of psychosocial development continues on in health toward the next crisis. However, if the crisis is not met and the ego has not adapted, the tensions and scars of that stage will continue to influence successive stages of psychosocial development.

Young Adulthood: Intimacy versus Isolation

The developing ego has had to cope with five crises in previous stages and now either builds on those successful adaptations or carries the unresolved polarizations into the new demands of the young adult years. We will explore the dimensions of intimacy that confront the individual at this point in the pilgrimage toward maturity.

INTIMACY: LOVE, MARRIAGE, FRIENDSHIP

The movement toward intimacy comes from within the human organism as an outgrowth of the maturing, integrated sense of identity. Intimacy is the need to share one's inner self with other selected persons on a deep, personal level—a revealing of one's true self. Erikson's concept of intimacy has a larger meaning than just sexual intimacy. Sexual intimacy is of the physical domain. Erikson is concerned with the intimacy of the social-emotional domains—friendships and small group and community involvements. Physical intimacy is but one facet of self-sharing, not the focus of it. Thus, one can have many intimate heterosocial and homosocial relationships without physical intimacy.

The question of intimacy is generally framed in the language of sexuality and romance to the extent that the rich variety of these facets of intimacy becomes lost. The question of intimacy includes friendships, family, church, and community life as well as dating and marital relationships. One of the most important questions the young adult faces is, "Who will be my friends, my community, my people?" Paul and Lanham [18] stress that "there is a further commitment each of us makes as we enter into relationships. We maintain a covenental commitment to the community as well. Our sense of fidelity must transcend the one-on-one relationship to include the larger community that is impacted by our lives. We do not make our choices in isolation, nor are the effects of our choices limited to one relationship"[18].

Erikson's approach to intimacy is expressed in psychosocial terms such as **affiliation** and **partnership** [7]. The psychic sharing of self is at the heart of this concept. The psychosocial history of the self comes together in the new crisis of intimacy. The positive psychic elements of trust, autonomy, initiative, industry, and identity enrich the meaning of intimacy to transcend a strict psychosexual interpretation. The friendships and partnerships of the mature adult are based on the quality of psychosocial intimacy. The sharing of oneself with a friend is mature when these psychosocial elements are active. This sharing is crucial to the establishment of a congenial social group;

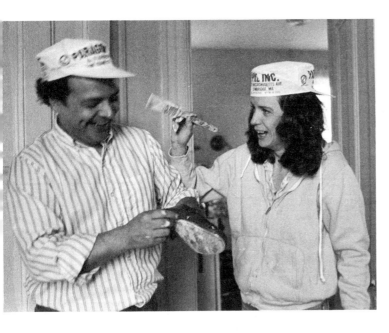

Figure 28-4. Intimacy is not restricted to physical exchanges but includes the mutual sharing of ideas and values that are central to one's self-identity. (Photograph by Ed Slaman.)

the cohesiveness of a small support group is dependent on the reciprocal sharing of one's identity with others. Civil responsibility is a task that the young adult can fulfill only with this strength. It is in sharing or losing oneself in others that one finds a new sense of personhood.

The term **affiliation** is used to indicate the meaning of intimacy as inclusive of friendships and partnerships. These friendships and partnerships are based on choice rather than the "blood bonds" of family. Erikson states, "From here on, ego-strength depends on an affiliation with others who are equally ready and able to share in the task of caring for offspring, products, and ideas" [6]. It is interesting to contemplate how this statement might be expanded to include the multiple facets of intimacy that are important to healthful personhood in marriage and friendship.

Howard and Charlotte Clinebell [4] have suggested that there are 12 dimensions to intimacy, which expand the meaning of intimacy in the directions indicated by Erikson as being important to the psychosocial crisis of the young adult years. **Emotional intimacy** refers to the capacity to perceive nondefensively the meaning and focus of the emotion that the other person is expressing. **Intellectual intimacy** is the sharing of ideas without polarization of the relationship. The capacity of a couple to share aesthetic facets of life and to act together in creative ways are two complementary dimensions of intimacy. These two facets are expressed as **aesthetic intimacy** and **creative intimacy.** Erikson, like Freud, stresses the importance of love and work in the healthy, mature adult. Clinebell brings these areas together in the capacity of a couple to be close in sharing common tasks and then adds the quality of relating in times of fun and play. **Crisis intimacy** involves a couple's coping with the problems and the painful situations in their life as a couple.

How a relationship manages the conflicts that come out of differences in interests, perspectives, and goals is an important test of a mature intimate relationship. The combined strengths of shared commitment and **ultimate concern** facilitate growth in the relationship and within each individual. The most important facet, on which the others depend, is the quality of **communication** intimacy [4].

There are dimensions of intimacy that are most meaningfully expressed within the extended family, friendship circles, and general community involvement. Intellectual intimacy provides us with a facet for ongoing growth in all of our relationships. This sharing of ideas challenges us to grow as persons throughout our development and thereby to positively affect the health of the surrounding community. The expression of one's creativity often demands friendships and circles of relationships that will nurture the aesthetic sensitivity. Play is a vital part of our lives, providing us with means of stress reduction and health. The family that plays together stays together, and the community that expresses itself in celebrative play provides a healthy climate for the next generation. The intimacy of work through sharing common tasks and goals is an important way for a community to express itself and to create a greater sense of unity and purpose.

ISOLATION: SEPARATION, LONELINESS

When the ego has not mastered an essential skill in prior psychosocial stages, the developmental lag will evidence itself in a new crisis in the young adult years. Erikson sees the individual as being caught in a conflict between a lack of readiness and the demands of a new stage in the psychosocial sequence. "The counterpart of intimacy is distantiation: the readiness to repudiate, isolate, and if necessary, destroy those forces and people whose essence seems dangerous to one's own" [6]. This process leads to a separation in a relationship that may have begun with some anticipation of success. The problem is that the lack of a sense of identity and fidelity leads to a defensiveness and fear that polarize the relationship. There is a risk inherent in intimacy that many individuals shrink from in fear, feeling that the demands for commitment, loyalty, and responsibility are too much.

Mature intimacy is founded on an identity strength that frees the individual to free others to be wholly themselves—not a dependent appendage. Identity strength allows one to appreciate the differences of others without a need to change them or their values into a common system. The differences of experience, education, values, or goals can enrich rather than destroy a relationship. The potential polarizations in any intimate relationship are overcome by these strengths. When they are missing, the polarizations dominate the relationship and often lead to separation, divorce, and loneliness.

Unresolved identity questions lead to major problems with tasks, such as selecting a mate and finding a congenial social group. These are individuals who cannot deal with the question of intimacy, whose progress toward self-actualization and maturity becomes truncated. Problems are evidenced through two patterns of isolation. The individual may function in **expressive isolation,** which is self-protective of the image the person shows to other people. This person can function within socially defined roles, always doing the right thing. He or she may be socially charming, but in close relationships, is shallow and subservient to the ideas and the values of the other person, unable to express true feelings, values, or opinions for fear of criticism. The ego strength depends on the approval of others in the surrounding culture regardless of the cost.

The characteristic of expressive isolation makes it unlikely that the tasks confronting the young adult will be managed successfully. This individual may aggressively function as though in charge or control of his or her life; the attempts to compensate for feelings of inadequacy may lead the individual into a pseudo-intimacy, which becomes manifest in forms of heterosexual conquest and control. Reciprocal sharing of identity and care is avoided. The "swinging single" pursues intimacies that protect the person from disclosure and responsibility. If such an individual should marry and bear children, it is unlikely that he or she will be able to expand a sense of care and commitment beyond the preoccupation with self-protective patterns of socialization. Thus the tasks of raising children and managing a home through responsible vocational endeavor will be most difficult for the individual to fulfill.

Although it is not considered pathological in nature, expressive isolation involves anxiety that inhibits and undermines the adjustments appropriate to young-adult life. It certainly blocks the possibilities for the individual to become a fully functioning personality; energies are invested in defensive rather than actualization processes. A more severe and pathological form of isolation is **receptive isolation.** In this pattern of behavior, the defensiveness is expressed in the distortion of social and environmental stimuli. Environmental events are translated to fit into the individual's expectations regardless of how contradictory the original stimulus may have been. Reactions are based on the perceived, rather than the actual stimulus. This person is deeply and emotionally invested in each experience and thus is unable to take the self-objective approach that would help clarify interaction patterns.

This type of isolation has a far more radical influence on the individual's capacity to differentiate and to integrate identity in relation to social and environmental expectations and demands. The individual is locked away in the isolation of self from growth-producing intimacies. Developmentally, the individual carries this isolation into midlife where it is expressed in dysfunctional ways. One of its characteristics is anxious self-absorption, which undermines healthy self-awareness and emotional development. The individual stagnates, failing to become creatively involved in the social order.

The individual's struggle with intimacy and isolation crises is further complicated by the ongoing task of relating the self to the surrounding culture. The process of differentiating and integrating a sense of identity prepares one for the task of integrating a sense of intimacy. However, the process is ongoing and expands to include the culture and its institutions. Where does one fit in, and how will one's values and purpose be expressed?

Finding One's Niche

The relationship between a sense of self and the culture holds significant implications for how one will handle commitments to marriage, family, work, and recreation. The intensity of the struggle for identity is often carried into the young adult years, during which time the task of adapting to the culture becomes a central issue. Kenneth Keniston has conceptualized a separate phase of development for many individuals in their twenties. They are caught in a conflict between their personality, their values, and the institutions of the culture.

The young adult in this phase of development has great difficulty in accepting society's demands and expectations. Keniston feels that "the awareness of the actual or potential conflict, disparity, lack of congruence between what one is (one's identity, values, integrity) and the resources and demands of the existing society increases. The adolescent is struggling to define who he is: the youth begins to sense who he is and thus to recognize the possibility of conflict and disparity between his emerging selfhood and this social order" [10].

According to Keniston, the young adult is very involved in three major tasks. First, there is the continuing quest to operationalize a sense of identity; this is often reflected in how the individual focuses vocational objectives. Many approach this task in economic terms. It becomes the means for meeting primary needs and also the secondary needs of socialization and recreation. Others approach work in the vocational sense, as an expression of who they are and what they value. Second, there is the quest for authentic or fulfilling intimacy. The nature of this crisis has been explored in the preceding discussions on Erikson.

The third task that Keniston develops is that of relating self to culture. The young adult may reflect problems with this task in a variety of ways. One style is that of radical activism, in which the individual seeks to change the culture in some dramatic and critical way. Keniston has studied radical activist groups and sees combinations of idealism, frustration, and an often unrecognized dogmatism operating in their response to the culture. The institutions of the social order become the focus of confrontation; basic to the confrontation is a conflict in values. Young adults who have

attained high levels of academic success may become polarized with the values of society. For example, during the 1960s, the focus of such polarization was the war in Vietnam together with the issue of civil rights, and young adults invested time and energies in attacking perceived injustices. The traditional young-adult tasks shrink in relative significance and may be postponed while these individuals seek to change the social order. The established order carries expectations of role and style that may be associated to such a degree with the opposed values that they express their point through a radical style change (e.g., clothing, hair style, language, use of drugs). If the tasks of marriage and family are pursued, the radical style may evidence itself in family life-style and in how the needs and crises of other members of the family are met.

Some young adults may be so ambivalent toward society that they make a choice to separate themselves in their life-styles. They may have tried the radical activist approach and have become disillusioned as to its efficacy. Inasmuch as their basic sense of identity has been focused, they often seek to establish their own community with other individuals who share this polarization with the values and expectations of the institutions of society. The in-grouping may be so strong that a separate communal life-style is established. Communes were springing up throughout our country in the 1960s and into the 1970s. The timetable for dealing with tasks of intimacy, including marriage, family, and community life, was important. However, the style or approach to these tasks departed from traditional ways. Communes generally had retention problems. The rapid turnover in membership evidenced failure in facilitating task fulfillment during the young adult years. Commune participation provided a moratorium period for many. Having served that purpose, the commune was abandoned as a structure for ongoing task fulfillment.

Perhaps what we are observing is in actuality more a cognitive conflict than a psychosocial problem. Young people are exposed to new information, ideas, and values, and these must be assimilated into their current value structures. The cognitive conflicts can be emotionally wrenching as individuals try to acknowledge differing viewpoints without violating their current value systems. Participation in communes and activist groups minimize the dissonance while they readjust value orientations. King Solomon warned us that with wisdom or knowledge one must also seek understanding. Perhaps as young people are able to embody their values within a larger structure, to establish firm identities, and to set priorities, the sanctity of the commune or focused organization becomes unnecessary.

The third approach to negotiating the relationship between self and culture is to compromise or adapt. This approach may follow the exploration of the first and second styles. The author thinks of a young man who spent 2 years as a member of a radical revolutionary organization following an initial involvement in the peace movement. Disillusioned with this group, and beginning to confront the demands of marriage and family life, he took his family into a communal setting. It was less than 1 year before his own values and interests led him away from the commune. At the age of 29, he rejoined the mainstream of society with a teaching position and a home in the suburbs.

The realization of one's identity within the community is a major task of this young adult crisis. The negotiation process involves some ongoing problems with time perspective. The individual's past experience and the present society demand renegotiations as to where his or her identity will connect; the individual seeks to preserve the integrity of values and goals while finding an avenue of creative expression within society. The investment of this young adult in a reexamination of the cultural inheritance is vital to society. If the renegotiation is achieved, the young adult will contribute to society the strengths of intelligence, ethical sensitivity, and energy.

This process of renegotiation and reinvestment is an outgrowth of the fulfillment of the tasks of identity and intimacy. Keniston's concept of the task of negotiating a relationship between self and culture is consistent with Erikson's emphasis on intimacy in tension with isolation in the young adult years. Whether or not to become an integral part of the community, and/or how to do so, are central questions of the young adult years. When positively accepted, this bonding leads to generativity in the middle adult years.

MAINTAINING POSITIVE MENTAL HEALTH DURING ADULTHOOD

The path to self-actualization and mature functioning is made smoother by the presence of loving support systems in one's life. The process of successful psychosocial maturation provides the individual with major strengths to enter the new crisis of intimacy. However, there are environmental and social forces that frustrate rather than facilitate this process.

We have selected Erikson's concept of the epigenetic principle to explore how failure in ego adaptation in the earlier psychosocial crises resurfaces again to make this transition to the young adult years difficult. It is important to recognize the critical role of family systems and cultural forces in this transition experience.

In defining the tasks, crises, and possibilities for the young adult years, it is important that we not overlook those who, for a variety of reasons, are regarded as "nonnormative." There are many young adults with disabilities, often lifelong ones, that handicap the transition into the young adult years.

Resolution of Psychosocial Crises

The positive elements of trust, autonomy, initiative, industry, and identity must be present in the individual before he or she can respond effectively to the psychosocial crisis of intimacy. Elements of unresolved psychosocial experience in one's life can move the individual in the direction of isolation.

The commitment of oneself to another demands a great act of trust. Many young adults find this to be an overwhelming challenge. They shrink back in fear of being hurt or rejected. Unconditional positive regard may not be reciprocated, or the details of an intimacy may be misinterpreted or misread. Heterosocial relationships may become diffused, as evidenced by a series of broken relationships. There are great numbers of persons who frequent singles' bars, where lasting commitments are not expected. Individuals are left feeling hurt, and they carry the scars of mistrust into the next relationship. When mistrust dominates, fear and the loneliness of adult isolation are the result.

The childhood years may have led to feelings of shame and doubt in some individuals. How one feels about oneself in terms of competence influences the response to a demand for emotional intimacy. To doubt oneself is a signal to others to doubt also, and establishes patterns of mutual rejection. To give oneself too completely to the other is seen as a loss of autonomy if the ego is fragile. It is easier for the individual to avoid emotional intimacies or to become extremely domineering in social relationships.

The childhood scars of guilt over being sexual may very well surface in an individual as an inability to make a meaningful heterosexual relationship work. The guilt may even be much broader and may include the fear of taking the initiative in relating to others and the environment. The pattern of shrinking back makes it difficult to begin to build a mutually caring relationship. The guilt and fear associated with autonomous opinions, value systems, or actions are minimized by parroting those of the partner and assuming a passive or dependent role in the relationship. The task of rearing children may lead to a pattern of parenting that is anxious; the children may experience the parent's guilt and fear in the unrealistic controls and compulsiveness that are imposed on them.

The middle childhood years serve to build a strong sense of industry, which becomes critical to productivity and creativity in later life. During these years, if an individual does not feel good about his or her performance and is low in motivation and successful achievement, the responsibilities of the young adult years can create a response of anxiety and indecisiveness. Usually, there is a pattern of signaling to others that the individual feels, or is, inferior to which others respond with various forms of rejection. Thus the industry that is essential to making intimacy work in practical care may be overshadowed by this lack of self-esteem and self-confidence. If one is not confident in one's own product, why should anyone else have confidence or respect? The industry essential to success in work is also missing; the individual lacks the confidence to express the self in civic affairs and in building a congenial social group. Industry is the basis of

loyalty and commitment. The interrelationship of work, play, and love in our earlier developmental experiences provides us with the foundation for the intimacies of the young adult years.

We have already explored the importance of identity consciousness to reduce the demands of the ego when meeting the tasks of intimacy. The young adult who has failed to integrate a sense of identity either retreats from emotional intimacy or violates the other person's dignity through promiscuous physical or social relationships (e.g., gossip).

Unresolved conflicts and poorly separated relationships with one's parents may get in the way of meaningful emotional intimacy. Sheehy notes that "a favorite way of twisting an intimate relationship out of shape is to invite our partner to replace our phantom parent and tell us what to do. Or what not to do, especially when it's something that we're looking for an excuse to avoid anyway" [21]. Sheehy feels that adolescence does not end until that time in the twenties when a "provisional identity" is achieved. These identity issues continue to influence us throughout our adult

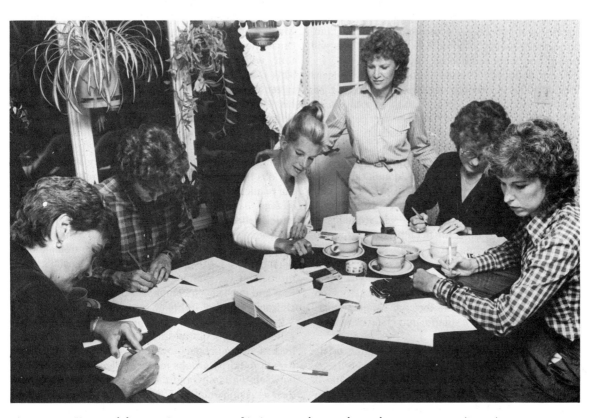

Figure 28–5. Young adults experience a sense of intimacy as they work together on a community project.

lives; thus intimacies are significantly complicated by ongoing struggles with identity [12, 17].

Preparation for Adult Responsibilities

The transition to adulthood is not only affected by the incompletely resolved tasks and crises of earlier experience; there are also forces operating in family life, educational experience, and subcultural affiliation that serve to either facilitate or frustrate the transition process.

The humanistic fulfillment models of Maslow, Allport, and Rogers provided us with the characteristics of fully functioning or self-actualizing mature personalities. Although these theorists gave minimal attention to the earlier developmental processes, they did recognize the importance of particular experiences in fostering self-actualization. The central emphasis on the emerging self and one's internal resources has to be balanced by what Rogers refers to as the need for "unconditional positive regard." This potential for maturity becomes actualized in a psychological climate of acceptance and empathy. An understanding communication between the developing child and the parent is crucial to this process of actualization. If the child is treated with conditional acceptance and faulty communication patterns, it is unlikely that he or she will develop a sense of positive self-regard.

Rogers' definition of unconditional positive regard in relationships is generally developed in terms of therapeutic or teaching relationships. In these contexts, he sees the helper as providing the necessary climate for change and self-actualization. It is in reference to these relationships that he writes: "By acceptance I mean a warm regard for him as a person of unconditional self-worth—of value no matter what his condition, his behavior, or his feelings. It means a respect and liking for him as a separate person, a willingness for him to possess his own feelings in his own way. It means an acceptance of and regard for his attitudes of the moment, no matter how negative or positive, no matter how much they may contradict other attitudes he has held in the past" [20]. The avenue to maturity is highly dependent on the availability of social forces of understanding communication through family experience or the presence of a significant person or persons in one's life.

The need for positive regard is not limited to the childhood years. The young adult has generally expanded life to the extent that he or she seeks life in more diverse experiences. Marital and family relationships are the most obvious of these expressions of need. Yet most of the time and energy involves work-related experiences and relationships. It is here that the need for positive regard and affirmation is critically important. The creative fulfillment of the worker and the productivity of the organization have a vital relationship. Roger Gould notes that "being able to do what we do well makes us feel vital and makes work a labor of love" [8]. The choices the young adult makes in relation to education and work hold significance for the rest of the life span. As Gould expresses it, "we must do work that confirms our talents and expresses a psychodynamic theme close to the core of us" [8].

One of the major factors facilitating the transition into adulthood is cultural continuity. Continuity is present when the experiences of childhood and adolescence are preparatory to what the culture expects and provides in later development. There is continuity when the gender-typing experiences of childhood prepare the individual for gender-role expectations in the marriage and family life experiences of later development. However, our culture goes through such rapid and dramatic changes that the child's experiences may be discontinuous with what is expected of him or her in later development. The most dramatic illustration of this phenomenon is in the changing roles of women. Many women are caught in a state of diffusion because the shaping they have had is now in discontinuity with what is expected of and available to them. This discontinuity serves to create polarizations between what the man had expected of the roles of both his wife and himself in marriage and family life fulfillment. The increase in marital and family life conflict is an understandable consequence of such discontinuity.

Society is going through one of the most significant periods in human history in regard to role changes in the relationships between men and women [17]. These changes have set in motion a consciousness of gender-typing patterns and their influence on both identity and intimacy issues in the adolescent and young adult years. The changing role of women has a tremendous potential to alter the nature of the psychosocial crises throughout development. The discontinuities in culture and experience complicate the nature of the psychosocial crisis of intimacy.

It is most difficult to interpret with reliability and validity the subcultural forces that are at work in the lives of young people growing up in our society. Members of minority groups may experience discontinuity between the family and the larger culture throughout their developmental experience; they may learn to cope with mixed cultural experience and varied role expectancy. The problems become more complex when marriage leads to further discontinuities of tradition and expectancy.

The Disabled Adult

Chapter 19 explored the developmental problems of the disabled child. Individual differences due to socio-emotional handicaps in early childhood have a continuous influence on psychosocial development. Neurological problems and the impact of disease processes or accidents complicate educational and social development. The experiences of early childhood and adolescence often leave unresolved psychosocial crises for the disabled individual. How do the forces for actualization or "becoming" function within the life of the disabled person? Are not the environmental factors that block the development of a fully functioning individual likely to be more complicating in the life of this person? What are the possibilities for the disabled person to realize potentials, given both the disability and the insensitivity of society? Is it likely that this individual will be locked into what Maslow identifies as "deficiency motivation," or the lower levels within the hierarchy of needs? Is it not more difficult for the disabled adult to arrive psychosocially prepared and able to cope with the new crisis of intimacy versus isolation? Perhaps a better understanding on our part of disabled persons is the first step in providing some answers to these important ethical questions.

We have been very preoccupied with the establishment of norms for physical development, intelligence, personality, and normal adjustment. In critique of this approach, Thompson writes that this process leads to the realization that great numbers of children are nonnormative and are responded to as different. To be responded to as not meeting the norms is to be cued to function with self-conscious low self-worth; this attitude undermines motivation and destroys hope. "A necessary condition of happiness in its broad sense is self-respect. Because the handicapped adolescent is seldom in a position where anything he says or does meets the impossible standard set for him, he is eternally denied the ingredients of self-esteem. At every turn he is told implicitly and explicitly that he does not meet the standard and is not likeable for his own sake" [22]. Applying Rogers' concept of the need for unconditional positive regard, one can see how difficult it is for such a person to actualize potentials or to become a fully functioning person.

The problems of low self-esteem have such historical significance in the disabled individual's psychosocial development that these problems of ego adaptation are brought into each new crisis. The transitional period from school to postschool experiences is a particularly crucial period, since the cumulative effects can be devastating to the development of initiative and industry, let alone the higher level of psychosocial skills. Thompson challenges the schools and institutions of society to work together to ensure that young people with neurological problems are given every possible opportunity to find the opportunities to set realistic goals and to achieve success by their own efforts in order to provide a sense of hope and self-worth. There is also a great need for assistance in learning social skills. Unacceptable patterns of behavior can be worked on by eliminating the forces that continue to block and to frustrate the possibility for positive self-regard. The most important positive force is the power of acceptance and encouragement. It is tragic that the already disabled individual should have to carry the additional complicating handicap of limited support and encouragement.

A further complication is the lack of availability of environmental and institutional resources. Those who meet the norms find these resources to be readily accessible; meanwhile, the handicapped individual often has to carry three additional problems, the lack of positive, encouraging love, the lack of availability of resources, and opportunities for independent work and living. Historically, we have seen many who in spite of their handicaps have overcome the obstacles and become models of courage and discipline for the nonhandicapped. New currents of support are increasingly in evidence; educational resources are being expanded to meet the needs of all disabled children and adolescents into the young adult years. The schools have been a leading force in building social and environmental support resources, and this concern has generalized to the other institutions and organizations in our communities. The mental health movement, rehabilitation programs, group homes and communities for the retarded, and adult organizations for the blind and deaf have been established to further the process of actualizing the potentials of these disabled persons.

Two major areas of preparation for the young adult years are the vocational and social areas. For the disabled person, the postschool years may become more problematical due to the inaccessibility of resources. Community organizations have to take up where the school systems leave off. Society is responding more specifically in making cultural and environmental resources available to a greater extent. Transportation, parking, and building facilities are being provided for the handicapped. Nonhandicapped persons find it difficult to imagine the experiential world of the handicapped. Some simple experiments can help to simulate the experiences of disabled persons: (1) Try to follow a television program with the sound off; (2) have someone help you to walk blindfolded around and through an area in which you live, study, or work for a 15-minute period, then have the person stand back for a moment to let you experience being on your own with such a disability; or (3) try to master access to a building, a vehicle, or a classroom while working from a wheelchair or crutches.

Many disabled individuals with excellent academic credentials are refused career opportunities because of the biases of employers and the public. As mentioned earlier, it is difficult to work toward self-actualization when one is unsure of the ability to provide adequate food, shelter, and clothing for oneself. Even the most stable and intelligent individual will begin to experience some undermining of self-confidence and self-worth.

There is a contradiction between the idealism of the actualization theories and the realities of life for the disabled. The challenge remains to express those ideals in a vital and practical way in the lives of the

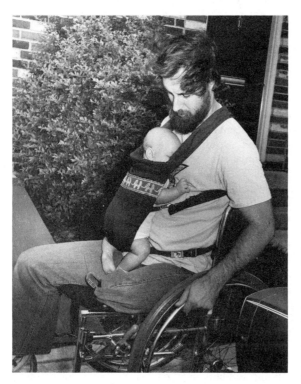

Figure 28–6. Physical impairments and disabilities need not interfere with one's ability to enjoy life's experiences fully.

disabled. If we fail to provide the support and the resources of the community to make the optimal level of functioning possible for these individuals, we need to reevaluate the degree of our own actualization and maturity as human beings and as a nation.

SUMMARY

There are multiple perspectives on the definition and characteristics of the psychosocially maturing adult. There are also differences in the emphasis on stress, conflict, or defensiveness in the dynamics of maturation. The nature and the degree of the influence of earlier childhood and environmental experiences are interpreted in various ways. For some, like Erikson, the early psychosocial crises are vitally involved in how the individual deals with adult tasks. It should be noted that, while less developed in their perspectives, the actualization humanistic theorists give some attention to the critical importance of affirmation, care, love, and support of significant persons in the individual's developmental experience. These approaches stress an idealistic and optimistic view of the individual as being capable of self-actualization. Other theorists enrich our understanding of the complex relationship between the personality and the environment. The emphasis on "activity levels" and on the individual's patterns of response to environmental feedback enlarges our understanding of unique styles of behavior in the adult personality.

As we summarize our discussions, we note that there are differences in emphasis that are not necessarily contradictory. These approaches enlarge our understanding, and each serves to balance and potentially to enrich the other perspectives. There are certain common denominators in most definitions of psychosocial maturation into the young adult years; three general areas of thematic consistency are evident.

First, there is a consistent emphasis on the processes of differentiation and integration in focusing the task of identity for the young adult. The process of differentiation involves the sorting out of experiences, both past and present. This capacity is important throughout the maturation process and evidences itself in the qualities of flexibility, openness, nondefensiveness, and spontaneity in the mature adult. The capacity to integrate these experiences into a stable sense of who one is provides the qualities of predictability, dependability, and stability in the young adult years. Thus differentiation and integration are complementary dynamics operating in the maturing personality. The processes of identity and intimacy demand this capacity.

psychosocial expressions of intimacy. This third theme addresses the coping capacity of the individual, which builds on the resources of the first two. The task here is to operationalize identity and intimacy in managing one's environment and the economy of one's life. This task involves the capacity to draw on the resources of the surrounding culture and the environment without being either overwhelmed into conformity or polarized into alienation. Coping with one's environment and culture in ways that are nurturing toward others, while preserving the integrity of one's sense of identity, is a central characteristic of the mature adult. At this point, review again the characteristics of a mature system according to Werner's theory in Chapter 2. Compare these key points to the theories given in this chapter. Although they are derived from very different perspectives, theories of maturity mesh beautifully.

It is evident that, with varying degrees of emphasis, most models for understanding the mature personality give attention to the importance of developmental history. What we have become as adults has been shaped to some degree by the presence or absence of significant persons and support systems in our childhood experience. Thus there are implications for ethical responsibility to provide resources that encourage positive, optimal development in the lives of society's children. We are challenged to function beyond the level of mere adjustment to those tasks that assure our own survival. Thus the young adult psychosocial crises serve to prepare us for the next task and crisis. As the individual successfully matures through the young adult years, the phase of creativity and "generativity" surfaces. The processes of developing authentic identity and intimacy prepare us for loving, caring for, and nurturing our own families. This process is preparatory to the expansion of those strengths into an expressed concern for the quality of life within the larger family of humanity.

Let us return to our opening analogy. Those hazy and sometimes threatening hills are inviting now, because the reward and fulfillment are in the climb. Fortunately, maturation is an ongoing process. Each hill and valley has its potential to enrich the life of the individual and through the individual to build a better world. There are even loftier hills ahead!

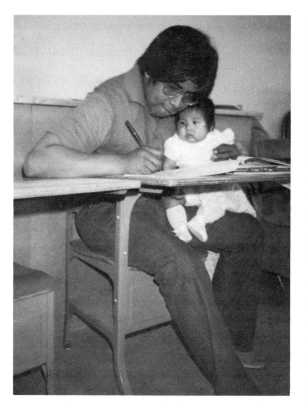

Figure 28–7. Young adults frequently are involved simultaneously in the dual tasks of continuing personal development and fostering the development of the next generation.

Second, whether expressed as a natural unfolding or an actualization or as a psychosocial process, the tasks and crisis of intimacy represent a core dimension of young adult experience. The basic emphasis here is on the capacity of the individual to enter into loving, caring, and nurturing intimacies. The strength to give and to receive love is a common emphasis in defining psychosocial maturity. The task of developing mutually satisfying experiences in sexual intimacy is a significant dimension of young adult life. The multidimensional facets of intimacy enlarge this experience beyond sexuality into the areas of work, play, and nurturing activities. The building of friendships and community with a sense of mutuality is characteristic of the mature young adult.

Third, there is an emphasis on the individual's capacity to cope with the environment and the challenges of external task fulfillment. The first theme emphasized the internal process of differentiating and integrating identity; the second theme focused on the

REFERENCES

1. Allport, G. W. *Personality, A Psychological Interpretation.* New York: Holt, 1937.
2. Allport, G. W. *The Individual and His Religion.* New York: Macmillan, 1960.

3. Combs, A. W., Richards, A. C., and Richards, F. *Perceptual Psychology: A Humanistic Approach to the Study of Persons.* New York: Harper & Row, 1976.

4. Clinebell, J. H., and Clinebell, C. H. *The Intimate Marriage.* New York: Harper & Row, 1970.

5. Erikson, E. H. *Childhood and Society* (2nd ed.). New York: Norton, 1963.

6. Erikson, E. H. *Insight and Responsibility.* New York: Norton, 1964.

7. Erikson, E. H. *Identity, Youth and Crisis.* New York: Norton, 1968.

8. Gould, R. *Transformations.* New York: Simon and Schuster, 1978.

9. Havighurst, R. J. *Developmental Tasks and Education* (3rd ed.). New York: McKay, 1972.

10. Keniston, K. *The Uncommitted: Alien Youth in American Society.* New York: Dell, 1970.

11. Keniston, K. *Youth and Dissent: The Rise of a New Opposition.* New York: Harcourt, Brace, Jovanovich, 1971.

12. Levison, D. J., et al. *The Seasons of a Man's Life.* New York: Knopf, 1978.

13. Maddi, S. R. *Personality Theories: A Comparative Analysis* (4th ed.). Homewood, IL: Dorsey Press, 1980.

14. Maslow, A. H. *Toward a Psychology of Being* (2nd ed.). New York: Van Nostrand, 1968.

15. Maslow, A. H. *Motivation and Personality* (2nd ed.). New York: Harper Brothers, 1970.

16. Maslow, A. H. *The Farther Reaches of Human Nature.* New York: Viking, 1971.

17. Mayer, N. *The Male Mid-Life Crisis: Fresh Starts After Forty.* Garden City, NY: Doubleday, 1978.

18. Paul, C. R., and Lanham, J. *Choices: In Pursuit of Wholeness.* Kansas City: Beacon Hill Press of Kansas City, 1982.

19. Rogers, C. R. *Client-Centered Therapy.* Boston: Houghton Mifflin, 1951.

20. Rogers, C. R. *On Becoming a Person: A Therapist's View of Psychotherapy.* Boston: Houghton Mifflin, 1961.

21. Sheehy, G. *Passages: Predictable Crises of Adult Life.* New York: Dutton, 1976.

22. Thompson, A. Moving Toward Adulthood. In L. E. Anderson (Ed.), *Helping the Adolescent with the Hidden Handicap.* Los Angeles: California Association for Neurologically Handicapped Children, 1970.

29
Changing Roles in Western Society

Clara S. Schuster and Helen J. Smith

> If I could never really be like other people then at least I would be like myself and make the best of it.
>
> —Christy Brown, *My Left Foot*

Introduction

Role Theory
Role assignment
Interdependence of roles
Necessity of roles for society

Factors Influencing Roles
Changes in family structure
Economic influences
Influence of the mass media

Gender-Role Expectations
Male roles—past and present
Female roles—past and present
Blending roles

Summary

Roles—the behavior patterns that culture assigns to particular social positions or situations—are such an integral part of each of our lives that we seldom give them much thought until they become a problem to our internal or external adaptation in meeting life's challenges. Roles, which are frequently associated with stages of development, serve as society's "road maps" for meaningful and satisfying life relationships by providing an orderly method for transferring knowledge, responsibility, and authority from one generation to the next [23].

"Roles are inescapable. They must be played or else the social system will not work" [10]. Roles provide individuals with ongoing "norms," models for behavior that not only establish expectancies, but provide a "gateway to the world" [5]. When behavior patterns are habituated, the choices are narrowed and fewer decisions and disagreements are required (if all agree with the rules of the roles) [2]; thus more energies are available for positive, productive, creative behaviors within the accepted limitations or foci.

Middle-class children generally see themselves as progressing through a series of increasingly more desirable and complex roles. This outlook implies that one must consciously work at attaining the behaviors, attitudes, and values associated with a particular cultural role. As such, each new role carries with it the potential for gratification and increased ego-identity if it is achieved; poor self-esteem and role confusion can result if the role is not mastered. The learning of new skills and behaviors can consume high levels of energy until the role is internalized; the component behaviors can then be used as means to achieve other goals. The potential for successful mastery of one or more roles is decreased if several roles are assumed at the same time, such as marriage and parenthood. The gradual addition of new roles allows for adjustment or acclimation to one role before energies are focused toward new tasks. The process of role achievement is also facilitated when an individual has a strong, stable role model with whom to identify and to imitate. For most children, this model is found in their parents.

During the childhood years, an individual has innumerable contacts with the values and the goals of other people. The child begins to internalize the values of those who are significant to him or her and observes how the other person achieves goals or translates values into action. When these goals are reasonably consistent and attainable, the individual is assisted to develop a lifelong sense of direction and purpose. A sense of self-esteem is achieved as the individual masters these roles.

When the roles portrayed by a significant other are consistent with the goals and the needs of the developing individual in a fairly stable culture, internal equilibrium is heightened and transitions to new roles are fairly smooth. However, when the roles, values, and goals of one generation are no longer seen as relevant by the new generation, serious external and internal disequilibrium can occur. Psychological security is threatened.

Western culture is changing rapidly; young adults face a different culture from that faced by their parents. Increases in technology and social mobility as well as economic changes have created marked changes in life-styles and values and their associated roles. "Getting ahead" has replaced survival, expressing one's life in a meaningful way has replaced earning enough money to live, and maximizing potentials has replaced adherence to strict cultural roles. If individuals feel that their parents' values of thrift, honesty, and industry are meaningless in this new world, then considerable anger may be felt by individuals toward their parents for preparing them for a world that no longer exists [23]. They may feel trapped into a set of behaviors to the point of losing contact with their real selves [10]. Fortunately, in spite of the differences in circumstances, there are usually enough common values and ideals that old roles can be successfully adapted to the new roles that are emerging.

ROLE THEORY

Social behavior is never instinctually determined. Behavior, or roles, are learned within the context of a culture. Roles are important but are not necessarily controlling, even though they involve "gender appropriate roles" reinforced since early infancy. "Technological and cultural progress has created considerable overlap and complexity in modern adult roles" [17]. Specific roles are assigned in two ways.

Role Assignment

Acquired roles are those based on characteristics over which we have had no choice, such as gender, race, and age. The interpretations, the behaviors, and the responsibilities associated with acquired roles vary widely among cultures. All human societies differentiate roles on the basis of age and sex [9, 17]. These roles are linked to power, privilege, and prestige. Within the last decade, the roles formerly expected of men and women have come into serious question. A brief look at some anthropological studies, such as Margaret Mead's classic study of three New Guinea cultures, calls into question the assumed inherent characteristics of males and females and what their resulting roles should be [14].

The individual exercises a measure of choice over the second method of role assignment. However, the choice of an **achieved role** (e.g., student, wife, athlete) is frequently made without careful evaluation of the ramifications or the role responsibilities. For example, the choice to marry and to become a spouse is seldom made on the basis of what duties this role brings with it. Each occupation has an accompanying set of role expectations that are inherited with the job. Some of these characteristics are formalized in a job description. Even the mention of a certain occupation usually brings to mind some expected ways of behaving, dressing, and even speaking. For example, ballet dancer, English teacher, truck driver, police officer, and nurse will conjure up different ideas in our minds.

Many roles are not clearly defined as being either achieved or acquired but may be a blend of both (for example, age roles). Although in some aspects one's age role is an achieved role, it is not a chosen role. It progresses through a sequential achievement of years with no reversals. Increased privileges and responsibilities frequently accompany each birthday, at least during the earlier years. However, for a variety of reasons, either physical, mental, or emotional, an individual may not behave in a lockstep fashion in carrying out age-role expectations. Most of us at one time or another have been told to "act your age"; seldom is this admonition used to denote a person performing above the complainant's age-role expectations—only below. Ashley Montagu points out that when people conform to age-role expectations, aging and rigidity occur much earlier [8].

Interdependence of Roles

In addition to identifying how roles are bestowed, that is, how they are acquired or achieved, it is important to consider the fact that roles are not mutually exclusive. No one can function, even for a short period of time in only one role. For example, a woman can be a student, a daughter, a mother, a wife, and a career person (and much more), all at the same time. Occasionally these layers of roles may require "peeling off" one layer at a time in order to look at them separately. Most of the time, there are few problems that arise from carrying a multiplicity of roles, and in practice, they may blend well with one another. Many roles depend on gender; for example, being female bestows the roles of daughter, sister, wife, and mother. As her gender allows the female to embrace certain roles, it also eliminates several other options, such as brother and father.

The roles that a person achieves or acquires are not always a harmonious blend. The role expectations for a father at any given moment may be in direct conflict with his career role, his role as the chairman of a civic organization, or as a member of an athletic team. One is forced to reassess values and priorities by sorting out which issues or needs are most pressing at the moment or have the most significant long-range effect.

Conflicting role expectations are not always on an individual, internal basis; frequently they are between two or more individuals. For example, what is a wife's role, both from her point of view and her husband's? Many of the frustrations experienced by people living together, particularly within a family, come from conflicting role expectations. Since the orientations of individuals to roles are seldom identical, no agreed-upon definitions are available. With societal needs changing so rapidly, the chances are that conflicting role expectations will occur. Role conflicts may occur from the most internalized personal level to a societal level, and the role expectations may be in direct conflict with an individual's ability or desire to implement these expectations.

There are a variety of subcultures within the major culture of every geographical area. Often it is assumed that persons who speak English or the dominant language of the area have been socialized into the same role expectations as others in the community. However, even with racial, geographical, and age factors being the same, ethnic background, religious upbringing, economic class, and individual family training will socialize individuals for different goals and expectations. When these factors are not recognized, miscommunication, misinterpretations, and even social conflict may result. A lack of knowledge regarding another person's cultural background often results in insults and hurt feelings.

As new waves of immigrants from Oriental- and Spanish-speaking countries as well as native Americans (American Indians) interface more frequently with the dominant U.S. culture, the need for information and understanding of different role expectations becomes more apparent [19]. The smallest communications can often be an initial source of misunderstanding; usually these are in the nonverbal range. For example, in the interpretation of what it means when a child does not look directly at an adult who is speaking, a middle-class white might conclude that the child is lying or shameful. A psychologist might interpret this behavior as "poor self-concept." An American Indian and an Oriental or a Spanish-speaking person would probably see this behavior as that of a polite child who is respectful of adults. Many other examples of cultural differences in nonverbal communication patterns that are a part of these individuals' socialized role expectations may be noted in daily transactions, behavior patterns, and value systems [19].

Conflicts also occur with the rapid influx of technology or with the changing economic conditions. The variety of new occupations and the resulting job descriptions have produced many conflicts between male and female role expectations. As a society or as individuals, we often are not prepared to incorporate these new job roles into our existing gender-role expectations. For example, is "computer programmer" a male or a female occupation, or is it neuter?

In addition to the tendency of roles to overlap and to conflict, roles may also be complementary like a lock and key. They may be complementary within or between the individuals of a system. For example, when a person is a husband, a complementary set of expectations is given to the wife. The larger societal implications and the benefits of these complementary roles are somewhat apparent; the result is usually the division of a certain set of tasks between the two persons (see Chap. 31), leading to the successful accomplishment of all the tasks. This is one reason why traditional roles are difficult to change. Complementary changes must occur at other or all levels of the system's functioning (family or society).

To summarize briefly, roles are culturally determined sets of expected behaviors bestowed on individuals because of acquired or achieved status and characteristics. Individuals carry numerous roles at any one time. These roles may fit together harmoniously, or they may result in conflict either within the individual or with others.

Necessity of Roles for Society

Although some individuals have found their specific roles to be a burden or a yoke, roles have continued in some form over the years. For society, it is a way of dividing up tasks, an essential prerequisite if people are to live together. The three primary functions of societal roles are to delegate economic responsibility, to orient new members, and to care for dependent members.

Many jobs are essential to keep society functioning and goods and services moving. Rather than each individual or family unit struggling on its own, a network of occupations has evolved to provide the various goods and services to help ensure that economic needs will be met. Many examples of unequal and unrealistic role assignments can be found in every society and almost every place of employment.

Every society must develop a system to orient and provide for new members. In western society, these tasks have been incorporated into various roles, such as mother and teacher. Most of these roles have traditionally been given to women, thus linking children to females with a far stronger bond than with males. It has also meant that males have traditionally been given the roles that are primarily for economic support.

A third societal purpose that is served by the assigning of roles is the care of the dependent members of society. In addition to needing orientation, children must have their economic and emotional needs met. Other dependent members of society include infirm older persons and persons of all ages with disabling conditions. The definition of who belongs to any of these dependent groups varies greatly from one society to the next. It might be noted that each of the various states of dependence carries with it specific role expectations. In addition, the designation of who is to be the caretaker varies. One of the simplest and most convenient methods society has found for choosing the caretaker is to attach the responsibility to other roles or to a specific occupation, many of which have been associated with women in western society.

These three major tasks of society have traditionally been delegated according to acquired roles. The convenience of using acquired roles instead of achieved roles can be demonstrated. First, society is guaranteed a ready and fairly consistent percentage of members in the role. Second, acquired roles, because they are readily identifiable, offer a quick reference for appropriate social behavior. Thus roles are convenient tools for the division and the accomplishment of tasks by society. The assignment of tasks according to some characteristic, such as age, gender, or race, provides individual members with readily identifiable ways of behaving. Society and individuals often use these acquired roles as a guide for interaction. **The danger is in using the external criteria rather than individuality as the basis for relating to others (stereotyping).**

FACTORS INFLUENCING ROLES

Roles are becoming less static in terms of both their numbers and their expectations. A variety of factors influence the changes that are occurring. As with many areas of societal change, the pace of change is increasing each year. Some of the factors that seem to be affecting role expectations most dramatically include economic conditions, the family structure, and the mass media.

Changes in Family Structure

Changes in family structure have created dramatic readjustments in role expectations. This factor, above all others, makes a difference in an individual's day-to-day living patterns. Predictions vary as to whether these changes are temporary or whether they are of a more lasting nature.

According to Bronfenbrenner [1], the extended family has almost disappeared from the American scene. Although most nuclear families do have extended families, they frequently do not live within close proximity. Three generations living within the same household is considered the rare exception. Not only are extended families no longer being incorporated within the same household, but the number of children per household has declined markedly. One or two generations ago, four- and five-children families were common; today, many families are limited to two children. This situation, of course, shortens the period of time when there are small children in the home. However, many families find themselves investing an equal amount of emotional energy in their two children as yesterday's parents invested in five children.

With the recent extended economic recession, many adult children are returning to live with their parents because of the loss of a job or a roommate, a divorce, or simply the expense of living alone. Sometimes a young adult will move in and out several times before finding it possible to be self-supporting. Many adjustments are required, including the redefining of the role relationships of parents to children. Further redefinitions and adjustments of role expectation must be made if the adult child also has children.

In the past, most women spent many years at home with the children, from the time the first child was born until the last child left home. Typically, this time span extended over a period of 30 to 35 years. In today's society, however, children are only in the home for about 20 to 24 years. This fact, coupled with the longer life span, means that the couple will experience a longer period of time in the "empty nest" stage. Therefore, even if she is employed outside the home, when the woman's career as a mother is completed earlier, she must find new roles to play and alternative ways of defining herself as a woman. She can fill her hours with individualized leisure time activities, volunteer work, or group leisure-time activities. However, many women have found these activities to be unfulfilling or impractical because of the need to support aging parents or to assist their children who are still partially dependent, although no longer living at home. Consequently, most women enter or reenter the job market.

A second phenomenon that was formerly a rarity is the childless couple. Many people, for a variety of reasons, are choosing not to have children at all, or the choice may be delayed until 30 years of age or more. In 1983, 49 percent of married couples in their twenties had no children, and 19 percent had only 1 child [22]. People feel less apologetic today for not having children, even for not wanting them. This attitude represents a dramatic break from the traditional progression of roles.

There are some indications that childless marriages are more satisfying in today's world, since different ideas of how to rear children can be one of the major causes of friction due to differing values of the marital partners. Very few people have formal training in child-rearing and thus must rely on the roles or methods remembered from their own childhood (memory traces). Children also increase the demands on the finances and the time of the parents. In addition, many women resent the interruption of their careers and do not want to be a full-time, housebound parent.

The third trend, the "blended family" (see Chap. 33), has created some new roles. The role of stepparent is not new, but there are few positive role models for the

stepparent or ex-spouse to imitate. Many people are very uncomfortable with these roles, yet struggle valiantly to fulfill them. Another set of people who must find some resolution to the role are the grandparents, particularly the parents of the individual who was not awarded custody. Many children end up being cut off from at least one set of grandparents, even though this may or may not be the wish of the children or of the grandparents. The child may acquire two new sets of step-grandparents. Again, these new roles may be difficult to assume; at best, they are awkward in the beginning.

Foster children are often lost in the shuffle of shifting families. Biological family ties may become severed, and role expectancies may change with each new family. The number of children being cared for by nonrelated persons runs from a high of 10 percent in New York City to an average of 5 percent or less in other areas of the country [11]. However, these figures do not reflect the total number of children who move in and out of foster care.

The biological parent or parents, the child, and the other care-taking adults must all reorient their self-identification in these roles; they are forced to find new ways to relate to each of the persons involved. Many biological parents find the situation so awkward that they prefer to stay away from the child rather than to endure the pain of not being the only parent [4]. Even the terms used to describe each of these roles, such as "natural" or "biological" parents, reflect the conflicts inherent in these roles. The child is placed in a vulnerable position because of the multiplicity of significant role models, each with differing values, behaviors, and expectations. Which model will he or she identify with in later years? Has there been enough consistency to form a stable internal image? If not, an acute identity crisis may result.

A fourth trend or change in the traditional American family is the increased number of unmarried, or single, adults. In the United States, 43 million (or one out of every three) adults are single at any one time [22]. since 95 percent of all persons marry at some point in their life, many of these have not yet married or are between marriages or are widowed. For generations, many of the traditional male and female roles have been based on the assumption that marriage is a normal state. Individuals who choose to remain single object to this assumption with the implied status it confers on the married, while conferring the role of second-class citizen on the unmarried.

Single persons are making a major economic impact. Food products and housing are now designed and marketed to meet the needs of the single person as well as those of larger families. The needs of single persons for social contact are different from those of the married person; this too is having an impact on the economy and is creating new enterprises, such as singles' bars and health salons. Some singles choose to fulfill their need to nurture in part by taking on a more intensive role as an aunt or an uncle. For some families, most often nonwhites, this is not a new role but in fact has been a part of the family system for many years [19].

Economic Influences

A number of changes have taken place in the economic sphere since World War II that affect role expectations. Some of these changes include the expected standards of living, the geographically mobile patterns of living, the types of employment available, and the

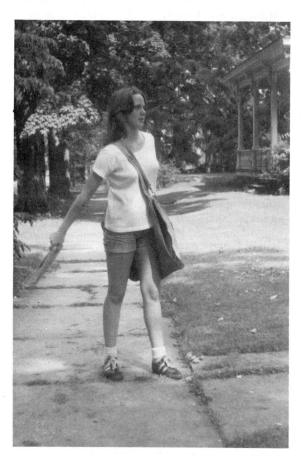

Figure 29–1. Many girls are handling paper routes today—a job formerly reserved for boys.

education required to meet these new standards. These economic changes have created new roles, some of which modify or conflict with long-standing roles, especially those based on gender.

When one examines the changes in the standard of living, it soon becomes apparent that expectations have risen considerably. Perhaps more important than the actual rise in living standards are society's accompanying expectations. The impression that very few people live in a state of poverty has made it even more uncomfortable for those who do. In order to obtain a higher standard of living (or even to maintain a middle-class standard of living), both spouses frequently are required to work outside the home. Thus some women are "forced" into a role for which their early years may not have prepared them. Other women work outside the home by choice because they feel this is an expression of their potentials.

It has been difficult for many families to integrate the reality of the wife's being employed away from the home into the traditional role for women. This situation has necessitated changes for everyone. Some families have attempted to continue the traditional male-female division of household duties, with the woman responsible for child-rearing and the indoor household tasks. Even with many modern conveniences, however, the wife frequently feels that it is unfair to her to have to work full time and still maintain full home responsibilities while the husband works only at his job and refuses to assist at home. On the other hand, some husbands feel it unfair that they continue to work full-time away from home while modern conveniences have decreased the wife's work load, giving her time for leisure while the husband works. Each couple struggles with these issues anew; often the redivision of labor and a redefinition of roles are sources of major disharmony in the marriage, although when resolved, they can also be sources of renewed vitality and satisfaction in life.

Raising the standard of living is hard to do in some situations, particularly for the single-parent family. Over 90 percent of single-parent families are headed by women [3]. Although most persons find it difficult emotionally and financially to maintain a single-parent family, it is considerably more difficult for most single female heads-of-household to maintain a middle-class standard of living than it is for single males to do so because of differences in salaries. The situation is even more tenuous for women of racial or age minorities, who find employment opportunities limited. Fortunately, women have directly benefited from the influx of men into certain professions, such as social work and schoolteaching. The wage scale has increased in these occupations significantly more quickly than in other traditionally female occupations.

A second significant economic influence has been the change in patterns of living. The continued movement from rural to urban and suburban living has once again meant changes in male and female roles. It is a common lament that if a woman is home during the day, she must become the chauffeur for the family, frequently not by choice but out of necessity [1]. Although this role has given the wife a certain amount of independence and has certainly reinforced the need for a driver's license, it becomes a difficult position because, once again, the woman may feel that she is a "gofer" rather than a partner in the adventure of marriage and parenthood.

Many of the employment options existing today were not available 10 years ago. These changes have forced a shift in the classification of jobs, which may not fit with traditional gender, race, or age expectations. Giving up the idea that mathematical concepts and logic belong only to males is a difficult task for many men and women; most occupations that call for these skills are still dominated by males. It should also be noted that it is just as difficult for society as a whole to adjust to the idea that males are equally competent in professions that involve the care of children or assistance with the activities of daily living. Critical changes are occurring; more males are entering the field of nursing, social work, and early childhood education.

Although many of the highly manual, skilled jobs have been traditionally filled by males, this concept also is being challenged. Many women are now demanding that their individual talents rather than their gender be considered as the primary criterion for employment. The equal rights movement has made considerable impact on equal employment laws and opportunities. However, male leadership still seems to predominate in many companies and in government bureaucracies. One must recognize, in fairness, that this situation may at times be due to insufficient numbers of adequately trained or experienced women as well as to cultural pressures.

Fair employment and education laws are also beginning to break through gender and minority discriminations based on traditionally acquired roles. Some occupations, such as law enforcement officers, lawyers, and physicians, have traditionally excluded many qualified women. In recent years, there have been many pressures in these professions to take a higher proportion of minorities of all categories. This pressure has forced the reassessment of professional roles, in terms of competencies rather than in terms of gender or ethnic values.

Recently a growing number of "househusbands" have been noted. Sometimes this decision to reverse traditional roles is welcomed by both partners. Frequently it begins as both a necessity (the husband is unemployed) and an adventure. Role reversal can lead to a better understanding of the spouse's frustrations. Thus far, few families have maintained this alternative style of living for a long period of time (e.g., 10 years).

Persons who are forced into role reversals due to unemployment may resent or feel threatened by the new responsibilities and relationships. Role reversal may be neither welcomed nor seen as an adventure. Consequently, unemployment may be devastating to the identities of the adults and subsequently have serious and negative effects on the development of children.

High schools have been forced to make curriculum changes in anticipation of the changing life-styles and family structures that are emerging. Many high schools now include classes to prepare young people for independent living and to orient them to the establishment of a family of their own.

Influence of the Mass Media

Differential treatment according to gender begins the minute a person is born. Research indicates that the amount of touching, the type of touching, and the amount of verbal interplay are closely related to the gender of the child [12]. These subtle influences also affect one's gender-role behavior very early in life. The early images we receive of male and female roles are often not examined until adolescence or beyond. In the past, the exposure to roles, goals, and value systems could be carefully monitored by the family and the society. Cultural mores required that people be discreet or discriminating with the images of men and women that were presented in the print media. With the advent of movies and television, however, a total picture and image became possible, and multiple events can be portrayed simultaneously. A wide variety of cultural life-styles, values, and roles can be presented. Not only is it possible to present an event more graphically, but dress, mannerisms, and attitudes can also be conveyed more readily. Intricate and intimate interactions between persons can be—and are—clearly depicted in movies and television.

Several studies have been conducted on the racial and gender-role models presented to children on television and in books. According to one research report, males were most often in the lead role, were more aggressive, and more often came out the winner. Females

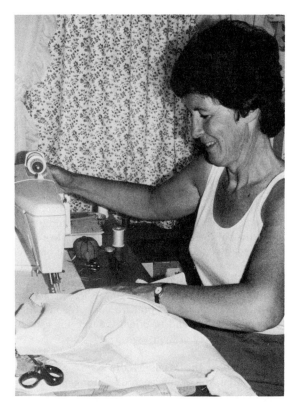

Figure 29-2. Some women find the role of housewife to be rewarding. It offers them opportunities to be organized and creative in their own way and at their own pace.

were less often the primary character; they were portrayed as being dependent and sometimes cunning [16]. A number of very deliberate efforts are currently being made to present alternative gender-role models to children. Monitoring the media to which a child is exposed will make a difference in the child's expectations.

As an adult, it is still difficult not to be caught up in the stereotyped role patterns presented by the media. Whether we are watching a commercial urging us to have "sex appeal," to be "more of a man," or to dress in today's fashion or a program showing a successful doctor, lawyer, or police officer, gender-role models are reflected. The effects of mass-role expectations are far-reaching. Even when conscious efforts are made to be more aware of and to eliminate the old cultural stereotypes of males, females, age groups, and races, society often ends up merely creating new role expec-

tations or stereotypes based on these characteristics (Fig. 29-3).

GENDER-ROLE EXPECTATIONS

Male Roles—Past and Present

To describe the concept of masculinity, either past or present, is a difficult task. No one definition is possible, partly because there are so many specific exceptions to any or all definitions. An attempt to describe the mannerisms associated with male role expectations often results in a series of negatives, such as men do not cry, men do not show their feelings, or men are never scared. Positive ways of describing masculine mannerisms include naming characteristics, such as physical strength, stoicism, aggressiveness, independence, ability to take command of situations, and other characteristics that are incorporated into the "macho" role. (One might note that even the term *macho* has a different meaning to different individuals or cultural groups.) The value of male characteristics is heavily influenced by ethnic group, socioeconomic level, individual goals, and educational level. Members of some subcultures, who find survival both tenuous and difficult, usually place high value on the macho attributes. Since these mannerisms of toughness and physical strength may not be necessary or even appreciated by some males, these males may experience some role conflicts with their cultural peers or even within themselves if they accept the idea that they are "less male" because they do not possess these characteristics [21].

The male role has experienced great changes in the vocational field. Traditional male occupations have included those requiring arduous physical skill or leadership and responsibility. Traditional male role models, or heroes, have stressed the physically rough man who did not acknowledge either emotional or physical pain. Much of the emphasis for male socialization has been the use of the military model. For many young males, this is still the primary role model. This model stresses independence while striving to become the one at the top. It places little value on individual differences or needs.

Until the early 1900s, very few fields of employment were closed to men because women were usually confined to the home and thus were unavailable to compete for positions. As new fields opened up that required specialized education (e.g., engineering, computer programming), these were also seen as male po-

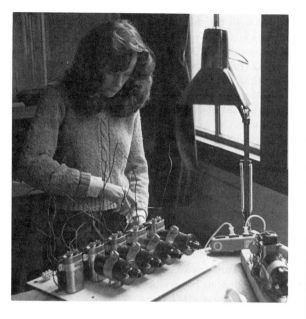

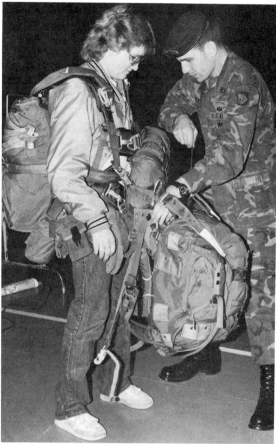

Figure 29–3. Women in today's world pursue activities and careers once exclusively reserved for men. (Photograph on right by Ed Slaman.)

sitions because they involved the use of machines and numbers. As service-oriented professions expanded (e.g., teaching, nursing), these were seen as feminine occupations, since they appeared to be extensions of the woman's role within the home. Today, however, most employers are required to use less discrimination on the basis of gender in their hiring practices. Employees should be and often are chosen on the basis of competence, individual talent, and interests rather than on the basis of gender. Intelligence is not limited to male physiology, but neither is empathy the sole prerogative of women! The changes in the male role have been gradual. It should be noted, as mentioned in Chapter 1, that these changes occur more slowly in the working class [21].

The role of the single male adult has often been seen as an enviable position, and a number of expectations have been assigned to this person. He is the "rich uncle" to some or the "nonconformer" to others. A man

in a specific career, such as medicine or the ministry, is expected to be very devoted to his work or to God. Sometimes a single man will be devoted to the care of an aging and infirm parent, usually his mother. Today the expectations seem to be less polarized. For both men and women, the single state is becoming more acceptable and valued in its own right. Society is recognizing that being single can be a conscious choice on the part of an individual for many reasons, which do not necessarily have to be explained. As a result, fewer specific role expectations are based solely on one's marital status. A single man is no longer stereotyped as a socially isolated man or as a "Don Juan."

Throughout history, role expectations for husbands in western societies have included those of protection and provision. Colonial as well as pioneer men were pushed into these roles with little question; brute physical strength was essential to daily survival. Along with these expectations was the premise that the man should hold the leadership position in the family and should be in charge of both the household and community affairs. Today many of these male role expectations have continued. Although there is less need for physical strength, many husbands still see themselves as the primary protector and provider of material goods. These role expectations may be reinforced by the wives.

Cultural role expectations for husbands are in a state of flux at this time, which is a potential source of anxiety and tension for both men and women. Both men and women often use the husband's economic ability to provide as a yardstick for measuring both the man's worth and his worthiness. (It is obvious that these qualities are not equivalent; think of what happens to human dignity in this value system if the man is unemployed, often through no fault of his own.) One of the authors, while counseling clients, has found that many husbands express total dismay and disbelief when they are told that providing economic security alone does not satisfy their wives. Wives also expect emotional warmth and stability, a satisfying sexual partner, interesting company, and many other characteristics, depending on the specific needs of the woman. These other role expectations seem to come as a surprise to some husbands.

Tension in marriages is quite often the result of different role expectations and the accompanying unfulfilled needs. The role behaviors and values learned during one's childhood may be entirely inappropriate in the new relationship, since circumstances and needs may be very different from those of the family of origin. New heroes, or role models, are emerging. Gerzon, in *A Choice of Heroes*, identifies five new masculine role models. He labels them as the healer, the mediator, the companion, the colleague, and the nurturer. These new role models may in fact be more appropriate for today's society [7].

The role of husband is frequently coupled with the role of father. In the past, fathers were expected to play a somewhat limited role with their children. Once the child was conceived, the father's role was often defined only in terms of supporting the mother both financially and emotionally. Often he was the reserve force for punishment. Any direct care for the child was seen as being over and above his duties; in fact, it was seen by some as a demasculinizing activity. The father's responsibility was to be a role model for male children and to impart whatever sexual knowledge was to be given them. He represented the stern, sober side of life.

Today a father is expected to be more actively involved with his children. Direct physical care of very young children is expected as well as continuous open, warm, emotional contact. Many men are finding these contacts to be both interesting and rewarding. One result is that more men are seeking custody of the children during divorce proceedings. Others, however, find the demands uncomfortable and do not allow themselves to become too involved. The divorced father is in a unique position. After having become emotionally involved, he then finds himself alone and cut off from his children. The adjustment to being a "weekend father" is often so painful that having no contact at all becomes easier for him to cope with.

Female Roles—Past and Present

To describe feminine traits is equally difficult. What are the mannerisms that distinguish a woman from a man? Each of us is too close to the question to be completely objective. Differences are taken for granted; only when a person seems to be out of character for his or her gender is attention focused on what is a gender-appropriate behavior or trait. Female mannerisms and characteristics are not the opposite of those possessed by males. Both are culturally defined and mediated. Some personality traits that people have come to expect of women include kindness, helpfulness, patience, gentleness, daintiness, gracefulness, seductiveness, emotionalism, and passivity as well as being a good listener and domestically oriented. Children's books and records are a fairly accurate indicator of what female as well as male role expectations have been and, to a degree, still are.

Today the traditional definitions of female behavior are being challenged, since these role expectations are generally limiting rather than proactive. Women are attempting to eliminate the limits and constrictions and to conform to fewer role expectations based solely on gender differences. Thus to attempt to define "typical" female mannerisms today is both impossible and foolish. Most limits are being challenged, but not all have been eradicated. Some people observe that most women more than 55 years of age are comfortable with the more traditional divisions of male and female roles while most women less than age 35 are uncomfortable with stereotyped roles [24].

The role of the single woman is undergoing marked changes. In the past, the single woman was usually cast as a spinster or an "old maid." Sometimes this role carried with it a heavy family responsibility, such as the care of elderly parents or infirm siblings. The role of career woman was somewhat palatable as long as the career was confined to a service profession, such as teaching, nursing, social work, or library work. The career woman was presumed to be asexual with no current interest in sex and little experience in the past. Generally it was assumed that with time the woman would mellow and "settle down" in marriage. Other career options were seldom entertained for the single woman.

Today a single woman's sexuality is more readily accepted. This acceptance, combined with advances in contraceptive techniques, has allowed more similarity in life-style between the single woman and the single man than was previously known. Career options are less limited than before, so that the single woman is often able to support herself comfortably and move away from her family of origin. However, being single is still frequently seen as a transitional state and not as a way of life. For many women there is still considerable pressure, both external and internal, to marry and to have children [18]. Even with all the cultural advances, the single woman may still be viewed with some suspicion as having a character flaw that makes her undesirable.

For many years the primary female role expectation was that of housewife, which included the wife role and the homemaker role. The role of housewife is frequently seen as being dreary, unrewarding, frustrating, and undesirable. This view is reinforced by much of the entertainment in the mass media; the housewife is portrayed as basically passive, unimaginative, uncreative, and unable to understand her children or her husband's work. Although this portrayal may be an accurate picture of some women, it is hardly a true picture for all or even most. Many women find parts of the housewife role to be very challenging and rewarding.

Helena Lopata studied 571 housewives in the Chicago area. The women in her study identified several major advantages of homemaking, including freedom from supervision, working at one's own pace, and the ability to make decisions. In addition, since the role is rather nebulous, it is possible to "do one's own thing" [13], to find time to pursue hobbies or friendships.

Lopata found that metropolitan American housewives do not form a homogeneous group, as implied in the mass media. Although many housewives accepted the concept that a woman's major responsibility is the home, they also saw the home as a place for expression of creativity and opportunity for multidimensional expansion. Many of those with higher levels of education and income found interest in supporting their husbands' careers as well as becoming involved with creative child care, community activities, and self-expression, whereas others felt that the only occupation worthy of intellectual identity was a career or a job. Lopata did find that housewives, as a whole, expressed a more limited view of life than did single or career women, regardless of age or of educational, financial, or social level [13]. The disadvantages of being a housewife included limited adult companionship, minimal mental stimulation, work that is never really finished, and limited time for self and self-expression.

The role of wife is one that is dependent on the accompanying role of husband. Wife and husband can be seen as complementary roles. In the past, the wife was often seen as an extension of her husband and his career. Some women continue to be comfortable with this arrangement. Many women, however, prefer to carve their own personality on the role of wife. One change is the tendency to expect more out of the relationship. For many women, this means that they expect more from the sexual relationship for themselves; they may also want more emotional support and companionship from the relationship. One conflict that frequently arises is the husband's assumption that "more" is simply a desire for more material rewards or more frequent sexual activity. Thus a gap in role expectations and fulfillment arises.

The maternal aspect of the housewife role is particularly challenging and rewarding for some women by offering an outlet for the nurturing needs. Some women find motherhood to be supportive of their need to be influential and to have some control and power; this can be seen as a compromise between the traditional aspects of what is considered female and the need to be aggressive. The importance of the mother role is recognized by psychologists and educators, and our culture gives verbal reinforcement to her value and efforts. However, in terms of financial remuneration and other concrete recognition, the rewards are few and far between. Child-care workers are among the most poorly paid, yet they control our nation's most valuable resource—our children. Demands are being made today to recognize the importance of this role. New issues are being raised, including that of the value of homemaking services and of mothering. Consideration of retirement credit for homemaking and higher wages for child-care personnel are only two aspects of this increased sensitivity.

A woman's basic orientation affects her attitudes and relationships with other people. Lopata identified seven distinct types of women based on the focus of their interests [13].

1. **The husband-oriented woman.** Whether motivated by respect, genuine love, admiration, insecurity, fear, or a sense of obligation to her source of income, the husband-oriented woman conveys to others that she is married to the most wonderful man in the world. He is usually successful in providing for the family needs. His word is law, his wish is her delight; no sacrifice is too great for him. When children arrive, they are not to bother him. Babysitters may be used frequently to allow the parents to pursue their social life together. For the wife, the roles of social companion and sexual partner to her husband take precedence over all others.

2. **The child-oriented woman.** This woman marries in order to have children. The basic family unit consists of the mother and her children. Although the husband is expected to provide for the needs of the unit, he is emotionally external to it, perhaps even seen as a necessary evil. He is tolerated, accepted, or appreciated, but he is never a full partner in the family adventure. For the wife, the companionship of her husband and other adults is secondary to her involvement in the world of her children. She may find herself without a meaningful role or identity when the children leave the family.

3. **The house-oriented woman.** The home is this woman's pride; it is kept spotless regardless of income level. Neither children nor husband are to mess it up. Her role is to keep things well-organized and clean. This type of woman feels that she can control her house—it stays the way she puts it, and it does not talk back. She frequently feels that other people impinge upon her, but her home is her stability, the concrete proof of her competence.

4. **The life cycle-oriented woman.** This woman observes that role changes occur with the entrance and departure of family members. She shifts her attention from the wife role to the mother role after the birth of the first child; the wife role does not assume the central focus again until after the children leave. She can only handle one major role at a time. To be a guide for the children and a companion for the husband at the same time is asking too much, even though she is aware of the shifts.

5. **The family-oriented woman.** This woman is able to blend all the roles in the family: wife-companion, mother-guide, home organizer. She may or may not be a college graduate, but she exhibits spontaneity and creativity in managing multiple roles. Frequently, her personal needs are secondary to or blended with those of the other family members. Her needs may be met only if they are compatible with the needs of other family members. Flexibility and enjoyment of life with others are her hallmarks.

6. **The self-directed woman.** This woman may also blend the three roles easily, but she sees each as a unique opportunity for self-expression, since her major focus is her own individuality. Learned roles may serve as guides, but her expectations are uniquely her own. She may sympathize readily with women's liberation movements.

7. **The career- or society-oriented woman.** This woman is rare among housewives, since the focus is on her role outside the family. According to Lopata's research, she is usually very young or no longer married. Children usually are not included in her life plan. Since childless marriages are more acceptable, this orientation is a more viable option for the woman who wishes to pursue an individual career within the context of marriage.

The role of housewife has been taken so much for granted in the past that little study has been done on the subject. Although it is a role most women experience at some time in their lives, little orientation is provided for it, except for the role modeling that a girl receives from her own home [13]. A number of changes appear to be taking place in this role with changes in technology and culture. It is likely that changes will continue to occur as the various aspects of the housewife role are examined more closely.

Blending Roles

Every society has had some form of family system [6]. The family has been the major socializer for gender and social roles. Three major orientations are observed [15]. **Postfigurative** societies emphasize continuity with the past. Custom is sacred and individuals rigidly adhere to roles. Because of great stability and resistance to change, the children are able to see their own futures in their grandparents' lives. Innovations are assimilated, not accommodated since they allow no alternatives to their life-style (e.g., Amish communities). **Cofigurative** societies allow the young people opportunity to adapt to cultural changes. The grandparents no longer serve as models. But a generational break is never complete, since both the past and the present influence development and attitudes. Most of us fall into this category. **Prefigurative** societies are those experiencing very rapid change. Because the future is unknown and past models are seen as inadequate, each young person creates an individual standard of behavior and a personal value system. Innovations are accommodated, not assimilated. Several post–World War

II countries faced (and are still facing) this dilemma. Children in urban areas feel the estrangement more quickly than those in rural areas.

Sociologists and others are increasingly aware that culture is not a static entity. Although this creates a barrier to role stability, it also provides the opportunity for role creativity—the opportunity to move from stereotyped to individualized roles. This opportunity presupposes, however, the ability to accept others in their new roles as well as the expectation that we ourselves will receive acceptance from others. Adherence to traditional roles tends to keep a husband and wife in their own worlds [6]. Working-class couples have the greatest difficulty with this issue. Since each becomes involved with his or her respective breadwinning and/or homemaker roles, the companionship role is underdeveloped. Each tends to turn to their gender peers for leisure-time activity, support, and advice, rather than to the spouse. Companionship, as mentioned earlier, is a foreign concept to them.

The basic orientation of an individual may encourage him or her to continue with traditional roles within the family and within society. This can still be rewarding.

"Instrumental and expressive orientation are not only encouraged by sex-role socialization and cultural norms, but they are chosen by people because of the rewards for each type of performance. Instrumental action tends to be rewarded with the recognition of achievement and personal approval, such as income, social honor, and high grades (as in education). Expressive leadership is rewarded by such personal qualifications as affection, social approval, love and concern. While each sex can respond to both types of rewards, men tend to find greater social support in their striving for instrumental rewards, and women in expressive gratifications. These preferences are, of course, socially learned, but that fact does not make either one any less gratifying to the people involved" [6].

Most of our daily contacts consist of formal, impersonal roles. Consequently, we need a private, relaxed, affirming relationship with another person(s). "We live much of our lives in roles—a student, worker, husband, wife, son or daughter. We live and act out these roles conventionally. They do not necessarily reflect our deepest selves. If we pretend we are only these roles, acting them out as if they reflected our deepest selves, then we have taken the path toward isolation, loneliness, and despair. We may reach a point at which we no longer know who we are" [20].

The family is one place where we need to be able to fully express ourselves as persons [9]. That is not to say that roles are inappropriate. Roles are still essential for the division of workload and the smooth functioning of the family as a whole (see Chap. 33). But the family is where rules are flexible enough to allow experimentation with one's interests, skills, and time in the face of life's exigencies. Flexibility and creativity help the

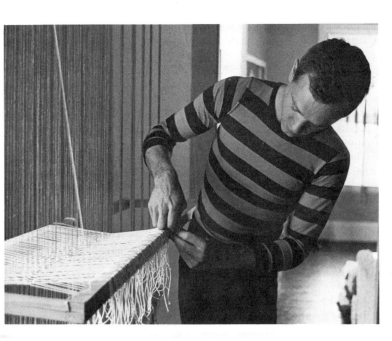

Figure 29-4. Many men today take pride in their handicraft skills as a way of expressing their unique interests. (Photograph by Ed Slaman.)

developing individual as well as the parents (also developing individuals!) to interface more effectively with the external world. When the rules governing the behavior expectations of roles are relaxed, everyone benefits.

When people experience the freedom to share themselves honestly with others, then both parties get to know each other more fully. As the person discovers the self, he or she is freed from externally imposed traditional roles and released to maximize potentials in creative ways. Old roles may be incorporated or released, but the new roles assumed by the authentic individual, are respectful of the needs and rights of others as well as the requirements of the moment. One no longer needs to rely on a "power structure" for security and the smooth orchestration of either a family or a business life. When the husband and wife share more egalitarian roles within the family, both find affirmation, richer companionship, and more appropriate role expectations [6, 20] because they respond to one another as total persons rather than stereotyped roles.

The healthy person is able to use the roles learned during earlier years as a foundation for growth while exploring his or her potentials and finding a niche. Eventually, there is a blending of old and new roles that satisfies the requirements of the situation without compromising the integrity of the individual.

SUMMARY

Social roles are sets of expectations tied to specific tasks and characteristics. Roles may be chosen or assigned because of certain characteristics, such as age, gender, or race. Each of us plays several roles at one time: Some of the expectations are harmonious with one another, some are dependent on one another, and others are in conflict.

Many roles still depend on gender. It is part of our basic orientation to life. But the devaluation of one gender limits the development of both! The elimination of restricting stereotypes is a task that concerns both men and women since gender roles are reciprocal [17]. Men frequently need to be encouraged to find their expressive self, while women need support in finding their instrumental self. Polarization of roles stifles the potentials of each. "Men and women should both retain the traits they prize and adopt cross-sex attributes, and thus move beyond sex role limitations" [17].

Whether one acknowledges, tries to break with, or goes along with role expectations, roles are important for both individuals and society as a whole. As challenges to these expectations occur, it is necessary to sort out specific out-dated role expectations that are still being applied. Roles need to be assessed in terms of their potential for the expression of individual values, which allow for the continued growth of the individual. One needs some assistance in preparing for roles in order to reduce role anxieties. In addition, the individual requires some assistance in the choice of roles, so that the roles are focused toward the attainment of personal goals. In this way, even changing roles will still allow for the sensitive blending of past, present, and future.

REFERENCES

1. Byrne, S. Nobody home: The erosion of the American family, a conversation with Urie Bronfenbrenner. *Psychology Today* 10(12):41, 1977.
2. Cherlin, A. Remarriage as an incomplete institution. *Am. J. Sociol.* 84(3):634, 1978.
3. Eshleman, J. R. *The Family: An Introduction* (3rd ed.). Boston: Allyn & Bacon, 1981.
4. Fanshel, D., and Shinn, E. B. *Children in Foster Care, A Longitudinal Investigation.* New York: Columbia University Press, 1978.
5. Garbarino, J. *Children and Families in the Social Environment.* New York: Aldine, 1982.
6. Garrett, W. R. *Seasons of Marriage and Family Life.* New York: Holt, Rinehart & Winston, 1982.
7. Gerzon, M. *A Choice of Heroes.* Boston: Houghton Mifflin, 1982.
8. Goleman, D. Don't be adultish: An interview with Ashley Montagu. *Psychology Today* 11(3):46, 1977.
9. Hutter, M. *The Changing Family: Comparative Perspectives.* New York: Wiley, 1981.
10. Jourard, S. M. *The Transparent Self* (Rev. ed.). New York: Van Nostrand Reinhold, 1971.
11. Kolhs, A. "New Directions for Hennepin County Family Services." Paper presented in Minneapolis, May 1977.
12. Korner, A. F. The Effect of the Infant's State, Level of Arousal, Sex and Ontogenetic Stage on the Caregiver. In M. Lewis and L. A. Rosenblum (Eds.), *The Effect of the Infant on Its Caregiver.* New York: Wiley, 1974.
13. Lopata, H. Z. *Occupation: Housewife.* New York: Oxford University Press, 1971.
14. Mead, M. Sex and Temperament in Three Primitive Societies. In H. L. Ross (Ed.), *Perspectives on the Social Order.* New York: McGraw-Hill, 1963.
15. Mead, M. *Culture and Commitment: A Study of the Generation Gap.* New York: Natural History Press/Doubleday, 1970.
16. Miles, B. *Channeling Children: Sex Stereotyping in Prime-Time T.V.* Princeton, NJ: Women on Words and Images, 1975.

17. Pitcher, E. G., and Schultz, L. H. *Boys and Girls at Play: The Development of Sex Roles.* South Hadley, MA: Bergin and Garvey, 1983.

18. Sheehy, G. *Passages: Predictable Crises of Adult Life.* New York: Dutton, 1976.

19. Staples, R., and Mirandé, A. Racial and cultural variations among American families: A decennial review of the literature on minority families. *J. Marr. and Fam.* 42(4):157, 1980.

20. Strong, B., et al. *The Marriage and Family Experience* (2nd ed.). St. Paul, West, 1983.

21. Troll, L. E. *Early and Middle Adulthood* (2nd ed.). Monterey, CA: Brooks/Cole, 1984.

22. U. S. Bureau of the Census. *Statistical Abstract of the U.S., 1985* (105th ed.). Washington, DC: United States Government Printing Office, 1985.

23. Wixen, B. N. *Children of the Rich.* New York: Crown, 1973.

24. Yankelovich, D. New rules in American life: Searching for self-fulfillment in a world turned upside down. *Psychology Today* 15(4):35, 1981.

X
The Family

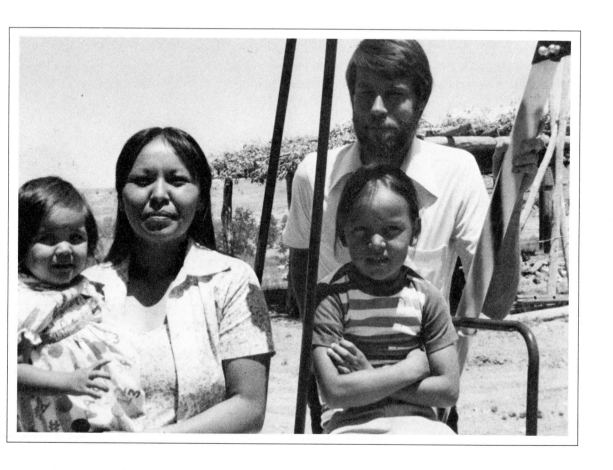

30
Initiating a Family Unit

Clara S. Schuster

> Coming together is a beginning; keeping together is progress; working together is success.
>
> —Henry Ford

Introduction

The Family as a System
Role of family in society
Significance of marital choice

Choosing a Partner
Social factors affecting courtship
Choice to remain single
Traditional steps leading to marriage
Dating
Courtship
Engagement

Establishing a Successful Adult-Adult Relationship
Honeymoon
Establishing the new family unit
Communication between partners
Balancing unity and separateness
Conflict management

Conclusion

The couples who are contemplating the initiation of a new family unit are dedicated to the concept of the "ideal" relationship. They are in love. In spite of the problems they may have observed within their parents' marriages or even in those of their peers, they are convinced that their relationship is unique and therefore immune to boredom and destructive conflicts. Many married couples **are** able to achieve a special relationship—not because they are free from cultural stressors, but because they recognize and work with their strengths and weaknesses. After 3, 12, 26, or 54 years of marriage, these couples will say that they are more in love than when they left for their honeymoon.

A successful union does not just happen because the individuals wish for it. A successfully functioning family unit requires a realistic appraisal of each situation. It requires sacrifice, forgiveness, commitment, and planning. In short, a good relationship is earned—it is worked for—and not automatic because two people love each other.

A good union begins long before a couple pledges their marriage vows. It starts with two people who have learned to know themselves, their goals, and their value systems. These factors become guidelines during courtship as they look for someone with compatible goals, values, and approaches to the exigencies of life. Gradually, through an honest and open sharing, two persons develop a mutual respect that cherishes the uniqueness of each one and yet binds them together in their understanding of life and hopes for marriage and family.

THE FAMILY AS A SYSTEM

The family is a social system comprised of two or more interdependent persons that remains united over time and serves as a mediator between the needs of its members and the forces, demands, and obligations of society. As a system, all the characteristics of open systems discussed in Chapter 2 are pertinent to describing, explaining, and assessing the levels of family functioning.

Role of Family in Society

As a system, the family experiences dynamic interaction with other families and social systems of the culture. Each family affects, and is affected by, this contact with the suprasystem. Society identifies specific responsibilities for families that when fulfilled enhance the total functioning of the society. Each family, however, functions independently and puts its own stamp on the task.

FUNCTIONS OF THE FAMILY SYSTEM

Companionship. The primary function of the family in society is to provide companionship. Humans are gregarious and need affiliation with other humans to fully realize their own potential. We each need to know and be known as an individual in order to appreciate and to value our own uniqueness. The world is too large for us to know and be known in detail by each person with whom we have contact. Consequently, we play a role or present a pseudoself to the world at large. It is only with a small, intimate group of persons that we have the time or inclination to reveal our true selves. Within the family there are a multiplicity of experiences that occur over an extended period of time that facilitate the required peeling away of roles and pseudoselves in order to extract full value from relationships and to promote optimal personal growth.

The consistency with which other persons respond enables us to develop a sense of trust, which lays the foundation for attachment, loyalty, and love—the bedrock of feelings of kinship and the springboard for personal development. Self-esteem is enhanced as family members affirm the presence and value of one another. No matter how badly we fail, in a **well-functioning family** the other members will value our efforts, sympathize with our pain, and continue to accept us.

Many observe that companionship is even more critical than sexual compatibility in marital satisfaction [3, 20]. Genuine companionship fosters an emotional intimacy that stimulates the growth of the individuals while binding them still closer together. When two people are true friends, they are able to share themselves on a personal level. They can share their dreams, disappointments, fears, values, reactions, triumphs, and failures openly without fear of reprisal, ridicule, or loss of face.

True companionship is predicated on an equality in the relationship between two persons. It requires an

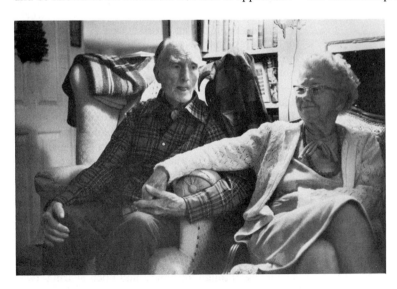

Figure 30–1. True love, mutual respect, and open, intimate communication foster a genuine companionship, a foundation for marital satisfaction, and a springboard for personal growth through the years.

intimate knowledge of both one's self and the other person, so that a sensitive reciprocity is established. It means responding to the total person, and not simply to the role or the concern of the moment. Such intimacy and companionship takes time—even years—to develop. It begins with courtship and can, if worked on, continue through the childbearing years and into the postchildrearing period. Unfortunately, some individuals may become so involved in their breadwinning, homemaking, or childcaring roles that their companionship roles may be underdeveloped, leading to antagonism because of a lack of understanding or appreciation for the other. Cultural and personal factors that advocate rigid gender-role stereotypes tend to keep husband and wife in their own worlds, spending time with same-gender friends for companionship and advice, thus decreasing spousal companionship [20]. As our society becomes more impersonal, the companionship role takes on more importance.

Sexual Relations. Human sexuality serves three functions, each of which can deepen the tie between the couple: reproduction, pleasure, and communication [35]. Every culture has developed its own set of rules to guide sexual expression. Infant betrothals, child marriages, and chaperones are all efforts to restrict premarital experimentation. Incest taboos and rules prohibiting intrafamily/clan sexual relations are also attempts to control potentially disastrous outcomes.

In most cultures, marriage legitimizes sexual relations and expression. The spouses now have free access to a sexual partner, except when medical conditions or religious beliefs prescribe brief periods of abstinence. In most cultures, the spouses are expected to be monogamous, that is, faithful to each other. However, in some cultures, a double standard may allow the husband (but not the wife) to seek other sources of sexual outlet in order to "relieve the wife of her burden."

Economic Cooperation and Protection. In the past, the greater physical strength of the male was essential to provide for the safety of the home and food for the table. The female offered protection by providing clothing and warm meals. Today it no longer takes adult males and females enmeshed in stereotyped gender roles to maintain the economic and social stability of the family. So many tasks have been automated (clothes-washing, transportation) or can be purchased (fresh meat, ready-made clothing) that one can live easily and successfully without an adult partner. However, in spite of this new freedom of life style, most persons still find they can live more cheaply or comfortably when there is a second person to share expenses and home maintenance responsibilities.

Legitimate Procreation. A universal and historical function of family life is the reproduction of the human race—the provision of future workers for the maintenance of society. Legitimacy assures responsibility for the child's care and socialization. "Society's concern with legitimacy is not an effort to brand or embarrass children born out of wedlock, but a well-intentioned attempt to ensure the welfare of the children in each new generation" [20]. Legitimacy provides for the orderly transfer of property, wealth, titles, or position. Blood kinship also assigns primary responsibility for the care of the ill, the disabled, and the elderly.

Socialization of Offspring. The family is the child's training ground for adult responsibilities. It is within the family that one develops self-discipline and a respect for other persons. The child gradually learns and internalizes rules, roles, and responsibilities through the models and guidance offered by the parents.

Enculturation of Citizens. The family teaches its members the traditions, taboos, and values of the culture. Each subculture or family has its own unique status and traditions within the community. Ordinal position, socioeconomic status, and ethnic or religious background give the family its unique orientation to the culture at large. The values and the identities learned during childhood shape our expectations of the adult years.

Social Control. Whenever two or more people interact, some common rules must be accepted by all parties for continued cooperative effort and maintenance of individual rights. Families are expected to help their members to learn and to abide by the rules of society. Successful adaptation to rules within the family is a prelude to successful adaptation to societal rules. When the family cannot, or will not, control the behavior of its members, then society is forced to impose sanctions.

FAMILY STRUCTURE
The family is universal because the needs to which it responds are universal. Its structure varies to meet the needs of a particular society and culture [20]. Agricultural societies tend to have **extended families.** A bride or groom may join the new spouse's household as an-

other member, both physically and psychologically, or the couple may set up a separate home contiguous to the family of one spouse. The extended family may function as an economically cooperative unit. Boundaries between the new couple as a separate unit and the parents may become blurred. Close kinship ties are fostered—a factor that can have both positive and negative aspects, depending on the people involved.

In industrial societies, small mobile family units are essential for economic survival. The new couple separates physically from their families of origin. The **nuclear family** (the couple and their children) comprises an economically and psychologically independent unit. This unit has been the typical family structure in the United States for the past century. Unfortunately, it also has tended to separate family members from significant role models, emotional support, financial assistance, and affirmation during times of crisis.

With the emergence of a technological society, family structure may change again. The nuclear family still appears to be the cultural ideal, but there is a revival of the concept of extended family. Advances in computer technology allow many persons to work at home at a terminal instead of moving from city to city when they change jobs [42]. This allows today's family to combine the best of both basic family structures. They maintain the economic and psychological integrity of the nuclear family while maintaining accessibility to the extended family for continued affirmation and support.

Significance of Marital Choice

In primitive, agricultural, and early industrial societies, families are held together by necessity [42]. Men and women need each other for survival. Gender roles are so rigidly maintained that one cannot survive without access to the services of the other. Today, in western society, marriages are held together by choice, or by consensus and mutual affection, rather than by formal, stereotyped gender controls [9]. For a marriage to survive successfully, the individuals involved must be able to relate to each other as people, not just as roles. Consequently, they need to establish not only a working partnership but a deep friendship as well [8]. Although it appears to be comparatively easy to obtain the dissolution of a marriage from a legal standpoint, an unhappy marriage or divorce is a severe, emotionally traumatic event. Therefore it is wise to be fully aware of the implications of one's marital decision and to know both one's self and the other person as well as possible before the final step is taken.

CHOOSING A PARTNER

Social Factors Affecting Courtship

To those of us raised with the individual freedom granted by western culture, the personal choice of a marital partner appears to be an inalienable right. Yet for much of the rest of the world, and for most of recorded history, people have had little personal input into this decision. Even if free choice appears to be a right, however, there are many factors that narrow the field of choice for us.

CULTURAL MORES

The mode of choosing a marital partner is frequently dictated by the culture. In some, it is strictly by **parental choice,** arranged to meet societal needs or religious goals, to prevent war, to distribute or to retain wealth, to honor ancestors, or to ensure purity of blood lines. Therefore, happiness is not a factor in determining the success of a marriage [22], and failure is not allowed. Gender roles are critical and strictly enforced. Some spouses may never meet before the wedding. In India, a female may be betrothed during infancy. In order to ensure compatibility (at least in skill performance), she assumes residence with her parents-in-law by 10 or 11

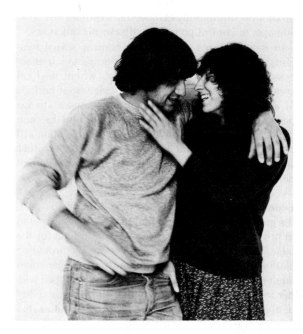

Figure 30–2. Each culture develops its own approved mores for courtship behaviors.

years of age, and the marriage occurs with the onset of menarche.

In other cultures, marital choice is a **joint adventure.** The parents exercise considerable influence, but the child also has a voice in the final choice. The final decision may be made by either party. Meanwhile, considerable effort is taken to prevent promiscuity. Males and females are segregated for all casual and formal social events, and chaperones are employed when dating begins.

Other cultures allow unlimited social and sexual access. The choice is left to the **individual,** but there may still be strong cultural overtones or parental approval may be required. In some cultures the male and/or the female must prove their eligibility for marriage by achieving pregnancy. In other cultures, premarital pregnancy is linked with religious or social depravity. Most individuals in western cultures today seek parental input, or at least approval, but make their own choice of marital partners.

SOCIOECONOMIC FACTORS

The choice of a partner may be a personal affair, but it is strongly influenced by the values and orientation of one's culture, family, and social class. Each class, ethnic group, neighborhood, or social circle has its own values and expectations [27]:

1. Upper class. Graceful living
2. Upper middle class. Career, education
3. Lower middle class. Respectability and stability of job
4. Working class. Financial survival, available job
5. Lower class. Physical survival

Upper-class families tend to maintain more supervision and control over their offspring's mate selection [16, 35]. The children often attend private school (a form of social isolation), and when they leave home for college, the exclusivity patterns tend to persist. Most upper-class young adults marry in their mid- to late twenties—after completion of college and the initial establishment of a career.

Middle/working-class families also provide supervision by encouraging group activities at church, school, or with the family. "Commercial" dating (e.g., skating, dancing, sports) is common. Formal engagement and wedding activities are important social events. Most middle-class young adults marry in their early to mid-twenties—often during or immediately following college or career training.

Lower-class families tend to provide little or no supervision of dating [35]. Engagements are generally informal, and marriage often occurs with pregnancy. Most of these individuals marry in their teens or early twenties before completing their education. We are reminded that such broad categorizations are used to observe trends and should not be used to stereotype specific individuals.

Choice To Remain Single

Some persons make a conscious choice to remain single. They recognize a singlemindedness in their approach to life, and find that their careers take precedence over any desire to marry. Others recognize a strong desire for independence and self-direction, which would be jeopardized by the unity of the marriage bond. Still others, recognizing their own unique personalities, goals, and values, decide that finding a suitable spouse to meet their unique needs is unlikely and consequently decide not to look. Some persons enjoy the freedom of multiple relationships and find the focus on one relationship a stifling experience. Others would like to marry, but are unwilling to take "just anyone." For these individuals, singlehood is far more preferable than marriage to the wrong person.

In a marriage-oriented society, it is difficult for the individual to admit to the self or to others that he or she does not want to marry, is afraid of marriage, cannot find a suitable partner, or would not make a suitable marriage partner. Since the unmarried person is still in the minority, he or she may interpret singlehood as undesirable and suffer episodes of low self-esteem. Between 1975 and 1990, the number of never-married men and women 25 to 29 years of age is expected to rise from 26 percent and 16 percent, respectively, to 46 percent and 28 percent, respectively [32]. Some persons may choose a temporary or permanent single lifestyle for very positive reasons. Others may avoid marriage for very negative reasons.

Emotional intimacy frightens many people [19]. These persons may have fears of: (1) losing personal boundaries or identity; (2) being known too well (the possibility of being revealed as weak, inadequate, or undesirable); (3) being attacked for personal values; (4) being abandoned by one to whom has been entrusted intimate thoughts and feelings; or (5) injuring another emotionally or of being injured, which inhibits singularly or collectively the establishment of emotional intimacy. Those persons who have been victims of incest or exploitation may have developed such a deep fear or hatred of the opposite gender that the idea of a gentle, considerate, loving relationship is incompatible with any previous experience. Some individuals who have previously experienced an intense, emotionally intimate relationship may feel so betrayed by the former partner that to place trust in a second person, or to become vulnerable a second time and chance the agony of another rejection, may be impossible for them. These persons can be greatly helped by good counseling. Unresolved conflicts of this nature will continue to affect all one's relationships, indeed, even the relationship with oneself.

The single person faces some unique social problems. Food packaging and housing options favor married persons and families. Most singles want to enjoy a relationship with peers but may not enjoy the singles' bar or the holiday ski-resort or beach atmospheres. If the single person engages in an honest, intimate exchange with a married person of the opposite gender, he or she is suspected of spouse snatching; if the exchange is with someone of the same sex, the individual is suspected of homosexuality. Consequently, many single persons are prevented from having growth-producing relationships, and feel very isolated from society. Parents frequently continue to relate to their unmarried son or daughter as if he or she were not yet fully adult. Single-parent adoptions help to offset some of this isolation, but they cannot make up for peer intimacy. However, many singles find greater acceptance by both family and married peers after an adoption.

Traditional Steps Leading to Marriage

The method of choosing a marital partner varies widely among cultures, and has changed radically in western cultures during the past two generations. Today, marriage is preceded by a period of increasingly intense social pairing, which offers the opportunity to gradually narrow the potential options for choice of a permanent partner.

DATING

Most individuals date several persons prior to marriage with no commitment beyond the actual agreement for the date itself. Many people date purely for the fun of it. In some cultures, it is considered unusual and immoral to date without a marriage commitment or without at least an interest in exploring that option [13].

The nature and character of a date is highly influenced by the age as well as the social position of the participants. Most persons begin dating in junior or senior high school and continue until they marry.

Younger daters frequently are involved in group activities, such as roller skating, school dances, or a spontaneous get-together at the local McDonald's. Older daters tend to prefer more solitary activities that allow them to explore a common interest (concert, boating) or that facilitate communication to enhance their knowledge of each other and themselves.

Functions of Dating. Dating serves several important functions:

1. Dating provides activity for leisure time. Dating offers opportunities for entertainment, recreation, even education, as the couple pursues a common hobby or interest together.

2. Dating can offer status to the persons involved. A date with the star football player or a cheerleader may offer as much status to the adolescent as a date with the community's leading attorney or TV newsperson would to a young adult.

3. Dating offers the opportunity to learn interpersonal skills. Individuals get to know how others think and react to events. They learn that there are differences in emotional responses and expression. They teach each other how to adjust their behavior to meet the other's needs and how to behave in a new situation. They learn negotiation, the give and take so essential in a working relationship.

4. Most importantly, dating helps the individual to learn about him- or herself by clarifying one's value system as it is applied to various situations. Dating lays a groundwork for courtship by helping one to identify what type of person is most compatible with one's personality.

5. Some persons date in order to pursue a friendship. They thoroughly enjoy the companionship of a particular person whom they date with no thought of a permanent relationship. Both individuals can mature as they share their lives, values, and goals with each other.

6. Still others may date to engage in sexual intimacy. It may be an immature but honest search for love and security, or it may be purely for exploitive reasons with no intention of follow-through and responsibility nor any idea of the long-range effects on the other person.

7. Dating also constitutes a form of courtship, especially as one matures. Each date holds the potential for meeting one's future partner. Dating permits the individual to select his or her partner on the basis of personal preference and paves the way for an eventual decision to marry a specific person or to remain single.

Process of Dating. Initiating a date increases vulnerability, thus it is very difficult for a shy or insecure person. Even a legitimate rejection may be interpreted as personal devaluation [2]. The first date with an idealized "special" person may be fraught with so much anxiety that communication is inhibited. Dates structured around group activities tend to reduce the strain on a couple by spreading the responsibility for conversation and activity and reducing the focus on the individuals involved.

On their first few dates with each other, individuals tend to use formal or stereotyped behaviors. Gradually, as each begins to know the other better, they move toward a more relaxed, individualized, and personalized behavior. The relationship becomes more meaningful as they dare to be honest with each other about feelings and values. The more affirming and committed they become to the relationship, the more they dare to be themselves [2].

Dating sharpens one's ability to see people as individuals. All men and all women are **not** alike. The ability to make fine discriminations between them enables one to make a marital choice that is based on identification of the most compatible factors.

Each relationship is a learning experience for future relationships. One needs several deep relationships to get to know one's self and how to negotiate conflicts of interest. The benefits of dating include learning how to deal with frustrations and difficult partners, learning how to communicate thoughts effectively, learning how to empathize with another's feelings, learning how to resolve a problem and come to a common decision, and learning how to commit one's self to another. In addition, dating provides an avenue for the emotional weaning from parents [2].

COURTSHIP
Courtship begins when both members of the dyad have marriage in mind whether or not this intention is verbalized [17]. Often there is no sharp line between dating and courtship.

The Filtering Process. Because people are socialized to value certain traits, they tend to marry someone who exhibits similar characteristics and values (homogamy). When a couple shares a similar background, they have "organized their stock of experience in a similar fashion" [40], a factor that facilitates communication and reduces conflict of values. The choice of a mate naturally begins with who is available. The individual's contact group tends to bring together persons of similar class, interests, education, and goals.

From this pool of eligibles, one tends to select or to eliminate potential partners on the basis of physical appearance, height, age, race, energy level, or social habits. Physical attractiveness and personality are primary components in the initial choice. As the relationship becomes more complex, lifestyle, aesthetic interests, hobbies, communication sensitivity, and leisure-time activities tend to maintain or dissipate interest in the relationship. As companionship is intensified, values, religious beliefs, goals, family relationships, and ethics are explored for compatibility.

Essence of Love. Eventually a couple decides that they are in love. Love is usually the only socially acceptable reason for marriage in western culture [36]. The religious institutions of the culture teach that love nurtures marital happiness and family solidarity and therefore emphasize that love must prevail in family relationships [12]. Immature persons view the experience from the standpoint of "being loved," rather than "sharing love," or "giving love." Consequently, these individuals may fail to learn "how" to love [18]. They assume that it is easy to love but difficult to find the right person to love. Once they fall in love they assume it is permanent and fail to extend the effort required to stay in love.

Although it is recognized that love makes a positive contribution to our lives, love is a very elusive concept because of its highly personal quality. Infatuation, puppy love, and crushes can elicit many of the same physical responses that are interpreted by the individual as true love. True love is variously defined as a deep and tender feeling of affection or devotion, an intense emotional attachment between two people. A crush is a one-sided love that is usually based on the idealized image of another. Puppy love may be quite genuine but immature as yet because of the developmental level and experiential background of the two people involved. Infatuation is a self-centered form of love that grows out of a need to belong to someone. "The other person is a hook on which these self-generated emotions are hung" [5].

Infatuation versus Love. The idea of love at first sight is a myth. True love is a gradually emerging emotion that is not possible until the uniqueness of the individual is recognized. Infatuation tends to ignore reality and to idealize the loved one while focusing on physical characteristics, limited experiences, and minimal emotional intimacy. The individual often has a blind sense of security or jealousy or refuses to look at the relationship or the other person more deeply for fear of losing the idealized image. The person is actually "in love with love" and is more concerned about self-enhancement and pleasure than about the welfare of the other or the long-range implications of the relationship.

Infatuation plays an important role in the courtship process in that people generally "fall in love with love" several times before they marry. Love may begin with infatuation, but real love arises from an appraisal of the total person. The deeper one knows the other, the more intense and committed the love and the relationship become. Real love also idealizes the loved one, but this image can be checked against reality without a sense of loss because real love can allow the partner to be wholly himself or herself without feeling a need to make the person fit into one's own image or value system. Eric Fromm shares that the paradox of mature love is that two persons become one while remaining separate [18].

Physical attraction is important, especially in the beginning, but it plays a relatively minor role in an evolving relationship where personality attraction assumes a significant role. Feelings of trust and a sense of security are fostered in a mutually affirming relationship, where each looks for ways to enhance the functioning of the other and to strengthen the relationship.

Fromm postulates that true love is an art that must be learned [18]. We **learn** to love a specific person as we get to know his or her strengths and weaknesses [23]. We accept and love the **total** person. Just as individuals must perform grief work (see Chap. 21) when they experience the loss of someone to whom they are attached, those individuals who are creating a new attachment may have to perform "love work" [24]. "Love is a constructed experience built with feelings, ideas, and cultural symbols" [37]. We allow ourselves to fall in love with persons who meet our cultural, social, and personal criteria for a potential partner.

True love expands the sensitivity and expression of all five domains. The physical domain is energized for activity. Love adds "wings to our feet," and craves satisfaction. The social domain finds expansion through a friendship and companionship that relaxes the mood and thus the body through a sense of security; one's horizons are also expanded through new acquaintances and experiences. The affective domain achieves heights never before experienced by enlarging one's emotional capacity [2]. A partner allows one to give of the self, providing opportunity for the centering of altruistic, allocentric behaviors. This love overflows in relationships with other people. Eric Fromm states that "Giving is the highest expression of potency. In the very act of giving, I experience my strength, my wealth, my power. This experience of heightened vitality and potency fills me with joy. I experience myself as overflowing, spending, alive, hence as joyous. Giving is more joyous than receiving, not because it is a deprivation, but because in the act of giving, lies the expression of my aliveness" [18].

The cognitive domain is involved through confirmation of the other's right to express, feelings, goals, and values wholly, and the reciprocal affirmation by the other of one's own self, feelings, goals, and values. This indicates that love must be a bidirectional relationship or else it will disintegrate. Each person must maintain control over his or her own life, actions, direction, and energy. With this foundation, problems can be identified, and the issues negotiated as necessary. Mature love includes responsibility, commitment, unselfish acceptance of the other person's strengths and weaknesses, and mutual respect. The spiritual domain is also sensitized by an increased awareness of aesthetic experiences and the miracle of finding "someone who loves me" and someone who is "worth the investment" of time, energy and intimacies.

Types of Love. As we travel through life, we experience one or more types of love.

Filial love. The love for one's parents is based on dependency, trust, gratitude, and appreciation for the care and sacrifices they have made for us.

Sibling love. The love for one's brothers and sisters is based on companionship, shared experiences, rivalry, and competition. The quality varies with the culture and the family, but there is a tendency to feel a genuine kinship and desire to support one another as necessary regardless of previous altercations.

Spousal love. This love takes many forms, which may be transient, fixed, or mixed in any single relationship. **Erotic** love focuses on the physical component. **Romantic** love idealizes the spouse and spawns selfless devotion. **Manic** love is a combination of erotic and romantic love that is characterized by obsessive feelings of jealousy, and the sense of a loss of control over one's own destiny. The individual often feels that life without the partner would be meaningless and goes to extremes to maintain the relationship. **Pragmatic** love is practical and realistic. The goal is mutual contentment with a focusing of energies toward compatibility and mutual problem solving. **Ludic** love avoids a deep emotional commitment. Fun, not rapport, is the goal. **Philos** love focuses on commitment, closeness, shared experiences, and friendship. There is a deep, enduring companionship expressed as mutual caring, affection, and support—the precious commodities of a solid relationship. **Stogic** love is an extension of friendship. Although a solid relationship exists, it is basically unexciting and uneventful. **Altruistic** love parallels parental love in that the need to provide nurturance to the other takes precedence over one's own welfare. **Agape** love is an intellectual or aesthetic love. It seeks not to possess but to give. It is a self-spending love. **Parental love.** This love is felt for a dependent person. Feelings range from a sense of power or control to that of humility, which is evoked by the honor of caring for another person.

Feelings of love may transfer or generalize from one person to another, but the uniqueness of each relationship modifies the character and the expression of those feelings.

Identifying Potential Partners. Many persons are frustrated by the inability to find suitable potential partners. Previous life experiences may have left the person "gun shy," or current social contacts may be too limited. One should not simply wait while continuing to be friendly, outgoing, warm, and enthusiastic but should seek opportunities to meet people with similar interests and values. Too often in the search for a potential partner, a person concentrates on "what I want." This self-centeredness shows in the individual's relationships. One must treat others with respect and concentrate more on "what I have to offer." This allocentric approach is both more appealing and more mature.

Premarital Sex. Sexual attraction is a normal part of any relationship. At some point, each couple must face the question of how fast and how far their physical intimacies should progress. They must decide on the meaning of sexual intimacies and how and when this is most appropriately achieved for them. This approach implies choice. "Unless freedom of choice is based on an understanding of the alternatives from which choice is to be made, it cannot be truly free. The fact that American society is pluralistic does not imply that the individual is without a point of view. It implies only that he or she works out his or her own point of view, one does not accept it ready-made from others" [5]. If our freedom of choice injures or deprives another of freedom of choice, then ultimately freedom of choice ceases to exist. Both parties must carefully think through the available facts and personal values and accept full responsibility for their own behavior [5]. This

is predicated on a mature understanding of one's value system and motivations.

One study indicates that 95 percent of men and 81 percent of women participate in intercourse before marriage [25]. However, sexual intercourse has a different meaning for each person involved. Males tend to focus on eroticism, whereas females are more concerned about romanticism. Consequently, the motivation may differ greatly, which is fertile ground for misunderstandings of intention and hurt feelings. When the female interprets a bid for sex in light of her own romantic notions of love, she may impart a more serious note to the relationship than is felt by the male.

For some individuals, intercourse may be seen as a way to prove one's masculinity or femininity. Thus, it is a means to an end. However, being a "real man" or a "real woman" involves more than the ability to copulate. The anticipation of sexual demands by one individual may put the other on guard and thus serve as a barrier to the development of a viable relationship.

The age of the participants is another factor that affects the character of a physically intimate relationship. For example, the 15-year-old seeking security, status, or identity will place quite a different meaning on an intimacy than the 35-year-old divorcée seeking companionship, recreation, or personal expression.

The individual's decision to participate in sexual intercourse appears to be consistent with a total outlook on life. "In conservative circles, those who think highly of themselves tend to refrain from intimacies that violate their convictions; conservative women who engage in sexual relations tend to be those whose self-esteem is so low that they are desperate for anything remotely resembling affection and acceptance from men" [2]. In liberal circles, those with low self-esteem are the least likely to have sex [2].

Religious affiliation does not appear to make a significant difference where premarital sexual behavior is concerned; however, the individual's degree of devotedness to a concept of God and participation in religious activities is highly correlated. The more "religious" a person is, the more internalized are the values of his or her religion, the more likely the individual is to avoid coitus before marriage [7, 39].

It is difficult to make an unbiased decision about premarital sex. Parental culture and religious affiliation give one standard; peer culture and mass media offer one at the opposing end of the continuum. Sex is a marketable commodity. "The mass media often function like a lens, dissecting out and magnifying small groups and making them appear to be entire populations" [5]. Adolescents frequently are led to believe that everybody is doing it and that sex is an essential part of adult life. What one believes about sexual need will affect behavior. If one believes it is a form of self-preservation and that dire consequences will result from the denial of basic urges, then one may feel it is acceptable to pressure another person into intercourse. The underlying questions are What controls whom? and Who controls what? Does the individual control sex or vice versa?

Sexual behavior tends to occur in a step-wise fashion. One begins with hand-holding, moves to kissing, various forms of light and heavy petting, and finally to intercourse. Once a barrier is broken, it is easier to engage in the same activity again. Fears and inhibitions are overruled, and sensual pleasure presides. The longer a person is at one level, the less interesting the activity becomes, and normal physical responses impel the person to engage in a more erotic activity.

At some point, the couple must make a decision on the limits of their behavior. They need to engage in a full and free discussion of their feelings, values, and the implications of each step. It is better to move too slowly than too fast because one of the partners (especially the woman) may become angry, disgusted, and disillusioned if pushed too fast [2]. Ambiguous standards tend to invite infractions by an eager partner, which is the reason a real love relationship is predicated on the emotional maturity of the persons involved. One must think through his or her personal values and standards and not leave the decision to the whims of another. Many persons believe that the negotiation and teamwork involved in making and implementing this decision are more significant than the nature of the decision.

The only way to preserve self-respect and personal integrity is by sticking to one's beliefs. If the experience evokes feelings of guilt, it will retard rather than enhance the relationship [27]. "A person who feels something must be done because others are doing it has sacrificed freedom of choice just as much as the individual who refrains from doing something because others have prohibited it" [5]. "A person who seeks mature, integrated behavior patterns seeks to be consistent in his value judgments, his personal and social relationships, and his sexual behavior" [27]. This means that one's relationships, decisions, and behaviors must be consistent with a core value system. The individual cannot override basic values and be at ease with self. "To remove sexual behavior from the ethical context is to oversimplify and dehumanize the individual" [27].

Some persons feel that they prefer to prove their love and respect for the partner by refraining from sex. This avoids any hint of exploitation and stresses the affective and cognitive aspects of intimacy. In one major recent study, only 4.5 percent of the males reported that sex strengthened interpersonal relationships with their partner [30].

ENGAGEMENT

With the announcement of a couple's plans to marry they enter a new world. The couple has confirmed for themselves and for others their commitment and intention. Their courtship has become public. Their relationship assumes greater seriousness and responsibility. They begin to be viewed and to be responded to by others as a single unit. This new label influences their concept of self and their relationship. While engagement offers greater security to the couple, it also affords numerous opportunities for increased tension and conflict as they begin to work together in earnest toward common goals.

The engagement period is ostensibly to prepare for the wedding: arranging for the official to perform the ceremony; developing a guest list; obtaining a marriage license; submitting to a blood test; and so on. However, the engagement is in reality the beginning of the couple's formal unity while it at the same time offers them the opportunity to assess their compatibility and to take appropriate action if necessary before the final step is taken.

Functions of the Engagement Period. The engagement period fulfills four major requirements. First, it allows the couple to strengthen their relationship. The increased commitment encourages heightened openness and intimacy. How well do they really know each other? The sharing of feelings, opinions, and values provides the opportunity for increased closeness, but it also risks the possibility of rejection by the other. This is the reason it is so critical that each person know him- or herself well before making a marriage commitment (see Chap. 28).

When one's identity is secure, then he or she brings a healthy, positive outlook to the relationship. One's values and goals are not tied to the whims, needs, or strengths of the other. The individual is able to be fully her- or himself, offering enough flexibility to be compatible and cooperative, yet with an individuality that brings stimulation and stability to the relationship. A secure identity means that one has the ability to be honest with oneself about one's own deep feelings and therefore can be honest with others [34]. Only through honesty in self-identify is there the ability to evaluate self and to hear the other person's view fully. Then love can spring from "being-love" (giving) rather than "deficiency-love" (taking) to create a healthy, growth-producing relationship [31]. Deficiency-love is a selfish love characteristic of persons with poor self-concept. These individuals must "borrow" from the other person to feel complete. Being-love shares a peer relationship—each partner can give reciprocally for the benefit of the other. Thus both are enhanced.

Pseudomutuality may develop when one person is unable to tolerate the unique interests, values, and goals of the other. When differences are recognized and appreciated, they can enrich the relationship. When one person feels threatened by the differences, then the couple may extend their energies toward meeting role expectations rather than exploring, developing, and integrating their unique identities [41]. The relationship becomes static because change is seen as a threat. Although the couple may feel unhappy, frustrated, or unfulfilled, they may refuse or may be unable to seek a real solution to their problems, which increase with marriage. If a husband and wife relate to one another only on the basis of roles, the marriage tends to erode.

During the engagement, the couple begins to develop their own traditions—the special song, place, activity, poem, phrases, pet words, and so on. These become a bond of uniqueness that helps to bind them together. They usually begin to think about finances more seriously.

Sometimes an individual feels the need to reveal his or her past in its entirety. If the partner is likely to learn of significant information through a third party, then it is best to share it honestly from the beginning [5]. However, indiscriminate sharing to obtain emotional release is both unwise and immature. Information should be shared because it can help the couple to develop a deeper understanding and appreciation of each other that will ultimately enhance their relationship as they work through issues together. During courtship, the couple should evaluate the emotional maturity and health of one another. The couple may need to seek counseling if they are concerned over these issues. A lack of emotional maturity or stability is highly associated with marital discord [27]. Marriage to an overly sensitive or neurotic person can be very difficult. This trait will not change after marriage; therefore, discord during courtship can serve as a warning.

A second function of the engagement period is to redefine one's social world. Psychologically and socially, the couple become a unit. The individual's orientation changes from the family of origin or a first marriage to the new relationship. If the emotional commitment and focus of energies do not change, the

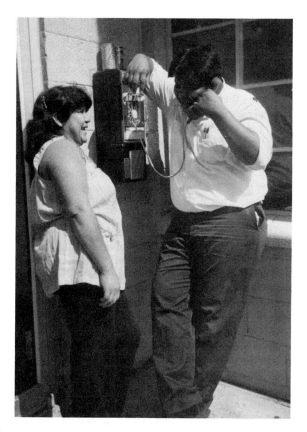

Figure 30–3. Maintaining contact with in-laws can provide support and encouragement during times of stress and excitement.

new relationship is at risk. Marriage is not just a union between two isolated people. It is a union between two families [41]. One must meet and become integrated (as much as possible) with the in-laws. The better the relationship with the future in-laws, the more support and encouragement the couple will receive in the years ahead. Parents can ease the normal anxiety and stress of the engagement period, as well as offer a hand (or a shoulder) when problems arise later. Parents generally begin to treat their child in a more adult manner and the espouser as a member of the family.

During this period one also has a chance to see how the intended mate relates to his or her own parents. This relationship can give clues to one's own marital relationship, since the modeled patterns tend to be replicated. The individual's relationship with the in-laws also gives a foretaste of the years to come. When in-laws disapprove of a potential mate, it is a sign of trouble ahead. Secret marriages to avoid parental censure-ship tend to aggravate rather than to alleviate the problem. The parents are hurt by the lack of trust and confidence expressed by the couple, and the individual now has two hurdles to overcome to reestablish a working relationship with the in-laws.

During this time the couple also becomes more intimately acquainted with the other's friends and social world. Adjustments begin to occur as each begins to drop some old acquaintances and make new friends with more compatible interests. Social habits begin to change as they assume a more serious stance. Each begins to see the other in more diverse situations and to project what marriage to the other person will be like.

The third function of an engagement is to prepare for married life. The couple begins to consider the types of responsibilities associated with the decision and to learn the skills deemed essential to their new roles (e.g., cooking, home repairs, gardening, housekeeping, shopping). Some of the ideas a couple should explore include money management, career goals, religious involvement, household work division, number and spacing of children, feelings about infertility/adoption, values and moral standards, role expectations, discipline of children, leisure-time activities, educational plans, and where to live.

Obviously, most couples are not going to agree on every issue, but this is part of the preparation for marriage: to learn how to negotiate an issue so that neither one feels subjected to the other's view. Issues of power and control will emerge as the couple shares information. This emergence is predicated on the individuals having sufficient time with each other to explore these issues. If one partner in the relationship is in military service or away at college, then communication may be carried out by letter and telephone. However, couples should be aware that it is relatively easy for a completely incompatible couple to have a smooth relationship when they are far apart most of the time [17].

One of the biggest dangers to a relationship is the overly agreeable couple. Often this is because one is always holding back until he or she knows what the other expects or wants. One person may be overly concerned about presenting a positive image of the self to the loved one. As a result, one (the weaker personality), in essence, becomes an extension of the other (the stronger personality). They become two strangers in love because of the lack of honesty, naturalness, and genuine mutuality. It is a superficial intimacy that is more concerned with the self being conveyed than the self one truly is! A wise friend once remarked, "If two

people always agree, one of them is unnecessary." Each relationship needs the stimulating, balancing input of both persons. Interaction patterns will become apparent only with time and exposure. The best marital success is enjoyed by those who have known each other at least 2 years, and have been engaged 6 to 12 months [17, 36].

Assessing Compatibility. A fourth function of the engagement period is the final assessment of compatibility prior to legalizing the relationship. The "halo effect" may mask behaviors that will be interpreted very differently after a few months or a few years of marriage. "Problems that present themselves during the planning stages will appear unmasked and more severe after the couple has been formally united" [17].

A similarity of affiliation needs and emotional stability will facilitate marital compatibility. The couple also must assess their authority/submission needs (see Chap. 17 on ordinal position). Conflicts may arise over who is "boss." The degree of participation in decision making during dating can give a person a feel for the partner's creativity and flexibility. One can be dominant without being domineering. There are many circumstances that require mutual decision making, such as washing the car, deciding which set of parents to visit for the holiday, where to spend the honeymoon, or who should change residence or jobs after the marriage.

Intelligence and educational level are critical factors in a long-term relationship [2, 44] because they effect the uniqueness of input, problem-solving skills, and the ability to work together as partners. A quick wit can sharpen the other's wit and increase life's enjoyment when it is equally matched, but it can be a sword that severs the relationship in a mismatched pair. The less educated or less intelligent partner may feel threatened or incompetent; the more gifted may feel the need to inhibit the expression of ideas that are not comprehended or misinterpreted. The gifted can stagnate without adequate challenge. This stagnation is especially true for the woman [44], who is more likely to remain at home during the child-rearing years with a subsequent decrease in adult peer contact. Playing table games is one way to assess intellectual and emotional compatibility. The **Ungame*** and **Reunion*** offer excellent mediums for getting to know another person.

Sexual expression and compatibility is another area of concern to many couples. Many who abstained during earlier courtship may now participate in physical

---

*Ungame Company, P. O. Box 6382, Anaheim, CA 92806

intimacies as an outgrowth of their new devotion and commitment. Most persons can make a sexual adjustment with almost anyone; therefore, one's spouse should be chosen for other reasons [27, 44]. "If sexual compatibility were a question of physique, this evidence would be crucial. However, this is not the case. Human beings of almost any shape and size can relate sexually. For this reason, it is not necessary to 'try each other out for size'" [2]. Since approximately 50 percent of engagements are eventually broken, some individuals may find that "physical intimacy prior to marriage can make an advisable separation difficult and painful to carry out, and leave the participants guilt-ridden" [36]. Other individuals, of course, may feel otherwise, depending on their value systems.

Another area frequently overlooked by a couple is the energy level or life tempo of the other. One's energy level can either intensify or dull the most routine activity. An individual's zest for life and living can exhilarate or exhaust and bore the partner as the years roll by. One needs a high degree of flexibility to keep up with a partner who has a high verve for life.

Many couples live together without marriage (cohabitation) as a way to assess their compatibility. This is usually an extension of the courtship process rather than an alternative to marriage [35]. Marriage changes the relationship so much that even living together cannot reveal some of the later relationship problems [44].

Prerequisites of a Successful Marriage. Most persons experience homogamous marriages (marriage within their same social group). Homogamy facilitates the compatible blending of interests, values, traditions, and experiences. Common social, religious, and leisure-time contacts tend to lend support to the stability of the relationship. Despite these pressures, many individuals choose a mate with a radically different background, which provides stimulation and novelty for years. These persons have defined their own set of values and can create a very rich, meaningful relationship.

Mixed marriages include not only interracial marriages, but intergeneration, interfaith, international, and interclass marriages. But in truth, every marriage is a mixed marriage, for it brings together two people of different family origins, traditions, experiences, kin relationships, and value systems. For any marriage to be successful, certain prerequisites are essential [2, 17, 33]:

Emotional maturity. A self-objective knowledge of one's own skills, weaknesses, values, goals, and feel-

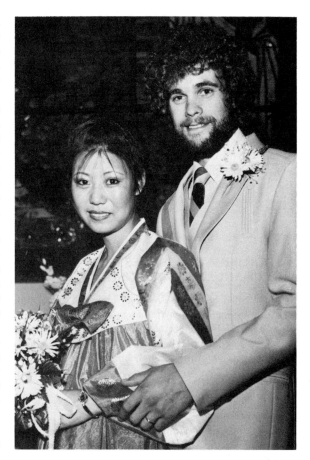

Figure 30–4. Intercultural marriages can provide a wide variety of family traditions for individuals to draw upon while developing their own along with childhood stories that can entertain the couple and their children for years to come.

ings. Maturity includes the characteristics of self-discipline, self-objectivity, and self-responsibility.

Love. Genuine, altruistic, being-love based on realistic appraisal of the total person. "An emotionally healthy person would rather risk the death of love than allow love to develop on an unreal foundation" [2].

Compatibility. Similarity of interests, values, goals, energy, intellectual skills, and lifestyles.

Skill. Communication and problem-solving ability, empathy, and compassion.

Effort. Willingness to sacrifice and to focus all energies toward resolution of problems.

Commitment. The determination to make it work, to "hang in there" during the tough times (all marriages have them). "The degree of their commitment to the marriage will be the measure of its stability while they are learning to cope with the problems plaguing them" [17].

Support. The affirmation offered by family, friends, and community.

Flexibility. The ability to adapt to changes in the other person or circumstances, and to meet life's problems. The couple may work together to create change through dialogue, reading, or counseling. Each should accept the differences of the other as stimulating, exciting, and helping to expand one's world.

Caring. The ability to be concerned about the welfare of the other, to want to care for and to make life better for the other person.

ESTABLISHING A SUCCESSFUL ADULT-ADULT RELATIONSHIP

In the United States, the average male is 25 years of age and the female 23 years of age at the time of their first marriage [45]. Eighty-four percent of couples will opt for a religious ceremony [38]. The wedding signifies the legal beginning of their oneness. A public ceremony allows family and friends to celebrate the event with the couple.

Honeymoon

The wedding is frequently followed by a vacation trip, which allows the couple time to concentrate on and invest in each other. The honeymoon needs to provide leisure, privacy, and novelty. Even if it is short, it will be a special memory later on [27]. The honeymoon serves two basic functions: It facilitates the establishment of marital sexual expression and encourages the couple to make the transition from dual independence to mutual interdependence.

MARITAL SEXUALITY

Both partners must develop sensitivity and competence as an intimate sexual partner if the couple is going to enjoy a satisfying sexual relationship [13]. Neither partner should expect instantaneous success. It may take 2 weeks to more than 9 years before a particular couple achieves a mutually satisfying sexual adjustment [21]. Prior knowledge about anatomy and techniques will facilitate adjustment. Some authorities observe that prior masturbation experiences may help the husband and wife to be more aware of their body sensations and to work with them toward orgasm [2]. The new husband may find that the stress of the moment overrides his eagerness, preventing the attain-

ment of a full or prolonged erection. The new wife may find old taboos interfering with her ability to relax and to appreciate the new freedom of marriage. The honeymoon is a time to become comfortable sharing each other's bodies. Light and heavy petting need to continue as preludes to copulation. When bypassed, sexual dysfunctions may occur [2].

The ability to communicate openly about likes, dislikes, and willingness to be creative also can enhance sexual enjoyment. The couple should remember that sexual freedom does not license exploitation or abuse. Continued mutual respect; flirting, dressing and grooming to please the other; and spontaneous smiles, hugs, kisses, and caresses throughout the day make the time in bed more desirable to both.

Young couples tend to have intercourse frequently. They may try several times daily during the honeymoon, and gradually taper off to three to four times per week. Frequency varies with the couple, but the average appears to be twice a week after several years of marriage [43]. Fifty percent of women experience orgasm within the first month of marriage, and 75 percent within the first year. Orgasm may not be associated with the sexual act, but may occur the next day [29]. Only fifty-three percent of women report orgasm almost every time they have intercourse [25]. Satisfaction, however, is more than orgasm: "The couple will not be able to find sexual satisfaction if they do not find happiness in other ways; but their companionship will find richer meaning and interpretation through their sexual union" [27].

MUTUAL INTERDEPENDENCE

Marriage is fraught with big and little decisions. The couple must merge their independent habits into a mutually compatible routine. Who fixes breakfast? Who uses the bathroom first, and what shelf holds whose paraphernalia? What time do we go to bed or get up? How often and when do we have sex, go to church, eat?

During the honeymoon, the couple begins to realign priorities so that the needs of both may be met, and they begin to turn first to each other rather than to parents or peers for support, stability, and encouragement. During this time, the friendship experienced prior to marriage can become even stronger. In a healthy marriage, the two will become the best of friends, mutually dependent on each other for advice and confidence. Gradually a new oneness emerges, and the marriage relationship becomes more important than the individuals within it [5]. This oneness does not mean an annihilation of the individuality of either but, rather, a respect for the needs of both for the good of the whole. They establish a duet where each blends in a balanced way with the skills and needs of the other. As they practice and get to know each other better, the harmony becomes even more evident to both themselves and others.

Establishing the New Family Unit

Once the bride and groom return from the honeymoon, they must get down to the serious business of establishing a home. The establishment of a home includes mundane tasks, such as cleaning out an apartment and setting up housekeeping; it also means the more complicated tasks of establishing their new roles as husband and wife. Some of these tasks or adjustments include [27]:

1. Establishing routines for daily living
2. Learning how to make purposeful decisions together
3. Building new friendships as a couple
4. Developing relationships with in-laws
5. Establishing a working family budget
6. Developing a "double-person" spending/shopping mentality
7. Establishing religious habits
8. Deciding on contraceptive methods
9. Learning how to negotiate conflicts
10. Learning the give and take of living together
11. Allocating responsibilities
12. Developing effective communication patterns
13. Establishing a shared core-value system
14. Identifying family "rules"
15. Creating common goals
16. Deciding on leisure-time activities and community involvement
17. Establishing financial credit
18. Developing a satisfying sex life
19. Establishing a balance between togetherness and respect for individuality
20. Establishing traditions as a family

The key to a satisfactory and successful negotiation of these and other tasks is the couple's ability to communicate openly and honestly with each other.

Communication Between Partners

There are several characteristics that are found in all successful adult-adult relationships: mutual respect, allocentrism, common interests, self-disclosure, and spontaneity. Self-disclosure is most critical to effective communication. Most of our relationships involve ful-filling a role (e.g., student, employee, neighbor, consumer, attendee, teacher). If we continue to relate to all people in a role capacity, then we relegate ourselves to the position of actor rather than person. As we hide our true feelings and responses from others, we also hide them from ourselves and as a result may lose the ability (or never gain the ability) to know our true feelings, values, and goals [26].

It is in the process of revealing ourselves to others that we discover who we really are [41]. "Alienation from one's real self not only arrests personal growth, it tends to make a farce out of one's relationship with people" [26]. When we fail to share ourselves, we become difficult to know or to predict, and therefore difficult to love. Self-disclosure by one partner encourages reciprocal disclosure by the other. Thus we "touch base" and enhance our appreciation for the uniqueness of ourself and the other. Self-boundaries become clearer and mutual respect is enhanced. When each partner remains emotionally isolated, untouched by the other, the couple retains a role relationship. They may be married, but they can experience an overwhelming sense of loneliness because there is no genuine contact. "The loneliest loneliness is to be alone with someone with whom one wants to feel close" [41].

Marriage survival depends partly on the development of clear and healthy identities [21]. Each partner must have achieved Erikson's earlier developmental tasks successfully [15] and have his or her self-identity firmly in hand (see Chap. 28). One must know who one is before fully appreciating the self or sharing that self with another. One must be honest with the self about deep feelings before one can be open and honest with others [34]. The individual must know who "I" is before he or she can say with genuine honesty, "I love you" [41]. Getting to know one's self and personal values, goals, preferences, strengths, and weaknesses is a task many people avoid or only partially fulfill. Yet self-knowledge is the bare foundation of all other relationships. If the individual knows and accepts the self, then he or she can accept the other, and both lives are enriched through the relationship.

If a person has not completed "identity homework," there may be a cloudy or poor concept of self. Erikson [15] identifies this person as one who tends to retreat or to withdraw from honest communication with others. The low self-esteem that began in childhood continues to color the adult life. "To be married to a person with a poor self-image is horrendous. Marriage does not produce this low self-esteem, but it can reinforce it" [21]. If one partner is constantly subjected to abuse, putdowns, and lack of respect by the other, then self-esteem can be eroded after marriage. If one partner has severe neurotic problems and is constantly rationalizing personal difficulties or projecting them onto others, this too will severely strain the relationship [27].

In both of these situations, the immature or disturbed partner may avoid discussing any problems as a way to avoid emotional discomfort. Facts may become heavily tinged with personal values and feelings. Consequently, mutually satisfying resolution of conflict may become impossible. If both persons are immature or neurotic, then their common inadequacies tend to compound their problems [27].

The partner's self-esteem can be enhanced through continual affirmation of his or her value and presence, reassurance, recognition of strengths and talents, minimization of weaknesses, and by signs of appreciation and encouragement. If one partner is building up the other partner, the partner doing the building should not tear her- or himself down. Each can continue personal growth through reading, acceptance of responsibility, reaching out to other people, continued openness, and involvement in activities that bring pleasure or satisfaction in achievement. Outside friends can reduce the burden of friendship on a marriage, but one must be careful not to allow them to intrude on the strength of the marital bond [21].

BALANCING UNITY AND SEPARATENESS
Families struggle with two opposing psychological forces: togetherness—the need for love, approval, agreement and sharing; and individuality—the need for autonomy, separateness, and recognition of uniqueness [4]. These two forces actually compose a single continuum, representing the ability of the family to see and to appreciate the boundaries between the subsystems of the family [19]. Families with low cohesion and inappropriately rigid boundaries comprise the "disengaged" end of the continuum. At the opposite "enmeshed" end, there is high cohesion and very diffuse boundaries. In the middle "normal range," boundaries are clear, differences are respected, yet appreciation is strong. The key to the continuum is the degree of personal identity mastered by each member and the ability to communicate this to others.

Disengaged Relationships. These family members adamantly assert their independence. They are so concerned about self-recognition and self-enhancement that there may be minimal bonding, or empathy, for others. They may demand their "rights," but do not acknowledge responsibilities to other members. They seldom share their true feelings or values in such a way that understanding is enhanced. Each member is an independent psychological subsystem. Communication is task-oriented, consequently each family member lives a role relationship. They do not really know one another because genuine intimacy is not fostered.

Enmeshed Relationships. Intimacy can become confused with an unhealthy togetherness or an extreme cohesion that results in a loss of personal boundaries and identity [19]. High self-disclosure and inappropriate disclosure (e.g., sharing with the wrong subsystem) can tie the members so closely that boundaries become blurred. Each member is required to be like the other, to have the same feelings and values. One person's business becomes everyone's concern. Reality and individual differences are submerged in the demand for self-confirmation, or reflection, in the lives of others. Such intimacy becomes smothering [19].

This kind of relationship occurs when none of the individuals has developed a strong or healthy sense of personal identity. Instead, each develops a pseudoself—an identity based on external pressures, or roles, instead of internalized assessment, values, and goals. The couple merges their pseudoselves in marriage. They become involved in playing their roles and being what the other person wants them to be. At the same time, each unwittingly demands that the other enhance the functioning of his or her self. However, since neither individual knows the self well enough to identify personal needs or to communicate adequately to the other who he or she is and what may be needed, neither individual truly develops identity even within marriage or takes full responsibility for personal development. The couple, and eventually their children, develop a "mass ego identity" in which all family members are expected to have the same feelings, reactions, needs, values, and goals as the other members.

These individuals feel that they cannot live without the other person because each needs the other for strength or direction. They have difficulty with independent problem solving and decision making. If one experiences injustice or anger, the partner is expected to feel the pain just as acutely as the aggrieved and thus help to dissipate some of the intensity of emotion. This "no-self" individual laughs when others laugh but without understanding. The person has no separate joys, goals, or independent value system and is unable to offer an objective or unique perspective to discussions. Such a person is **very** adept at getting along with others and is well liked, even sought out, because of the tendency to affirm and to support the views of others. Consequently, the no-self person may be very successful at business and in social life, where he or she can play a role. But in the deeper intimacy of marriage, where each must carry part of the responsibility for decision making and value clarification, this individual may be a complete failure. The poor differentiation of self makes him or her merely an extension of the other person. He or she lives vicariously.

The no-self person can be a strong, demanding, flamboyant individual who draws strength and courage from the partner to face the world with confidence; or he or she can be a quiet, hard-working "backseater" or a friendly, joke-filled alcoholic. They all have one thing in common: the strength to face each day and its problems is external to themselves. These individuals do not face stress well, tend to blame other people for their failures, and may retaliate quickly if they perceive support is decaying.

The person who provides the emotional strength, who "gives in," finds it very draining to be the decision-maker and the guide for two people. Many of these persons experience high stress or dysfunction because of the erosion of their emotional strength [4]. Other persons may thrive on the sense of importance and power the relationship gives them.

Demeshment can occur when one partner begins to more clearly define and openly state inner convictions, values, principles, and goals and begins to take responsible action based on these convictions. He or she must be able to maintain a separate sense of self in the face of emotional pressure from the other and to assume responsibility for his or her own emotional reactions. The individual must be able to emotionally step back from an interaction and observe the interplay, much as a third person might do, and concentrate on the process, not just the product, of the interaction. He or she must get beyond feelings and emotions in order to look at the situation realistically and differentiate between facts, beliefs, opinions, and convictions. In this way the dynamics of the situation can be analyzed.

An individaul can extricate her- or himself from an unhealthy relationship by trying to develop a person-to-person relationship, in which discussions are about one's own values, ideas, and opinions, rather than people, events, and things. As one becomes aware of personal feelings and reactions, they can be brought under control. One broadens perspectives by listening to all sides, refusing to align oneself with another's position, or defending one's own. Counterattack is counterproductive. An emotional distance is essential to think about the events of a relationship. Emotional is-

sues are best discussed at a nonemotional time when the facts and the communication process can be more clearly evaluated.

Normal Range. Marital adjustment and balance are closely related to the couple's ability to communicate. The more open they can be and the more areas they are free to discuss, the closer their relationship will be. Two factors facilitate intimacy. The most important is self-disclosure, which requires a balanced, reciprocal sharing of feelings, reactions, perceptions, values, and goals. This sharing of information, which is difficult to obtain from other sources, tends to escalate and become deeper with time. Self-disclosure is the foundation of appreciating individuality. Affirmation, the second factor that facilitates intimacy, is the foundation for togetherness. It is expressed through the many ways one recognizes the existence of the other: responding relevantly to communications, accepting the other's self-experiences, involving oneself in the other's interests, and personalizing one's interactions.

The fear of rejection and other barriers to emotional intimacy can be overcome by the affirming support offered by a warm, sensitive partner. Each person has a right and a responsibility to personal feelings and to differentiate the self from others. We cannot find ourself in other persons, we cannot live life for them, nor use them for our own selfish purposes or self-affirmation [6]. We must show appreciation for the right of other persons to determine their own direction.

Conflict Management. No two people will see eye-to-eye on every issue. It is ironic that the relationship that produces the greatest satisfaction in life also produces the greatest conflict. In fact, the more intimate a relationship, the more prone a couple is to conflict [37]. As they relate to more issues and involve deeper layers of their personality, conflict is inevitable [2]. As they reveal more of the self to the other, each becomes more vulnerable to hurt and affirmation. But it is only as each one discloses personal feelings, preferences, construction of reality, priorities, and limits that personal space is defined and mutual respect fostered.

Cultural tradition encourages the suppression and repression of conflict. This tradition can put a secondary strain on a couple who feel that the marriage is deteriorating when differences emerge. The avoidance of conflict through suppression of self-disclosure leads to the isolation of the individuals, misunderstanding, resentment, anger, hostility, bitterness, hatred, and scapegoating [10]. The couple may develop "pseudomutuality" to decrease the occasions of conflict. They retreat to roles and decrease their intimate exchanges, which merely blurs the problems and moves the couple toward one or the other end of the togetherness-separateness continuum. On the surface, they have a good relationship, but in reality, they miss a healthy relationship (see Chap. 33). Other couples may develop a "pseudohostility." They bicker over trivia and discharge the negative energy that comes from the tension of covering up the real conflicts. Intimacy is again thwarted.

If two people live together and are honest with each other, the uniqueness of their individual needs will clash. Conflict in and of itself is not destructive [10]. In fact, conflict is essential to growth, for it "necessitates the continual negotiation and renegotiation of values, beliefs, and goals" [14]. It is the handling of the conflict which is constructive or destructive. When conflict is successfully negotiated, the individuals have a decrease in anxiety that can lead to growth and personal optimism. Conflict does not dull love. It is an indifference to the partner's frustration, needs, and values that kills love. The honest, even heated sharing of conflicting needs is growth-producing. The avoidance of conflict only compounds the issue by storing up tensions from unresolved conflicts. These tensions will erode the relationship or emerge as a single large explosion at some later point ("gunny sacking").

When two people have healthy self-identities, they can share without fear of losing face or power in the relationship. They meet as equals, each trying to enhance the other.

Many arguments are worthwhile because they (1) enable a person to get in touch with the real self before arriving at a solution, (2) expose the underlying problem, (3) clear the air, (4) enable one to reevaluate the self or one's partner, (5) foster the mutual facing of a problem, and (6) encourage the creation of joint solutions that can draw the couple closer together [27]. If an argument is to be constructive, however, it must be part of the problem-solving sequence. "Hit and run" tactics are destructive and no growth is possible. Conflict, if resolved, helps to assure that neither individual will be "swallowed up" by the other [41]. A good argument can sharpen one's wit and provide a source of healthy stimulation.

Successful family conflict moves through five stages [19].

Prior condition stage. In addition to differences of personality and experiences, prior conditions, such as ambiguous roles and responsibilities, scarcity of essential resources, unhealthy dependency/independence, poorly defined rules, and inadequate information all set the stage for tension. Consequently, self-disclosure and communication are critical factors in reducing surprises and thus the occasion for conflict.

Frustration awareness stage. Individual perceptions will affect sensitivity to tension or conflicts. Inaccurate perceptions can create conflict where none exists. It is critical at this stage to share and to validate perceptions. Couples miscommunicate about 20 percent of the time [41]. Clarification can avoid unnecessary conflicts. Conflict also can be avoided if one decides the negative consequences outweigh the positive outcomes. "Backing off" does not resolve the issue but may be the better part of valor under the circumstances. Getting caught up in the minor issues of life can block one's view of, and appreciation for, the whole picture.

Active conflict stage. Nothing can be resolved if a couple refuses or is unable to communicate with each other effectively. To remain constructive, the couple **must** communicate, which includes listening and empathizing as well as honest self-disclosure. The ground rules for fair fighting are: (1) Make allowances for circumstances; (2) do not confront the other when ill or tired; (3) both persons need to consent to confrontation; (4) meet face-to-face; (5) keep the subject current; (6) keep it private; (7) separate fighting and lovemaking; (8) use "I" statements; (9) listen without interrupting; (10) deal with negative feelings; (11) be honest—why are you really angry?; (12) do not blame; (13) do not generalize (always, never); (14) try humor; (15) be creative; (16) stick to resolvable issues; (17) do not leave scars by accusations or verbal or physical abuse.

When the differences are not negotiated satisfactorily, one of the persons may resort to coercive efforts to obtain compliance. Tradition and Judeo-Christian teaching support male leadership in the family. Many persons quote Saint Paul's admonition to wives to "submit yourselves unto your own husbands" (Ephesians 5:22). They use this as a foundation for unmitigated authority, which demands compliance and obedience. In essence, the wife becomes an extension of the husband's needs, desires, values, and goals.

By taking this statement out of context, people forget that Saint Paul goes on to say that husbands are to "love their wives as their own bodies" (Ephesians 5:28). This means a mutual respect for her needs and values as if they were his own. There is no room for coercion or dictatorship here but the emphasis is on a genuine partnership where both respect the needs, values, and goals of the other. Each is nourished, cherished, and enhanced in such a relationship. The will of the other is sought as a valued contribution to the partnership.

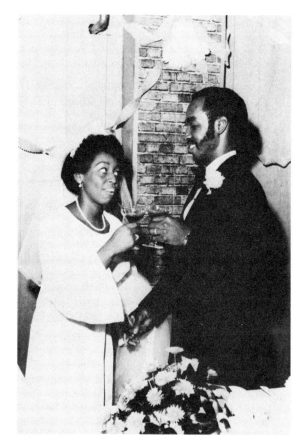

Figure 30–5. Individuals who have taken time to get to know themselves and to develop their own skills generally make wiser choices of marital partners and experience higher marital satisfaction.

The more egalitarian the relationship, the better the communication and the better the conflict resolution. If a couple suppresses hostile feelings and avoids the conflict and satisfactory resolution, then resentments compound to poison the relationship. Loss of self occurs as the relationship erodes.

Solution stage. Rationality must replace subjective, paranoid, authoritative feelings if a mutually satisfactory solution is to be found. Both must participate in the brainstorming of alternative solutions and potential consequences. It is too heavy a burden for one person alone to carry. When both participate, there are no losers—both win, and self-esteem is enhanced. The steps to effective resolution include: (1) defining the problem (they may see it differently), (2) trying to understand underlying causes, (3) considering possible

solutions, (4) agreeing on the best approach, and (5) demonstrating a willingness to implement the solution. The couple does not need to agree on everything or every issue, but they do need to be able to work out a mutually satisfactory compromise. If personal desires, selfish whims, and hurt feelings take precedence over the success of the marriage, then perspective is lost, compromise is impossible, and the marriage is jeopardized. The parts have become more important than the whole. Poor conflict resolution leads to warfare or withdrawal, both of which are self-defeating.

Each person must have sufficient commitment to the relationship to carry him or her over the difficult times. The involvement of either individual in extramarital affairs tends to undermine trust in the relationship and to divert energy away from a resolution of the couple's conflicts [33]. Consequently, it erodes the unity of a couple toward a common goal and mutual satisfaction.

Follow-up stage. For conflict resolution to be successful, both partners must follow through with their end of agreed-upon behavior changes or responsibility. The patterns of conflict negotiation used in earlier confrontations tend to be repeated. Consequently, the early months of marriage are critical to establishing healthy approaches to communication and conflict management. If a couple finds that their confrontations are destructive rather than growth-producing, then marital counseling should be sought early, before permanent scars are left by sharp tongues and immature behaviors.

CONCLUSION

There is no rational reason why anyone needs to marry in the United States today. Roles, responsibilities, and job opportunities are no longer dependent on gender. With technological advances, all needs can be purchased or performed oneself with simplified devices. However, "the very technological advances that have made it possible to live as an unattached individual have created a cold, impersonal world that makes us crave intimate relationships. At the same time, these conditions make it hard to find and sustain them" [37]. Consequently love, companionship, and good communication are essential ingredients in initiating and maintaining a meaningful, long-term working relationship. If a marriage is to last, it must be approached carefully, for such a relationship is all-embracing.

Marriage is a new reality. It is a constantly emerging, developing relationship, which is constructed by the unique interaction of the partners. "Two strangers come together and redefine themselves" [1]. A healthy marriage begins with two people with strong personal identities. This comfort with one's self is discreetly shared with family and close associates. There is no need to continue to play a role in intimate interactions. As one shares inner values, opinions, hurts, and ecstasies, mutual respect and appreciation are developed. Love springs from a desire to share the self and to enhance the other (being-love) rather than from a need to fulfill one's self in another (deficiency-love) [31].

The "responsible I" assumes responsibility for one's own happiness and comfort, and does not blame others for failure or unhappiness. It is in the context of two people with healthy identities that true intimacy evolves into a rich, lasting marriage that fosters the continued growth of each member. Conflict actually helps the couple to grow closer together while it more clearly defines the individual boundaries. Marriage is not an easy relationship. At its best, it is an intense relationship between two very separate people. It takes hard work and compromise to develop a mutually respectful and enhancing relationship. It will inevitably involve the total personality of both partners in face-to-face contact [44].

REFERENCES

1. Berger, P., and Kellner, H. Marriage and the Construction of Reality: An Exercise in the Microsociology of Knowledge. In P. J. Stein, J. Richman, and N. Hannon (Eds.), The Family: Functions, Conflicts and Symbols. Reading, MA: Addison-Wesley, 1977.
2. Blood, B., and Blood, M. Marriage (3rd ed.). New York: Free Press, 1978.
3. Blood, R. O., and Wolfe, D. M. Husbands and Wives: The Dynamics of Married Living. Westport, CT: Greenwood Press, 1978.
4. Bowen, M. Family Therapy in Clinical Practice. New York: Jason Aronson, 1978.
5. Bowman, H. A., and Spanier, G. B. Modern Marriage (8th ed.). New York: McGraw-Hill, 1978.
6. Buscaglia, L. Personhood: The Art of Being Fully Human. New York: Fawcett Columbine, 1982.
7. Cannon, K. L., and Long, R. Premarital sexual behavior in the sixties. Journal of Marriage and the Family 33(1):36, 1971.
8. Caplow, T., et al. Middletown Families: Fifty Years of Change and Continuity. Minneapolis, MN: University of Minnesota Press, 1982.
9. Cherlin, A. Remarriage as an incomplete institution. Am. J. Sociol. 84(3), 1978.
10. Crosby, J. F. Conflict Resolution: An Entrée into Self. In

E. A. Powers et al. (Eds.), Process in Relationship: Marriage and Family (2nd ed.). St. Paul, MN: West, 1976.
11. Dahms, A. M. Intimacy Hierarchy. In E. A. Powers et al. (Eds.), Process in Relationship: Marriage and Family (2nd ed.). St. Paul, MN: West, 1976.
12. D'Antonio, W. V. The family and religion: Exploring a changing relationship. Journal for the Scientific Study of Religion 19:89, 1980.
13. Duvall, E. R. M. Marriage and Family Development (6th ed.). New York: Harper & Row, 1985.
14. Eisenman, E. P. The Origins and Practice of Family Therapy. In P. J. Stein, J. Richman, and N. Hannon (Eds.), The Family: Functions, Conflicts and Symbols. Reading, MA: Addison-Wesley, 1977.
15. Erikson, E. Childhood and Society (2nd ed.). New York: Norton, 1963.
16. Eshleman, J. R. The Family: An Introduction (3rd ed.). Boston: Allyn & Bacon, 1981.
17. Folkman, J. D., and Clatworthy, N. M. Marriage Has Many Faces. Columbus, OH: Merrill, 1970.
18. Fromm, E. The Art of Loving. New York: Harper, 1956.
19. Galvin, K. M., and Brommel, B. J. Family Communication: Cohesion and Change. Glenview, IL: Scott, Foresman, 1982.
20. Garrett, W. R. Seasons of Marriage and Family Life. New York: Holt, Rinehart & Winston, 1982.
21. Garrett, Y. The Newlywed Handbook: A Refreshing, Practical Guide for Living Together. Waco, TX: Word Books, 1981.
22. Goode, W. J. The Contemporary American Family. In P. J. Stein, J. Richman, and N. Hannon (Eds.), The Family: Functions, Conflicts and Symbols. Reading, MA: Addison-Wesley, 1977.
23. Hendrick, C., and Hendrick, S. Liking, Loving and Relating. Monterey, CA: Brooks/Cole, 1983.
24. Horschild, A. R. "Attending to, Codifying and Managing Feelings: Sex Differences in Love." Paper presented at American Sociological Association: San Francisco, CA, 1975.
25. Hunt, M. Sexual Behavior in the 1970s. New York: Dell, 1975.
26. Jourard, S. M. The Transparent Self (Rev. ed.). New York: Van Nostrand Reinhold, 1971.
27. Kelly, R. K. Courtship, Marriage and the Family (3rd ed.). New York: Harcourt Brace Jovanovich, 1979.
28. Kinsey, A. C., Pomeroy, W. B., and Martin, C. E. Sexual Behavior in the Human Male. Philadelphia: Saunders, 1948.
29. Kinsey, A. C., et al. Sexual Behavior in the Human Female. Philadelphia: Saunders, 1953.
30. Kirkendall, L. A. Premarital Intercourse and Interpersonal Relationships. Westport, CT: Greenwood Press, 1984.
31. Maslow, A. Toward a Psychology of Being. New York: Van Nostrand, 1968.
32. Masnick, G., and Bone, M. J. The Nation's Families: 1960–1990. Cambridge, MA: Harvard University Press, 1980.
33. Masters, W. H., and Johnson, V. E. The Pleasure Bond: A

New Look at Sexuality and Commitment. Boston: Little, Brown, 1975.

34. Rogers, C. R.   *On Becoming a Person.* Boston: Houghton Mifflin, 1970.

35. Saxton, L.   *The Individual, Marriage and the Family* (4th ed.). Belmont, CA: Wadsworth, 1980.

36. Sell, C. M.   *Family Ministry: The Enrichment of Family Life Through the Church.* Grand Rapids, MI: Zondervan, 1981.

37. Skolnick, A. S.   *The Intimate Environment: Exploring Marriage and the Family* (3rd ed.). Boston: Little, Brown, 1983.

38. Smith, H. I.   *More Than "I Do," A Pastor's Resource Book for Premarital Counseling.* Kansas City, MO: Beacon Hill Press of Kansas City, 1983.

39. Spanier, G. B.   "Sexual Socialization and Premarital Sexual Behavior: An Empirical Investigation of the Impact of Formal and Informal Sex Education." Doctoral dissertation, Evanston, IL: Northwestern University, 1973.

40. Stein, P. J., Richman, J., and Hanson, N.   *The Family: Function, Conflicts and Symbols.* Reading, MA: Addison-Wesley, 1977.

41. Strong, B., et al.   *The Marriage and Family Experience* (2nd ed.). St. Paul, MN: West, 1983.

42. Toffler, A.   *The Third Wave.* New York: Morrow, 1980.

43. Westhoff, C. F.   Coital frequency and contraception. *Family Planning Perspectives* 6:136, 1974.

44. Whipple, C. M., and Whittle, D.   *The Compatibility Test: How to Choose the Right Person and Make Your Marriage a Success.* Englewood Cliffs, NJ: Prentice-Hall, 1976.

45. U.S. Bureau of the Census, September 1985.

31

Decision To Be
or Not To Be Parents

Clara S. Schuster

To be a good parent you have to believe in the species—somehow.

—Benjamin Spock

The decision (or lack of it) of whether or not to have a child is probably one of the most significant decisions in an individual's life, since that decision will profoundly influence the lives of many other persons, including the life of the child produced. Although parenthood is a statistically normative phenomenon in the lives of young adults, it is a singularly momentous event to the individuals involved.

Most couples want or plan to have children "someday," but feel a need to complete other tasks and goals (e.g., education, career, financial obligations, personal development) before assuming the responsibilities of parenthood. Subtle—and not so subtle—pressures are placed on the couple if they wait too long. The in-laws want to see their grandchildren before they die. The husband's friends may tease him about his virility, and the dedication of the wife to her "feminine role" may be in question. Some couples may even receive subtle questions about consummation of the marriage. Friends and family members may pressure the couple to become a "complete" family by having children—inferring that the couple is not a family by itself.

On the other hand, concern about zero population growth has created pressure for the couple who have or want to have three or more children. "Don't you know when to stop?" "Did you ever hear of birth control?" "What else do you and your husband (or wife) do in the evening?" are all common questions to which the couple may be subjected. Some parents indicate that they are treated as if they have committed a crime by producing a large family, even though they may be socially, emotionally, and financially able to provide for their own and the children's needs.

Some individuals choose to become parents because it will offer another outlet for their own creativity and psychosocial-sexual development; they see parenthood as another opportunity to share themselves intimately with others. They may view parenthood as an art—the chance to become actively involved in the creation of another person, not just physically, but socially, cognitively, and emotionally. Parenthood offers the potential of another exciting adventure in life—another avenue for self-actualization and psychological fulfillment.

Some individuals feel that children will offer them the opportunity to fulfill their own life goals. They may receive emotional satisfaction in doing things for others or may feel that they are obtaining a second chance to accomplish (through the child) what they wanted to do or felt they missed the first time through. Some women have children to dissipate loneliness or to provide a face-saving escape from unsatisfying employment.

The quality of the parent-child relationship and the emotional satisfaction received by the parents will depend heavily on the individual parent's level of development and motivation for parenthood. The child demands and needs much personal attention during the early months of life; the interdependent relationship is heavily skewed toward dependence on the part of the infant. Parents who are expecting more positive feedback may find parenting a disappointing or draining experience. Other priorities, goals, and concerns may cause the parent to begin resenting the amount of time and energy demanded by the child.

An individual couple may want children because they feel that the child gives them a common goal—a shared interest—that will help to solidify and to maintain the union. Conversely, a couple may decide against becoming parents because they feel a child would add too much stress or interfere with their current relationship.

Some couples may become parents because they feel that children help to bond the three generations: Through pregnancy and parenthood, the couple shares a common experience with their own parents, and grandparents may become more willing to accept the young couple as adults. Unfortunately, some individuals find that parenthood evokes the memory of painful experiences with their own parents, which in turn can negatively affect the new parent-child relationship.

Some couples and cultural groups feel that children offer security for the later years of life, while others may see children as their hold on immortality—someone to carry on the family name, traditions, or business or to receive the inheritance. Children may be seen to offer the couple status: they may be a sign of success, or they may be a means of displaying the parents' financial success through the quantity or quality of the child's clothing and toys.

Deciding to have a child is a family affair that should be thoughtfully considered, both individually and collectively. One minister, when counseling young engaged couples about marriage, frequently asks them, "Will this union add or subtract from your ability to meet your personal goals?" This is a very astute question; perhaps couples should ask themselves the same question when considering the addition of another family member. If a child prevents the other members of the family from reaching their personal goals, resentment may develop and interfere with the total family dynamics. If the child allows the individual family members to expand the alternatives for goal achievement, then the enriched family system can enhance its cohesiveness, joy, and maturity level.

DECISION AGAINST INCREASING THE FAMILY

The decision for voluntary childlessness has become an increasingly popular option among American couples. Concern over population increases and personal development of the individuals involved are major factors in the decision.

Voluntary Childlessness

During the 1970s, 5 to 7 percent of couples chose a childless lifestyle [56]. Unfortunately, the proparenthood mentality of society may stigmatize the childless couple—treating them in subtle ways as social deviants, intimating psychological maladjustment, emotional immaturity, immoral character, or marital instability [56]. They, at best, may be seen as selfish and self-indulgent [44]. In actuality, they often have an above-average education and intelligence, share a more egalitarian relationship, and have high marital satisfaction and good communication skills [17, 56].

One-third of childless couples decide prior to marriage to remain childfree [56]. In fact, many of them make the decision during their teenage years. It is not until they are older that they realize the rejection of parenthood is not synonymous with the rejection of marriage. The other two-thirds slip into a childless marriage because of permanent postponement [56]. Children are postponed for a definite period while the couple accomplish a goal, such as travel, home purchase, or schooling. In the second stage, they still plan to have children someday, but postpone the event for an indefinite period until they can "afford it," or "feel more ready." During the third stage, the couple begin to deliberate on the pros and cons of parenthood. They realize that it is an irrevocable decision. There are no periods of trial parenthood. There is no choice of the type of child. They decide to make the decision later when their lives will suffer less disruption. In the final stage, they accept the state of permanent childlessness. They have weighed the pros and cons and have decided parenthood is not the right decision for them. As a couple, they may feel that their contribution to society is more constructive by pursuing a career rather than raising children. This is not necessarily a selfish decision or a reaction to parenthood per se. It may be a very realistic evaluation of the couple's strengths, weaknesses, values, and goals.

Factors Affecting the Decision

Parenthood demands a long-term commitment of energy, time, and material resources. The financial obligations involved in child-rearing are increasing. A 1981 estimate indicated that it would cost $134,000 to raise one child from birth to 18 years of age [42]. These figures do not include college expenses or the indirect cost of the parent's lost income if a decision is made to stay at home (which may be $100,000 or more). If the parent returns to work, there is the added expense of child care. Second and third children cost proportionately less than the first child because of shared resources, but the additional expense may still discourage large families in today's society.

For those concerned with population trends, an average of 2.5 children per female is considered to be the replacement rate [38]. The current rate of 1.8 children per female places us below zero population growth. Although the United States can support a much larger population than its current one of 245,000,000 people, there is a concern that the potential problems (e.g., environmental pollution, population density) may dilute the quality of life to an unacceptable level [32].

Many couples begin to recognize that the parenthood mystique is "not all it is cracked up to be." They see the sacrifices made by their parents and peers and realize that their own lives are happier as they are, which does not mean they dislike children. Many of these individuals are successful nurses or school teachers. They are merely aficionados of their adult-centered lifestyle [56].

In 1975 Ann Landers asked her readers a simple question: "If you had it to do over again, would you have children?" She received an unprecedented 10,000 letters, 70 percent of which responded "No!" [32]. The myth of parenthood was shattered; it became clear that the fairy tale "and they lived happily ever after" might have ended with the birth of a baby. The "no" mail fell into four categories:

1. Some parents were concerned about world tensions and the effects of overpopulation on quality of life.
2. Other parents felt that the children had ruined their relationship with each other. Many felt that personal time and energy were so heavily drained that they were no longer free to experience life as an individual in their own right. Mothers expressed more concern over this aspect than fathers did. Fathers may resent the financial cost; mothers are concerned with the personal cost. One survey of stress and life satisfaction indicated that the parents of young children feel significantly more stressors than individuals in other phases of life. The results also indicated that satisfaction with life (especially for women) drops with the birth of the first child. Stressors decrease and general life satisfaction increases as the children become older, and many parents express marked increase in life satisfaction when the children leave home [9].
3. The saddest letters came from parents whose children had left home and had essentially broken their emotional ties. The parents felt that the children had forgotten them. Some older persons want their children to express gratitude to them for having devoted years of labor to their upbringing; other older persons seek and need the companionship of their children; still others feel they have lost a friend. This last attitude is perhaps the most painful. Whether real or perceived, lack of attention is interpreted as rejection.
4. Bitter letters were received from disenchanted parents whose children did not match their dreams; they felt that the children had failed them. Their children did not possess a prized skill or physical attractiveness, or they were delinquent, colicky, or had crooked teeth requiring expensive dental work. These parents found it impossible to relive their own lives through the children's social activities. They felt

they had done "all the right things," had even "lived by the book," but they were disappointed by the results.

Although one must acknowledge that such a survey is biased by the intensity of the feelings of those who responded, their reactions to parenthood are, nevertheless, significant and should be considered by couples who are assessing their assets, liabilities, and motivations for parenthood. Parenthood is not all fun and games or even a job that can be laid aside at the end of the day. It may be that the results reflect the immaturity of the parents who responded, and highlight the need for education/counseling about the realities of parenting. Successful parenting requires dedication of oneself to another, a task that demands considerable maturity. Joys are frequent when expectations are realistic and motivations are not self-serving. The pleasure comes from a job well done, but concrete evidence of the success of one's efforts may not be clear until the child's adult years.

Contraception

Although couples have attempted to control conception for centuries through techniques such as the ingestion of special herbs, religious rituals, or timing coitus with the phases of the moon, effective methods of contraception have been available only since 1930 [38]. Reliable, efficient methods emerged in the late 1950s when "the pill" was released.

Many doctors and psychologists feel that a minimal interval of 2 to 3 years between children is beneficial to both the mother and the child. Effective family-planning techniques are essential in order to space children and to avoid having unwanted children who may cause additional stress on the family unit. The mother of an unwanted child may avoid getting adequate prenatal care and may give minimal attention to the child after birth. Unwanted children are more likely to be battered, they experience a higher mortality rate, and they have a higher juvenile delinquency rate.

CHOICE OF METHOD

There is no single ideal method of contraception; every method has its drawbacks. Each couple must weigh the advantages, disadvantages, and side effects of each method, taking into account religious and moral ideals and personal and aesthetic factors when making the decision. The safest and most effective method of birth control is abstinence. However, most people do not find this method personally appealing.

The sexually active couple needs to have a clear understanding of the reproductive system and the ovar-ian cycle (see Chap. 3), both to enhance their satisfaction and to increase their success in the use of the method they choose. The single most critical factor in the success of a method is conscientious acceptance of responsibility for implementation. The method chosen may be very effective, but it cannot be expected to be efficient if it is used haphazardly.

METHODS

When choosing a method of contraception, the couple needs to consider (1) the mechanisms of action (i.e., how and when the method works), (2) undesirable side effects of the method (and what to do about them), and (3) the effectiveness rate of the method. The medical profession has devised a scale by which effectiveness of contraceptive methods can be compared. The scale indicates the number of pregnancies per 100 years of use; this number can be translated into a percentage. The natural fertility rate (if no method of contraception is used) is 80 (i.e., a woman has an 80% chance of becoming pregnant if sexually active). Of course, there is frequently a difference between the theoretical and the actual effectiveness of a contraceptive method. For instance, the pregnancy rate for women who use an oral contraceptive is theoretically close to zero. However, in actuality, effectiveness is reduced because many women forget to take the pill. The six most frequently used contraceptive methods are compared in Table 31–1.

Prevention of Ovulation. Ovulation can be prevented through hormonal control of the menstrual cycle (see Chap. 3 for a review of this subject). About 40 percent of women in the United States rely on the contraceptive pill for birth control [23]. Hormonal contraceptives are composed of a combination of estrogen and progesterone. The artificial maintenance of estrogen and progesterone levels suppresses the maturation of primary follicles, interferes with the release of luteinizing hormone (LH) by the pituitary, effects changes in endometrium development, and effects cervical mucosa changes. Ovulation may still occur when estrogen dosage is too low. The sudden drop in progesterone level that occurs when the pill is stopped simulates the normal hormonal drop preceding the menses and usually precipitates degeneration of the endometrial lining.

The side effects or undesirable effects from the contraceptive pill are determined by the balance of estrogen and progesterone in any given woman. Every pill has a different ratio of these two hormones, and in addition, every woman has her own natural balance. If a woman has a naturally high level of estrogen and is taking an estrogen-dominant pill, she may develop

Table 31-1. Comparison of Birth Control Methods

Method	Percent Chance of Pregnancy*	Advantages	Disadvantages	Contraindications
Chance (sexually active)	80			
Oral contraceptives Combined pill Minipill	 0.2 4.3	May eliminate cramps, acne; no action required at coitus; regularity of menstrual cycle	Must be taken every day; requires prescription; increased risk of blood clotting	Smokers Sickle cell anemia Hepatitis Breast-feeding Over age 35 Diabetes Hypertension Severe renal disease
Intrauterine device (IUD)	1.9	No need to take pill every day; separated from coitus	May cause cramps or longer menses; may need to check for "tail" of device before coitus	Women who have long, crampy periods Cervicitis Venereal disease Endometriosis Anticoagulant therapy
Diaphragm with jelly or cream	2.4	Nothing ingested; may be inserted several hours before coitus; no major side effects or dangers; used for coitus during menses	Cream must be reapplied within 1 hour before coitus; must be left in 6–8 hours after coitus; requires professional fitting and prescription	Severely displaced uterus Cystocele
Condom with foam	4.3	May be purchased at any drugstore; protects against venereal disease	Must be removed carefully to prevent spilling; dulls penile sensation	
Foams, jellies, creams	14.8	May be purchased at any drugstore	Must be used within 1 hour before coitus; messy; must be deposited at entrance to cervix	Allergy to solution
Rhythm (calendar)	20	Nothing has to be purchased	Not as safe as Basal Body Temperature (BBT) or cervical mucus check	Irregular periods

*Pregnancies per 100 woman years

symptoms of estrogen excess or progesterone deficiency or both. The reverse may also be true. If symptoms develop, the solution is to switch to a pill with a different balance rather than to discontinue the pill. The pill is a set of choices, not one choice.

Hormonal suppression of ovulation can also be achieved by subcutaneous implant of time-release hormone capsules. The minute, sustained release of estrogen allows for lower doses and fewer side effects. It is more effective and efficient, since it removes the human error of forgetting. Hormone-impregnated vaginal rings and intrauterine devices also are available at some clinics and negate the need for daily remembering.

The contraceptive pill is generally contraindicated (not recommended) if a woman is breast-feeding, since some women find that it interferes with milk production. Some women find that the menstrual period is greatly shortened and the flow lightened when they are taking the pill. Occasionally, the menses will disappear altogether, and the woman may be temporarily infertile following use of the pill. Diabetes and sickle cell anemia may also be aggravated by the pill. Since oral contraceptives may increase the blood-clotting factors in some persons, their use is not advisable for women with a history of phlebitis or other clotting problems. The results from recent research have prompted the U.S. Department of Health and Human Services to advise women who use oral contraceptives not to smoke [16]. There is evidence of a decreased risk for developing ovarian and endometrial cancer in women who have used oral contraceptives [12].

Prevention of Spermatogenesis. Male contraceptives are still in experimental stages of development. Current hormone-therapy regimens achieve significant oligospermia but may not achieve azoospermia. Since sperm take 71 ± 4 days to develop, an implant or injection may take 6 to 8 weeks before fertility is decreased. The same delay is observed when therapy is discontinued. Because current hormone therapy affects libido (sexual desire) and potency, it is considered undesirable [23].

A compound, gossypol, extracted from cottonseed has been used in China and demonstrates potential for reducing the sperm count without reducing libido [23]. However, its effects on the cardiac and respiratory systems may prove it undesirable.

Prevention of Union of the Sperm and Egg. If the couple prefer not to tamper with the hormonal balance, they may elect a method that prevents the sperm from reaching the egg. As mentioned earlier, abstinence is an extremely effective method. However, if the couple engages in other noncoital sexual activities, sperm can be accidentally transferred from the male to the vaginal area, and pregnancy, although unlikely, could still occur. Some couples rely on coitus interruptus. In this method, the penis is withdrawn just prior to ejaculation. The couple should be aware that ejaculation may be hard to control or to predict, and that sperm may be present in the preejaculatory secretions. Couples also find this method to be psychologically frustrating. The pregnancy rate is 15 to 25 percent [49]. Those who plan to use this method should become familiar with the squeeze technique popularized by Masters and Johnson to prevent imminent ejaculation.

The "rhythm" or "natural" family planning method combines knowledge of the ovarian cycle with abstinence. The aim is to avoid intercourse on the days surrounding ovulation. Predicting ovulation by the calendar alone (see Chap. 3) has a pregnancy rate of 14 to 30 percent; the rate decreases slightly when using the basal temperature records.

In the calendar method, the woman keeps a record of the menses for at least 6 months and then performs the following calculations: she subtracts 18 from the number of days of the shortest cycle (this represents the first unsafe day) and then subtracts 11 days from the number of days in the longest cycle (this represents the last unsafe day). Unprotected intercourse should be avoided during the interval between those two days of the cycle.

The basal temperature usually remains below 98°F during the follicular phase of the cycle and rises with ovulation. Unprotected intercourse should be avoided for 3 days before ovulation is expected and can be resumed 3 days after the temperature rises. Many women subtract six from the earliest recorded day of temperature elevation just to be sure (if the first day of temperature elevation is day 17, then the first 11 days are considered to be safe).

Assessment of the cervical mucus can add further accuracy to pinpointing the day of ovulation. The Billings method, used by physicians, can identify more accurately when ovulation actually occurs. Advocates of the method indicate that it can be used effectively with irregular cycles and that it allows more "safe" days than the other two methods [8]. As ovulation approaches, the mucus begins to thin. **Spinnbarkeit** is the term used to describe the stretchability of the mucus. Ovulation occurs at, or within, 1 to 2 days of maximum spinnbarkeit. By removing some of the mucus with a speculum, an applicator, or her finger, a woman can learn to assess her degree of spinnbarkeit.

There are three other things a woman can do to pinpoint the day of ovulation: (1) judge the consistency of the cervical os by touch (it is soft, like the lips, at ovulation and firm, like the nose, soon afterwards); (2) touch diabetic test tape to the cervix (it turns from yellow to dark blue at the time of ovulation); and (3) look at the cervical mucus under a microscope (at ovulation the pattern will resemble a fern, but this pattern disappears in 2 or 3 days).

Douching is generally considered to be an ineffective method because sperm can enter the cervix after intercourse much more rapidly than the woman can administer the douche solution.

Mechanical barriers to contraception are the condom for males and the diaphragm, cervical cap, and vaginal sponge for females. These methods are effective if they are used in combination with chemical contraceptives. The condom serves as a barrier to both sperm and venereal disease. It is the only reliable temporary male contraceptive. The man should put on the

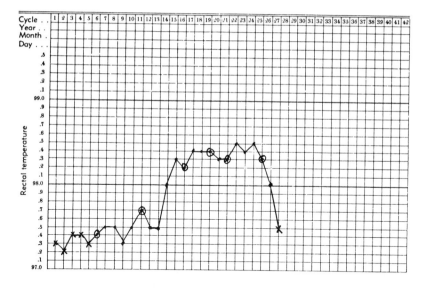

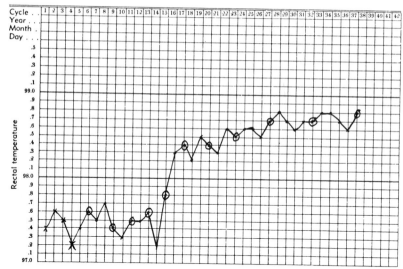

Figure 31–1. Basal temperature chart. Cross marks indicate menses; circles indicate intercourse. Upper chart: Ovulation occurred on day 14, no pregnancy occurred. Lower chart: Ovulation occurred on day 15. Continued elevation of temperature beyond 16 days after ovulation indicates a possible conception.

condom during foreplay and after erection but before inserting the penis into the vagina. There should be a space between the end of the condom and the penis for receiving sperm. A condom should be used only once.

Diaphragms require a vaginal examination for fitting and a prescription. The client must be taught how to insert and remove the diaphragm properly. If it is inserted improperly, the cervix may actually be pushed into a position that will facilitate entrance of the sperm into the uterus. The client is usually advised to insert the diaphragm regularly each evening as a part of bedtime routine or within an hour before coitus. It must be left in place for at least 8 hours after coitus. Many women do not like to manipulate the genitalia for insertion, but users indicate that the diaphragm does not interfere with enjoyment of intercourse. A woman needs to be refitted after each pregnancy or after any pelvic surgery or weight change of 10 pounds or more. The diaphragm can be used during menstruation.

The cervical cap fits directly over the cervix, blocking the opening by suction adherence. It is difficult to insert, but can be left in place between menses.

The vaginal sponge provides both a mechanical barrier and a spermacide. There is some concern about pelvic infections if it is used improperly or left in place beyond the recommended length of time.

Spermacides prevent union of the sperm and ovum by immobilizing or killing the sperm. Creams, jellies, foams, suppositories, or collagen sponges can be used alone or with a mechanical barrier. To be effective, they must be applied near the cervix and within 1 hour before coitus. Some people feel that spermacides are messy; others may experience burning, irritation, or even allergic reactions. Spermacides also provide some protective action against venereal diseases [23].

Interference with Implantation. The intrauterine device (IUD) is a small object that is placed inside the uterus by a physician or nurse midwife. The pregnancy rate is 1 to 3 percent [23]. The IUD prevents implantation of the blastocyst. Copper- or progesterone-treated IUDs have even greater effectiveness. Cramps may occur with insertion of the IUD and even afterward. An over-the-counter aspirin substitute may be recommended. The first menses may be heavier than usual, and subsequent menstrual periods may also be longer and heavier than those prior to the IUD insertion. Special attention should be paid to vitamin C and iron in the diet, a lack of which is associated with increased menstrual flow.

Clients may be taught to feel for the IUD tails in the vagina to make sure it is in place, since the expulsion rate is high (4 to 18 percent) [23]. However, the tails may be coated with vaginal discharge, so the fact that they are not felt does not always mean that the IUD is not in place. The placement can easily be checked by a health practitioner and should be checked as soon as possible if the client suspects that the device has been expelled. The client will need to return for a checkup every year. Some IUDs must be changed every 1 or 2 years, while others may be left in place for an extended period of time. In order to be sure that she is aware of any spontaneous expulsion of the IUD, the woman should check all tampons or sanitary pads before disposal. Expulsion of the device is most likely to occur in the first 3 months of use and during menstruation.

Sterilization. Surgical contraception, or sterilization, is designed to provide permanent birth control. So far, the attempts to reverse these procedures have not had a very high rate of success; however, it is anticipated that by 1990 reversibility will be a valid option. The majority of the current permanent methods are designed for women; however, none of these compare in safety, effectiveness, or cost to the one method available for men—vasectomy.

Vasectomy involves the severing of the vas deferens, the two tubes that carry sperm from each testicle. Patients report some pain the day of the procedure and the day after. At least three successive ejaculations must be free of healthy, mature sperm before other methods of contraception can be discontinued. Contrary to the beliefs of some men, vasectomy does not interfere with ejaculation, orgasm, or sex drive. In fact, many men indicate an increase in sexual arousal because of the perceived freedom from impregnation of the partner.

A variety of sterilization methods are available to women. Most of these methods involve abdominal tubal ligation and cauterization by laparoscopy or mini-laparotomy. These methods generally require hospitalization; however, they are increasingly performed on an outpatient basis.

Abdominal tubal ligation, which is often performed immediately postpartum, involves the tying and cutting of the fallopian tubes. It is a relatively simple surgery if performed postpartum or by laparoscopy. Because the incisions are so small, they can be covered by Band-Aids.

Some physicians are using chemicals or plugs to block the tubes, but these methods are as yet not as effective.

Involuntary Pregnancy

In spite of the advances in contraceptive techniques and the ready availability of information and equipment, 18.4 percent of babies born in 1980 were to single mothers [40]. One study estimates that two-thirds of pregnancies among married couples are unplanned, and one-half are unwanted [25]. Unplanned pregnancies are the result of three major factors: naiveté, ignorance, and ineffective birth control practice.

Some women, especially young adolescents, may not connect coitus with pregnancy until after conception. This attitude is more typically found in the younger woman who developmentally is caught up in the interests and concerns of the immediate environment rather than those of the future. Such women may believe that it cannot happen to them or that because of their age they are sterile. Many young people receive minimal or no family planning information because the discussion of sex is still a taboo topic in many families and cultural groups.

It is not uncommon for a woman to continue using the same ineffective method of birth control that she practiced before an unwanted conception [25]; this practice may be related to the helplessness syndrome (see Chap. 14). Some women do not use contraceptive methods because of perceived religious or social guilt. Others use alternative "old-wives'-tale" methods based on inadequate understanding of anatomy and the process of conception. They may feel that conception cannot occur the first time, or that sitting on the toilet will "drain it all out" [25]. Some women (and men) may secretly or unconsciously desire a pregnancy, leading them to use contraceptive methods erratically.

POSTCOITAL BIRTH CONTROL

Prostaglandins, a group of naturally occurring fatty acids, can interfere with implantation of the blastocyst by increasing uterine activity. This will decrease the blood supply to the uterus and consequently decrease the oxygen available to the young embryo. Prostaglandin therapy is especially effective the first 2 weeks— prior to the onset of the menses [23].

Postcoital contraception also includes the "morning-after" pill. Diethylstilbestrol (DES) is a synthetic estrogen that must be taken twice daily for 5 days. Contraindications to its use are the same as those to estrogen in the contraceptive pill. If a woman is more than 2 weeks pregnant when DES is taken, serious malformations may occur on an unaborted fetus. The full dose must be taken to be effective.

BIRTH CONTROL VACCINE

The development of a vaccine has been plagued with many problems. Such a vaccine, when available, would work on the antibody-antigen principle discussed in Chapter 22. It is difficult to develop antibodies specific to the reproductive system that are also safe, effective, and reversible.

Abortion

Birth control may be extended beyond conception through the use of abortion. Advocates for or against abortion may base their stand on philosophical, religious, ethical, eugenic, social, political, psychological, or medical issues. Opinions regarding abortion can be divided into four major viewpoints [24], as discussed in the following sections.

NO GROUNDS FOR ABORTION

Some people feel that there are no grounds for termination of a pregnancy; each life is considered sacred and every human has a right to live. Advocates of this view indicate that they do not know when an individ-

ual becomes uniquely human in the spiritual or emotional domain versus being purely animal in the physical, cognitive, or social sense.

There are many opposing views on the beginning of a valued human life, which these individuals have considered and questioned. Is it (1) during the preschool years, when the child begins to develop a concept of right from wrong; (2) during the toddler years, when the child begins to use language or to develop autonomy from the mother, or (3) at the moment of birth? If birth, then physical separation from the mother would apply to a fetus of any age. However, birth is generally thought of in terms of a full-term infant; thus premature infants may be viewed differently in terms of humanness! (4) Others feel that "life" begins at the point when the fetus is mature enough to sustain extrauterine life. In the medical field, this is usually considered to occur between 24 and 28 weeks of gestation (see Fig. 5–10). However, with advances in medical science, much younger fetuses are now beginning to survive. (5) Some mothers acknowledge individuality of the fetus when they experience "quickening"—fetal movement at about 20 to 24 weeks. However, fetal movement has been occurring freely since the third month of gestation. (6) Others advocate that since the criteria for death is now based on "brain death," the criteria for life should be based on "brain life." Brain function appears to be present by 8 weeks of gestation based on electroencephalographic readings [20]. They feel the fetus, which is dependent on placenta at this point, is as much a human as an 80-year-old on a ventilator. (7) Another view is that human life begins when the heart begins to beat (22 days after conception), which is less than 1 week after the first missed menstrual period. It is the ambiguity of these commonly held views on the beginning of human life that leads advocates of this viewpoint to believe that (8) the child is a human entity from the moment of conception.

MEDICAL GROUNDS FOR ABORTION

When the life of the mother is threatened, those who hold the first view may be forced to reassess priority of right to life. Continuation of a pregnancy may cause the death of both mother and child. Others feel that if there is strong evidence that the child will be born with a severe physical or mental abnormality, termination is desirable. They feel that the quality of life of the individual and the family is as significant as the principle of life itself.

SOCIAL GROUND FOR ABORTION

Circumstances (e.g., out-of-wedlock pregnancy, rape, extramarital conception, maternal age, shaky marriage) or other priorities (e.g., financial needs, education, career) may make child-rearing unacceptable. The quality of family life is considered to be significant in this view. Unplanned and unwanted babies have a higher incidence of social and emotional problems that seem to be related to rejection by the mother.

Advocates of the earlier views may feel that social grounds are unacceptable criteria for abortion and would encourage the woman to respect the human life through childbirth and then to release the child for adoption. However, even going through the pregnancy may cause serious social difficulties that are deemed detrimental to the woman's emotional health.

GENERAL AVAILABILITY OF ABORTION

Many persons feel that abortion should be freely available at the request of the woman for any reason. Women who believe that all babies should be wanted support the view of "abortion on request" when other methods of birth control have failed. The woman feels that she should have the right to terminate the pregnancy before she has developed a personalized image of the fetus.

Most women undergoing abortion indicate a tremendous sense of relief; a few indicate emptiness or regret. Counseling prior to and after an abortion is essential to help a woman to explore the issue honestly and holistically, to identify her true reasons for desiring the abortion, and to discuss alternatives. Feelings of grief, exhibited as mild and self-limiting guilt and depression, are normal and common following abortion. A few women indicate having nightmares and guilt feelings many years after an abortion when the issues have not been adequately resolved. The abortion may become a ghost of the past she must deal with in a subsequent pregnancy, labor, and delivery [22, 53].

Studies indicate that the incidence of serious postabortion emotional disturbance is highest when the woman (1) is ambivalent about the decision, (2) is coerced into the decision, (3) is forced to have the abortion because of medical problems, or (4) already has symptoms of severe personality disorganization [14]. In most cases, "the abortion appears to be genuinely therapeutic" for the woman who honestly desired the procedure [50] and has resolved the questions discussed above.

Research indicates that some women who have had elective vaginal abortions with cervical dilation have twice as high a risk of losing subsequent pregnancies as a result of cervical incompetence. There is also a higher rate of complications during pregnancy and higher prematurity and perinatal death rates [15, 35] in subsequent pregnancies.

DECISION TO INCREASE THE FAMILY

Biological procreation is not synonymous with true parenthood. Children whose parents choose to have them as an outgrowth of their own abundance, life satisfaction, and creativity are fortunate indeed. Unfortunately, many parents ignore or are grossly ignorant of their influence on their child's development [2]. A parent who is still involved in his or her own identity crisis may not be sufficiently flexible to meet the child's changing needs. Parents who have not yet resolved their own identities may experience much more difficulty in allowing their child to have a separate identity. Developmental level rather than chronological age, then, becomes a critical factor in parenting success.

As indicated earlier, a couple's decision to have children may be strongly influenced by cultural standards—they feel that it is the thing to do after marriage. Such a decision is based on roles rather than goals for the couple. A new family member will change the direction and reciprocity of communication, which can lead either to firmer commitments or to rivalries. Insecurity or weak identity in one parent can be compensated for by the strength of the other, but if the interdependence of the couple is so lopsided that it approaches dependence on the part of one member, it may threaten the success of both the marriage and the potential parenthood [27]. "The optimal condition for parenthood is marriage based on a compatible partnership, which can reduce the frustration, anxiety and anger of everyday life to a tolerable minimum and which at the same time can provide a creative reciprocity and spontaneous solidarity" [27].

It is obvious that a couple should assess their financial resources. Will they be able to live on only one income? If both parents want or need to continue working, who will care for the child, and how much will it cost? Will the individual parents be able to complete their own education or career goals? Parenting is easier when these questions have been successfully resolved. A planned pregnancy that has been achieved after careful weighing of both family and personal resources can offer a period of great joy, excitement, anticipation, and strength for the couple.

Pregnancy

Pregnancy is a biologically normal but exceptional period in the life of a woman. The first sign that a woman has become pregnant is usually a missed menstrual period. Both her physical and psychological responses to this event may be colored by whether it was planned or "accidental," whether she is married or single. The pregnancy may declare her adulthood and indepen-

individuals may be erroneously diagnosed as pregnant by competent physicians [3]. The symptoms of pseudocyesis are psychogenic in origin; some studies indicate that psychological factors acting on the anterior pituitary can initiate maintenance of the corpus luteum even though conception has not occurred [3].

The **positive signs** of pregnancy are dependent on confirmation by a qualified health professional. These signs are usually not discernible until the second trimester.

The signs of pregnancy are summarized in the following list:

Presumptive signs
Amenorrhea
Fatigue
Frequency of urination
Morning sickness
Enlargement and tingling of breasts
Weight gain (although some women may lose weight during the first trimester because of nausea and vomiting)
Increase in BMT
Probable signs
Quickening—movement of the fetus felt by the mother
Abdominal uterine enlargement
Positive pregnancy test
Positive signs
Auscultation of fetal heart—felt heart sounds can be identified around the twentieth week with a stethoscope. The Doptone (electronic stethoscope) can pick up fetal heart sounds as early as the fourteenth week
Palpation of fetal parts and movement by a health professional
Visualization of the fetus by ultrasound or x-ray. Ultrasound can identify the presence of a fetus as early as two weeks

PHYSIOLOGICAL CHANGES
Pregnancy affects almost every system of the woman's body.

Endocrine System. Increased levels of progesterone and enlargement of the thyroid increase the basal metabolic rate of the body to 20 percent above the nonpregnant state. The increased caloric needs may be responsible for hypoglycemia (low blood sugar), which can lead to fainting and nausea. Having frequent, small meals and eating crackers before arising to activity in the morning or after a nap can reduce the symptoms. Nutritional intake needs to be increased to meet the needs of both the mother and the fetus.

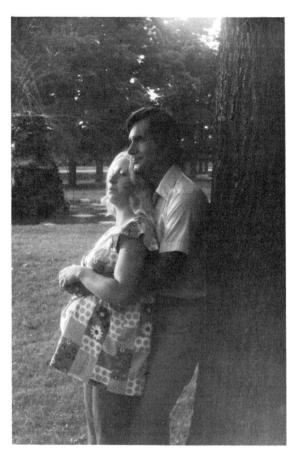

Figure 31–2. Both the father and the mother experience dreams, aspirations, and fears of the future with a new baby. Pregnancy can help to draw the couple closer together.

dence, verify her feminine role, confirm her love, extend her dreams, confer status on her, engender fear, or present major physical, social, or psychological problems.

SIGNS OF PREGNANCY
The **presumptive signs** of pregnancy, which appear during the first trimester, are mainly the result of changes in the hormone balance. Other factors, including birth control pills, can cause one or several of the same signs. Consequently, these signs are not definitive indicators of pregnancy.

The **probable signs** of pregnancy usually appear in the second trimester. Since these symptoms may occasionally appear without a pregnancy, they also are not considered confirmatory. Pseudocyesis (false pregnancy) can replicate the presumptive and probable signs of pregnancy so closely that one-third of these

Integumentary System. Adrenal and placental hormones can cause darkening of areas of the skin. The nipple and areola are universal targets for darkening. Many women also develop a line between the umbilicus and the symphysis pubis, known as the linea nigra. Pigmentation of the cheeks and forehead is known as chloasma or the "mask of pregnancy." Some women merely become more freckled.

The sebaceous and sweat glands become more active, increasing hygienic needs and reactivating acne problems in some women. The increase in total body hair growth may make some women self-conscious. Many women become aware of an increased rate of hair loss after the birth of the baby; this phenomenon is due to a sudden decrease in the number of active, growing hair follicles in the scalp following birth.

Increased activity of the adrenal cortex may lead to the development of striae (stretch marks). Unfortunately, creams do not appear to prevent or to remove these marks, which appear as reddish-purple, wavy, shiny, depressed streaks on the abdomen, buttocks, thighs, or breasts. Many of the stretch marks will disappear after pregnancy, but some will remain as smaller, pale, shiny stripes.

Cardiovascular System. Blood volume increases 30 to 40 percent by the end of the first trimester in order to meet the needs of the enlarging breasts and uterus. This change increases the work load of the heart. The pulse rate may increase about 15 beats per minute, but the blood pressure should not change. This blood volume change may be responsible for lightheadedness on arising. Increased blood volume can also precipitate headaches. Persistent headaches—especially toward the end of pregnancy—should be reported to the physician. Redness of the palms and soles as well as nosebleeds are also attributed to the increased blood flow. Increased blood flow to the vocal cords may cause deepening of the voice and hoarseness.

The increased blood volume, combined with increased uterine size and pressure, can reduce return flow of blood from the legs and lower areas of the body, which in turn can lead to edema and varicose veins. Elevation of the legs and the use of support hose can alleviate discomfort and prevent problems. Persistent edema, especially toward the end of pregnancy, should be reported to the physician.

Hematocrit and hemoglobin levels may drop quite low during pregnancy because of the increased volume and subsequent dilution of the red blood cells. Iron intake should be monitored to ensure that the needs of both mother and fetus are met.

Respiratory System. The total air volume of the lungs is increased during pregnancy, facilitating the exchange of oxygen and carbon dioxide without increasing the respiratory rate. During the third trimester, pressure of the uterus against the diaphragm and rib cage may make the woman feel uncomfortable and short of breath. "Lightening" (tilting and lowering of the uterus during the last weeks of pregnancy) greatly alleviates the discomfort.

Gastroinestinal System. Progesterone appears to relax the walls of the gastrointestinal tract as well as the uterus. Consequently, motility is slowed, and the sphincters are relaxed. As a result, stomach emptying occurs more slowly. Escape of stomach contents into the esophagus may cause heartburn. Increasing uterine size may prevent large meals and interfere with evacuation of the bowels during the last trimester. Increased fluids and dietary bulk can help to alleviate the difficulty.

Genitourinary System. Pressure of the uterus on the bladder during early pregnancy and again during late pregnancy after lightening may necessitate frequent urination and thus disrupt sleep. The relaxing effect of progesterone on the urinary tract sphincters may allow passage of bacteria into the bladder, leading to bladder and kidney infections.

Bed rest allows the fluid accumulated as leg edema to return to the circulatory system, where it can be excreted by the kidneys. The woman's salt intake may be limited by some physicians with the intent of reducing the work load of both the heart and the kidneys. Side-lying positions reduce the pressure of the uterus against the ureters (such pressure can trap the urine in the kidney and cause pain) and against the inferior vena cava (this pressure can slow the return of blood to the heart and cause faintness).

Musculoskeletal System. Progesterone also causes softening of the cartilages, especially of the hips and symphysis pubis. Toward the end of pregnancy the mother may appear to "waddle" as a result of loose joints. This loosening allows for expansion of the birth passage during the birth of the baby. The increasing size of the uterus creates strain on the support ligaments, but it also changes the mother's posture as the center of gravity changes. The resultant backache can be alleviated by mild exercises, low-heeled shoes, and good posture. Muscle cramps of the lower extremities can be stopped by straightening the leg and pressing the toe upward toward the knee.

The few research studies that are available offer contradictory evidence on the effect of exercise on the fetus, the woman's body, and labor and delivery [30]. Loosened joints, a shifting center of gravity, and changing body space predispose the woman to accidental injuries. Strenuous, weight-bearing exercises can decrease uterine blood flow by as much as 70 percent [30]; consequently, any exercise needs to be individualized and monitored.

PSYCHOSOCIAL CHANGES
IN THE EXPECTANT COUPLE

Pregnancy is a critical phase in the life cycle of the couple, requiring psychological adaptations leading to new levels of integration that normally represent development. As with any new experience, the couple usually find the adaptive and integrative tasks to be more difficult with the first child. This situation may be compounded by a lack of exposure to child care during their developmental years. Parenthood offers an opportunity for personal, psychosocial, and psychosexual growth. However, it can also be traumatic to those who have not accomplished successfully the earlier developmental tasks.

If the pregnancy was planned, and if the child is wanted by both parents (not all planned pregnancies are really wanted), "the oneness of the pregnant woman with her mate encompasses their yet unborn child, creating the psychodynamic foundation of the triad: father-mother-child" [4]. This confirmation of the couple's love can deepen the bond between them. Both of them will begin to fantasize and to identify with a dream of their child to be. On the other hand, ambivalence toward the pregnancy may undermine the meaning of the marriage and affect the emotional climate awaiting the unborn child. Since parenthood implies a lifelong commitment, the parents may feel trapped, unable to return to their own childhood and interests. Other expectant parents may "revive their memories of childhood and discover a new order of reconciliation with their parents within their own experience of becoming parents" [27]. Interests and social relationships may change as the couple assumes a new family identity.

Psychosocial Changes in the Pregnant Woman. The pregnant woman is frequently described as being moody and emotionally labile. The constant redefining and integrative tasks absorb much of her emotional energy. The task is easier if the pregnancy was planned and she has a supportive, encouraging family [22]. Women need such support and emotional input during

their pregnancy; it is as if they are storing up emotional energy to share later with the neonate. Stressors and anxieties can interfere with this process. Fortunately for the pregnant woman, many other people who accept her pregnancy positively also become protective of her. They are concerned about fatiguing work, her diet, and her comfort. They may even treat her as if she were marginally ill, encouraging her to rest and to avoid bad news and generally pampering her. People she has never met may strike up a conversation centering on her pregnancy. Some women resent this personal intrusion; others welcome the attention.

The classic studies of Grete Bibring [5] on psychological processes during pregnancy indicate that pregnancy is a crisis precipitating profound psychological as well as somatic changes. Bibring observed that many women exhibited symptoms of "borderline psychosis" during pregnancy even if they appeared to have had good mental health prior to pregnancy and wanted the baby very much. A first pregnancy becomes the central focus of the woman's life. "They are the pregnancy, and the pregnancy is them" [22]. It is a very cosmic experience. Most women are in awe of the conception. Pregnancy heralds a point of no return [6]; the woman can no longer return to her nonpregnant, never-pregnant self. Acute disequilibrium may accompany her attempts to reorganize her self-concept. This phenomenon should be viewed as a normal developmental process that is essential to assuming a new identity and a new role. This disequilibrium is especially poignant in the change from "Mary" to "mother," or with the first pregnancy.

Prior to quickening, the woman must accept the pregnancy as a part of herself. After quickening, she is forced to recognize the separateness of the growing body and to invest herself emotionally in the infant while preparing herself for their physical separation. Most women grossly underestimate the development of the fetus in the first trimester [34]. Fantasies about the baby are common during this period, as well as tension or anxiety about the labor and delivery process.

The pregnant woman emerges from this phase with a new relationship to herself. Pregnancy can reactivate previously unresolved or partially resolved developmental conflicts. The reintegration of the past, present, and future can lead to maturation. However, the person who has not worked through these crises may find the parent-infant relationship unsatisfying. The pregnant woman needs extra support and encouragement during this time in order to recognize, to resolve, and to enjoy the developmental phenomena peculiar to pregnancy. The course of the postpartum period is based on the ego strength of the woman, her relationship to her mother, and the quality of the mental support she receives [22]. A sensitive marital partner offers support during this period of change and crises. An unhappy marriage increases the probability of postpartum depression [22]. The more egalitarian marital styles increase the flexibility of roles and therefore ego strength and comfort.

Psychoanalytical studies indicate that increases in the progesterone levels during pregnancy cause the woman to have an increased sense of relaxation and well-being. This phenomenon is also associated with a decrease in anxieties and a retentive tendency, leading to increases in self-centeredness, primary narcissism, and fantasies [4]. A spontaneous interest in her own past, other children and babies, and looking at baby books helps the woman to develop a more concrete image of her fantasized child.

Reva Rubin has identified two mutually independent but highly correlated questions that modify perception of stimuli and behavior throughout pregnancy [46]. The first deals with the woman's perception of time within the life space, presupposing that the woman wants a child "someday." The second question is concerned with the woman's personal sense of identity—her femininity or womanhood, which is established by the biological fulfillment of pregnancy. These two questions can be followed through five separate stages of the childbearing process, as discussed in the following sections.

Prepregnancy. "Someday" is seen in the abstract future. A woman who has never achieved a pregnancy may question her sexual and procreative ability. Even a woman who has achieved one pregnancy may feel that it was accidental and may want a second pregnancy to prove her functional ability.

First Trimester. The first missed menses and the awareness of potential pregnancy come as a shock. "Who, me? Now?" Even the woman desirous of the pregnancy may become aware of other priorities that need to be attended to before the addition of a family member. Financial resources, educational and career goals, and other plans suddenly assume major importance. The ramifications of childbirth and parenting may suddenly seem overwhelming, and the woman may question her motives, wondering if it is too late to back out. The pregnancy offers proof of her sexuality and reassurance against the fear of infertility. However, the wish to be pregnant may not be synonymous with the desire to have a child or to become a

mother. The lack of positive signs at this stage makes the woman look inward for evidence of proof of the pregnancy. The lack of concrete evidence may prevent her from telling others for fear that just the telling will prevent its occurrence, or she may proudly announce that she is pregnant, yet secretly fear (or hope) that she is not. She may be ecstatic, afraid, disbelieving, or resigned. Each woman is unique in her reaction and her level of acceptance.

Second Trimester. When the baby begins to move, it becomes a physical reality to the woman. The movement signifies a form of communion between them, and mothers-to-be begin the process of attachment to the fetus [10]. The abdomen enlarges to the extent that maternity clothing becomes necessary. Others become aware of her pregnancy, whether she has told them or not. "Yes, it has happened to me! Now!" The woman who is unable to accept her pregnant state may refuse to wear maternity clothes until the third trimester.

This stage offers several tasks that are unique to pregnancy [27]:

1. The woman becomes acutely aware of herself as a link between the past and the future. Life-cycle time assumes a new perspective.
2. She needs to redefine femininity and body image.
3. Reassessment of life-cycle role and maturity level leads to a new self-identity.
4. Personal and family goals will need to be reassessed in light of resources and new responsibilities.
5. Marital and parental relationships are reassessed. Some wives (and husbands) become acutely aware that they will never again be alone with their spouse.

Third Trimester. The fantasy image of the unborn child becomes very real during the third trimester. The woman may fear the baby's loss and may become very protective of herself both physically and psychologi-

Table 31-2. Psycho-Social Changes of Pregnancy

Stages of the childbearing process	"Life space" (timing)	Personal sense of identity
Prepregnancy	Someday (abstract future)	Can I?
First trimester	Not now! (someday)	Who—me?
Second trimester	Now!	Yes, me!
Third trimester	Make someday now!	Me–us
Labor	Now?	Who—me?
Delivery	Questions resolved	

cally. "Me" changes to "us." She wants the "someday" to be "now"! Time seems to pass slowly. The woman keeps herself busy to keep from thinking about the baby, but her thoughts are constantly there. Mothers are noted to touch and rub their abdomens during the third trimester. Those who make this gentle massaging and stroking a daily occurrence show greater comfort with, touching of, and talking to their babies after birth [10]. Such activity appears to strengthen the bonding process by facilitating recognition of the reality of the child's growth [54] and individuality. Many mothers prepare themselves for childbirth and motherhood by attending classes; others are unable to project themselves beyond the delivery. Lack of preparation for the baby may signify a disbelief on the part of the woman in her ability to produce a child, or an unconscious rejection of the child [27]. Women in some cultural groups do not obtain baby supplies until after the birth, feeling that it would bring bad luck.

The woman may fear the birth of a defective child or may fear her own death during childbirth. As delivery draws closer, these thoughts may increase or may become submerged under thoughts of the immediacy of her child to be. Toward the end of pregnancy, some mothers may feel that the fetus is an enemy. They find the kicking painful, and breathing is difficult. The antagonism may be aggravated by lack of sleep caused by the movement of the fetus when the mother lies down to rest.

During the last month, most mothers become impatient and anxious for the physical separation. They want to see their baby, to hold it in their arms, to assume a new form of love and communication. Many express the idea that they feel like a child waiting for a Christmas gift. Many mothers have a burst of energy toward the end of pregnancy and often spend considerable time cleaning and preparing the home as if a significant guest is about to arrive.

Labor and Delivery. The woman frequently returns to the same three questions during labor and delivery. During the early stages she again asks, "Who, me? Not now—someday." After waiting so long, it is hard for her to believe the time has finally arrived. When labor is active she becomes very assured that "It is **me** and it is **now**!" Toward the end of labor, the mother is saying, "Make it now! Let there be a separation of us!" The questions are resolved with the reality of the delivery.

Psychosocial Changes in the Expectant Father. Fatherhood is not synonymous with motherhood. Fatherhood is socially and emotionally significant in its own right. Fathers indicate that their mate's pregnancy touches virtually every facet of living, including their self-image, their role as a husband, their social contacts, and even their work relationships [52]. Even though it may engender fears regarding the financial security of the home, the woman's pregnancy is almost always a source of pride to the man; he sees it as evidence of his power to share in the creation of life and of his masculinity. Many men become more health conscious (e.g., a decrease in smoking). They feel the need to take care of themselves so they will be ready for the new responsibility [41].

Changes in gender-related, culturally imposed roles and physical removal from the extended family both allow and require the man to become more involved in his wife's pregnancy. Many men try to forge a special relationship with the fetus by going shopping with the wife (especially for baby things), increasing participation in home care, and readying the baby's room [41]. The tough, domineering, unemotional "real man" portrayed by the mass media may put the father in conflict with how he really wants to act and to react. He may question his own gender identity, feeling that he will be seen as effeminate or even homosexual if he is "soft" [9]. This reaction may prevent him from giving his wife the tenderness she needs during this time.

One study indicates that there are three basic orientations of men that can strongly influence their response to an involvement in pregnancy [7, 27]:

1. The man with an immature romantic orientation to his union may experience a sharp maturational crisis with the advent of pregnancy. The need to assume more and new responsibilities may leave him with a sense of awe. He is frightened by the threatened loss of a carefree adolescence. His casualness may precipitate marital and in-law crises. Juvenile notions of masculinity may be reassessed. The integrative task of evolving a new self-identity may be extremely difficult. He may find his wife's changing figure less attractive, even repulsive.

2. The career-oriented man may resent the intrusion of the pregnancy, feeling that "it" is a burden that will interfere with his life goals. This is especially true if he is still engaged in educational preparations. His more ritualistic approach to life makes him want to retain the locus of control. He may see his old self to be quite adequate and will resist changes in his self-identity, especially when imposed by his wife, in-laws, and friends. He tends to continue old habits including motorcycling and camping with his wife. A detached attitude is common.

3. The family-oriented man accepts pregnancy as a divine gift. He feels that fatherhood is another goal in the fulfillment of life and assumes anticipatory fatherhood behaviors during the pregnancy. He thrills at the changes in his wife. Together they watch and feel the baby move, look at and read books, and attend parenting classes. Like the mother, he begins to watch other children more, to seek out couples with children, to talk to other people's babies, and to ask questions of his own parents. He also may fantasize an infant. His integrative task is made easier by his participation in the pregnancy and his anticipation of new responsibilities. A very close bond with his wife may evolve into a new and richer partnership.

Regardless of their orientation, some men feel that they lose their own identity as the woman's pregnancy becomes the focus of attention and conversation by friends and relatives as well as of their lifestyle. "The American culture reinforces a pregnant woman much more actively than it does an expectant father" [19]. He may feel left out and insignificant unless health care agencies, family, and friends consciously include him in the preparation and interests. He may feel that the obstetrician has replaced him in importance to his wife and may come to resent the pregnancy and the child. Some men will cover up or deny their reactions by becoming overinvolved in work or hobbies. Participation in prenatal classes or father's groups that explore men's feelings and the couple's relationship can help men to work through any problems during pregnancy, improve marital quality, and enhance bonding to the baby [19, 57].

The Couvade Syndrome. Twenty to 25 percent of men may identify so closely with the woman's pregnancy that they develop psychosomatic symptoms mimicking pregnancy or other physical problems [30, 55]. Loss of appetite, toothache, nausea, vomiting, and weight gain are common—even abdominal pain and distension. Some professionals feel that the symptoms are an unconscious bid for equal time and attention or a result of envy of the woman's ability to conceive. Other professionals feel that the majority of symptoms appear to be caused by anxiety (usually unperceived) felt by the man for the woman [55]. Still others see the couvade syndrome as a positive identification on the part of the man with what the woman is experiencing. Occasionally, other relatives, including siblings of the baby-to-be, may experience an increase of physical problems. The man may be very sensitive to any teasing about his symptoms and needs a warm and accepting approach from anyone helping him to handle his symptoms. Medical personnel need to take the couple's pregnancy into account when planning any medical care for the father.

Sex during Pregnancy

Most couples experience changes in their sexual relationship after the advent of pregnancy. Changes in hormonal balance cause some women to desire more sexual activity (especially around midpoint) [36] and others to want less. Fear of disturbing the pregnancy may cause other couples to avoid coitus. Some men feel it is immoral, improper, or unclean to have sex during pregnancy. Superstitions and fears of fetal loss or damage discourage some men. Their concerns over possible birth defects are as great as women's during the pregnancy [41, 48]. For some, abstinence may be seen as an excuse to seek extramarital affairs. For others, it may be the "ultimate sacrifice" of the man to ensure a successful birth [41]. Intercourse becomes increasingly awkward as the pregnancy advances. A broad repertoire of techniques and alternatives as well

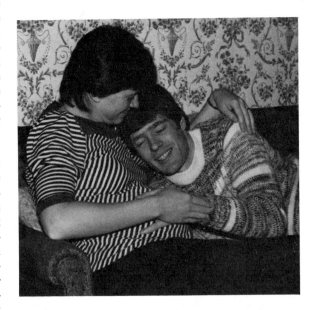

Figure 31–3. The father can be an active member of the pregnancy. Both the father and the mother begin to know their baby before it is born by noting its activity level and response to stimuli. Such shared experiences help to prepare them for the emotional investment that is essential to the infant's (and their own) socioaffective development in the months ahead.

as a sense of humor can help the couple through the later months.

The woman's changing body shape requires a redefinition of body image and sexuality for both the pregnant woman and her mate. Some men find the pregnant woman to be attractive and desirable; others find her grossly repulsive. The latter attitude can create great strain on the union. The woman likewise may feel herself to be very attractive, or she may feel "like an elephant." Her self-concept will affect the relationship with her partner.

Most physicians place no sexual restrictions on their clients as long as they are comfortable and there are no cervical changes. Most women (over 80%) report no pain during intercourse [51]. Other pregnant women may experience a sense of fullness or even pain for as long as 30 minutes after sexual arousal [21]. Orgasm in the female is associated with uterine contractions. Consequently, women who are prone to spontaneous abortion in early pregnancy may be advised to avoid orgasms. Research indicates that orgasm in late pregnancy may increase Braxton-Hicks contractions or even lead to premature labor [21]. In fact, some cultures use the stimulation of orgasm as a method to induce labor.

Abstinence may be recommended by some physicians for the last 2 to 6 weeks of pregnancy. Although rare, there is some evidence that air may be introduced into the vagina during sexual foreplay, which can lead to death of the mother as a result of air embolism [21]. The introduction of bacteria may lead to infection. These dangers may require reassessment of priorities and sexuality for the couple. Other physicians recommend no restrictions; this approach is appreciated by the couple who experience heightened sexual drive with the onset of early labor.

INFERTILITY

Infertility, "the inability to achieve a pregnancy after one year of sexual relations without contraception, or the inability to carry a pregnancy to a live birth" [39], is a problem for 15 percent or one out of seven couples [18]. Thirty-five percent of infertility problems are of male origin, and 50 percent of female origin [47]. Couples who have never produced a child are said to have **primary infertility.** Couples who have had at least one child are classified under **secondary infertility.** The term **sterility** is reserved for those conditions producing irreversible infertility.

Females usually achieve maximum fertility at about 24 years of age and males at 25 years of age. Fertility rates begin to diminish rapidly in females after age 30 and in males after age 45, although men in their eighties have been known to father children [26].

Response of the Couple to Infertility

The inability to conceive a child—especially primary infertility—can be devastating to a young couple. Infertility constitutes a critical and complex life crisis. The individuals involved feel as if the future is out of their control. This forced helplessness is a grave threat to ego-identity and integrity. Infertility may also pose a threat to the individual's sexual integrity, necessitating a redefining of sexuality as well as of roles, goals, and worthiness [33]. These internal stressors, combined with the external social pressures to have children, may precipitate a psychological crisis that can be severe enough to interfere with functioning in all four domains. The woman may feel that she has been "cheated" out of her career. The man may feel guilty for "theft" of the woman's rights [37]. The couple who seek help with their problem may find it financially and emotionally expensive. Their initial hope and enthusiasm give way to despair and depression as the months pass by.

Causes of Infertility

Fifty to 60 percent of infertile couples can be "cured"—often by gaining a better understanding of anatomy and the process of conception. Others may require medical or surgical assistance or even psychotherapy. During the first visit for infertility assistance, the husband and wife are usually counseled about male and female anatomy (see Chap. 3) and coital techniques. Occasionally couples are identified who have not achieved full male penetration, even after several years of marriage. Some women routinely douche immediately before coitus; the resulting change in pH may prevent conception by killing the sperm.

The couple is also counseled on the ovarian cycle (see Chap. 3) and the viability of the ovum. Some couples have thought that the fertile period occurred at the end of the menses, like the estrus cycle of a cat or a dog. A clear understanding of the timing of coitus in relation to ovulation may be sufficient to achieve a pregnancy. The woman is usually given a chart to keep a record of her early morning temperature. A rise of 0.5 to 1.0°F indicates that ovulation has occurred (the increase in progesterone causes the elevated temperature). The woman is asked to keep the chart for several months in order to identify an ovulatory pattern (see Fig. 31–1).

The husband and wife are asked to apply any new information they may have obtained at the interview. The couple should also obtain a complete medical checkup and examination of the reproductive system to rule out any obvious organic causes of infertility. Subsequent visits are under the direct supervision of a medical doctor.

MALE FACTORS

The doctor will usually request a semen analysis to check male fertility. This specimen is easily obtained from the man by wearing a condom during intercourse or through self-stimulation and ejaculation into a clean receptacle. The average volume is 3 ml per ejaculate (less than 1 teaspoon), with about 100,000 sperm per cubic centimeter [58]. All the sperm are not completely or well formed (morphology), but at least 60 percent must be so in order to achieve a pregnancy (Table 31–3). If the results from the semen analysis are poor, some changes in environmental factors may lead to improvement. Attention to adequate diet and vitamins may improve morphology. Thyroid extract can improve the concentration [43]. Heavy alcohol consumption is suspected of causing some types of infertility.

Motility of the sperm can be affected by heat. The testes develop in the fetal abdominal cavity and descend into the scrotal sac before or shortly after birth. The scrotum is a physiologically active muscle covering the testes and spermatic cords that maintains the testicular temperature approximately 2.2°C lower than the abdominal temperature [43]. As body temperature increases due to exercise or environmental temperature, the scrotum relaxes and allows the testes to be lowered and cooled. In cooler conditions, the scrotum draws the testes close to the body to maintain their temperature. Exposure to heat can damage developing sperm; recovery may require several weeks. Repeated exposure to high temperatures can cause permanent

damage [43]. Counseling can frequently identify heat-related causes of decreased motility; for example, the man may have been taking frequent very hot baths or wearing jockey shorts or an athletic support.

Common preventable causes of male sterility include postpubertal mumps, exposure to x-rays, undescended testicles, and venereal disease.

FEMALE FACTORS

One of the first goals of the physician is to discover whether or not the woman is ovulating. Evaluation of the temperature chart can give some clues: The first and last half of an anovulatory cycle may show minimal change in average temperature. Most women experience one or two anovulatory cycles per year [43]. Two medications are available to stimulate the ovulatory function of the ovary. Injections of menotropins (Pergonal) followed by HCG stimulate growth and maturation of the graafian follicle. Chlomiphene citrate (Clomid), taken orally, stimulates the pituitary to release FSH. Both treatments, especially Pergonal, are associated with a higher than average multiple birth rate due to multiple ovulation [28].

A second major cause of female infertility, blockage of the fallopian tubes due to a previous infection (especially gonorrhea), can be identified through relatively simple procedures. The success rate of surgical repair is variable, depending heavily on the extent of the damage.

Women who are able to conceive but have difficulty maintaining the pregnancy may be assisted by hormonal therapy (progesterone) during the first trimester. Spontaneous abortion due to an incompetent cervix may be prevented by suturing of the cervix until term.

MALE-FEMALE PROBLEMS

Some infertility problems result from the unique combination of two otherwise normal individuals. Forty to

Table 31-3. Normal Semen Analysis

Factor	Normal Values	Lowest Value Needed To Achieve Conception
Volume	1.5–5 ml	1.0 ml
Motility		
Percentage	Over 60%	50%
Rate (evaluated on a scale of 1–10)	8–10	5
Concentration	40–160 million/ml	20 million/ml
Total sperm count	Variable	50,000,000/ejaculate
Morphology	Over 70% normal and mature sperm	60 percent normal and mature sperm

60 percent of joint fertility is due to an antigen-antibody reaction: The woman's cervical mucosa may form antibodies against the husband's semen, thus killing the sperm [43]. Diagnosis is made by microscopic evaluation of semen removed from the vagina approximately one hour after intercourse. The antibody level can be reduced by preventing contact for 3 to 12 months (most couples prefer to use a condom rather than abstinence). The cervical mucosa can be bypassed by artificial insemination with the husband's sperm (AIH).

Faulty understanding of spermatogenesis may also decrease the chances of pregnancy. A couple may attempt to "save up" sperm by avoiding intercourse until the time of ovulation. Since sperm have a high mortality rate after 3 weeks of storage, the couple may actually be implanting only dead sperm. On the other hand, the couple may have intercourse daily or several times daily around the time of ovulation. Because of inadequate opportunity to build up a reserve supply, the total sperm count may be too low to achieve a pregnancy. Couples are usually encouraged to maintain a normal pattern of sexual activity throughout the month and then to have intercourse every other day around the time of ovulation as indicated by the temperature chart. The woman is also encouraged to remain on her back for at least 30 minutes after intercourse to facilitate bathing of the cervix with the semen [43].

PSYCHOGENIC INFERTILITY

Occasionally, infertility can be the result of an unconscious desire to avoid parenthood, even though on the conscious level the individual may express an intense desire for pregnancy. Emotional factors can produce physiological changes (e.g., tubal spasm, anovulation, reduced sperm count), which can prevent conception [45]. Some individuals may subtly avoid coitus during potentially fertile times. Counseling can be very helpful in identifying their true feelings. Women may fear dying in childbirth or having an abnormal child; they may also be afraid of losing their mate during pregnancy because of decreased attractiveness and after the birth because of competition. Both male and female infertility may stem from hostility or marked ambivalence toward one's own mother [45] as well as weak self-identity. Psychotherapy and reeducation in interpersonal relationships may help such persons to resolve old conflicts and resulting guilt, thus enabling the individual to achieve pregnancy and meet parenthood responsibilities more successfully.

Alternatives

ARTIFICIAL INSEMINATION

Artificial insemination with the husband's sperm (AIH) can be used when the man's sperm count or concentration is low. The husband's semen is centrifuged to increase the concentration and then frozen in nitrogen vapor until needed. Pregnancy may be achieved if sperm from three or four ejaculates are concentrated and combined. Frozen sperm may maintain motility indefinitely; a woman in England conceived a child through AIH 8 months after her husband's death [1].

If the husband's semen analysis is very poor, the couple may choose artificial insemination with donor sperm (AID). Twenty thousand children are conceived each year by AID [1]. Because of the religious, ethical, and legal issues involved, intensive counseling should accompany this form of semiadoption. The physician usually chooses a donor who is physically similar to the husband. Mixing of the husband's semen with that of the anonymous donor frequently helps to offset adverse psychological reactions.

Sperm banks have been established as repositories for donor sperm. One of these banks specializes in storing sperm of Nobel Prize winners and other eminent, intelligent men. Nine percent of AID recipients are single women [1].

IN VITRO FERTILIZATION

The advances in medical science now allow a physician to remove a ripe ovum from the ovary, mix it with sperm, allow it to grow briefly (8- to 60-cell stage), and then place it in a woman's uterus (test tube babies). Each year, more children are conceived and born by this method [1].

The processes of marital unity, procreation, childbearing, and childrearing no longer need to be seen as one. The links can be substituted at any point. This raises ethical, religious, medical, and legal issues for each couple and even for society. A husband's sperm may fertilize a donor's ovum and be implanted in the wife. A husband's sperm and a wife's ovum may even be implanted in a surrogate mother after conception to bypass the problem of habitual abortion. The medical possibilities for infertile couples are endless. Some medical centers are now freezing young embryos for implantation at a later date. What is the legal status of a frozen embryo if the parents die before implantation?

ADOPTION

The other alternative for infertile couples who want to increase their family is through adoption. Again, intensive counseling is advised in this situation. "Infertile couples seeking to adopt a child are often plagued by unresolved feelings of grief, low self-esteem and threatened sexuality" [39].

Couples who do not achieve a pregnancy may be financially and emotionally exhausted when they apply for adoption. They frequently feel lonely and isolated. Individuals who have children (or who do not want children) do not understand the emotional pain the couple is experiencing and may offer platitudes rather than real support. Couples are often embarrassed to discuss their infertility even with each other, let alone with parents or friends. Misinformation may prolong the delay in seeking professional help. Friends and family may suggest that the infertility is "all in the head" or that the couple just needs a change of pace or a second honeymoon. The woman may feel shame and guilt that she is "not fulfilled" and the man because he is "not virile." These reactions need to be resolved.

Couples (and some single persons) can legally adopt children through agencies or private sources. The decline in the number of children available for adoption, however, may constitute still another threat to the psychological health of the infertile couple, because this situation once more places them out of control of their own destiny.

All states designate a division of the welfare department or children's services to handle adoptions. Private agencies also offer adoption services. Although each agency sets its own policies, procedures, and price, each is subject to state law. Private adoptions are legal in some states and may be arranged through a lawyer or a physician. The cost of private adoptions is generally higher. State agencies usually offer the couple greater security; occasionally private adoptions may be challenged because of legal loopholes or inadequate release procedures.

Most states require an adjustment period of 6 months to 1 year before the adoption can be finalized. The couple may see this as another anxiety-producing situation, fearing that the child with whom they are falling in love may be removed from their home (which is, however, very rare).

Couples who are unwilling to wait 3 to 5 years for an infant may choose to adopt an older child, a biracial child, or a "handicapped" child. Some states have subsidized adoption plans that will assist the couple with the medical expenses of the physically disabled child. International adoptions are also becoming increasingly popular.

Adoption presents an emotional barrier to some cou-

ples who feel strongly about blood lines or whose concept of sexuality is tied to their ability to procreate. Such a couple may need to redefine their concept of sexuality as well as their values, priorities, and goals. Unsound motives for adoption and unresolved conflicts about infertility may affect the quality of the parent-child relationship. The chances of success in adoption are as great as those with natural-born children when the parents have accepted their infertility realistically, without guilt or other anxiety, and when the child is accepted unreservedly as an individual to be loved, nurtured, and guided.

SUMMARY

Procreation is not synonymous with parenthood. Successful parenthood requires sufficient personal maturity to become unselfishly involved in facilitating the growth and development of another person. But parenthood is only one avenue for achieving Erikson's tasks of generativity. Many couples achieve generativity through their careers, community service, and hobbies. Veevers states that, "It is in everyone's best interest to make having children the result of a deliberate choice, rather than of sexual happenstance" [55]. The childless marriage is equally viable and satisfying to a couple if it is a **chosen** lifestyle [17]. It can be devastating if it results from involuntary infertility. The decision to have a child should be jointly resolved by the couple through a weighing of personal and family assets, values, goals, and priorities: "Every pregnancy, no matter how enthusiastically welcomed and experienced, requires the prospective parents to perform a significant amount of psychological 'work' in order to prepare themselves physically and emotionally for the arrival of their new child. This work consists of personal change and growth and necessarily causes some amount of anxiety" [22]. Different maturity levels, degrees of involvement, and social pressures may influence the reactions of the couple individually and jointly.

The pregnant woman tends to become introverted and to have wide changes in mood as she attempts to integrate the new experience with her past, present, and future self-identity. The social and emotional support of the expectant father and the extended family can influence her acceptance of the pregnancy and the smoothness of her transition to parenthood after the birth.

Pregnancy and childbirth provide one more avenue of emotional involvement between the husband and wife. The experience tends to bring out the "hidden side" of masculinity. Expressions of caring, concern, and tenderness emerge, and feelings of empathy, fear, weakness, and sympathy are expressed [40]. Both the mother and the father find pregnancy a sobering and maturing yet exciting and fulfilling experience when a child is wanted and planned for.

The options for both inhibiting and facilitating conception allow most couples marked control in the process of family planning. The issue is no longer how and when to become pregnant but if and why. Many moral, legal, and religious issues are raised by the medical options available today.

REFERENCES

1. Anderson, J. K. *Genetic Engineering.* Grand Rapids, MI: Zondervan, 1982.
2. Anthony, E. J., and Benedek, T. (Eds.). *Parenthood: Its Psychology and Psychopathology.* Boston: Little, Brown, 1970.
3. Barglow, P., and Brown, E. Pseudocyesis. In J. G. Howells (Ed.), *Modern Perspectives in Psycho-Obstetrics.* New York: Brunner/Mazel, 1972.
4. Benedek, T. The Psychobiology of Pregnancy. In E. J. Anthony and T. Benedek (Eds.), *Parenthood: Its Psychology and Psychopathology.* Boston: Little, Brown, 1970.
5. Bibring, G. L. Some Considerations of the Psychological Processes in Pregnancy. In *Psychoanalytic Study of the Child,* Vol. 14. New York: International Universities Press, 1959.
6. Bibring, G. L., et al. A Study of the Psychological Process in Pregnancy and of the Earliest Mother-Child Relationship. In *Psychoanalytic Study of the Child,* Vol. 16. New York: International Universities Press, 1961.
7. Biller, H. B., and Meredith, D. *Father Power.* New York: David McKay, 1975.
8. Billings, J. J. *The Ovulation Method: Natural Family Planning* (4th American Ed.). Collegeville, MN: Liturgical Press, 1978.
9. Campbell, A. The American way of mating: Marriage si, children only maybe. *Psychology Today* 8(12):37, 1975.
10. Carter-Jessop, L. Promoting maternal attachment through prenatal intervention. *MCN* 6:107, 1981.
11. Chez, R. A. Sex in pregnancy. *Contemp. Ob./Gyn.* 6(2):99, 1975.
12. Child, M., et al. Oral contraceptives and cancer risk. *Morbidity and Mortality Weekly Report.* Centers for Disease Control 31:393, 1982.
13. Coleman, S., and Piotrow, P. T. Spermicides—Simplicity and Safety Are Major Assets. *Population Reports,* Series H. Barrier Methods H–79–H–118, 1979.
14. Donovan, C. M., Greenspan, R., and Mittleman, F. The decision-making process, and the outcome of therapeutic abortion. *Am. J. Psychiatry* 131:1332, 1974.
15. Effects of abortion on later pregnancy. *Contemp. Ob./Gyn.* 8(3):66, 1976.
16. *FDA Drug Bulletin* 8(2):12, 1978.
17. Feldman, H. A comparison of intentional parents and intentionally childless couples. *J. Marr. and the Fam.* 43:593, 1981.
18. Friedman, B. M. Infertility workup. *Am. J. Nurs.* 81:2041, 1981.
19. Gearing, J. Facilitating the birth process and father-child bonding. *The Counseling Psychologist* 7(4):53, 1978.
20. Goldenring, J. M. Letter to the Editor. *New Engl. J. Med.* 307(9):564C, 1982.
21. Goodlin, R. C. Can sex in pregnancy harm the fetus? *Contemp. Ob./Gyn.* 8(5):21, 1976.
22. Grossman, F. K., Eichler, L. S., and Winickoff, S. A. *Pregnancy, Birth, and Parenthood.* San Francisco: Jossey-Bass, 1980.
23. Harper, M. J. K. *Birth Control Technologies: Prospects by the Year 2000.* Austin, TX: University of Texas Press, 1983.
24. Howells, J. G. Termination of Pregnancy. In J. G. Howells (Ed.), *Modern Perspectives in Psycho-Obstetrics.* New York: Brunner/Mazel, 1972.
25. Hubert, J. Belief and Reality: Social Factors in Pregnancy and Childbirth. In M. P. M. Richards (Ed.), *The Integration of a Child into a Social World.* London: Cambridge University Press, 1974.
26. *Infertility.* Columbus, OH: Ohio State University Hospitals, 1975.
27. Jessner, L., Weigert, E., and Foy, J. L. The Development of Parental Attitudes during Pregnancy. In E. J. Anthony and T. Benedek (Eds.), *Parenthood: Its Psychology and Psychopathology.* Boston: Little, Brown, 1970.
28. Johns, M. P. *Pharmacodynamics and Patient Care.* St. Louis: Mosby, 1974.
29. Kee, B. L., and Schult, M. O. Maternal Development. In E. J. Dickason and M. O. Schult (Eds.), *Maternal and Infant Care.* New York: McGraw-Hill, 1975.
30. Ketter, D. E., and Shelton, B. J. Pregnant and physically fit, too. *Am. J. of Matern.-Child Nurs. J.* 9:120, 1984.
31. Lamb, G. S., and Lipkin, M. Somatic symptoms of expectant fathers. *MCN* 7:110, 1982.
32. Landers, A. If you had it to do over again, would you have children? *Good Housekeeping* 182(6):100, 1976.
33. Love, V. *Childless is Not Less.* Minneapolis, MN: Bethany House, 1984.
34. Lumley, J. M. Attitudes to the fetus among primipares. *Aust. Paediatr. J.* 18:106, 1982.
35. Madore, C., et al. A study on the effects of induced abortion on subsequent pregnancy outcome. *Am. J. Obstet. Gynecol.* 139:516, 1981.
36. Masters, W., and Johnson, V. *Human Sexual Response.* Boston: Little, Brown, 1966.
37. McKee, L., and O'Brien, M. The Father Figure: Some Current Orientations and Historical Perspectives. In L. McKee and M. O'Brien (Eds.), *The Father Figure.* New York: Tavistock, 1982.
38. Mears, E. The Control of Conception. In J. G. Howells

(Ed.), *Modern Perspectives in Psycho-Obstetrics*. New York: Brunner/Mazel, 1972.

39. Menning, B. E.   The infertile couple: A plea for advocacy. *Child Welfare* 54:454, 1975.

40. National Center for Health Statistics.   *Advance Report on Final Natility Statistics, 1980.*

41. Richman, J.   Men's Experience of Pregnancy and Childbirth. In L. McKee and M. O'Brien (Eds.), *The Father Figure.* New York: Tavistock, 1982.

42. Rising costs for raising children. *U.S. News and World Report* 91(21):9, 1981.

43. Roland, M.   *Management of the Infertile Couple.* Springfield, IL: Thomas, 1968.

44. Rosenthal, T.   Voluntary Childlessness and the Nurse's Role. *MCN* 5:398, 1980.

45. Rothman, D., and Kaplan, A. H.   Psychosomatic Infertility in the Male and Female. In J. G. Howells (Ed.), *Modern Perspectives in Psycho—Obstetrics.* New York: Brunner/Mazel, 1972.

46. Rubin, R.   Cognitive style in pregnancy. *Am. J. Nurs.* 70:502, 1970.

47. Rutledge, A. L.   Psychomarital evaluation and treatment of the infertile couple. *Clin. Obstet. Gynecol.* 22:255, 1979.

48. Schuster, C. S.   Unpublished research, 1980.

49. Shapiro, H. I.   *The Birth Control Book.* New York: Avon Books, 1982.

50. Smith, E. M.   A follow-up study of women who request abortion. *Am. J. Orthopsychiatry* 43:574, 1973.

51. Steege, J. F., and Jelousek, F. R.   Sexual behavior during pregnancy. *Obstet. Gynecol.* 60:168, 1982.

52. Support for expectant fathers. *Pediatric Nursing Currents* 23(6):26, 1976.

53. Tipping, V. G.   The vulnerability of a primipara during the antenatal period. *Matern.-Child Nurs. J.* 10:61, 1981.

54. Trabert, C.   Prenatal tactile intervention can be encouraged. *MCN* 6:108, 1981.

55. Trethowan, W. H.   The Couvade Syndrome. In J. C. Howells (Ed.), *Modern Perspectives in Psycho-Obstetrics.* New York: Brunner/Mazel, 1972.

56. Veevers, J. E.   *Childless by Choice.* Toronto: Butterworth, 1980.

57. Woolery, L., and Barkley, N.   Enhancing couple relationships during prenatal and postnatal classes. *MCN* 6:184, 1981.

58. Ziegel, E., and Cranley, M. S.   *Obstetric Nursing* (7th ed.). New York: Macmillan, 1978.

32

The Expanding Family

Clara S. Schuster

Common concern for the helplessly dependent infant promotes an integrating union of the prospective parents; and this solidarity strengthens the endurance of anxieties and frustrations as much as it fosters dedication to the child and his future.

—Lucie Jessner, Edith Weigert, and James Foy, *Parenthood*

Preparation for parenthood begins long before the birth of a new baby, in fact, even before conception; it begins with one's own infancy and relationship with one's parents [31]. Pregnancy and childbirth merely intensify the process. A number of significant decisions need to be made when a couple is expecting a child. One decision concerns employment: How long will the woman continue to work, and when will she return to the job market—if at all? Should she return to work while the husband remains at home for child care? If both parents return to work, what arrangements are available for child care—should they use grandparents, a babysitter, or a day care nursery? Is the cost of child care adequately offset by the woman's salary to make her return to work worthwhile? Can part-time work, home-based work, or alternating hours for husband and wife be arranged? Though innocuous on the surface, these decisions may be critical to the optimal development of the child, and they can be a source of crisis and conflict for couples who feel that the woman's place is in the home, while financial conditions still require her assistance in supplementing the family income.

Another major decision involves the method of infant feeding. For some women the commitment to breast-feeding or bottle-feeding is established long before pregnancy is confirmed [6]—by previous experiences, psychosexual development, and the meaning of the breast to the woman. However, even though the decision is hers finally, it is not hers alone. The support of her mother, the attitude of the husband, and even the opinion of friends become significant in both the woman's decision and her success at breast-feeding [6] should that be her choice. Some women are greatly repulsed by the idea of breast-feeding, feeling that it is "animalistic." Some husbands are very possessive of the wife's breasts and do not want them shared by the baby. Other children in the family may feel that breast-feeding is degrading, "weird," or "sick." The negative attitudes of others may be conveyed to the breast-feeding mother in both overt and covert ways, which can undermine her commitment to this form of nurturing. Because of all the adjustments she is making to new responsibilities and relationships, the new mother is vulnerable at this time to the opinions of others.

A third major decision centers around health care for the childbirth experience. Twenty years ago mothers found a physician through family or friends and then followed his or her advice exclusively. Today, the decision regarding the amount of active involvement the couple will have in the birth process belongs to the woman and her partner. How much do the woman and her partner want to participate in the birth experience? Do they want to have the baby at home [60], at a childbirth center [51], or in a hospital? Today, couples are encouraged to choose a physician who supports their views on the childbearing process.

It is essential at this time that the woman (and her partner) have absolute confidence in the skill and integrity of the physician. The doctor's role is more than physical support; it involves emotional support of the entire family during this crisis event. Because of their commitment to the family-centered approach while offering high-quality care to the healthy expectant couple, midwives are gaining more acceptance in the United States. For most couples, pregnancy and childbirth should be approached as a normal process and as a social event rather than as an illness or disease state requiring extensive medical direction and intervention to maintain or to regain high level wellness.

PREPARATION FOR CHILDBIRTH AND PARENTING

Almost all couples engage in some preparation for childbirth and child care. For many it will involve only the purchasing of essential clothing and supplies; others may discuss the upcoming childbirth experience with their friends and family members. Unfortunately,

these sources frequently have various "horror stories" to tell, which may increase the pregnant woman's fears rather than help her to prepare realistically and constructively for the event of childbirth. Many pregnant couples read pamphlets from the physician's office, but what is shared by friends has more reality than the contents of an impersonal booklet. Some women systematically write down questions to ask the obstetrician. Others find the public library to be a rich source of information on fetal development, childbirth, and child care. A growing number of parents take advantage of formal classes offered in the community.

Instruction in Child Care and Parenting

Many communities offer a variety of classes on preparation for parenthood. Recently, more public school systems have been including parenting courses as a part of their health education series [92]—a trend the author highly supports. Adult education programs, volunteer community groups, and some doctors sponsor classes for expectant parents. The American Red Cross offers, free of charge, an excellent preparation-for-parenthood class that encourages participation of the father as well as the mother. A number of hospitals have successfully inaugurated innovative prenatal education classes for children that help prepare them for the arrival of a new sibling. [85]. The processes of pregnancy, childbirth, and sibling rivalry are all covered in detail. Some hospitals make provisions to allow siblings to attend the birth [63].

Many parents-to-be are unable to project themselves beyond the birth experience and consequently obtain very little knowledge about the techniques of child care. These individuals depend on the hospital staff, their mothers, or friends to tell them what to do and how to care for the baby. The information that parents want and need is covered in other sections of this text (e.g., characteristics of neonates, Chap. 6; common concerns, Chap. 7; safety, Chap. 8; and interactional tools, Chap. 9). Practitioners working with new parents need to be aware that the parents' knowledge of infant care and infant development is probably quite limited [47], and should offer assistance by teaching infant care and parenting skills as well as providing information on other community resources, such as public health nurses, Child Conservation League (CCL), extension courses from colleges and universities, adult education courses sponsored by the local school systems and the American Red Cross. The American Red Cross First Aid Course is also recommended to parents because it can help prepare them to handle some

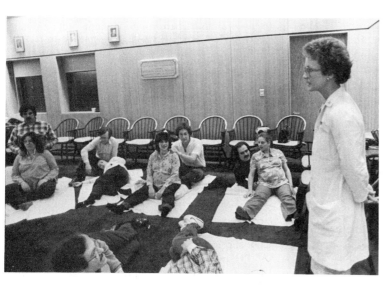

Figure 32–1. Parents who participate in childbirth classes find themselves better prepared for the experience. Childbirth can be as encompassing for the father as it is for the mother when the couple works together in the birth of their child. (Courtesy of Beth Israel Hospital, Boston. Photograph by Michael Lutch.)

of the minor injuries all children receive in the process of growing up.

Preparation for Childbirth

Many communities now have one or more organized programs to help parents acquire knowledge and skills that assist the woman to remain relatively comfortable and in control of herself during labor, and to allow both the woman and her partner to participate actively in her labor and the delivery of their baby. These classes usually include information on anatomy and the birth process as well as special techniques of relaxation and breathing. Participants indicate they have reduced anxiety, heightened concentration, and decreased pain during the childbirth process, all of which help to foster enjoyment of the experience. The psychophysical (Dick-Reed) method encourages mental dissociation from the body with relaxation and breathing activities. Education and exercises are used effectively to break the fear-tension-pain cycle. The psychoprophylactic (Lamaze) method applies classic Pavlovian conditioning to childbirth. Through conditioning, discipline, and concentration, new responses are taught to block out the perception of pain. In both these methods, and in the Bradley method, the couple learn a new appreciation for the functioning of the body during labor. All these methods teach the couple how to work with, rather than against, the body in order to facilitate the labor process. "The woman learns how to integrate the physical, emotional and intellectual aspects of her personality so that she can work as a harmonious and fo-

cused unit throughout the complex demands of labor" [15]. The unprepared woman finds that the physical domain begins to dominate her responses, blocking rational and effectual integration of the cognitive and affective domains.

The provision of a physically and socially supportive environment by the husband or other meaningful person reduces the woman's stressors and facilitates her ability to work cooperatively with her labor process. Fatigue is minimized, and the sense of being in control is maximized. Women left alone for long periods during labor may experience sensory deprivation and confusion [49]. The woman's favorable response to labor seems to depend on the presence of the father rather than the ease of the labor [49]. If the father of the baby is present in the delivery room, she reaches out to share this historic moment [14].

Although the purist would advocate that the use of these "natural childbirth" methods be substituted for medication during labor and delivery, most instructors of the methods, doctors, and mothers themselves see the use of these methods as a way to reduce, not to eliminate, medication—as a way to remain in control of the labor, rather than to be controlled by it. Research indicates that prepared women have shorter labors, need less medication, and enjoy the birth experience more [38, 59].

Classes in parenting and preparation for childbirth also give the parents an opportunity to meet with other young couples and thus to share ideas and fears under the guidance of a knowledgeable person. The emotional and social bond of the expectant parents may be strengthened as they pursue a common interest. Contact with other expectant couples can help them to assess their own changing roles and goals. The peer group can offer a support system that substitutes for the guidance and socialization formerly offered by the extended family.

Not all parents attend classes, although they may be available in the community. Factors, such as lack of time, previous knowledge and experience, lack of interest, or cultural conditioning, may prevent attendance. Some mothers feel that they do not need preparation (childbirth is a "natural event"); some are afraid that classes will increase their fear (they want to avoid the experience); others do not believe that anything can really help (the helplessness syndrome). It should be strongly emphasized that classes can and do help even the most fearful, the most naive, and the most unbelieving to experience easier, more satisfying childbirth and child-care experiences. Even multiparous parents have stated that preparation-for-childbirth classes offered them the opportunity to be more intelligent health care consumers.

THE BIRTH PROCESS

Several events may occur toward the end of gestation that give the mother and her physician clues that labor is imminent:

1. Descent of the baby's head into the pelvic cavity causes a slight forward tilt of the uterus ("lightening"). This movement greatly relieves pressure on the rib cage and diaphragm, so that breathing is easier; however, it increases the pressure on the bladder.
2. "Ripening," or softening, of the cervix occurs in response to both the pressure of the fetus and hormonal influences. Most women have effacement (thinning of the cervical walls) and some dilatation (opening of the cervix) prior to the onset of labor.
3. Changes in hormonal levels may make the woman alternately very tired or full of energy. The instability of her energy level may be confusing to both the woman and those around her.
4. The frequency and strength of Braxton-Hicks contractions (the irregular uterine contractions experienced throughout pregnancy) will increase. Occasionally, these contractions may be regular enough and strong enough to cause the mother to believe she is in early labor. She may be hospitalized

for several hours before the phenomenon known as "false labor" is identified. Although painful, these contractions are not strong enough to cause the essential effacement and dilation. The disappointed mother is sent home to await the onset of true labor.

Initiation of Labor

The initiation of labor is dependent on a "constellation of interrelated events." No one factor is responsible for the total process of initiating labor. One factor may remain stable while the levels of other elements change. It is the critical change of several components that appears to trigger labor. The major components appear to be [82]:

1. The secretion of adrenocorticotropic hormone (ACTH) by the fetal pituitary stimulates the fetal adrenals to increase cortisol production, which in turn initiates uterine events.
2. A rise in maternal estrogen levels increases the vascularity of the uterus and the responsiveness to oxytocin. Estrogen may also stimulate prostaglandin production.
3. The decidua (endometrial lining) begins production of prostaglandin, which, in turn, sustains estrogen levels and has an oxytocic effect on the uterus. Semen also has a high prostaglandin level and may play a role in initiating labor following intercourse in late pregnancy [16].
4. The aging process results in the production of less progesterone. The sensitivity and reactivity to oxytocin by the uterine muscle has been kept in abeyance throughout pregnancy by the presence of high progesterone levels.
5. Cervical and vaginal distension leads to reflex release of oxytocin by the mother (Ferguson's reflex).
6. Oxytocin appears to be the main hormone that stimulates uterine contractions. It is produced by the posterior pituitaries of both the mother and the fetus.

There are three classic signs of the initiation of labor. An individual woman may experience one, two, or all of them. The three signs are as follows:

1. The appearance of bloody discharge ("show") due to the loosening of the mucoid plug that has sealed the cervix during pregnancy.
2. The occurrence of uterine contractions, gradually increasing in frequency and intensity. Tightening may be felt in the back and lower abdomen, similar to that felt with menstrual cramps.

3. The rupture of the "bag of waters" enveloping the fetus, allowing passage of fluid through the vagina. This fluid may seep slowly, or a large amount may be emitted at once. The woman may confuse this event with urinary incontinence. There is no warning or pain. Women are encouraged to cover their mattress with a plastic protector during the last month of pregnancy and to wear a sanitary pad when they are out in public.

Labor and Delivery

As discussed in Chapter 5, labor is divided into three stages. Each woman's labor is uniquely her own. To compare experiences is unfair, but certain common elements do emerge. Many factors can influence both the duration of each stage and the mother's psychological response to that stage. During the first stage, the cervix is dilating to allow extrusion of the fetus; during the second stage the fetus passes through the birth canal (vagina); during the third stage the placenta is delivered. Some nurses call the first hours after delivery the "fourth stage," when the mother is still evacuating large amounts of blood and fluids from her body.

The first stage of labor is subdivided into three phases. The mother usually enters the health care system or calls for her childbirth assistant during the first phase. The contractions in this phase are not painful or prolonged (20 to 45 seconds). The rest periods between contractions gradually shorten from 20 minutes to about 5 minutes. The woman is usually comfortable and can walk around or even keep herself busy with household activities, reading, or sewing. She is generally excited and talkative. ("Who me? Now? Maybe it is only false labor.") There is an element of disbelief and ambivalence. ("Am I ready?")

This is a good time for the birth attendant to review the birth process and the relaxation and breathing techniques to be implemented in the next phases with the mother and her primary support person. If possible, the mother should be encouraged to rest between contractions in order to conserve energy for the work to come. During this phase, the cervix becomes effaced and dilates to about 4 cm.

As the contractions become stronger, longer, and more frequent, there is no longer any doubt ("Ready or not, it is **me** and it is **now!**") In the second phase, the woman loses her mood of excitement and entertainment; she becomes serious and introverted, concentrating on herself and her contractions. There is not much time for rest when the contractions occur every 3 to 5 minutes. However, the prepared mother is able to focus her energies to work with the contractions and

to relax and refresh herself between them. A strong, quiet, supportive environment greatly improves her confidence and her ability to concentrate. If the mother has chosen a hospital setting, fetal monitors (see Chap.5) are frequently attached at this point to assess the fetal response to the stressors of labor. Each contraction of the uterine muscles causes a temporary decrease or cessation of blood flow to the placental site. Consequently, monitoring of the duration of contractions and the fetal heart rate is recommended to assess the oxygen status of the fetus (see Fig. 5–4).

Contraction patterns have four distinct phases. The onset of the contraction is characterized by a gradual increase in intensity. The uterus can be felt to harden as the muscles contract. During the acme, or peak, of the contractions, the uterus appears to raise itself upward, away from the vertebrae. If the woman is fearful, she will tighten her body, including her abdominal muscles, thus counteracting the effectiveness of the uterine activity and increasing the pain. The intensity of the contraction is released during the decrement phase. Associated pain disappears, and blood flow returns to the placental site. The rest phase between active contractions is essential for both fetal and maternal recuperation.

The contractions of the second phase of the first stage of labor bring about complete effacement and dilate the cervix to 7 cm. These first two phases last approximately 10 hours for the primiparous woman (having her first baby) and are considerably shorter for the multiparous woman. Fortunately, the transition or third phase of the first stage of labor is brief (30 minutes to 1 hour). The 60- to 80-second contractions are intense and frequent (every 2 to 3 minutes), and the final dilation (8 to 10 cm) is hard work. A prepared partner (usually the spouse) can greatly facilitate the mother's ability to work with her body and to remain in control of the birth process. The close support of the father can be very meaningful to both of them at this time. The most effective focal point for the mother is her partner's eyes. The mature, well-prepared couple will function as a symbiotic team—a factor that helps to strengthen their commitment to each other and to the new baby.

Pain medication, if administered, is usually given just prior to the transition phase. Intense concentration on breathing techniques can increase oxygen to the fetus and decrease pain perception by the mother. The unprepared, uncooperative mother frequently recalls this phase with fear and embarrassment and as a point of disintegration. The prepared mother recalls it as having been difficult, but feels proud that she was able to maintain control. These two alternative responses can leave their mark on the woman's concepts of her self-identity and sexuality. They may even affect her relationship with the baby and/or the father.

Once the cervix is completely dilated, the baby begins to pass through the pelvic canal (see Fig. 5–3). Contractions during the second stage remain long (60 to 90 seconds) but are further apart (3 to 4 minutes). Up to this point, the mother's main task was to concentrate on breathing patterns that would facilitate relaxation and increase the oxygen available to the fetus. Now, as she feels the descending baby press against the lower colon, she takes a deep breath and pushes downward with all her strength to help push the baby along. The pain of the last phase of stage 1 is gone and is replaced by physically hard work. During the first stage, there was nothing the mother could do to stop the contractions or to speed the delivery; now she can actively work with the contractions to assist the process. The woman is generally advised against pushing as the baby "crowns" (passes through the perineal opening). Gradual stretching of the tissues and an episiotomy (a short cut made to enlarge the opening) can reduce pain and prevent problems following delivery. This second stage generally lasts 30 to 60 minutes for the primipara but may take only 10 minutes for the multiparous woman. Although concentrating heavily on the task in which she is involved, the woman in this stage frequently engages in conversation between contractions. Her birth time is close. Her excitement is contained.

When medications have been minimal and involvement high, the signs of stress are eased with the birth of the baby. Joy floods the mother's face; her eyes sparkle; her excitement is no longer contained. The prepared mother seems infused with a new pride and heightened self-esteem ("I did it!"). She exchanges conversation with her partner and the doctor. The focus is no longer herself, but the baby. The unprepared mother may express relief ("It's over—I survived!").

While the mother is talking and watching or holding her baby, the uterus resumes contractions. Within 5 to 20 minutes the placenta is expelled—a rather anticlimactic event, which many mothers say hurts more than the birth itself, since their attention is no longer focused on working with their body.

The mother and father who have participated actively in the childbirth process experience an indefatigable elation. They will talk to anyone and everyone, reliving the experience with enthusiasm and joy. Days, week, even years later, the woman and her husband will revel in the richness of the experience they shared. A new dimension has been added to their relationship. Even the child will be told of the details of his or her own birth.

Because of the pioneer work performed by the physicians J. H. Kennell and M. H. Klaus [40], many hospitals and most birthing centers encourage close contact between mother and infant during the hour after birth. When the father is also involved during this period, enriched family relationships can develop that appear to have substantial positive long-range effects on family relationships and the child's development. Allowing the father to be present during Caesarean

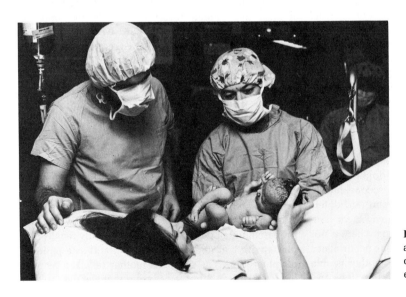

Figure 32–2. Early introduction to the alert infant facilitates the establishment of interactional synchrony between parents and baby.

childbirth and/or to have close contact with the baby immediately after delivery also fosters the greater bonding and involvement of the father [55, 75].

THE PUERPERIUM

The puerperium, sometimes known as the "fourth trimester," is the 6-week period following delivery of the baby. During this time the uterus gradually returns to its prepregnant state. Uterine involution (a process thought to take about 6 weeks) is most rapid during the first 2 weeks after delivery. During this time the lochia (bloody discharge) gradually changes in color from bright red to creamy white. Some discharge may continue for 2 to 4 weeks after delivery. Couples are usually advised against intercourse for 2 to 6 weeks after the birth (depending on both the physician and the mother) in order to avoid infections or an unplanned pregnancy. Ovulation may resume in 14 days or may be delayed several months. Most women will reinitiate menses 4 to 8 weeks after delivery unless they are breast-feeding, in which case the menses may be delayed until weaning [56]. However, anovulation is not assured, and women are advised to consult their physician about appropriate methods of birth control.

Many women are concerned about "flabby belly." The stretched abdominal muscles take time to resume good tone, although the process can be facilitated through specific postpartum exercises and tightening of the abdominal muscles. Many mothers continue to have an enlarged abdomen for several months after delivery. The existence of weak abdominal muscles 6 months later is due to lack of exercise; they are not a natural consequence of pregnancy.

Postpartum Depression

DEPRESSION DURING THE FIRST WEEK ("POSTPARTUM BLUES")
Eighty percent of mothers experience a letdown or depression during the hospital stay [38]. Several theories are offered to explain this depression; one factor appears to be the rapid decrease in estrogen and progesterone levels following delivery. Temporary imbalance of the hormonal system appears to reduce energy levels and to foster emotional lability. A second theory indicates that the mother may be experiencing sleep deprivation syndrome [89]. The expectant mother needs more sleep toward the end of pregnancy, but she frequently finds it difficult to assume a comfortable resting position; she may be kept awake by the move-

ment of the baby or the excitement of her own thoughts. The mother may go into labor after a full day awake; she may then be awake and working hard for 12 or more hours of labor. After the baby is born, her euphoria and need to relive the experience verbally may prevent sleep. Other factors, such as hospital routines, physical discomfort, or concern over the baby or herself, may also prevent the mother from obtaining adequate sleep. It is not unusual for a new mother to have gone 36 to 48 hours without sleep in the period of time surrounding her labor and delivery. When she returns home to resume responsibility for household tasks, care of the new baby (who may want to be fed every 3 hours), and her own physical recuperation, she may be in a serious state of sleep deprivation; thus it is not surprising if she becomes irritable, headachy, restless, emotionally labile, or depressed. Health-care facilities and family members can be very helpful by assuring uninterrupted periods of sleep and assuming routine responsibilities for the woman so that she can devote her energies to her own restoration and the process of bonding with her new baby.

A third theory on postpartum depression is offered by Klaus and Kennell, advocates of early mother-infant contact [35, 37, 38, 40]. They feel that the phenomenon may be due to inadequate contact wth the infant during the hospital stay. The mother is given inadequate opportunity to channel her emotional energies toward forming affectional ties to her new baby. Hospital routines and other persons caring for the infant can deprive the mother of opportunities to get to know her baby and to develop competence in child-care techniques.

This theory is also supported by James and Joyce Robertson [71]. They theorize that heightened anxiety is a normal phenomenon accompanying the hormonal changes following birth. The intensity of maternal anxiety would be identified as psychotic at any other time but serves to direct the mother's attention toward the baby immediately after birth. This heightened anxiety assures close proximity of the mother and attention to the infant's interactional cues—essential ingredients for the infant's survival and normal development. The Robertsons observe that it is abnormal if a mother does not experience heightened anxiety. Practitioners need to help the mother to realize that this anxiety is normal, and help her to direct it into effective child care. They also feel that mother-neonate separation interferes with the effective focusing of the heightened anxiety, which leads to depression and can become a barrier to sensitive bonding with the infant, since it is the mother's frequent contact with the infant and her repeated experience with success in care and comforting that increase self-confidence and facilitate bonding [71]. By the fourth month after birth, the heightened anxiety has decreased, but because confidence in her own skills is increased, sensitive interaction is maintained by the empathy developed by the mother during the early months.

T. Berry Brazelton offers a fourth theory about postpartum depression, which indicates that the mother is experiencing a conflict between the idealized image of motherhood and the reality of her own competencies [38, 39]. She may experience unrealistic expectations of herself as a mother, and the conscious or subconscious recognition of this credibility gap can elicit feelings of helplessness or self-criticism, which lead to depression.

The author has heard many new mothers express that they were upset or depressed because their husband was not able to share this very special time with them. His working hours or hospital policies prevented adequate contact time. For some mothers, this was their first experience with hospitalization, and for a few, the first time ever to be separated from the family overnight (they had never gone to a summer camp or spent the night at a friend's home). Therefore, the depression may actually represent a form of separation anxiety.

DELAYED DEPRESSION

Many mothers experience a postpartum depression or disturbance several weeks or months after delivery. Fatigue may also play a role in this type of depression. The mother seldom obtains more than 5 consecutive hours of sleep, and she may find it difficult or impossible to nap during the day.

Ramona Mercer observes that a mother may go through a period of grief as she relinquishes the fantasies and expectations of pregnancy and adapts to the realities of the baby, the associated workload, and her physical appearance (her figure may not return instantly with fashion-model curves) [52]. In some cases, the mother may not be able to adjust her prenatally formed mental image of the infant (e.g., coloration or gender) with the real baby [14, 35]. Her dream may have consisted of a fat, happy, cuddly baby who slept all night, was fed four times daily, and enjoyed a bath every day. Instead, the baby may appear thin, cry frequently, stiffen when held, wake twice during the night, demand to be fed every 3 to 4 hours, and cry all through the bath! She may be very critical of her performance during labor or may view having had a Cae-

sarean birth as a failure. Her identity as a woman may be threatened.

The learning of new skills is draining; the redefinition of herself as a mother and changes in the relationship with her husband require energy investment [62]. Physical recovery is slowed when adequate rest is not obtained. The maintenance of ongoing responsibilities while assuming new ones may seem overwhelming. Most new mothers are unprepared for how tired they will feel and how much assistance will be needed these first weeks as they make the transition to motherhood [52, 62]. The initial 4 to 6 weeks appear to be the period of peak adjustment. After that (when the baby begins to sleep longer at night), parents begin to focus beyond immediate needs to the growth and developmental needs of the infant [83]. Postnatal classes during this time to discuss parental concerns can be very supportive [83].

Other mothers may have experienced inadequate coping patterns prior to pregnancy and motherhood. The responsibility for another person who demands and needs her constant attention may prove to be overwhelming. Building on Brazelton's idea, some mothers experience an abrupt confrontation with reality after bringing the baby home. The small nuclear family of today may have failed to provide her with adequate experience in the care of young children. The mother may not have enough knowledge to know what behaviors are normal or enough experience to be comfortable in handling the baby. She may not have extended family or even friends nearby to help answer questions or to relieve some of her anxieties and responsibilities. Her anxieties are translated into body language and transmitted to the infant, increasing the infant's anxiety (see Sullivan's theory in Chap. 9). The harder she tries, the more upset the baby seems to be. She begins to doubt her own ability to be a mother. This baby does not match her dreams. Fortunately, most mothers are able to readjust their dream to approximate reality.

Motherhood itself may also fail to match the woman's dreams. When the novelty wears off, she may find herself feeling tired, bored, and unchallenged. Attempts to breast-feed may be aborted; the baby may be colicky. The lay literature abounds with articles and books about the bounties of motherhood. A woman may expect to have instant, overpowering love for the infant; she is surprised to discover that the birth experience did not suddenly turn her into a knowledgeable and loving mother. She may begin to question her sexuality, her motives, her ability to love. A mother or father frequently does not begin to feel love or a feeling of emotional reciprocity until the baby begins to socialize overtly with others [73]. A deep relationship takes time to develop—it evolves slowly, and many factors can block or facilitate that process (early contact after birth appears to facilitate the process). The bonding process is discussed later in this chapter.

One of the major precipitating factors of postpartum depression, especially for the primiparous woman, is the dramatic change in life-style. During her pregnancy (and perhaps all her life), she has been cared for. Others concerned themselves about her safety, her emotions, and her diet, catering to her whims and needs. Now she is the caretaker. She is no longer the recipient but the giver of nurturance.

Perhaps for the first time in her life, the new mother is responsible for someone else—not for just a few hours or a few days, but for a year, five years, 15 years, or more. This fact may have overwhelming ramifications for the woman if she feels that the child will continue to require as much care as has been necessary during the first few weeks or months of life. She may feel a loss of her own identity in the press of all the responsibility.

During pregnancy she was the center of attention. (How did she feel? Was she comfortable? Could anything be done to help her? How much longer did she have to go?) Now the baby is the focus. (How is his health? How much does he eat? Is he warm enough? How much does he weigh now?) The mother takes a back seat. The attention she does get is tangential to the infant's health and development.

If the mother was working before the baby was born, she enjoyed a fixed schedule or routine. She could plan her day or her week. Now her schedule is unpredictable and out of her control. When she wants to sleep, the baby wants to eat; when she wants to watch television or spend time with her spouse, the baby demands attention. During the first months, she may feel that she is controlled by her offspring which is especially true for parents of twins [21]. Fortunately, most infants begin to establish a predictable wake-sleep pattern by 3 months of age.

Another dramatic change in life-style that may be precipitated by the birth is the loss of adult contact, especially for the woman who had previously worked outside of the home. Her world now centers around the home and the baby. As the novelty wears off, the mother may experience sensory deprivation. She may feel isolated and depressed by the lack of adult contact. She needs stimulating conversation to keep her mind

active and satiated; she needs to voice her own opinions in order to maintain a sense of self-identity and to test reality.

Another major precipitating factor of postpartum disturbance may be the mother's preception of her own time within the life space. To many women, childbirth signifies the point of transition from youth to adulthood. The new mother may suddenly realize that she is no longer looking ahead to what her life will be— she is there. She suddenly realizes how rapidly the preceding years have passed and may telescope the future. She is at a crisis point in life. Time seems to be passing too quickly (or, in some cases, too slowly). Thoughts of her own death are common, even though she realizes with gratitude that she survived the childbirth experience. She must face her own mortality and integrate this concept into her approach to life; she must complete the crisis of reintegration of her past, present, and future that was initiated by the pregnancy.

There are many potential emotional hazards for the new mother. The older mother (30's or 40's) may find the change especially difficult. Her self-identity is undergoing dramatic modifications as her role, responsibilities, and relationships change. Even the well-prepared mother of a much-wanted child faces these critical adjustment tasks. She needs time and much support as she is making these adjustments. It helps her to realize that her questions, anxieties, and self-doubts are normal. The transformation in self-identity to the role of a competent mother does not occur overnight. Good family and community support systems can greatly facilitate the transition and bring very positive long-range benefits to the child and family [27]. Most mothers begin to feel comfortable with their new role within 3 to 4 months [73].

Lactation

The American Academy of Pediatrics and several other leading medical societies strongly recommend the promotion of breast-feeding in the United States and throughout the world [64] because of the physiological advantages of breast-feeding for both the mother (e.g., decreased uterine involution time) and the infant (e.g., reception of antibodies in early breast milk). In the long run, however, except in situations where it is difficult to maintain a sterile, fresh supply of milk, the attitude of the mother toward herself, her infant, and her choice of feeding technique is more significant than the actual method she uses to provide physical nourishment to the infant.

Today, sixty percent of mothers choose to breast-feed [1]. The reasons against breast-feeding were cited in the introduction. The educated woman from a middle- or upper-income level is most likely to choose breast-feeding [80]. She may see breast-feeding as a natural part of her role as a mother and a normal extension of her psychosexual development. Her extended family may offer supportive encouragement, and her husband may express pride in her desire and ability to nurture the infant in this way. Some mothers choose to breast-feed because of peer pressure or as a status symbol. Others may breast-feed because their mothers, best friends, or husbands expect them to do so. The mother herself may feel that breast-feeding is the only way to be a "real" mother. However, if she harbors unconscious reservations about the exposure and touching of her breasts, her attitude will be transmitted to the baby, and the experience will prove to be un-satisfactory for both.

Some mothers may choose to breast-feed because it is easier, more convenient, and cheaper than bottle-feeding. However, dietary intake is important to the mother's health; she needs to add 130 calories to her intake for every 100 ml of milk she produces. At full lactation, she will produce 850 to 1200 ml of breast milk per day [30]. Adequate protein, fluids, calcium, and vitamins must be provided.

About 50 percent of breast-feeding mothers continue to nurse their babies through the sixth month [1, 6]. To be successful, the mother must first of all really want to breast-feed. Second, she must believe in her own ability to produce milk. All new mothers have some doubt about this phenomenon (and there are no ounce markers on the breast to help her evaluate how much milk the baby is actually receiving). Her best assurance that the baby is adequately fed is the baby's response. Is the baby satisfied after feedings? Is the baby sleeping between feedings? Is the baby wetting diapers and gaining weight? If so, then the baby is getting enough to eat. Weighing after each nursing is unnecessary.

Many mothers say that they stopped nursing be-cause their milk was "not rich enough," their breasts were not large enough, or they did not have enough milk. In reality, the size of the breasts has no correla-tion with the amount of functional breast tissue. Most of what provides the breast contour is fat and connec-tive tissue, not functional tissue. Breast milk is nor-mally a bluish-white, watery fluid. Adequate production depends on adequate fluid intake and ad-equate suckling. However, in our culture it is more ac-ceptable to blame a physical malfunction than to admit self-doubt, embarrassment, or sexual anxiety as the real reason for failure [80].

The third factor facilitating successful breast-feed-ing is that the woman needs to have enough knowl-edge about the process of lactation to be able to understand and work with her body. The breast under-goes preparation for lactation during pregnancy. There is growth of breast tissue and frequently some secre-tion of colostrum, the precursor of breast milk. This yellowish fluid is high in protein, fat, sugar, salts, and antibodies. Following delivery, psychic factors and the suckling of the breast stimulate a neurohormonal re-flex of the nipple, which in turn causes the posterior pituitary to continue production of oxytocin. Oxytocin appears to stimulate production of prolactin by the an-terior pituitary. Prolactin, in turn, stimulates the se-cretion of milk by the cells that line the mammary alveoli. Oxytocin, the hormone that caused the con-traction of uterine muscles during labor, continues to help the uterus to return to prepregnant size. During the first week after delivery, many breast-feeding mothers experience uterine cramps while nursing the infant. Oxytocin also causes contraction of the mus-cles surrounding the milk glands and ducts, which ac-counts for the "milk let-down reflex" experienced by mothers and facilitates the flow of milk from the nipple.

The marvelous reflexive process of milk production allows the mother to breast-feed under very unusual circumstances. Occasionally, because of maternal ill-ness, neonate illness, or a late decision to breast-feed, the mother may not nurse for 2 weeks or more after delivery. But, even in the absence of any previous stim-ulation, lactation can be established successfully at this late date. In fact, even the mother who has not deliv-ered a baby but is increasing her family through adop-tion can initiate the same neurohormonal reflex and cause her breasts to begin lactation. Although it may take her several weeks of persistent nursing effort, she can stimulate production of enough milk to meet much of the baby's nutritional needs [45, 93].

Continued production of milk depends on emptying at least one breast at each feeding. Milk is produced continually in the alveoli during lactation. The milk is transported through tiny ducts to 15 to 20 large sinuses behind the nipple, which function as reservoirs for the milk until suckling occurs. Emptying of the reservoirs depends on both suction and compression during nursing. The infant will empty the breast of milk in 5 to 10 minutes of vigorous suckling, but mothers usu-ally suckle the baby longer after the nipples "toughen"

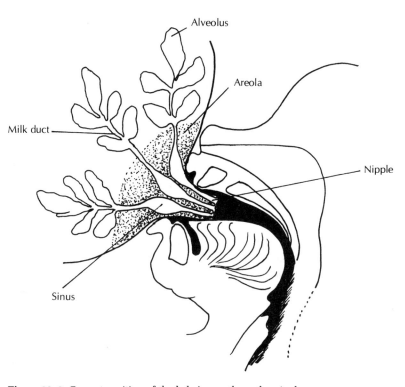

Figure 32–3. Correct position of the baby's mouth on the nipple.

in order to satisfy the baby's need to suck as well as to provide nourishment. This suckling period also offers a special time for the mother and infant to communicate with each other.

Complete emptying of the breast appears to stimulate continued production of milk. Frequent emptying increases the speed of production, whereas infrequent nursing will slow down production. By this mechanism, a mother can successfully breast-feed twins or even triplets. She may also find that her other children or even her husband may want to suckle. These are normal events and will not reduce the amount of milk available to the infant. Women can continue to lactate for years if they are adequately stimulated [45], although many mothers prefer to transfer the baby to a cup by the time the child is 10 to 12 months of age. Weaning should be a gradual rather than an abrupt process for both the mother and the infant. Abrupt cessation of nursing will cause an excessive and painful accumulation of milk in the lactiferous sinuses. A woman may continue to excrete small amounts of milk for 4 to 5 years after cessation of breast-feeding.

The mother and baby are most ready to nurse immediately after delivery. The infant in state 4 is able to respond eagerly and to coordinate sucking and swallowing reflexes. The licking and suckling stimulation of the nipple encourages early production of milk (within 2 to 3 days). When the mother is forced to wait 12 to 24 hours before nursing, the infant is frequently too sleepy or too agitated to take the nipple easily, sucking and swallowing reflexes may be poorly coordinated, and the nipple inadequately stimulated. Milk production, therefore, may be delayed until the fourth or fifth day after delivery.

Many breast-feeding mothers experience nipple tenderness. One of the most critical factors is the "latching on" process. The infant must have sufficient nipple in the mouth to be able to compress the milk sinuses and to extract the milk. It is necessary that a large part of the areola be included in the "bite." If only the nipple is inserted, vigorous sucking action is required to obtain milk, resulting in excessive friction on the nipple as well as incomplete emptying of the sinuses.

Mothers are usually encouraged to alternate breasts at each feeding to assure adequate emptying and to prevent soreness of the nipples. Changing the position of the baby during nursing (e.g., lying down versus sitting up) can also help to prevent or alleviate tenderness. Rubbing the nipples gently with a towel during pregnancy and limiting nursing time to 10 minutes during the early feedings may also help to avoid soreness. Even with these precautions, however, many others experience some soreness or even nipple bleeding between the sixth and tenth day after delivery. These symptoms disappear as the nipples toughen. Release of the suction by inserting a finger into the corner of the baby's mouth before removal from the breast can help to avoid nipple irritation throughout the nursing period.

Both lactating and nonlactating mothers experience primary engorgement 2 to 3 days after delivery, which is caused by increased blood flow to the breasts in preparation for milk production. Woman may complain of tenderness in the breasts and in the armpits. Although postdelivery medication can help to reduce the intensity of primary engorgement, there is little that can be done to offer relief for the discomfort except to take pain medication. Primary engorgement subsides gradually after 2 to 3 days. The breasts of nonlactating mothers will return to normal size about 3 weeks after delivery.

Secondary engorgement occurs when the breasts begin to produce milk. Prior to this time, the baby receives colostrum during nursing. When the milk "comes in," the mammary ducts and lactiferous sinuses may fill rapidly. Discomfort due to secondary engorgement can be relieved through frequent brief nursings to prevent overdistention of the sinuses. Once the sinuses have been stretched, the filling preceding each nursing is no longer painful, even though the breast may feel firm to the touch.

Lactating mothers also experience a decrease in breast size in 2 to 3 weeks. This phenomenon, combined with the baby's needs for more milk, may cause the mother to believe that her milk has "dried up." Adequate rest, fluids, diet, and frequent nursing will ensure continued production. Supplemental bottles are usually discouraged during the first month, since they may interfere with the establishment of the balance between supply and demand. Supplemental bottles are also discouraged because a different type of sucking action is required to extract the milk. Some believe the binipple experience can be confusing to the young baby.

Milk production is very sensitive to psychic influences. Suckling, sleep, and sexual intercourse increase prolactin production [45]. Fatigue, fear, pain, anxiety, or emotional stress can inhibit the "let-down reflex" and decrease milk production. Thinking about nursing or hearing the baby cry can elicit the let-down reflex, causing a tingling sensation and release of milk. The oxytocin-induced let-down reflex can actually cause the milk to squirt 3 to 4 feet from the uncovered breast. Gentle pressure against the nipple effectively stops the leakage. (If the mother is out for a formal evening, crossing of the arms will effectively and discreetly apply pressure against the nipples.)

Breast-feeding is an exciting and positive experience for the woman who is secure in her own psychosexual development and views nursing as a natural sequela to pregnancy. Such a woman finds breast-feeding emotionally satisfying and an aid to communication with,

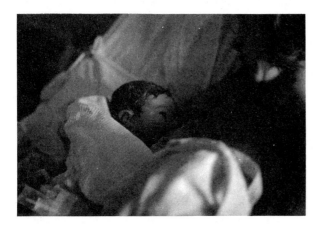

Figure 32–4. When offered the breast within the first hour after birth, the baby is usually alert and able to coordinate the sucking and swallowing reflexes. Immediate breast-feeding not only fosters earlier production of milk but also facilitates the mother-infant bonding process.

and attachment to, her new baby. Relaxin, a hormone released during the suckling, can also help the mother to feel more relaxed and secure in her role as primary caretaker, nurturer, and mother of the neonate.

La Leche League International (9616 Minneapolis Avenue, Franklin Park, Illinois 60131) is an organization established by mothers to evaluate and to disseminate information on breast-feeding to new mothers and professional persons. This organization has branches throughout the United States and even overseas where young mothers can meet together to offer mutual support and understanding to one another and exchange ideas about their babies. Their book, *The Womanly Art of Breastfeeding* [44], contains valuable information and practical advice on breast-feeding from the family perspective. Another book entitled *Nursing Your Baby* by Karen Pryor [65] is also very valuable to the woman who is considering breast-feeding.

THE NEW FAMILY

Most parents experience a feeling of awe and reverence at the birth of their child. They are overwhelmed by the miracle of birth and gaze in amazement at the tiny creature they were instrumental in creating. Prepared parents who participated actively in the birth experience talk to anyone and everyone who will listen for days and weeks after the birth as if trying to validate and absorb the reality of the event. They experience a "high" that extends beyond the birth experience and helps in the establishment of a positive relationship with the baby. The maturing individual who is successfully integrating past, present, and future is able to transfer the love for the fantasy child to the real child. The new infant is seen as a part of self, a part of the mate, and yet as an individual entity [7].

Bonding

The early verbal and nonverbal experiences between infant and parents create a pattern of mutuality that subconsciously establishes the tone for interpersonal relationships and their intrapsychic coloring throughout life. Attachment of the infant to the parent has been discussed in Chapter 9. Because dependence during infancy is almost absolute, it is essential that strong affectional ties also be established by the parents toward the infant in order to ensure adequate physical and affectional nurturing during the early months of life. Parents exhibit their affectional ties to the infant

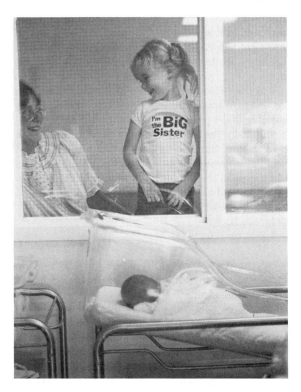

Figure 32–5. Many hospitals now encourage siblings to visit to facilitate bonding and to decrease rivalry.

through nonverbal behaviors such as vocalizing, rocking, touching, attending promptly, body and breath warmth, closeness, and gazing. These parental behaviors appear to be essential to the early security and thus to the development of the infant [38, 71, 90] (see Chap. 9).

Bowlby, Spitz, and Mahler have written quite profusely and elegantly of the mother-infant dyad or bonding process—the intimate attachment of each to the other—which is characterized during the early months by a mutual focusing on the infant's needs. This is followed by a gradual decentering, with mutually reciprocal or symbiotic interaction. The individuation of the two members of the system is usually complete by 3 years [50], but they continue to maintain a heavy emotional investment in each other throughout life [6]. This ability of the mother to become and to remain socially attached to the infant ensures the survival of the young [23, 71]. Current research is beginning to indicate that infantile autism, nonorganic failure-to-thrive, and the battered child syndrome may be related to inadequate attachment of the mother to her infant [13, 22, 71].* Unfortunately, little research has, as yet, centered on the father-infant bonding process.

Early interaction appears to be facilitated through the possession of specific characteristics, or "tools," on the part of both the parent and the infant. When functioning optimally, the reciprocal use of these tools can lead to an intense, mutually satisfying relationship. Infant tools have already been described in Chapter 8. The infant's use of these tools helps to endear the child to the parent and to encourage continued investment of her time and energies to meet the infant's physical and social needs.

PARENTAL TOOLS

Contact with an appealing baby appears to elicit specific responses from the parents, even when previous contact with babies has been minimal or absent. Whether these responses are imitated by watching others (learned), remembered from mothering received as a child (memory traces), or instinctual in nature (innate), no one knows. The stability of these characteristics across cultures and centuries leads one to believe that they are innate. However, humans are so strongly influenced by culture, experience, and preconceived views of others that innate behaviors are easily submerged or extinguished by traditions or perceived roles. Some behaviors appear to help make the infant more alert and to foster increased quantity and quality of interaction.

The use of a **high-pitched voice** by the parents is the most fascinating of all phenomena to observe. When an adult, especially the mother, is facing and talking to an infant, her voice immediately softens and elevates. In the middle of a sentence, she may turn to an adult in the room and, without taking a breath, suddenly drop to normal-pitched speech. She can reverse the episode just as rapidly. Data clearly indicate that infants have a strong preference for the high-pitched

female voice [23]. Many mothers also have an insatiable desire to talk to the baby, especially to repeat the name frequently as if to connect the two, to reassure themselves of the reality of this new life in their care—to confirm the miracle. With the neonate's ability to turn to sound and to synchronize movements with speech rhythms, the mother is reinforced to repeat the behavior [17].

Rocking behavior is usually engaged in when a baby is held even if the child is asleep. Those with strong parental instincts are even noted to rock and "jiggle" a baby doll in child-care classes when learning infant care. This rocking behavior, in addition to soothing the child and significantly increasing visual scanning behavior up to 71 percent when accompanied by elevation to the shoulder [42], is thought to excite vestibular stimulation, thus facilitating coordination and voluntary control of movements. Harlow has shown that monkeys raised in isolation with a stationary, nonmovable "mother" develop severe autostimulatory behaviors, including self-cuddling, self-rocking, biting, scratching, and hair pulling. When approached by another monkey or a human, they withdraw in marked fear. If physical contact is made, they react with immediate, uncontrolled, aggressive, hostile behaviors [74]. Monkeys with movable "mothers" did not exhibit these behaviors. Rocking activity, then, appears to be essential to the coordination and development of the physical, affective, social, and cognitive domains. Evidence derived from growth patterns of premature infants indicates that weight gains are accelerated when the infant is stimulated by regular rocking or movement in moderate amounts (e.g., use of waterbeds).

Attending is another characteristic observed in parents who are bonding to their infant. They literally cannot take their eyes off the baby; it is as if they are visually engulfing the child—making him or her a part of themselves. Since infants prefer a facial pattern, they are stimulated to return the attending behavior. Assumption of the **en face position** (the full-face eye-to-eye position) is also characteristic of parents who are developing an attachment to their infant. Eye-to-eye contact holds the infant's attention for longer periods of time and helps the parent to feel accepted by, and closer to, the infant. When the adult's and infant's faces are at cross planes rather than parallel to each other, the infant does not attend as easily or as long.

Smiling and **mouth movements** also elicit longer fixation responses from the infant—especially after the neonatal period [72]. This is another mutually reinforcing activity, especially when combined with adult vocalization.

*This does not mean that the mother does not love her child, nor does it rule out organic or attachment-tool deficits on the part of the infant that may set up barriers to parental bonding. It takes two persons to establish the synchrony of interaction. Many of these infant-parent dyads fail to establish this critical synchrony during the early weeks after birth, when maternal heightened anxiety is at its peak. Negative experiences or faulty expectancies on the part of either parent or infant can lead to maladaptive behaviors and inappropriate cueing and responding on the part of either or both.

Enfolding is a more complex behavior, incorporating several other patterns that are more difficult to identify, such as touch, muscle tone, and body blending. Infants become quiet with a gentle, relaxed touch. They also are quieted by the low, rhythmic beating of the heart heard when they are held close to the caregiver's chest. This close contact also allows for stimulation of the olfactory sense and provision of warmth. Ashley Montagu speaks of the importance of touch in communication. Tactile-kinesthetic stimulation, appropriately given, facilitates relaxation in the neonate. This relaxation of infant muscle tone is a tactile as well as an affective reinforcer to the caregiver.

The parent, then, like the infant (as described in Chap. 8) is in possession of critical tools that facilitate parent-infant interaction and bonding. As the baby uses a tool, the caregiver reciprocates with a reinforcing tool that encourages the infant to repeat the behavior or to continue the interaction; thus a ballet of interaction can be observed and objectively recorded. The foundation is established for a mutually rewarding relationship that supports the development of the infant. The development of parental attachment can be facilitated by helping parents to become aware of, and sensitive to, the interaction cues emitted by the infant and to use reciprocal behaviors appropriately to elicit infant responses [10, 53]. Too much or too little use of parental tools can tire or understimulate the baby (see Chap. 15).

MATERNAL BONDING

With the advent of birth and the physical separation of the mother and the baby, the mother must accomplish the critical task of establishing a mutually satisfactory symbiotic affectional relationship with the baby. Contrary to popular thought, this task often is not accomplished instantaneously nor easily. The attachment process begins during pregnancy. During the early months of pregnancy, most mothers, even those with unplanned conceptions, begin to accept the growing fetus as an "integral part of herself" [6]. When fetal movements begin to be felt, a form of communication is sensed by the mother, and even the unwanted baby usually begins to be accepted [37]. "The mother's initial reaction to holding her baby or being at least allowed to inspect him is obviously a moment of profound significance for her; an observer who is not too preoccupied with making detailed observations will recognize from the mother's silent tears, her look of awe, and the tenderness with which her arms reach out, that he is participating vicariously in one of woman's most intimate experiences, and at such a moment will find it difficult to intrude on her privacy" [91].

Mothers are noted to progress through an orderly sequence of behaviors upon introduction to their new baby after delivery. Klaus and Kennell describe the first step as "looking." The mother seeks eye-to-eye contact with the infant; she assumes the en face position and appears to "engulf" the baby visually. This behavior continues throughout the hospital stay and is noted to be present in some mothers for months. It is as if they are visually reassuring themselves of the reality of the infant's presence. Mothers who are attaching express the feeling that they cannot seem to satiate their need to look at the child; every movement and every breath are noted. The bonding process is facilitated when this introduction occurs immediately after birth, since both the mother and infant are in heightened states of alertness and receptivity. The infant's open, alert eyes associated with state 4 enhance the mother's feeling that the infant is looking at, accepting, and getting to know her.

When the naked baby is placed in close proximity to the mother, she begins to touch the infant's extremities with her fingertips for about 4 to 8 minutes [40]. The fully clothed and wrapped baby may be "finger-tipped" for a longer period of time, thus institutional procedures and policies may interfere with normal progression to the "palming" stage, in which the mother begins to touch the baby with her whole hand, starting first with the arms and legs and then moving to the trunk with caressing and massaging movements. Reva Rubin identifies these behaviors as being associated with the "taking in" phase of attachment [77]. Even when the mother is physically separated from the baby, her thoughts are constantly with the baby. She talks to anyone who will listen about the unique characteristics of her offspring. She is in awe, trying to absorb her new experience; the whole miracle of birth has overwhelmed her. The advent of motherhood is not yet a reality.

During the "taking-hold" phase (lasting about 10 days), the mother begins to enfold the baby and to mold more easily to the infant's contours. She is beginning to recognize the little signs that indicate discomfort, hunger, or the desire to be held. During this phase, the mother is full of questions and is receptive to teaching: She needs encouragement and support in feeling competent to care for this new life. All her attention and energies are focused on the needs of the infant. The mother may focus so much attention on the infant that she ignores her own needs for rest. She is usually discharged from the health care facility during this time.

Family members need to provide adequate care and support to prevent overtiring, especially if there are other children in the home.

Although still in Mahler's autistic period, the mother gradually begins to "let go" about 2 weeks after delivery [77]. She begins to regard the infant as a separate individual and to attend to some of her own unique needs (for example, she may have her hair done at the beauty parlor or fix a special dinner for her husband). Some mothers take longer to reach this third phase. Mothers who continue with this high intensity responsivity begin to show signs of "burn out." It is important to the development of both the baby and the mother that she take the initial steps toward separation.

The affectional attachment process is very fragile and tenuous. "While the bonds of affection are still forming, they can be easily retarded, altered or permanently damaged" [37]. Minor problems during pregnancy, a difficult labor and delivery, a premature birth, or minor problems after birth can interfere with the bonding process of the mother. She may resent the child who has caused her so much pain and anxiety or may resist attachment for fear she will lose the child. This feeling is a normal defense against the pain of loss.

At the turn of the century, Budin noted that premature infants were frequently abandoned by their mothers if they were not allowed to see the baby or to participate in their care [11]. Cooney made the same observations in the 1930s. Klaus and Kennell observed that an inordinately high proportion of healthy premature infants from their hospital became victims of parental abuse and neglect. A search of the literature revealed that 13 to 36 percent of children who are severely neglected or abused were premature or experienced prolonged separation from the mothers [36]. They postulated the existence of a biologically determined "sensitive period" for attachment and bonding by the mother.

Klaus and his associates set up an experiment involving 14 mothers of normal newborn infants [40]. The mothers were given 1 hour of private contact time with their nude infant in bed during the first 2 hours after birth; they were also given the nude baby for 5 extra hours per day on each of the next 3 days of life for a total of 14 extra hours of contact time during the hospital stay. The interaction of these mothers with their infants was then compared to the interaction of control mothers who did not experience this extra time. Mothers who had early and frequent contact with the infant showed more attachment behaviors (looking at the infant; smiling at the infant; holding the infant closely; rocking, talking to, and caressing the infant) at 1 month after discharge than mothers who experienced minimal contact or prolonged separation [40]. These mothers were also much more reluctant to leave the infant with another caretaker in order to go out for an afternoon or an evening. Not all replications of this study have supported the "sensitive-period" theory [38]. Other potentially significant variables within the populations (such as breast- versus bottle-feeding, level of education, and economic level) need to be further evaluated [30]. But for high-risk babies and/or mothers, the early contact appears to make a profound difference in the quality of mother-infant interaction.

Early maternal contact appears to be highly correlated with the later exploratory behavior of the infant [40]. When the children from Klaus's study were 2 years old, the mothers offered fewer verbal commands but asked more questions of their children [69]. When these same children were 5 years old, they had significantly higher IQs and advanced scores on two language tests [70]. Thus the child's cognitive, affective, social, and even physical development may be indirectly facilitated by early and extended mother-infant contact.

Lee Salk also identifies a statistically significant difference in holding behaviors of mothers who had contact with their infants within 24 hours of life versus those whose introduction was delayed beyond 24 hours. He postulates that separation interferes with the establishment of a "natural" mother-infant response [78]. Studies by Brazelton, Gil, and Kennell and Klaus all support his hypothesis. Klaus and Kennell identify a very high incidence of failure-to-thrive, battered-child syndrome, and unwarranted maternal concern about infant health in children who experienced prematurity, minor health problems, or separation from the mother [37]. Although it is recognized that multiple factors are involved, evidence is strong that "the formation of close affectional ties may remain permanently incomplete if extended separation occurs and anticipatory grief becomes too far advanced" [37].

The rooming-in experience in the hospital allows both the mother and father frequent and prolonged contact with their baby. Lactation induces an emotional state that intensifies the receptive and retentive tendencies that are experienced during pregnancy and heightened with a positive childbirth experience, thereby facilitating affectional symbiosis. "Frequent and intimate contact with a thriving infant has a stimulating and integrating effect on motherliness" [5]. It is evident that early contact with an alert baby promotes positive feelings. In addition, knowledge of infant care and characteristics offsets maternal insecurity.

Now that amniocentesis and ultrasonography are

available, parents frequently know their infant's gender prior to birth. Bonding theorists have begun to explore the effects of this information on the parent's attachment process. Current evidence indicates that there is an increase in feelings of well-being and in attachment to the fetus after viewing the infant by sonography and the assurance that the baby appears to be healthy [41, 54]. However, a study of the effect of this knowledge on the mother's behavior 2 to 5 days after delivery indicates no significant difference in the bonding behaviors exhibited by the knowledgeable mothers [28].

The confident, secure mother who has established solid and healthy emotional ties with her infant is able to retain her own individuality while meeting the needs of her infant. Motherliness is a dynamic reciprocal state that requires changes in the quantity and quality of the relationship with age, situation, and maturation of both the child and the mother.

PATERNAL BONDING

In western culture, the father has found it more difficult to identify with the infant and to express his true feelings than does the mother. Traditionally, the culture and the practices of health care agencies have kept the father much less involved—in fact, they have shut him out of the "woman's domain." The image of "manliness" portrayed by the mass media does not usually include the warm, tender, affectionate father. If these characteristics are portrayed, it is often with humor or a hint of weakness. It is unfortunate that being an affectionate father has been seen as a character flaw that robs the man of his ability to think objectively or to retain power or respect. Pregnancy and childbirth provide men with an avenue for increased emotional involvement with their mates and with life in general. It allows the man to get in touch with the "hidden side" of masculinity by eliciting expressions of empathy, fear, and sympathy, and by encouraging expressions of caring, concern, and tenderness [68].

Fatherliness is not synonymous with motherliness nor is it a substitute. Benedek offers the idea that they are "complementary processes which evolve within the culturally established family structure to safeguard the physical and emotional development of the child" [4]. The father's participation in child-rearing is related to both his gender-role concepts and to the time available [18]. The nurturing aspect of fathering is influenced by the culture and the man's experience with his own father [18] as well as by his participation in the birth.

Nurturance—the provision of affective support and physical caretaking tasks—can be and is being provided more frequently by both parents in today's so-

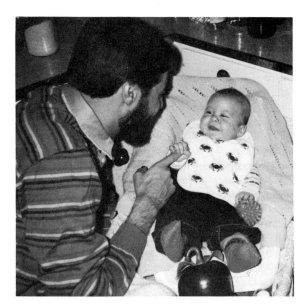

Figure 32–6. Feelings of tenderness and gentleness are human characteristics—not the prerogatives of women. (Copyright ©1985 Lindsay E. Easter.)

ciety. Fathers indicate a strong desire to become involved, even staying home from work in order to spend more time with the baby and to help the mother. The extent of the father's involvement is often determined by what the mother is willing to relinquish [67].

The second aspect of fatherhood is the emotional involvement—the bond or affectional tie. Feelings of warmth, devotion, protectiveness, and pleasure at physical contact are expected of mothers. However, these qualities have not been culturally fostered in men. A father, insecure in his new role or identity, may feel confused as he tries to sort out these new feelings, his masculinity, and his new responsibilities. The capacity to enrich and to actualize one's life through the experiences of another is not the prerogative of women. Feelings of tenderness and gentleness, the capacity to empathize and to respond emotionally to others, and the ability to value a love object more than the self are **human characteristics** [31]. Such attributes can enrich each person's relationships. One study reports fathers spending less than 1 minute per day talking with the young infant [66]. Another reports 3.2 hours with older infants [43]. The age and sex of the child influence the father's participation.

When fathers have been involved, accepted, and supported during the pregnancy, delivery, and postpartum periods, their involvement in and attachment to their neonate appears to be as strong as the mother's [29, 67]. There is no support for a hormonal basis for responsivity in either parent. Sensitivity appears to be a consequence of contact with the baby rather than a precursor to involvement [24]. Fathers have been found to be just as sensitive and responsive as mothers to infant cues and equally competent in providing affection, stimulation, and physical care [26, 79]. Studies indicate that the father's behaviors are almost identical to the mother's when he is left alone with the infant. When the mother, father, and infant are together, the father clearly plays a more active role in interacting with and caring for the neonate [57, 58, 79].

When fathers are present at the delivery, they go through a period of "engrossment"—intense involvement and absorption, or preoccupation with thoughts of the infant—similar to that experienced by the mother [29]. They are able to identify their infant readily and tend to feel more comfortable in caring for their infant.

Paternal contact and caregiving is greatly increased during the first 3 months of life if the father is allowed to undress the infant and to establish eye contact with the child for 1 hour during the first 3 days of life [46]. Strong paternal affectional bonds are enhanced by early contact with the open-eyed, alert infant in state 4. The period immediately after delivery is especially conducive to the development of affectional ties. Like the mother, fathers who are separated from their offspring during the early days, weeks, or months of life have more difficulty developing strong emotional ties and in showing affection to their offspring [29].

Although we speak of maternal attachment and paternal attachment as separate entities, they appear to be one and the same—parental attachment. In the past, cultural factors have prevented the emergence of the father's true feelings and role. With the greater involvement of the father in the pregnancy process (seen in the expression "We are pregnant") and in the delivery as well as the increased opportunity for infant-father contact in the hospital setting, the nurturant skills and affectional bonds of the mother and father will begin to blend even more closely. In today's small nuclear family, the father's physical involvement is essential; with the emphasis on the individuality and development of the woman as well as the man, the father's emotional involvement is liberating. Shared nurturing allows both partners to enjoy the child while promoting fulfillment of the individual goals. The parents begin to model each other in greater family unity as well as responsiveness and tenderness toward the baby [67].

ADOPTIVE PARENTING

The question has been raised about whether or not it is the delay in the introduction of a child to adoptive parents that may account for some of the difficulties adoptive parents express in completing the bonding process successfully [29, 38]. The key is the adoptive parents' commitment to the new child [88]. Adoption does present some unique barriers, but most components parallel those of bonding in biological parents:

1. A healthy parental attachment depends on a sense of entitlement to be a parent to the child. Those who see kinship limited to blood ties will experience more difficulty admitting the child to the emotional bond of the family. Once a child is legally and morally free for adoption, the parents can invest themselves without fear of loss. Most biological parents never face the entitlement crisis. However, some women face this in out-of-wedlock pregnancies.

2. Couples need a validation of parenthood. The pregnant couple of a wanted child find that friends and family offer support. After the baby is born, announcements are circulated and the child is greeted by the community. Adoptive parents need this same reassurance of acceptance by significant other people.

3. Adoptive parents need assistance with preparation for parenthood as much as pregnant couples do [48]. They also need opportunities to talk about the feelings and the role changes that emerge with an expanded family [87].

4. When a new baby is born, the relatives engage in "claiming behaviors" that help to identify the child as a family member: name choosing, pointing out family resemblances, religious ceremonies—all facilitate bonding. Some of these same events occur with adoption. Pictures are placed on walls and stories are shared to help claim the adopted child into the nuclear family [88].

5. Love develops gradually over time as synchrony of interaction is established. When the other criteria are satisfied, 75 to 87 percent of adoptive parents will feel that the child (even an older child) is their own within 1 month after placement [20].

ATTACHMENT PATTERNS

So far we have spoken as if attachment always occurs immediately and in the hospital setting. Lest we be accused of perpetuating the "motherhood or parenthood myth," a few more observations need to be made. Bonding, or the degree to which a parent feels the child occupies an essential position in his or her life [73], is a gradual process. What we have discussed so far are the precursors to that process and the environmental conditions that appear to influence the strength of the bond.

Components of parental attachment or bonding include feelings of warmth; a sense of possession; feelings of devotion, protectiveness, and concern; acceptance of inconveniences; a positive anticipation of prolonged contact; pleasure in the interaction; and a sense of loss over real or imagined absence [73]. These feelings are not automatically present with the birth or adoption of the baby or child; they develop over time in a fairly regular pattern.

Research by Robson and Moss [73] indicates that, at first contact, 34 percent of mothers reported having no special attachment feelings at all. (This finding is not necessarily contradictory to the observation that new mothers frequently experience a great sense of awe on first contact with their offspring; one can feel awe without having a feeling of belongingness). Seven percent of the mothers reported negative feelings, and 55 percent reported positive feelings. Only 4 percent indicated experiencing a real "love" at first sight. During the first 4 days, many mothers reported experiencing a feeling of estrangement. The neonate was seen as inanimate or subhuman. The mothers attempted to make contact and often personalized the infant's behaviors. Flailing of the arms was interpreted as "waving at me"; eye-to-eye contact was interpreted as "waking up for me."

During the first month, the mothers were tired and often felt insecure and unable to control the crying, eating, sleeping, and stooling patterns. They were unable to communicate with their infants and looked for the little signs of fleeting smiles, eye-to-eye contact, and vocalization efforts as reinforcers for being a good mother. Many questioned their decision to have a baby during that first month. As the infant tools strengthened, positive feelings began to emerge. Between the fourth and sixth weeks, the infant became a **person** to the mothers. They felt that their efforts were being rewarded with reciprocal attention, which increased their feeling of rapport.

The mothers began to feel important and needed when they observed the differential response of the infant to them versus other people. By the end of 3 months, most felt very strongly attached to the infant. One mother who had experienced very negative feelings toward the infant during the first 6 weeks began to feel just as strongly in a positive way once the infant began to respond more definitively.

The attachment process in this study appeared to be affected by (1) the mother's personality and level of emotional development, (2) the mother's life experiences and preparation for the birth, and (3) the infant's behavioral characteristics or use of tools. For mothers experiencing early attachment (during the first 2 days of life), the infant's social behaviors were insignificant; the critical factor was that the mothers really wanted their babies. These mothers were very calm, secure, and competent; were experienced in child care; and saw the infant as a part of themselves and yet as a unique entity. The infant's social skills did become critical to maintaining the attachment, however. Late attachers typically had ambivalent feelings about having a baby or becoming a mother and exhibited much anxiety. Many of their babies were difficult to care for and gave little cause for love or inadequate response to the mothers' caretaking efforts. Others simply did not want the baby. The attachment bond became stronger as the infant responded to care. The infant's ability to smile and to give eye-to-eye contact appeared to have central importance in the mother's development of attachment [73].

Rivalry in the Family

The addition of a second, third, or fourth (or more) child to the family makes the communication system infinitely more complex. Each member of an interaction must become aware of the relationship each has with other members of the family. When a relationship is particularly close and meaningful or is perceived as essential to one's own well-being, competition for attention may lead to jealousy (fear of losing to the competitor) or rivalry (hatred or dislike of those with a perceived advantage) [33]. This antagonism, usually one-sided, results from fear of losing the attention or love of the esteemed other person. There is a feeling of replacement, a loss of status in the previous relationship. The aggrieved family member may begin to make unreasonable demands for time and attention in order to regain or assure status.

Although we usually think of rivalry as occurring between siblings, it can occur with any relationship at any age when friendships expand and change. Even animals may express increased needs for attention when a new baby arrives [2]. Rivalry exemplifies a desire to maintain the security of the status quo. Rivalry is very commonly expressed by the husband or wife when a new baby arrives. Each needs to remain sensitive to the continued emotional needs of the spouse as a separate individual—not just as a parent. Sometimes parents become so involved in the novelty and thrill of parenthood that all their attention and emotional energies become focused on the new baby. Even parents who desparately wanted and planned for the baby may begin to feel some resentment at the need to consider the new baby when they are making a decision to go out for the evening or just to spend some time alone together. As a result, marital happiness may

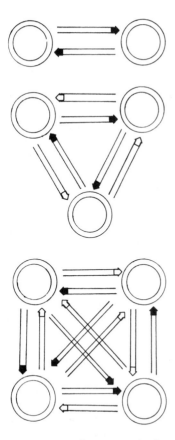

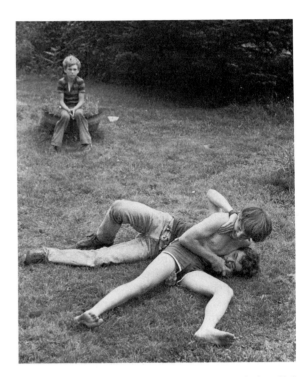

Figure 32–8. Sibling rivalry that is inadequately handled during the early years may continue to create interactional problems in the years ahead.

Figure 32–7. The communication system within a family becomes infinitely more complex each time a new member is added.

decline. It takes time for the parents to adjust to the idea of being a larger family, not just a couple. They need to be reminded to continue to spend time alone with each other, even if only for a 20-minute walk.

Children between the ages of 18 months and 3½ years are most likely to feel and to express rivalry with the new baby, especially if the parents have been oversolicitous or inconsistent in discipline [84]. Children of this age are beginning to realize that the mother is not a part or an extension of themselves, but she is still essential to their security and independence. It is difficult for them to comprehend the need to wait until later for attention. Sibling rivalry may be expressed by avoiding any form of contact with the new baby, by verbal rejection, or even by physical abuse of either the baby or the mother. Some children become destructive of property or abusive to pets—a form of scapegoating.

Rivalry can be prevented by including the current family members in the birth preparations as much as possible [85]. The age and comprehension level of a young child will require modification of when and how he is told. Storybooks can facilitate this process [25]. The new baby should be thought of and spoken of as "ours" rather than as only the mother's; this prevents a feeling of being "shut out" from the event—a precipitator of jealousy for both husband and children. Switching of rooms, beds, and so on should be accomplished as long as possible before the new baby arrives so that younger children do not feel physically displaced by the baby. Some families and hospitals are including children in the birth experience [63]; others include the child in postpartum visits to the hospital [86]. There is a marked reduction in noncompliant, restless, clinging behavior, and a marked increase in filial attachment when children are included and spared separation experiences. The father's active involvement with the older child (or children) also helps the child to adjust more easily [9]. When the mother returns from the hospital, her first concern should be to let the older child know how much he or she was missed and to renew the bond between them. After the older child is ready, the new baby can be introduced.

After the baby arrives home, unity is fostered by involvement of the other family members. Children who share in the infant care and household chores (according to age) are elevated to the status of "competent helpers." Both the father and siblings should have the opportunity to assist in showing off the new baby and should be allowed to participate in the conversations with guests. Younger children often enjoy imitating child-care activities with a special doll. Role playing helps them to understand and to integrate the new experience into their own lives. Dramatic play with bathing, bottle-feeding, and even attempts to breast-feed are common and therapeutic.

A new baby does require a lot of time and attention. Laughing about the inconvenience of diapering and the messiness helps older children to take these in stride. Emphasizing that the mother performed the same tasks for the older children when they were young takes the sting off the perceived extra attention given to the baby and offers a foundation for emphasizing how much the older ones have grown up in skills, interests, and communication abilities. The birth of the sibling thus heightens the distinction between self-nonself, but the feelings evoked by this distinction can be channeled into a warm, affectionate tie between the siblings by the understanding and continued affirmation shown by the parents [19]. It is essential to find time to maintain the closeness of the previous one-to-one relationship, especially with young children. This can be done by reading to the older child while feeding the baby or walking to the park with the baby in a carriage.

The parents will need to consider the young child's concept of a baby. All that an older sibling often sees is a head and a blanket. What is underneath? Children may pinch, pull and pick at a baby during the first week—not because of jealousy, but from curiosity. A parent should show the child the new baby—naked, and state that "you looked just like that when you were a baby." Children are usually fascinated to learn that they were once attached to the mother by the umbilical cord [85].

A child may become jealous of the mother's role and develop a "little mother" complex characterized by possessiveness and a desire to give all the child care. Possessiveness in early childhood is natural. The school-age child may see the baby as a real live "baby doll"—a dream come true. The adolescent may wish to assume an adult role early. Parental handling of such situations depends on the age of the child. All should be allowed to participate in the care of the baby, but relationships must be kept very clear, and the child should be encouraged to develop skills and interests

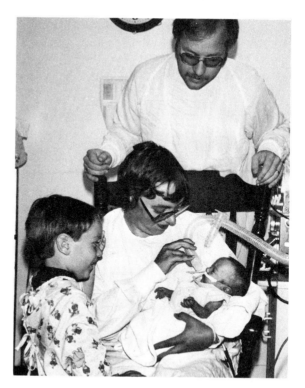

Figure 32–9. The first meeting. Sibling rivalry can be reduced by the introduction of the older child to the new family member at a pace and in a way suited to the child's interactional style.

that are age-appropriate. Usually the novelty wears off and family relations begin to assume normalcy.

Some mothers allow a teenage sibling to assume a mother's role, since it reduces their work load and they have a built-in babysitter. The baby may become more attached to the older sibling than to the mother. However, when the sibling leaves for college, marriage, or a job, the separation can be very traumatic for all three: The teenager leaves a part of the self, the young child may feel abandoned and forced to develop new emotional attachments, the real mother has to assume a new role that she may resent.

When love and acceptance are contingent on the child's ability to meet a parent's need, and when self-worth becomes relative by frequent comparing of children to one another, then validation of individuality and worth are arbitrary, which is fertile ground for severe sibling rivalry [76]. Severe sibling rivalry can continue into adulthood, affecting the quality of the sibling relationship [3, 76]. If parents are psychologically unavailable to the children, the children can form such

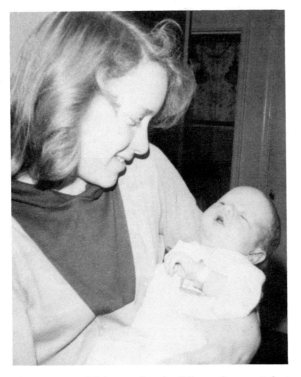

Figure 32–10. Adolescent female siblings of a new infant may develop a "little mother" complex. While the desire to be actively involved in the care of the new baby is typical for children of all ages, it must not prevent the pursuit of activities that are more normal and growth-producing for their ages.

a tight, loyal, mutual support group that the development of a healthy individual identity may be impeded by the closeness [3]. Other persons, even spouses, may be shut out later in life. Parents are in a key position to help children learn how to negotiate differences, to appreciate one another's strengths and weaknesses, and to affirm the value of others. In this environment, siblings can become supportive friends for a lifetime.

CONCLUSIONS

The period of transition to parenthood begins prior to the birth of the baby. The attitudes of parents are affected by both the culture and their individual values and goals. Self-identity is reassessed in light of past, present, and future experiences. Shared experiences and responsibilities help to foster family unity and facilitate integration of new self-identity.

Health care agencies and cultural mores are en-

couraging participation of the father in the childbirth experience and expressing acceptance of his capacity for gentle tenderness toward his wife and baby. The addition of a new child by birth or adoption places stress on the family relationships as new lines of communication are established; family members must retain their individuality while taking into account the needs of others. The first and most critical task of the parent is the establishment of interactive synchrony with the new child. From this sensitive mutual responsivity emerges the infant's attachment and the foundation for the healthy emotional, cognitive, and social development of the child.

Parenthood is potentially another step in the psychosexual ladder of development. It is exciting and growth-producing for individuals who have successfully accomplished previous psychosexual tasks. However, it can be traumatic for the individual who is not yet secure in a personal identity. Consequently, parenthood should not be entered lightly or by accident. Parenthood should be a planned event if each family member is to thrive and mature optimally.

REFERENCES

1. American Academy of Pediatrics. The promotion of breast-feeding. *Pediatrics* 69:654, 1982.
2. Bahr, J. E. Canine and feline rivalry: Another form of sibling rivalry. *Pediatric Nursing* 7(4):18, 1981.
3. Bank, S. P. and Kahn, M. D. *The Sibling Bond.* New York: Basic Books, 1982.
4. Benedek, T. Fatherhood and Providing. In E. J. Anthony and T. Benedek (Eds.), *Parenthood: Its Psychology and Psychopathology.* Boston: Little, Brown, 1970.
5. Benedek, T. Motherhood and Nurturing. In E. J. Anthony and T. Benedek (Eds.), *Parenthood: Its Psychology and Psychopathology.* Boston: Little, Brown, 1970.
6. Beske, E. J., and Garvis, M. S. Important factors in breast-feeding success. *MCN* 7:174, 1982.
7. Bibring, G. L. Some Considerations of the Psychological Process in Pregnancy. In *Psychoanalytic Study of the Child.* Vol. 14. New York: International Universities Press, 1959.
8. Bibring, G. L., et al. A Study of the Psychological Process in Pregnancy and of the Earliest Mother-Child Relationship. *Psychoanalytic Study of the Child.* Vol. 14. New York: International Universities Press, 1959.
9. Bittman, S. J., and Zalk, S. R. *Expectant Fathers.* New York: Hawthorne Books, 1978.
10. Brazelton, T. B. The remarkable talents of the newborn. *Birth and Family Journal.* 5:187, 1978.
11. Brazelton, T. B. *On Becoming a Family: The Growth of Attachment.* New York: Delacorte Press, 1981.
12. Budin, P. *The Nursling.* London: Caxton, 1907.
13. Campbell, B. K. "The Psychotic Child: Early Identifica-

tion of Psychosis in the First Years of Life." Address presented at the conference entitled An Interdisciplinary Approach to the Optimal Development of Infants: The Special Child. Ann Arbor, MI, April 4, 1979.

14. Carek, D. J., and Capelli, A. J. Mother's reactions to their newborn infants. *J. Am. Acad. Child Psychiatry* 20:16, 1981.

15. Castor, C. R. Education for Childbirth. In E. J. Dickason and M. O. Schult (Eds.), *Maternal and Infant Care*. New York: McGraw-Hill, 1975.

16. Chez, R. A. Sex in pregnancy. *Contemp. Ob./Gyn.* 6(2):99, 1975.

17. Condon, W. S., and Sander, L. W. Neonatal movement is synchronized with adult speech: Interactional participation and language acquisition. *Science* 183:99, 1974.

18. Cordell, A. S., Parke, R. D., and Sawin, D. B. Fathers' views on fatherhood with special reference to infancy. *Fam. Rel.* 29:331, 1980.

19. Dunn, J., and Kendrick, C. *Siblings: Love, Envy and Understanding*. Cambridge: Harvard University Press, 1982.

20. Feigelman, W., and Silverman, A. R. Preferential adoption: A new family formation. *Social Casework* 60:302, 1979.

21. Foley, K. L. Caring for the parents of newborn twins. *MCN* 4:221, 1979.

22. Fraiberg, S. "Clinical Issues in Infant Assessment." Address presented at the conference entitled An Interdisciplinary Approach to the Optimal Development of Infants: The Special Child. Ann Arbor, MI, April 4, 1979.

23. Freedman, D. G. *Human Infancy: An Evaluationary Perspective*. New York: Halsted Press, 1974.

24. Frodi, A. M. Paternal-baby responsiveness and involvement. *Infant Mental Health Journal* 1:150, 1980.

25. Gates, S. Children's literature: It can help children cope with sibling rivalry. *MCN* 5:351, 1980.

26. Gearing, J. Facilitating the birth process and father-child bonding. *Counseling Psychologist* 7(4):53, 1978.

27. Goldstein, S. "Primary Prevention: A Federal Perspective." Address presented at Primary Prevention Programs: Models for a Hopeful Future. Pittsburgh, PA, April 29, 1978.

28. Grace, J. T. Does a mother's knowledge of fetal gender affect attachment? *Matern.-Child Nurs. J.* 9:42, 1984.

29. Greenberg, M., and Morris, N. Engrossment: The newborn's impact upon the father. *Am. J. Orthopsychiatry* 44(4):520, 1974.

30. Herbert, M., Sluckin, W., Sluckin, A. Mother-to-infant bonding. *J. Assn. Child Psychol. and Psychiat.* 23:205, 1982.

31. Jessner, L., Weigert, E., and Foy, J. L. The Development of Parental Attitudes During Pregnancy. In E. J. Anthony and T. Benedek (Eds.), *Parenthood: Its Psychology and Psychopathology*. Boston: Little, Brown, 1970.

32. Josselyn, I. M. Cultural forces, motherliness and fatherliness. *Am. J. Orthopsychiatry* 26:264, 1956.

33. Katz, L. G. Brotherhood/sisterhood begins at home: Notes on sibling rivalry. *J. Can. Assn. Young Child.* 7:20, 1981.

34. Kennell, J. H., and Klaus, M. H. Caring for the Parents of Premature or Sick Infants. In M. H. Klaus and J. H. Kennell (Eds.), *Parent-Infant Bonding* (2nd ed.). St. Louis: Mosby, 1982.

35. Klaus, M. H. The biology of parent-to-infant attachment. *Birth and Family Journal* 5:200, 1978.

36. Klaus, M. H., and Kennell, J. H. Mothers separated from their newborn infants. *Pediatr. Clin. North Am.* 17:1015, 1970.

37. Klaus, M. H., and Kennell, J. H. Mothers Separated From their Newborn Infants. In J. L. Schwartz and L. H. Schwartz (Eds.), *Vulnerable Infants: A Psychosocial Dilemma*. New York: McGraw-Hill, 1977.

38. Klaus, M. H., and Kennell, J. H. Labor, Birth, and Bonding. In M. H. Klaus and J. H. Kennell (Eds.), *Parent-Infant Bonding*. St. Louis: Mosby, 1982.

39. Klaus, M. H., Leger, T., and Trause, M. A. (Eds.). *Maternal Attachment and Mothering Disorders: A Round Table*. Sausalito, CA: Johnson & Johnson, 1975.

40. Klaus, M., et al. Maternal attachment: Importance of the first post partum days. *N. Engl. J. Med.* 286:460, 1972.

41. Kohn, C. L., et al. Gravidas responses to realtime ultrasound fetal image. *J.O.G.N. Nurs.* 9:77, 1980.

42. Korner, A. F., and Thoman, E. B. Visual Alertness in Neonates as Evoked by Maternal Care. In L. J. Stone, H. T. Smith, and L. B. Murphy (Eds.), *The Competent Infant: Research and Commentary*. New York: Basic Books, 1973.

43. Kotelchuk, M. The Infant's Relationship to the Father: Experimental Evidence. In M. Lamb (Ed.), *The Role of the Father in Child Development*. New York: Wiley, 1976.

44. LaRossa, R., and LaRossa, M. M. *Transition to Parenthood: How Infants Change Families*. Beverly Hills, CA: Sage Publications, 1981.

45. Lawrence, R. A. *Breast-feeding: A Guide for the Medical Profession*. St. Louis: Mosby, 1980.

46. Lind, J., Vuorenkoski, V., and Wasz-Hacket, O. In N. Morris (Ed.), *Psychosomatic Medicine in Obstetrics and Gynaecology*. Basel: Karger, 1972.

47. Linde, D. B., and Engelhardt, K. F. What do parents know about infant development? *Pediatric Nursing* 5(1):33, 1979.

48. Lockhart, B. When couples adopt, they too need parenting classes. *MCN* 7:116, 1982.

49. MacFarlane, A. *The Psychology of Childbirth*. London: Open Books, 1977.

50. Mahler, M. S., Pine, F., and Bergman, A. *The Psychological Birth of the Human Infant*. New York: Basic Books, 1975.

51. Maloni, J. A. The birthing room: Some insights into parents' experiences. *MCN* 5:314, 1980.

52. Mercer, R. T. The nurse and maternal tasks of early postpartum. *Matern.-Child Nurs. J.* 6:341, 1981.

53. Meyers, B. Early intervention using Brazelton training with middle-class mothers and fathers of newborns. *Child Dev.* 53:462, 1982.

54. Milne, L. S. and Rich, O. J. Cognitive and affective aspects of the responses of pregnant women to sonography. *Matern.-Child Nurs. J.* 10:15, 1981.

55. National Institutes of Health. *Caesarean Childbirth.* Concensus Development Conference Summary. Bethesda, MD, Vol. 3, No. 6, 1980.

56. Ojofeitimi, E. O. Effect of duration and frequency of breast-feeding on postpartum amenorrhea. *Pediatrics* 69: 164, 1982.

57. Parke, R. D. Father-Infant Interaction. In M. H. Klaus, T. Leger, and M. A. Trause (Eds.), *Maternal Attachment and Mothering Disorders: A Round Table.* Sausalito, CA: Johnson & Johnson, 1974.

58. Parke, R. D. The father's role in infancy: A reevaluation. *Birth and the Family Journal* 5:211, 1978.

59. Parke, R. D. *Fathers.* Cambridge, MA: Harvard University Press, 1981.

60. Pearse, W. H. Trends in out-of-hospital births. *Obstet. Gynecol.* 60:267, 1982.

61. Pederson, F. A. (Ed.). *The Father-Infant Relationship: Observational Studies in the Family Setting.* New York: Praeger, 1980.

62. Pellegram, P., and Swartz, L. Primigravida's perceptions of early postpartum. *Pediatr. Nurs.* (November-December 1980):25.

63. Perez, P. Nurturing children who attend to birth of a sibling. *MCN* 4:215, 1979.

64. Promotion of breast feeding. *Pediatr. Res.* 16:264, 1982.

65. Pryor, K. W. *Nursing Your Baby.* New York: Pocket Books, 1980.

66. Rebelsky, F., and Hanks, C. Fathers' verbal interaction with infants in the first three months of life. *Child Dev.* 42:63, 1971.

67. Reiber, V. D. Is the nurturing role natural to fathers? *Matern.-Child Nurs. J.* 1:366, 1976.

68. Richman, J. Men's Experience of Pregnancy and Childbirth. In L. McKee, and M. O'Brien (Eds.), *The Father Figure.* New York: Travistock, 1982.

69. Ringler, N. M., Trause, M. A., and Klaus, M. H. Mother's speech to her two-year-old, its effect on speech and language comprehension at 5 years. *Pediatr. Res.* 10:307, 1976.

70. Ringler, N. M., et al. Mother-to-child speech at 2 years— Effects of early postnatal contact. *J. Pediatr.* 86:141, 1975.

71. Robertson, J., and Robertson, J. "From Birth to Three: The Vulnerable Years." Address at the conference entitled An Interdisciplinary Approach to the Optimal Development of Infants: The Special Child. Ann Arbor, MI, April 5, 1979.

72. Robson, K. S. The role of eye-to-eye contact in maternal-infant attachment. *J. Child Psychol. Psychiatry* 8:13, May, 1967.

73. Robson, K. S., and Moss, H. A. Patterns and determinants of maternal attachment. *J. Pediatr.* 77:976, 1970.

74. *Rock-a-Bye-Baby,* film (BBC-TV, 1975; Time-Life).

75. Rodholm, M. Effects of father-infant postpartum contact on their interaction 3 months after birth. *Early Hum. Dev.* 5:79, 1981.

76. Ross, H. G. "Adult Perception of Severe Sibling Rivalry." Paper presented at nintieth annual convention of The American Psychological Association, Washington, D.C., Aug. 26, 1982.

77. Rubin, R. Maternal touch. *Nurs. Outlook* 11:828, 1963.

78. Salk, L. The Critical Nature of the Post Partum Period in the Human for the Establishment of the Mother-Infant Bond: A Controlled Study. In J. L. Schwartz and L. H. Schwartz (Eds.), *Vulnerable Infants: A Psychosocial Dilemma.* New York: McGraw-Hill, 1977.

79. Sawin, D. B., and Parke, R. D. Father's affectionate stimulation and caregiving behaviors with newborn infants. *Family Coordinator* 28:509, 1979.

80. Schmitt, M. H. Superiority of breast-feeding, fact or fancy? *Am. J. Nurs.* 70:1488, 1970.

81. Silverman, W. A. Incubator-baby sideshows. *Pediatrics* 64:127, 1979.

82. Speroff, L. What initiates labor? *Contemp. Ob./Gyn.* 7(5): 113, 1976.

83. Stranik, M. K., and Hogberg, B. L. Transition into parenthood. *Am. J. Nurs.* 79:90, 1979.

84. Sutton-Smith, B., and Rosenberg, B. G. *The Sibling.* New York: Holt, Rinehart and Winston, 1970.

85. Sweet, P. T. Prenatal classes especially for children. *Am. J. Matern.-Child Nurs.* 4:82, 1979.

86. Trause, M. A., et al. Separation for childbirth: The effect on the sibling. *Child Psychiatry Hum. Dev.* 12:32, 1981.

87. Walker, L. O. Identifying parents in need: An approach to adoptive parenting. *MCN* 6:118, 1981.

88. Ward, M. Parental bonding in older-child adoptions. *Child Welfare* 60:24, 1981.

89. Williams, B. Sleep needs during the maternity cycle. *Nurs. Outlook* 15(2):53, 1967.

90. Winnicott, D. W. The Mother-Infant Experience of Maternity. In E. J. Anthony and T. Benedek (Eds.), *Parenthood: Its Psychology and Psychopathology.* Boston: Little, Brown, 1970.

91. Wolff, P. H. Mother-Infant Relations at Birth. In J. G. Howells (Ed.), *Modern Perspectives in International Child Psychiatry.* New York: Brunner/Mazel, 1971.

92. Zeyen, D. D. *Healthy Mothers, Healthy Babies: A Framework for Curriculum Development in Responsible Childbearing Preschool Through High School.* Reston: VA: Association for Supervision and Curriculum Development, 1981.

93. Zimmerman, M. A. Breast-feeding the adopted newborn. *Pediatr. Nurs.* (January-February, 1981):9.

33
Maintaining Family Unity

Clara S. Schuster

The family is our refuge and springboard;
nourished on it, we can advance to new horizons.
In every conceivable manner, the family is link to
our past, bridge to our future.

—Alex Haley

The headline reads: "Man kills parents, two brothers, and himself." The media commentator reflects the whispers of the shocked suburban neighbors: "The neighborhood is paralyzed tonight by this grisly event. Teachers describe the alleged murderer-suicide as a quiet, well-behaved, honor student coming from a **good** family. The parents, both professional people, were actively involved in community as well as church activities. Just last week the father was honored . . . ." We all know this scenario, yet are stunned anew with each recurrence.

A less familiar, yet more common vignette, centers on lonely, aging parents—people who have raised one or more children to adulthood only to see them swallowed up by peer groups, cultural enticements, and the exigencies of daily life. With sad, bitter hearts they protest to sympathetic ears, "I did everything for them when they were little. Why can't they remember me now? We had such a **good** family."

How often do we hear the words, "It was such a **good** family," repeated? Yet **good** families have children who become heavily involved in drugs or other delinquent or criminal activities. **Good** families have children who run away from them. **Good** families suffer the pains of separation and divorce. Each time a **good** family experiences one of these tragedies, we wince, realizing our own vulnerability and not knowing quite how to predict or to prevent these devastating plights.

On the other hand, we are also aware of individuals of historical reknown or even within our own communities, who, in spite of growing up in adverse circumstances, such as single parentage, poverty, social disadvantage, or inadequate cultural modeling, turn out to be "giants" in society through their allocentric (other-centered), mature, self-sufficient, and warm human approach to life.

The family, as a system, is a prototype of society. Through its hierarchical relationships, rules, values, and communication patterns, children learn and test skills that they will utilize when relating to the larger society. The family is the bedrock of society. It is the garden in which personalities germinate, grow, and mature. The family supplies the nation with citizens—workers, consumers, taxpayers, and leaders. The health of the nation depends on the health of its citizens [17]. The health of the citizens depends on the health of the family [3, 4, 5, 9].

If these suppositions are valid, then we must safeguard the health of the family as a whole, with as much vigor as we support the development of the individuals within it. We must identify ways to foster the unity of the family without neglecting the individuals within it. We must reevaluate our criteria of **good** families. We must begin to identify the characteristics of **healthy** families. Only then will the potentials of family life be maximized as well as the quality of life for the individuals who comprise the family system.

MAINTAINING THE ADULT-ADULT RELATIONSHIP

When a couple marry, they promise to love, cherish, and honor each other "till death do us part." They are caught up, as they should be, in the joys of physical and social intimacies. They are enveloped in the task of "becoming one." But unity does not refer to the fusion of selves that may occur between poorly differentiated spouses. Nor does it refer to the development of a pseudoself where one (or both) depends on an attachment to the other person for self-identity [3]. Both situations are potentially disastrous. In the first, both parties become involved in being what they think the other expects them to be, yet each demands changes in the other in order to enhance his or her own functioning. Neither person assumes full responsibility for self [3]. In the second situation, one person becomes an extension of the other. There is no sense of goals

or power or even strength for daily living except as ego strength is borrowed from the other (fused ego boundaries).

Genuine unity recognizes, cherishes, and safeguards the individuality of each member. Because ego boundaries are clear, the partners are able to share a comfortable, nonthreatening emotional closeness without fear of loss of self or submersion into the ego deficiencies of the other. The couple who negotiates this early task successfully is well on the way to a lifetime of family unity.

The good feelings and lofty intentions of honeymooners do not ensure a good family unit. Reality soon sets in, and egocentric idealistic thinking is confronted with new tasks, relationships, and challenges. Since families are no longer held together by necessity (i.e., a man and a woman needing each other to perform the tasks of life that could not be accomplished alone), the establishment of companionship is imperative for the health of the union and for vibrant survival in the years ahead. Today, when families are "held together more by consensus and mutual affection than by formal, institutional controls" [8], the longevity of a marriage, as well as the joy and the strength derived from it, is enhanced when the couple are the best of friends and not just role partners.

Adjusting to the Expanding Family

The early years of marriage offer the couple the opportunity to get to know each other more deeply and to learn how to meet and resolve problems when they arise (see Chap. 30). The couple can direct their energies toward accepting, defining, and refining their roles as husband, wife, and companions. Because these years usually are fairly free of responsibility, the couple can share many hours of uninterrupted companionship and spontaneous leisure activities; it is a time in which to bond.

The arrival of the first child creates marked changes in life-style, time availability, and priorities for the couple. For many individuals, not only is this the first time they have had anyone else depend on them, but it is for 24 hours a day, 7 days a week. Studies consistently indicate that marital happiness and adjustment decreases with the birth of the first child [28, 34, 36]. Some of the factors that decrease marital happiness are obvious, such as a lessening in the leisure time a couple has together, increased tiredness, increased concerns over the financial integrity of the family, and even a rivalry between partners as discussed in Chapter 32.

Other factors are more subtle, such as increased time

cerned with their own life-styles and development than that of others will find the adjustment most difficult.

However, **marital satisfaction and family satisfaction are not synonymous** [33] and the decrease in marital satisfaction after becoming parents is not sufficient to destroy most marriages. When both parents are secure in the love of the other and have a good sense of personal identity, parental satisfaction will offset marital disappointment. In fact, many marriages become even more satisfying after children are born because of a sense of achievement and pride [25], a sense of fulfillment, a new way to share their love together. Children give parents the opportunity to "reaffirm and rejuvenate their basic commitments to love, life, work, and play" [16]. The couple has a common goal toward which to strive—to raise their children to successful adulthood.

Mature individuals who have achieved a sense of unity are able to expand their concept of the family system to include the new members as unique individuals. The readjustment of priorities can be seen either as a temporary inconvenience or as a growth-producing challenge that accompanies the transition from being a couple to being a family, which can lead toward higher levels of both personal and family functioning.

Maintaining Vitality

Some couples can become so engrossed in the joys and/or responsibilities of parenthood that they forget the original purpose of their union—permanent, in-depth companionship. After children arrive, they may find that the husband gets caught up in earning sufficient money to provide for the needs of the family; the wife becomes involved in child care, homemaking, and/or her own career. As the years progress, they become strangers sharing the same bedroom. Each is involved in his or her separate responsibilities. If both spouses work, they may feel that there is even less time to spend together. They begin to relate to each other as roles rather than as people. There are so many interruptions when they are together that it gradually extinguishes their sharing behaviors. They begin to treat the family in a global manner, as a single unit rather than recognizing the unique needs and contributions of each member as a separate individual. Suddenly, parents may feel a loss of their own identity within the family system. They play a role, but they do not feel that they are recognized or appreciated for the contributions they make. Thus, the family system can become less mature rather than more mature over time, using Werner's system criteria (see Chap. 2).

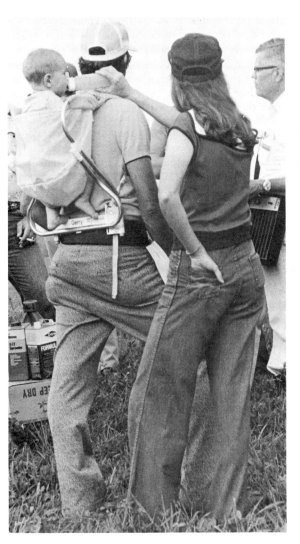

Figure 33–1. Each family defines its own concept of relaxation and leisure-time activity. (Courtesy Gene Hettel, Department of Public Information, Ohio Agriculture Research Development Center.)

with in-laws (who may have much unsolicited advice), decreased time for conversation and social intimacy, delayed plans, decreased spontaneous lovemaking because of tiredness or fear of interruptions, and decreased contacts with the "outside world" because of all the paraphernalia that must accompany travel with the baby. Many couples find they have outgrown their friends who do not yet have children or who live more spontaneous life-styles. The couple who is not yet ready to settle down or individuals who are more con-

The nuclear family, as a system, is self-limited. It has a beginning, a period of growing, and then a shrinking as it begins to release members to society [2]. Eventually, the two senior members will die and the family will cease to exist. If the couple do not maintain the vital companionship of earlier years, the family will self-destruct when the children leave home (or even earlier). The couple will live very separate lives and in very different worlds. They may be lonely and sexually frustrated [7]. The parents may literally find themselves strangers to each other with no common goals or meanings to life. Because wives are usually more personally involved in the management of the home and children, they are more vulnerable to family problems [28].

In the midst of childrearing, the parents need to separate the spousal subsystem from the parent-child subsystem [33]. The elusive yet all-vital quality of marital love must be maintained. This love does not survive merely because it existed when vows were exchanged. It survives and grows because the couple works at nurturing each other. Successful marriages have husbands and wives who are not tied to traditional roles [16]. Each respects the individual needs, talents, and interests of the other and works these into the division of responsibilities. The lover-companion relationship is enhanced when the husband is more interpersonally oriented [28], so that he is able to provide solace and spiritual nourishment to his wife and family.

In a vital marriage, the partners look for opportunities to spend time alone as a couple. Even though both of them may work and feel swamped with responsibility, they **make** time for each other. They may share family chores, such as shopping, doing dishes, or wrapping Christmas gifts, or they may merely sit and talk, watch television, or jog together. The sharing of a joke or incidents from the day and brief exchanges of affection indicate a recognition of, and appreciation for, the presence of the other person. But the couple also needs special time alone to enjoy their relationship without interruption, to renew their commitment, to rejuvenate their relationship. Depending on the couple's financial resources, this can take many forms. Attending a concert, a sports event, or an auction can help to relieve the stresses of everyday life. Most women appreciate the opportunity to eat at a restaurant. An evening at a motel or a week-end away from home can provide the time to revitalize a relationship. Some counselors recommend that a married couple continue to "date" once a week. It may only be a picnic or long walk to the park topped off by an ice cream

cone, but it is time alone together. There should be a minimum commitment of time each month to spend exclusively with each other in a mutually pleasurable activity. When planned ahead, both partners can look forward to the break from everyday routines and responsibilities. Children grow to appreciate and to respect their parents' time alone.

Adjusting to the Decreasing Family

A satisfying marriage takes years to develop [7]. The couple who have maintained a vital, caring, open, sensitive relationship during the childbearing/caring years will find that they not only cope more effectively with the normal psychological tensions of family living, but they will still be friends after the children leave home. Since there will probably be another 20 years of living together as a couple after the children leave home, the time spent in getting to know each other becomes an investment in life itself. The love shared in the early years takes on a new and deeper meaning with the sharing of experiences, crises, and memories. If mutual respect has been developed, then each can rise to new heights of personal fulfillment. This time of life is one of new beginnings, not of the "empty nest" [17]! Each partner will have more energy to pursue his or her career. For those women who saw motherhood as their career, the change can be frightening, but the loving support of a lifelong companion can make her transition easier and more exciting.

The postparental period allows a couple to focus on their relationship to each other. Some may even experience a "honeymoon" period and an enriched relationship and deeper tolerances [21]. Because they no longer feel the need to be models for the children or to be alert to their children's needs for guidance, the parents tend to relax in their roles and expectancies of each other, a phenomenon known as "mellowing."

PARENTAL RELATIONSHIPS WITH CHILDREN

Most of us have had an intimate acquaintance with only one or two families prior to initiating our own: our family of origin and perhaps that of a good friend. Other families are seen only as they present themselves to the outside world. And it is here that we get to the heart of the question, "What is a **good** family?" We can look around and identify those families who are financially secure in the community, yet affluence is not enough if the relationship is devoid of social meaning to the individuals within that family [16].

Family satisfaction was actually increased during the Depression years because the members of families had more time to spend with one another [7]. Many persons from the poorest states (Southeast) report the most positive affects [6]. Although abject poverty may increase stressors, wealth beyond necessity does not ensure conjugal peace.

The fundamental determinant of the quality of subjective human life is the presence or absence of meaningful interpersonal exchanges that provide psychological support [6]. Many families experience pseudomutuality. They look good to others, not because of financial security, but because of their altruism, or their social sophistication. They participate in community, educational, civic, and religious organizations and are friendly to neighbors, but there is little if any honest interaction among the family members [9]. These families may avoid conflict by suppressing negative reactions and behaviors. The members do not share personal feelings or values with one another because of fear of censure or the anxiety such sharing causes other family members. Their lives may become painful because of a lack of mutual respect, which robs them of the energy to face even the simplest of daily tasks. When people experience true companionship (see Chap. 30), they are freed to create an even more satisfying existence.

Because our culture places so much emphasis on material goods and social position, we are tempted to use these artificial standards to assess a **good** family. As we examine these criteria more critically, however, we begin to realize their superficiality. We also realize the limitations on our ability to establish evaluative criteria based on personal experience. We may judge our own family as good or bad based on our subjective experience within it, yet a sibling may have an opposing opinion. The quality of family functioning can be assessed by four major approaches:

1. Developmental approach. Assesses the ability to accomplish specific tasks and responsibilities
2. Interactional approach. Assesses the quality of interaction between members
3. Systems approach. Assesses the degree of system maturity
4. Structural-functional approach. Assesses role differentiation and relationships

The first method was proposed by Evelyn Duvall, and the second has been developed by Dolores Curran. Both of these researchers had extensive experience with families and were involved in major research projects before presenting their ideas. Each set of characteristics was developed in conjunction with the cul-

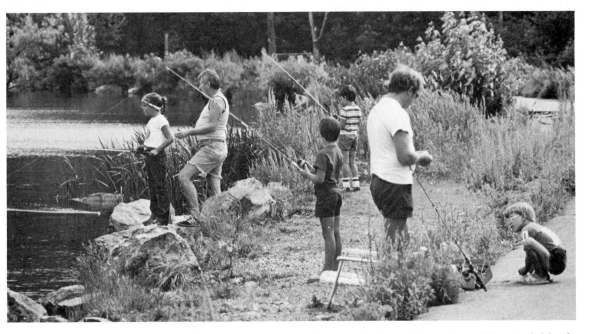

Figure 33–2. In some communities, neighbors take on the roles that were previously held by members of the extended family.

ture of their era. Although Duvall's frame may be seen as too traditional by some, it is hard to deny the necessity for the successful completion of the tasks she outlines. Curran's frame was developed when society was moving from an emphasis on roles to an emphasis on goals.

The third, more theoretical approach uses both Werner's dimensions presented in Chapter 2, and Tapia's frame from Chapter 34. The fourth approach, also discussed in Chapter 34, is heavily biased culturally and frequently is not flexible enough to be used in a situation where roles are being questioned and are changing rapidly. As in most situations, the practitioner must be committed to pluralism when working with individuals and families. Each approach makes a contribution to our understanding of family functioning.

Responsibilities of the Family

The family is a dynamic system. The members within it are in perpetual change as they progress through physical, cognitive, emotional, and social development. Changes in one member of the family necessitate changes in other members and, consequently, in the total family system. Duvall identified eight discrete family stages. The needs and experiences of each stage are distinctly different from those that precede or follow it. The stage is usually based on the age of the oldest child in the family. Consequently parents may find themselves in two or more stages simultaneously if they have more than one child [11]:

1. Beginning family
2. Childbearing family
3. Family with preschool children
4. Family with schoolagers
5. Family with adolescents
6. Family as a launching center
7. Family in middle years
8. Aging family

Successful parents exhibit flexibility and resiliency as they meet the needs of their rapidly developing children. But parents change, too, as they meet new challenges. As families progress through these developmental stages, Duvall proposes that the basic responsibilities remain constant. Although these tasks were developed for the western culture, in some manner, every culture must provide a means for mastering them. Duvall's family tasks may be assumed by the extended family or the commune. In the nuclear family, the responsibility for orchestrating the mastery of tasks

falls on the shoulders of the adult members or the administrative head of the family system.

FAMILY TASKS [11]

Physical Maintenance. The family must provide for the basic life support needs of its members. This includes provision of food, shelter, clothing, health care, and so on. The quality of these services will depend on the cultural context as well as the financial status of the family. When the nuclear family is unable to provide these services, the local welfare department may become involved to assist the family in ensuring that survival needs will be met.

Allocation of Resources. The family apportions possessions, space, time, and affection to its individual members based on a perception of the individual's needs and the value assigned to that member. Some parents do not realize their children's need for toys or even for their own bed. The parents themselves may have grown up in deprived environments and now give their children only what they have to or have left over after meeting their own needs. Other parents provide the children with "what I never had." The children, unaware of the sacrifices involved, become demanding of more.

Mature parents share resources equally with the children, helping them to become aware of financial and time limitations and expecting reciprocal sacrifices on the part of the children. The children may not have the same toys or jackets as the children down the street, but they realize that the parents share freely and fairly of what they have. Because the parents share affection with their children and respect their children's personhoods as well as their belongings, self-esteem is enhanced and unity is fostered.

Division of Labor. This task is frequently a source of friction in today's families. Each of the parents, coming from differing families of origin, may have different concepts about the husband's or the wife's role within the family. The traditional roles of the culture may be in conflict with the individual parent's opinions or the needs of the family. Together the couple must decide on the responsibilities of procuring an income for the family, managing household chores, and caring for the children. Under these headings would come mundane tasks, such as washing out the bathtub after use, changing the baby's diapers, polishing shoes, or fixing breakfast.

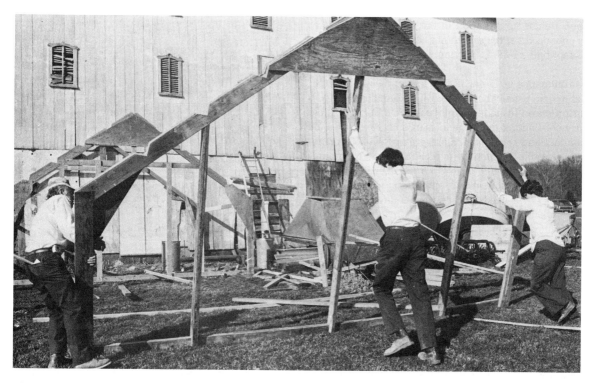

Figure 33–3. Working together at difficult tasks promotes egalitarian relationships that enhance respect for the value of each person.

When the parents can discuss these issues openly, match needs with skills or interests, and show flexibility and fairness in the division of tasks, unity is enhanced. As children mature, they are given responsibilities commensurate with their understanding and level of skill. They participate as partners in the business of making the family work smoothly. Unity is not enhanced if they feel that the parents are shirking their fair share. When all members participate fairly in the division of work, then there is more time available to share leisure-time activities.

Socialization of Family Members. Parents gradually guide children into increasingly mature patterns of behavior that become internalized and self-monitored. Aggression, sleep habits, elimination, and sexual drive are gradually brought under voluntary control. The norms and expectations of the community as well as those of the family set a standard for behaviors. The more complex behaviors that involve attitudes, social orientation, biases, and involvement are learned through observation. Parents cannot expect behaviors

from their children if they are not exhibiting the desired characteristics themselves. It is difficult for a child to value hard work or a good use of time if the parents watch television all evening while the child studies.

Reproduction, Recruitment, and Release of Family Members. Parents increase the family size through birth and adoption. The goal of the child-bearing family is to release self-sufficient, productive individuals into society at maturity. Temporary increases may occur through caring for foster children or accepting an exchange student.

Circumstances may necessitate the inclusion of in-laws or friends. Rules have to be established that protect the boundaries of the family system and the relationship among members. If boundaries are not clearly contained, unity will be jeopardized. Unity thrives on continuous relationships with a stable group of people, where identity and relationships are clearly differentiated and articulated. When new members are accepted (e.g., daughter- or son-in-law) and valued for their unique contribution to the family system, unity is enhanced. At the same time, a new couple needs to accept both of the in-law families as their own [25].

Maintenance of Order. Every family has a hierarchical system usually based on age, sex, and skills. A decision-maker (usually one of the parents) is responsible for coordinating the exigencies of daily life. Rules for conduct and relationships are present even if unspoken. Smooth functioning is facilitated when communication is open and clear. Each member is respected for his or her unique needs, opinions, and goals. When a conflict over needs occurs, the persons involved are able to share their points of view freely. Negotiation and mutual compromise is encouraged. When alternative solutions can not be identified, then the decision-maker considers what is best for the total family. Because of mutual respect, the members of the family accept the decision, even though it is not the most desirable one for some of the members. Mutual respect enhances unity.

Placement of Members in the Larger Society. Parents provide a "minisociety" that prepares children to interface with the broader culture. The family teaches children how to interact with both vertical and horizontal relationships. The parents introduce the child to the community's parks, stores, entertainment facilities, and transportation system. They prepare the child for school and influence his or her adjustment to it by their own attitude and the amount of support they extend to both the child and the school system. The parents' attitude toward, and involvement in, church, community organizations, and political systems influences the child's attitude toward the institutions and the values of the broader culture. Parents who are interested in news events, value systems, and their cultural heritage and who discuss these with their children help them to become more aware of their own identities and value system within the culture. Sharing and preparation enhances unity and offers security to children by minimizing surprises when they are confronted with the realities of "life in the big world."

Maintenance of Motivation and Morale. All persons need to be recognized for their uniqueness. When family members affirm one another's efforts, confidence is enhanced, and creativity is encouraged. When support and affection are given routinely, unity will be maintained during crises. Family rituals, gatherings, and festivals help the members to appreciate their heritage and to anticipate their future. A sense of kinship

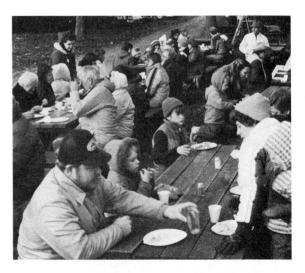

Figure 33–4. Participation of the family members in community activities enhances their sense of belonging to the broader culture.

and loyalty is fostered. These periods of sharing help family members to refine their philosophy of life and to identify their commonalities. The good feelings engendered by mutually enjoyed work and leisure activities help to carry the family through the difficult times that are common to all families.

EVALUATION OF FUNCTIONING

The success of a family, according to Duvall, is based on how well the family: (1) meets its short-term aspirations; (2) attains the goals society sets for it, and (3) masters the developmental tasks at each stage.

Although Duvall's tasks concentrate on specific, identifiable behaviors of the family system as orchestrated by the administrative subsystem, one must acknowledge that successful meeting of these tasks can facilitate the intangible bonding, or unity, that occurs among its members. Unity will be enhanced not only across generational lines but also between members of sibling subsystems as well.

Many families, however, appear to meet all these tasks with success and still do not achieve genuine unity among their members. These are the **good** families portrayed in the introduction. Something is still missing.

Characteristics of Healthy Families

Both the task (Duvall) and the systems (Werner, Tapia) approaches to family assessment share a significant philosophical view: Both approaches assess the family as a total unit. The task approach emphasizes the ability of the family system to accomplish the four main functions of open systems: containing, obtaining, maintaining, and disposing (see Chap. 2). It concentrates on output, or the interface with the supersystem. Throughput is secondary to the output. Goals appear to be heavily influenced by external sources.

The systems approach presented in Chapter 34 emphasizes the degree of differentiation attained by a system: the differentiation from the supersystem as well as the differentiation of its component parts. Werner's continuums allow for an objective assessment of the degree of differentiation attained. This approach also concentrates on the system's interface with the supersystem. Whereas the family task approach deals with five domains (physical, intellectual, social, emotional and spiritual), the systems approach focuses mainly on the affective and social domains.

The intrafamily-dynamics approach focuses not on the total unit, but on the interaction among the subsystems (adult-adult, adult-child, child-child). The health of these interactions is assumed to reflect the degree of differentiation and articulation achieved by the system. The healthier the interaction, the more success the family-as-a-whole will experience in meeting family tasks. This approach concentrates on throughput and is concerned with the affective, social, and spiritual domains. Goals are determined by internal sources.

Psychologists and family development specialists today are realizing that the evaluation of families according to their ability to meet the expectations of culturally determined roles is an anachronism. Families no longer are held together by necessity. Women are able to earn a living through gainful employment, and men are able to cook and to launder clothes. "Today the major function of family is relational. Our needs are emotional, not physical" [9]. The fractionalization of a family was formerly due to the failure of its members to fulfill roles. Today it is due to a failure to achieve goals, usually in the social and emotional domains.

A Harris survey in January 1980 found that family success was more important than financial success to 96 percent of the American population surveyed [9]. Most of our daily contacts involve using a formal, impersonal "role" self. Consequently, each person needs a small, intimate, private group that accepts idiosyncrasies and allows relaxation and the "peeling away" of these multiple impersonal roles. If Maslow's [29] lower-level needs of survival, safety, and security are met, individuals begin to search to meet their needs

for belongingness and affection, esteem and self-respect, and self-actualization, through the structure of family relationships.

Several persons have attempted to identify the characteristics of healthy families [9, 28, 39]. The most complete listing was developed by Dolores Curran from a survey of professional persons (e.g., doctors, scout leaders, school personnel, psychologists, ministers) who had daily, intimate contact with families. From their observations, Curran identified 15 traits of psychologically and socially healthy families—families who release healthy, productive citizens into society. She consolidated these characteristics into 12 major areas representing the interactions among members of families [9]. No family is perfect, but these traits provide information and guidelines for distinguishing between "healthy" and "good" families.

Open Communication. Every commentator on healthy family dynamics identifies communication as a key to family health. Through honest, open communication, the members are able to solidify their own individuality and that of others. Healthy individuals not only express their values and feelings but listen sensitively to those of other family members. They encourage independent thinking and feelings. When confrontations arise, they develop approaches not only to resolve the conflict, but to restore the mutuality of the relationship. These family members value the time spent conversing with one another and use every opportunity to share events, aspirations, disappointments, and feelings. The television is not allowed to usurp their relationship time. Nonverbal messages are decoded, and members are careful not to use turn-off words and put-down phrases that would stifle free and creative expression of the authentic self.

Affirmation and Support. The members of a healthy family make opportunities both to affirm and to support the value and uniqueness of each member. They like one another and say so. They extend appreciation for the efforts of other persons even if the final product is not commendable. They support the other members' goals even when it may require some sacrifice on their part (e.g., listening to a third-grader learning to play a violin, or shifting schedules and responsibilities to accommodate a parent returning to school). The basic mood of this family is positive. They know that even if they fail to achieve a personal goal, the other members will extend sympathy and understanding rather than criticism or ridicule. The whole family suffers if members cannot affirm one another [16] because self-esteem is lowered. The healthy family extends support to community institutions, but not automatically, for they expect the same open communication, affirmation, and respect from the institution as is found in their own family.

Mutual Respect. The healthy family values and respects each member regardless of age, disability, or eccentricity. Because of the respect shown and the affirmation offered, each person grows in self-respect—a self-respect that fosters the cherished care of one's own physical and psychic selves. This respect generalizes and transfers to institutions and persons outside the family and not only to those with whom they agree or find commonalities. Sex, creed, color, career, disability, or social orientation do not interfere with the respect that is afforded each person with whom they have contact. These individuals show respect but are not obsequious. They respect people, not positions. Each member has learned within the context of the family to approach every person with the same gentleness, tenderness, and respect that they themselves cherish and thrive upon. This respect extends to the personal property of other persons as well as each person's right to solve his or her own problems, to make mistakes, to identify friends, or to experience periods of solitude. These individuals do not invade the "personal space" of another person. In short, the subsystems are clearly delineated and members do not try to make others an extension of their own ego. They demand respect for their own selves by their deportment and their authenticity of interaction. Mutual respect is one of the strongest aspects of family unity [21].

Trust. Trust is recognized as a precious possession. It is the foundation of intimate relationships. The husband and wife trust the commitment of the other to the marriage. The children trust the parents' intentions and guidance to keep them safe (socially, emotionally, and spiritually, as well as physically), even though it may mean the frustration of a particular goal. The parents trust the ability of the child to gradually assume more self-direction. Members also recognize the essence of confidentiality. Confidences are cherished and maintained.

Share Time. Lack of time is probably the most pervasive enemy the healthy family has [9]. The activities of daily living, work, and community commitment may encroach on this precious, limited commodity. A strong sense of family rests on the time spent together; the experiences and responsibilities shared; and the goals, values, and priorities developed in tandem. If members do not make time for one another and for family activities, they become "ships passing in the night." Consequently, allegiance, socialization, and the establishment of values are turned over to other sys-

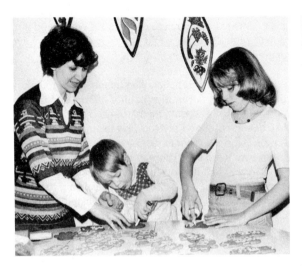 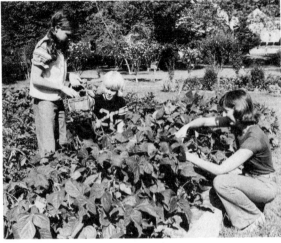

Figure 33–5. Assisting with household tasks helps to socialize children, refines their sensorimotor skills, prepares them to assume adult responsibilities, and increases their sense of self-worth. (Courtesy *Mt. Vernon News*.)

tems, such as the school, clubs, church, scouts, neighbors, or peers.

The high fractionalization rate of families today may actually be an artifact of society more than it is a conflict of personalities. The family that values its unity must take an assertive stance against intruding pressures. Each member must find a balance among extrafamilial, intrafamilial, and personal commitment times. They must not allow business or civic responsibilities to infringe regularly on family life. There comes a point where an individual must reassess priorities. If maintaining family integrity and unity is important, then the courage must be summoned to use that small but emphatic word, "No." The decision must be made as to what is more important: a public image or family relationships. If external forces are allowed to direct the individual's time, he or she in essence is saying "No" to the family and offering its members

---

Cat's in the Cradle

By Sandy and Harry Chapin

My child arrived just the other day
  he came to the world in the usual way—
But there were planes to catch and bills to pay
he learned to walk while I was away
  and he was talkin fore I knew it and as he grew
                                            he'd say

    I'm gonna be like you, Dad
    you know I'm gonna be like you.

and the cat's in the cradle and the silver spoon
Little boy blue and the man in the moon
when you comin' home, Dad
          I don't know when
          but we'll get together then—
    you know we'll have a good time then

My son turned 10 just the other day
  he said, Thanks for the ball, Dad, com'on let's play
Can you teach me to throw?
I said not today, I got a lot to do
He said, That's okay
        and he walked away
          but his smile never dimmed
    it said I'm gonna be like him, yeah
        you know I'm gonna be like him

and the cat's in the cradle and the silver spoon
Little boy blue and the man in the moon
when you comin' home, Dad
          I don't know when
          but we'll get together then—
    you know we'll have a good time then

Well he came home from college just the other day
  so much like a man I just had to say
Son, I'm proud of you, can you sit for awhile
He shook his head and said with a smile—
  what I'd really like, Dad, is to borrow the car keys
  see you later, can I have them please?

When you comin home, Son?
        I don't know when
        but we'll get together then
    you know we'll have a good time then

I've long since retired, my son's moved away
  I called him up just the other day
  I said I'd like to see you if you don't mind
  He said, I'd love to, Dad—if I can find the time

You see my new job's a hassle
  and the kids have the flu
  but it's sure nice talkin to you, Dad
  It's been nice talking to you

And as I hung up the phone, it occurred to me—
  he'd grown up just like me; my boy was just like me

and the cat's in the cradle and the silver spoon
Little boy blue and the man in the moon
when you comin home, Son?
        I don't know when
        but we'll get together then, Dad,
    we're gonna have a good time then

Figure 33–6. Cat's in the Cradle. Words and music by Sandy and Harry Chapin. Copyright © 1974 Story Songs, Ltd.

"left over" time. Sandy and Harry Chapin's "Cat's In The Cradle" poignantly catches the rhythm of this lifestyle. Sometimes a career, or at least an employer, may need to be changed, so that the individual is able to work to live and not live to work.

Men and women can "burn out" as they juggle home, work, and family responsibilities and activities. It is only as they develop a clear sense of their own boundaries and priorities that they can balance their stressors and assets and proceed on a relatively smooth course. Adults also have to be careful not to overload children in the push to maximize potentials. A child should be involved in only one activity at a time that requires practice [9] (e.g., piano, ballet, football, or band). That activity should have intrinsic value to the child, so that parental time is not "zapped" by forced spectatorship or supervision.

Healthy families structure time for each interactional subsystem to develop appreciation for the other. They prize time alone with individual members. Charles and John Wesley, outstanding humanists and theologians of the 1700s, came from an impoverished family of 19 children. When Suzanna, their mother, was asked how she accounted for her sons' self-confidence, personality, and spiritual success, she replied that she scheduled 1 hour each week to be spent alone with each child and engaged in activities he or she wanted or needed to do. This individual time was respected and jealously guarded by each member of the family. No intrusions were allowed except for emergencies [43]. Time was made for the parent and the child to get to know and like each other. **Special time with each child is not a luxury but a necessity** [9]. Parents must keep time in balance for each child even if one is gifted or disabled. Time cannot evolve disproportionately around any one member of the family.

The family needs to plan group time together. Work activities can be turned into play (e.g., yardwork, car wash, redecorating, food preparation). A sprinkling of humor throughout the activities of daily living relieves drudgery, depression, and conflicts. Pure play activities should be planned regularly into the schedule, such as trips to museums, a picnic (even in the snow), a trip to the beach, volleyball games, bike trips, bowling, or fishing. These excursions need not be expensive; they are only the mediums that provide the time together to share ideas. Window-shopping after the stores have closed for the day can be more fun than the actual purchasing of goods. Brief activities can be worked into the daily schedule. Memories are made from the sharing of simple, fun events. (Parents who need ideas might start with *Let's Make a Memory* by Gloria Gaither

and Shirley Dobson [14].) A weekly ethnic meal can provide variety and much discussion around the table. Reading a book or watching a special television program together also provides fuel for animated, authentic conversations that center on feelings and value systems. It can be enlightening and entertaining to speculate how one would allocate monies received from a hypothetical sweepstakes or inheritance.

In the midst of sharing time with one another, family members must respect the need of each to share time with the self. Private time is essential for unwinding and processing events. The individual must have the opportunity to get to know and to like the self.

Foster Responsibility. Genuine happiness and contentment result from the confidence of knowing that one has mastered difficult skills and situations and can continue to do so. Children need challenges to grow. Because the parents understand the relationship between responsibility and self-esteem, they gear responsibilities to the child's capabilities and then support the child's efforts. They do not remove the obstacles in their children's lives that can foster growth. They do not cover up for the child's neglected or forgotten responsibilities, but allow the child to live with the natural consequences of irresponsibility. They help the child to recognize the self as a partner in the tasks and responsibilities of the family system. In this way, children learn not only the psychomotor skills essential to successful independent adult living, but also the problem-solving and self-discipline skills essential to successful goal-setting and achievement.

Teach Morals. Curran observes that too many people emphasize "doing your own thing" over an evaluation of the effect of the behavior on one's long-range lifestyle and goals or the effect of the behavior on the lives of others. This tends to create a self-centered, hedonistic culture [18]. The source of authority becomes the person alone. Parents need to teach specific guidelines about right and wrong and to share with their children values and principles to believe in and to guide behavior. At the same time, parents need to realize that intent is crucial in judging behavior and must take time to understand the child's frame of reference. Both autonomy and unity are fostered when parents have clearly defined values and standards that are comfortably integrated into their own behavior and openly shared with their children [31].

Share Religious Beliefs. Religious participation correlates positively with increased marital satisfaction,

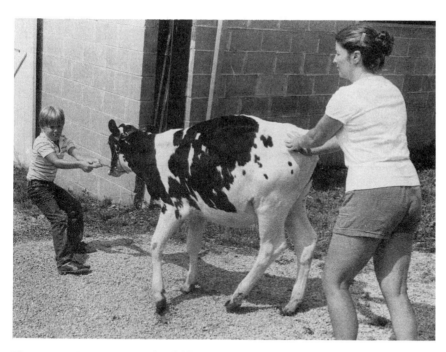

Figure 33–7. Parents support the child's burgeoning skills and sense of responsibility by assisting as necessary, but not by assuming the responsibility for the job.

happiness, and adjustment [22]. Sharing religious beliefs is more than teaching the nuances of church doctrines or institutionalized faith as practiced through rituals, memorized prayers, and participation in corporate worship. Healthy families share their religious beliefs because of the difference it makes in everyday family life. A vital religious core provides common values and a sense of meaning and purpose, or direction, to life. Families, like individuals, need the hope and strength that come from a belief in something higher than self. The family that pursues only material objects or goals, may be a candidate for self-destruction either from the eventual boredom of material pursuits or the inability to meet a crisis when it arises [9].

The healthy family does not have a rigid set of rules and prohibitions [16]. Rather, the internalized principles are woven comfortably into the fabric of daily living. The members recognize the difference between breaking conventions and breaking convictions. The peace of mind enjoyed by those who have made a commitment to something higher than themselves and have internalized a positive value system enables them to extend more energy toward other people, affirming and supporting their growth.

A 1981 Gallup survey of youth found that parents who placed a high value on religion were more likely to (1) help children with their homework, (2) share physical affection with their children, (3) tell them they were loved, (4) praise them, and (5) talk with them about their daily activities [15]. Children are more likely to embrace the parents' value system if they see that it sustains their parents through crises. Curran observes that "we must ask ourselves if those drawn to the cults are not really seeking a sense of family, complete with its traditions and value systems, which may have been missing in their own childhood families" [9].

The way we translate our values and religious beliefs into everyday living is the way we pass on our faith, or lack of it. Many religious doctrines teach that love must prevail in family relationships, thereby nurturing marital happiness and family solidarity [10]. However, some doctrines also prescribe gender-role behaviors that may actually undermine family relationships by failing to recognize the individuality of the members.

Enjoy Traditions. The healthy family views itself as a link between the past and the future. It shares stories both funny and sad about the history of the family. Grandparents are seen as valuable sources of family history, folklore, and cultural preserves. The family leans heavily on its religious and ethnic traditions for a sense of identity as well as its relationship to the broader culture. It also develops its own unique traditions based on rituals learned in the family of origin, spontaneous events, or personal desires. Young couples frequently experience conflict over rituals surrounding significant events, such as Christmas (e.g., whether to open presents on Christmas eve or on Christmas morning). As the family develops its own traditions, the members eagerly anticipate the next occurrence of the event, jealously guarding against any changes in the rituals or intrusions on the family time. The anticipation of holidays and other periodically recurring special events relieves the boredom and drudgery of routine events and responsibilities. The sharing of ethnic customs, rituals, food, or even language provides a sense of kinship that sustains during periods of crisis. Such close, shared experiences provide a lifelong base of love and support.

Respect Privacy. The healthy family protects and encourages the right of each member to be their own person. Each member can choose their own friends, follow their own fads, keep or dispose of their own material possessions, and be alone. Permissiveness does not mean indulgence, but freedom to be one's self. Mutuality is still expected and fostered.

Value Service. Healthy families stress cooperativeness, not competition, in relationships. Because members are at peace with themselves, they enjoy sharing their abundance of ego with others. The empathic and altruistic orientation developed within the family impels them to serve others in concrete ways. Neighborhood children, foster children, exchange students, lonely college students—all are made to feel welcome in their home. There is always enough love, affirmation, and good will to include another. (Conversely, new members or visitors may serve as distractors or substitute gratifiers in a dysfunctional or unhappy family system.) Members of healthy families donate blood, time, and/or expertise to improve the quality of life in the community. However, even volunteer time is kept in balance with family responsibilities and relationships. Through giving of the self in service to others, the individual actually receives more ego strength.

Seek Help. The healthy family is aware of its own limits and seeks help when necessary (see Chap. 34). It recognizes that no family is perfect and does not strive for an impossible, self-imposed standard (a self-defeating mentality [2]). Family members expect problems and consider them a normal part of intimate,

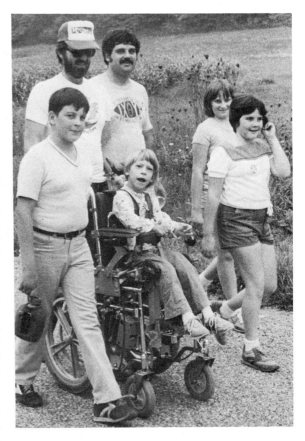

Figure 33–8. Parents model a spirit of community responsibility by participating in walk-a-thons, car washes, Red Cross Bloodmobile, and so forth. When the children are included, it enhances their self-esteem and facilitates the development of concern about the welfare of others.

honest relationships. They develop problem-solving techniques for identifying and dealing with specific problems as they arise. They seek help in the early stages of a problem before it reaches unresolvable dimensions [5]. Unity is enhanced because each member feels a responsibility to contribute to the resolution of problems and conflict-of-need situations.

When Children Become Adults

In spite of the aesthetic appeal of Curran's major areas of family interaction, there is no magic formula for assuring a positive outcome to the efforts of childrearing. The unique personality structure and ego intensity of the individuals who are involved will dynamically interact, creating a different relationship among the members of each separate interactional subsystem of the family. Biological factors, health status, educational and cultural opportunities, cultural standards, peers, adult role models, kinship contacts, and financial security are all factors that make a contribution to the final outcome. However, despite these potential influences, "the family, more than any other single agency lays the foundation for mental health or illness, for good or poor adjustment in life" [5]. Even the early parent-child relationship continues to affect the relationship of grown children with their parents [17], partly because the quality of the interaction tends to endure over time [25]. Parents continue to influence the child's adult development and interactions because of the value system the child has internalized and his or her identification with the discipline-reward system used by the parent [17].

One of the most difficult tasks of parenthood is the pacing of efforts to foster independence. When parents release the authority and the responsibility for guidance too early in a child's life, it makes it more difficult for the maturing offspring to accept the rules and regulations of other persons and institutions [27]; it also decreases the sense of caring between parents and child and thus the bonding with one another. On the other hand, independence and self-esteem are decreased and conflict is increased when parents continue to rule adult children.

Bowen, an outstanding psychiatrist, observes that families are constantly balancing two opposing forces: (1) togetherness (the need for love, approval, acceptance, and agreement), and (2) individuality (the need for autonomy, productivity, and creativity) [3]. If togetherness predominates, an undifferentiated family ego mass or fusion of selves prevents the independence and the maximization of the potentials of individual members. This kind of family expects everyone to hold the same opinion or to feel equally disturbed when one person perceives an insult from an outside source. Alternate viewpoints or even a clarification of the facts are not easily tolerated; subjective, self-effacing overtones color both intra- and extrafamily relationships. A severe pathology of the family as well as its individual members can develop. If individuality prevails, then perspective is lost: The parts become more important than the whole, and the bond is weakened. Among the members of this family, there is no sense of belonging to, or caring for, one another. Mutuality is lost.

The healthy family supports autonomy and gradual assumption of responsibility for problem solving by keeping communication lines fully open. Through careful listening, the parent gives the child permission to express what he or she is feeling and helps to clarify problem situations. Since the feeling system links the affective and cognitive domains [3], this technique facilitates greater self-understanding and autonomous problem solving. Thomas Gordon's approach to family communication facilitates this process. He advocates an **active listening** technique for parents to use with their children in which they listen for the feelings and meanings of a communication from the child without inserting judgmental overtones [20]. This approach fosters self-disclosure and identification of the specific underlying problem when conflict surfaces.

Gordon states that it is critical to identify the "ownership" of a problem in order to remain objective and protect individuality. He also emphasizes the use of "I messages"—statements that explain how a behavior or situation makes the speaker feel or affects the speaker's life (e.g., "If you get a cold because you don't wear a rain coat today, I will have to stay home to take care of you. That means that I will not get paid for that day of work and we will not be able to. . . ."). This honest, open approach allows two persons to develop an authentic relationship, which fosters negotiations for a mutually acceptable solution. Conflict-of-needs is no longer a power struggle where one person "wins" while the other capitulates. It is a "no-loser" approach that enables both parties to know and to respect each other better [20]. Their mutual respect thus leads to an increased differentiation as well as an increased integration of the parent-child subsystem, which fosters unity.

Grown children tend to reproduce the parents' culture if they have had a close relationship with good identification [17]. They continue to use the parents as a resource for decision making. Superordinate/subordinate roles are released. The relationship becomes one of friendship or mentorship over time because mutual respect has been established and each individual's uniqueness has been recognized and fostered. When contact between the generations is rewarding, it will continue over time [21].

VARIATIONS IN THE FAMILY EXPERIENCE

The traditional family has consisted of a working father, a homekeeping mother, and one or more children. This societal tradition may subconsciously create stress for those who fail to achieve it, straining their reserves to face realistically and positively the family situation in which they find themselves.

Single Parent Homes

600,000 babies (17.1% of all births) are born to single mothers in the United States each year [41]. Another 1 million children enter single-parent families each year because of the divorce of their parents [30]. Almost 20 percent of today's families are single-parent families, and 50 percent of children spend some part of their lives in a single-parent home [13]. Over 10 million children are being raised in father-absent homes [12]. Single-parent homes are generally a transitory state, since 80 percent of divorced persons eventually remarry [30].

The quality of family functioning following a divorce depends on the circumstances surrounding the divorce and the maturity of the persons involved. "For children to maintain healthy images of themselves, they must have healthy images of both parents. Blaming one parent for causing the divorce is harmful. A child identifies with both parents and feels the blame [32]. How can a child say "I am good" if he feels that he comes from "bad stock" [34]?

Children often feel they are not free to love whom they wish following a divorce [35]. The younger child experiences fewer adjustment problems at the time of a parental separation [35] but may exhibit a cumulative effect of stress during the adolescent years, experiencing substance abuse and academic and sexual problems [24]. The children maintain a strong loyalty to the predivorce family structure [26]. Loyalty or commitment conflicts are avoided when divorced parents maintain a positive relationship with each other [38]. Shared parenting, when possible and appropriate, can greatly facilitate the children's adjustments and identities. Children are able to distinguish and to accept the differences in their parents' personalities, behaviors, and values [38]. The negative feelings of children that accompany a divorce have usually become positive again by the time 2 years have passed [1, 26].

The new family, as a system, is greatly stressed. The children may actually belong to two-family systems and thus feel they are only part-time members of either family. The sense of not wholly belonging to a family

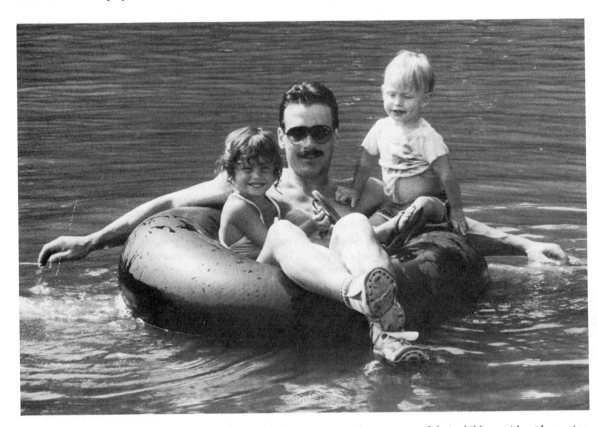

Figure 33–9. Noncustodial parents are challenged to find ways to enjoy the company of their children without becoming a perpetual source of entertainment or gifts.

may dilute their loyalty and hence their willingness to assume responsibility to make either of the new families work at optimal levels. The custodial parent may feel so overburdened and thus overwhelmed by the responsibility for orchestrating family life, that the children may be asked to assume a decision-making responsibility for which their experience and understanding have not prepared them [1, 12]. Single-parent families frequently experience difficulty meeting Duvall's tasks because of financial limitations. Family health is also jeopardized by the need to share holidays with either both or alternating parents. Traditions become difficult to establish or to maintain.

Though difficult, healthy families are still possible in single-parent homes. Communication becomes a critical factor, and mutual respect for feelings, time constraints, and values is essential. The continuity of parenting needs to be assured for each child, since fractionalization of the love relationship is more devastating than fractionalization of the legal bond between the parents. Trust must be regained and affirmed [4].

Blended Family

Although painful, divorce often allows an adult the opportunity to experience much personal growth. Two to 4 years after a divorce, an individual begins to feel more confident as a new self-identity emerges [40]. Remarriage is viewed as a second chance at happiness, and it can be. However, establishing a new family unit with children requires much planning and hard work. Second marriages have a higher divorce rate than first marriages because of an individual's unresolved problems from the previous marriage, the resistance of children to the formation of a new family system [30], and the misunderstandings that can arise from differing rules and expectations. The increased feelings of individualism that are spawned by a divorce may interfere with a couple's ability to establish marital satisfaction [19] through unconditional trust and bonding. Problems may arise as individuals find themselves financially as well as emotionally obligated to more than one nuclear family.

Two people usually marry because they are "in love." But the children may not share their parent's opinion of the new family member. The remarriage of a parent destroys the children's fantasy of a reunion of their biological parents. Since the children's relationships with a parent predates the adult companionship relationship, the stepparent may feel like an outsider [42]. There is no legal relationship between the stepparent and the stepchildren, a factor which may precipitate

discipline problems, financial-support problems, and even sexual problems. Incest, exploitation, and sexual abuse are much more common with stepchildren because cultural taboos may be more lax [12, 23].

Maintaining contact with all the relatives for the sake of the children may prove to be most difficult while establishing new relationships with the stepparent's family. This family, which struggled so hard to reorganize following the death or divorce, must now face reorganization once more [30]. The children, who have just experienced a loss of a significant person with the inevitable accompanying grief, must now learn the new rules and roles incumbent in the new family structure. In essence, they may feel a loss of their comfortable roles, which can lead to a loss of self-confidence with all of its correlates.

The parent and stepparent must work together to create a new sense of family solidarity [40]. The stepparent can never replace the biological parent. The family, consequently, must face and acknowledge the "ghosts of the past," but must live in the present [35]. This process requires good communication.

New patterns, rules, and expectations will take the place of old ones, creating a sense of "we-ness," mutuality, and shared values. The increased experience and maturity of the remarried couple can enable them to learn from past mistakes and to set more realistic expectations.

Active listening, respect for individuality, sharing responsibility, and planning for family leisure-time activities can facilitate the bonding process among members. Understanding and fairness are critical issues. If this trust is violated, a them-us split occurs along kinship lines or along adult-child lines, leading to a second divorce or to behavioral problems. The adults need to weave love, caring, and fairness into the fabric of daily life. When conflict does occur, family conferences can open doors to new levels of understanding and respect. Gradually, new rules and expectations will consolidate, and behavior patterns will become habituated. At this point, choices are narrowed so that fewer decisions are necessary—a point that reduces disagreements and increases family unity [8].

Cultural Variations in Family Relationships

The United States is not really a melting pot of cultures as we are led to believe. It is more like a painter's palette where colors blend at random along the edges but maintain their uniqueness at the center. Many families do blend into the larger culture, but others prefer to retain the flavor of their ethnic heritage. These families may have differing views on kinship ties, hierarchical structure, roles of individual family members, and premarital or extramarital sex [37]. Although the family structure or value system may differ from the "traditional" life-styles of the prevailing culture, the family can still be highly adaptive and healthy. Staples and Mirande offer an excellent overview of many cultural differences in the United States [37].

SUMMARY

The **good** family is not synonymous with the **healthy** family. A definition of the former typically employs culturally imposed external status symbols, such as wealth, education, and/or position. A definition of healthy families, on the other hand, is based on the interpersonal dynamics within the family—an internal factor observed only by persons with intimate contact with the family.

Since children have a tendency to emulate parental behaviors, interaction patterns are transmitted from generation to generation. Thus, the microculture of the family system provides a medium for "inheriting" mental health or mental illness [3, 4, 36]. Family unity is not a given because two people fall in love and marry: They have to work daily at maintaining respect and communication. It involves the reciprocal activi-

ties of open sharing and active listening. A healthy family shares a mutual respect and an open communication that lead to deeper understanding and appreciation of each individual's feelings and value system. Respect and communication lead to greater unity, or bonding, among the members, enabling them to transfer this same respect and allocentrism to persons outside the family system. The success of parenting often depends on the quality of the social environment and the community support [16]. The involvement in too many community activities or extracurricular activities connected with one's employment can overburden the family system, while the availability of support resources can help to relieve family conflict.

Divorce is frequently the result of a couple's inability to establish an open communication with each other. Divorce usually does not completely sever the relationships with a former spouse, however, especially if there are children involved. The parents must continue to cooperate for the sake of the children. When a child has free access to both parents, the long-term negative effects of a fractionalized family are minimized. The postmarital relationship can be enduring and amazingly resilient—much like a kinship relationship [40].

The paradox of family unity is that it is strongest when family members recognize and appreciate the uniqueness of one another.

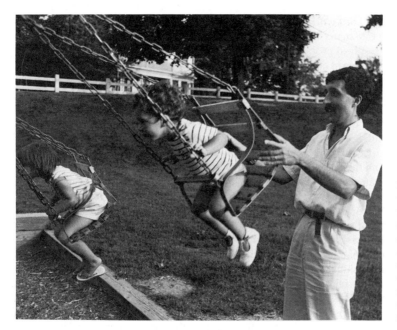

Figure 33–10. The quality of the relationship between a parent and child is more critical than the quantity. The quality will be determined by the parent's ability to participate in activities at the child's level of development. The synchrony established during these early years is the foundation of solid family relationships that emerge into close friendships during later years. (Photo by Ed Slaman.)

REFERENCES

1. Allers, R. D. *Divorce, Children, and the School*. Princeton, NJ: Princeton Books, 1982.
2. Birdwhistell, R. L. The idealized model of the American family. *Social Casework* 51:195, 1970.
3. Bowen, M. *Family Therapy in Clinical Practice*. New York: Jason Aronson, 1978.
4. Bowlby, J. *Attachment and Loss*. Vol. 2. *Separation, Anxiety and Anger*. New York: Basic Books, 1973.
5. Bowman, H. A., and Spanier, G. B. *Modern Marriage* (8th ed.). New York: McGraw-Hill, 1978.
6. Campbell, A. Subjective measures of well-being. *Am. Psychol.* 31:117, 1976.
7. Caplow, T., et al. *Middletown Families: Fifty Years of Change and Continuity*. Minneapolis: University of Minnesota Press, 1982.
8. Cherlin, A. Remarriage as an incomplete institution. *Am. J. Sociol.* 84(3):388, 1978.
9. Curran, D. D. *Traits of a Healthy Family: Fifteen Traits Commonly Found in Healthy Families by Those Who Work With Them*. Minneapolis, MN: Winston Press, 1983.
10. D'Antonio, W. V. The family and religion: Exploring a changing relationship. *J. Sci. Stud. Relig.* 19:89, 1980.
11. Duvall, E. R. M. *Family Development* (4th ed.). Philadelphia: Lippincott, 1971.
12. Eshleman, J. R. *The Family: An Introduction* (3rd ed.). Boston: Allyn and Bacon, 1981.
13. Furstenberg, F. K., and Nord, C. W. "The Life Course of Children of Divorce: Marital Disruption and Parental Contact." Paper presented at the Annual Meeting of the Population Association of America, San Diego, April 29–May 1, 1982.
14. Gaither, G. and Dobson, S. *Let's Make a Memory: Great Ideas for Building Family Traditions and Togetherness*. Waco, TX: Word Books, 1983.
15. *Gallup Youth Survey*. George Gallup Jr., Associated Press, 1981.
16. Garbarino, J. *Children and Families in the Social Environment*. New York: Aldine, 1982.
17. Garrett, Wm. R. *Seasons of Marriage and Family Life*. New York: Holt, Rinehart and Winston, 1982.
18. Glasser, L. N., and Glasser, P. H. Hedonism and the family: Conflict in values. *J. Marr. Fam. Counsel*. (October 1977):11.
19. Glenn, N. D., and Weaver, C. N. The marital happiness of remarried divorced persons. *J. Marr. Fam.* 39:331, 1977.
20. Gordon, T. *P.E.T., Parent Effectiveness Training: The Tested New Way to Raise Responsible Children*. New York: Wyden, 1970.
21. Hess, B. B., and Waring, J. M. Changing patterns of aging and family bonds in later life. *Family Coordinator* (October 1978):304.
22. Hunt, R. A., and King, M. B. Religiosity and marriage. *J. Sci. Stud. Relig.* 17:397, 1978.
23. Hutter, M. *The Changing Family; Comparative Perspectives*. New York: Wiley, 1981.
24. Kalter, N., and Rembar, J. The significance of a child's age at the time of parental divorce. *Am. J. Orthopsychiatry* 51(1):85, 1981.
25. Klemer, R. H., and Smith, R. M. *Klemer's Marriage and Family Relationships* (2nd ed.). New York: Harper & Row, 1975.
26. Kurdek, L. A., Blisk, D., and Siesky, A. E. Correlates of children's long-term adjustment to their parents' divorce. *Dev. Psychol.* 17:565, 1981.
27. Lasch, C. *Haven in a Heartless World: The Family Besieged*. New York: Basic Books, 1979.
28. Lewis, J. M., et al. *No Single Thread: Psychological Health in Family Systems*. New York: Brunner/Mazel, 1976.
29. Maslow, A. H. *Toward a Psychology of Being* (2nd ed.). Princeton, NJ: Van Nostrand, 1968.
30. Messinger, L., and Walker, K. N. From marriage breakdown to remarriage: Parental tasks and therapeutic guidelines. *Am. J. Orthopsychiatry* 51:429, 1981.
31. Murphey, E. B., et al. Development of autonomy and parent-child interaction in late adolescence. *Am. J. Orthopsychiatry* 33:643, 1963.
32. Novak, J. C. Children vs. divorce. *Ped. Nurs.* 8(1):33, 1982.
33. Reiss, I. L. *Family Systems in America* (3rd ed.). New York: Holt, Rinehart and Winston, 1980.
34. Rollins, B. C., and Feldman, H. Marital satisfaction over the family life cycle. *J. Marr. Fam.* 32:20, 1970.
35. Satir, V. *Peoplemaking*. Palo Alto, CA: Science and Behavior Books, 1972.
36. Spanier, G. B., Lewis, R. A., and Cole, C. L. Marital adjustment over the family life cycle: The issue of curvilinearity. *J. Marr. Fam.* 37:263, 1975.
37. Staples, R., and Mirandé, A. Racial and cultural variations among American families: A decennial review of the literature on minority families. *J. Marr. Fam.* 42:157, 1980.
38. Steinman, S. The experience of children in a joint-custody arrangement: A report of a study. *Am. J. Orthopsychiatry* 51:403, 1981.
39. Stinnett, N., Chesser, B., and DeFrain, J. *Building Family Strengths: Blueprint for Action*. Lincoln, NE: University of Nebraska Press, 1979.
40. Strong, B., et al. *The Marriage and Family Experience* (2nd ed.). St. Paul: West, 1983.
41. U.S. Bureau of the Census. *Statistical Abstract of the United States, 1983*. Washington, DC: U.S. Government Printing Office, 1983.
42. Visher, E. B., and Visher, J. S. Major areas of difficulty for stepparent couples. *Int. J. Fam. Counsel.* 6:71, 1968.
43. Wesley, John. *The Works of John Wesley*. Vol. 9, *Letters and Essays*. Kansas City, MO: Nazarene, 1958.

34
Fractionalization of the Family Unit

Jayne A. Tapia

... I wish we felt free to hug and laugh, talk and be ourselves and tell the truth. I wish we knew what it is to be a family.

—Judith Mattison, *I'm Worried About Your Drinking**

Introduction

Study of the Family
Theoretical approaches
Levels of family functioning
   Level I: Infancy, or the chaotic family
   Level II: Childhood, or the intermediate family
   Level III: Adolescence, or the family
     with problems
   Level IV: Adulthood, or the family
     with solutions
   Level V: Maturity, or the ideal family

Stressors to the Family Bond
Acute stressors—crisis situations
Chronic stressors—long-term situations
Cultural stressors in contemporary life

Results of Family Stress
Physical abuse
Separation or divorce

Maximizing Family Potentials
Assessment of and approach to families
Facilitating intrafamily communication

Conclusions

The family is a frequent topic of seminars, workshops, books, magazine articles, and radio and television talk shows as people debate the "crisis in the family" and the "survival of the family." Intensive interest and concern have been generated as we have proceeded from an era in which the family was considered sacred and not to be criticized, to one in which it was blamed for all the ills and maladjustments of our youth and society as a whole, and then to the current era, which is characterized by a fear that the family as a basic unit of society will not survive. As discussed in Chapters 2 and 30, there are many different groupings that can be called a family. One author, after studying 250 different societies, concluded that the nuclear family is universal. The family exists because it meets human needs; it is a biological, psychological, social, and cultural necessity [14].

We are living today in a rapidly changing world. The family is changing also; many of its traditional roles have been taken over by other agencies of society. However, there is one essential function of the family that no other agency can fulfill and to which all other functions are ancillary: that is, to facilitate the formation of loving, mature, and flexible individuals who can adequately adjust to an ever-changing future [35].

*J. Mattison, *I'm Worried About Your Drinking*, (Minneapolis, Augsburg Publishing House, 1978). With permission.

The family is a very complex organism, which makes it difficult to study, to understand, or to conceptualize. The family must be viewed as a system that requires adaptive, integrative, and decision-making processes in order to survive and to provide for the continuity and growth of both the system and its individual members [25]. The family unit and its members are faced with many changes over time to which they must adapt. The health of a family depends on the manner in which it performs these processes. Thus the family is more than the sum of its parts. It is a basic unit of society in which members have definite relationships with one another and responsibilities toward one another that affect and are affected by their role and relationships in the community and in society at large.

Fractionalization of the family refers to the decreased interdependence of family members that occurs when various stressors, forces, or pressures are exerted on the family that cause it to split apart or to become less unified, less able to interrelate adaptively with the community, and less able to meet each member's needs and expectations. Families may be fractionalized even when the members are not physically removed from the family unit. Family members can be emotionally alienated from each other, causing emotional interactions that can be disruptive to the well-being of all the family members, the family group, and even the community. If one or both parents are unable to communicate effectively, for example, this can cause minor or major difficulties for some of the family members individually and for the group as a whole as it relates to society. Juvenile delinquency is often a symptom that something is maladaptive within a family; this problem obviously has a profound effect on society as well. Alcoholism and child abuse are other symptoms of the alienation of individual family members.

Social changes are having a profound effect on the family and its ability to maintain is equilibrium. Before the twentieth century, social change was more gradual and less extreme. Family structure was more enduring, and family members retained a feeling of belonging to one another and to society [42]. Families have always been threatened with disruption by forces over which they have no control, such as the illness or death of a member. The families in our contemporary society, however, face additional factors that have profound effects on family development, such as the decline of the male role as head of the household, the increase in the number of working wives, the isolation of the nuclear family, the increase in individualism and individual freedom, the increase in premarital and extramarital sexual relationships, the decline in religious observances, and the transfer of many traditional functions of the family to other institutions in society [29]. Some families and their members are better equipped than others to handle the changes and pressures that are continually exerted upon them, but all families are somewhat vulnerable.

Compared with other associations in society, the average family is organizationally inferior. Its age composition is heavily weighted with dependents, and it cannot freely reject its weak members and recruit more competent teammates as do other associations. Its members receive an unearned acceptance, for there is no price for belonging. Because of its unusual age composition and its uncertain sex composition, it is by no means ideally manned to withstand stress. Yet the family is the bottleneck organization through which almost all troubles of modern society pass. No other institution so reflects the strains and stresses of life. The modern family experiences recurrent tension precisely because it is the great burden-carrier of the social order [20].

STUDY OF THE FAMILY

Research activity over the past two decades has resulted in an increased body of knowledge about the family. This empirical data has been utilized to develop a conceptual approach to intervention and prevention of some of the complex problems confronting many families today. Case loads in family counseling centers have risen dramatically as changes in family life have created an increased need to seek help with family problems. One counseling center located in the greater Boston area reported that 60 percent of the agency's clients requested counseling for marital problems and 20 percent for parent-child problems [38]. A study of community human service needs in metropolitan Boston reported that 50 percent of the 1043 families interviewed had one or more problems in the following categories: child behavior, 23 percent; employment, 21 percent; family personal, 17 percent; financial, 13 percent; elderly, 12 percent; alcohol, 12 percent; homemaker, 6 percent; home nursing, 4 percent. Thirteen percent of the families interviewed experienced problems in three or more of the above categories [47]. In the future, as more families seek help in the resolution of family problems, more trained and experienced counselors who are well grounded in family theory will be needed. As individuals study family relationships, personal attitudes, experiences, and values are generally reassessed in an effort to increase their ability to develop a satisfying family life.

Theoretical Approaches

Many theoretical approaches to the study of the family have been delineated. Four approaches appear to be especially useful in developing an understanding of the family as a conceptual whole.

THE DEVELOPMENTAL APPROACH

The developmental framework for study of the family has come from several fields of inquiry: sociology, anthropology, psychology, and home economics. Much of the work in this framework has been summarized by Duvall [11]. In this framework, the family as a unit passes though several developmental stages. Successful development of the family depends on the satisfactory blending and mastery of biological requirements, cultural imperatives, and personal aspirations and values. The family is neither entirely independent of other social systems nor entirely dependent on them. (Duvall's position was discussed in Chap. 33.)

Although the developmental approach integrates some very distinct concepts about the family and helps us to understand the family as a group that grows and develops over time, it is sometimes difficult to apply this approach to all families, especially to those without children and those in which there is only one parent. It is also somewhat difficult to develop a holistic concept of the family as a unit when there is so much emphasis on the individuals within the family group.

THE STRUCTURAL-FUNCTIONAL APPROACH

The structural-functional approach of study views the family as one of several subsystems in society, with the relationships between family and society or family and other subsystems as the focus of investigation. Within the family, each member occupies a position or positions to which a number of roles are assigned. The individual defines role expectations in a given situation in terms of the reference group and his or her own self-concept. The individual family members engage in role playing, and the family is studied through analysis of its interactions. Three major functions have been particularly emphasized: (1) the functions of the family for society; (2) the functions of the subsystems within a family for the family or for each other; and (3) the functions of the family for individual family members, including the development of personality. Various family members have certain recognized roles that are dependent on age, gender, generation, and economic and political factors.

Two different types of role-differentiated activities have been identified: one is an instrumental or masculine behavior, and the other is an expressive or feminine behavior [36]. This approach can aid in developing an understanding of the family as a group with structure and functions that define its relationship in society. However, the functions of the family are not well defined in this approach and are subject to cultural stereotypes.

THE INTERACTIONAL APPROACH

The interactional framework is a system for viewing the family by means of the interaction of its members. The unique characteristic of the interactional approach is that it is based on the quality of the communication process. This approach has been widely used because, among other factors, it is able to focus successfully on the family as a small group, and thus it has been possible to study family interaction in great detail. This approach does not focus on the family's relationship to society [51]. However, the family with healthy interactions will identify with the "broad" family, or society (the research by Curran in this area is discussed in Chap. 33).

GENERAL SYSTEMS THEORY

The systems framework is a very viable method of studying the family (see Chap. 2 for a review of systems theory). In this approach, the family is seen as a dynamic social system that is constantly evolving in structure and function. It has subsystems (mother-child, husband-wife) and a suprasystem (community) that can be objectively identified and analyzed. Families have four main structural characteristics: organization, boundary, differentiation and specialization, and territoriality. The main family functions are considered to be support, regulation, nurturance, and socialization of its members. Family functions change as input from the suprasystem requires the family to modify goals or behaviors. In order to survive and grow, the family is required to utilize adaptive, integrative, and decision-making processes [25]. The application of general systems theory to the family extends some of the concepts that are integral to the structural-functional framework. It assists the student in developing a concept of the family as a unit, its relationship to other systems, and its dynamic, changing state.

OTHER EMERGING THEORIES

Two other emerging theories are also gaining recognition as being useful in analysis and study of the family. The conflict theory includes concepts about competition, consensus, negotiation, bargaining, power, influences, aggression, threats, promises, conflict management, and the consequences of conflict. These concepts can be used to analyze a wide range of family relationships [52]. The other emerging theory concerns choice and exchange; this theory is beginning to be employed extensively by scholars who study the family [40].

Levels of Family Functioning

The theoretical frameworks just discussed are helpful because they are (1) descriptive—they have been built from the practice of working with families—and also because they are (2) prescriptive—they can be utilized in helping families to meet the demands of modern life. One model that can be utilized to understand the ways in which families differ has been developed from concepts common to the developmental, structural-functional, and systems frameworks. It is based on an assessment of how the family meets the tasks that are assigned to it by society [56].

Four family tasks—sexual, economic, reproductive, and educational—are universal to all cultures [39]. A modified and expanded version of these tasks [13] can be used to describe and analyze the level of family functioning. The first and most basic task is to provide for physical survival and security. The family must have the means to provide a home, food, clothing, and sanitation in order to survive. Only after these needs have been provided, can the family secure other material goods that offer comfort or convenience.

The second basic task is the provision of social experiences and emotional expression. The family provides the milieu for sound emotional development. It is responsible to society for providing an atmosphere of love; protecting its young from emotional turmoil; and instilling values, standards, and ethical attitudes that will enable the individual to manage relationships with others outside the family, such as at school or work.

The third main task involves sexual differentiation and training of the children. Every family, regardless of its culture or uniqueness, has the task of helping children to know who they are and training and socializing them. This task includes the recognition of individuality and gender-related identity as well as assistance in the development of competencies and mastery of individual developmental tasks (discussed in previous chapters).

The fourth and final main task is the support and the growth of individual family members. Each family must continually struggle with the conflict between growth of individual members toward greater independence and the desire for its members to remain a cohesive part of the family. It must help its members to develop individual identity and ego-strength while at the same time having the ability to conform to the best interests of the family group. The roles and responsibilities of individual family members become more distinct yet more interdependent for the benefit of the total family as the family matures. A healthy family is one in which the individuals have a strong bond with the family group, which in turn supports each of its members in their pursuit of individual skills and abilities [13].

In addition to viewing a family's ability to meet these essential tasks, one may also utilize Werner's general systems theory (see Chap. 2) to help delineate and assess the family's developmental level. The factors become:

1. Individualization and role independence of the subsystems in the family
2. Efficiency of the family in allocating resources and making decisions
3. Interfamily organizational patterns for communication and cooperation
4. Interpretation and processing of events, and the resultant interface of the family with the environment/culture
5. Generation and utilization of alternative means for goal achievement
6. Independence of the family from other persons or agencies in goal setting and the ability to focus energies toward goal achievement [59]

If one were to examine every family in America for their ability to meet these tasks, one would find families at all levels along a continuum, from those unable to meet any of the tasks to those who could meet all of them in the most healthful and ideal manner possible. Five developmental levels can be identified that represent the family's ability to function adaptively with society to meet its needs. These levels, discussed in the following sections, are similar to the stages of development described by Erikson.

LEVEL I: INFANCY, OR THE CHAOTIC FAMILY
The least mature level of family functioning is characterized by disorganization in all areas of family life.

Roles are undifferentiated and adaptive skills are limited. This type of family barely meets its needs for security and physical survival; its members are characterized by their inability to secure adequate wages or housing; to budget money; or to maintain adequate nutrition, clothing, heat, and cleanliness. Family activities are geared toward immediate gratification and are highly dependent on sporadic environmental events. The patterns of communication and cooperation are diffuse. This family lives from day to day without orientation to the future. The members rigidly cling to the limited skills available to them regardless of their adaptivity.

The limited skill repertoire decreases the family's ability to provide for healthy emotional and social functioning of its members, which is reflected in the family members' apparent alienation from the community. They distrust outsiders, are unable to utilize community resources and services, and become hostile and resistant to offers of help. The immaturity of the parents are shown in their inability to assume responsible adult roles—a factor that often results in socially deviant behavior, including child neglect and abuse.

The children suffer in other ways, too, because their parents are unable to act as the effective role models that children need if they are to mature into capable, socialized adult men and women. Because of this lack of differentiation, there is much distortion and confusion of roles in the family. The children, sometimes at a young age, may be forced to take over many of the tasks and roles of their nonfunctioning parents. Such situations perpetuate the family's pattern of chaos and disorganization into the next generation. The total family, not just its individual members, exhibits the helplessness syndrome.

This type of family obviously fails to provide support for the growth of its individual members. The family exhibits feelings of depression and failure with no hope of success either for individual members or for the family unit. The basic insecurity of the family members prevents change; ritualism, defensiveness, and distortion are used as devices to keep other persons and agencies from getting near enough to assist the family toward growth and self-sufficiency. Although we generally associate this family with situations of abject poverty, the real key is in the intrafamily relationships. The dynamics of relationships of persons within the Ewing family of the "Dallas" television series strongly exhibit level I characteristics (e.g., lack of trust, diffuse communication patterns, uncertain family composition, inability to identify, let alone share, true feelings and values).

LEVEL II: CHILDHOOD, OR THE INTERMEDIATE FAMILY

The second level of family functioning is characterized by slightly less disorganization than in the level I family, and its members exhibit slightly more skill in meeting their needs for security and physical survival. Although still alienated from the community, they have more ability to trust and, subsequently, more hope for a better way of life. They exhibit autonomy, but little initiative as a family. The parents are immature, however, and socially deviant behavior may occur. Distortion and confusion of roles exist, but the parents are more willing to work together for the benefit of the whole family. There are rudimentary patterns for communication and cooperation, and the children are not neglected to the extent that they must be removed from the home, as is often the case in a level I family.

This type of family is still unable to support and to promote the growth of its members. Role differentiations may be present, but family members exhibit a rigid adherence to age and gender roles to preserve individual identity, rather than to promote family integrity or family goals. There is confusion in the identification and independence of the family subsystems. The family members appear unable to change, are defensive and fearful, and lack the resources to gain a sense of accomplishment. The level II family also possesses a limited repertoire of adaptive skills. The family does not actively seek help and requires much assistance before the members are able to acknowledge their problems realistically. This family, like the aggressive toddler, feels powerful as it begins to recognize its individuation and separation from other families, yet is unable to exercise self-control or mature judgment. The family's financial income may be adequate, but it is not able to plan and to utilize its resources well; this results in impulse buying and the inability to meet financial obligations.

LEVEL III: ADOLESCENCE, OR THE FAMILY WITH PROBLEMS

The level III family is essentially normal but has more than the usual or healthy amount of conflicts and problems. As a unit, it is more capable of physical survival and of providing security for its members than the level I and level II families, but these abilities may vary greatly. Socially and emotionally, this family functions better than either of the two previous types. Family

Table 34-1. Ability of Families to Meet Basic Family Tasks

Four Basic Tasks (see p. 700)	Family Level				
	I	II	III	IV	V
1 Survival	Bare	Minimal	Adequate	Good	Excellent
Security	—	Some	Adequate	Good	Reasonable
2 Social	Unclear	Rigid	Clear	Good	Excellent
Emotional	—	—	Limited	Good	Excellent
3 Sexuality	—	Barely	Rigid	Adequate	Excellent
Training	—	—	Limited	Good	Excellent
4 Support	—	—	Rarely	Adequate	Excellent
Growth	—	—	—	Adequate	Excellent

members demonstrate greater trust in people, have the knowledge and ability to utilize some community resources, and are less openly hostile to outsiders. Frequently one parent is more mature than the other, and the children have less overall difficulty adjusting to changes in the family, the school, and the environment. Although many of the members are industrious, the identities and the roles of members and the identity and the goals as a separate family unit may still not be clearly defined.

This family may have more difficulty in the task of providing sexual differentiation and training of children than they have in the first two tasks. Although the children are cared for physically, there may be many emotional conflicts, resulting in affective and cognitive confusion for the children. In addition, because one parent may be quite immature, difficulties for one or more of the children may result. The parents are often unsure of their own identity and are therefore unable to help the children find theirs. Very often individuals in the family experience success and achievements outside the family, and members may even deliberately seek outside achievements to replace some missing satisfaction within their family life.

On the positive side, this family shows an increasing ability to face some of its problems and to look for solutions. They may seek and use outside help much more effectively and appropriately than a level I or II family. Members are future-oriented, even though the present may be painful.

LEVEL IV: ADULTHOOD, OR THE FAMILY
WITH SOLUTIONS
A family at this level may be described as stable, healthy, and happy, with fewer than the usual number

of problems or conflicts. This stability is a result of the family's ability to handle most problems as they arise. This family capably provides for survival and security and emotional and social expression. The parents are usually quite mature and confident in their roles as spouses, parents, wage-earners, and members of society. The identity of individual family members and of the family unit is clearly defined and protected. Parental roles are clearly defined but flexible, to allow for goal mastery rather than just role mastery. The parents have fewer difficulties in providing for sexual differentiation and training their children, although they may have difficulty with achieving true intimacy.

The main problems of this family center around the stages of growth and the various developmental tasks of the children. If problems arise in this area, the parents often refer themselves to outside sources for help. However, they may show excessive anxiety over these problems. In general, the needs of individual members and group needs and goals are usually brought into harmony by this family. Although crises may temporarily immobilize the family, they have the ability to adapt, to change, to enjoy the present, and to plan for the future.

LEVEL V: MATURITY, OR THE IDEAL FAMILY
This family is only a short step above level IV. This type of family can be described as truly homeostatic, with a healthy balance of individual and group goals, activities, participation, and concerns. The integrity of each member is highly respected and protected, yet well articulated within the hierarchical organization of the dynamic system. Adaptive flexibility is a hallmark. All tasks are met by this family, and all supplies are provided. Identity and intimacy are secure. Generativ-

Table 34-2. Relationship of Werner's Systems Development Theory to Level of Family Functioning

Continuum Factors (see p. 35)	Family Level				
	I	II	III	IV	V
1	Mass ego identity	Confused relationships	Some individuation	Clear identities	Differences respected
2	No real leadership	Autocratic leadership	Authoritative leadership	Flexible leadership	Cooperative leadership
3	Poor communication	Rudimentary efforts	Weak patterns	Cooperative milieu	Integrated interdependent
4	Everything personal attack	Weak differentiation	Family-other clear	Focused on stimulus	Discrete responses
5	Limited, rigid skills	Rigid approaches	Limited flexibility	Adaptive approaches	Flexible, creative approaches
6	Highly suggestible	Labile goals	Weak self-direction	Independent	Stable goals

ity tasks are the focus of the family. Integrity of both the unit and the individuals is maintained; the only exception is in times of extreme or multiple crises. The family may then be temporarily immobilized, but they can still ask for, and use, help from appropriate sources.

A well-organized level V family has been defined by researchers as one in which there are stability of goals, agreement on role structure, subordination of personal ambitions to family goals, satisfaction with the family because it meets the physical and emotional needs of its members, and collectively perceived and shared goals toward which the family as a group is moving [19].

STRESSORS TO THE FAMILY BOND

The traits that a family develops depend on the way it individually and collectively responds to the myriad of pressures of modern life. Many problems are a result of economic and technological pressures, which may involve striving for advancement, denser living conditions (larger population competing for limited resources), and new life-styles. In this section we will examine some of these pressures more closely.

Acute Stressors—Crisis Situations

A family crisis may be defined as any situation for which the usual adaptive skills of family living become inadequate. Crises may result from the loss of a member, a loss of social status, the addition of a member, or a combination of factors [11].

DETERMINATION OF A CRISIS

Several variables intertwine to determine if an event becomes a crisis for any given family [20]. The first factor is the hardship of the situation or event, which involves not only what physically happens to the family but also how suddenly the crisis occurs and whether or not the family has had time to prepare. Families who give birth to a disabled child or who lose possessions or family members as a result of a sudden natural disaster, such as a fire, earthquake, or flood, will all classify the event as a crisis, regardless of the level of family functioning during noncrisis times.

The second variable involves the resources of the family itself—how well it has adapted to its roles and functions, at what level the family can be found on the continuum of family functioning, and how it has responded to crisis situations in the past. A level IV or V family is better able to define and to confine a crisis situation rapidly and to utilize the necessary resources to promote a rapid recovery.

A third variable is how the family defines the event. What is a crisis to one family may be only a slight problem to another. Loss of a job, for example, may not be defined as a crisis in a level I or II family but may produce severe and lasting effects in a level III or IV family. As a matter of fact, level I and II families live in a world of multiple adverse circumstances that level III families would almost always define as crises.

The last major variable is the type of response given by the community or society. This response can either be accepting or rejecting by helping the family and its members through the crisis, or it may create further crisis for the family by punishment or persecution. The response of the community is formulated from its values and standards in relation to the various crisis events. Chronic drunkenness may be a way of life among the poor in our cities' ghettos and may not be defined as a crisis in such communities, although it most certainly would be considered a crisis in a middle-class suburban or rural society, especially when the behavior of the individual results in nonconforming behavior.

REACTION TO CRISIS

The reaction of the family members to crisis is also an important consideration. Each person's developmental level and unique personality affect both the perception of a situation and the reaction to it. Personality changes take place during a crisis as each individual member experiences stress caused by change in the normal role and interaction patterns, and the family is forced to work out new patterns. Depending on the type of crisis, family members may suddenly find that their old patterns of relating to one another

and of meeting their economic and social needs do not work. All of the family's energy is directed toward coping with the crisis and finding other ways to meet ongoing demands on the family unit. Usually there is no energy left over for recreation, affection, or sexual enjoyment. The parents are frequently more abrupt with each other and with the children, shifting their anger with the crisis onto the other family members [20].

The resolution of a crisis occurs in stages. At first the family is numbed by the blow. It takes time for the implications of the impact to be realized: "Then as facts are assimilated, organization slumps, roles are played with less enthusiasm, resentments are smothered or expressed, conflicts develop or are converted into tensions that strain relations" [20]. As the tension and disorganization increase and peak, the family is open to help and assistance. They will try new approaches until something works and some equilibrium is established. The new level of equilibrium will be fragile or solid, depending on how the problem was managed [20].

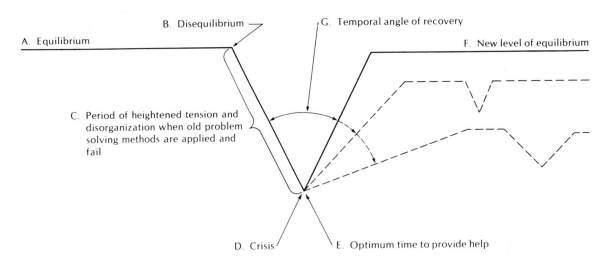

A. Signifies the state of being, functioning, or balance that exists in the daily life of the individual or family.

B. A problem occurs, bringing an initial disruption of the state of equilibrium.

C. As attempts to solve the problem fail, tension and disorganization increase.

D At the point that all known resources and problem solving methods are exhausted, a crisis occurs.

E. More receptivity to help at the point of crisis, since other avenues for problem solving are not available.

F. Equilibrium reestablished, the level depending on how the problem was managed. The lower the level of equilibrium, the more fragile it is.

G. Represents the relative amount of time for reestablishing equilibrium.

Figure 34–1. Longitudinal responses to a state of crisis. (Developed by Dr. William Glenn Morgan. Used with permission.)

A family's final adjustment to a crisis can bring the family back to its previous level of organization or to a higher or lower level, depending on the support it received through the crisis, its integration (bonds of coherence and unity), and its adaptability (capacity to meet obstacles and shift course). Many studies have indicated that well-organized families are better able to prevent situational crisis formation and are more able to mobilize personal resources to recover from a crisis [20].

Chronic Stressors—Long-Term Situations

A chronic stressor may be an acute stressor that has not been resolved over time or that was resolved in a manner that continues to cause disruption to the family. Many acute crisis situations become long-term or chronic situations.

ALCOHOLISM

Alcoholism is one of the largest health and social problems in this country, yet it often goes unnoticed or untreated. Five stages can be identified in chronic alcoholism. The first stage is one of denial. Drinking episodes are intermittent, and both spouses attempt to normalize drinking and to explain away early symptoms. In the second stage the spouse of the alcoholic attempts to solve the problem with his or her own resources. When the husband is the one with the drinking problem, the wife reasons that she can force him to stop because he lacks the willpower; she engages in behaviors, such as nagging, threatening to leave, hiding bottles of liquor, and attempting to control money.

She also attempts to conceal the extent of her husband's drinking from the outside world, avoids social situations that might cause the drinking to be exposed, and covers up with the husband's employer.

The third stage is one of disorganization and chaos. At this stage, the spouse begins to look for help outside the family circle. Since the problem is already chronic, there is usually much disruption and disorganization within the family, such as severe financial problems, sexual problems, and problems with the children. Usually, alcoholics alternately indulge, ignore, and abuse the children, while the spouse becomes increasingly harassed and irritable. The spouse usually holds the alcoholic responsible for all of their difficulties. The family is caught in a vicious circle: The alcoholic's behavior causes anxiety to the family, and their reaction to the drinking usually gives the alcoholic further reason to drink.

In the fourth stage, if the husband is the alcoholic, the wife assumes authority and responsibility for all family decisions and activities. Often she becomes the sole wage earner; the alcoholic takes the role of another child in the family. At this point, there are two possible outcomes to the situation. The first possibility is that the situation will continue indefinitely at stage 4. The family has adapted to the stress of living with an alcoholic, and although the situation is less than healthy or happy, it is at least tolerable. The second alternative is that the marriage will be terminated by divorce or permanent separation. The wife who chooses this alternative is often subjected to more physical abuse, infidelity, and economic deprivation

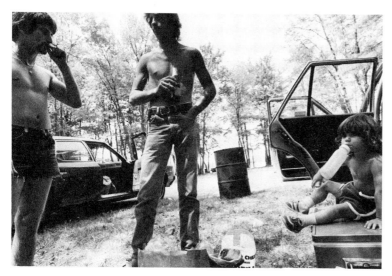

Figure 34–2. Affective and social development come to a halt when individuals turn to alcohol or drugs as a solution to problems instead of identifying and working through alternative solutions. The entire family is affected by an increase in stress when one member fails to carry his or her load.

but has stronger ego-strength than the wife who continues to live with the alcoholic spouse in stage 4. Regardless of the wife's (or husband's) initial personality, the spouse often becomes emotionally ill through the stress of living with an alcoholic [1].

When the wife is the alcoholic in the family, the husband will usually ignore or cover up her drinking for a longer period of time than the wife does in reverse circumstances, but he is also more likely to terminate the marriage than to continue living with the problem. The alcoholic mother is more detrimental to the development of the children because they experience greater exposure to the situation [30]. The children are victimized by a desire to believe their parents in the face of continued broken promises. They begin to withdraw reliance on verbal communication, depending only on actions and deeds. They learn from the model presented by their parents to act out their impulses; they also learn to rely on themselves and not to develop trust in others. Because of the inconsistency of the alcoholic parent, the children have great difficulty in learning rules and regulations. Children are often ignored in the family because the alcoholic is at "center stage." Studies have shown children of alcoholics to be more prone to delinquency, anxiety-neurosis, depression, hostility, and gender confusion [22]. They eventually tend to become alcoholics themselves.

UNEMPLOYMENT

One study of 25 families faced with unemployment found that they all went through stages similar to those described in acute crisis resolution. None sought help until they reached the stage of disorganization [2]. Research indicates that men of higher socioeconomic levels and older men suffer most acutely from unemployment. The higher the family's income before unemployment, the more difficult is the adjustment for the entire family [5]. Adjustment to unemployment involves not only finding another means of support, but perhaps altering one's job outlook and career identity, minimizing expenditures, decreasing involvement in community associations and activities, altering priorities and plans for the future, and rationalizing the family's place in society. Recent studies of unemployed men, many of whom had worked steadily for the previous 20 years, revealed that most men felt "small" and "insignificant" as a result of their unemployment; they also felt confused and disillusioned by traditional values. Some even felt that they could be replaced in their families [5]. All these feelings are characteristics of the helplessness syndrome.

LONG-TERM ILLNESS

In instances of severe illness, the major implication for the family is that basic roles can no longer be filled by assigned family members but must be taken over by other members. The family must again go through the same stages of disorganization, recovery, and reorganization before the adjustment is complete. When the husband is seriously ill, it usually means that he must first adjust to the patient role and can no longer do the things he normally did before the illness. His wife must also adapt to his new role, and often she must become the wage earner as well. The role reversals may be very difficult for both to accept. Frequently there are severe financial problems associated with medical bills as well as loss of the husband's income. Because serious illness is something to be avoided in our culture, the patient often suffers a social stigma that results in further loss of contact with persons with whom he was previously involved.

When the wife is the patient, the adjustment is equally difficult. The wife-mother must accept the fact that she is physically part of the family but is unable to perform her normal functions. If she is physically separated from the family, the situation may be even more difficult, especially if the children are not allowed to visit. When either the husband or the wife is chronically ill, there may be an alteration or ending of their sexual relationship, which may cause additional stress on the marriage.

There is little research concerning the possible effects of the parent's illness on the roles played by children in the family; they may regress as a result of one parent's getting all the care, or they may mature faster. Obviously the way in which the children are affected depends on their gender and developmental level as well as their relationship with the parent who is ill [3].

When the child becomes the long-term patient, the parents usually go through a period of initial disbelief and lack of acceptance of the problem. However, they must eventually face the problem and grieve for the loss of what the child could have been. Working through this grief process is difficult for families with troubled relationships. In level I, II, and III families, the child may become the center of the family's conflicts, or the illness may serve to intensify already existing problems. As the physical needs of the child change, the family must change its way of reacting, which can further increase the stress on the family (see Chap. 35).

The child's reaction to illness is often a reflection of the parents' and siblings' reactions, as well as a result of the physical and social limitations placed upon the child and his or her level of comprehension of events. In one study of juvenile rheumatoid arthritis patients, it was found that children with severe physical disability experienced retardation in emotional and social growth. This study suggests that the more physically disabled the child is, the more psychosocial difficulty may be experienced [10] (see Chap. 19).

Cultural Stressors in Contemporary Life

Many parents today were raised in traditional families and tend to value many of the mores of traditional families [43]. At the same time, American families face pressures from inflation, mass media, government policies, and a cultural change in values that was unknown to previous generations. Consequently, they find the need to alter or to discard many traditional views in order to meet the unique needs of their contemporary family. This transitional generation is attempting to preserve the best of traditional family life while eliminating unsatisfactory elements and assimilating new interactional patterns [43]. When these families fail, they tend to blame themselves. However, the larger forces assailing families today may create stressors beyond a family's abilities to cope; such stress can cause fractionalizations too ragged to mend without aggressive outside assistance—an assistance the community often fails to offer or the traditional upbringing of some individuals has taught them to avoid.

DUAL-CAREER FAMILIES

The term **dual-career families** was coined to designate a type of family structure in which both heads of household pursue active careers outside of their home and family lives [45]. A career designates a type of employment that requires a high degree of commitment and has a continuous developmental character. The stress of commitment to a career was first studied in 1968 and reexamined a decade later. Some progress has been made in resolving the stresses and dilemmas created by this life-style, such as overload, conflict with cultural ideals, identity issues, social networking and role cycling [45].

Overload may occur because of the lack of time to perform domestic chores, to oversee children's activities, to meet the demands of a career, and to engage in leisure-time activities in which both partners or the entire family can participate. Chores tend to be equally divided in dual-career families more than in families where the wife merely works to help out with finances.

Dual-career families tend to rely on some form of domestic help. Leisure-time and day-to-day activities are planned ahead of time [32].

The discrepancies between personal goals and prevailing cultural ideals or parental examples also can produce stress. Families can resolve this dilemma by evolving ways to emphasize the positives that derive from their life-styles and to ignore external pressures that stifle full expression and development. In most studies of dual-career families, both spouses report that their careers are worth the demands and the strains [32, 45, 48].

Identity dilemmas still exist. The main "tension lines" for men center on how much responsibility to take in the home and how much occupational achievement to tolerate in their wives. For women the "tension lines" usually stem from self-perceptions of their roles as good wives and mothers and criticisms from others about these roles. The dual-career wife may develop a "work personality" and a "home personality," deemphasizing her cognitive and organizational skills at home [45].

Social network dilemmas may arise when extended family members need help. With a full-time career, there is little time to help others outside the nuclear family. In fact, the dual-career family often relies on the extended family to help them [32]. Friendships with other couples are often limited because the dual-career couple has to deal with so much overload that friends are chosen carefully with an eye to what they can do for one another [45].

There are two basic types of role-cycling conflict in the dual-career family: (1) conflicting demands that arise from the occupational and family roles of the couple (career versus family) and (2) those that arise solely from their occupational roles (career versus career) [45]. Even if both careers are important, the man's career is typically given higher value [24]. Many professional women give up their careers, at least while their children are young, because of the enormous pressures involved [24]. Any decision to move to another city so that one of the partners can accept a promotion is usually made jointly and is usually contingent on the other partner being willing or able to find a satisfactory position in the new location [44]. This decision is usually very complex and difficult to make because the advancement of one partner's career may be detrimental to the other's. Consequently, some couples, even with young children, end up employed in two distant locations, which necessitates the establishment of a second residence with weekend commuting.

MOBILITY

Mobility represents a very important stressor in contemporary American life. Every year more families change residence because of a job promotion (i.e., upward mobility) or a job change, or a job transfer. Some families are required by their employer to move as often as every 2 years. Current estimates indicate that one out of five families moves each year. Moving is a significant stressor, even if it is the result of a promotion. Reestablishing the household in a different location is relatively simple, but developing new community ties, social peer group relationships, and school adjustments can be very difficult. Every family that has had to make such a change will testify to the problems created both for the family as a whole and for the individual family members.

JOB-RELATED ABSENCE OF THE SPOUSE

The absence of a spouse due to employment constraints also places stress on the family. This absence may result in loneliness and having to manage as a single-parent family sometimes for short periods of time such as when the husband is a salesman, or for long increments of time, such as when the husband is in military service. This second type of separation causes problems for the wife, who often experiences social ostracism while her husband is away, and who must learn both independence and good management of family affairs. If the wife is forced to live with relatives for economic reasons, she may be faced with additional stressors. When the husband returns, the stress may be even greater because the marriage essentially must be started anew or because both partners have changed considerably during the separation and roles must be redefined. This problem is probably greatest for young couples who marry just before the husband goes on a remote assignment, or the separation occurs when a child is expected. When the husband returns, he will be instantly expected to assume a father role for which he may not be prepared. When there are other children, there may be problems with discipline and estrangement when the father returns. The control of family expenditures is another area in which problems may arise [18]. Each time a family experiences a lengthy separation of one or more of its members, no matter what the reason, there will be stress caused not only by the separation but also by the reunion.

SEPARATION FROM THE EXTENDED FAMILY

The isolation of the nuclear family from the extended family is an indirect but important stressor. With so many families moving regularly, many are unable to maintain continued contact with their families of origin. This situation places a greater burden on the nuclear family to be all things to its members, especially to the children. Whereas a few generations ago extended family networks provided babysitters and helpers to the parents, today the family must hire strangers and seek help from community agencies when problems arise. In addition, children today are often not exposed to older generations on a regular basis. Many children do not see their grandparents more than once a year and are thus missing an important tie with the past and the valuable emotional and social experiences this contact provides.

ECONOMIC PRESSURES

The economic pressures on contemporary families are tremendous. How well families provide their members with material goods is seen as a measure of their worth in contemporary society. The pursuit of happiness through the purchase of more and more goods is a fairly common phenomenon. It is one of the reasons why more and more mothers are entering the work force and why many male heads of households have more than one regular job. The pursuit of affluence can have a negative effect on family life, however, if the parents are constantly working and are not using their energy to participate in the family unit and the children do not feel needed and do not learn responsibility. According to one psychiatrist, "Affluence inappropriately utilized can deprive the child of the needed experience, success, and support that stimulates a positive self-concept" [31].

MARITAL DISCORD

Marital discord begins with the disenchantment that results when a person first discovers that the spouse is incapable of meeting all of his or her expectations. The gap between the dream and reality can be both shocking and painful. Each partner brings to the marriage not only preconditioned male-female expectations but also an entire series of internalized customs, attitudes, and values that are frequently extremely important emotionally, whether the individual is aware of it or not. The spouse may not agree with the expectations and more often than not may find some of them unreasonable. Each partner must learn to adjust to the other; problems arise when one or both of the partners are unwilling to make adjustments. Inflexibility steals the romance from the marriage. The development of change-resistant patterns of relating to one another may be the result of personal problems or of inadequate psychosocial maturation. Each partner must resolve or work through personal problems before adequate energies are available to work through mutual problems in the marriage. Sometimes the most difficult adjustments come several years after the honeymoon [29], when the partners begin to evaluate the accomplishment of personal goals within the existing family system.

If one were to ask all the unhappy marriage partners in the world why they could not adjust to each other, one would probably get as many specific answers as there are marriages. However, if one inquired more deeply, certain patterns of maladjustment would emerge: (1) winning the "who's right" argument and destructive quarreling, (2) disguised feelings and passive resistance, often generated by unresolved resentments that have been allowed to fester quietly, and (3) blackmailing, brainwashing, or subtle pressure techniques used to manipulate one's spouse [29].

One study of Americans who had been married for 10 years and who considered their marriages to be satisfactory and likely to continue indicates that there are five distinct patterns of husband-wife interaction [9, 29]. The first is the **conflict-habituated** pattern, which is characterized by almost continuous verbal conflict between the partners. In the second or **devitalized** pattern, the partners have lost the close sharing identification and deep feeling that they had at the outset of the marriage. This pattern often begins to be felt with the birth of the first child. Interaction is characterized by resignation, apathy, and acceptance of any modest gratification that can be obtained. Each partner then turns to other facets of life for basic fulfillment. The third type, called **passive-congenial,** is similar to the devitalized pattern except that the relationship has never been vital, even during courtship. In **vital marriages,** the man and woman deeply invest their total personalities in one another, emphathize with each other, spend a good deal of time together, and adjust easily and well to each other. The final pattern, the **total marriage,** is rare and has all the strength of the vital pattern, but the psychological investment of each spouse in the other more nearly encompasses the total needs and fulfillments of each of the partners.

DIFFERING MATURATIONAL LEVELS
Stress is often placed on the marriage relationship, and later on parenting relationships, when one partner is emotionally unprepared for the husband/wife role or the mother/father role. All humans grow, develop, and change over time, but they do so at different rates. As individuals go from one developmental task to another, they master some tasks better than others. In their interpersonal relationships, individuals are often operating on old patterns of behavior that date back to some earlier point in the developmental cycle (see Chap. 17); sometimes people are "stuck" in these previous sets and have not successfully worked them through (see Chap. 28). This situation can be very damaging to the family because it is difficult to maintain a mutually satisfying emotional relationship with one's spouse under these circumstances. A spouse may feel that his or her deepest, most meaningful thoughts and feelings cannot be shared because of the partner's lack of understanding or empathy and may feel very lonely within the marriage.

DIFFERING VALUES AMONG FAMILY MEMBERS
Marital unity and family harmony depend on a reasonable amount of consensus on values. Family members may be in conflict among themselves or with conditions or systems outside the family. When there is conflict in both areas, dissonance is maximized. External family conflict comes when its members hold values that are different from the general culture or the reality of their situation; internal family conflict occurs when various members of the family hold values that are essentially different from one another. This latter situation can often be found when adolescent members of the family ascribe to values that differ markedly from those of their parents [7].

There are many types of value conflicts facing contemporary families: (1) freedom in family experience versus order and efficiency, (2) work achievement versus love-reproduction, (3) personal self-expression versus devoted childrearing, (4) flexible, general training versus rigid, specific training, (5) high aspiration level for children versus realistic expectations, (6) family loyalty versus community loyalty, (7) extensive casual association versus restricted association, (8) love experience versus love safety, (9) free sexual expression versus sexual restraint, (10) early marriage versus mature, discriminating partner selection [7].

This list of stressors is not intended to be complete; rather, it is intended to give the reader an increased understanding of why families have problems in contemporary society. Any one of these stressors alone may or may not become a problem to a family. Often it is the combination of stressors that may occur at any given time, or the accumulation of stressors over time, that inhibits the family from coping successfully. The family may even regress to function at a lower level as a result of these stressors.

RESULTS OF FAMILY STRESS

All families at the first three levels of functioning on the continuum are fractionalized to some degree, since they are not well integrated as a system and do not function at optimal levels.

Physical Abuse

It has been hypothesized and supported by some research that "in a society such as ours in which aggression is defined as the normal response to frustration, we can expect that the more frustrating the familial and occupational roles, the greater the amount of violence" [53]. Thus, the more stressors there are on the family at any given time, the more likely the family is to use violence as a response to frustration. In the first comprehensive national study done on violence and the American family, it was found that as the amount of conflict increased, so did the rate of violence, and as the amount of verbal aggression increased so did the physical aggression [54]. Families who reported 10 or more stressful problems had higher rates of abusive violence. A conflict over the children was most likely to lead a couple to blows. Spousal abuse was low in households with no children and increased with each additional child up to six children. Statistics show that each generation learns to be violent by being a participant in a violent family. There is probably not an increase in violence today, but there is a greater awareness of it as values and social expectations change [54].

Family abuse may occur between parents, siblings, parents and children, or parents and grandparents. Either the husband or the wife may initiate abuse. Three characteristics of families with wife abuse tend to include: a dominant husband who makes the family decisions, a full time housewife, and a wife who is worried about economic security [54]. The less education the husband has received, the greater the chance will be that he will physically abuse his wife [46]. Alcohol is frequently associated with abuse.

Battered wives come from all social classes, and they tend to marry younger. Women have reported that violence started early in their marriages and was worse when they were pregnant [17]. These men tend to exhibit rivalry in relationships and immaturity in responses to frustration. When wives are abused, they are more likely to pass abuse on to their children (scapecoating) [46].

Three characteristics of those families where the wives abuse the husbands include growing up in a family where the mother hit the father, being physically punished beyond 13 years of age, and being employed outside the home as a manual worker. Although abuse by wives is fairly common, it is not brought to light as frequently as abuse by husbands because males can generally do more damage than females [54] and males are more ashamed to admit the situation to others.

The abuse of children is a phenomenon of maladjustment that can be diagnosed and treated. Assault on a child often has fatal consequences. When death occurs, the father is most frequently involved [17]. Violence once expressed seems more likely to be repeated [17]. Those who batter infants show evidence of deep hostility and psychiatric disturbance, and have a history of childhood neurosis, unhappiness, and lack of success as well as a family history of psychiatric illness [46]. Children who experience violence, experience it over and over again. It is rarely a "one shot" event. In families that were studied in 1975, children who were pushed, grabbed, or shoved had these experiences 6.6 times over a 12-month period; kicks, bites, and punches happened 8.9 times and beatings 5.9 times over a 1-year period [54].

The pattern of violence is cyclical. Children who have been abused or neglected grow up lacking trust and are unable to form a close relationship with their spouse when they marry. They frequently lack a sense of positive self-esteem and competence; in other words, they exhibit the helplessness syndrome. Such individuals often want children, but when they become parents they have no knowledge of appropriate child-rearing practices or of normal growth and development. As a result, as parents they make unreasonable demands on the child; for example, they may punish a 6-month-old child for crying when this is the child's only means of communicating needs. Battering usually occurs during a crisis, when parental anger and frustration are multiplied and the parent interprets the child's behavior as being accusatory and rejecting [60]. A family in which children are abused is at level I or II. Because of the modeling of their own parents, these parents may feel that firm discipline is the appropriate and only way to redirect the child's behavior. They often exhibit the "little adult" concept of children that was characteristic of the Middle Ages.

Elderly abuse can generally be found in one of three situations: (1) The family is initially loving and quite happy to make a home for a parent, but the increased disability in the parent sours the relationship; (2) an elderly person is taken in reluctantly because the disability interferes with independent living; or (3) the family is already in stress, and violence is likely to break out whether or not the elderly person is there [46]. Frequently, the elderly parent feels useless and unwanted in another household. It may mean a move to another city where the parent has no friends or connections. When the children reach retirement age, they may not welcome the stress and the additional burden that care of their elderly parents may place on them. It is not difficult to see how the violence can begin.

One study of elderly persons reported that 40 percent of adult children screamed and yelled at the parents; 14 percent forced medication; 8 percent used physical restraints; 7 percent threatened to send them to a nursing home; 5 percent threatened physical force; 4 percent withheld food; and 1 percent confined them to a room or slapped, shook, or hit them with an object [16].

In the same study, the adult-aged children reported the following about their parents: 54 percent tried to make them feel guilty; 43 percent manipulated other family members; 37 percent cried; 36 percent screamed and yelled; 33 percent used their disability to win sympathy; 18 percent slapped, shook, or hit them with an object; 16 percent refused food; 15 percent refused medication; and 5 percent called the police [16].

Most people take on the job of caring for an elderly parent or family member with no previous experience and may need help in order to give proper care. They also need counseling. With emotional and physical support from community agencies, individuals can learn to manage this very trying period of life. This aspect of abuse is one that will continue to be studied as more ways are sought to improve the quality of life for older persons who are now living longer.

It should be obvious by now that the level of family functioning is not synonymous with the family's economic status but with its socioemotional maturity level. However, families that are unable to meet needs in one area often experience difficulty in meeting other tasks as well.

Separation or Divorce

Families that are fractionalized by divorce, separation, or desertion usually have a history of disturbance leading up to the event. Many of the stressors already discussed in this chapter are among the reasons for family dissolution. Divorce can occur in families at any of the first four levels of functioning, although it would be less common at level IV. Regardless of the reasons that lead to the dissolution, it is an event that is characterized by disequilibrium that approaches severe disorganization. Although this period of disorganization may extend over several years [27], the children may

be unprepared for the separation when it occurs and usually suffer some adverse effects, such as confusion, difficulty in school, or health problems. Many children feel humiliated at being abandoned by their parent; they go through a process of sadness and grieving for the lost parent and the lost family structure. Depending on their age, the children may exhibit a conscious, intense anger directed at one or both of the parents; divided loyalties, such as when the parents use the children as pawns in their desire to hurt each other or to seek revenge; or a strong desire for the remaining parent to remarry. Children are keenly aware of being different from other children and often experience feelings of extreme loneliness [12, 27, 28, 50].

When a marriage has ended, whether by death, separation, desertion, or divorce, the remaining parent must face a complete reorientation of his or her life. The single parent must now make all major decisions alone, with no partner to present another viewpoint. Financial problems often force the woman to return to work. Parents without partners must struggle with enormous personal difficulties while at the same time trying to be a stabilizing influence for the children. Many single parents and their children still find stigmatizing experiences in their communities. Even after the adjustment has been made, the family may have considerable difficulty in meeting all its roles and tasks. Although the burden is greater for the parent, the family can still function at a fairly high level, depending on other factors associated with the individuals in the family and the commitment of the family as a system to work together to meet its tasks. One study, which compared child behavior in 16 intact families with that of 16 divorced families, found that the relationships among family members appeared to be a more potent influence on child behavior than marital status. The negative effects of divorce were mitigated when positive relationships with both parents were maintained [23].

MAXIMIZING FAMILY POTENTIALS

A professional person comes in contact with many different families in the course of work, whether such a person is a social worker helping a family to procure food stamps, a neighborhood aide helping a family to get to medical care, a dentist explaining good oral hygiene to a child and parent, a teacher having a family conference about a child's reading problem, a funeral director helping the family to make plans for the immediate future, or a doctor trying to decide whether it is best to hospitalize a mother or to treat her at home.

In order to work successfully with an individual or a family unit, the practitioner will need to know what kind of orientation the family has to the particular situation, what their strengths and weaknesses are as individuals and as a family unit, and what their particular needs are. In other words, the practitioner will need to make an assessment of the individual and the family.

Family assessments can be involved and detailed (for example, when a social worker takes a social history of a family seeking aid), or they can be very simple, examining only one particular phase of a family's ability to function. Usually each profession develops its own tools for assessment that help the practitioner to decide which problems the family needs assistance in resolving. One interdisciplinary method is to assess the level at which a family is able to meet the four basic tasks assigned to families in our society, as described earlier in this chapter. Once the family's level of functioning has been ascertained, the practitioner can maximize the assistance provided to that family by modifying the approach of the intervention to the level of functioning.

Assessment of and Approach to Families

As previously explained, families vary in their ability to function, and this ability can be measured and evaluated along a continuum. The practitioner who is working with a family will best be able to assist them if approaches are used that are appropriate to the family's level of functioning. These activities can also be put on a continuum. All of the key activities to be discussed are inherent in the helping process, but they will be more effective if the practitioner can concentrate efforts on the activity appropriate to the family's level of functioning. In doing so, measures can be initiated that are meaningful and economical in time and effort, and these in turn will lead to greater success in helping families to reach their highest level of functioning.

Since the family's level of functioning is an indication of its state of health, any change in that level also indicates a change in its health status. Thus the degree of family movement from one level to another can serve as a yardstick with which the practitioner can measure and evaluate the effect of intervention and service [53].

LEVEL I FAMILY

Establishing a trusting relationship with a level I family is the most important activity in the therapeutic process, but it is also the most difficult one. The practitioner must develop a caring, freeing relationship with one or more members of the family and help the family to feel that the practitioner cares about them, accepts them as they are, and understands their difficulties. Effective interaction requires extreme sensitivity on the part of the practitioner to the cues emitted by the family. The facilitator must move in synchrony with the pace the family sets. A practitioner who cannot establish this relationship with family members cannot help them to grow. Although this activity is basic for a level I family, it is difficult for the family members to accept because of their fear and distrust of people outside of the immediate family. Acute helplessness syndrome immobilizes them.

This task will demand much of the practitioner—consistency, maturity, patience, endurance, limit setting, and clarification of his or her role. The family may see the practitioner as a "good parent" and will test the practitioner for consistency and try to be dependent. The practitioner, seeing him- or herself as a partner working with the family, cannot allow the dependence to go beyond the trust relationship. The practitioner must be constantly alert to the subjective factors that operate within the self as well as the other factors operating in the family, the community, and the environment in order to evaluate progress toward the development of mutual trust. When the practitioner has ascertained that a relationship is developing, and that the family, like the newborn infant, has had its need for security met within an interpersonal relationship, the practitioner and the family can move into level II activities. The development of trust takes time; the practitioner should be cautioned not to force growth to level II. This growth will emerge on its own as a result of consistent, warm, concerned support.

LEVEL II FAMILY

With the level II family, the practitioner needs to continue to maintain the warm and accepting support of the trust relationship but now uses it as a stepping-stone to help the family to begin to understand itself more clearly and thus to begin to define its problems. Because of the trust established between the two, the family can begin to venture forth in self-discovery with help from the practitioner, who will clarify and reflect their words, actions, thoughts, and responses. The practitioner should be honest in sharing his or her observations and personality with the family, so that the family members can feel more willing to be honest with themselves. The problems identified by the practitioner may not be accepted by the family. Intervention is most effective when the family identifies its own needs and priorities and the practitioner then helps the family to meet these perceived needs. This process strengthens the trust bond and can eventually lead to the more realistic evolution of needs and the establishment of priorities characteristic of level III families.

The counseling relationship demands even more of the practitioner than the previous trust relationship; interpretations and diagnoses must be accurate, behavior consistent, and concerns genuine. The practitioner must very accurately understand subjective feelings about the family and his or her relationship with the family. The goal is to help this family grow to the point (level III) at which the members can assume the initiative to work independently on solutions to some of their problems. Progress is seen when the members begin to feel more like a family and to experience the practitioner as a "sibling"—that is, they will vacillate between dependence and independence and will compete for attention and control. The practitioner, acting as a partner with this family, helps them to understand that he or she shared personal thoughts and actions so that they could better understand themselves and their interaction as a family unit.

LEVEL III FAMILY

A complex of activities is required to help the level III family solve its recognized problems. The practitioner assists them by providing teaching, information, coordination, referral, teamwork, or special technical skills that enable the family to establish realistic priorities and to seek help independently. Often they must move backward to a previous level of activities and then forward again as more difficulties are looked at and worked on. In order to facilitate success, the family should be encouraged to start with the easiest of the most pressing problems.

Working with this family demands from the practitioner a wealth of technical and interpersonal skills as well as knowledge of community resources and the ability to lead, to coordinate, and to cooperate with other team members. The practitioner is seen by the family as an adult helper with expertise in the solution of problems. The practitioner provides the needed teaching, referral, and coordination to assist the family but continually emphasizes the importance of their making their own decisions. The practitioner assists the family in trying out their decisions and evaluating outcomes, thus helping the family to improve their ability to manage their roles and tasks as they proceed from one problem to another.

LEVEL IV FAMILY

The practitioner's main activity with the level IV family is preventive teaching to enable the family to main-

tain its health. The practitioner helps the members to anticipate problem areas, to work through possible alternatives, and then to study the consequences of these alternatives. Since prevention is stressed, he or she teaches the family about the resources that are available in times of need or crisis. The practitioner is also in a unique position to help this family grow and to increase the members' self-understanding and effectiveness in group functioning. Such intervention requires much maturity, foresight, knowledge, and experience on the part of the practitioner. If he or she is able to serve the family at this level, the family will be able to use community services appropriately when there is a need. This family sees the practitioner as an expert teacher and partner.

LEVEL V FAMILY

Intervention is not necessary for this family unless there is a crisis, and at such times, the family would seek help from the appropriate community source. If services are required, the practitioner would probably use activities appropriate to the situation—either level III or level IV—in assisting the family to regain its equilibrium.

Facilitating Intrafamily Communication

One of the most critical needs in today's society is for people to learn to communicate meaningfully with each other. Many of the troubles that plague the family grow out of, or are aggravated by, ineffective communication. Communication is learned within the family, and certain patterns of communication are passed on from one generation to another through the family [37]. When a child becomes an adult, he or she will experience difficulty in social relationships if adult patterns of communication have not been developed. When individuals have learned this skill, they will be able to establish satisfying relationships with family, peers, co-workers, acquaintances, and friends.

Usually family members do not deliberately set out to hurt, annoy, or frustrate one another. Misunderstandings often happen, however, because they have not made their feelings clear to themselves or to others. One author has compared the process of communication in the family to radio broadcasting when it was in its infancy, because the radio signals were frequently overwhelmed by static, interference from other stations, and fade-outs [35]. The adult can learn to improve communication skills first by analyzing which interactions are effective and which ones are not; second, by getting in touch with true feelings; and

Table 34-3. Model for Assessment of and Approach to Families

Helping Activities	Trust	Counseling	Complex of Skills	Prevention	None
Continuum of Skills / *Practitioner and Family—Partners* / *Partnership* / *Partnership Stressing Family's Ability* / *Practitioner—Expert and Partner* / *Family Independent*	Acceptance and trust, maturity and patience, clarification of role, limit setting, constant evaluation of relationship and progress	Based on trust relationship, uses counseling, and interpersonal skills to help family begin to understand itself and define its problems. Practitioner uses honesty, genuineness, and self-evaluation	Information, coordination, teamwork, teaching; uses special skills, helps family in making decisions and finding solutions	Anticipated problem areas studied, teaching of available resources, assistance in family-group understanding, maturity, and foresight	
Continuum of Family Functioning / *Practitioner—Good Parent to Family* / *Practitioner and Family—Siblings* / *Practitioner—Adult Helper to Family* / *Practitioner—Expert and Partner with Family* / *Help Not Needed*	Chaotic family, barely surviving, inadequate provision of physical and emotional supports. Alienation from community, deviant behavior, distortion and confusion of roles, immaturity, child neglect, depression-failure	Intermediate family, slightly above survival level, variation in economic provisions, alienation but with more ability to trust. Child neglect not as great, defensive but slightly more willing to accept help	Normal family but with many conflicts and problems, variation in economic levels, greater trust and ability to seek and use help. Parents more mature, but still have emotional conflicts. Do have successes and achievements, and are more willing to seek solutions to problems, future-oriented	Family has solutions, are stable and healthy with fewer conflicts or problems, very capable providers of physical and emotional supports. Parents mature and confident, fewer difficulties in training of children, able to seek help, future-oriented, enjoy present	Ideal family, homeostatic, balance between individual and group goals and activities. Family meets its tasks and roles well, they are able to seek appropriate help when needed
Family Levels	I Infancy	II Childhood	III Adolescence	IV Adulthood	V Maturity

Source: J. A. Tapia, The nursing process in family health. *Nursing Outlook* 20:267, April 1972. With permission.

third, by a conscious attempt toward more meaningful adult communication.

TRANSACTIONAL ANALYSIS

A frame of reference that is easily understood, analyzed, and used is transactional analysis (TA), created by Berne and popularized by Harris and others [4, 21]. TA defines three basic ego states: the Parent, the Adult, and the Child. At any given moment, an individual is in one of these three states: When thinking, feeling, perceiving, and behaving in a censorial, judgmental, rule-oriented manner, the individual is in the Parent ego state; when objectively defining issues, gathering information, deciding on various outcomes, and making choices on the basis of current reality, the individual is in the Adult ego state; when thinking, feeling, or behaving as does a young child, the individual is in the Child ego state.

TA offers the observer a method of analyzing the transactions between people. A transaction can be complementary when the initiator gets the desired response. An example of a complementary Parent-Parent transaction is an exchange of prejudices:

John: He should know better than to do that!
Rick: You're absolutely correct!

An example of a complementary Adult-Adult transaction is an exchange of information:

John: Do you know where my baseball is?
Rick: It's in the closet.

An example of a complementary Child-Child transaction is an exchange of feelings:

John: I hate what Jane did to you!
Rick: Yeah, I'm through with her forever!

An example of a complementary Parent-Child transaction is adapting to a demand:

Rick: You'd better put your things where you can find them.
John: I'm sorry. I'll try harder.

A transaction becomes crossed when the stimulus fails to get the desired response. Crossed transactions usually precipitate interpersonal conflict, but they can also be used constructively if the sender tries to "hook" the other person out of a Parent or a Child ego state and into the Adult state. An example of a crossed transaction that is disruptive is the following:

John (in the Adult state): Do you know where my baseball is?
Rick (in the Parent state): You'd better put your things where you can find them!

An example of a constructive crossed transaction is the following:

John (in the Child state): I hate what Jane did to you!
Rick (in the Adult state): I suppose we all have to take rejection once in awhile.

Another type of transaction is called duplex. It occurs when the stated meaning (verbal) does not match the unstated meaning (nonverbal behavior). An example of a duplex transaction is the following:

John (in the Adult state): Do you know where my baseball is?
Rick (Parent to Child): It's in the closet with the rest of your mess!

The theory behind transactional analysis is that memories of past transactions are stored in the brain and can be unconsciously replayed in new transactions when the stimulus of the new situation is familiar or similar to that of the old one. By studying their own behavior, people can learn about their predominant ego state and can analyze their transactions and their basic ego position in life, develop more satisfying relationships with others, and mature and grow as individuals. A professor once told the author that if you can figure out what your Parent is saying and what your Child really wants, you can use your Adult to satisfy both [58].

COMMUNITY AGENCIES

Because communication patterns are learned within the family and because family communication is often a major contributor to family problems, more and more professionals are treating problems within the context of the family. In family therapy, one or more professionals work with the family group in order to build the bridge of family understanding of problems and to assist the family to find solutions. The family unit or individual members may seek and find help from many different sources in the community: the family's clergyman is often trained in counseling techniques; the local mental health center, family life center, or family service agency employs professionally trained persons who are often called on for help; schools usually have counselors and social workers who are available to work with children and their families; hospitals, health centers, and public health agencies have trained personnel; and finally, there are many family counselors in private practice, as well as self-help groups, such as Parents Anonymous.

The important point is that families who are unable to solve their problems in a manner that is acceptable and healthful for all the members should not hesitate to utilize the resources that are available to them in the community. Too often, independent-minded people think that if they have a difficult problem, it is their fault and they must suffer with the problem or find the solution without outside help. They are unable and unwilling to seek assistance. This attitude is negative and self-defeating, and these people should be encouraged by their friends and acquaintances to seek professional help. Often it is only when someone from outside the situation is able to take an objective look at all the facets of the problem that the family members can be helped to become more objective about the problem and its possible solution.

CONCLUSIONS

This chapter has covered very briefly some of the theories about the family and how it functions. It has shown some of the ways in which families differ and how one can identify and assess those differences, and it has given guidelines for assessing malfunctioning families and a tool to use in working with them based on their developmental or functional level. The chapter has also briefly discussed some of the stressors in contemporary society that cause problems for many American families, and the need for improving communication within families in order to develop a healthier, more satisfactory family life.

It is the author's belief that individuals as well as the family system can be assisted to grow, to develop, and to mature by trained, caring, helping persons. Maturation is a lifelong process; it does not stop when an individual graduates from school, gets married, has a child, becomes a grandparent, or is widowed. As discussed in earlier chapters, there are developmental tasks all through a person's life and all through a family's life. The more successful a person is at meeting the challenges of each developmental task the greater is the possibility that the next task will also be met successfully and that the person will have a satisfying life. An individual's emotional maturity is indicated by "the extent to which he expresses his own feelings and convictions, balanced with consideration for the thoughts and feelings of others, without being threatened by the expression of feelings, either his own or others'" [49].

There is no doubt that marriage and family life in today's society are changing. The approaches that work successfully for one family may not be at all relevant to another one. It is important that people be willing to look at all the pressures on the family and to consider alternative ways to alleviate them. Marital styles are also changing as more couples discover that they can open up their marriage into a creative sharing between two people who deeply love and are deeply committed to one another. Some authors call this a "relationship marriage" because great emphasis is placed on the relationship of the couple and their interpersonal communication. It can also be called a "total marriage" because it is held together by internal cohesion. This type of marriage is not easy to achieve but is the most rewarding of all marriage styles. Both partners must be aware of their individual responsibilities, and both must be committed to work at the relationship. To make a marriage successful takes as much intelligence and skill as succeeding in a career or any other major enterprise [33].

Some couples naturally develop a relationship marriage because they are mature, knowledgeable, and committed enough to make the relationship a way of life for themselves. Others may be helped through marriage counseling. Another option that is available to help couples explore and expand the dimensions of their marriage is the "Marriage Encounter" movement, which began in Spain more than 20 years ago in the Catholic Church and has spread to include Jewish and Protestant religious denominations. This encounter is usually held over a weekend. Thousands of couples are currently rediscovering each other and their commitment to each other through these encounters, and they are discovering how to open up lines of communication with their own feelings.

The key to high level family functioning is the maturational level of the major adults in the family unit. These adults establish the tone and the communication style within the family system as well as the relationship of the family with the community. Education and therapy must focus on the development of the individual members as well as that of the members as a system. Fractionalization can be prevented. When fractionalization is unavoidable, each family member still has the right to emerge from the relationship with a high level of social and emotional health.

REFERENCES

1. Bailey, M. B. Alcoholism and the Family. In M. B. Bailey (Ed.), *Alcoholism and Family Casework*. New York: Community Council of Greater New York, 1968.

2. Bakke, E. W. The Cycle of Adjustment to Unemployment. In N. W. Bell and E. F. Vogel (Eds.), *A Modern Introduction to the Family.* Glencoe, Ill.: Free Press, 1960.

3. Bell, R. R. Impact of Illness on Family Roles. In B. W. Spradley (Ed.), *Contemporary Community Nursing.* Boston: Little, Brown, 1975. P. 333.

4. Berne, E. *Transactional Analysis in Psychotherapy.* New York: Grove Press, 1961.

5. Braginsky, D. D., and Braginsky, B. M. Surplus people, their lost faith in self and the system. *Psychology Today* 9:68, 1975.

6. Broderick, C. D. (Ed.). *A Decade of Family Research and Action, 1960–1969.* Minneapolis: National Council on Family Relations, 1971.

7. Christensen, H. T. The Intrusion of Values. In H. T. Christensen (Ed.), *Handbook of Marriage and the Family.* Chicago: Rand McNally, 1964. P. 969.

8. Cook, J., and Munce, S. Group Treatment for Abusive Parents: Creating a New Family System. In R. C. Jackson and J. Morton (Eds.), *Family Health Care: Health Promotion and Illness Care.* Berkeley: Public Health Social Work Program, School of Public Health, University of California, 1976.

9. Cuber, J., and Haroff, P. *Sex and the Significant Americans.* New York: Penguin, 1977.

10. Dirks, P. Juvenile Rheumatoid Arthritis: Effects of Illness and Disability on the Parent-Child Relationship. In R. Jackson and J. Morton (Eds.), *Family Health Care: Health Promotion and Illness care.* Berkeley: Public Health Social Work Program, School of Public Health, University of California, 1976.

11. Duvall, E. R. M. *Family Development* (4th ed.). Philadelphia: Lippincott, 1971.

12. Gardner, R. A. *The Boy's and Girl's Book About Divorce.* New York: Bantam Books, 1981.

13. Feldman, F. L., and Scherz, F. H. *Family Social Welfare—Helping Troubled Families.* New York: Atherton Press, 1967.

14. Geddes, J. B. Will the Family Survive the Twentieth Century? In C. C. Barbeau (Ed.), *Future of the Family.* New York: Bruce, 1971. P. 11.

15. Geismar, L., and Charlesworth, S. Parsimonious practice research, or, have your diagnosis and research it too. *Aust. Soc. Work* 29:5, 1976.

16. Gilbride, N. Study says home care urgently needed. *Home Health Journal* (Nov. 1982).

17. Gregory, M. Battered Wives. In M. Boland (Ed.), *Violence in the Family.* Atlantic, NJ: Humanities Press, 1976.

18. Greenwald, J. (Ed.). Family separation. *Times Magazine Handbook for Military Families* (May 1977):67.

19. Hanford, J. New pressures on family life. *Soc. Casework* 50:3, 1969.

20. Hanson, D. A., and Hill, R. Families Under Stress. In H. T. Christensen (Ed.), *Handbook of Marriage and the Family.* Chicago: Rand McNally, 1964.

21. Harris, T. A. *I'm O.K.—You're O.K.* New York: Harper & Row, 1969.

22. Hect, M. Children of alcoholics are children at risk. *Am. J. Nurs.* 73:1764, 1973.

23. Hess, R. D., and Camara, K. A. Post-divorce family relationships as mediating factors in the consequences of divorce for children. *J. Soc. Issues* 35(4):79, 1979.

24. Holmstrom, L. L. *The Two-Career Family.* Cambridge, MA: Schenkman, 1973.

25. Horton, T. E. Conceptual Basis for Nursing Intervention With Human Systems. In J. E. Hall and B. R. Weaver (Eds.), *Distributive Nursing Practice: A Systems Approach to Community Health.* Philadelphia: Lippincott, 1977.

26. Kanter, R. M. Jobs and families: Impact of working roles on family life. *Child. Today* 7(2):11, 1978.

27. Kelly, J. B., and Wallerstein, J. S. Effects of parental divorce: Experiences of the child in early latency. *Am. J. Orthopsychiatry* 46:20, 1976.

28. Kelly, J. B., and Wallerstein, J. S. Effects of parental divorce: Experiences of the child in later latency. *Am. J. Orthopsychiatry* 46:256, 1976.

29. Klemer, R. H. *Klemer's Marriage and Family Relationships* (2nd ed.). New York: Harper & Row, 1975.

30. Krimmel, H. *Alcoholism: Challenge for Social Work Education.* New York: Council for Social Work Education, 1971.

31. Levey, R. Twenty-four family varieties. *Boston Sunday Globe,* January 30, 1977.

32. Leiber, E. K. The professional woman: Coping in a two-career family. *Educ. Horiz.* 58:156; 1980.

33. Mace, D. R., and Mace, V. *We Can Have Better Marriages if We Really Want Them.* Nashville, TN: Abingdon, 1974.

34. Max, P., and Quensnell, J. Family Life: The Agony and the Ecstasy. In C. C. Barbeau (Ed.), *Future of the Family.* New York: Bruce, 1971.

35. McGinnis, T. C., and Ayers, J. V. *Open Family Living.* Garden City, NY: Doubleday, 1976.

36. McIntyre, J. Structural Functional Approach to Family Study. In F. I. Nye and F. M. Berardo (Eds.), *Emerging Conceptual Frameworks in Family Analysis.* New York: Macmillan, 1966.

37. Milloy, M. A look at the family and family interviewing. *Child Welfare* 1:40, 1971.

38. Miller, M. Family counseling's own family expands. *Boston Globe,* July 4, 1977.

39. Murdock, G. P. The Universality of the Nuclear Family. In N. W. Bell and E. F. Vogel (Eds.), *A Modern Introduction to the Family* (Rev. ed.). New York: Free Press, 1968.

40. Nye, F. I., and Berardo, F. M. Introduction in *Emerging Conceptual Frameworks in Family Analysis.* New York: Praeger Publishers, 1981.

41. Parsons, T., and Fox, R. C. Illness, Therapy and Modern Urban American Families. In N. W. Bell and E. F. Vogel (Eds.), *A Modern Introduction to the Family* (Rev. ed.). New York: Free Press, 1968.

42. Peterson, C. A. A house divided cannot stand: The tragedy of the generation gap. *Parent's Magazine* 48:46, 1973.

43. Pogrebin, L. C. *Family Politics: Love and Power on an Intimate Frontier.* New York: McGraw-Hill, 1983.

44. Pogrebin, L. C. Working woman. *Ladies' Home Journal* 91:50, 1974.

45. Rapoport, R., and Rapoport, R. *Dual-Career Families Re-Examined.* New York: Harper & Row, 1976.

46. Renvoize, J. *Web of Violence: A Study of Family Violence.* Boston: Routledge and Keagan, 1978.

47. Rochman, M. *Report on Community Human Service Needs, Use and Awareness in Metropolitan Boston.* Boston: United Community Planning Corporation, Report No. 142, 1977.

48. St. John-Parsons, D. Continuous dual-career families: A case study. *Psychol. of Women Q.* 3:30, 1978.

49. Saxenian, H. Criterion for emotional maturity. *Harvard Bus. R.* 36:56, 1958.

50. Schlesinger, B. *The One-Parent Family* (4th ed.). Toronto: University of Toronto Press, 1978.

51. Schvaneveldt, J. D. The Interactional Framework in the Study of the Family. In F. I. Nye and F. M. Berardo (Eds.), *Emerging Conceptual Frameworks in Family Analysis.* New York: Macmillan, 1966.

52. Sprey, T. Conflict Theory and the Study of Marriage and the Family. In W. R. Burr, et al. (Eds.), *Contemporary Theories about the Family.* Vol. II. New York: Free Press, 1979.

53. Steinmetz, S. K., and Straus, M. A. (Eds.). *Violence in the Family.* New York: Dodd, Mead, 1974.

54. Straus, M. A., Gelles, R. J., and Steinmetz, S. K. *Behind Closed Doors: Violence in the American Family.* Garden City, NJ: Anchor Press/Doubleday, 1980.

55. Sussman, M. B. The family today: Is it an endangered species? *Child. Today* 7(2):32, 1978.

56. Tapia, J. The nursing process in family health. *Nursing Outlook* 20:267, 1972.

57. Thomas, D. Assessment of Family Functioning: The Transactional Analysis Model. In R. C. Jackson and J. Morton (Eds.), *Family Health Care: Health Promotion and Illness Care.* Berkeley: Public Health Social Work Program, School of Public Health, University of California, 1976.

58. Weber, R. J. "An Introduction to Transactional Analysis for Managers." Unpublished work.

59. Werner, H., and Kaplan, B. *Symbol Formation.* New York: Wiley, 1963.

60. Younes, R. Child abuse and neglect: Incidence, historical perspective, detection and treatment. *Health Values: Achieving High Level Wellness* 1:34, 1977.

35

The Family with a Disabled Member

Clara S. Schuster

Sorrow fully accepted brings its own gifts.

—Pearl S. Buck, *The Child Who Never Grew*

Throughout pregnancy most parents, especially the mother, invest extensive amounts of energy in physical and psychological preparation for the new baby [11]. "Nest building" activities, such as preparation of the infant's room, collecting a layette, and making articles by hand for the baby, all imply a joyful anticipation of the event. Grandparents, other children in the family, and friends frequently contribute to the preparation, indicating the high social value of the addition of another member to the family.

The parents, especially the mother, begin to fantasize about the new baby. They may begin to formulate, consciously or unconsciously, a concept of the baby's appearance, behavior characteristics, gender, special talents, intellectual potential, and even future contributions to the family or society. These daydreams create an "ideal child"—a unique combination of each parent's self, loved ones, past experiences, present values, and future goals. The parents dream of giving the child what they did not have during their own childhood, and they see the child achieving the same or higher levels of life-style or values.

The mother may come to view the child as an idealization of herself [11] or an extension of herself [33] because of her close association with the fetus. Most parents also entertain at one point or another the fear that the child may have abnormalities. Whether the pregnancy is desired or rejected, this appears to be a universal concern. Many parents are reluctant to mention these anxieties lest the very expression of the fear precipitate the event [22]. Most parents are able to minimize these fears and to anticipate a happy outcome. The ability of the parents to produce an unimpaired child is psychologically and culturally critical to their sense of personal adequacy [4]. They want to produce a miniature composite of themselves. When this occurs, the two initial tasks of parenthood are made infinitely easier: (1) to become attached to the child (it is hard to reject what is perceived as a part or extension of the self), and (2) to develop a new self-image as an adult responsible for another life—a parent. The mother may see the infant as something she has made, a gift that she presents to her husband or to society [32, 41, 42]. This narcissistic investment in the infant predisposes her to dream of a "perfect child" because the baby becomes so closely tied to her own feelings of achievement and self-worth.

The birth of an infant, especially the first one, is a crisis event for any family. When the new infant does not match the ideal infant, the parent is challenged to blend, or to bend, the ideal to meet the reality. Sometimes the gap involves a very superficial factor; for example, the author and her husband expected a brown-haired baby but had a very blonde one instead. We were not even aware of our preconceived expectation until after her birth, when we recognized our shock reaction. It was a small, superficial difference, but one that nevertheless required an adjustment of our concepts about "our baby." At other times, the gap between the ideal and the real is so great that every coping skill a parent possesses is called upon, and even then these skills may not be sufficient to bridge the gap readily or comfortably. The gender of the child sometimes falls into this category. The parent (or parents), for one reason or another, may have planned or counted on one gender. When the infant turns out to be the "wrong" gender, it may take days, weeks, months, or even years for the parents to accept the disparity with their ideal. Some parents are never able to forgive the child for defying their dreams.

Almost 14 percent of neonates have one or more minor malformations [18]. Three to 4 percent of infants are born with severe congenital abnormalities [31]. There are 250,000 impaired babies born annually in the United States, and over 1005 different birth defects are recognized [10]. Since the "cuteness" of a baby is a factor known to aid in the parents' positive feelings toward an infant, an atypical physical appearance or behavior can present a barrier to bonding [18]. When an infant is born with a defect that is obvious at birth

or shortly thereafter, the crisis of the birth and the necessity of bridging the gap between the real infant and the ideal one may present seemingly insurmountable obstacles to the parents. The psychological pain of the parents can be a fractionalizing factor in the parent-child relationship that can interfere with the bonding process, a factor that will ultimately affect the development of both the child and the parents. While parents are still in the process of getting to know their new child as a separate individual, their emotional energy may be diverted from external relationships and used for internal relationships in order to enable them to cope with the "pain gap."

To be successful both as individuals and as parents, the parents must accomplish the two initial tasks of parenthood in spite of the gap between the ideal infant and the real one. Unless they are able to cope with their own narcissistic injury, a healthy attachment to the infant will be difficult if not impossible. This lack of attachment can reduce the amount of warm, consistent, and nurturing attention the infant will receive during the critical early months of extrauterine life. Parental grief over the disability may inhibit synchronized responses to the infant and thus will effectively prevent the child's ability to predict events, to master effective signaling systems, to imitate, and to learn [18]. According to theories of early infant development and recent research on attachment and bonding, the child is potentially a high-risk candidate for physical, emotional, social, or cognitive deficits that can negatively influence the child's ability to maximize his or her innate potentials (see Chap. 19).

If this hypothesis is true, then educational intervention for the physically disabled child must be instituted as soon as it is apparent that the disability exists. Since the family is the socialization and educational system for the young infant, educational intervention must begin with the administrators of that system—the parents—in order to prevent or to ameliorate the fractionalization of the parent-child relationship as well as to offer them information on the disability and special intervention techniques. The parents, however, will find it difficult to meet even the most basic nutritive needs of the infant, let alone the socialization and specialized needs of the child, if their energies are completely invested in identifying and supporting their own identity and self-esteem. Many, if not most, parents need counseling to help them put roles, relationships, and identities back into a healthy perspective.

The practitioner must have a broad empirical knowledge of typical parental reactions before counseling or working successfully with parents of physically disabled children. From this knowledge one can develop a sensitivity to the individual reactions and needs of each parent being counseled. One must reach the parents as people before one can teach them as parents. The practitioner must understand both the quantity and the quality of coping patterns associated with this unique stressor before accurately interpreting the coping behaviors exhibited by individual parents. As mentioned in the preface, it is easy to be critical of what we do not understand or to perceive as abnormal what is foreign to us. Many parents have been erroneously labeled "hysterical," "overprotective," or "nonaccepting" by insensitive professionals. In their eagerness to analyze the parents' behavior, the practitioners' attitudes can convey to the parents a feeling of being "inappropriate" or "pathological." Such negative labeling of an intense, but normal, response can increase parental stress and reduce effective coping during the crisis as well as in the years ahead [43].

REACTIONS OF PARENTS

Birth of an Impaired Infant

When the parents learn that their baby is impaired in some way, their dream of living "happily ever after" is shattered. New goals may need to be established for the child, themselves, and for the total family. The couple, individually and collectively, assumes a new self-image. They may feel an intense isolation from the infant, from each other, or even from people in general. There is a heightened sense of aloneness and vulnerability. The normal period of disequilibrium following birth and adjustment to new roles is intensified. The parents find that their relationships with family, spouse, friends, and professional agencies change. The spontaneous joy and atmosphere of celebration following the birth of a healthy child may be sharply muted by the parents, family members, and friends.

The task of integrating past, present, and future becomes exceedingly difficult for the parents. They ask themselves questions such as, "Why me?" and "Could this have been prevented?" Guilt lies heavily on them. There are usually no answers, and usually no guidelines or models to emulate. These factors heighten the parents' sense of isolation and anxiety as they attempt to establish a semblance of equilibrium. The mother, because of her greater narcissistic investment, usually reacts more strongly than the father, at least outwardly. The fact that the father usually has a job to which he can "escape" helps him to retain some stability of schedule and emotional distance from the event. Very

few studies have included the father's responses, but indications are that he feels the pain as greatly as the mother but handles it differently. The culture may have socialized men to handle stress in a different manner. Many men are less willing to talk about the disability. Frequently they are not as actively involved in their child's care and may not be included in counseling sessions. Consequently, they may lack an understanding of their child's needs [28]. This may be a potential source of contention between the parents, since the mother may interpret the father's more stoic approach as a lack of concern.

However, the ego-identity of both parents is severely threatened. Their concept of their own sexuality or that of their spouse may be questioned. They may feel personally responsible for the child's existence and interpret the loss of the perfect child as a defect in their own humanness, in their own integrity, or in their ability to produce a "whole child" [9, 12]. The birth of a defective child may be seen as an ineradicable stigma and a reflection on their own adequacy, identity, procreational ability, and ancestral background [6]. This is a point of no return; they cannot "make right" what has happened. The father may feel overwhelmed with the financial responsibilities involved in caring for the child, and may wonder if he can now continue to provide for the needs of his family. He may resist asking for financial aid because this is a further acknowledgment of his inadequacy. The mother may also feel overwhelmingly inadequate, especially if she saw her career as that of being a mother. At the onset of her career, she has created a "bad child"; she has failed. She has lost status in her own eyes at a time when she was expecting a "promotion." She may have felt somewhat unprepared but challenged by the idea of learning to care for a normal infant; she is overwhelmed and devastated at the idea of caring for a disabled infant. She has failed before she started; she does not understand why and feels that the situation is unfair. Both parents may suffer from acute helplessness syndrome. The presence of a chronically disabled child may precipitate or aggravate health problems in the parents (see Chap. 42). Parents often experience duodenal ulcers, headaches, chronic fatigue, hypertension, obesity, or menstrual difficulties [28]. Moreover, realization that a pregnancy may result in the birth of another disabled child can have a very negative effect on the parents' sex life.

The birth of a defective infant appears to be less devastating if there is already one normal child in the family [20]. The couple have already proved their soundness of body, adulthood, and sexuality, and they have also been inducted successfully into the status of parenthood. Now they are merely expanding their responsibilities—not changing them. Many parents may not have the courage to risk another pregnancy, if the first child is impaired; thus the issues of soundness and sexuality may never be completely or adequately resolved.

Disability After the Neonatal Period

LATE-APPEARING CONGENITAL ANOMALIES

Many hereditary traits and congenital disabilities, such as deafness and cerebral palsy, do not become apparent until several months after a child's birth. Others, such as diabetes or mental retardation, may take several years before the parents recognize a problem, and professionals document it. In these cases, the parents have had an opportunity to bond to the infant. They have been able to integrate some of their ideal infant with the real infant in their arms. They still hold to their idealistic hopes and dreams for the young child but begin to modify these in the exigencies of daily living. Gradually, the parents become aware that something is wrong as they observe that the child is not achieving the expected milestones, fails to respond in an expected manner, or begins to develop an unexpected behavior.

Unfortunately, many of the parents' initial observations and concerns are ignored or treated lightly by the professionals as being the projections of overanxious, neurotic parents [44]. Even if a professional suspects a problem, many parents report that they are told "Don't worry, everything's fine," or "He'll outgrow it." Many feel forced into an aggressive advocacy role for their child, a stance that precipitates personality changes [19, 44] as they "fight the system," trying to secure diagnosis, treatment, or information. The search for assistance for their child may consume most of their energy and time, cutting into a healthy relationship with the child or between the spouses. Parents have to be strong to cope. They are forced to tell their story repeatedly as they seek assistance. Once the diagnosis has been made, rather than devastating the parents, most express a tremendous sense of relief to know what they are dealing with [44]. The truth sets them free to focus their energies on treatment for the child's welfare. The parents have a sense of accomplishment in having fought a battle for their child and having won. No longer do they fear being stigmatized as neurotic parents. Their efforts and behaviors have been vindicated!

TRAUMATIC INJURY OR ILLNESS

The immediate effects of a serious injury or illness in a child cannot be disputed by either parents or professionals. The parents deeply fear the loss of a child they knew and loved. They also have intense fears about whether the child will recover to full functioning or be left with a permanent disability, emotional problems, or cognitive deficits because it is frequently difficult to predict the sequelae of an injury. When disastrous consequences result, the parents feel the loss of their normal child just as acutely as if the child had died. It is probably as difficult for the parents to make the adjustment to the loss of a normal child as it is for the parents to accept the congenitally impaired child.

When an older child or adolescent is injured, the parents may face having a dependent child once again at a time in their lives when they were beginning to enjoy more freedom from active parenting skills. The dependent child may seriously interrupt the parents' goals and life-style—a factor that can lead to marked resentment.

When a child or adult family member is temporarily or permanently disabled, there are role changes in all other family members. The responsibilities of the disabled family member must be assumed by other members of the system. When an adult is disabled, the family may need to seek alternative sources of income to maintain living expenses. The additional responsibility may lead to fatigue, anger, or depression if the disability continues too long without external relief or support. Chapter 34 discusses some of the sequelae.

The question that the parents of any impaired child may ask is "Why?" When the disability is due to an accident or illness, the parents may assume the guilt, identifying ways the trauma could have been prevented, "If only I had. . . . " Guilt, whether directed at one's self, the spouse, or a sibling, can devastate the family unit. Crisis counseling is essential.

Factors Affecting the Response of Family Members

The response of the other family members to a disabled member depends on many variables. Most of the responses are attempts to maintain psychological equilibrium and ego-identity. One major factor that affects the parents' reaction is whether or not they have become attached to the child. In general, the older the child when the disability becomes known, the stronger is the attachment bond and, therefore, the greater is the resistance to fractionalization. Loving attention continues to be showered on the child in spite of the

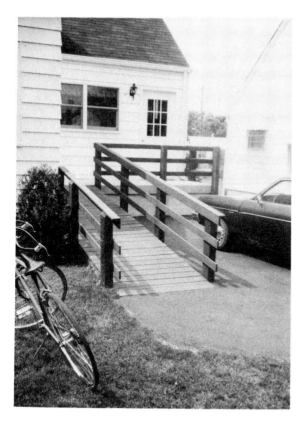

Figure 35–1. Families may be reluctant to make the unique adaptations to their home that are essential for meeting the needs of a disabled family member. Such changes not only increase the financial burdens of the family but also announce to the world the presence of a disabled family member—points that must be weighed against the individual's increased independence or the greater ease in caring for him.

child's limited responsiveness or ability to reinforce parental behaviors.

TELLING FAMILY MEMBERS
How family members are told about a disability and the type of affective support given them at the time are crucial to the family members' future relationships with one another, the disabled person, and professional persons [44]. In many cases, individuals may not remember exactly what was said to them but will vividly recall years later how they were told (or not told) about the disability of a family member. The brisk, hurried, impersonal practitioner can leave an individual feeling even more isolated and angry. People desire the

truth, sensitively presented; hope must be maintained and new roles simply and gently described. New situations may need to be explained several times, because shock and grief may prevent a clear understanding the first time an individual is informed about a disabled member of the family.

People indicate that anxieties are frequently reduced after seeing a deformed baby or an injured family member because the infant, the child, or the adult does not look as bad as their imaginations may conjecture. Family members appreciate staff members who make themselves available to answer questions, to listen, and to talk about the disabled person's positive aspects. This approach demands great maturity and a solid empirical foundation on the part of the practitioner. The practitioner must be able to recognize the limitations of preventive medicine and not harbor feelings of guilt because he or she cannot cure the problem. The practitioner must be able to handle his or her own grief and have a realistic perspective on the situation before solid, effective support to family members can be offered. The furtive looks; avoidance behavior; whispers, or tightly drawn faces of embarrassed, grieving, curious, or insecure staff members can increase the family members' sense of stigma and isolation. The feeling of stigmatization and isolation may be more incapacitating, for example, to the parents of a disabled child than the child's defect.

TYPE OF DISABILITY
The type of disability will affect the family members' responses. Have the members had contact with a person exhibiting this disability before, and if so, was it negative or positive? Are there other primary or extended family members with the same or other problems? This second factor may increase the intensity of family grief, since it can reactivate old wounds or intensify the feeling of personal responsibility or inadequacy. On the other hand, although family members may be disappointed, they may feel that they have coped successfully once and can do it again.

The degree of deformity or disability may intensify the family members' response. However, there is no clear correlation. It is the meaning of the disability to the family rather than the degree of involvement that is significant. One parent may be more disturbed by a facial birthmark than by a metabolic imbalance or a club foot. A mentally retarded child often creates more psychological stress and stigma than a physically impaired child [45]. Consequently, when parents have a child with both physical and cognitive defects, they tend to use the physical handicap as an excuse for the developmental delay [39]. Orthopedic anomalies and blindness appear to create the greatest barriers to maternal bonding because of an obvious discrepancy from the normal, anticipated inability of the child to perform self-help skills, or the inability of the infant to establish eye-to-eye contact, which is a significant reinforcer for maternal caretaking [1, 13]. The correctability or life-threatening nature of a defect may affect the intensity of responses. Parents may experience marked difficulty bonding to a child they expect will die. Investing heavily now will hurt intensely later. Anticipating grief may prevent continued investment in or emotional commitment to a person with Alzheimer's disease or a stroke.

The value system of the family will also affect their response to disability or to congenital anomaly, in part because the couple's reasons for marrying or having a baby are incorporated into this value system. Those who place high value on physical perfection and beauty may find a facial scar or a cleft lip especially difficult to accept. Mental retardation is frequently difficult for the highly educated couple to accept, and an uncomplicated cerebral palsy, an amputation, or a paralysis may be difficult for the physically oriented family.

DEGREE OF MATURITY

An individual's degree of maturity at the time of the entrance of a disabled person into the family heavily effects acceptance and coping skills. Younger children

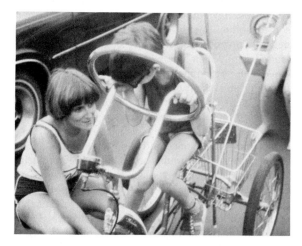

Figure 35–2. Honest, realistic acceptance of a child's disability allows both the child and the parents to advance to higher levels of affective and social maturity and to invest their energies in creating alternative approaches for the accomplishment of normal developmental tasks.

tend to accept the disability, although they may be disappointed in the loss of a potential playmate. The preschooler, with incomplete concepts of causality, may attribute the anomaly or injury to negative feelings stemming from sibling or parental rivalry. School-agers and adolescents may experience embarrassment from the perceived stigma associated with a disabled person. They may also resent the increased workload associated with the reallocation of responsibilities. Many individuals will become more serious and mature as they become more sensitive to the needs of someone besides themselves.

The emotional maturity of the parents is critical in their response to disability. Those who have not yet successfully resolved Erikson's task of identity (e.g., very young parents) may be especially vulnerable to experiencing intense or pathological reactions and will need much assistance in separating their personal integrity from the event. Some very young or immature parents may still be too involved in their own development to recognize the significance of their child's impairment. Role confusion and accompanying feelings of worthlessness or naivete may prevent the individuals from seeking appropriate assistance for themselves or the child. Some persons are likely to accept as true whatever is told them by the practitioner, since they are extremely vulnerable to the attitudes of others. Sensitive, synchronized assistance from the practitioner can give young adults an insight that can facilitate the growth of the family. This growth can lead to new depths of self-understanding and value clarifications that family members never knew were possible; they may even feel thankful for what the experience has taught them about life and living [5]. The severe injury or chronic illness of a spouse may precipitate an annulment or divorce when a partner feels cheated out of companionship, sexual relations, or a shared work load.

The ability of a couple to give mutual support to each other and to their other children is often critical in their ability to mobilize coping strategies. Yet parents frequently find they are not united in efforts to solve a disabled member's problems [28]. The communication patterns established prior to the event may facilitate or hinder their ability to express their grief and to mitigate a sense of personal isolation. When the parents are able to share how they feel without criticism from the partner, it can help to strengthen their marital commitment and facilitate their personal growth. The couple often feel that no one else can really understand or share their burden—they are alone, but at least they have each other. However, if each person retreats into his or her own private world, the burden is compounded and the chance of fractionalization of the family is increased. Many persons may want and need to be left alone for short periods of time while they attempt to absorb the reality of what has happened to themselves or the child and begin to gain some new internal perspectives. However, to "crawl into a shell" is unhealthy and is an indication of the need for intensive professional counseling.

Narcissistic hurt can cause the parents to attribute a birth defect to "the other side of the family." Sensitive genetic and social counseling may be essential to prevent the hostility and rejection inherent in this response. Families who are able to support the integrity of each member can emerge from the situation as a more cohesive unit.

The family members' ability to communicate their thoughts and feelings becomes a valuable tool for identifying stressors and resolving the pain. This skill may need to be encouraged and fostered in individuals who are not yet comfortable with Erikson's task of intimacy. The practitioner may need to assure family members of the acceptability and the normalcy of their thoughts and feelings before they will feel free to disclose reactions toward the disabled family member, and life in general that are socially taboo. The sensitive counselor may even need to identify typical reactions for people before they are able to identify or to admit, even to themselves, their true feelings.

Feelings of alienation may temporarily impair communication between husband and wife [27]. Although they may share food and space, they may become virtual strangers because of the inability to share their thoughts and feelings. Couples who are able to reestablish the bridges of communication find that they can develop "emotional bonds of great depth and enduring strength" [27].

RELIGIOUS ORIENTATION

A serious illness or the birth of a defective child almost always awakens questions involving the spiritual domain. The religious orientation or values of the individual may either hinder or facilitate coping skills. People universally ask, "Why me?" If their concept of God is that of an overseer, judge, and punisher, they may search their own background for a serious sin that they committed. Premarital sex frequently becomes the identified behavior for which they are being punished; this concept evokes high levels of guilt and is very difficult for the individual to deal with. Frequently a person feels that the "sin" cannot be shared or discussed with anyone, not even the spouse; the burden is carried alone in secret. Very sensitive counseling may be required to help such an individual put events into a realistic perspective and to alleviate the guilt. Counseling by a clergyman may be very helpful.

People may experience much conflict over how God fits into the picture. Friends may comment on how lucky a child is that God provided a specific, capable set of parents. Although on the surface, the friend's comment is offered as a compliment, and it may be helpful to some parents, it raises several critical philosophical questions: (1) Does God deliberately create a defective child and then look for suitable parents? (2) Does God have a certain number of "flawed models" which are bestowed on the most worthy (or the most sinful)? (3) Does God deliberately test our strength and tolerance levels through pain, illness, and deformity?

Other well-meaning friends, attempting to offer a glimmer of hope, will share the idea that "If you live close enough to God and really have faith, then the person will be cured." This is an exciting thought to family members who may also seek the assistance of faith healers on this basis. Although the author is aware of many miraculous cures and would not negate the power of a living, loving God, what happens if the person is not cured? Would it be a result of a person's lack of closeness to God? This would mean that one's own spiritual health is in jeopardy, or that the parent's inadequate spiritual growth is keeping the child from being cured. This kind of belief leads to too much guilt for any person to live with. Persons of this persuasion are cautioned to pray, "Thy will be done," and leave the matter in God's hands.

At the other end of the continuum are those who feel that God is a companion, a helper, or a guide in times of stress. They feel that God does not purposefully create a defective child or deliberately cause a serious accident or allow illness; this idea, to them, would imply a cruel God. They feel that as human animals, people are subject to natural disasters, developmental problems, and genetic mutations. Being human offers no immunities or special privileges over any other species, except that it provides the ability to think creatively and to communicate with God. Some may feel that God could and would cure if He wanted to. But why would God cure one person and not another? The issue is resolved by accepting the fact of the disability and the philosophy that God will give inner strength each day to face the responsibilities and sorrows, not just somehow, but triumphantly and confidently.

Each of us is influenced by the attitudes of the larger culture as well as by our own experiences and education. When a child has an impairment devalued by the community, the parents frequently hold the same biases. They will need to resolve this conflict before they can interact freely with the child. Juxtaposition of values is not an easy task and requires much sensitivity from practitioners while the parents are reassessing their values.

Some parents may experience extreme conflict regarding the decision to institutionalize a child or adult family member. They are caught between what is best for the person involved and their own feelings of what is best for the family as well as the reaction of family members (immediate and extended), friends, and the community. Each situation must be handled individually. Some children do require specialized care, but a premature or inappropriately timed placement may result in adverse long term psychosocial effects to both the child and the parents. Most developmentalists recommend caring for a child at home as long as possible in order to develop a sense of selfhood and security in the child, since this is the essential foundation for learning about one's own potentials and the environment.

COMMUNITY ATTITUDE

The support of the community and friends is vitally important. Friends, not knowing what to say and coping with their own disappointment and vicarious grief, frequently avoid the family with a disabled member or the couple with a disabled child. When they meet on the street, eyes are averted and faces become rigid. Feelings of isolation are reinforced. The couple suddenly feels as if they have done something terribly wrong, that they are contagious or grossly inferior. Families are fortunate indeed who have friends that are still able to see them simply as John and Mary, not as the couple with the defective baby, or as if one member had ceased to exist.

Response Patterns of Parents

Even though the parents have not seen their baby, attachment has already been made to an idealized infant [21]. With the birth of an impaired infant or the injury of a child, the parents' fears of having a damaged child are realized. The parents are consequently presented with two major problems: (1) to resolve the loss of their dreams, and (2) to accept the reality of their new child. The highly charged longings for the normal child are recalled and intensely felt while they are gradually released, with reinvestment in the real child [40]. The release of the idealized infant or injured child requires strenuous "grief work"—a process that some parents may never complete because of the pain involved. It

is also difficult to both release and reinvest at the same time [12]. Each contact with the child may serve as a reminder of the lost "ideal" child.

IMMEDIATE BEHAVIORS

Although there is wide variation in the magnitude of expressed behaviors and in their duration, the grief process progresses rather predictably through five stages [3], which are discussed in the following sections. Somatic complaints are frequent during the earlier stages. Unless good supportive guidance is available in the early months, the parents may not be able to complete each stage successfully and may continue to exhibit behaviors typical of an early stage for many years. Many parents do not complete stage 4 for about 4 to 6 months or longer, depending on the type and degree of disability as well as on the quality of support offered. Some parents may never resolve the first four stages. A parent may also exhibit behaviors of more than one stage or may return to an earlier stage while attempting to complete grief work. Asynchronous movement of the parents through the stages may cause tension by creating communication barriers between them.

Stage 1. When the parents learn of the disability, they characteristically exhibit symptoms of shock and denial. ("It can't be true." "Are you sure it's the right baby?") Numbness and disbelief set in; the whole world seems unreal; feelings of detachment and unreality predominate. The parent listens but does not hear what is said; it is too much to take in all at once. The parents may put the existence of their baby's disability out of their minds, repressing it as a defense against emotional pain. They may need to have the situation explained a third, fourth, or fifth time, simply and honestly, before the reality begins to have meaning to them.

This stage includes feelings of sorrow, emptiness, and helplessness. Uncontrollable spontaneous weeping or complete apathy may be observed. The parents' thoughts and behaviors are still directed toward the loss of the idealized child. They may deny the existence of the disability while mourning the death of the child of their dreams. Their thoughts focus on their own personal loss. Denial is healthy in that it allows the parents to absorb the reality slowly, at their own pace. It is wise for the physician to recommend or obtain for the parents a second opinion or consultation during this period. This second opinion helps to confirm the reality of the situation and also helps to engender confidence and trust in the physician. Parents seeking a consultation on their own may hesitate to return to the first physician.

The phase of shock and denial may last several days to several months. Some families continue in the denial aspect for years; they may exhaust themselves physically, emotionally, and financially searching for a doctor who will deny the diagnosis or promise a "miracle cure." Stage 1 is characterized by both cognitive and affective denial.

Stage 2. Stage 2 is characterized by cognitive awareness of the deviation from the dream child but continued affective denial. This awareness results in intense anger, hostility, and the need to fight anything or anyone who is connected with the disability or who imposes confrontation with reality. As a result, expressions of hostility are frequently directed toward the doctor or the hospital staff. As parents continue to search for an answer to "Why me?" and to affix blame to an event or person, they may become angry with each other, other (normal) children, or themselves. Anger toward God may be expressed through refusal to attend church or to pray. Anger toward the child and toward God may be felt but is difficult to express, and thus other adults in the environment may be used as emotional scapegoats for the displaced hostility. Professional persons who are able to recognize that the anger is not a personal attack (even though it may be thus verbalized) find it much easier to deal constructively with parents who are expressing acute hostility due to grief. Counterattack on the hostile parents may increase their feelings of guilt and intensify or prolong their grief.

Some parents may blame the doctor for poor obstetrical practice, even when the disability is a result of a genetic or an environmental factor. Warm, open, honest support at this time can facilitate the grieving process and lay a foundation for realistic, constructive adaptation to the circumstances and healthy, cooperative relationships with health and educational practitioners.

Anger may also result from a perceived incompetence to produce a whole child or to prevent an accident as well as the incompetence to care for a child with special needs. Both are a threat to self-esteem. The parent may feel hatred toward the child as the source of the threat to self-esteem. Hatred in turn may precipitate feelings of anger and guilt. Encouragement of physical activities that simulate a normal routine and help the parents to learn any special procedures essential to the care of their child may increase feelings of competence and help to offset some of the excessive

energy generated by their feelings of helplessness and anger.

Stage 3. Stage 3 is characterized by appeals for help. Cognitive rebellion is moderated by affective awareness of the reality. The parents may begin to reach out to the physician (provided the relationship is still intact) to explore other diagnostic possibilities or to find a new cure. Others may spare no expense in their search for an "educational cure." They cling unrealistically (to the observer) to the hope of cure. The mother may feel that if she gives the child enough love and attention, the problem will resolve itself—an attitude reminiscent of the magical thought powers of the preschooler.

The parents may also begin bargaining with God through increased prayer and church attendance. Pleas are made to God to cure the child and remove their shame. Promises may be made and even money offered. Disenchantment may ensue when no cure is forthcoming.

The positive aspect of stage 3 is that the parents' energies are now focused toward the real child rather than toward the lost child or their own narcissistic hurt.

Stage 4. Stages three and four are frequently interchanged and revisited. When all active coping strategies have failed to remove the problem, the parents may lapse into deep depression, withdrawal, despair, and disorganization. This stage represents the family's complete exhaustion. They have not yet accepted the reality, but the facts have imposed themselves on the parents, and they can no longer resist them [37]. Defensive retreat—a dulling of reality—appears to be an essential prelude to reorganization and mobilization of constructive coping strategies. There is a final letting go of the dream child in this stage; this activity is very painful. Olshansky indicates that many parents are never completely able to release the idealized child and continue through life in a state of chronic sorrow [30]. Most parents eventually are able to acknowledge the impairment even if they are unhappy about the child's disability. They are able to mobilize and to reorganize priorities, values, and coping strategies sufficiently to be able to cognitively and effectively accept the disability (stage 5).

Although complete acceptance of both the child and the disability represents the ultimate goal, some families are never able to reorganize their self-system completely so that their energies are totally directed toward the real child. Most parents experience residual elements of stage 4 when the child enters a new developmental stage or is faced with new tasks. Periodic grief reactions are normal in the "best adjusted" parent [23, 46]. It is not a denial but a facing of reality to feel sorrow for the child who (1) experiences difficulty with new tasks (e.g., the tying of shoes by a blind child); (2) is unable to join in an activity enjoyed by the parents (e.g., inability to enjoy a rendition of Handel's *Messiah* by a deaf child); or (3) faces a developmental milestone (e.g., menarche in a Down's syndrome daughter).

The critical times for parents are (1) when they first suspect or discover a disability, (2) when the child enters public school (5 to 6 years of age), (3) when the child leaves public school and seeks employment or independent living (18 to 21 years of age), and (4) when the parents are unable to continue caring for a child because of age or illness [36]. Even parents of normal children feel a sense of loss and stress at these times. Parents of disabled children are forced to face the widening gap between the ideal and the real child once more and make appropriate adjustments without role models, and usually with inadequate professional assistance.

Stage 5. Even though parents may retain residual feelings or behaviors from previous stages, most are able to adapt constructively to the realities of life with the less than ideal child and begin to find joy in the relationship and pride in the child's accomplishments. They learn to appreciate what the child can do and love him or her in spite of the impairment [10]. Acceptance does not mean resignation to the impairment. The parent in this stage is characterized by the ability to appreciate realistically the child's abilities and to develop these abilities while making modifications for the child's limitations. The focus becomes the child's progress toward maximization of potentials rather than the parent's disappointment that the child is abnormal. Goals and approaches are appropriately modified to the child's functioning level. This parent

can function as an active member of the professional habilitation team. In fact, parents who are unable to reach this stage may be the casualties of insensitive, inept handling by practitioners during earlier stages rather than representing an inherent inability to accept imperfection in their offspring.

The complete resolution of stage 5 may take many months, or even years. How can one realistically accept an uncertain, unpredictable future? Extensions of the grief process beyond 6 months may indicate a need for more intensive professional counseling. Sensitive counseling at a later time can still help parents to resolve earlier thoughts and feelings so that stage 5 can be successfully reached. However, rearing a disabled child is a dynamic process in which the parents may need to renegotiate their acceptance of the child and the disability at each major new challenge [29]. Many become extremely competent paraprofessionals who can be rich resources for the new (and old) practitioner.

LONG-RANGE REACTIONS AND ADAPTATION

Successful completion of the grief process requires not only the release of the idealized child but also acceptance of (1) the personhood of the real child, and (2) the limitations of the disability. Various combinations of acceptance and denial lead to different long-term parent-child relationships (see Table 35–1).

When the idealized child is not released, the parents (or parent) may continue to reject the real child because of the unresolvable discrepancies. The disability may also be denied. Synchrony of communication is not established, and professional assistance may be resisted. Children of these parents are the most likely candidates for the syndrome of neglect and failure to thrive. The child may be related to more as a bothersome pet than as a respected, cherished person.

Some parents may continue to retain the idealized image of the child and transfer these dreams to the real child. The disability is denied or ignored. The parents' expectations may remain the same for the child even

Table 35–1. Long-Range Parental Reactions to Child with a Disability

Type of Reaction	Attitude toward Child	Attitude toward Disability	Manifestation of Reaction
Rejection	Rejected	Denied	Neglect of Child
Idealization	Accepted	Denied	"Pushing" the child
Pity	Rejected	Accepted	"Smothering" the child
Realistic acceptance	Accepted	Accepted	Constructive guidance

though the disabled individual is unable to fulfill them. The parents may feel that the social stigma of having a disabled child is unbearable, and may focus their energies toward retaining their own self-esteem rather than maximizing the child's potentials. They may be very hostile toward the child and use abusive methods of discipline in trying to make the child meet their goals. These parents may continue to seek a miracle cure and refuse special educational assistance.

A third group of parents completely lose contact with their idealized child. They accept the disability to the point where it becomes the focus of all interaction with the child ("**We** have a **defective** baby"). The disabilities outweigh the child's normal aspects, and the child as an individual is lost. The child's uniqueness and individuality are not acknowledged in the parents' sorrow over the child's defect and in the stereotyped behaviors or responses they attach to the defect. Their own feelings of guilt regarding the cause of the defect may also cause them to concentrate on the disability, or they may be attempting to cover up for conscious or subconscious feelings of disgust or rejection toward the child. The end result is intense pity for the child and smothering, overprotective behaviors to hide or to atone for their own negative feelings. The parents attempt to remove all further problems and frustrations from the child. They may become so devoted in their attention that they do not allow the child challenging opportunities for growth; they make the child dependent on them and thus create a handicap. The parents also lose their own identity as they become slaves to the disabling condition. They may feel the disability with its attendant special care needs gives them special status and, thus, relate to the child as paraprofessionals rather than as loving parents.

The parent who is able to release the idealized child and to accept fully both the child and the disability is in the best position to deal with the circumstances realistically and constructively. This attitude does not imply that all grief over the loss is eradicated, but it does mean that the parent is able to identify both the assets and the liabilities of the child and to extricate the self from narcissistic delusions and personal guilt. This parent may still become irritable from fatigue, depressed by financial concern, or discouraged by slow progress. This milieu allows for the personal growth of both the child and the parent. They are able to work around the disability to achieve tasks. Joy is found in small progress. The child is gradually included as an active part of the team, with the parent giving help and guidance only as necessary.

LIVING WITH A DISABLED FAMILY MEMBER

Disabled Child

Approximately one out of every seven families has a handicapped child. Entrance of a disabled child into the family alters almost every aspect of family life. The parents face much more than the process of mourning the loss of the dream child and accepting the real child with a disability—parents wish it were that simple. The level of family functioning (see Chap. 34) may temporarily disintegrate or further compound perceived stressors and feelings of helplessness. Essential medical care increases the financial burden of the family. The family expenses may also be increased by extra laundry, damaged clothing and furniture, extra heating, or the need for additional domestic help, baby sitters, or respite care [42].

The mother may feel compelled to stay at home with the child, although she had planned to return to work. Consequently, the financial base is eroded as well as the potential for career fulfillment. The father may need to find a second job in order to meet the additional expenses. Some parents may decide to change jobs in order to obtain a higher income even though the employment may not meet their own actualization needs. Other families may feel the need to move or to remain in an area where more appropriate medical or educational resources are available. The travel time to and from doctors' offices and hospitals can be physically exhausting.

Hoping against the odds and facing the uncertainty of the future can be emotionally exhausting. Caring for a child who requires special care or exercises or who is frequently in pain will exact its toll even from an exceptionally stable and mature parent. It is frequently the mother who must absorb the pressures of day-to-day care of the severely disabled child. The father usually maintains a fairly routine schedule of employment outside the home, but the mother's responsibilities gradually increase as she must drive the child to clinics, ongoing therapy programs, and preschool programs. It is usually the mother who remains at the hospital with the child if surgery is scheduled, or serious complications require specialized care [23, 28]. It is also usually the mother who searches the stores for special food products or equipment to meet the child's needs; implements a therapy program at home; cooks the special diet; or performs the dressing, toileting, and general activities of daily living that the child is unable to perform. All these activities are added to the mother's other responsibilities of managing the home and caring for the other children. Unless the father is able to give her some relief from these responsibilities, she may have little or no time for the development of her own interests or for meeting her own needs as an individual.

When a family member needs extensive care at home, responsible family members may experience "burn out" [44]. Families need referral to respite care centers that offer temporary relief [32]. Unfortunately, there are not enough care centers available. Extended care facilities and nursing homes can offer some relief while family members take a well-earned vacation or parents recuperate from their own illnesses.

The delay in the infant's use of interactional tools may discourage the parents who need reinforcement to indicate that they are "being good parents." Personal goals may be thwarted and family interaction time reduced. Leisure time activities are also altered and reduced. When outings are planned, the parents of the severely disabled child may have to pack a wheel chair, special eating utensils, extra clothes, medications, special toys, and other accoutrements essential to the functioning or independence of the child. Physical and emotional exhaustion, fear of another pregnancy, and limited amounts of time available for intimate solitude may interfere with the parents' sexual life, again increasing their sense of personal isolation [27]. All these factors and more contribute to the increased incidence of marital problems, divorce, suicide, and alcoholism found in parents with disabled children [2]. Parents need to be encouraged to find some personal "release" time and to continue to engage in activities that allow them to enjoy each other's companionship.

The parents who have only one child, and the child is disabled, also need to consider the kind of life they will have, for example, in 20 years. Some parents will so involve themselves in the needs of their disabled child that other aspects of their life as a family are neglected. Personal accomplishments may be eclipsed by the needs of the child. If the child dies or is institutionalized later on, the parents may suddenly feel abandoned, that they have fought against the odds through the years and are now left with nothing. The parents may find they are strangers to each other or even may feel their lives have been wasted on an individual who could never adequately repay their efforts by becoming more independent. They are left without an identity or a future, and may feel alienated again—or still. A second child can give them a sense of personal worth and accomplishment, help to main-

tain a sense of normalcy in family life, and offer relief from the intensity of care and entertainment the severely disabled child may require. A physically and mentally normal child can draw out and challenge the disabled child in ways the parents never dreamed. There can be healthier lives for everyone with a second and a third child. Siblings can have a normalizing effect on the whole family [38]. If the risk of another disabled child is too great, children can be added by adoption. The family with a disabled child may find life difficult, but life can also be enormously enriched by the child's presence.

Up to this point, the discussion has been limited to the mother-father-child triad. However, the family does not live in a vacuum. Relationships with others within the extended family or the community can also facilitate or hinder the parents' long-range adjustment.

REACTION OF GRANDPARENTS

At a time when the parents need someone strong and wise to confide in, they may find that their own parents may increase rather than share the burden [26]. The grandparents may continue to deny the problem, or they may offer suggestions for care and guidance that may be contrary to professional advice and can interfere with the parents' ability to cope realistically with the child's limitations. Occasionally grandparents may become so distraught that role reversals occur— the parents end up comforting the grandparents.

Some grandparents may feel embarrassed by the situation and may seek to prevent the news from leaking out to friends and neighbors—especially if the child has a hereditary disorder. One family kept their secret from both sets of in-laws and all friends for more than 10 years by institutionalizing the impaired child. Grandparents may also react with anger and attempt to affix the blame to the other side of the family. ("I told you not to marry ——." "You might have expected your child to be blind because your wife wears glasses" [even though both the father and grandmother may also wear glasses].) These grandparents appear to suffer from even more narcissistic hurt than the parents do.

Fortunately, there are also those grandparents who care more deeply about the child than about their hereditary pride and thus attempt to support the parents. The grandparents' pain can be reduced and their support capabilities strengthened if the parents are able to include them in all the information shared by the physician and in the working through of plans. If they live close enough, they can provide significant help to the parents by assuming some of the home care activities and by providing transportation and babysitting relief for the parents. Parents who are isolated from extended family members may find that the emotional and physical burdens of raising a severely disabled child without ready assistance can be very taxing on their physical and emotional health and that respite care is essential.

REACTION OF SIBLINGS

The brothers and sisters of the disabled child will know sooner or later that something is wrong. If the parents attempt to hide the fact of the disability, the truth may be distorted by youthful imaginations working overtime. The siblings may begin to wonder if the disability is their fault, or if it might happen to them also [27]. Honest, simple explanations can help to alleviate a great deal of fear and misunderstanding. When the disability is the result of a genetic factor, the parents and the siblings should have genetic counseling made available to them. Genetic counseling is also essential for the family planning of extended family members.

The siblings' attitude is usually a direct reflection of the parents' **true** reaction to the disabled child [19]. Some siblings are able to take life with a disabled family member in stride and include the disabled individual as much as possible in the normal activities of

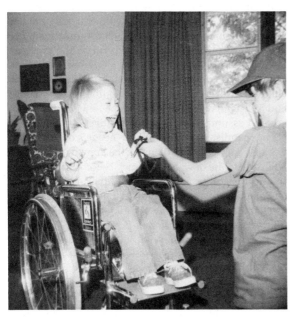

Figure 35–3. The sibling relationship as well as the disabled child's self-concept is usually directly correlated with the parents' true reaction to the disability and their acceptance of it.

family life and daily living. Others are embarrassed by the disability and may refuse to have friends visit the home or refuse to accompany the family to social events when the disabled child is included. Sibling rivalry can be intense. The "normal" child may resent the abnormal home life or the extra time the "handicapped" child extracts from the parents. The disabled child may be jealous of the normal child's skills and opportunities [8]. Mutual sharing of grief, mutual planning for the future, and mutual involvement in the habilitation program can help siblings to develop mature responsibility and respect for human rights and human dignity. It should be emphasized again that the total family can be drawn closer together by the event when communication lines remain open and individuality is respected. If the child is hospitalized, siblings can be encouraged to maintain daily communication through telephone calls, tape recordings, pictures, and notes [8].

A potential source of problems is the sibling who becomes overinvolved in the care or responsibilities for the disabled child. Some siblings may change their life plans in order to continue to care for the disabled member. Parents should encourage each child to continue to seek out individual talents and interests in order to maximize potentials. Some siblings may also try to "take over" for the disabled child, hindering efforts toward independence. They need to learn to share in the joy of helping the disabled member to become more independent. By including the disabled sibling in games of pretending and in the normal bantering that occurs in families, and by allowing the disabled sibling opportunities for both winning and losing at games, the other siblings can help prepare the disabled child to face the adult world with greater flexibility and stronger coping skills. Individuals who have grown up in such an environment frequently possess great sensitivity to the needs of disabled persons and may seek careers in which they can advocate and protect the rights of disabled individuals.

REACTION OF FRIENDS

Close friends may experience a grief process similar to that experienced by the parents, grandparents, and siblings. Because of greater distance, however, the reaction is usually not as intense. Some friends are able to empathize with and offer support to the parents. Many others, however, may be so consumed by their own grief, or so concerned that they will increase the parents' grief if they say the wrong thing, that they may avoid the couple in order to avoid an awkward situation. Again, the parents may suddenly find themselves alone. Their friends are avoiding them, and they are too stunned to reach out for help. Their sense of alienation is too intense for words. Sometimes, all the parents may need is a shoulder to cry on, not words of comfort.

More distant friends and community members are frequently curious—a normal phenomenon, but one that is distressing to the parents, who suddenly feel that they are on public display. Parents may avoid leaving the home except for essentials, such as grocery shopping; thus they may feel imprisoned in their own home, another factor that increases feelings of alienation and depression. The drastic change in the family's life-style may also create stress and increase stigma and fear.

Although friends and community members are curious at first, the parents' attitude becomes critical to the child's acceptance by the community. "The child must depend on his parents to take a stand, to assert his identity as a worthwhile individual" [27]. The parents function as role models for the rest of the community in relating to the child. This may be easy to

say, but it is very difficult for parents who have no guidelines for themselves. The parents' personal identity must be strong and their acceptance of the child's disability must be high to help change the attitude of the public from one of curiosity and stigma to one of respect, understanding, and acceptance. This change becomes a lifelong process. The parents' modeling changes with the child's developmental and skill level.

Disabled Adult

When a parent is disabled, the responsibilities for maintaining the family system must be reassigned. Depending on the degree of disability and dependency, the nondisabled parent may feel the responsibilities too great to maintain the family as a separate system, which may force the disabled member back to the family of origin or into a nursing home. Sometimes children feel obligated to abbreviate their educational pursuits because of limited financial resources and the need for baby sitting or homecare assistance while the nondisabled parent works.

The extent of disability, the financial security, the age of the children, and the availability of extended family or close friends to assist with the reassignment of family tasks (as well as the new responsibilities) are critical components in the ability of the family to adapt to the new circumstances. Children may become very resentful of the usurpation of their time or may rally to the task, achieving new levels of self-understanding and maturity. Their reactions depend on the previous child-parent relationship as well as parental handling at the time. Professional counseling is valuable as the children grieve the loss of the old (the known parent and life-style) while adjusting to the new (disabled parent and assumption of responsibilities).

The nondisabled parent also needs counseling to work through the grief of losing the known partner and adjusting to the new: Sex life may become nonexistent; financial stability may be eroded; the individual may feel inadequately prepared to assume the necessary responsibilities; social contacts may be curtailed while interaction with professionals is increased. The parent may try to manage the grief, fear, or questions of the children without having resolved them personally. In spite of all these barriers, most families with disabled adults find highly adaptive life-styles. Some may even emerge enriched by the experience as they undergo major adjustments in their value systems and priorities, which in turn enables them to appreciate in a new way the value of health, family, and friends as well as a deeper purpose in life.

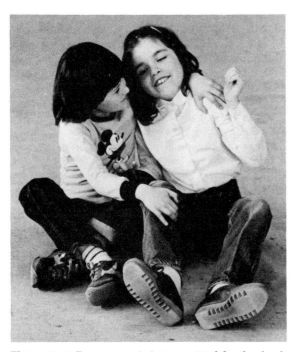

Figure 35–4. Peer contact is just as critical for the development of the disabled child as it is for the physically and mentally "normal" child. Such relationships benefit all persons involved.

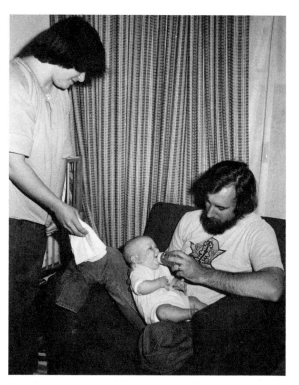

Figure 35–5. Disabled family members need to be included in family responsibilities. The disability does not negate the individual's ability to love, parent, discipline, or share.

MAXIMIZING FAMILY POTENTIALS

Too often the focus of professional intervention for the family with a disabled member becomes the disability—the individual's limitations and the corresponding therapeutic measures to prevent complications, to ameliorate the deficiency, or to correct the impairment. This approach is erroneous because the impairment is only one facet of the person's life. The client must be approached from a holistic perspective—as a total person and as a member of a family system. The family is the child's first and most effective teacher. Including the parents as integral respected members of the habilitation team is financially judicious and can elevate parental competence in performing essential skills, enhance parental self-esteem, facilitate the parent-child bonding process, and, in the long run, foster greater independence in the child. The mother's major concern is usually interpersonal relationships—hers and the child's. The father's major concerns generally center around financial independence—his own

as well as for the child's adult years [16]. If an adult member of the family is disabled, practitioners need to consult with the entire family to help them reassess roles and responsibilities. Education on sexuality and sexual techniques may become a critical issue [7]. Timely, effective counseling can help maintain family integrity and the personal growth of the individual members.

Immediate Assistance to Families

Whether the professional counselor is a physician, nurse, psychologist, minister, social worker, or teacher, two fundamental concepts of successful counseling must be offered:

1. Acceptance of the feelings, perceptions, and cultural values of the client. This does not mean that the practitioner agrees with these feelings, but one must acknowledge that the feelings are real and painful to the client and accept them on that basis.
2. Assistance for the client to see the reality of the situation in a healthy, constructive way. This may require reassessment of values and priorities, which is a difficult task that involves a disequilibrium before the reintegration of the self-system.

The counselor cannot force a client to agree with new views; neither can the practitioner help the client to see reality if the practitioner does not openly accept and deal with the client's feelings. The client must feel accepted and understood before there is sufficient energy available to accept and understand what the counselor has to offer.

The practitioner working with the family needs to be honest and open in discussing the disabled person's status. Explanations should be simple and repeated as necessary. Discussions should show acceptance and concern for the people who have lost a precious family member. Negative predictions for the future should not be offered, since no one can predict with complete accuracy, and these predictions tend to increase anxiety unnecessarily. However, family members should be informed of realistic alternatives and the critical factors, such as education, that can influence the disabled person's future. The practitioner should discuss the disabled person's condition in terms of the present and the near future, emphasizing the family's role in maximizing the person's current potentials.

The practitioner can offer the family members support in their expressions of grief, reassuring them that such feelings are normal can be very therapeutic. To label a parent "hysterical" is stigmatizing and can aggravate grief (stoicism may be a pathological behavior, not a healthy one). Occasionally a family member may need a mild tranquilizer for assistance through the early period. Acceptance of reality may be difficult for some family members. Physical symptoms, such as fatigue, weakness, aching, emptiness, headache, frequent sighing, or shortness and tightness of breath, can all be closely related to grief and need to be treated accordingly [26].

Family members need encouragement and support in the difficult process of accepting the disabled person, the diagnosis, and their own feelings. If they feel that their own reactions are abnormal or a sign of weakness, this feeling may stand in the way of successful completion of the grieving process. Guilt is the most difficult feeling to work through. If people can identify the source of their guilt response, it will frequently resolve without further assistance. However, the affective domain is not always easily controlled by the cognitive domain. Showing one's acceptance of the disabled person and of family members can be very supportive. The realistic identification of the positive qualities of an infant or a disabled person can also facilitate acceptance by the family.

Two very helpful hints can be shared with family members. The first is to take one day at a time. When people try to see the whole future at once, it is overwhelming. Many anticipated problems never materialize when the needs of each day are met successfully. Second, in the case of a disabled child, the parents should see the child as a baby or as a child first and interact on that basis, at times pretending a bit if they must (e.g., it may make the parents feel better to hang a mobile over the crib of a blind infant). The parents should be encouraged to play with the child and talk to him or her (even the deaf child) and to vary their care and attention only as absolutely necessary. In short, the parents should enjoy the child.

The parents may need much support in recognizing the emotional needs of the infant or child. Although disabled, the infant still exhibits more normalcy than deviancy. Families are frequently told to "treat him (or her) as you would any other baby." Although this is true in many situations, this concept may be difficult for parents to understand or to accept. The infant still needs food, shelter, clothing, and protection. Most of all, the child needs the same discipline, challenges, playtime, warmth and love that is offered to every other child. The individual will continue to grow up with or without the parents' help, and the disability may still be there when the individual reaches adulthood. How-

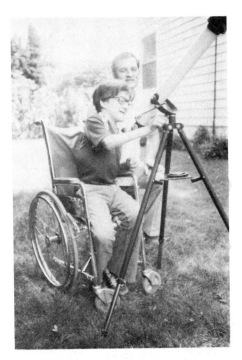

Figure 35–6. Parents are challenged to find unique yet normal activities that enable them to enjoy a common interest with their disabled child.

ever, a child will grow up more successfully and better able to face life independently if he or she has had the parents' love, acceptance, and realistic guidance as an infant and young child. Inadequate parental acceptance and support may prevent realization of the child's full potentials.

Long-Range Assistance for Family Members

The competence and coping skills of family members are increased when they feel secure in the elements of basic care. Consequently, family members need to be taught the special procedures and exercises to maintain or help to regain maximal functioning levels for the disabled person. Informing parents about Havighurst's tasks may help them to understand their role in the child's development. The disabled person may need to use an alternative strategy for achieving a certain task (see Chap. 19). Finding alternative strategies can offer a challenge to the creativity of family members, and can be a source of increased self-esteem when they can take an active part in formulating a successful approach. Parents may be encouraged to keep a diary or to record the occurrence of specific behaviors in order to help them to see progress in a child, since the day-to-day progress may be so slow that discouragement sets in. The ability to evaluate the progress made in a concrete way can be a reinforcer for the parents.

The most difficult or distressing period for many family members may be the time span between diagnosis and the identification of sources of assistance in establishing plans for habilitation or rehabilitation. The family needs to be put in touch with the appropriate agencies that can give them specific ideas or support in meeting the disabled person's special needs or can assist them in meeting financial needs. The person or persons who give the family members a diagnosis also have a moral responsibility to offer them referral to potential sources of assistance in helping them to maximize the disabled person's potentials. Too many families are left to find these limited sources on their own.

The parents of chronically ill or disabled children need support at the time of crisis but may also continue to need support counseling periodically throughout the years [24]. Many support groups have grown out of a concern for a specific disability, such as cystic fibrosis, cerebral palsy, Down's syndrome, or paraplegia. To list all of them would be impossible and impractical, but it is important to note that new parents and newly disabled persons and their families can receive very real support from someone else who has been through the same experience, and their sense of isolation can be greatly reduced. The following agencies can function as central clearing houses that can refer families to interested groups that can provide specific reading materials or lend support:

1. Closer Look, National Information Center for the Handicapped, Box 1492, Washington, DC 20013
2. Council for Exceptional Children, 1920 Association Drive, Reston, VA 22091
3. Local Mental Health Associations
4. Local Public Health nurses
5. Local public schools' departments of special education
6. Local Head Start programs (ages 3 to 5 years)
7. National Association of the Physically Handicapped, 76 Elm Street, London, OH 43140
8. National Paraplegic/Quadriplegic Foundation, 333 North Michigan Avenue, Chicago, IL 60604

The parents of blind or deaf children are in particular need of very early intervention. Assistance with blind children can be obtained without charge through the local state's bureau of vocational rehabilitation or bureau of services for the blind and for deaf children

from the John Tracy Clinic, 806 W. Adams Blvd., Los Angeles, CA 90007 (Telephone: [213] 748-5481). The local Social Security Administration provides financial support (supplemental security income) to many eligible children and adults.

Several books may prove very helpful to parents who are struggling to understand themselves and a child's special needs. Six books that are exceptionally well written and have wide applicability are the following: Pearl Buck, The Child Who Never Grew (New York: John Day, 1950); Marie Killilea, Karen (Englewood Cliffs, NJ: Prentice-Hall, 1962); Audrey McCollum, Coping With Prolonged Health Impairment in Your Child (Boston: Little, Brown, 1975); Eugene McDonald, Understanding Those Feelings (Pittsburgh: Stanwix House, 1962); Elsie Wentworth, Listen to Your Heart (Boston: Houghton Mifflin, 1974); Bonnie Wheeler, Challenged Parenting, A Practical Handbook for Parents of Children with Handicaps (Ventura, CA: Regal Books, 1983).

Parents in the United States should be reassured that Public Law 94-142 guarantees their disabled child a free, appropriate public education (see Chap. 19). Section 10 of the Education Act of 1976 guarantees similar educational services to British citizens [43]. Early contact with the local school system can facilitate the early planning for appropriate services, placement, and equipment. Some communities offer educational programs to children as young as 1 month of age. The state Bureau of Vocational Rehabilitation offers training/educational services for disabled adults.

CONCLUSION

The entrance of a disabled member into the family is one of the "most stressful experiences that a family can endure" [19]. The event will ultimately influence almost every aspect of family life. The disabled person needs to be challenged and supported in efforts to become or remain an active member of the family system. Complete dependency is oppressive and demoralizing. The inclusion of the disabled member's opinion in decision-making processes will enhance self-esteem and can ease the burdens of leadership. Active participation in division-of-labor can also aid the disabled individual to maintain self-esteem.

Grief for the loss of the idealized child must occur before the parents can begin to attach to the real child. Barring unusual circumstances, the disabled child will continue to grow and develop toward adulthood. Except in cases of very severe disability, the degree to which the child will be able to cope with life will depend more on parental attitudes, guidance, and support than on the degree of the disability per se. The parents will need to accept the disability before the child can accept it; the child will need to accept the disability before he or she can accept the self, he or she will need to accept the self before he or she can enjoy the environment, and he or she will need to enjoy the environment before he or she can learn effectively from it.

The practitioner's role is to support the family's expressions of grief while helping members to identify strengths in both themselves and in the disabled family member. Many families find it helpful to have contact with an older child or adult with the same disability who is adapting successfully to the activities of daily living. It helps both the family members and the disabled person to realistically identify ways that the disabilities can be minimized (not eliminated) by maximizing abilities (see Chap. 19).

When a severely disabled person enters the family, it interrupts both family life and the functioning of the individuals within that family [17]. Effective counseling can help families in establishing effective coping patterns and the new directions and meanings to life that are critical to the successful long-range adaptation of each family member. Each member can bring unique pleasure and rewards to the family—but only if given the chance.

REFERENCES

1. Baum, M. H. Some dynamic factors affecting family adjustment to the handicapped child. *Except. Child.* 28:387, 1962.
2. Bloch, J. Impaired children, *Children Today* 7(6):2, 1978.
3. Bowlby, J. Grief and mourning in infancy and early childhood. *Psychoanal. Study Child* 15:9, 1960.
4. Branson, H. K. When a defective infant is born. *Bedside Nurse* 3(11):18, 1970.
5. Buscaglia, L. (Ed.). *The Disabled and Their Parents: A Counseling Challenge.* Thorofare, NJ: Slack, 1983.
6. Butani, P. Reactions of mothers to the birth of an anomalous infant. *Matern.–Child Nurs. J.* 3:59, 1974.
7. Cornelius, D. A., et al. *Who cares? A handbook on sex education and counseling services for disabled people* (2nd ed.). Baltimore; University Park Press, 1982.
8. Craft, M. J. Help for the family's neglected "other" child. *MCN* 4:297, 1979.
9. Daniels, L. L., and Berg, C. The crisis of birth and adaptive patterns of parents of amputee children. *Clinical Procedures, Children's Hospital* 24(4):108, 1968.
10. Darling, R. B., and Darling, J. *Children Who are Different: Meeting the Challenges of Birth Defects in Society.* St. Louis: Mosby, 1982.
11. Deutsch, H. *The Psychology of Women, Vol. II, Motherhood.* New York: Grune & Stratton, 1945.
12. Engel, G. L. Grief and grieving. *Am. J. Nurs.* 64(9):93, 1961.
13. Evans, S., Reinhart, J., and Succop, R. A study of 45 children and their families. *J. Am. Acad. Child Psychiatry* 11:440, 1972.
14. Fraiberg, S. Blind Infants and Their Mothers. In M. Lewis and L. A. Rosenblum (Eds.), *The Effect of the Infant on Its Caregiver.* New York: Wiley, 1974.
15. Graceley, K. A. Parental attachment to a child with a congenital defect. *Pediatr. Nurs.* 3(5):15, 1977.
16. Gumz, E., and Gubrium, J. Comparative parental perceptions of a mentally retarded child. *Am. J. Ment. Defic.* 77(2):175, 1972.
17. Harris, S. L. *Families of the Developmentally Disabled: A Guide to Behavioral Intervention.* New York: Pergamon Press, 1983.
18. Hildebrandt, K. A., and Fitzgerald, H. E. The infant's physical attractiveness: Its effect on bonding and attachment. *Infant Mental Health Journal.* 4:3, 1983.
19. Howard, J. The influence of Children's Developmental Dysfunctions on Marital Quality and Family Interaction. In R. M. Lerner and G. B. Spanier, *Child Influences on Marital and Family Interactions: A Life-Span Perspective.* New York: Academic Press, 1978.
20. Howell, S. E. Psychiatric aspects of habilitation. *Pediatr. Clin. North Am.* 20:203, 1973.
21. Kennell, J., Slyter, H., and Klaus, M. The mourning response of parents to the death of a newborn infant. *N. Engl. J. Med.* 283:344, 1970.
22. Klein, H. R., Potter, H. W., and Dyk, Ruth B. *Anxiety in Pregnancy and Childbirth.* New York: Hoeber, 1950.
23. Knafl, K. A., Deatrick, J. A., and Kodadek, S. How parents manage jobs and a child's hospitalization. *MCN* 7:125, 1982.
24. Kornblum, H., and Anderson, B. "Acceptance" reassessed—A point of view. *Child Psychiatry Hum. Dev.* 12(3):171, 1982.
25. Lax, R. F. Some aspects of the interaction between mother and impaired child: Mother's narcissistic trauma. *Int. J. Psychoanal.* 53(Part 3):339, 1972.
26. Lindemann, E. Acute grief: Symptoms and management. *Child and Family* 4:73, 1965.
27. McCollum, A. T. *Coping With Prolonged Health Impairment in Your Child.* Boston: Little, Brown, 1975.
28. McKeever, P. T. Fathering the chronically ill child. *MCN* 6:124, 1981.
29. Murphy, M. A. The family with a handicapped child: A review of the literature. *Developmental and Behavioral Pediatrics* 3(2):73, 1982.
30. Olshansky, S. Chronic sorrow: A response to having a mentally defective child. *Soc. Casework* 43:190, 1962.

31. Pi, E. H. Congenitally handicapped children and their families: Short- and long-term intervention. *Pediatric Basics* 31:10, 1981.

32. Powell, T. H., and Hecimovic, A. *Respite Care for the Handicapped: Helping Individuals and Their Families.* Springfield, IL: Thomas, 1981.

33. Ross, A. O. *The Exceptional Child in the Family.* New York: Grune & Stratton, 1964.

34. Schuster, C. S. "Disabled Child Without a Handicap." Unpublished paper, 1975.

35. Schuster, C. S. *Selected and Annotated Bibliography on the Reactions of Parents to Physically Disabled Infants* (ERIC Document Reproduction Service No. ED 125 177), 1976.

36. Seligman, M. *Strategies for Helping Parents of Exceptional Children: A Guide for Teachers.* New York: Free Press, 1979.

37. Shontz, F. C. Reactions to crisis. *Volta Review* 67:364, 1965.

38. Simeonsson, R. J., and McHale, S. M. Review. Research on handicapped children: Sibling relationships. *Child: Care, Health and Development* 7:153, 1981.

39. Simpson, A. Personal communication, 1977.

40. Solnit, A. J., and Stark, M. H. Mourning and the birth of a defective child. *Psychoanal. Study Child* 16:523, 1961.

41. Tischler, C. L. The psychological aspects of genetic counseling. *Am. J. Nurs.* 81:733, 1981.

42. Tisza, V. B. Management of the parents of the chronically ill child. *Am. J. Orthopsychiatry* 32(1):53, 1962.

43. Topliss, E. *Social Responses to Handicap.* New York: Longman, 1982.

44. Turnbull, A. P., and Turnbull, H. R. *Parents Speak Out: Views From the Other Side of the Two-Way Mirror.* Columbus, OH: Merrill, 1978.

45. Wilson, J. L. The Effects on the Whole Family of a Child with a Severe Birth Defect. In M. Fishbein (Ed.), *Birth Defects.* Philadelphia: Lippincott, 1963.

46. Winkler, L., Waslow, M., and Hatfield, E. Chronic sorrow revisisted: Parent vs. professional depiction of the adjustment of parents of mentally retarded children. *Am. J. Orthopsychiatry* 51:63, 1981.

47. Wheeler, B. *Challenged Parenting: A Practical Handbook for Parents of Children with Handicaps.* Ventura, CA: Regal Books, 1983.

XI
Middlescence

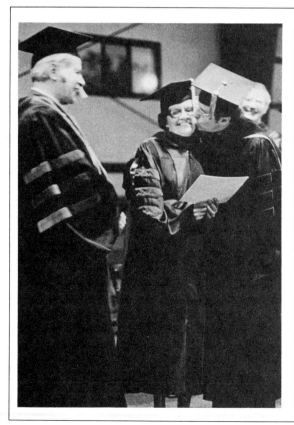
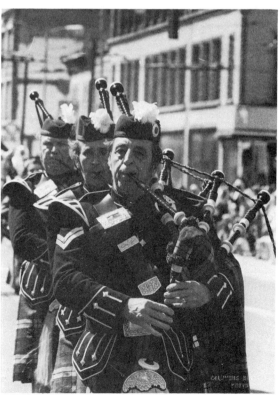

36
Biophysical Development During Middlescence

Leona A. Mourad and Shirley S. Ashburn

Every man desires to live long, but no man would be old.

—Jonathan Swift, *Thoughts on Various Subjects*

Introduction

Theories of Aging
Genetic theory of aging
Random error theory of aging
Autoimmune theory of aging
Theory of DNA cross-linkage and aging
Free radical theory of aging
Cycling to noncycling cells model
Wear-and-tear theory of aging

Somatic Changes Through Middlescence

Maintaining Health During Middlescence
Nutrition
Sleep and rest
Dental health
Effects of the environment on maintaining health
Stress
Health maintenance activities

Alterations of Health During Middlescence

Implications

The physical vigor of youth may have passed and the purported tranquility of old age has not yet arrived, but the middle-age years are among the most productive years of the life cycle. This span of time is frequently referred to as the "prime of life" [2]. "Middlescent" means being in the middle of the age continuum. Our arbitrary definition of human middlescence is that period of life between 35 and 65 years of age. Again, as for other age periods, these chronological parameters are flexible, but specific ages do offer some concrete guidelines for discussion. This 30-year period comprises almost one-half of an individual's entire life span.

The middle-adult years are often characterized by noticeable changes in the way the body works and looks. The subtle changes that began in young adulthood progress steadily. Middlescents should be able to cope with these changes if they have learned to compensate for them.

This chapter will focus on the biophysical development and changes that occur during middlescence. Some of the intrapersonal (affective and cognitive) and interpersonal (sociocultural) aspects will be indicated as they influence or are influenced by the internal and external changes inherent in the biophysical aging process.

Many of the generative tasks of middlescence are concerned with the "production" of a unique biophysical self whose particular needs for food, shelter, warmth, safety, oxygen, rest, and elimination are affected by that person's cellular age. The **biological** age of one's cells and organs is unique to each person as a function of **chronological** age. One's life expectancy is partially dependent on the responses of the various body organs to the aging processes. Therefore, before discussing the unique middlescent productive self, various theories of cellular aging will be presented. As we age, we each experience some or all of these changes.

THEORIES OF AGING

Aging is a process that occurs over time in which the effects of the process (age) are evident in specific physiological changes. A physiological phenomenon must meet four criteria before it can be considered an unequivocal component of the overall aging process [6]:

1. Universality. Identifiable in all members of one species, although the degree of its effects on an individual may vary from person to person (e.g., baldness).
2. Intrinsicality. A restriction of acceptable aging factors to those changes that are of endogenous origin (e.g., gray hair).
3. Progressiveness. A factor that develops rapidly and progressively with increasing age and has a higher incidence above a certain age (e.g., atherosclerosis).
4. Deleteriousness. Generally associated with more cross-bonded collagen fibers (a ground substance of cells that will be discussed more fully later in this chapter), causing increased rigidity of the collagen molecules. Some theories indicate that many of the physical characteristics of old age appear to be due to the increasing rigidity of collagen molecules that contain a greater number of cross-bonds. Although the concept of deleteriousness is accepted for all aspects of the aging process, the existence of cross-bonding alone cannot be regarded as the sole cause of true age effects. Degradative changes must ensue when senescence sets in, and even though the degree to which these changes occur may be dependent on the degree of cross-bonding, the crossbonds themselves have only a secondary role to play in aging.

Genetic Theory of Aging

The genetic theory explains why, but not how, aging occurs. Human longevity is governed to a large extent by genetic factors and can be predicted with a fair de-gree of accuracy for any person by calculating the average of the ages of the two parents, and four grandparents at the time of their deaths [6]. Furthermore, the cells of various tissues of the human body divide and multiply at different rates. The average life span for any one species appears to be determined by genetic factors transmitted from parents to offspring. Each organism may contain certain genes that control the "genetic clock," thereby determining the speed at which metabolic processes are performed and thus the length of time that elapses before death occurs [6]. Cell divisions appear to cease after a certain age; this phenomenon may be due to a preprogrammed intrinsic factor, the exact nature of which is yet to be determined. The reader will recall from Chapter 3 that in living organisms, "cell growth is under the control of tissue hormones, which either repress mitosis or, by their absence, permit cell division to proceed" [6]. It is also assumed that certain genes control nucleic acid repair and are capable of transcription by the removal of an appropriate repressor substance. The control of the production of these repressor substances is mediated by regular genes, which may control overall cellular function. Thus some of the phenomena of aging are preprogrammed or genetically determined. Some believe that "in the absence of such programmed events, aging would not occur at all or it would occur later" [14].

Random Error Theory of Aging

The random error theory states that spontaneous random error occurs in the synthesis or transmission of genetic information from mother to daughter cells during cell mitosis. These genetic mutations and chromosomal alterations lead to modifications or loss of cellular control of growth and function. One known cause of mutations is radiation, but all such mutations are not directly related to radiation exposure. Since some radiation changes do not increase the rate of aging, the use of genetic mutation as a definitive theory of aging is questionable [14].

Autoimmune Theory of Aging

The autoimmune theory states that autoimmunity with its associated autoantibody formation is critical in causing cellular death and cellular changes that lead to the aging process [14]. Aging cells may synthesize and release antibodies with specificity to self-tissues or serum components. With aging there is decreased synthesis of normal antibodies, leading to less effective immune functions, prolonged infections, and increases in immune complex diseases and cancer.

However, researchers have not currently identified a direct causal effect of the autoantibody process on aging.

Theory of DNA Cross-Linkage and Aging

The theory of deoxyribonucleic acid (DNA) cross-linkage is one "by which the smallest amount of interference can produce the greatest amount of damage" [14]. Cross-linkages between the double strands of the DNA molecule or within one or both strands separately result in damaged chromosomes (see Chap. 3). Repair of the damaged strands may be accomplished incompletely, not rapidly enough, or not at all, resulting in a DNA molecule that is incapable of "correct" transmitting properties. Cross-linking is thus the principal reaction in the initiation of irreparable spontaneous damage to DNA and consequent spontaneous cell death [14]. Those individuals who are able to repair DNA most efficiently would thus enjoy the longest life spans.

Free Radical Theory of Aging

The free radical theory is a special application of the cross-linking theory. Free radicals are highly reactive cellular components derived from atoms or molecules in which an electron pair has been separated into two electrons that exhibit independence of motion [14]. Oxygen is a molecule that commonly generates free radicals. In relation to aging, free radical-induced alterations of vital molecules create malfunctions that accumulate during a person's lifetime, resulting in inadequacy of cellular functions and regenerative mechanisms. Accumulation of such damages in cellular cytoplasm during aging produces cells with altered permeability to electrolytes. It also leads to reproductive alterations affecting the synthesis and transport of vital substances across cell membranes; these alterations are characteristic of aging organisms.

Cycling to Noncycling Cells Model

The cycling to noncycling cells theory is another model used to explain the aging process. Cellular aging is described as a progressive conversion of cycling to noncycling cells. Noncycling (resting) cells accumulate metabolic debris (aging debris), which lessens their ability to grow and reproduce. This accumulation also decreases their capacity for rapid, sustained growth in response, for example, to tissue injury or infection. Some noncycling cells may not be able to reenter the cycling (growth) phase, and those cells will age and ultimately die. Cycling is thus vital, positive, and productive, whereas noncycling is negative and destructive for many cells.

Wear and Tear Theory of Aging

The wear and tear theory assumes that an organism "wears out" with use. This theory does not take into account a living organism's mechanisms for self-repair, or the fact that such an organism may actually benefit from wear, tear, and repair. This theory does show that increased metabolic function accelerates the rate at which cells "wear out" and die, being exhausted of adaptation energy. Aging may be regarded as a "breakdown or impairment of performance" by endocrine and neural control mechanisms [14], not just cellular wear and tear over time. Some data are now beginning to point in this direction and will be discussed under specific organ systems later in this chapter. Loss of control, whether intracellular, enzymatic, or from extracellular hormonal regulators, appears to be a major factor in aging mechanisms.

In summary, theories on aging are focused on the genetically determined "normals" of the species; on the checks and balances of the species (e.g., enzymes, hormones, electrolytes, minerals); on cellular membrane functions, intracellular DNA, and ribonucleic acid (RNA) replications, and cross-linkings; and on the general wear and tear interactions between and among all of the above factors in utero, in vivo, and trans vivo. The influence of one's environment throughout life will be discussed in the section on biophysical system growth and development and thus has not been included as a theory of aging.

Although there are many theories describing how and why aging occurs, there is as yet no **one** theory that is universally accepted by researchers. From infancy to old age, all types of aging changes take place. It is not only that the body ages overtly, but that a variety of covert aging changes are constantly occurring (e.g., blood cells go through approximate 120-day life cycles; the epithelial cells lining the intestines and the skin go through their own specific cycles) [5]. All individuals go through similar aging processes, but it is not known as yet why some persons show marked age-related changes at much earlier ages than others, nor why there may be such wide variations in aging among persons in the same family and in similar environments and societies. It may be difficult to ascertain which are intrinsic and inevitable changes and which are changes imposed on the tissues by common or uncommon external factors (e.g., drugs, smoking, solar exposure, nutrition).

SOMATIC CHANGES THROUGH MIDDLESCENCE

The various tissues, organs, and systems of the body age in similar but varying stages or degrees. These changes are, at first, microscopically evident, and then grossly visible with increasing years and age. The use of the electron microscope has been most useful for determining the fine details of age-related changes in tissue structures. Biophysical changes in tissues due to aging are very evident in those connective tissues that hold the cells of the body together. As a person approaches middle age, and the connective tissue growth reaches a plateau, the individual no longer adds skeletal height and the tissues begin to show the common signs of aging.

Collagen and Elastin

Collagen fibers and elastin fibers make up the greatest percentage of connective tissues, and changes in these fibers (primarily increased cross-bonding and loss of water content) appear to be directly age-related. Thus some explanation of the characteristics of collagen and elastin should clarify their relationship to aging in tissues. Collagen, elastin, and ground substance provide support to cells. They also serve as a means of exchange for metabolites between blood and tissues, provide storage for fuel in adipose (fatty) tissues, protect against infection, and help to repair injuries [18]. Collagen is a large protein structure consisting of three intertwining chains, each chain containing 1012 amino acids and amino acid residues. These three strands are flexible but offer great resistance to a pulling force. They are stable and resist deforming, making them excellent fibers for connective tissues. The three strands are held together through electrostatic bonds (hydrogen, sodium, nitrogen, and calcium ions). With increasing and advancing age, there is increased cross-bonding between and among the three chains, making them less resilient and less able to maintain their water (hydrogen-oxygen ratio) content. When the collagen fibers age in vital organs, such as heart muscle, lung, brain, or kidney tissues, these organs are less able to perform their normal functions, making them vulnerable to injury or death of some or all of their cells.

Elastin is the second of the major connective tissue fibers. Elastin fibers are strands found in and among collagen fibers that serve similar functions of maintaining flexibility and strength of connective tissues. The relative percentage of elastin fibers gradually decreases after age 50 [6], resulting in less flexible, "stiffer" tissues. Thus the flexibility, strength, and water content of collagen and elastin fibers are age-related.

Skeletal System

Growth of the bony skeleton ceases by early adulthood when full height has been reached. From 40 years of age until the end of middlescence, bone mass begins to decrease. Calcium loss from bone tissues becomes pronounced during and following menopausal changes, with osteoporosis (calcium loss leading to decreasing bone density and mass) being a truly age-related or age-determined process [6]. Thirty-five to 40 percent of all females will develop osteoporosis, which increases the incidence of fracture from minimal trauma [4]. Males also lose calcium from their bones, but male bone loss may start 15 to 20 years later and occurs at a slower rate than in females. (The male is not subject to the same hormonal changes that women experience during menopause; the male skeleton contains more calcium and is heavier than that of a female of the same size). Consequently, middlescent males possess more bone strength than middlescent females. Osteoporosis is most common in Caucasians and least common in Blacks. There is degeneration of the intervertebral discs, disc spaces become narrowed, and the vertebrae become wedge-shaped, increasing the curvature; as bone density decreases, the weight-bearing vertebrae of the back become compressed, accentuating the roundness of the upper back.

The most rational measure to prevent or to slow bone demineralization and other joint degenerative changes is an adequate calcium, vitamin D (aids in calcium deposition), and protein intake throughout life combined with physical activity and regular exercise (force on bone decreases demineralization). Hormonal replacement therapy should be considered for menopausal women [3, 4].

A loss of skeletal height gradually becomes more noticeable in middlescent persons due to this "hump" and a change in the normal 130- to 135-degree angle of the hip-femur joint (Fig. 36–1). With aging, the angle becomes more acute, resulting in a slight height decrease. This height decrease is more pronounced in women. The skeletal changes in the vertebral column and hip joints are also due to lessening of the elasticity of the cartilages between the bones of those tissues. Loss of elasticity of cartilage is due to hardening or thickening of the collagen fibers. Inflammatory or degenerative changes in joint cartilage also affect overall height.

Muscular System

Muscle strength and mass are directly related to active muscle use. Muscle growth or hypertrophy continues through middlescence in proportion to muscle use. Young middlescent persons (35 to 45 years of age) usu-

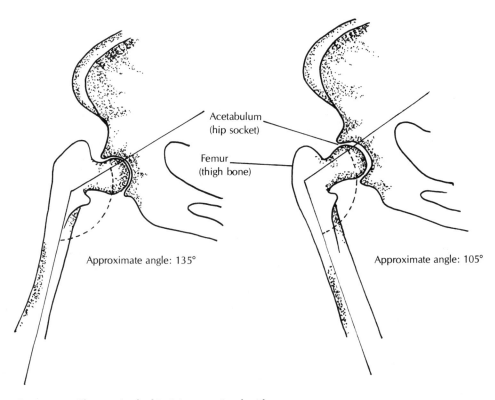

Acetabulum
(hip socket)

Femur
(thigh bone)

Approximate angle: 135°

Approximate angle: 105°

Figure 36–1. Changes in the hip joint associated with age.

ally maintain the pattern of muscular activity established during young adulthood through their occupation or work, home upkeep and repair activities, and their hobby or recreational activities. Some middlescent adults may become more sedentary, decreasing strenuous work or occupational behaviors and changing to less demanding recreational activities; thus, the muscles begin a slow decline in mass, structure, and strength. Muscle loss is also caused by changes in the collagen fibers, which become thicker and less elastic, causing sagging or drooping of muscles as evident in the drooping of facial, breast, and abdominal muscles. Lower back pain among middlescents may be related to impaired flexibility of the hip and back and reduced elasticity of the hamstring muscles. The smaller waistlines and trimmer lines of clothes designed for younger people will not always fit the enlarging torsos of middlescent men and women. Many clothing manufacturers have attempted to solve this problem by designing clothes that are more tailored to the middlescent body (half-sizes). Prudent diet and regular exercise will aid in maintaining (or regaining) muscle tone and decreasing intramuscular fat [1].

Integumentary System

The tissues of the integumentary system maintain a healthy, intact, glowing appearance until 50 to 55 years of age if the individual is receiving adequate vitamins, minerals, nutrients, and fluids, and maintains appropriate cleansing habits. Wrinkles gradually begin to become more noticeable due to DNA changes and to increased cross-bonding of collagen fibers (see Chap. 39). From 25 to 70 years of age the water content of the body decreases from 61 to 53 percent, and fat content increases from 14 to 30 percent [17]. Much of the water loss is from the integumentary tissues, accounting for the dry skin of middlescent and older persons. An increased exposure to the sun over prolonged periods of time can accelerate the appearance of dry skin and wrinkles. Wrinkling tends to be less marked and to occur later in life in Blacks and Orientals [6].

As integumentary tissues lose water, they become thinner and drier and more easily bruised, cracked, or lost through cuts or burns. Skin wounds have slower rates of healing in middlescent persons, possibly as a result of decreased rates of resynthesis of cells needed for wound healing and collagen formation [6]. After 45 years of age, females have less skin thickness and less

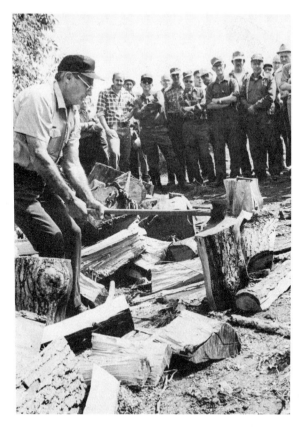

Figure 36-2. Many persons retain their neuromuscular strength throughout the middlescent years. Selye's theory of stress response helps to explain the surge of energy experienced under the stress of competition.

total skin collagen than males [6]. Both males and females, however, have lost some subcutaneous fat by this time (even in the obese), and this can usually be seen over the tibia (shin). After their climacteric, females may have increased fat deposits along skin fold lines (e.g., under the arms and breasts and in the groin area) [4].

During the early adult years, the skin is relatively elastic and will follow the receding tissues from which excess fat tissue disappears with weight reduction. Around the age of 40 years, however, an individual who has just completed a significant, and often too rapid, weight reduction may feel (and act) younger but will actually appear older. This phenomenon is caused by the loose skin folds that cannot recede as readily to accommodate the loss of fat. This flabby skin connotes the presence of an aging integumentary system [13].

"Bags" under the eyes also often accompany mid-

dlescent aging. They are caused by weakening of the underlying muscle and fibrous tissue. Consequently, the lower eyelid falls in folds, the subcutaneous fat herniates the weakened muscles, and the skin balloons.

Gray hair is simply hair without pigmentation; the melanocytes that provide pigment granules to the hair eventually are depleted. Many view it as a symbol of distinction.

Hereditary tendencies toward baldness become more apparent with age. Some possible causes of baldness include a gradual decrease in scalp circulation and a decrease in adrenal secretion. Males are more frequently affected than females.

Central Nervous System

The functioning of the central nervous system through the early middlescent years is normally maintained at the same high level achieved in young adulthood. Physiologically, middlescent persons may engage in intellectual functioning of a highly complex nature; many are concerned with fiscal, economic, social, environmental, and governmental issues. Experience and affective maturity may give them advantages over younger adults when critical decisions or organizational skills are needed. However, some individuals may experience a gradual decline in mental functioning and mood with advancing or increasing age (over age 50) due to changes in the biological functioning of enzymes, hormones, and motor and sensory functions. The individual may evidence a slight slowing of reflexes and a slower response to sudden changes in environment. Despite an increase of brain-cell loss, there are a large number of functioning cells in the human brain. Many cells seem to have no identifiable function and perhaps are to be regarded as a contingency reserve [5].

Special Senses

Visual changes become noticeable during early middlescence, primarily the development of **presbyopia,** or impaired vision, as a result of loss of elasticity in the crystalline lens of the eye. Presbyopia begins at about 40 years of age for many people and usually is correctable with eyeglasses or contact lenses. The lens of the eye may gradually become more opaque after age 45; thus various degrees of cataract formation can become a common age-related condition.

The senses of hearing, smell, taste, and touch are generally maintained at high levels during early middlescence. Noticeable losses in hearing and smell may begin around 50 years of age [18].

Cardiovascular System

Heart size does not increase beyond the normal "fist" size in the average middlescent person. However, as middlescence progresses, changes in heart size may be noted in some individuals, with hypertrophy occurring primarily in the left ventricle. Left ventricular hypertrophy may occur independently or may be caused by arterial hardening (the left side of the heart must increase its size and muscle mass to force the blood through the narrowed [atherosclerotic] or less resilient [arteriosclerotic] systemic arteries). The atria (upper heart chambers) gradually become stiffer and more collagen-filled after age 40 [6].

The functions, rate, and rhythm of the heart are maintained in the early middlescent years through active work and recreational activities. After age 45, especially if work and leisure activities become more sedentary, the heart begins to lose its tone, and rate and rhythm changes become evident. It is desirable to keep the blood pressure under 150/90. [3]. Refer to Appendix E for other biophysical parameters.

Respiratory System

The functioning of respiratory tissues in middlescent persons may be predicated on whether or not the person is a cigarette smoker, and if so, the extent and duration of smoking activities. Smoking increases the risk of respiratory disease and decreases respiratory efficiency. The respiratory tissues maintain full vital respiratory capacity (maximum breathing capacity) throughout early middlescence, barring repeated contact with respiratory illnesses, such as pneumonia, asthma, bronchitis, and the common cold. Of these diseases, the first three may cause some residual loss of functioning lung tissues. As the years advance, lung tissues become thicker, stiffer, and less elastic, resulting in gradually decreased breathing capacity by 55 or 60 years of age. Respiratory rates increase in response to decreasing pulmonary function to maintain adequate cellular and tissue perfusion of oxygen.

Renal System

The normal mechanism of renal filtration of blood for the collection and elimination of wastes in urine is usually maintained at full capacity through early middlescence. Adequate daily fluid intake helps to ensure proper kidney functioning. With aging, there is a gradual decrease in the number of nephrons, the functional units of the kidney, but the kidneys contain reserves of functional tissue.

More aging females than males suffer from stress incontinence (intermittent leakage of urine from sudden strain). This form of inconvenience, or embarrassment, may occur when the person sneezes, coughs, or is suddenly startled. It is caused by the gradual change in the urethral muscular support resulting in weakening of the sphincter control. It can be either alleviated or reduced in frequency by performing pelvic floor tightening exercises and/or pessary. Surgical correction may be required for some persons.

Gastrointestinal System

Normally, secretions from the gastrointestinal tract are maintained at high levels through early middlescence. From 30 to 60 years of age, there is a steady decline in gastric juice secretion as well as decreases in free acid content, total daily acid production, and pepsin content in the stomach. The middlescent may begin to eliminate certain foods from the daily diet that "disagree" with him or her. In addition, ptyalin (the starch-digesting enzyme) in saliva production declines sharply at about 60 years of age. Pancreatic digestive enzymes gradually decrease in production from 20 to 60 years of age [18].

Metabolic System

Secretions of hormones and vital digestive fluids are usually maintained in early middlescence. Secretions of the endocrine glands (e.g., insulin, glucagon, epinephrine, norepinephrine, thyroxine, estrogen, progesterone, testosterone, glucocorticoids, and mineralocorticoids) are normally maintained at the individual's norms during early middlescence. Age-related changes become more noticeable after age 45.

Blood Sugar Levels and Acid-Base Balance

The blood-sugar level and the acid-base balance have a number of alternate control mechanisms; thus at rest they remain relatively stable into old age. However, exercise and stress alter their balance and levels, which correlates with the decreased ability of aging persons to withstand or respond to stressful situations as well as they did when younger. Stress may contribute to the increased incidence of adult onset diabetes mellitus.

Hormonal Changes

As people progress through middlescence, sex hormone alterations result in marked biological changes. One of the major health alterations during middlescence concerns climacteric changes, those changes brought about from decreases in the production of male or female sex hormones, specifically testosterone, estrogen, and progesterone from the gonads.

THE FEMALE CLIMACTERIC

The productive period of estrogen/progesterone production in the female through early adulthood and early middlescence results in ovulation followed by menstruation or by pregnancy with fertilization of the ovum.

During the climacteric period, the ovaries cease to liberate ova, and the uterus gradually abandons the monthly process of shedding and regenerating its lining. Many women equate their capacity to produce children with their femininity; thus a loss of or alterations in this capacity may be seen as a loss of their feminine worth. As a result, the climacteric period with its accompanying menopause (cessation of menses) can be a particularly traumatic period in the life cycle. In some women the change is easy; it is accepted as part of the normal course of events and is adjusted to as another life experience. In other women, however, this period may result in neuroses and frank psychoses with severe depressive reactions. Approximately 80 percent of menopausal women experience some symptoms [4]. The most severe symptoms occur in women who lose their ovaries through surgery or radiation when they are premenopausal. Because of the complete and sudden loss of female hormones, their bodies have no time to make the normal, gradual transition. Fortunately, as more and more data accumulate, therapeutic measures for the symptoms and changes have become available, lessening the severity of the symptoms and easing the passage through this period of change.

The cessation of menstruation may occur in a number of different ways, all of which are regarded as normal. It usually assumes one of four patterns:

1. Sudden cessation of menstruation.
2. Regular cycles with a gradual diminishing of the menstrual flow.
3. Loss of menstrual regularity, with the periods coming farther apart, although with a fairly normal amount of flow.
4. Shorter cycles with a profuse flow.

At the present time, there is no known way to predict which pattern a woman will follow. The average age at which menopause occurs in females in the United States is approximately 51 years of age [4], but it may occur much earlier or much later. If menopause occurs earlier than this, a woman may have only one or two cycles that are different from her usual pattern; the woman whose menopause is later may have several years of marked menstrual irregularity. Symptoms vary with the individual, but the classic symptoms appear to be breast tenderness, increase in breast size, and, occasionally, the development of fibrocystic breasts. These symptoms, like many others, are caused by hyperactivity of the pituitary gland. No longer under the normal cyclic influence of the ovarian hormones, the pituitary produces excessive amounts of gonadotropins, which lead to a disturbance in endocrine balance and alterations in metabolism. Two symptoms that are known to have a physiological basis are listed below [4].

1. "Hot flashes." The aforementioned glandular imbalances are a source of instability in the vasomotor system, causing an irregularity in the diameter of the blood vessels. This produces a hot, tingling sensation over the whole body, lasting from a fleeting second to several minutes each time. Hot flashes can occur several times over a 24-hour period.

2. "Flushes." Another vasomotor symptom involves a visible blushing of the head, neck, and upper chest and back. Flushes are caused by an expansion of the peripheral blood vessels and are followed by "sweats" (profuse perspiration) and a feeling of chilliness. These flushes may occur as often as once or twice a day, or sometimes as often as every half hour. They interfere with daytime activities and with sleep when they occur at night. They are intensified in women who are experiencing concurrent excitement or stress.

Other symptoms associated with menopause include nervousness, depression, melancholia, feelings of hopelessness, frigidity, memory impairment, insomnia, vertigo, headache, tachycardia, palpitations, fatigability, muscle or joint pains, abdominal distention, constipation or diarrhea, spots before the eyes, ringing in the ears, and sensations of choking and suffocation. Headaches, of which approximately one-third of menopausal women complain, are usually of the nervous tension type, rarely migraine [4].

Some clinicians feel that many of the above symptoms are not totally the result of physiological causes (i.e., estrogen and progesterone decreases) but are due to psychological causes that produce the physiological reaction. They attribute anxiety to the loss of childbearing potential or child-rearing activities and functions, or to thoughts of becoming old. Since many women experience relief from the majority of the severe symptoms with the administration of estrogen and progesterone compounds, the authors believe that the symptoms are more likely to be physiological than psychological in origin [3, 4].

Menopause should not attentuate a woman's sexual capacity, performance, or drive [7]. However, some body tissue and organ changes accompany menopause, such as thinning of skin tissues, loss of normal skin turgor, scaling and wrinkles, reduced secretions from mucous membranes, and atrophy of the reproductive organs. Vaginal tissues shorten and become less elastic (loss of elastin fibers). Vaginal secretions and circulation decrease, which may lead to itching and dryness of the perineum and vulva with easy bleeding and the erosion and ulceration of the perineal tissues. Decreased estrogen levels also change the vaginal secretions to alkaline, thus increasing susceptibility to infection [4].

After menopause, the breasts lose some of their subcutaneous fat and glandular tissues, which may cause them to droop or hang. The palms and the soles of the feet develop hardened plaques (keratoderma climactericum) and the bones lose calcium, becoming osteoporotic and decalcified. The development of back symptoms, such as backache, low back pain, and thoracic kyphosis (hump) is evidence of the osteoporosis that is correlated with menopause. Thus many symptoms referable to nearly all the organs and tissues in the body may accompany menopause.

THE MALE CLIMACTERIC

The male climacteric, which occurs at a much slower rate and over a relatively longer span of time than the female climacteric, may include decreased libido, headaches, weight gain, mood swings, alterations in concentration span, and memory lapses. The extent of these symptoms within the male population is difficult to ascertain, possibly because of reluctance on the part of males to admit to these symptoms openly.

Alterations of testosterone production result in changes in sperm production, although sperm appear to be produced in sufficient quantities for conception throughout a long life span, as evidenced by the phenomenon of a few 90-year-old men becoming fathers. Decreases in the amount of testosterone cause decreased sex drive, which may result in impotence or failure to achieve erection. Impotence may be a problem in males over 50 years of age, but again, the extent of the problem is difficult to determine, since it tends to affect the same population as those undergoing climacteric changes.

As aging proceeds, males experience changes in the frequency, strength, and duration of erection and sex drive, leading to concern for their "maleness." Several health alterations may influence erectile power, including iliac and pelvic vessel arteriosclerotic changes that cause decreased blood supply, atrophy, or pressure on pelvic nerves from intervertebral disc protru-

sions; diabetes [10]; and tumor growth in the bowel, pelvis, or prostate. Some medications, especially antihypertensives, muscle relaxants, and tranquilizers, may also cause impotence. Prostatic hypertrophy, with its subsequent surgical resections, has profound effects on erectile power and potency (see Chap. 39).

As a result of aging, the male may take longer to attain an erection or may notice a reduction in seminal fluid volume and a decreased ejaculatory pressure, but he should not lose his facility for erection at any time, presuming general good health and no psychogenic blocking, well into the 80-year-old age group. Masters and Johnson's research indicates that the male's loss of erective prowess is not a natural component of aging but may be more related to lack of understanding, fear of performance, or disuse [11].

MAINTAINING HEALTH DURING MIDDLESCENCE

Nutrition

Middlescents are responsible for their own well-being. Each has some control over the aging process. During middlescence, one continues to need complete proteins in the diet to maintain cell function and repair. Complete proteins, such as milk, cheese, eggs, meats, poultry, and fish, should be eaten daily in moderation, with modification for saturated fatty acids and cholesterol intake (skim or lowfat milk should be used, as opposed to whole milk; egg substitutes or egg whites to help decrease the cholesterol intake from egg yolks, since egg yolks are the major source of cholesterol intake in the diet). Poultry and fish also contain less cholesterol than red meats or liver, and both should be substituted frequently for red meat. Cholesterol and saturated fatty acid intake are of concern primarily because of the end result of their metabolism in the body. Excess intake may lead to deposits in vital organs and tissues, thus affecting health and longevity.

Cholesterol is a white, waxy substance related to fats that is commonly found in foods, such as liver, egg yolk, and kidney. It is a normal part of body tissues and is especially important for proper functioning of nervous tissues and liver cells. It is closely related to the sex hormones and hormones from the adrenal gland. Daily cholesterol needs are met through intake of carbohydrates, fats, and amino acids. Excess cholesterol is removed from the body in the bile. However, high intake of cholesterol-rich foods may result in deposits of cholesterol in some organs or tissues, namely, in the heart, arteries, brain, and gallbladder, posing increased risks of cardiovascular accidents and gallstone formation. Foods that contain large amounts of saturated fats also contribute to degenerative cardiovascular conditions. A high intake of foods that are cholesterol-rich and high in saturated fat markedly increases the risk of cardiovascular conditions and premature death. The use of polyunsaturated (vegetable) fats and oils should be substituted for saturated (mainly animal) fats for dietary and metabolic needs to help maintain healthier tissues throughout one's life.

Incomplete proteins, such as those in dried beans, peas, legumes, peanut butter, cereals, and breads, supply vitally needed raw materials and vitamins for cellular metabolism. Minerals and vitamins are also supplied by daily intake of green and yellow vegetables, fruits, and fortified seasonings (iodized salt). Iron-rich foods, such as raisins, fruits, organ meats (liver), egg yolk (in moderation—limit to three per week), oysters, legumes, and nuts, should also be included. Dark leafy vegetables help to keep hemoglobin production high for proper oxygenation. Adequate fluid intake and bulk in foods assist in the elimination of fecal wastes and lessen constipation problems. The quantity of food

ingested daily should be sufficient to maintain normal weight but not to cause weight gain. Many persons find a natural decrease in appetite accompanies a decrease in energy expenditure; others merely gain weight and must use willpower to reduce calorie intake to maintain their desired weight. Carbohydrate and fat rather than protein intake should be reduced when weight maintenance or reduction is essential.

The average basal metabolic rate (BMR) for an adult is approximately 40 calories per hour (960 per 24 hours), depending on age and gender. The BMR is the amount of energy (calories) expended for maintenance of body functions when the body is at rest. Some persons (50 to 60 years of age) may require only one-half the calories per day recommended for younger persons because of decreased activity or mobility. Lowered BMR appears to be intrinsic with advancing age [18], but it may be further reduced by decreased thyroid hormone production [9]. The BMR changes that result from hypothyroidism lead to a metabolic rate that is 15 to 40 percent lower than normal. Adult hypothyroidism (myxedema) affects women five times as frequently as men, occuring most often between the ages of 50 and 60 [18].

Sleep and Rest

Middlescent persons have the same individual needs as younger persons for rest and quiet, requiring on the average 6 to 8 hours of rest and sleep per night. Frequently, the reduction of physical energy expenditures as the individual approaches retirement age is accompanied by a decrease in sleeping time to 5 to 6 hours per night. Quiet times or naps during the afternoon or evening often take the place of nighttime sleep (especially in the middlescent person who attempts to continue at a pace approximating the level of activity as a younger person), so in actuality the overall time spent in napping and sleep approaches that of earlier years.

Dental Health

Dental problems with loss of teeth are a continuing concern during the middlescent years. Through proper care and adequate fluoride exposure, a person should be able to retain natural teeth throughout the lifetime. However, many persons currently over age 55 have lost most or all of their teeth. Periodontal disease, which damages tissue surrounding a tooth and eventually erodes the bone that forms its socket, is a major cause of lost teeth during the middlescent years. Lost teeth may be replaced with bridges, plates, full dentures or dental implants, but many individuals remain without dentures (edentulous). Ill-fitting, missing, or irregu-

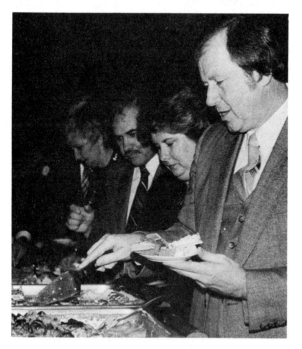

Figure 36–3. Food continues to be a major attraction at social events. Middlescents with sedentary jobs need to be sure to get enough exercise to offset the extra calories and to use self-control to avoid extra strain on the circulatory system.

larly shaped teeth or dentures contribute to decreased intake and mastication of food, decreased fluid intake, oral disease, and diseases of the face, jaws, and head.

Effects of the Environment on Maintaining Health

Maintaining high level health throughout middlescence is a constant challenge and is becoming more and more difficult due to environmental influences. Health is internally maintained through cell metabolism, hormonal secretions, intake, and the body's ability to process nutrients and fluids. Health maintenance is also influenced externally by many factors, including urban living, climatic factors of temperature, environmental carcinogens, adequacy of intake, and environmental stressors (which increase the energy needed to cope).

Rural living is healthier than urban living. More and more environmental conditions are being implicated in the development of cardiovascular and cancerous conditions. The exposure to external air that is heavy with the fumes of trucks or factory smoke or to internal air that is heavy with fumes from plastic raw materials, dyes, or tobacco smoke has been associated with the development of carcinomas of the lung, liver, bladder, and pancreas as well as blood disorders. Maintaining one's health under the external influences from the environment is becoming increasingly more difficult. However, further subjection of oneself to the intake (internalization) of substances that are known to be harmful to health (e.g., cigarette smoke, alcohol, excessive vitamins, unprescribed medications, illicit drugs) requires no comment for the intelligent person. The increasing rate of lung cancer is directly correlated with cigarette smoking [12]. Lung cancer is the leading cause of cancer death in males [3]. In 1985, it also surpassed breast cancer to become the leading cause of death in females and is correlated with the increase in female smoking. Cancers of the colon and rectum, which are the leading types of internal cancer in both males and females, have been attributed to the refined foods and lower roughage intake in highly industrialized countries. Early diagnosis and treatment can cure (by removal of the offending cell or body part) 75 percent of the persons affected [3].

The exposure to communicable diseases, such as flu, common colds, hepatitis, and other contagious diseases, is more prevalent in crowded, urban populations. The marital status also appears to influence health maintenance, with married women living longer than single women or those who are widowed or divorced. Married men also live longer than men who are single, widowed, or divorced [19]. Finally, one's gender influences longevity, with the average female outliving the average male [20].

The additives in foods have been accused of making it more difficult to maintain an optimum level of health. The processing of foods to retard spoilage requires the addition of preservatives, such as nitrites, benzoates, and other substances. Taste, color, or other additives increase exposure to potentially harmful substances.

Some environmental conditions affect the health status in a positive way. For example, a low incidence of some types of cancer has been noted in the residents of Utah. Several factors, including limited use of tobacco and alcohol and the presence of trace metals (which appear to be essential for normal cellular functioning) in the area, may contribute environmentally to their healthful lives.

Stress

A major internal and external influence on health throughout one's life is one's adaptation to stressful situations. No discussion of middlescent health states would be complete without correlating them with the stress response. Stress can be defined as a syndrome of changes in the biological system resulting from a stressor (threat). **Stress response** is the sum of the changes brought about as the biological system adapts to the stressor (e.g., injury, illness, physical or psychological threat).

The physiological stress response is composed of several stages and steps. According to Hans Selye, the "father" of stress syndrome theories, the general adaptation syndrome has three stages [15]:

1. Alarm stage. This stage consists of the neuroendocrine responses to the threat to the system. These responses involving the autonomic nervous system and the adrenal medulla, result in increased production of norepinephrine and epinephrine, which increase cardiac rate and output, increase blood pressure, increase the respiratory rate, decrease the blood supply to visceral organs, increase the blood supply to vital organs (heart, brain, liver, peripheral muscles), and dilate the pupils. These responses constitute a physiologic "call to arms"—the fight, flight, or fright responses to the stressor. This stage may last from a few minutes to up to 24 hours or longer.
2. Resistance stage. This stage is the period of adaptation to the stressor. It is a result of adrenal cortical production of antiinflammatory or proinflamma-

tory hormones in order to adapt to or cope with the stressor. The purpose of the adrenal cortical activity is an attempt to confine the effects of the stressor to the smallest area of the biological system that is capable of overcoming the stressor. The resistance stage may last a very short time, or it may last for months or even years (e.g., as in recovering from tuberculosis).

3. Exhaustion stage. In this stage, the "adaptation" energy of the biological system is exhausted, and the person becomes severely ill. When the body functions can no longer be maintained, the person dies. If the stressor is overcome, the adaptation energy is used to effect recovery, with return to healthier states. Repeated assaults from stressors and the stress responses required to cope with them may exhaust all adaptation energy, and death will result.

Each individual's stress responses tend to follow the pattern given above. A person's responses may be mediated by his perception of the stressor. By learning what causes threats to himself, a person can modify his responses to conserve his adaptation energy. It also behooves each person to identify his characteristic responses: Does he act outwardly ("fight" response); does he act inwardly ("flight" response); or does he ride the fence, not knowing which way to turn ("fright" response)? Identification of stressors and individual responses is the first step in learning to predict and control both stressors and responses.

Selye also identified some conditions that he referred to as "diseases of adaptation" (more properly "maladaptation"). He labeled diseases of some tissues and organs as "inappropriate" adaptations to stressors. Some diseases of adaptation as identified by Selye include collagen diseases (rheumatoid arthritis, progressive systemic sclerosis), allergic conditions, asthma, and ulcers [15]. Finally, Selye identified the "local adaptation syndrome" (LAS), an attempt by the body to keep the response in the smallest area. An example of the LAS is the circumscribed area of inflammation around a cut on a finger; it is a localized response with no (or only slight) systemic involvement.

Illness or altered health states may result from lack of successful adaptation. A stressor can overwhelm a person's total adaptive capabilities at any particular time (see Chap. 42).

Health Maintenance Activities

As each individual approaches middlescence, there are several steps that can be taken to assist in maintaining or retaining the body in an optimal state of health. The most important step is to engage in preventive health measures. After 40 years of age, each person should have an annual complete physical examination, including rectal, pelvic, blood, and urine chemistry examinations, and dental and oral examinations every 6 months. The eyes should be examined every 1 to 2 years by an ophthalmologist or optometrist. Females should continue breast self-examination every month and should have a baseline mammography between 35 and 40 years of age. Pap tests should be performed at least every 3 years. Immunizations should be kept current (see Table 7–3).

In addition to the above-mentioned check-ups, after 50 years of age, females should have a mammography every 2 to 3 years, and both females and males should have their bowel movements checked for occult (hidden) blood annually. After age 50, men should have a proctoscopy (viewing of rectum and sigmoid area with flexible tubular instrument) performed every 3 to 5 years after two initial negative tests 1 year apart.

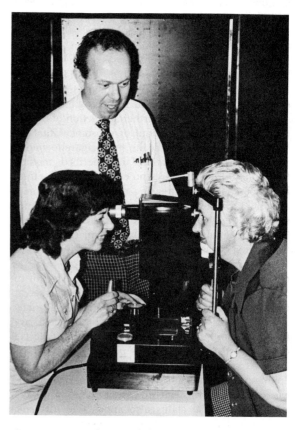

Figure 36–4. Regular visual checkups should include a test for glaucoma for all persons over 30 years of age.

Regular exercise (daily, if possible) promotes high level wellness if it is individualized to the person's needs. No exercise regimen (even at a well-known gymnasium or health spa) should be initiated by a middlescent until a physician has been consulted. Most people over 30 years of age or overweight should have a stress electrocardiogram to assess the consequences of beginning a jogging program [1]. However, walking is a very valuable exercise to maintain physical strength and health and can usually be undertaken without medical prescription. The distances walked should be increased gradually over time.

Medical examinations allow for health education and early identification of problems with initiation of prophylactic or ameliorative measures to prevent the progression or the complication of a disease process.

ALTERATIONS OF HEALTH DURING MIDDLESCENCE

Only a small number of middlescent persons are affected by ailments so disabling that they bring about a drastic change in life-style [8]. Middlescent persons do, however, frequently encounter stressors through illness, accidents, and other events. Middlescent persons must not only contend with the usual alterations that affect humans living in society but must also deal with the effects of aging cells influencing recovery. Aging lengthens the recovery time as a result of slower and more prolonged responses to stressors, more pronounced reactions (i.e., more severe illness), and (frequently) the existence of more than one illness at a time. Aging persons are less active and less mobile, making them prone to degenerative or chronic conditions. Thirty-eight percent of persons less than 65 years of age have one or more conditions that involve a chronic illness [17]. The most common major disorders in otherwise healthy middle-aged persons are obesity, hypertension, and arthritis [5], all of which contribute to accelerated aging.

Some degenerative alterations are gender-related and are fairly common to large numbers of middlescent groups. In males, deposits of uric acid and gout become a problem after 30 years of age, being 10 times more common than in females. Urinary conditions that affect frequency or urgency in urination affect one-third of older persons, with urinary complaints being more common in females [17]. Females tend to have more obesity problems, dizziness, and pain in their feet than do males, whereas males have more difficulty in hearing [17].

IMPLICATIONS

A major task of middlescence is to adapt oneself and one's behavior to the signals of accelerated aging processes. Middlescent persons can positively influence their longevity by avoiding unnecessary stressors or by finding coping behaviors to minimize stress adaptation requirements. They can also take various precautions to decrease the risk of injury, as discussed in the following paragraphs.

1. As the eye ages, hyperopia and presbyopia occur, leading to farsightedness. Caution must be taken to prevent falls, cuts, and other injuries that result from sight or distance changes in the aging eye. Obtaining and wearing prescription eyeglasses can help to decrease such injuries.

2. As collagen fibers lose their elasticity and contractility with aging, the muscles and joints respond more slowly, leading to falls, bruises, and fractures. Therefore, all loose rugs should be anchored firmly to prevent tripping, and long cords should be taped down or placed behind furniture to prevent catching of heels. Shoes should be low-heeled to prevent ankle, knee, or hip and arm injuries from turning, tripping, or falling. Sports activities should be matched to physical skills and limitations.

3. As atherosclerotic plaques and arteriosclerotic processes (hardening of arteries) progress with aging, there is a decreased tolerance for heat and cold, and the blood supply to vital organs and tissues may be decreased. Rising slowly from a lying or a sitting position to a standing one allows for vascular adjustment in order to prevent fainting from cerebral anoxia. Care should be taken to prevent injury to feet and legs from temperature extremes: for example, testing the temperature before stepping into a tub of water, wearing woolen socks to maintain steadier foot circulation, and wearing slippers and well-fitting shoes to prevent ulcerations or gangrenous areas due to ischemic tissues, which can be caused by pressure points. Persons with decreased peripheral arterial circulation should not wear support hose, constricting garters, or sit with their legs crossed over their knees, since these behaviors further decrease arterial perfusion. Venous stasis and edema may also be concerns for middlescent and older persons. Decreasing salt intake (and thus lessening water retention) lessens stasis edema. Varicose veins are more common in older individuals because of valvular changes. Persons with varicosities may wear elastic support hose to increase venous return, thus lessening venous stasis. The performance of specific exercises, such as alternately raising and lower-

ing the legs, increases arterial flow; by increasing muscle action, one also increases return of venous blood to the systemic circulation. Keeping as active as possible and spending as much time walking as one's health and time permit are also positive health habits that should be encouraged through middlescence.

4. As middlescence proceeds, one's resistance to infection decreases due to errors in replication and changes in immune cell functions. The exposure to infectious agents, such as cold viruses or bacteria, that could lead to infections, such as pneumonia, should be avoided if possible. Wearing warm clothing helps to prevent chilling.

5. A wide variety of other injuries and conditions, such as burns, heart conditions, lung diseases, ulcer development, and constipation problems, are common in middlescence. Burn trauma can be avoided through caution when handling matches, flames, or hot fluids or foods. The best "prevention" against ulcers, heart conditions, and constipation is to recognize and externalize one's concerns in responding to stressors. It appears that such action provides a focal point for energies elicited by the stressor and can decrease emergence of destructive internal responses.

At this point, the reader may feel discouraged about the biophysical aspects of middlescence. However, most middlescent persons experience very good health, especially if a good foundation of wise health care has been laid during the young adult years. Inadequacies in health care or inappropriate health care practices during the developmental and early adult years can affect one's health status during the later adult years. Many of the processes discussed become more pronounced and prevalent with increasing age, but precursors and early changes begin during young adult or early middlescent years. It is interesting to note that scientists initially working with the United States space program chose middlescent individuals to be the first astronauts on the moon. These men, whose ages ranged from 38 to 45 years, were chosen because they were mentally alert, physically sound, and emotionally stable individuals. Sally Ride, the first U.S. female astronaut to travel to outer space, was 32 years old.

Responses to illness during middlescence are not different in character from those of younger or older persons, but they do differ in the extent or degree of reaction. As one ages, the stressors encountered "add up," and the sum saps the amount of available adaptation energy. As the years proceed and stressors are encountered, the individual responds more slowly and possibly in a more pronounced way to stressors, as evidenced by more chronic, long-term health alterations

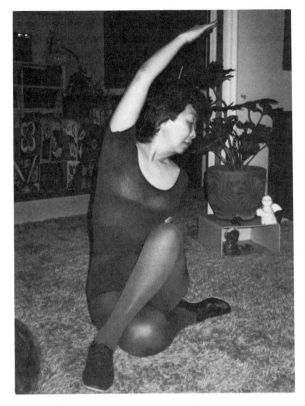

Figure 36–5. Middlescents should begin an exercise regimen sensibly. Stretching is one form of activity that increases range of motion and tones the muscles before more vigorous exercises.

of greater severity and with involvement of more than one system. Thus several factors must be considered by practitioners when they are counseling or caring for middlescent persons with health alterations:

1. Biological age
2. Previously encountered and resolved stressors of physical origin (trauma, illness, the climacteric) or psychological origin (e.g., emotional problems, impotence, depression, anxiety)
3. Previously encountered stressors that were not resolved (or could not be "cured"), resulting in long-term alterations (e.g., diabetes, obstructive lung disease, surgical loss of organs or tissues) with a superimposed acute stressor (e.g., cold, pneumonia, urinary tract infection, heart failure, cerebrovascular accident, toe gangrene)
4. Usual coping behaviors of the individual in response to a stressful situation (e.g., denial, seeking medical attention immediately)

5. Availability and past utilization of support systems, such as significant others, religion, economic resources, and residence facilities
6. Amount of adaptation energy available

Selye states it thus [15]:
"Strive to achieve the highest attainable aim
But do not put up resistance in vain."

REFERENCES

1. Bailey, C. *Fit or Fat?* Boston: Houghton Mifflin, 1978.
2. Bromley, D. B. *The Psychology of Human Aging* (2nd ed.). Baltimore: Penguin, 1974.
3. Brunner, L. S., and Suddarth, D. S. *Textbook of Medical–Surgical Nursing* (5th ed.). Philadelphia: Lippincott, 1984.
4. Budoff, P. W. *No More Hot Flashes and Other Good News.* New York: Putnam, 1983.
5. Burnside, I. M. (Ed.). *Nursing and the Aged* (2nd ed.). New York: McGraw-Hill, 1981.
6. Hall, D. A. *The Aging of Connective Tissue.* New York: Academic, 1976.
7. Harris, J. *The Prime of Mrs. America; The American Woman at Forty.* New York: Putnam, 1975.
8. Hunt, B. K., and Hunt, M. *Prime Time: A Guide to the Pleasures and Opportunities of the New Middle Age.* New York: Day Books, 1974.
9. Jacob, S. W., and Francone, C. A. *Structure and Function in Man* (5th ed.). Philadelphia: Saunders, 1982.
10. Kintzel, K. C. (Ed.). *Advanced Concepts in Clinical Nursing* (2nd ed.). Philadelphia: Lippincott, 1977.
11. Masters, W. H., and Johnson, V. E. *Human Sexual Inadequacy.* Boston: Little, Brown, 1970.
12. Morbidity and mortality weekly report. *Smoking and Cancer* 31(7):77, 1982.
13. Parker, E. *The Seven Ages of Woman.* Baltimore: Johns Hopkins Press, 1960.
14. Rockstein, M. (Ed.). *Theoretical Aspects of Aging.* New York: Academic, 1974.
15. Selye, H. *The Stress of Life* (Rev. ed.). New York: McGraw-Hill, 1976.
16. Smith, E. Exercise for prevention of osteoporosis: A review. *Physician and Sportsmedicine* 10(3):72, 1982.
17. Steele, H. C., and Crow, C. B. *How to Deal With Aging and the Elderly.* Huntsville, AL: Strode Publishers, 1970.
18. Timiras P. S. *Developmental Physiology and Aging.* New York: Macmillan, 1972.
19. Troll, L. E., et al. *Families in Later Life.* Belmont, CA: Wadsworth, 1979.
20. Walford, R. L. *Maximum Life Span.* New York: Norton, 1983.

37

Cognitive and Psychosocial Development in Middlescence

Robert Bornstein

If you would not be forgotten as soon as you are
dead and rotten, either write things worth reading
or do things worth the writing.

—Benjamin Franklin

The philosophical roots that gave rise to the scientific, psychological study of human development caused research to focus on the infantile and childhood determinants of adult behavior. Conditions arising out of the industrial revolution provided impetus in the early 1900s for serious study of the adolescent stage of development. A number of forces first combined in the mid–1940s and then coalesced in the 1960s, 1970s, and 1980s to make old age and aging a major concern. Having focused on the two extremes of the life span, it was finally inevitable that developmentalists would look to the midlife phases (young adulthood and middlescence) for the links and bridges between these extremes.

This emerging interest in middlescent development among social and behavioral scientists has also been mirrored within the general population, where there has been a recent increase in the number of "midlife crisis" articles appearing in the popular press, and an enthusiastic reception given to books, such as Gail Sheehy's *Passages*.

The links and bridges uncovered thus far suggest that cognitive and psychosocial development during middlescence is characterized by a unique type of developmental bipotentiality. On the one hand, the processes and events that constitute middlescence can, and sometimes do, result in decreases in self-concept and esteem, personal adjustment, life satisfaction, and overall cognitive and psychosocial functioning. Furthermore, these negative shifts of middle age may be continued into, or exacerbated during, the later years of life. On the other hand, these same processes and events appear to provide other individuals with the opportunity to develop previously untapped sources of strength and satisfaction, thus resulting in a fuller, broader, and more enriching way of life that can then be maintained well into old age. Obviously, such developmental bipotentiality must also characterize the individuals who confront these processes and events. The outcome of such confrontations will to a large extent depend on the individual's reactions to, and utilization of, the opportunities presented.

THEORIES OF RELEVANCE TO THE STUDY OF MIDDLESCENCE

Biological Theories

Only passing reference will be made here to biological theories of middlescence, since they have been amply covered in the preceding chapter and their relationship to psychosocial development is neither well documented nor understood. To preview a point that will be made in Chapter 40, a graph drawn to represent biological functioning across the life span is not equally effective in communicating the course of psychological and social development, especially during middle and old age. For example, the biologically based degenerative change referred to as the menopause has been focused on by professionals and lay people alike as an event of middle age that has potentially traumatic overtones. Later in this chapter it will be demonstrated that the menopause results in a variety of individualistic responses ranging from the highly negative to the highly positive. This wide range of individualistic responses to biological events in general has directed social scientists to a growing consensus that an individual's progression through adulthood is more clearly defined or marked by psychosocial events and processes than by biological ones.

Psychological and Social Theories

JUNG'S ANALYTIC THEORY
Jung states that those aspects of one's personality that are the most basic are the very ones that are most difficult to deal with. Therefore, dealing with these aspects is postponed until such time as the individual has developed sufficient coping skills to handle them. During the "easier" stage of personality development, the ego, which serves to link the individual to external

reality, is being formed. The first 40 years or more of life are spent in this process, which is designed to optimize the individual's relationship with external environmental forces. The second and more difficult stage of personality development begins at approximately age 40 and continues throughout the remainder of the life span. This second stage is devoted to the development of the inner or true individual; hence the term **individuation** given to the process involved. The aim or goal of individuation, which presumably can only be approached but never fully attained, is the achievement of full and complete self-realization.

It is important to note that, according to Jung, the tasks of discovering one's real self and of striving for self-integration have been reserved for the second half of life, when the individual has acquired enough strength and coping skills to deal effectively with these basic issues of self-identity. Sufficient strength and coping skills are prerequisites because the individual must be able to integrate and to accept the most basic and primitive aspect of his or her personality, that is, the collective unconscious. When, or if, all goes well during this second stage of personality development, the individual approaches a self-realization in which the collective unconscious has revealed the accumulated wisdom and experience of countless eons of human existence. The major point is quite clear: The realization of one's full human potential, including wisdom, can only be achieved late in life because the process of individuation leading to this realization begins only in middlescence. The negative side of the bipotentiality inherent in Jung's theory is that the middle-aged individual may be unable to move toward realization of his or her full human potential.

ERIKSON'S STAGE OF GENERATIVITY
VERSUS STAGNATION
The concept of generativity denotes a concern with the establishment and guidance of future generations (see Appendixes B and C for the complete theory). Although the act of producing offspring may serve as one means of expressing generativity, the fact of having children per se does not guarantee that the individual has achieved a generative orientation. True generativity is a movement away from self-concern and self-indulgence and toward the welfare of those who are to follow us. According to Erikson, the mature individual is deeply involved with the welfare of future generations (his or her own as well as the children of others), is concerned about the kind of society future generations will have to live in, and is motivated to repay the world in some way for that which he or she has taken

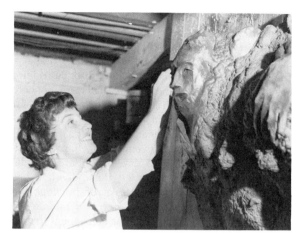

Figure 37–1. Erikson's task of generativity takes many forms as the individual tries to improve the quality of life for those around him or her or to leave something of value for future generations.

from it. Repayment typically involves meeting one's social and civic responsibilities (one of Havighurst's developmental tasks of middle age), and is often expressed through volunteer work. Many middlescents serve on community agency boards or citizens advisory boards; they may campaign for candidates for political office or solicit during fund-raising drives for charity. Others will participate in Little League, Scouting, or school activities. Red Cross, churches, and YMCA and YWCA offer other opportunities to express one's generative tendencies. The "Gray Lady" is encountered about as often as the "Candy Striper" in many settings. This desire to remain involved and productive in at least part-time work, including volunteer work, remains high even throughout old age [32]. In contrast, the concept of stagnation denotes a total absorption with the self and its needs to the exclusion of any concern about the welfare of others.

According to Erikson, the healthy resolution of the generativity versus stagnation dichotomy consists of possessing an abundance of generativity and just enough stagnation to guarantee that the individual will be sufficiently concerned with his or her own needs to ensure basic survival. Any resolution that deviates from this optimal or ideal ratio is associated with maladjustment. Thus bipotentiality exists in the possibility of either the healthy development of a primarily future-oriented world concern or the unhealthy development of a basically present-oriented self-absorption. An important aspect of Erikson's theory is the concept that the proper resolution of this seventh life-stage task is

contingent on, but not guaranteed by, the degree to which proper or optimal resolutions have occurred for all six previous developmental tasks. In turn, an optimal and healthy resolution of generativity versus stagnation will be important not only to the quality of psychosocial functioning during the middle years but also to the quality of life in the later years.

PECK'S DEVELOPMENTAL TASKS OF MIDDLE AGE
While Erikson theorizes that there is only one developmental task to be resolved during middlescence, Peck [57] hypothesizes that there are four. One of these tasks is "valuing wisdom versus valuing physical powers." The general course of biological development dictates that there will be a decline in general physical functioning and attractiveness (according to western society's youth-oriented criteria) throughout most of middle age and all of old age. Those individuals whose self-definition (identity) and value system place biophysical characteristics in a position of dominance and salience are quite likely to grow increasingly dissatisfied and unhappy as they grow older. To the extent that they rely on their physical powers in their social and work roles, these individuals are also likely to become less efficient and productive. A more positive alternative is needed, and one is provided in the form of wisdom. Defined as the ability to choose the most effective alternative of those available in any given decision-making situation, wisdom tends to increase with the accumulation of experience that accompanies growing older. Hence, greater life satisfaction, happiness, and psychosocial efficiency are made possible by the movement away from valuing physical powers and toward wisdom during middlescence. (Note the congruence of this position with that of Jung, who states that the acquisition of true wisdom begins in middle age.)

Peck's second developmental task is that of "socializing versus sexualizing in human relationships." Menopause may enable one to perceive a loved one more clearly as a total individual and companion rather than merely as a sexual object. As concerns with sexuality and sexual motivations decline with both age and years of marriage (this decline is not caused by the menopause per se), they can and should be increasingly replaced by concerns about the deeper and more meaningful aspects of interpersonal relationships.

A third developmental task of middlescence is "cathectic flexibility versus cathectic impoverishment." Peck defines cathectic flexibility as "the capacity to shift emotional investments from one person to another, and from one activity to another." Cathectic impoverishment is the lack of this same capacity. Flexibility rather than impoverishment becomes increasingly important during middle age because this is the time of life when most adults begin to experience the death of their own parents, the departure of their children from home, and various sources of social and friendship disruptions. Since both community and work involvements are at their peak, there also exists the greatest potential and need for the establishment of new emotional ties to people and activities.

A fourth and final developmental task of middle age is that of "mental flexibility versus mental rigidity." Because many of the major life decisions have already been made by middle age (e.g., whether or not to marry, choice of spouse, choice of career, whether or not to have children), the possibility exists that individuals will become increasingly set in their ways; that is, dogmatic in both opinion and ideas, closed-minded toward new experiences, and inflexible in seeking solutions to life's questions. According to Peck, such individuals can be said to be governed by the particular patterns of their past life history experiences. Since the general developmental processes and the particular events of middlescence may be relatively novel, behavior that is controlled by past responses may be less efficient than behavior that is guided by the individual's previous experience in problem solving. This latter description is that of mental flexibility.

HAVIGHURST'S THEORY OF DEVELOPMENTAL TASKS
Havighurst [33] proposed seven developmental tasks for the middle adult years (see Appendix C).

The particular order in which these developmental tasks are listed does not imply a predetermined hierarchy; the tasks are to be mastered as they are presented by society to the middle-aged adult—one at a time, in various combinations, or all at once. Failure to master these developmental tasks will result not only in exposure to social disapproval, high anxiety, and maladjustment but also in a decreased likelihood of mastering the developmental tasks to be presented during old age. In a similar vein, the likelihood of successful mastering of these developmental tasks depends on the degree to which the individual has mastered the developmental tasks of previous life stages. Thus the adaptations required in middle age result in another bipotentiality for adjustment that is, to some degree, preordained by previous adjustment history and foretells future adjustments. Several of Havighurst's developmental tasks have been or will be mentioned in conjunction with other theories, and several others will be discussed in conjunction with the effect of midlife events and institutions on self-esteem, happiness, and life satisfaction.

LEVINSON'S THEORY
OF INDIVIDUAL LIFE STRUCTURE
Levinson [48] hypothesizes that the life span can be broken down into five major eras, each lasting approximately 20 years. The first period is preadulthood, extending from birth to about 20 years of age, which is followed in turn by early adulthood from age 20 to 40, middle adulthood from age 40 to 60, late adulthood from age 60 to 80, and late-late adulthood, which ex-

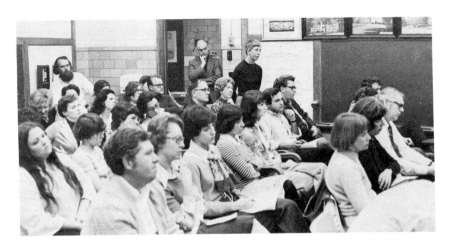

Figure 37–2. Energies formerly invested in improving individual relationships are now invested in improving community relationships as middlescents attend and participate in town and school-board meetings.

tends beyond the age of 80 years. Each era has its own particular flavor that is determined by the particular set of developmental tasks with which the individual is confronted; by the particular set of psychological characteristics that the individual possesses, such as motives, values, and attitudes; by the particular sets of social groups and institutions to which the individual belongs; and by the particular set of roles in which the individual engages. Levinson refers to both the style and the form of the interrelationships among all of these components as the "individual life structure." He also hypothesizes that there are transitional periods of approximately 5 years that serve to link together as well as overlap adjacent life eras.

The intent of the present chapter is best served by concentrating on the midlife transition, which represents the end of early adulthood and the onset of middle adulthood. Examination of the ages given above indicates that the midlife transition occurs at approximately 40 years of age.

As mentioned previously, individuals tend to make most of their major life decisions during the period of early adulthood. During the midlife transitional period, these prior decisions and commitments are reevaluated in an attempt to build a fuller, more balanced life structure. If this attempt is to succeed, these middle-aged adults must outgrow a number of youthful illusions, must accept the futility of attempting to stay young, and must cease worrying about growing old. In addition, discrepancies between one's present life

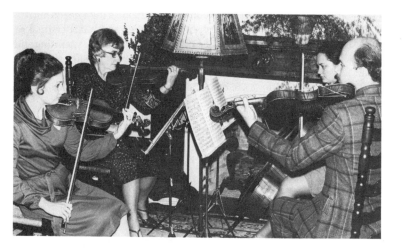

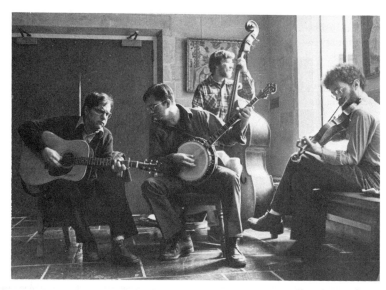

Figure 37–3. Interests, talents, and skills continue to be influenced both by past experiences and by one's current associations to provide a basis for social relationships and for aesthetic expression.

circumstances and the aspirations and expectations that existed when the original commitments were made must also be taken into consideration and reevaluated since it is quite likely that several discrepancies will have arisen during that time period.

For example, because younger workers often set lofty and somewhat unrealistic goals for themselves, they may perceive themselves as failing in their careers even when conventional and more objective measures might indicate otherwise. Although he or she is successful by all the yardsticks applied, the middle-aged worker may still feel alienated because the job or career that was chosen when other motivations were more salient is now found to be inappropriate to his or her newly developed sense of generativity. Such discrepancies also frequently occur with regard to marriage [11]. This process, which has been labeled "disenchantment" [58], consists of both a "cooling off" of the marriage relationship and a progressive loss of compatibility between a husband and wife. Even though disenchantment is not directly related to either marital dissatisfaction or divorce rates, it does provide grounds for "second guessing" during this period of reevaluation (see Part IX, especially Chaps. 30, 33, and 34 for a more detailed presentation of these family processes).

When the transitional period is concluded, a new life structure, which may assume a variety of different forms, is begun that ushers in the era of middle adulthood. For some individuals, the new life structure is a continuance of the previous total life-style, accompanied now by a commitment, an enthusiasm, and a sense of fulfillment that was missing in the previous life era. For others, there may be differing degrees of shifts in career, marriage, or social groups and roles. For relatively few individuals, there will be a total reorganization of such commitments. Although the smallest in numerical terms, this last group has received the most notoriety in the mass media; they have come to represent the epitome of change during the midlife crisis.

DISENGAGEMENT, ACTIVITY, AND IDENTITY CONTINUITY THEORIES

The major concern of the disengagement, activity, and identity continuity theories is with the cognitive and psychosocial changes that take place during the later years of life. For this reason, fuller and more detailed discussions of these three theories are reserved for Chapter 40. However, each theory either implicitly or explicitly says something of relevance to the cognitive

and psychosocial behavior of individuals during middlescence.

The major assumption of the disengagement theory [17] is that individuals must be removed from the mainstream of society (disengaged) prior to the time of their death in order to minimize any possible disruption to society. Since the likelihood of dying increases with age and older individuals tend to hold positions of greater wealth, power, and influence, the major focus of this theory is on society's need to disengage the older or aging adult and the possible mechanisms (such as retirement) for doing so. However, a second assumption states that some individuals undergo a self-disengagement process that has its beginnings during the middle years of life. This process is said to be characterized by a reduction in general energy levels, an increased preoccupation with one's own needs and desires, a reduction in social roles and interpersonal relationships, and a reorientation from counting the number of years lived to counting the years of life that may remain. It should be noted that some of these projections are consistent with previous characterizations

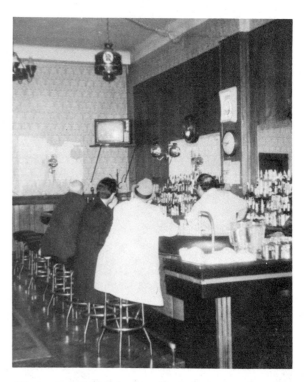

Figure 37–4. Each subculture has its own ideas about how adults should spend their leisure time.

of middlescent change, whereas others appear to be inconsistent.

Activity theory is primarily concerned with the explanation of why some individuals age more successfully than others, the degree of successful aging being evaluated in terms of life satisfaction or morale. The theory itself assumes that the level of one's life satisfaction and morale is directly tied to the level of general activity engaged in by the older adult, as represented by the totality of physical, psychological, and social activities and functions. Several of the theoretical positions already discussed either explicitly or implicitly point to several areas in which a decline in activity may take place during middlescence; many other areas become salient only in old age.

It is assumed that high life satisfaction and morale can be achieved through the substitution of new activities for lost or declining ones. Therefore, any of the biophysical declines discussed in Chapter 36 that result in a slowing down of physical activity will need to be compensated for by increases in either the cognitive, the psychological, or the social realms of activity. Similarly, the "empty nest" phenomenon of middlescence represents a source of lost functions and activities related to the parenting role that may require replacement. Theorists, such as Havighurst, have pointed out that it is during middlescence that the individual needs to prepare for the future loss of activities and roles that will occur in old age. For example, success in mastering the developmental task of cultivating adult leisure-time activities will have a positive effect in old age in terms of one's ability to adjust to the reduction in or loss of activities that are associated with the advent of retirement.

The identity continuity theory [2] assumes neither a necessary reduction in the individual's general activity level (disengagement theory) nor the necessity of maintaining high activity levels (the activity point of view). It assumes that successful aging is associated with the ability of the individual to maintain whatever patterns of behavior previously existed. From a practical point of view, the bipotentiality dealt with in this theory is whether or not the individual can maintain his or her previous style of life or patterns of behavior in the face of the particular set of processes and events that characterize middlescence in our society. The biophysical changes discussed in Chapter 36 represent some of these processes, and the developmental tasks proposed by Peck, Havighurst, and others represent some additional events that are peculiar to middlescence. Answers to this question are to be found in the data from empirical research on the cognitive and psychosocial development of middlescence.

FUNCTIONAL CAPACITIES IN MIDDLESCENCE

Cognitive Functioning in Middlescence

Two measures of cognitive functioning are usually reported in the literature: changes in intellectual abilities and intelligence per se, and changes in the performance of subjects in laboratory-created problem solving or learning situations. Intelligence test scores provide a quantitative estimate of cognitive capacity or capacities, but they provide little or no information about the actual quality of the thought processes or problem-solving strategies that are utilized in the achievement of that score. This latter point will be expanded as we pursue the data that are relevant both to the course of intellectual development during middlescence and to the learning and problem-solving skills of middle-aged adults.

THE COURSE OF INTELLECTUAL DEVELOPMENT
Most studies of intellectual development during adulthood have utilized a cross-sectional research strategy. The earliest of these studies concluded that the peak of intellectual development was achieved in the early teenage years; somewhat later studies placed the asymptote for intelligence in the individual's late twenties or early thirties; and the most recent ones place it well within middle age [12].

These results are highly consistent with the concepts of generational differences and the secular trend in human development. In the cross-sectional research strategy, groups of subjects of different ages are compared to one another. Since different subjects are studied at each age level, it is quite likely that the differences that are noted in intelligence are due less to age per se than to the differences in the life experiences of the different groups of subjects. Fifty-year-olds and 20-year-olds are born into different generations, which means that there are concomitant differences in many of the life history variables that are known to be related to measurable intelligence. Therefore, the later cross-sectional research studies that place the asymptote for intellectual development well into middle age are probably reflecting the life history advantages that these generations of subjects have relative to those that were measured in the earlier studies of intellectual development. This same phenomenon of generational differences has been documented in a number of developmental areas; it has been demonstrated that more recent generations tend to be taller, heavier, stronger, and healthier than previous generations, as well as being more intelligent. This generational shift has been termed the **secular trend.**

There is some evidence to indicate that in addition to being more intelligent, more recent generations tend to be more stable in their intellectual performances over at least a 14-year period [63]. One interpretation of these data is that more recent generations have been increasingly exposed to a modernized society that places a greater demand on individuals for heightened intellectual performance. It is further assumed that the continued use of intellectual functions results in their greater stability or at least less decline in these abilities throughout the latter portion of the life span. A great deal of the data to be presented later in the chapter clearly supports this set of assumptions.

Studies of intellectual development that utilized either the longitudinal research strategy or a strategy that combines both the cross-sectional and longitudinal strategies into a single research design, permit conclusions to be drawn about the actual age changes that take place in intellectual development. Taken together, these studies indicate that the intelligence quotient (IQ) is maintained or even increases slightly up to about 55 to 60 years of age [18, 55]. Although there is some controversy regarding the possibility of a slight intellectual decline after age 60, one point is quite clear: Even in those studies indicating a decline in intellectual performance after 60 years of age, the magnitude of the decline is such that the performance of a 70 to 75-year-old is still about equal to that of young adults [7, 37, 64]. Thus we can conclude that intellectual development peaks during the late middle years, or more conservatively, that it remains stable and superior to that exhibited by younger adults throughout the period of middlescence and into the beginnings of old age [7, 62, 64, 65].

Thus far, this discussion has dealt with general intellectual development during middlescence. An additional body of data has been accumulating that indicates that different forms or types of intellectual abilities apparently undergo different patterns of developmental change. It has been argued [39] that two broad classes of intellectual abilities become distinguishable from one another as intellectual development proceeds through adolescence and into adulthood. One class, **fluid intelligence,** consists of those abilities that are believed to be basically determined by the status of an individual's neurological and

physiological structures and functions as well as by the accumulative effects of negative learning experiences, such as those that produce mental rigidity and negative transfer. Fluid intelligence includes abilities, such as figural relationships, memory span, general reasoning, and associative power.

The other class, **crystallized intelligence,** is believed to be primarily determined by positive learning experiences, including any and all of those factors that tend to create and promote individual differences in general knowledge, motivation, and personal adjustment. It includes abilities, such as verbal comprehension, general information, number facility, and formal reasoning. Fluid intelligence would be expected to decline during the course of middlescence, since numerous degenerative biological changes are also taking place during this time period. On the other hand, the opportunity for learning and enculturation clearly increase with age, thus creating the expectation that crystallized intelligence would tend to improve with age.

According to the data from several studies, these predictions are fairly accurate. Fluid abilities tend to decline from a peak in early-to-middle adulthood while crystallized ones tend to remain stable or even to improve throughout the middle years and into old age [4, 38, 63].

The data also clearly indicate that the challenge of a complex and variable environment probably contributes to the overall stability or improvement (or both) in certain (crystallized) aspects of intellectual performance [61]. A high IQ, as assessed early in life, and the number of years of formal education are also positively correlated with this pattern of intellectual change [40, 56]. Individual differences in personality may also be influential, with those individuals who are more forceful, intense, and relatively strong in interpersonal relationships tending to have intelligence scores that increase with age [42].

LEARNING, PROBLEM SOLVING, AND PRODUCTIVITY
The overall conclusion drawn from laboratory-based research on the learning and problem-solving skills of subjects of different ages is that both types of performances tend to undergo slight declines during the latter half of middlescence. The difficulty in interpreting these kinds of data stems from the distinction that must be made between learning and problem solving per se and the measures of performance that are typically reported in the literature. One's performance on laboratory-created tasks is affected by a broad range of variables that may be relatively independent of the real

status of the performer's learning and problem-solving capacities.

One such variable is the motivational status of learners and problem solvers of different ages. Several studies suggest that when older adults are compared to younger ones they are less likely to respond in problem-solving situations unless they are relatively certain that their responses will be correct. This tendency toward greater cautiousness on the part of older subjects often results in their earning poorer scores, and it creates a hindrance to their own problem-solving or learning activities [9, 13, 25].

The exact nature and source of this cautiousness is still open to speculation. One author concluded that adults 40 years of age or less tend to have an "active mastery" orientation toward their environments [29, 30]. They perceive that boldness and risk taking will be rewarded, and they feel confident that they can achieve their goals by means of their own actions. However, starting at about age 40, there appears to be a reorientation toward a more passive mastery of the environment. The environment is now seen as being somewhat more complex and dangerous than it was at earlier ages, and the self-perception is that of having to conform and to accommodate. These proposed motivational shifts are consistent with an expansion-constriction view of the life span. According to this view, during the first half of the life span, individuals are characterized as "expansion-oriented"; that is, individuals tend to be externally oriented and to be driven by achievement, growth, and acquisition-oriented motives. In contrast, individuals during the latter half of the life span are "constriction-oriented"; that is, they become increasingly internally oriented and increasingly concerned about holding on to that which has already been gained as well as satisfying self-serving needs [47].

Regardless of the exact nature of the motivational shift being postulated, the effect on the performance of learning and problem-solving tasks would appear to be relatively straightforward. On the one hand, young adults who are still relatively attuned to the procedures of formal education and who are still oriented toward general achievement motives are more likely to be highly motivated to perform well on the problem-solving and learning tasks presented to them. On the other hand, middle-aged adults might perform more poorly than their younger counterparts simply because the performance of such laboratory-structured tasks is totally irrelevant to their personal motivations and concerns. More often than not, the motivational variable is linked to one or more characteristics of the task employed in such a way that the effects of each cannot be carefully evaluated. A prime example of this type of confounding interrelationship occurs between motivation and those memory processes that are critical to efficient problem solving.

Although research findings suggest that little or no long-term memory deficit occurs during the period of adulthood [23] and that significant short-term memory losses occur only at quite old ages [39], it has also been concluded that the more important or relevant the information is to the older adult, the more likely it is to be remembered [12]. More will be said about this particular topic in Chapter 40.

Other task characteristics may also place the older learner or problem-solver at a relative disadvantage. The pacing of a task is one such factor, since it interacts with age changes in reaction time. **Reaction time** is measured as the interval between the onset of the stimulus and the subject's response to it; this interval becomes increasingly greater from about age 20 and is greater for more complex tasks than simple ones. Older subjects, whose reactions are slowed down, are clearly at a disadvantage in the vast majority of laboratory-based studies of learning and problem-solving capacity because of the inclusion of a highly constrained time factor. Indeed, in the several studies in which such time constraints have been removed, it has been demonstrated that the performance of middle-aged and elderly subjects tends to become more congruent with that of the younger adults [1, 20, 21].

Even when learning and problem-solving capacity variables have been clearly and directly indicated as being contributors to the decline in performance, a difficulty in interpretation is often still present. For example, a number of studies indicate that middle-aged and elderly subjects utilize inadequate or inefficient mediational techniques during problem solving in comparison to younger adults [21]. However, the cross-sectional methodology employed in most of these studies leaves open the possibility that such deficits in performance are due to cohort-generational effects rather than to pure age-related declines in mediational skills. The mediational variable and three others for which generational differences have been found are discussed in some detail in Chapter 40.

Because it is so difficult to untangle the effects produced by generational differences, task characteristics, and motivational status from those produced by true age-related changes in learning ability and problem-solving capacity, it would seem logical to move away from laboratory-based research findings in order to gain an additional perspective. It has been stated previously that many aspects of intellectual performance peak during the middle years and that, in general, adults exhibit a greater fund of general knowledge during the midlife period than they do at younger ages. There is also a clear consensus that measures of general productivity, achievement, and community and work involvement reach a peak during middlescence. Such real-life measures of performance, when contrasted to the performances given in laboratory settings, clearly imply that middle-aged adults are at the height of their competence with regard to the type of learning and problem solving that applies to their everyday lives. The competence exhibited in real-life situations by middle-aged adults is the core precept in the analysis of psychosocial functioning, the topic to which we now turn.

Psychosocial Functioning During Middlescence

Although numerous definitions of personality can be found in the literature, all tend to have three elements in common: (1) Personality is a structure consisting of a particular grouping of traits, characteristics, values, attitudes, motives or behavioral styles; (2) this structure represents an individual's relatively unique interaction with his or her total environment (as such, it represents the totality of an individual's psychosocial functioning); and (3) once formed, this structure remains relatively stable across situations and endures over time. There is a great deal of controversy over the third point. The arguments for and against stability and a representative sample of the data gathered in support of each position are covered in some detail in Chapter 40. It will suffice for the purposes of this chapter to say that longitudinal research data indicate that there

are patterns of stability as well as patterns of change or instability in psychosocial functioning over the adult years.

Some psychosocial characteristics, such as general activity level; vocational interests; gender-expression; and life-style themes that include intellectualism, humanitarianism, practicality, and aestheticism, apparently tend to remain highly stable from the ages at which they are first developed [31]. Other characteristics show varying patterns of change, some changing in a similar direction for most adults while others change idiosyncratically. For example, the attitudes that subjects felt toward specific institutions, such as church, marriage, housekeeping, and childrearing were among the least stable and enduring aspects of personality measured in another longitudinal study [37].

Some of the changes that occur in the psychosocial functioning of middle-aged adults are a pure reflection of ontogenetic processes—universal or near universal developmental progressions that are relatively uninfluenced by specific past and present sociocultural forces. Although the exact nature of the midlife ontogenetic developmental progression is still open to speculation, a variety of possibilities have been suggested by the proposed shift from active to passive mastery, the expansion-constriction view of life span development, and the theoretical writings of Jung, Erikson, Levinson, and many others. It is also likely, however, that some midlife changes in psychosocial functioning are a reflection of the individual's immediate response to some current, and perhaps even traumatic, life situations. The third possibility is that such changes reflect the cojoint influence of ontogenetic processes interacting with current life events.

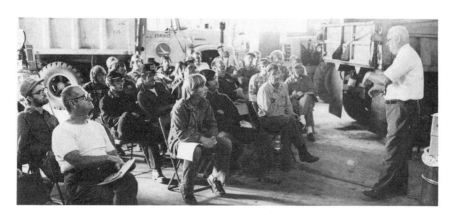

Figure 37–5. Learning experiences continue in many forms throughout the adult years.

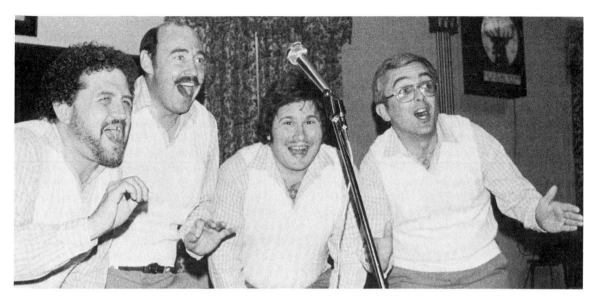

Figure 37-6. Middlescence is a wonderful period in the life cycle. The person has enough experience to provide competence and confidence and enough physical energy to invest with enthusiasm.

IMPACT OF MIDDLESCENT EVENTS, SITUATIONS, AND INSTITUTIONS ON LIFE SATISFACTION

Chronological Age and Gender

Many persons question whether or not middlescence is an age or stage of life that is more or less happy and satisfying than any other. Others wonder if there are any differences in the reported happiness and satisfaction of middle-aged men and women. Unfortunately, studies of self-esteem, self-concept, happiness, and life satisfaction have yielded somewhat contradictory results. Although some studies found little or no age-related change [15] and others reported decline in life satisfaction with age [46], an age-related increase in these measures was reported in a number of other studies [28, 35, 43, 51]. These and a series of somewhat related studies demonstrate that an individual's perception or evaluation of his or her particular life circumstances are a greater determinant of his or her self-esteem, happiness, and life satisfaction than is the individual's age or stage of life per se. Therefore, the most obvious conclusion is that each age or stage of life can be as positive (or negative) as any other; and that the self-esteem, happiness, and life satisfaction of middle-aged adults can be as positive as those of either younger or older adults.

A point needs to be made about the proper interpretation of the self-report data just alluded to. When chil-

dren, adolescents, and young adults are asked to evaluate middle age and several of its more pertinent situations, they tend to do so in negative terms. Middle age and the situations attendant to it are only slightly less negatively evaluated by middle-aged adults themselves. Such evaluations take on a positive tone only when middle-aged adults are asked to judge their own life circumstances. These findings can be interpreted in two different ways: The first interpretation is that middle age is in reality a troublesome and nonsatisfying stage of life, a fact that is denied and distorted by middle-aged adults when asked about their own life circumstances; the second interpretation is that everyone, including middle-aged adults themselves, are only assuming that middlescence is a troublesome and nonsatisfying stage of life for everyone but themselves. Such an assumption is not unreasonable, given the current youthful orientation of the society in which we live. According to this interpretation, the actual rather than the assumed state of affairs can be known only when individuals evaluate their own particular life circumstances. Fortunately, there is some evidence to indicate that such self-reports of life satisfaction and happiness are both reliable and accurate [72].

Also, no conclusion can be drawn with regard to the possibility of gender differences during middlescence. Thus one author states: "No one knows nor does anyone claim with reasonable proof that adult men are more adjusted or satisfied with life than adult women or that the reverse is true. Satisfaction is sexless; it is not the province of being male or female" [10]. There are, however, significant differences in the bases upon which each gender makes these judgments of self-esteem and happiness.

Although some feel it may be socially or economically mediated, many women apparently shift the basis for their self-image during middlescence away from relationships and towards their own abilities and feelings, whereas men remain relatively more occupationally minded [3]. It is quite possible that the shift noted for women is either reflective of, or caused by, the occurrence during middlescence of two major life events—the menopause and the "empty nest" phenomenon.

MENOPAUSE
During the first half of this century, **involutional melancholia** was a psychiatric label commonly applied to menopausal and severely depressed women. On the assumption that the menopause signified to these women that their childbearing days were over, their sexuality was in a state of decline, or their attractiveness was diminished or all three, it was further assumed that the depressed behavior of the patient was a clear reaction to the psychological significance of menopause. We now know, however, that involutional melancholia as a psychiatric diagnosis may occur at anytime during adulthood, that it applies equally to the depressed state of men and women, and that it has little or nothing to do with the menopause in particular or the climacteric in general.

In this regard, younger women see the menopause as a more significant life event than do either menopausal or postmenopausal women; only about one-half of menopausal women agree that the menopause is an unpleasant, disturbing, or generally negatively toned event, and approximately two-thirds of menopausal and postmenopausal women report positive changes once the menopause has been passed. Feeling better physically, having more confidence, and being freer to do things for oneself are some of the positive changes reported by postmenopausal women [54].

In another study, only 4 out of 100 women mentioned the menopause as the middlescent change that worried them the most. In contrast, widowhood was mentioned by 52 of these same women. Several other negative stereotypes were also unsupported; for example, 68 percent of the women reported either no effect or a positive change in physical and emotional health as an accompaniment to menopause, whereas only 32 percent reported a negative change. In addi-tion, 83 percent reported either no effect or that sexual relations had become more important, whereas only 18 percent reported that sexual relations had become less important [52].

None of the data reported above are intended to deny the fact that the menopause may be a potentially devastating event for some middle-aged women. The women studied in this latter report consistently rated themselves more favorably than they rated women in general, a fact that led the author to conclude that the attitudes of women toward menopause are both complex and ambivalent (a clear indication of bipotentiality). Furthermore, clinical findings suggest that the menopause does contribute to the formation of a midlife depression in some women, especially those who totally predicate their self-image and feelings of self-esteem on their biological femininity and the social roles that directly derive from it. For the vast majority of women, however, this does not appear to be the case.

THE "EMPTY NEST" PHENOMENON
The effects of the "empty nest" are quite similar to those of menopause; that is, having one's children leave home may be the occasion for decreases in life satisfaction, happiness, self-esteem, and general mental health in both men and women, or it may usher in a new and more positively toned stage of adult life.

The fact that the departure of children from a home may either aggravate an already existing middle-aged depression or may serve as the most prominent cause of that depression has been well documented in the context of clinical case studies. The process or dynamics through which the departure is translated into parental depression, however, is still open to clinical conjecture. One study [6] reports that "women who had overprotective or overinvolved relationships with their children were more likely to be depressed in their postparental period than were women who did not have such relationships" [71]. In this same study, it was also noted that homemakers were more likely to become depressed than were working women (presumably because this latter group of women were able to maintain another role in which they were active).

The first finding seems to offer support for two somewhat different dynamics: One is that overly maternal women are likely to interpret the child's departure from home as a form of personal rejection; the other is the existentialist notion that life without children becomes meaningless for such women. In either case, the additional evidence that homemakers are more likely than working mothers to become depressed lends support to the more general thesis that such depressions are a culturally based phenomenon caused by confining women to a constricted range of life choices and behavioral roles (see Chap. 29).

Although most studies focus on mothers, it is noted that fathers also experience emotional changes when their children leave home. Both parents may miss the child's company and the time he or she occupied in their lives. The parents may suddenly realize that they have missed hundreds of opportunities to have participated more actively in the child's development. In an attempt to cope with the loss or as an effort to compensate for earlier failures, some parents will now try to become more deeply involved in their child's life—a factor that may either enhance or frustrate the life of either. While the "empty nest" is associated with negative states in some parents, the data indicate that the majority of middle-aged people view this event quite positively. Most parents look forward to this event with anticipation and report positive feelings about being relieved of the restrictions that accompany childrearing [26, 50]. Furthermore, most postparental couples report improved marital relationships after their children leave; after honeymooning couples and the elderly, those couples whose children are leaving home report the greatest degree of satisfaction with their marriages [19, 23].

These findings should be encouraging to middle-aged adults whose children are about to leave home, since it is estimated that such couples will spend 20 or more postparental years together before either partner dies. The emptying of the nest does not mean, however, that family relationships and ties are ended or broken at this time. These same middle-aged adults will remain in close contact with their own aging parents and will provide economic help, emotional gratification, personal health care, and household management for them when and if it becomes necessary [36, 66, 67, 68]. They usually will also remain in close contact with their own children and will provide similar services whenever they are required [32]. In addition, a new and perhaps substitute family role often becomes available to these middle-aged adults—that of being grandparents.

Grandparenthood

Although we tend to assume that grandparenthood occurs in old age and at a time when most persons have retired and are more or less disengaged from many of their other roles and commitments, in actuality it is far more likely to occur during middlescence when work and other role involvements are at their very peak. This observation may partially explain the fact that grand-

parenting is associated with a variety of psychological meanings, that individuals differ in their styles of grandparenting, and that grandparents also report varying degrees of satisfaction or dissatisfaction with the role. For example, in one study [53] it was found that approximately 33 percent of the grandparents studied viewed grandparenthood as a form of psychological immortality or continuity; another 23 percent perceived it as a source of emotional self-fulfillment that was different from that experienced during parenthood; and an additional 8 percent saw grandparenthood as representing the creation of a new role, that of teacher or resource person. In contrast, 28 percent of the grandparents interviewed attributed little, if any, meaning to the role of grandparenthood. They reported feeling remote from their grandchildren and indicated that their grandchildren had little or no effect on their own lives. In congruence with the point made earlier, the vast majority of the grandmothers in this category indicated that they lacked the time to devote to grandparenting because of prior commitments to both work and community affairs.

Five grandparenting styles were discernible within the data of this same study:

1. The formal grandparents are those who do no parenting whatsoever. They follow what they regard to be the proper and prescribed role for grandparents, one that includes the provision of special treats and indulgences to their grandchildren.
2. Grandparents as a reservoir of family wisdom represents an authoritarian and patricentered relationship style, in which authority lines are maintained and emphasized, so that the relatively young parents occupy a subordinated position. The grandfather dispenses special skills and resources to the parents and grandchildren.
3. The distant-figure style of grandparenting is characterized by infrequent and short-duration contacts with the grandchildren. These contacts are usually confined to the celebrations that take place on holidays and other ritual occasions.
4. The surrogate parent style of grandparenting arises whenever a grandparent assumes actual child caretaking responsibilities for a parent who works.
5. The fun-seeking grandparents have a relationship with their grandchildren that is characterized by informality and playfulness and in which lines of authority are totally irrelevant. These grandparents participate with the child in a wide variety of activities for the express purpose of having fun.

The data offer some evidence that the grandparenting role may itself be affected by the general psychosocial status of the grandparents; thus the formal grandparenting style occurred more frequently in older grandparents than in younger ones, whereas the reverse was true of the fun-seeking and distant-figure grandparenting styles. The researchers themselves point out that the data may be reflecting a secular trend in which grandparenthood in middle age is qualitatively different from the grandparenthood that occurs in old age.

Additional support for this position is seen in the data from another study [49] in which it was found that young widowed grandmothers who led busy lives of their own often resented the demands made on them to care for their grandchildren. These women did not see babysitting as an enjoyable opportunity to interact with their grandchildren, and they reported being glad to return to the quiet of their own homes.

Although 60 percent of the subjects in the first study reported experiencing comfort, satisfaction, and pleasure from the grandparenting role, an additional 33 percent of grandparents reported discomfort or disappointment with the role. It would thus appear that grandparenthood, like the other midlife events and institutions previously discussed, is accompanied by its own kind of bipotentiality for life satisfaction and happiness.

General Health Status

A full discussion of health maintainence during middlescence has been presented in Chapter 36. It is being mentioned here because health status turns out to be one of the two or three most consistently accurate predictors of life-satisfaction and morale among both middle-aged and elderly adults; good health is associated with positive self-reported ratings of well-being, while poor health is predictive of negative ratings. Health status appears to affect well-being both directly and indirectly. In the latter case, poor health often necessitates a reduction in general activity level and an increased dependency on others—two conditions that, in turn, serve to directly reduce overall satisfaction and morale.

An often overlooked point is that poor health in the form of chronic illness and/or disabilities not only adversely affects the well-being of those individuals so afflicted; but it also has a correspondingly negative impact on the well-being of their spouses even when the health status of the spouse is relatively good [24]. Given the typical age differential of most married couples, we can anticipate that more late middle-aged women than men will experience a decline in their own life-satisfaction and morale as a result of the declining health status of their aging partners.

Loss of Spouse

The first and second ranked of life's stressors are the death of a spouse and separation or divorce. The negative impact of these events has been documented elsewhere in this volume (see Chaps. 21, 34, and 38), and need not be repeated here. Some findings from research in these areas, however, are worthy of particular note within the general context of middlescent well-being; and more importantly, such a discussion will serve to bring the other side of bipotentiality into focus. We have a tendency to overlook the fact that personal growth and development are also possible outcomes.

The negative impact of separation or divorce appears to be greater for middle-aged couples than for those either younger or older; presumably because middle-aged couples are at the peak of involvement

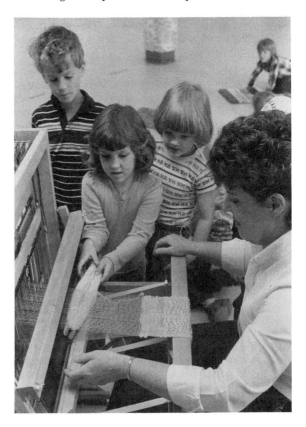

Figure 37-7. Generativity is expressed by sharing one's skills and interests with the next generation.

with their families and associated systems. While middle-aged divorcees are more disadvantaged than their male counterparts in terms of role loss, readjustment, social isolation, and economic deprivation, it is the men who seem to experience the greater reduction in well-being, presumably because they are ill-prepared to handle the daily routines involved in running a household. Women, on the other hand, seem to experience relatively more emotional turmoil prior to the actual separation or divorce [16].

In spite of the many difficulties associated with divorce, most divorced individuals experience a general sense of relief and report that their lives are more manageable than they were under conditions of continual tension and hostility [45]. Furthermore, husband-absent women appear to be less likely than their husband-present counterparts to see themselves as the second or more submissive sex. They are also reported to be more efficient, more ambitious, and better able to manage finances [8].

The death of one's spouse appears to be more stressful when it occurs in middlescence than later in life, since several studies have noted that older widows adjust more easily than do younger ones [49]. This effect may be due, in part, to the fact that the family system is less disrupted by death after the advent of the empty nest than prior to it; it is certainly due, in part, to the fact that death is more likely to have been anticipated, expected, and rehearsed for by the old. Thus, one study [27] found that those women who possessed long term knowledge of their spouses' inevitable deaths were better able to "pull themselves together" afterwards.

Although the death of a spouse is reported to be more stressful than separation or divorce, some of the long-term repercussions of the former actually appear to be less severe. Divorced individuals usually retain vestiges of personal guilt along with mixed feelings of longing and bitterness over the perceived role that each spouse played in the failure of the marriage; and the failed marriage can, in some communities, continue to be a source of social stigma. In contrast, loss of one's spouse through death is usually viewed as one of life's normal vicissitudes, one that merits the empathic and supportive behavior of family and friends in response to the surviving member's noble attempt to cope with his or her personal grief and loss.

In addition, the actual impact of the spouse's death depends on the degree to which the marriage role was central to the survivor's identity and value system. In all candor, one's status on the career ladder may take precedence over family involvement for many men and some women; and parenthood may be more important than the role of spouse, especially among women. Regardless of the actual hierarchy of roles involved, it is also true that some husbands and wives will have failed to establish close, meaningful, and intimate relationships with each other; not all dissatisfied and unhappy couples opt to separate and/or divorce. The death of one's spouse under either of these conditions would not be nearly as devastating and might even have positive consequences for the surviving spouse. Whatever the reason or reasons, a surprisingly large percentage of older widows not only appear to grow accustomed to living alone but also report actually preferring to do so [70].

Even the death of a deeply loved partner can have its positive aspects. Many such individuals come to realize for the first time that they do possess the personal strength and resources to cope with any and all of life's vicissitudes. Initially, they may be forced to pause and to reexamine the current flow of their lives, but it then becomes possible to strip away both the humdrum and the superfluous, leaving revealed that which is personally relevant and meaningful. The individual can then begin to live life to the fullest of his or her potential [5, 41].

Occupational Status

It seems most appropriate to conclude this discussion of midlife events and institutions with an examination of occupational status. For example, it has already been noted that the reaction to midlife events, such as menopause, the empty nest phenomenon, and grandparenthood, is often colored by the working or nonworking status of the individuals involved. Furthermore, one's career or job may serve as the vehicle through which identity and generativity are expressed (see the section on Erikson, preceding), or it may become a focal point in the reevaluation of one's entire life structure (see the section on Levinson, preceding).

A final justification for placing occupational status in a position of prominence is the sheer force of its prevalence—almost all adult males work, and at any given time, approximately 50 percent of adult females are also employed. In this latter regard, it is estimated that 90 percent of women are employed outside the home at some time in their lives. The trend, however, is toward relatively high employment rates for women in their late teens and early twenties and then again in their midforties. While the interim period of relatively low employment can be attributed to marriage and the onset of family demands, it is not clear that the upswing in employment for women during the middle years stems from any one particular cause. The

finding that increasing numbers of women are returning to college and then seeking employment after the
age of 30 [73] may reflect an adjustment to the empty
nest; a necessity brought about by general financial
difficulties, separation, divorce, or early widowhood;
or a generational difference in which the woman of
today is more career-oriented. For many women,
working simply represents a return to an earlier source
of self-expression and satisfaction in addition to that
already derived from family life.

In this regard, it has been pointed out that work may
have different connotative meanings for different persons [69]. For any given individual, the work being performed may come to symbolize one or more of the
following: a way of earning a living, a form of creative
self-expression or definition, a source of prestige and
recognition, a basis for feelings of worth and self-respect, a way of being useful, or an enjoyable activity
in and of itself. It is thus evident that the degree of
satisfaction or dissatisfaction derived from one's job,
work, or occupational status varies according to both
the meaning assigned to the work being performed and
the characteristics of the job per se. In this regard, one
writer concludes that "those most likely to experience
poor working conditions and least likely to experience
the delights of working—unskilled workers, minority
groups, and women—are likely to emphasize those aspects of their job that make the difference between its
being miserable and being okay" [69]. Although different individuals emphasize different aspects of their
jobs, American workers as a whole express highly favorable attitudes toward their work. Contrary to the
stereotype of wholesale job dissatisfaction, a fairly recent survey found that 75 percent of workers 21 years
of age or less reported being satisfied with their jobs,
whereas a full 90 percent of workers 30 years of age
or older expressed satisfaction [59].

Since the work role is the focal source of feelings of
self-esteem, satisfaction, and happiness with life in
general for almost all men and for an increasing number of career-oriented women, the relationship to one's
work produces an effect that extends well beyond the
confines of the work situation and into other life areas.
Some men become increasingly absorbed in their work
as they grow older, and there is a concomitant decline
in the degree to which these men are involved with,
and particiate in, family affairs [11, 23]. This distancing between an increasingly "workaholic" father and
his family may cause, contribute to, or simply reflect
the process of disenchantment. Whichever the case
may be, everyone is familiar with the wealth of negatively toned self-reports and clinical-case study data

coming from both wives and children who complain
bitterly of having husbands and fathers who are too
busy to provide the personal attention that is so vital
to their own happiness.

Furthermore, preoccupation with work, or any other
single role, to the exclusion of leisure time and other
role commitments tends to be associated with a less
than successful life-style. Another somewhat unsuccessful life-style is that in which individuals place a
great deal of emphasis on their leisure activities as a
form of compensation for the deficiencies experienced
in their work (or homemaker, parental) role. The most
successful life-styles encountered are those characterized by a balance between the use of leisure time and
the participation in major social roles, such as that of
worker, homemaker, and parent. Sometimes the leisure activities remain home-centered; for others, they
spread out into the larger community [34].

CONCLUSIONS

Three basic themes seem to stand out as reasonable
summary statements of the cognitive and psychosocial
development that occurs during middle age.

The first theme is that contrary to popular stereotypes, the middle years of life do more than just reflect
the accumulated effects of previous years of development; these are years that are themselves characterized by development and change. This change is both
inherent in the process of growing older and is necessitated by the events, situations, and institutions that
are commonly associated with middlescence in our
society but that are not necessarily an intrinsic part
of it.

The second basic theme is that of developmental bipotentiality during middlescence. Middle-aged adults
may evolve a future-oriented concern for society, or
they may become increasingly self-absorbed and
preoccupied; they may begin to reap the benefits of
wisdom, or they may be cut off from their true natures
forever; they may experience an increase in cognitive
proficiency or a decline in intellectual ability; they may
also experience an increase in self-esteem, happiness,
and life satisfaction, or they may suffer serious declines in all three.

The third and final observation is that generally
speaking, middle-aged adults appear to be "at the peak
of their form." Although the range of individual differences is quite large, the preponderance of data appears to indicate that cognitive skills tend to peak
during the late middlescent years as do work and com-

munity involvement and general productivity. Furthermore, feelings of self-esteem, happiness, and life satisfaction are at least as positive during this life stage as during any other.

The spirit of the full-productivity, peak-capacity, and high life satisfaction of middle-aged adults, as reported in this chapter, is captured in an anonymous quote in which the word **maturity** should be equated with **middlescence:** "Maturity is the time of life when, if you had the time, you'd have the time of your life."

REFERENCES

1. Arenberg, D. Age differences in retroaction. *J. Gerontol.* 22:88, 1967.
2. Atchley, R. C. *The Social Forces in Later Life* (3rd ed.). Belmont, CA: Wadsworth, 1980.
3. Back, K. W. Transition to aging and the self-image. *Aging and Human Development* 2:296, 1971.
4. Baltes, P. B., and Schaie, K. W. On Life-Span Developmental Research Paradigms: Retrospects and Prospects. In P. B. Baltes and K. W. Schaie (Eds.), *Life-Span Developmental Psychology: Personality and Socialization.* New York: Academic, 1973.
5. Barrett, C. J. Intimacy in widowhood. *Psychol. of Women Quarterly* 5:473, 1981.
6. Bart, P. Depression in Middle-aged Women. In V. Gornick and B. K. Moran (Eds.), *Woman in Sexist Society.* New York: Basic Books, 1971.
7. Bayley, N. Cognition and Aging. In K. W. Schaie (Ed.), *Theory and Methods of Research on Aging.* Morgantown, WV: West Virginia University, 1968.
8. Bendo, A. A., and Feldman, H. A. Comparison of the self-concept of low-income women with and without husbands present. *Cornell J. Soc. Relations* 9:53, 1974.
9. Birkhill, W. R., and Schaie, K. W. The effect of differential reinforcement of cautiousness in intellectual performance among the elderly. *J. Gerontol.* 30:578, 1975.
10. Bischof, L. J. *Adult Psychology* (2nd ed.). New York: Harper & Row, 1976.
11. Blood, R. O., and Wolfe, D. M. *Husbands and Wives: The Dynamics of Married Living.* Westport, CT: Greenwood Press, 1978.
12. Botwinick, J. *Cognitive Processes in Maturity and Old Age.* New York: Springer, 1967.
13. Botwinick, J. Disinclination to venture response versus cautiousness in responding: Age differences. *J. Genet. Psychol.* 115:55, 1969.
14. Bradbury, W. *The Adult Years* (Rev. ed.). Alexandria, VA: Time-Life Books, 1978.
15. Cameron, P. Stereotypes about generational fun and happiness vs. self-appraised fun and happiness. *Gerontologist* 12:120, 1972.
16. Chiriboga, D. "Marital Separation in Early and Late Life: A Comparison." Paper presented at the 32nd annual meeting of The Gerontology Society, Dallas, Texas, 1979.
17. Cumming, E., and Henry, W. E. *Growing Old: The Process of Disengagement.* New York: Basic Books, 1961.
18. Cunningham, W. R., and Owens, W. A. The Iowa State Study of Intellectual Abilities. In K. W. Schaie (Ed.), *Longitudinal Studies of Adult Psychological Development.* Guiford Press, 1981.
19. Deutscher, I. The quality of postparental life: Definitions of the situation. *J. Marr. and Fam.* 26:52, 1964.
20. Eisdorfer, C., Axelrod, S., and Wilkie, F. L. Stimulus exposure time as a factor in serial learning in an aged sample. *J. Abnorm. Soc. Psychol.* 67:594, 1963.
21. Elias, M. F., Elias, P. K., and Elias, J. W. *Basic Processes in Adult Developmental Psychology.* St. Louis: Mosby, 1977.
22. Erikson, E. H. *Childhood and Society* (2nd ed.). New York: Norton, 1964.
23. Feldman, H. *Development of the Husband-Wife Relationship: A Research Report,* Ithaca, New York: Cornell University, 1964.
24. Fengler, A. P., and Goodrich, N. Wives of elderly disabled men: The hidden patients. *The Gerontologist* 19:175, 1979.
25. Fozzard, J. L., Nuttal, R. L., and Waugh, N. C. Aged-related differences in mental performance. *Aging and Human Development* 3:19, 1972.
26. Gass, G. Z. Counseling implications of woman's changing role. *Personnel and Guidance Journal* 37:482, 1959.
27. Glick, I., Weiss, R., and Parkes, C. *The First Year of Bereavement.* New York: Wiley, 1974.
28. Gurin, G., Veroff, J., and Feld, S. *Americans View Their Mental Health: A Nationwide Interview Survey.* New York: Arno Press, 1980.
29. Gutmann, D. Female Ego Styles and Generational Conflict. In J. M. Bardwick et al. (Eds.), *Feminine Personality and Conflict,* Belmont, CA: Brooks/Cole, 1970.
30. Gutmann, D. The Cross-Cultural Perspective: Notes Toward a Comparative Psychology of Aging. In J. E. Birren and K. W. Schaie (Eds.), *Handbook of the Psychology of Aging,* New York: Van Nostrand, Reinhold, 1977.
31. Haan, N., and Day, D. A longitudinal study of change and sameness in personality development, adolescence to later adulthood. *Aging and Human Development* 5:11, 1974.
32. Harris, L., et al. *The Myth and Reality of Aging in America.* Washington, D.C.: The National Council on the Aging, 1975.
33. Havighurst, R. J. *Developmental Tasks and Education* (3rd ed.). New York: McKay, 1973.
34. Havighurst, R. J., and Feigenbaum, K. Leisure and Life-Style. In B. L. Neugarten (Ed.) *Middle Age and Aging.* Chicago: University of Chicago Press, 1968.
35. Hess, A. L., and Bradshaw, H. L. Positiveness of self-concept and ideal self as a function of age. *J. Genet. Psychol.* 117:57, 1970.
36. Hill, R. Decision Making and the Family Life Cycle. In E. Shanas and G. F. Streib (Eds.), *Social Structure and the Family: Generational Relations.* Englewood Cliffs, NJ: Prentice-Hall, 1965.
37. Honzik, M. P., and MacFarlane, J. W. *Personality Development and Intellectual Development from 21 Months to 40*

Years. APA Symposium on Maintenance of Intellectual Functioning with Advancing Years, Miami Beach, Florida, 1970.

38. Hooper, F. H., and Storck, P. A. "A Life Span Analysis of Fluid Vs. Crystallized Intelligence." Paper presented at the 25th annual meeting of the Gerontological Society, San Juan, Puerto Rico, 1972.

39. Horn, J. L. Organization of Data on Life-Span Development of Human Abilities. In L. R. Gowet and P. B. Baltes (Eds.), *Life-Span Developmental Psychology.* New York: Academic, 1970.

40. Hoyer, W. J., Labouvie, G. V., and Baltes, P. B. Modification of response speed deficits and intellectual performance in the elderly. *Hum. Dev.* 16:232, 1973.

41. Imara, M. Dying as the Last Stage of Growth. In E. Kübler-Ross (Ed.), *Death: The Final Stage of Growth.* Englewood Cliffs, NJ: Prentice-Hall, 1975.

42. Jarvik, L. F., Eisdorfer, C., and Blum, J. E. (Eds.). *Intellectual Functioning in Adults: Psychological and Biological Influences.* New York: Springer, 1973.

43. Kaplan, H. B., and Pokorny, A. D. Aging and self-attitude: A conditional relationship. *Aging and Human Development* 1:241, 1970.

44. Kelly, E. L. Consistency of the adult personality. *Am. Psychol.* 10:659, 1955.

45. Kitson, G. C. Attachment to the spouse in divorce: A scale and its application. *J. Marr. Fam.* 44:379, 1982.

46. Kogan, N., and Wallach, M. A. Age changes in values and attitudes. *J. Gerontol.* 16:272, 1961.

47. Kuhlen, R. G. Personality Change with Age. In P. Worchel and D. Byrne (Eds.), *Personality Change.* New York: Wiley, 1964.

48. Levinson, D. J., et al. *The Seasons of A Man's Life.* New York: Knopf, 1978.

49. Lopata, H. Z. *Widowhood in an American City.* Cambridge, MA: Schenkman, 1973.

50. Lowenthal, M. F., and Chiriboga, D. Transition to the empty nest. *Arch. Gen. Psychiatry* 26:8, 1972.

51. Lowenthal, M. F., and Chiriboga, D. Social Stress and Adaptation: Toward a Life-Course Perspective. In C. Eisdorfer and M. P. Lawton (Eds.), *The Psychology of Adult Development and Aging.* Washington, DC: American Psychological Association, 1973.

52. Neugarten, B. L. A New Look at Menopause. In C. Gordon and G. Johnson (Eds.), *Readings in Human Sexuality: Contemporary Perspectives.* New York: Harper & Row, 1976.

53. Neugarten, B. L., and Weinstein, K. K. The Changing American Grandparent. In B. L. Neugarten (Ed.), *Middle Age and Aging.* Chicago: University of Chicago Press, 1968.

54. Neugarten, B. L., et al. Women's Attitudes Toward the Menopause. In B. L. Neugarten (Ed.), *Middle Age and Aging.* Chicago: University of Chicago Press, 1968.

55. Owens, W. A. Age and mental abilities: A second adult follow-up. *J. Educ. Psychol.* 57:311, 1966.

56. Palmore, E. B. (Ed.). *Normal Aging II.* Durham, NC: Duke University Press, 1974.

57. Peck, R. C. Psychological Developments in the Second Half of Life. In B. L. Neugarten (Ed.), *Middle Age and Aging.* Chicago: University of Chicago Press, 1968.

58. Pineo, P. C. Disenchantment in the latter years of marriage. *Marriage and Family Living* 23:3, 1961.

59. Quinn, R. P., Staines, G. L., and McCullough, M. R. *Job Satisfaction: Is There a Trend?* (Manpower Research Monograph No. 30). Washington, D.C.: U.S. Department of Labor, Manpower Administration, 1974.

60. Richards, A. Personal Communication. 1984.

61. Schaie, K. W. Age Changes in Adult Intelligence. In D. S. Woodruff and J. E. Birren (Eds.), *Aging: Scientific Perspectives and Social Issues.* New York: Van Nostrand Reinhold, 1975.

62. Schaie, K. W. The Seattle Longitudinal Study: A Twenty-one Year Exploration of Psychometric Intelligence in Adulthood. In K. W. Schaie (Ed.) *Longitudinal Studies of Adult Psychological Development.* New York: Guilford Press, 1983.

63. Schaie, K. W., Labouvie, G. V., and Buesch, B. Generational and cohort-specific differences in adult cognitive functioning. *Dev. Psychol.* 9:151, 1973.

64. Schaie, K. W., and Strother, C. R. The effects of time and cohort differences on the interpretation of age changes in cognitive behavior. *Multivariate Behavioral Research* 3:259, 1968.

65. Schaie, K. W., and Strother, C. R. A cross-sequential study of age changes in cognitive behavior. *Psychol. Bull.* 70:671, 1968.

66. Shanas, E. The family as a social support system in old age. *Gerontologist* 19:169, 1979.

67. Shanas, E., et al. *Old People in Three Industrial Societies.* New York: Atherton Press, 1968.

68. Sussman, M. B. Relationships of Adult Children with Their Parents in the United States. In E. Shanas and G. Streib (Eds.), *Social Structure and the Family:* Englewood Cliffs, NJ: Prentice-Hall, 1965.

69. Troll, L. E. *Early and Middle Adulthood: The Best is Yet to Be—Maybe* (2nd ed.). Monterey, CA: Brooks/Cole, 1984.

70. Troll, L. E. *Continuations: Adult Development and Aging.* Monterey, CA: Brooks/Cole, 1982.

71. Williams, J. H. *Psychology of Women: Behavior in a Biosocial Context* (2nd ed.). New York: Norton, 1983.

72. Wood, V., Wylie, M. L., and Sheafer, B. An analysis of a short self-report measure of life satisfaction: Correlation with rater judgments. *J. Gerontol.* 24:465, 1969.

73. Zatlin, C. E., Storandt, M., and Botwinick, J. Personality and values of women continuing their education after thirty-five years of age. *J. Gerontol.* 28:216, 1973.

38
Midlife Crises

Nancy M. Whitacre

And let today embrace the past with remembrance and the future with longing.

—Kahlil Gibran, *The Prophet*

The midlife period presents unique challenges to each individual. It is the period when one expects to achieve maturity and to be most productive [21]. The middlescent is in a pivotal position. The individual, through introspection, can look back on successes and failures and look forward to options and assurances. "Is this all I am going to do?" and "Do I have enough time to accomplish everything that I want and need to do?" are two questions with which the middlescent struggles. The introspection and questioning help the middlescent to reassess values and relationships and to place tasks and goals into perspective.

Crises can be viewed as events or circumstances that challenge the individual's normal coping patterns and generally require the generation and adoption of new behaviors and philosophical approaches to the exigencies of life. A crisis involves a transitional period with the opportunity for further personality growth as well as the danger of an increased vulnerability to more serious consequences [5]. Thus, a crisis can become a stepping stone to either greater maturity or to personal disintegration. This chapter will address some of the unique stressors of middlescence and some techniques for maintaining psychological integrity through the transitional periods.

CRISIS THEORIES

Persons generally adopt behavior patterns that minimize self-awareness and self-strain. Since we are constantly facing situations that call for problem-solving techniques with a minimum of delay, habituated responses enable us to work through these daily tasks with minimal energy expenditure [5].

Caplan

Caplan [5] postulates that people develop a repertoire of coping skills that generally requires little or no adaptation to resolve problems. A crisis arises when these techniques are inadequate to meet the unique needs of the situation. In crisis, the individual initially attempts to use a known mechanism to help solve the specific problem within a reasonable length of time. As the person employs new approaches for resolution of the problem, a new pattern of behavior may emerge. Consequently, crises present opportunities for either disintegration or growth.

In crisis, the individual's functioning is interrupted. Unpleasant subjective feelings, such as anxiety, fear, guilt, or shame, often accompany a physical upset. Feelings of helplessness may also result in the disorganization of function. Individuals in crisis appear to be less effective than usual, and the activities in which they engage may appear to be unrelated to the external situation.

The individual may pass through four phases: (1) There is a rise in tension, which calls for the bringing forth of previous problem-solving methods; (2) if these methods fail, the stimulus will continue to evoke tension and disorganized functioning; (3) a mobilization and reorganization of internal and external resources may then occur, and various aspects of former goals may be released, the situation redefined, and the problem solved; (4) if the situation continues or cannot be resolved, an inner tension will mount that results in an anxiety and a disorganization of function that culminates in emotional upset [1].

Three factors affect the outcome of crisis resolution. The first factor deals with the goals and the experiences of the individual and whether situations are defined as problematic, stressful, or merely annoyances. The same event is not uniformly stressful to all persons. The second factor is the individual's ability to explore the link, real or symbolic, between a present crisis situation and situations of the past. If the same types of problems recur, the individual may continue to utilize ineffective methods of coping, or depending on the level of maturity, may explore a creative, novel means of crisis resolution. A third factor is the amount of affective energy available to invest in active resolution of the crisis. The availability of adequate support systems may influence this factor.

Erikson

Erikson's [11] seventh stage of ego development, generativity (expansion of ego interests and the sense of having made a contribution to the future) versus a sense of ego stagnation, defines the focal crisis of the midlife stage. Erikson sees generativity as a commitment and a concern for the next generation. The commitment is usually in the form of an acceptance of the tasks to be completed by this generation, such as providing leadership; exercising authority; making decisions that influence others [20]; guiding members of the younger generation; and making an artistic, scholastic, or political contribution. The process is equally applicable to a farmer, a factory worker, an educator, a musician, or a political leader.

Although Erikson delineated six developmental phases that occur before midlife, each factor must be renegotiated during the midlife period [12]. The individual benefits from past experiences, which serve as guides through new developmental crises. Although each situation is different, the person is now more mature and more experienced in handling similar stressors. The young person reacts with self-blame, hurt feelings, and bewilderment when experiencing rejection. The individual who has successfully worked through other stages of intimacy can more accurately assess another's motives and conclude, with some objectivity, that the real problem may be within the other person and thus achieve a successful internal resolution of the conflict.

The middlescent's life experiences and the manner in which earlier crises were resolved are important considerations in determining the successful resolution of generativity. The questions of which contributions to make or whether there is sufficient time left to make contributions (making a mark on society) are critical issues in midlife. The middlescent is confronting, once again, the value of his or her life and the purpose for living. The realization that "this is it" or the awareness that the dreams of youth will never be fulfilled or will require compromise weighs heavily on the ego of the middlescent. The fact that most individuals weather this critical period and develop new appreciation of their ego strengths is encouraging to the middlescent.

Kardener

Kardener [18] states that a crisis occurs when an individual's existing coping skills are unable to maintain the desired level of functioning. Many times, the coping skills utilized by the individual in crisis are maladaptive because of emotional regression. The emotionally regressed person actually may view the world with a childlike perception, and although many years separated from childhood, may still be heavily influenced by the early developmental years. If the skills modeled and encouraged by the parents were of a maladaptive nature, the individual, now an adult, will often retain only maladaptive coping patterns. The positive means for coping with crisis situations may be permanently lost to this person.

There is both a danger and an opportunity in coping with a crisis. There is a danger that the person may use only old coping skills in the face of unique problems. Flexibility is limited, and the creative resolution of a problem may present more of a threat than the problem itself.

Most of us cannot tolerate long periods of crisis without relief. Two weeks appears to be the maximum. Within a period of 4 to 6 weeks, a resolution of the problem must begin to occur. The results may not be the resolution hoped for and may be fraught with severe consequences. It is therefore imperative that the person in crisis is helped to realize that prompt attention to the problem is of the utmost importance. Professional assistance should be sought to aid in the development of coping options.

STRESSORS UNIQUE TO MIDDLESCENCE

Family Restructuring

AGING PARENTS

People are living longer, a fact that may have significant implications for middlescents. There are more four-generation families than ever before. The middlescent (male or female), no matter how old, how powerful in business, or how well established, with his or her own family, remains a "child" in the eyes of parents. Although many middlescents with elderly parents state, "I feel as if I'm the parent and they're the children," the fact remains that parents will always view their children as children, and most middlescent "children" recognize their subordinate role when relating to parents.

The middlescent may lose a major source of emotional support when a parent becomes debilitated. While coping with one's own developmental problems, the loss of a parent confidant increases the stress. Generally, the individual has no readily available solutions for the care of aging parents. Trial and error, full sibling cooperation, and "making the best of it" are coping approaches. The middlescent may opt to care for the parents when they are no longer able to care for themselves: The parents may be accepted into the home, even if problems between the grandparents and the rest of the family may be accentuated. Guilt often accompanies the decision to place a parent in a nursing facility. The middlescent also may suffer guilt over having to make decisions for, and about, parents or from the complaints of the younger generation who feel that their needs are overlooked. The stress of the middlescent may increase if an aging parent remarries after the death of a mate or if the parents are chronically ill, senile, emotionally labile, or die.

SANDWICH GENERATION

At the present time, many middlescents find that they are caught in the unique situation of having to help their aging parents as well as their own growing or grown children [23]. Elderly parents who are no longer able to live alone but do not require a sheltered home may move in with a middlescent son or daughter. There is usually some readjusting of schedules. If only two generations are under one roof, the problems tend to be fewer. However, when the middlescent's son or daughter returns home because of divorce or financial difficulties, the middlescent begins to feel "sandwiched" between the two generations. The middlescent finds it almost impossible to remain neutral in discussions, and finds that the leisure time spent with the spouse before this change in circumstances has all but vanished. The younger generation is asked to keep the stereo down because it bothers the older generation, and the older generation asks why the middlescent is so lenient on house rules for the younger generation. It requires much skill in interpersonal relationships and patience to resolve this dilemma. If grandchildren are involved, the situation potentially becomes even more labile. The middlescent may become so involved in meeting the needs of the other generations that personal needs and aspirations are once more submerged in the exigencies of living.

ADDITIONS TO THE FAMILY STRUCTURE

The care of young children may no longer be a major responsibility for the middlescent, but most children

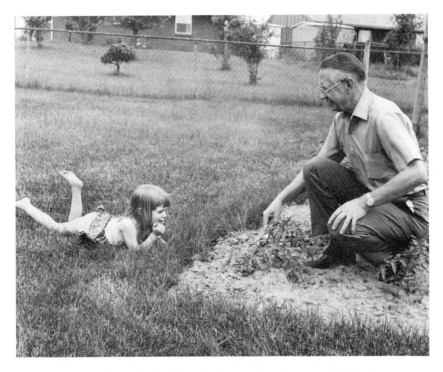

Figure 38–1. Grandparenthood adds a whole new dimension to one's life. Many grandparents say that they enjoy the privileges of parenthood without the responsibilities.

remain an integral part of the extended family. Adult children are flattered and pleased to be taken into their parent's confidence. Problems are discussed, and the children's advice is sought on family matters. Some parents find it difficult to make the transition from a parent-adolescent relationship to a friend-friend or mentor relationship, thus the development of both generations can be retarded. When a son or daughter marries, the parent is wise to welcome the new in-law into the family as an important member of the family. There are many adjustments to be made on both sides, and if these are dealt with in an honest, forthright manner, the difficulties can be minimized.

The arrival of the first grandchild may be viewed with some ambivalence on the part of the middlescent. First, grandparents are thought of as old, but the middlescent does not feel that old. Second, it may be difficult to realize that a son or daughter is mature enough to be a parent. It becomes difficult to remain silent about differences in infant and child care. As the grandchildren grow older, the grandparents tend to indulge them and to tolerate behavior they never tolerated with their own children. It is valuable for children to spend time with the grandparents to learn about the

"good old days" as well as to gain a sense of generational continuity, a sensitivity to other viewpoints, and the aging process. Grandchildren usually furnish a source of interest for the grandparents. Middlescent males frequently find more satisfaction in nurturing activities. Caring for grandchildren often allows grandfathers an opportunity to give the kind of nurturing they were too busy to give to their own children. This reciprocal arrangement is rewarding for both generations.

Physical Changes

CLIMACTERIC

Benedek and Deutsch [28] postulate that a woman's reaction to menopause is similar to her reactions to puberty and pregnancy even if menopause is thought of as a loss rather than a change. If women regard menopause as a loss, the chances of developing depression may be greater. Women seem to have an easier time accepting middle age and menopause when their lives have not been totally child-centered, if they are still married, and if their children remain close and gratifying to them. However, women who have centered their lives on their children may feel useless when the children leave home and are more likely to become depressed [28]. These women may feel as if they have been dismissed or retired from meaningful employment.

As women grow older and look back on middle age, they admit that menopause did not produce the problems they had anticipated. A woman should anticipate an improvement in physical status rather than dread hot flashes, crying, insomnia, and depression [16].

Recent studies indicate that men also experience a phenomenon called "male menopause" [27] or metapause, which may include self-doubt, insomnia, worry, tension, loss of appetite, or hypertension during middlescence. For some males, the transition is smooth, but for others it is a time of crisis. Unlike the female menopause, the outward changes are subtle and may go unnoticed [17]. A sense of urgency, fear, and loneliness may begin to plague the middlescent male. The recurring self-questions that are asked by these individuals appear to be "Who am I?" and "Where am I going?". The threats to the physical well-being of the male may evolve from insidious weight gain, decreased physical prowess, or panicky feelings of impending heart attacks. Marriage, family, sex, and work may all be affected by the male menopause syndrome [17].

OTHER HEALTH ALTERATIONS
Levinson states that "At mid-life, the growing recognition of mortality collides with a powerful wish for immortality and the many illusions that help to maintain it" [20]. One of the first indications of change is the fact that newspapers must be held at arm's length, and telephone books are almost impossible to read. Bifocals become a necessity. However, since this happens to so many individuals at the same age, it is not viewed with much alarm. The hair becomes grayer, and for males (more frequently than for females) it becomes more sparse. Facial wrinkles appear, sometimes almost overnight. The middlescent female is aware that body fat is more difficult to shed; therefore, visits to a health spa fill a need not only to tone up the body but also for a place to receive reassurance that one can still be attractive. In the male, lifting heavy objects becomes more difficult, and the discovery that he cannot run as fast or as far may be a source of concern.

An awareness of changes in body functioning can influence the patterns of life on a conscious as well as unconscious level. There may be pain from arthritic conditions or from old war or athletic injuries. Some individuals will succumb to the change with reduced

activity. Others seem to increase their activity levels to "make the most of what I've got" [21].

Career Reorientation/Reassessment
Active employment helps one to develop and to maintain personal, social, and economic security [35]. Too often we evaluate work only from the economic standpoint and forget that work provides structure in our lives. Social contacts frequently are continued outside the work place. Bowling teams, bridge tournaments, and social outings expand one's link with coworkers and their families. Occupational responsibilities also allow one to express and develop an area of expertise. Consequently, work commitments are related to feelings of self esteem. Many persons who are financially secure and do not need to be employed frequently engage in volunteer work, which allows them to contribute to the welfare of others and to meet their own generativity needs.

WOMEN ENTERING OR REENTERING
THE WORKFORCE
Many of today's women work outside of the home most of their adult lives. The proportion of married women and young mothers in the work force is increasing. The reasons are legion: In an era of inflation, economic factors play a significant role in the work decision; it has become socially acceptable for women to work; and women are becoming more aware of their own needs for self-fulfillment and development.

The most common employment history for middle-class women is to work until marriage or the birth of children. When the children are old enough to manage on their own for a few hours, many women reenter the work force [24]. Middlescent women reentering the work force may find their skills rusty or obsolete, and few positions may be available for which they feel competent. Secretaries today work with more sophisticated equipment, teachers' positions may require new competencies, and nurses who have not worked for over 5 years find that new techniques and skills are needed to function safely.

The women who are newly employed outside the home are likely to find increased stressors emerging within the home: The children may be ambivalent about the mother's time away from home; the children and the husband may be given increased responsibilities within the home; and the mother's attention is not readily available. A woman may experience guilt feelings as children and/or husband complain about the role shifts. She may feel conflict over traditional versus practical roles. The husband, who is also in middlescence, may find the enthusiasm that the wife has for her job is a threat. If he is bored with his work or thinks that opportunities for advancement are slim, a husband may feel threatened by a wife's increased financial and social independence. These factors can lead to serious disruption in the marriage [24].

CHANGE IN WORK STATUS

It is estimated that 60 to 80 percent of male identity evolves from work relationships [17]. Throughout their developmental years, males are asked with more seriousness and more frequency than females, "What are you going to be when you grow up?" Consequently, as adults, when asked to describe themselves, males are more likely to list their career affiliation before their gender, coloration, or height.

Many job changes during middlescence are for upward mobility within a career. The person has been groomed for the change over a period of time and it is an eagerly anticipated event. However, there are some who are content to remain at a given position where activities become routinized. One executive stated, "I've climbed rapidly up the corporate ladder, but I know the promotions aren't going to come as fast from now on. The funny thing is, I'm not even sure I want them to" [29]. Many forty- to 50-year-old individuals find that they are caught between career aspirations and social, financial, and personal realities. The competition for a position may create more stress than the middlescent feels can be dealt with successfully [17].

Unemployment is traumatic at any stage in adult life, but for the middlescent it can be catastrophic. Many are just beginning to develop retirement plans when the employer says, "Since our merger, ... " Unemployment may be precipitated through increased technology, the replacement of the middlescent with a younger person who can be paid less or who has more current information, or severe economic factors within the system. The attempt to survive in the employment market until retirement age, with the knowledge that mergers, computers, or younger people are coming into the ranks, can produce a crisis. The thought of trying to live on an early retirement income is also crisis-producing. Individuals may focus their energies on maintaining their current positions rather than seeking more lucrative or creative ones. Moreover, fear may force individuals to hide their feelings of resentment when they are passed over for promotion, and they may find virtue in patience [21]. The pressures of holding on to a position may lead to stress reduction through drinking, gambling, or depression. If it be-

comes financially necessary for a wife to continue working, or to obtain a paying position for the first time, a husband's feelings of despair, inferiority, and low self-worth may become overpowering. For anyone who has found identity within the employment context for 30 to 40 years, unemployment by layoff or retirement can be overwhelming.

An interesting phenomenon of the work world is that which is termed "promotion depression." The most common reaction to promotion is, for example, "I deserve it and I'm ready to tackle the new job. It's a challenge." However, a depression that follows promotion is also quite common. The new position may require more work than an individual is willing to assume at this point in life; he or she may have viewed the promotion as a haven or an easier position than the former one. But, promotions usually encompass more responsibilities, decision-making, as well as power. The individual may feel unable to meet or to avoid promotion responsibilities without losing face or self-esteem, thus a crisis occurs. The spouse may be used as a scapegoat, for example, "She always wanted me to be a vice-president. I hope she's happy now."

The psychoanalytical school offers an alternative explanation of promotion depression in males. The promoted person is caught in a psychological pattern with its genesis in early childhood—he feels vulnerable in surpassing his father [21]. The son's thought that he can now take the place of the father and win over the mother creates a fear that the father will take vengeance on the son, and the son is punished by feelings of depression.

Another explanation for "promotion depression" could be the "Peter principle" [30]. The individual consciously or unconsciously recognizes that the job is "too big" for his or her professional skills. A fear of failure may lead to depression.

REEVALUATION OF CAREER GOALS

When one reaches middlescence, it is essential to look at successes and failures. If the individual has not realized a life's dream, he or she must make other choices to make life fulfilling. If the individual is successful and content with a particular position in life, he or she needs to consider the meaning of success. When some people achieve their goals, they experience a feeling of entrapment or disappointment. The challenge was in the pursuit of the goal. If they come to this point, then they must reevaluate both the satisfactory and the disappointing events in their lives. Accepting the limitations and considering the possibilities ahead are essential to resolving generativity. To become generative, one must know what it is to stagnate [20].

Citing midlife crisis as the reason for his dissatisfaction, a 47-year-old mayor in Ohio announced he would not run for reelection [2]. The mayor implied he was tired of everything and would leave office for an uncertain future. Disinterest, feelings of abuse, and feelings of entrapment are all symptoms of a midlife crisis. Feelings of helplessness may ensue if no positive solutions can be identified. Stress from the job itself may become intolerable [7]. After a midlife evaluation, a person may change careers, capitalizing on dormant inner resources. Some individuals may find themselves for the first time in their lives and may surprise themselves by doing something totally different from previous expectations. The new career may have no real connection to previous jobs or financial status. For some this is a successful move, and their creativity and level of functioning is heightened. For others, a change in occupation does not relieve the dissatisfied feelings, and they feel trapped. Others may recognize that they have unfulfilled dreams but realize they are content with their work, their families, and their positions in life. Perhaps the dreams were unrealistic.

Freedom from Childrearing Responsibilities

There may be some negative consequences when a husband and wife are finally alone together. When the children are gone, so are all the diversionary activities, such as participation in school organizations, Scouts, Little League sports, and church activities or transporting children to various school functions. There is no one to take to the zoo, talk to, or play a game with in the evening. The main topic of conversation no longer revolves around the children's activities at school or at home. The couple whose communication had centered around these activities may feel that there is nothing left to talk about. Thus the potential for conflict from negative stressors is more likely to occur [21], since energies cannot be diverted elsewhere. Boredom may result from too much time alone together with too few common interests. In some cases, the result is separation or divorce.

Many mothers who have reached middlescence are confronted with the fact that the nurturing functions of motherhood are coming to an end or have already ended. In many instances, the mothering role has engrossed her activities for two decades or more. She is now essentially retired—ready or not. Two middlescent mothers [14] summed it up by saying, "As for the future, we are ill-prepared for it. We failed to understand that a good mother puts herself out of business—and we are out of business." The mother whose children have left home now focuses her concerns for the children in the form of thoughts and feelings rather than expending her time and physical effort [21].

With more mothers in the work force, the release of the children from the family system may be less of an emotional crisis than in the past, since the mother can spread her affective energies. For many, however, the feeling that their major life function is over may produce serious consequences. The fact that children must now pursue their own development in a family of their own, an education, or a successful career must be recognized. These parents may wish to continue the more dependent relationship, creating damaging crises for the children as well as themselves.

Many families experience an increase as well as a decrease in family size during middlescence. Children who have graduated from college, who have lost their jobs for a variety of reasons, or who recently have been divorced and have small children of their own are returning to their family of origin to "find themselves,"

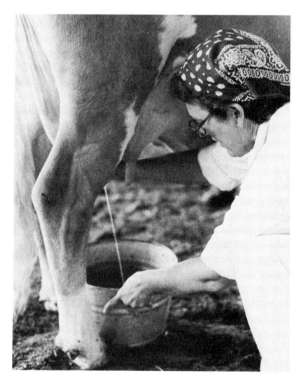

Figure 38–2. Family responsibilities must be reassigned when children leave home.

to save money, or to receive emotional as well as financial assistance from their parents [23]. The middlescent may be forced to cope with a change in daily routines, including two and perhaps three generations in the planning for meals, leisure time, privacy, and space. The crisis may not be the empty nest but rather the overcrowded, or unexpectedly full nest. These changes may come at a time when the middlescents were planning to have more freedom. Creativity and a spirit of cooperation are needed to guide those involved through the period of readjustment.

Widowhood is occurring later in life [26]. There is now an average period of nearly 15 years after the children leave home when the husband and wife are alone together. The fact that the husband and the wife are now able to spend more time alone together may have both positive and negative aspects. This "time of freedom" [25] generally includes freedom from financial responsibilities, freedom to be mobile, freedom from housework and other chores, and freedom to explore one's inner self. Many people at this time in their lives become introspective and redefine themselves as well as their marital relationships. Many individuals identify a better relationship with their spouse and a sense of accomplishment, or a job well done, and refer to life after the children have gone as a time of contentment and satisfaction. Studies indicate that upper-middle-class spouses have an appreciably more positive outlook on life after the children are gone than do those from less favorable circumstances [25].

Hobbies, volunteer activities, and sports may become important to some middlescents as they discover more time to spend in leisure activities [35]. The demands of caring for children, preparing meals on time, or attending school functions decrease dramatically. When a person is satisfied in an employment situation, work and leisure tend to blend together. There are many positive, supportive aspects about employment. However, when persons are working in positions that they dislike, satisfying leisure time takes on more significance, and they may live for these times [35]. However, many middlescents are unprepared for an increased amount of leisure. In the past few years, colleges and universities as well as community groups have been offering evening courses designed to help the middlescent cope with an increased amount of free time. A boredom-loneliness crisis can be averted if persons are able to structure their leisure time beneficially. The unprepared middlescent finds that the time wished for just a few short years ago now looms as an unwanted predicament.

MIDDLESCENT RESPONSES TO CRISIS

Self-Reflection

Around 40 years of age, the middlescent becomes more aware of the distance between self and the younger generation [25]. It is jolting to realize that the young people with whom one works are approximately the age of one's own children. The sense of identification with the older generation is stronger than with the younger generation because the middlescent feels that the older person understands the responsibilities that the middlescent is carrying.

The perception of time changes in the middlescent [25]. Life is viewed from the perspective of the time remaining to live rather than the time from birth to the present. Interestingly enough, most middlescents report that they are content to be where they are and do not wish to be young again. Most appreciate the maturity that they gained through adolescent trials and errors and the improvements they have made in problem solving through the successes and failures in early adulthood. Middlescents appear to appreciate the command that they now have over the life situations with which they struggled to cope in the past. Experience has given them confidence.

SELF-CONFRONTATION

Self-confrontation is a critical task in the life of the middlescent, since it helps the person to place life in perspective. Crisis occurs only if the gap between the reality and the ideal is too great to bridge or the person is unable or unwilling to modify values and goals.

Self-confrontation involves all aspects of life. The middlescent is beginning to develop an awareness of mortality, which may precipitate a reorganization of the value system or a reevaluation of his or her spiritual development. The period prior to this has been occupied with "making it"—establishing one's self in the world of work, making money, providing food and shelter, establishing a family—with little time to confront the self about the significance of any one part of life. When the "time left to live" becomes the orientation, self-confrontation is inevitable [20]. Many people feel that they are the only one wrestling with this phenomenon. It is important to share these concerns with significant others while critically viewing the past and setting goals for the future: Sharing helps to deepen the bonds with others [31].

An evaluation of the career situation may precipitate a major shift in occupational goals as discussed earlier. The realization that this may be the last chance to change jobs motivates some individuals to do what they had always wanted to do with their lives.

REORIENTATION OF VALUE SYSTEM

During the critical period of adolescence, one of the tasks was to formulate attitudes, beliefs, and values that could serve as guidelines to help the individual find direction and to make sense out of life. This structure often continues until midlife. Change is rarely dramatic. A gradual shift begins with doubt about a trivial matter. This doubt may be on a subconscious level. It is not until several unresolved doubts have accumulated that the person realizes the conflict and the need for revamping the value system.

Some middlescents may hold the belief that their bodies will not betray them and their physical strength will continue as it was 20 years earlier. When asked to participate in a baseball game at a family outing, the middlescent readily joins in. After a few minutes of strenuous activity, however, the middlescent finds him- or herself with a shortness of breath and aching muscles and may want to quit the game. The belief in his or her physical prowess is severely wounded.

Middlescents become skeptical about those things that they may always have accepted at face value. In order to achieve some harmony between the old beliefs and the new revelations, they must adopt a different point of view. Life is dynamic and these new values are continually tested. If the new ideology offers continuity and long-term meaning, the individual will be content with the new values and beliefs. However, if the new values and beliefs fail, more skepticism sets in and the process begins again [9]. The individual is fortunate who has adopted a value system during adolescence that transcends time.

Many middlescents, as they become more competent in their personal and professional lives, are looked up to by younger persons as role models or mentors. A mentor is usually 8 to 15 years older, and has extensive experience and seniority in the younger person's chosen career field or in practicing a valued philosophical orientation. A mentor is more than a teacher, although this is the most common definition. A mentor needs to be defined in terms of the character of the relationship and the function it serves. Some of the functions include serving as a facilitator to improve the younger person's skills, stimulating his or her intellectual development, or helping the younger person to sort out and establish a value system that will aid in meeting life's experiences. A mentor may use his or her influence to open new doors for advancement and

may initiate the protege into a new occupational or social environment. The most crucial function from a developmental view is that the mentor encourages the dreams that the younger person has, giving space to the younger person, but at the same time, encouraging clear thinking and risk taking. The mentor believes in the novice and helps him or her to define the self in a new world of responsibility and independence.

When the novice has successfully passed through the successive stages of development in the work world, with family relationships, or in social settings, and becomes a middlescent, then he or she is ready to assume the role of a mentor. When middlescents realize that they are no longer peers to the persons with whom they work, they can use their life experiences to enrich relationships with their younger associates.

Mentoring is part of that developmental process Erikson identified as generativity. A middlescent begins to acknowledge the flow of generations, using the experience, the leadership skills, and the decision-making capabilities he or she has developed to provide the counsel and the support that he or she once needed and received. A mentorship is not a one-way relationship, because the trust and the respect offered by the younger person helps to build the self-esteem and confidence of the middlescent. At a time when the middlescent's physical skills or appearance may be declining, social, emotional, and cognitive skills are refined and assume greater value in the eyes of both self and society.

EFFECTS OF REORIENTATION
OF PARENT-CHILD RELATIONSHIPS

A redefinition of self within the family is reflected in the care and the concern that the middlescent is able to offer the children. Healthy middlescent parents do not try to live their lives through their children nor foist on their children the things and opportunities they wanted but never received. Rather, developmentally healthy parents continue to allow their offspring to be individuals with their own values, hopes, and opportunities and allow them to fail at some things and to succeed in others. They allow the child to set the pace of the relationship. Parents are there to support, not to interfere.

Marital Relationship

Most middlescents weather early marital adjustments, children, and financial problems with one spouse over a period of approximately 20 years. The crises that surface in midlife can result in separation and divorce or in new understandings of one another and an improvement in the marriage.

Sometimes, one of the partners of a couple who has lived through two decades of corrosive togetherness will suddenly begin to withdraw and to act as though the past no longer mattered. The other partner of course feels insulted, hurt, bewildered, and denied [15], and resentment and alienation result. If both the husband and the wife are going through a midlife crisis at the time, the stress is greater for both. The middlescent may seek intimacy with someone other than the spouse as an answer to the crisis. Experience, however, leads the reality-oriented middlescent to the realization that there are tomorrows and there are mornings after the night before.

A separation from a spouse creates its own crisis. Although armed with the determination to make everything work out, the individual finds that furnishing an apartment, cooking for one, learning how to date again, and doing as one pleases do not provide the satisfaction and the contentment that was expected. A separation may place the children in situations where they are asked to side with either mother or father. Fathers are hurt that the children aren't eager to visit or even to call them. Mothers are hurt when children refuse to get involved, indicating that the issues have to be resolved by the parents.

Divorce is generally a wrenching experience, the tearing apart of a couple and usually a family. It is the conscious release of a dream and the admission of failure in the choice of a marital partner or of the ability to get along with someone. (Even battered spouses feel some responsibility for the situation.) Divorce can represent a future of loneliness and frustration. However, divorced women today have more opportunities for successful careers, are able to establish relationships with others in similar circumstances, and are able to adopt healthier coping mechanisms than the middlescent of a generation ago. Anger, hurt feelings, and guilt are usually predominant in divorces, however, and the scars from these feelings and emotions may be a long time in healing.

Many middlescents find that they are able to work through the stressors of marriage to a greater satisfaction with themselves and their marriages. Some spouses need to realize that if only one partner has been making the major decisions in their family life, now is the time for a more interdependent relationship. When this fact is acknowledged, both husband and wife are able to be more realistic in their marriage. Daily sharing becomes a cohesive factor in their marriage. Improvement in a sense of self is inherent in personal growth. If the individual is able to accept his or her own strengths and weaknesses, it is easier to accept the strengths and, more importantly, the weaknesses of others.

Communication is another important aspect of improving the marital relationship. A breakdown in communication is the foremost problem of couples who have been married for a long time [16]. Many years may have been spent with each partner communicating only with the people in his or her own "worlds." When the children leave home, the parents may suddenly discover that they are "alone", although still together. They have nothing to share. Counselors recommend that couples with communication problems use specific techniques aimed at alleviating the problem. One suggestion is to set aside 15 minutes per day for talking and listening to each other. Another strategy is to consciously inventory their communication patterns and jointly develop positive adjustments. One wife was astounded to find that the only time she initiated conversation with her husband was when she had a complaint, and that was usually about him.

Community Relationships and Responses

As the middlescent husband and wife find themselves with more leisure time, they tend to participate more in community activities [35]. Interest in their immediate neighborhood spurs the middlescent to become involved in action against (or for) school levies, city zoning regulations, or community safety programs. Neighborhood crime watches and looking after elderly neighbors are usually initiated by the middlescent. Membership in organizations on the local level are expanded to include leadership on a regional or statewide level. This interaction with the community may represent leisure-time activity for some people. For others, community-centered activity is a complement to their occupations. Businessmen frequently join Kiwanis, teachers may join service organizations, such as Sertoma, and nurses and physicians may become members of the boards of community health centers. Middlescents are called power brokers, decision makers, "The Establishment" [23]. Although our society places much value on youth, it is the middlescent who services the community and thus wields the power in the decision-making arena.

The middlescent may expand his or her sphere of influence to the national or international level [35]. Politicians, heads of national and international corporations, and senior faculty members at schools and universities, are some of the examples of middlescents

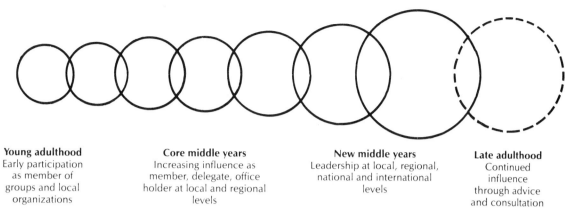

Young adulthood
Early participation
as member of
groups and local
organizations

Core middle years
Increasing influence as
member, delegate, office
holder at local and regional
levels

New middle years
Leadership at local, regional,
national and international
levels

Late adulthood
Continued
influence
through advice
and consultation

Figure 38–3. Progressive broadening of community participation during the adult years. (From J. S. Stevenson, *Issues and Crises during Middlescence.* New York: Appleton-Century-Crofts, 1977. With permission.)

who influence the younger generation and care for the older generation. It is interesting to note that although some members of this group of people conduct a major portion of the research on the young and the elderly, they have ignored for the most part carrying out research on their own generation.

The middlescent is viewed as assuming a supportive role for the young and the elderly in the community. The isolation sometimes experienced by both groups is understood, and the attempts to alleviate it become a focal point for the middlescent. Many middlescents renew their involvement in church activities, where

their experience energizes a church council or governing group that is suffering from repetitious leadership and membership. The end result of community participation by middlescents is that a group of qualified people join, produce, and lead activities that have a profound effect on many other community members.

STRESS MANAGEMENT

Anxiety, a diffuse feeling of apprehension or dread, is present to some degree in all of us. Some use anxiety as a motivator, while others become immobilized [37].

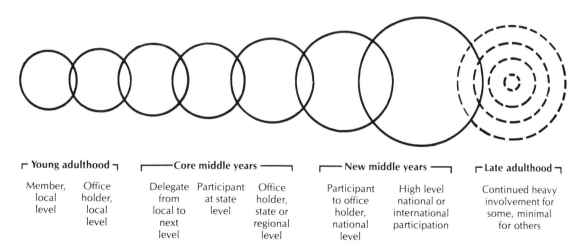

┌ **Young adulthood** ┐

Member, local level	Office holder, local level

┌─────**Core middle years**─────┐

Delegate from local to next level	Participant at state level	Office holder, state or regional level

┌── **New middle years** ──┐

Participant to office holder, national level	High level national or international participation

┌ **Late adulthood** ┐

Continued heavy involvement for some, minimal for others

Figure 38–4. Broadest participation in community affairs during the new middle years and variations of late adult participation patterns. (From J. S. Stevenson, *Issues and Crises During Middlescence.* New York: Appleton-Century-Crofts, 1977. With permission.)

A crisis occurs when a person is unable to deal effectively with an emerging problem, and the anxiety becomes unbearable [3]. The individual or his or her behavior may signal to others that something needs to be done to relieve the distress. Old conflicts symbolically linked with the present problem are revived and compound the perceived stress [29].

Classic Response Patterns

There are several major approaches that individuals can take when facing a crisis: They can call on old skills; create new approaches to master and intergrate the stress, which leads to further maturing; or they can use ineffective approaches, increasing the conflict and their sense of helplessness until, exhausted, they give into events and become dependent on others, which leads to regression. Other individuals may perpetuate a conflict by using only partially successful approaches. Since the conflict is never completely resolved the anxiety may become chronic [6]. Crisis at its best can be liberating by allowing the person to take a fresh look at the self, so that new wisdom, maturity, and insight may emerge. At its worst, crisis can result in destructiveness toward self and others [32].

FLIGHT

The first response to crisis, considered by many to be the least effective, is avoidance of confrontation [8]. As the crisis looms larger and longer, the person denies the existence of a serious problem. For example, the middlescent male with increasingly longer periods of unexplained absences from home will not be confronted by his spouse. She may make excuses or rationalize for her husband. For this wife, the avoidance of any conflict seems to be the successful way to deal with the situation. The term "problem" is not used by this individual because a person who avoids confrontation will not own up to a problem. The person who denies actual facts is difficult to work with; the denial is so strong that it is almost impossible to determine what is wrong. The individual who uses this approach has learned that avoidance may give the situation time to resolve itself or at least postpone the hurt and the grief that are surely going to occur. If suspicions do arise, the wife may use projection to further avoid the situation and to protect her ego. Projecting that someone else is responsible for the vague uneasiness or distress that she is experiencing is more acceptable than meeting the situation head-on. Avoidance is also associated with regression. The person reverts to a less mature level and earlier patterns of behavior in an attempt to cope with stress. The pitfall with avoidance is that

eventually there must be a showdown or confrontation.

Crisis intervention focuses on helping people to recognize their patterns of behavior and how to work through, not around, their problems. During times of crisis, people feel a loss of control over their lives, and helplessness sets in. Reestablishing a feeling of control is essential to rehabilitation and successful resolution. Individuals who have difficulty accepting long-term marital counseling may stay with a crisis intervention program because of the limited time factor and the fact that it provides a more direct control over their lives [13].

FIGHT

The second response pattern is that of direct confrontation to stressful situations [8]. The studies of coronary disease in hospitals, laboratories, and consultation rooms indicates that even though habits, such as smoking, poor diet, and a lack of exercise, are causative factors in heart disease, the major contributing factors involved are an excessive competitive drive, aggressiveness, impatience, and a tormented sense of urgency and time [36]. The behavior called "type A" was found not only in the corporate executive but also in most urban dwellers, including male and female librarians, florists, typists, and policemen. The "type A" behavior, which at times appears frantic, includes participating in too many activities at once, doing more and more in less time, creating deadlines where none exist, and displaying an aggressive drive that borders on hostility. Waiting in lines at the bank or the grocery store precipitates an exaggerated sense of urgency. Driving in heavy freeway traffic incites these individuals to swerve from lane to lane, honk their horns, or flash their lights frequently.

Stressors become an enemy to be met head-on and dealt with immediately. The "type A" person finds it difficult to relax; in fact, most feel guilty when they do. These individuals have few hobbies or diversions, and vacations are postponed rather than enjoyed. A longitudinal study of 3500 persons for a period of 10 years indicates that "type A" personalities are three times more likely to suffer coronary disease.

When the individual meets stress with stress, it creates even more stress, and physical changes occur such as rapid heart rate, high blood pressure, high cholesterol levels, and tense muscles that produce headaches and low back pain. Alcohol abuse is common among these people as they attempt to blot out awareness of stress. Anger appears to be an underlying feeling tone and, when confronted, the hostility is apparent. Projection, the blaming of others for their own mistakes, is common. The individual attempts to repress unpleasant, unwanted thoughts into the unconscious, having no time or energy to cope with them.

The young middlescent may suddenly realize that in order to stay on the promotion spiral, he or she must exhibit a competitive drive and become aggressive. These traits are valued by some as essential to "get ahead." The toll of these behaviors is evident in the rising heart disease and sudden-death statistics in males in their forties. The dilemma is that although people may understand the results of pressured behavior, this understanding may be eclipsed by the motivation to realize their dream.

FIXATE

An unspoken fear of some middlescents is that they do not have the courage to meet stressors head on. They withdraw all efforts toward identifying and resolving conflicts. Instead of expanding their social contacts and efforts to make the world a better place to live, they tenaciously hold on to familiar routines and literally stagnate. Stagnation means not growing, being stuck, or bogged down, in all relationships and feeling devoid of self-fulfillment. Unable to cope with the normal vicissitudes of life, the individual allows stressors to pile on top of what already cannot be managed. The stress level is increased by the individual's realization that contemporaries are reaching out to the community in more or less successful endeavors. The resolution of Erikson's task of generativity is so critical to the self-esteem of the middlescent that an ability to find or to accept suitable service outlets can send the individual into a spiral of depression. To remain fixated in a personal position that has little satisfaction and from which one is unable to move forward becomes a sentence for this individual. Inwardly, these individuals may wrestle with the dreams born in their twenties; outwardly, they continue as before. The pain and the struggles generated by the conflicts between internal dreams and exterior inaction is ignored. The stagnant person plods along unfulfilled and living in the shadow of death.

FAWN (FLATTER)

Some individuals, recognizing their insecurity and lack of direction, attach themselves to another. This happens when a person feels unsure of how to act in situations or never takes a stand on issues. The individual unconsciously receives vicarious satisfaction from the success of another whether a spouse, an employer, or an offspring. It becomes impossible for this person to state how he or she feels about almost anything because obsequious behavior has been used continuously to avoid stress. These people fade into the background. It is interesting to watch the "yes" men in plays, on TV, and in our own lives. They are portrayed as humorous characters who have no original thoughts but are always ready to affirm another. They feel that their employer values them because they always share the employer's point of view. These people frequently work for employers who need this type of affirmation and thus create a mutually reinforcing relationship. Their co-workers, however, do not share their enthusiasm to please the boss. Consequently, conflict avoided at one level can emerge at another. One cannot please both sides in either employment or family disagreements. The fawning individual becomes confused and hurt when the realization occurs that rather than earning respect and love, most associates find him or her spineless and weak. The fawning individual may become the scapegoat in the family.

Destructive Responses to Stress

SUICIDE

There are many other patterns of response to stress, several of which can be destructive to both self and others. Middlescent suicide is common, especially among males, although women make more attempts [10]. People who talk about suicide should be taken seriously. It was thought at one time that as long as people talked about suicide, they would not follow through. We now know that these persons give out many clues before the actual act. They may talk about it, give away prized possessions, or have a preoccupation with death. Persons going into, or coming out of, a depression are high suicide risks [19]. Physical signs may include insomnia, constipation, anorexia, and lack of sexual interest. The greater the self-depreciation, the greater the risk of suicide. Persons who are at risk for suicide are those who have a family history of suicide, have made repeated attempts, are worried about financial matters, experience real or imagined illness, or have suffered changes in significant relationships, such as separation, divorce, or death. Many of these factors are commonly found in the middlescent.

SUBSTANCE ABUSE

We are inundated with stories concerning drug and alcohol abuse in the young, especially teen-agers. However, the incidence of alcohol and prescription drug abuse among middlescents is staggering. Sleeping aids, appetite suppressants, and valium are commonly abused drugs. Alcohol consumption is considered socially acceptable in our society, but the person becomes dependent on it when the one cocktail before dinner gradually becomes two before, one during, and several after dinner. Some middlescents try to recapture their fleeting youth by emulating the youth culture. Sometimes this is limited to a mode of dressing or a hairstyle; unfortunately, they may also accept the use of hard drugs. Any time a person turns to chemical means to face stress, he or she robs the self of the opportunity for personal growth that is possible by accepting and facing a challenge. Each time one retreats, it makes it easier to withdraw the next time. Each time an issue is resolved, it makes it easier to face the next challenge.

Constructive Response Patterns

When an individual finds that a particular method is successful in reducing or alleviating stress, the method is incorporated into a repertoire of coping mechanisms. Some individuals may sit alone in a quiet place to think through a problem [1] or may talk a situation over with a friend. Others find that crying relieves tension. Others kick furniture, or slam doors (Spitz, stage II). For some, swearing or engaging in verbal battles with friends, spouse, or other family members may relieve tension (Spitz, stage III). But, tension relief is not synonymous with resolution.

Developing an awareness of stress-producing situations and assessing the sensations that accompany stress require focused, conscious effort. When people recognize head pressure, muscle tightening, and increased pulse rate, they need to stop and take time to determine the causative factor. Many will argue that they cannot stop; that they are in the process of meeting a deadline, on their way to an important appointment, ready to teach a class, or some other activity that precludes lending themselves to an analysis of the problem. **This refusal to look at the situation is part of the problem.** An individual **must** ask the self what the problem is, what is making him or her feel tense. Learning to assess the situation and to recognize some of the factors that may be causing the stress is therapeutic and the first step in problem solving. Recording daily priorities, deliberately slowing down the pace of life, or completely changing life-style may have to be instituted in order to reduce stress [36].

Biofeedback, or visceral learning, has proved to be successful for some people. They can learn to control their own irregular heartbeats, high blood pressure, nervous stomachs, or chronic headaches. While attached to a biofeedback machine, the individual responds to flashing lights or audible sounds that indicate the tension state of the muscles. Changes in the visual or auditory signals indicate that the person is learning to mentally control the autonomic nervous system. The control of autonomic bodily reactions or stress responses has been successfully mastered by some individuals through meditation. Reports of persons who have reduced pulse rate and blood pressure are common.

Unfortunately, biofeedback and meditation are not readily available methods for many people. Practical stress-reducing methods can include simple exercises. However, some middlescents may take up exercise with the passion of a 20-year-old, tire immediately, and then report that exercise doesn't work for them. Other activities may include sitting in a tub of warm water for one-half hour, reading, gardening, learning to play a musical instrument, sewing, knitting, fishing, stamp collecting, bird watching, kite flying, or becoming an arm-chair traveler. Obviously, this list is not comprehensive. Creativity and imagination will yield many more hobbies.

Many times, middlescents find that they are ill-prepared to deal with stress-reducing techniques. Work and the pressures that lead to the stress seem to be fixed behavior patterns that are difficult to extinguish. Their energy is exhausted by the stress of living. What they fail to realize is that the exhilarating feelings that accompany stress reduction are energy-producing, liberating, and well worth the effort to both mind and body.

Simple relaxation is singled out as a stress reduction method because it can be accomplished in a short period of time and can be done by everyone. Setting the environment by choosing a quiet place should be followed by assuming a comfortable position. Closing the eyes reduces attention to external stimuli, and inhaling slowly through the nostrils and exhaling slowly through the mouth is followed by concentrating on relaxing the head, neck, shoulders, arms, trunk and so on down to the toes. The entire procedure, with regular practice, takes approximately 5 minutes. Some individuals find they can do this on buses to and from work, in the classroom prior to a test, at their job, in the kitchen, or almost anywhere.

Drawing up a schedule for 1 week and tracking everything done at intervals of one-half hour results in an accurate picture of how one spends time. It is usually surprising to note how certain activities are followed by smoking or eating. When the person is able to determine what activities are causing the stress, elimination of those stressors is indicated.

The quality of interpersonal relationships is usually contingent on the amount of time and effort put into them. Although the middlescent has had years to develop relationship skills, specific relationships may be taken for granted. When an upset occurs, the person may be shocked to discover that he or she has been inadequately aware of the other person's sensitivities, values, attitudes, and ideals. Taking stock of relationships with others is one of the tasks of the middlescent. Couples who have weathered the early years of marriage and childrearing now find that they can realize a deeper, even more comfortable feeling that comes with genuinely knowing each other by the sharing they have experienced in their years together. They can be one another's best friend. The middlescent finds that an awareness of one's own faults facilitates making allowances for the shortcomings in an other.

An increased relaxed, meaningful time with one's spouse or another significant person helps to prevent and to alleviate stress and conflict. When middlescents lose their spouse through divorce or death, they may benefit by attending meetings and social functions sponsored by Parents Without Partners or widow-support groups. As individuals work through each stressful situation, they become aware that crisis can be a growth-producing experience. Helplessness is averted. The next crisis is met with the conviction that "this, too, can be resolved."

CONCLUSION

Although crises can and do strike at any point during life, the middle years appear to be a phase with a disproportional number of both predictable and accidental events that cause one to confront identity, value systems, and goals. Each crisis is faced separately, yet the cumulative experiences of events that have occurred from childhood through adolescence and young adulthood influence the individual's resolve and approach to a new situation [34]. Each encounter offers the potential for further remorse and withdrawal from the mainstream of life with a surface survival and a denial of one's true feelings and goals, or it can serve as a stepping stone for further development. The individual can break away from the fetters of past responses and relationships into new depths of self knowledge and heights of interpersonal relationships.

As middlescents face the empty nest, career crises, illness or death of parents, changes in physical prowess, and the advent of grandchildren, they are forced to confront issues, such as advancing age, the time left to live, goals, mortality, and the purpose and meaning of life—in short, they are confronted full face with reality.

Poorly and marginally adaptive persons tend to use psychological defense mechanisms that deny and repress the seriousness of events. They continue to use adaptive techniques developed during earlier years, regardless of their efficiency. Consequently, the emotional resolution of a crisis may be indefinitely delayed or even prevented, and personal development is truncated.

Some persons, however, are able to rise above the circumstances. Through deep, sometimes brutally honest introspection, they identify the need for reorientation. They accept the challenge and find a resolution of the pain of crisis, a new direction in life, and a release of energies toward goals found in meanings beyond their own existence. New levels of well-being and life satisfaction emerge from the creative handling of crises [34]. The middlescent of high well-being will simultaneously foster his or her own growth while

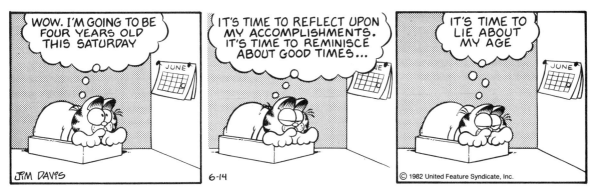

Figure 38–5. *Garfield.* Copyright © United Feature Syndicate, Inc., 1982. With permission.

contributing to the welfare of others. There may be regret over poorly handled events, but not recrimination—one learns from earlier mistakes. Meriweather Lewis, the explorer, expressed honest self-confrontation and generativity resolution by writing [4]:

"I view with regret the many hours I have spent in indolence and now sorely feel the want of that information which those hours would have given me had they been judiciously expended. But since they are past and cannot be recalled, I dash from me the gloomy thought and resolve in the future to redouble my exertions and at least endeavor to promote those two primary objects of human existence by giving them the aid of that portion of talents which nature and fortune have bestowed on me: or in the future to live for 'mankind' as I have heretofore lived for 'myself.' "

Gail Sheehy's book, *Pathfinders,* offers excellent examples of how midlife crisis is in truth a midlife challenge to those who have the courage to risk change.

REFERENCES

1. Aguilera, D. C., and Messick, J. M. *Crisis Intervention: Theory and Methodology* (4th ed.). St. Louis: Mosby, 1982.
2. Bitter mayor won't seek Bellefontaine post again. *Columbus (Ohio) Dispatch.* Jan. 30, 1983.
3. Bloom, B. L., and Parad, J. (Eds.). Definitional Aspects of the Crisis Concept. In *Crisis Intervention: Selected Readings.* New York: Family Service Association of America, 1978.
4. Bradbury, W., and the editors of Time-Life Books. *The Adult Years* (Rev. ed.). Alexandria, VA: Time-Life Books, 1978.
5. Caplan, G. *Principles of Preventive Psychiatry.* New York: Basic Books, 1964.
6. Cath, S. H., and Parad, J. (Eds.). Some Dynamics of the Middle and Later Years. In *Crisis Intervention.* New York: Family Service Association of America, 1978.
7. Cooper, C. L., and Payne, R. (Eds.). *Stress at Work.* New York: Wiley, 1978.
8. Cox, T. *Stress.* Baltimore: University Park Press, 1978.
9. Davitz, J. R., and Davitz, L. *Making It: 40 and Beyond.* Minneapolis: Winston, 1979.
10. Dixon, S. L. *Working with People in Crisis: Theory and Practice.* St. Louis: Mosby, 1979.
11. Erikson, E. H. *Identity and the Life Cycle; Selected Papers.* New York: International Universities Press, 1959.
12. Erikson, E. H. *Childhood and Society* (2nd ed.). New York: Norton, 1963.
13. Ewing, C. P. *Crisis Intervention as Psychotherapy.* New York: Oxford University Press, 1978.
14. Frankel, F., and Rathvon, S. *Whatever Happened to Cinderella? Middle-aged Women Reveal Their True Stories.* New York: St. Martin's Press, 1980.
15. Fried, B. R. *The Middle-Age Crisis* (Rev. ed.). New York: Harper & Row, 1976.
16. Gorney, S., and Cox, C. *After Forty.* New York: Dial Press, 1973.
17. Hallberg, E. C. *The Gray Itch: The Male Metapause Syndrome.* New York: Warner Books, 1980.
18. Kardener, S. H. A methodologic approach to crisis therapy. *Am. J. Psychother.* 29(1):4, 1975.
19. Kliman, A. S. *Psychological First Aid for Recovery and Growth.* New York: Holt, Rinehart and Winston, 1978.
20. Levinson, D. J., et al. *The Seasons of a Man's Life.* New York: Knopf, 1978.
21. Ldiz, T. *The Person: His and Her Development Throughout the Life Cycle* (Rev. ed.). New York: Basic Books, 1983.
22. Lindemann, E. Symptomatology and management of acute grief. *Am. J. Psychiatry* 101:141, 1944.
23. Maloney, L. D., and McCann, J. Middle age, the best of times? *U.S. News and World Report,* 93(17):67, 1982.
24. Mogul, K. Women in midlife: decisions, rewards and conflicts related to work and careers. *Am. J. Psychiatry* 136:1139, 1979.
25. Neugarten, B. L. *Middle Age and Aging: A Reader in Social Psychology.* Chicago: University of Chicago Press, 1968.
26. Neugarten, B. L. Time, age, and the life cycle. *Am. J. Psychiatry* 136:887, 1979.
27. Nolen, W. A. Male menopause: Myth or mid-life reality? *McCall's* (June, 1980):84.
28. Notman, M. Midlife concerns of women: Implications of the menopause. *Am. J. Psychiatry* 136:1270, 1979.
29. Parad, H., and Caplan, G. A Framework for Studying Families in Crisis. In H. Parad (Ed.), *Crisis Intervention: Selected Readings.* New York: Family Service Association of America, 1978.
30. Peter, L. J., and Hull, R. *The Peter Principle.* New York: Morrow, 1969.
31. Rice, B. Midlife encounters: The menninger seminars for business men. *Psychology Today,* 12(11):67, 1979.
32. Rogers, D. *The Adult Years: An Introduction to Aging* (2nd ed.). Englewood Cliffs, NJ: Prentice-Hall, 1982.
33. Sheehy, G. *Passages: Predictable Crises of Adult Life.* New York: Dutton, 1976.
34. Sheehy, G. *Pathfinders.* New York: Morrow, 1981.
35. Stevenson, J. S. *Issues and Crises During Middlescence.* New York: Appleton-Century-Crofts, 1977.
36. Tanner, O., and the editors of Time-Life Books. *Stress.* New York: Time-Life Books, 1976.
37. Zetzel, E. R. Anxiety and the capacity to bear it. *Int. J. Psychoanal.* 20:1, 1949.

XII
Older Adulthood

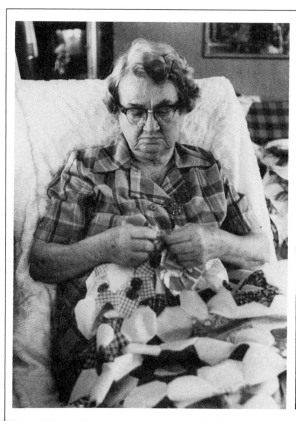
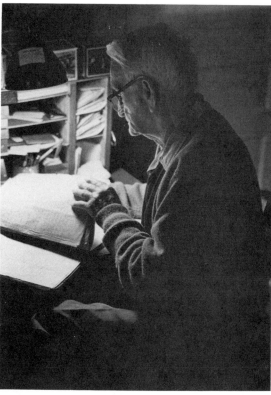

39
Biophysical Development of Later Adulthood

Johanna E. Flynn and Elizabeth R. Mabry

Old age is more apparent to others than to the subject himself. It is a new state of biological equilibrium and if the aging individual adapts himself to it smoothly, he does not notice the change.

—Simone de Beauvoir

Introduction

Old Age: Statistics and Terminology

Somatic Alterations of Later Adulthood
Cardiovascular changes
Pulmonary changes
Integumentary changes
Musculoskeletal changes
Genitourinary changes
Neurosensory changes
Endocrine and metabolic changes
Hematopoietic changes
Gastrointestinal changes

Alterations of Health in Later Adulthood
Skeletal and joint problems
Cardiopulmonary problems
Visual problems
Renal problems

Maintaining Health in Later Adulthood

Summary

The process of aging is not limited to those over 65 years of age; it actually begins during fetal development and continues until death. The rate of the process of aging becomes progressively more rapid in adulthood and affects different tissues at different rates. The biophysical changes of aging are inevitable, yet there is no formula that can determine precisely when the change will begin, the rapidity of the process of aging, or the severity of the alterations that a given person will experience. The theories about the aging process that are discussed in Chapter 36 indicate the complexity and interrelatedness of people and the environment.

The aging process varies greatly from one person to another. Not all people over age 65 look or feel "old." Mrs. T. is a spry, neatly attired woman with a pleasant smile and attractively coiffured gray hair. She walks with a quick step, her head held high, seemingly ready to face the world. Mrs. M. stands next to her, resting on her cane for support. Mrs. M. has little facial expression, her eyes look sad, and she walks with her head bent downward. Her clothes do not fit her ample body, and her hair is thin and straggly. Her head and arms shake periodically in a rhythmic pattern. Mrs. T. looks younger than her 75 years; in comparison, Mrs. M. looks older than her age. Mrs. T. may consider herself young-old, while Mrs. M. would probably consider herself old-old. A knowledge of the biophysical

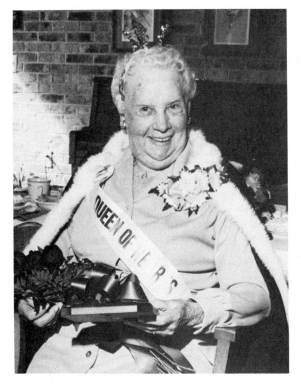

Figure 39–1. Each age has its own hallmarks of beauty.

changes of aging can help practitioners to understand and meet the multiplicity of needs of the older adult.

OLD AGE: STATISTICS AND TERMINOLOGY

The Aged in the United States

The people in western cultures are living longer, which is demonstrated dramatically by the present number of older adults in the United States. In the past decade, persons 65 years of age and older have increased from about 9 percent to over 11 percent of the total population, with an ever-increasing proportion of persons living to 75 years of age or more [66]. Likewise, the life expectancy at age 65 is an additional 18 years for females and 14 years for males. Although indicators are that females will still outlive males, the greater longevity for both sexes points to the survival of more older couples [38], with an accompanying shift in living arrangements and responsibility for their care [6]. The evidence indicates that marriage insulates people against premature death [25]. This implies that the health status of older persons who live with one or

more persons is higher than that of persons who live alone.

The health status of the aged population shows a very wide range, and differences in physical health appear to influence functioning far more than chronological age [6]. The age-related changes that are not associated with disease tend to occur slowly throughout life, with most persons remaining relatively healthy [48].

Although chronic conditions are more prevalent in those over age 65 and older persons do have more visits to physicians and hospitalizations per year than their younger counterparts, the adaptive potential for the older adult to the high structural and functional changes of age not only vary from one individual to another but also within any one individual. The growing interest in health promotion and maintenance among health care providers as well as programs in exercise, good nutrition, personal involvement, and self-care are helping the elderly to maintain their health and often to improve their well-being [3, 6, 48, 63].

Old age can be a healthy, satisfying time of life as the older adult adjusts to the changes of the aging process and maintains optimal function within these changes. The older adult can utilize a lifetime of learning to adapt and to adjust to the changes and losses that occur during the process of aging if emphasis is placed on maintaining optimal functioning.

Terminology of Later Adulthood

Many euphemisms have been introduced to paint a rosier picture of later adulthood, including "senior citizen," "golden age," "maturing years," and "age of serenity." The current emphasis on health care from a holistic perspective views aging as a developmental process of constant change wherein the individual learns new ways of relating biologically and psychosocially to self and environment. The aging person is assumed to be more diverse, more enriched, and to require more complex interactions for accommodating those changes that do occur [30]. A philosophy of care that defines health and wellness in terms of individual potential and needs reduces evidences of "ageism." Ageism behaviors are based on the prejudices and stereotypes attributed to older chronological age [11, 23].

Aging may be defined as "the regular changes that occur in mature, genetically representative organisms living under representative environmental conditions as they advance in chronological age" [5]. The distinction must be drawn between biological changes and those which result from disease. When this distinction is made, negative labels, such as "senility," will be limited to a precise description of organic brain disease. Too often, any person who tends to forget frequently, has decreased interaction with the environment, withdraws, or becomes confused is labeled "senile." In reality, many become less adaptive because the environment fails to provide meaningful, stimulating, synchronized stimuli. It is the deterioration of the environment, not the person, that creates the problem. When an appropriate environment is provided, signs of senility often disappear.

There appears to be some point in life when the efficiency of the body begins to decline and the ability to cope and to react to life situations is diminished. However, nurses and other health care workers who recognize the expected biological changes of aging and the relationship of societal influences to personal adaptation to these changes can and will support positive aging behaviors.

SOMATIC ALTERATIONS OF LATER ADULTHOOD

The successful adjustment to the changes in body structure and function as one ages results in a "healthy old age." The changes that occur with aging are often due to a complex interaction of intrinsic and external factors. Individuals age at different rates, and there is no known single process that people uniformly follow as they age. It is almost impossible to describe any spe-

cific elderly person because of the diversity of individual differences among the aged. Overall, the body of the older adult strives to maintain homeostasis even in the presence of some functional decline of each organ system. Body functions that involve only one organ system may change little from youth to old age. However, functions that require integrated activity of several organ systems appear to decrease at a more rapid rate. For example, there is little change in the fasting blood sugar from 30 to 80 years of age, whereas renal blood flow decreases by 50 percent from age 30 to age 80 [52].

As the body ages there are external changes that everyone can see; but it is the internal changes, which cannot be seen by the onlooker, that have a marked effect on the organism and its functioning. The aged person who is under stress is biologically more vulnerable than a younger person who has a greater reserve of energy to cope with stressors. The reader is reminded that the alterations in body systems discussed in the following sections vary in their expression from individual to individual. Some of these changes can be mediated by various planned interventions, such as stress reduction, diet, and exercise.

Cardiovascular Changes
The cardiovascular system of the older adult is able to provide adequate function and is capable of maintaining cardiac and circulatory activities that meet the

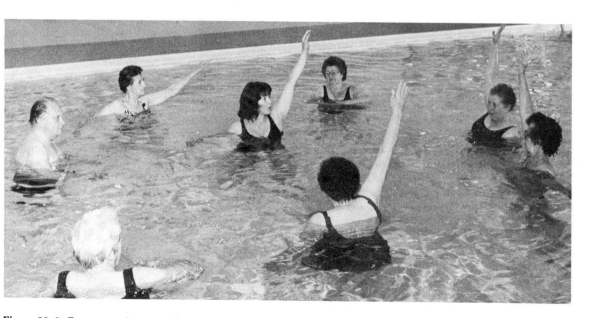

Figure 39–2. Group exercises provide supervision as well as socialization opportunities.

needs of the unique life style of the older adult. Decreased energy demands and a moderate degree of body atrophy place less stress on the cardiac functioning in the aged [46]. The cardiovascular system is subjected to numerous stressors throughout life and physiologic manifestations will eventually appear. The risk factors that have been identified as causative agents of heart stress and strain include cigarette smoking, drug and alcohol abuse, poor exercise regimen, air pollutants, obesity, poor diet, internalization of emotions, and chronic disease. The structural changes that the heart undergoes with aging are not spectacular. The heart remains the same size or becomes slightly smaller, resulting in a decreased cardiac output and stroke volume [2].

The age-related changes of heart and blood vessels are a result of the alteration of collagen, which becomes less soluble and stiffer with aging. As one ages, collagen increases in amount at the expense of muscle. Fat deposits appear at various areas, causing changes in the gross appearance of the heart. The efficiency of the heart muscle is decreased by endocardial thickening and the sclerosis that occurs throughout the heart. The valves become thicker and more rigid as a result of the sclerosis and fibrosis, which leads to a less adequate function of the heart when stressed. During rest, the function of the aging heart appears to differ little from the heart of a middle-aged adult.

By 60 years of age, the maximum coronary artery flow provides the cardiovascular system with 35 percent less blood than earlier years [24, 44]. Consequently, cardiac output and reserve diminish as one ages, taking longer for the heart to accelerate to meet the demands placed on it and to return to a normal level. Thus, sudden demands for more oxygen and energy brought on by biophysical, psychosocial, or environmental stresses are poorly tolerated by the cardiovascular system of the aged [24, 44].

Changes in the vascular system are similar to those that occur in the heart. Fatty plaques called **atheromas** are deposited in the innermost lining of the blood vessels and affect their ability to supply blood to tissues [24]. A fibrous tissue growth occurs in the middle layer of the blood vessels and causes increased rigidity, known as "**hardening of the arteries,**" or **arteriosclerosis** [44]. After 60 years of age, peripheral vascular resistance increases 1 percent per year, resulting in an increased diastolic blood pressure [24]. There is some question as to whether this increased resistance is due to a decrease in the size of the arteriolar bed or a decreased capacity of the small arteries and arterioles to

dilate. Hypertension is higher in aging black males than in other ethnic groups [59].

Pulmonary Changes

There is much evidence that the respiratory system also undergoes a number of structural and functional changes with aging. However, in the absence of disease, these changes do not interfere to any great degree with adequate gaseous exchange in the older adult. Biophysical pulmonary alterations include the following:

1. A reduction of bronchopulmonary movements occurs as a result of an increase in fibrous connective tissue and lymphoid elements. This increase of tissue causes the bronchopulmonary tree to become more rigid.
2. The ventilatory function is reduced due to obstruction of the pulmonary airways and decreased ability to expand and contract the lungs.
3. The vital capacity decreases with age.
4. The air remaining in the lungs following maximum expiration (residual air) increases with age.
5. The maximum breathing capacity, which is the largest volume of air moving in and out of the chest, is reduced as one ages.
6. The respiratory gaseous exchange is impaired due to underventilation of the alveoli or overventilation of parts of the lung that receive less blood.
7. There is altered intrapulmonary mixing of air due to decreased elasticity, regional obstruction in air flow, and decreased expansibility of various lung areas.
8. There is a decreased respiratory rate, a decrease in the amount of expired carbon dioxide, and a decrease in the amount of oxygen transferred to the blood. However, compensatory factors, such as increasing the number of red blood cells, help to maintain oxygen saturation levels.
9. There is an impairment in pulmonary elasticity and a decreased mobility of the rib cage.
10. The ability to cough decreases as a result of the diminished muscle tone and decreased sensitivity to stimuli that ordinarily elicit this reflex.
11. The effectiveness of the ciliary mechanism is reduced due to drying and atrophy of the epithelium lining the lungs.

The changes that occur with age in the pulmonary system decrease the mechanical efficiency of the lung under stress. Consequently, additional respiratory ef-

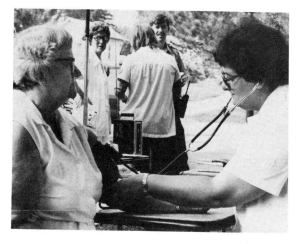

Figure 39-3. Many communities provide free health screening for high blood pressure, glaucoma, and diabetes.

fort is required by the older adult to obtain the oxygen necessary to maintain body homeostasis. The older adult is prone to lower respiratory tract infections, whereas upper respiratory infections tend to occur more frequently during the younger years [44].

Integumentary Changes

The integumentary alterations that occur with age are readily visible to the elderly person as well as to others. These external signs of aging are the clues by which most people judge aging. Some of the external signs of aging are a result of individual genetic and environmental interplay. Young persons are subject to graying hair, sagging muscles, and loss of subcutaneous fat, and yet are not thought of as growing old. The mass media have done much to deemphasize some of the negative aspects of aging; nevertheless, there remains a significant emphasis on a beautiful body and a youthful look. The aged person often does not feel old until he or she suddenly recognizes and acknowledges that the mirrored image reflects more gray hairs, wrinkles, sagging muscles, and an overall different appearance than is recalled from youth.

Permanent infolding of epithelium and subepithelial tissue causes wrinkling of skin [47]. These wrinkles are most pronounced on the face due to the repeated stress produced by the activity of muscles or as a result of atrophic (wasting or shrinking) processes that occur in the subcutaneous tissue. The predominant mood of a person, as expressed in facial muscles, may be permanently etched on the face in the form of wrinkles

above the eyebrows, around the lips, over the cheeks, and around the outer edges of the eye orbit. These wrinkles tend to give the impression that the person is continuously frowning or smiling. Exposure to the sun also produces and hastens the formation of wrinkles. In the black- and yellow-skinned races, wrinkling is less marked because the pigmentation of the skin offers protection from the sun [47]. Beauty creams, oils, and products that promise the disappearance of wrinkles do little for this normal aging phenomenon. Wrinkling of the neck is produced by shortening of the platysma muscle. This muscle becomes obvious in the fifties, when it creates the appearance of "railroad tracks" running from the clavicles to the chin. Aging women may attempt to cover up these markings with scarves or high necklines.

The smooth roundness of the trunk, face, and extremities is lost in old age because of the loss of fatty layers. Consequently, there is a deepening of hollows and an increase in joint size throughout the body. The bony prominences and muscle masses seem more visible. The hands vividly exhibit prominent veins, knuckles, and tendons that are covered over by a layer of dry, somewhat wrinkled skin.

Many persons who are more than 65 years of age have a thin, dry, relatively nonelastic skin that tends to remain elevated after it has been pinched as a result of degeneration of the collagen and elastic fibers. Elderly persons often complain of dryness and itchiness of the skin when the epithelial layer shrinks in thickness and the sweat glands diminish in number [47]. This condition may or may not be helped with various skin preparations.

Extremes of temperature are difficult for the elderly. Body temperature may elevate easily as a result of the loss of sweat glands. An extra sweater may be needed at other times due to the loss of body fat and diminished peripheral circulation.

The small blood vessels of the skin become so fragile that bruises are commonly seen. A slight bump on any part of the body can lead to the development of a large ecchymotic (bruised) area. Localized pigment plaques are also typical of advancing age. "Liver spots," moles, and various growths, usually benign in nature, appear on the body. These skin afflictions may occur on any skin surface. Although alarming to some persons, they are generally harmless in nature. Other benign lesions that occur in the aged include seborrheic keratosis, cherry angiomas, nevi (common moles), warts, spider angiomas, and scrotal angiomas [40].

Skin cancer in the aged is attributed to altered skin

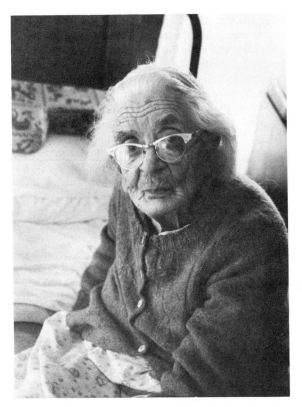

Figure 39–4. The elderly feel the cold more readily than younger persons and frequently need a sweater or shawl to maintain comfortable body temperature. It is also important to provide adequate sensory stimulation (at the individual's own pace) to help elderly persons maintain meaningful interaction with the environment.

function, excessive skin dryness, the aging process, the long-term effect of environmental hazards, and overexposure to the sun and ultraviolet rays. Basal cell carcinoma is the most common skin cancer. Skin cancer appears as a slowly enlarging tumor that smooths away skin markings and destroys the skin structures. The curative rate for skin cancer is high if early treatment is obtained.

The skin loses melanocytes with age [47]. Since the melanocytes contribute to the pigmentation of the skin, the skin of the elderly person becomes paler or lighter, giving the observer the impression that the person is anemic. The hair begins to turn gray, and a loss of hair is also common [47]. Hair loss occurs earlier in males than in females, evidenced by the appearance of visible bald patches; however, there is thinning of scalp hair of both males and females. Loss of hair is also evidenced in the pubic and axillary areas, and most of the hair over the extremities is lost. In contrast to the loss of hair over other body areas, there is an increased growth of hair on the face due to a change in the androgen-estrogen ratio. The facial hair on older women is often bristly and becomes a cosmetic concern. The skin of the older adult reflects the overall blood oxygen saturation, hygienic care, nutritional status, psychosocial stresses, and the climate or work environment to which the individual has been exposed over time.

Musculoskeletal Changes

The posture of the elderly person becomes a stance of general flexion [33]. The head is tilted forward, and the hips and knees are slightly flexed. The muscles in the torso are held somewhat rigidly. There is a wide base of support, with the feet placed far apart; shorter steps are taken. These changes create a shuffling gait.

A shortened stature is caused by shrinkage in the fibroelastic discs between the vertebrae of the spine. By age 55, a loss of one-half to three-fourths of an inch can occur. Further shortening can be produced by osteoporosis, which tends to shorten the spine, or by kyphosis, which bows the vertebral column [10].

A decrease in the skeletal mass affects all the bones of the skeleton [20]. Decalcification occurs in both the skull and the bones of the extremities. The bones become more porous, resulting in a decrease in the normal quantity and quality of bone structure. As the demineralization of bone proceeds, bones become brittle and fractures may be common.

Men and women frequently experience a weight loss of approximately 20 pounds around 70 years of age [22]. This weight loss is due to a loss in the number of body cells, changes in the composition of cells, and a decrease in body tissues. The decrease in skeletal muscle mass leads to decreased strength. The tissues of the joints and bones stiffen; thus movement and range of motion become markedly decreased. The oxygen supply to the muscles may also be decreased as a result of the reduced cardiac output. Mobility is lessened, and the elderly person is forced to move more slowly. The aged should be encouraged to maintain optimum levels of range of motion of all joints and muscles through planned exercise and activity. The changes that occur in the musculoskeletal system are progressive, but with modifications in the manner of living, the aging person will undergo little limitation of movement and activity.

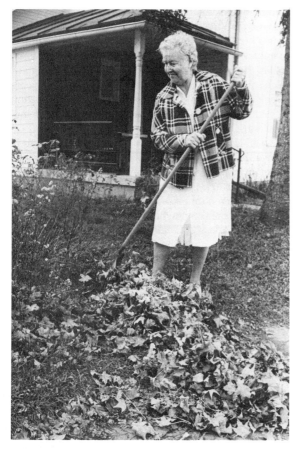

Figure 39-5. Elderly individuals should continue to participate in home maintenance activities as long as possible.

Genitourinary Changes

Renal function is slowed by both the structural and the functional changes that accompany age. As some of the nephrons of the kidney become nonfunctional and the aging kidney loses its ability to replace or to regenerate the injured or destroyed renal cells, major functions of the kidney will be decreased due to the reduction in the number of functioning nephron units [32]. As the heart gradually pumps less blood to the renal system, there may be as much as a 50 percent decrease in the blood flow through the kidneys. Renal plasma and blood flow in the kidney are reduced, and the renal tubular functions decline [32] due to an increase in renal vascular resistance as well as tubular narrowing. In general, there is a decrease in the filtration rate and in the concentrating and diluting abilities of the kidney. Wastes can be effectively processed by

the aged kidney, but more time is required to accomplish this task.

The kidneys of older individuals are still capable of maintaining the acid-base balance of tissue fluids, but the response time is prolonged [1]. Nocturnal frequency is common in the older adult who may awaken two, three, or four times during the night to empty the bladder. Nocturia occurs in 50 percent of elderly males and in 70 percent of elderly females [8]. The bladder of the aged retains its tone, but the volume capacity decreases. Many healthy aged persons are annoyed by the frequency and urgency they encounter during the night, since it disturbs their rest.

A common concern of the elderly male is enlargement of the prostate gland. This hypertrophy is present in three-fourths of the males over 65 years of age [28]. As the prostate enlarges, the contractions of this gland become weaker; therefore, there is a reduction in the volume and viscosity of the seminal fluid, and the force of ejaculation is diminished [62]. Urethritis and incomplete emptying of the bladder also occur as a result of the enlargement of the prostate.

The testes become smaller and less firm. The testicular tubes thicken and begin to degenerate, with the result that sperm production is reduced or inhibited. However, males are frequently capable of fathering children into their eighth or ninth decade. The changes in the genitourinary tract are gradual and very individual; thus intercourse may still be enjoyed by either gender regardless of chronological age. Problems of impotence in the male can be caused by an androgen deficiency, poor nutrition, physical debilitation, conditions, such as diabetes and prostate surgery, or emotional problems [28].

The female between 60 and 70 years of age continues to have sex steroid depletion, which results in some atrophy of the uterus, vagina, genital tissue, and the breasts [62]. Decreased skin elasticity causes decreased glandular tissue and tone of the breast. Loss of vulvar substance causes the mons pubis to flatten and the labia majora to appear less full. Uterine prolapse may result from relaxation of supporting musculature. Stress incontinence can also occur when an elderly woman laughs, coughs, or sneezes, leaving her in a rather embarrassing situation. However, good obstetrical care and controlled deliveries can prevent overstretching of tissues during the reproductive years, which in turn helps to decrease the incidence of uterine prolapse in aging women.

The vaginal mucosa thins and decreases in length. The cervix, uterus, and ovaries tend to shrink toward the prepubertal state (involution). There is a modest reduction in the size of the clitoris, but there is little loss in the sensations received. The lubrication from the Bartholin's glands decreases with age, but the application of a water soluble lubricant can help to reduce dryness. Atrophy of tissue and muscles is also seen in portions of the urinary tract, urethra, and the bladder surface. Since the urethral mucosa is subject to infection, good perineal hygiene should be encouraged to reduce the chances of developing an infection [28].

Neurosensory Changes

With advancing age, the body appears to become less efficient in receiving, processing, and responding to stimuli. The elderly person experiences neurological changes related to temperature regulation and ability to perceive pain. The older person feels cold more easily; it is common to see an older person wrapped in blankets and keeping the room quite warm. Pain perception and reaction to painful stimuli are decreased with age. A burn from an iron may not be discovered for a few hours, or frostbite may occur without the elderly person being aware that it has happened [9].

The central nervous system experiences a decrease in electrical activity rather than a loss of circulation or a decline in cell metabolism. This decrease in electrical activity may cause slowed or altered sensory reception and decreases in reaction and movement times for the older person [16]. The aged person takes longer to respond in a given situation; for example, when a cashier announces the amount of a purchase, it seems to take the older person forever to count out the proper payment. Drivers over 65 years of age are involved in a higher percentage of accidents than are younger drivers and are more likely to be found at fault, because it takes them longer to react and to initiate motion [36]. An older adult in a healthy state exhibits EEG readings that correlate closely with good levels of learning ability, memory status, and perceptual and sensory motor functions [16].

It becomes difficult for the aged person to identify objects by touch alone, since the number and sensitivity of sensory receptors are reduced in the aging process. Higher thresholds of stimulation are required for vision, hearing, tastes, and smell perception [31]. The progressive physiologic changes that alter hearing as one ages include degeneration of auditory nerve fiber, thickening of the ear drum, and decreased production of cerumen (ear wax). The exposure to high noise levels has been implicated as a cause of hearing loss, and preventive measures should be taken early in life to

diminish this risk factor. Older females have better hearing than males at the higher frequencies, but older males hear better than females in normal speech frequencies. Black males have better hearing than white males. Hearing acuity diminishes with increasing age at about the same rate for those who are 70 to 79 years of age as for those 60 to 69 years of age [18]. Distortion in sound sometimes makes the elderly person think that others are talking about him or her.

Visual acuity usually decreases with age. One study shows that 40 percent of males and 60 percent of females over age 65 have an uncorrected visual acuity less than 20/70 [31]. The incidence of cataracts (clouding of the lens) increases with age. The lenses of the eye also become somewhat rigid; therefore, the eye accommodates less efficiently. Adaptation to darkness decreases with age. The pupil is slower to react and adjusts poorly to changes in light. Peripheral vision also lessens as one advances in years.

The lens of the eyes tend to yellow as an individual ages. This yellowing of the lens makes vision less clear, glare more of a problem, and blue-green and yellow-white color distinctions more difficult. Sufficient illumination and diffuse lighting, rather than bright light from one direction, will decrease glare and improve vision. The inability to distinguish between green and blue or between yellow and white medications can present a health threat. Other modes of differentiation may have to be utilized.

The sense of balance and the ability to use fine movements are affected by the aging process. The aged person is seen to reach for doorways, chairs, and hand railings to maintain balance and ensure stability. For the elderly, writing and working with their hands as they once did can become an arduous task. A 72-year-old, who at one time produced beautiful crocheted handiwork easily, may now find it difficult to complete projects as rapidly and neatly as during earlier years. The general aging process of an individual is affected dramatically by the aging of the central nervous system. Since the central nervous system is closely related to the cardiovascular system because of its dependency on oxygen, low oxygen saturation can cause a disequilibrium that could endanger general body homeostasis [16].

Endocrine and Metabolic Changes

A wide variety of biophysiological processes are regulated by the endocrine glands. The endocrine system mediates body processes, such as cellular metabolism, fluid and electrolyte balance, diameter of small blood vessels, supply of blood to various tissues, and regulation of hormones. In the older person, cellular metabolism is affected by a decrease in the basal metabolic rate to 84 percent of that of a young male, a decrease in the overall utilization of glucose, and a decrease in adrenal activity under stress [54].

Fluid and electrolyte balance is harder to maintain in stress situations encountered by the older adult. Acid-base balance and blood pH shifts are more difficult to correct in the older person because it is difficult to predict how the aging body will react or the length of time required for any individual to respond to fluid therapy.

There is a decrease in both female and male hormones. The female may experience hormone imbalance as a result of estrogen depletion. Deficiency in the male hormone testosterone leads to decreases in physical reserve, sexual energy, muscular strength, and the number of viable sperm. Associated changes in the female reproductive system have already been discussed.

Hematopoietic Changes

Research on the hematopoietic (blood producing) system of the aged person is a relatively new area of investigation. Minimal changes are found in the hemoglobin level, red blood cell count, and circulatory blood volume for elderly persons who are relatively active, well, and socially involved [39]. Blood is normally on the alkaline side of neutrality, but with stress and exercise, excessive acid is produced and acidity increases. The speed at which the older individual's blood values return to normal limits is decreased 17 percent [54].

Immunology is an important facet of aging. Research indicates that with age (1) autoimmune phenomena increase in frequency; (2) cell-mediated immunity and humoral antibody immunity decline; (3) autoantibody formation increases; (4) the erythrocyte sedimentation rate increases; and (5) the percentage and number of lymphocytes in the peripheral blood decrease [12].

Gastrointestinal Changes

Although the digestive juices are decreased in the elderly person, they are still adequate for functioning. There is a lowered absorption rate, which results in decreased absorption of nutrients or drugs. Absorption is diminished by a rise in gastric pH and a decreased number of absorbing cells [27]. Reduced muscle tone causes slower peristalsis and slower elimination. Decreased digestive juices coupled with a low-

ered muscle tone and activity of the intestines may lead to indigestion and constipation in the aged.

A number of changes occur in the mouth during aging, which may have a marked effect on the nutritional status of the individual. Tooth decay, loss of teeth, degeneration of the jaw bone, progressive gum recession, and increased reabsorption of the dental arch make eating and chewing a difficult task for the elderly person. Reduced chewing ability, a decrease in salivation, and perhaps poorly fitting dentures compound the problem of poor nutrition in the aged. Atrophy of the taste buds occurs; therefore, food may have little flavor, so that one may see a 70-year-old adding excessive seasoning to food or much sugar to beverages. Taste sensitivity to sweet, sour, and bitter is lost earlier than taste sensitivity to salt. Aged persons have a characteristic unpleasant, bitter taste in their mouths called dysageusia [50].

Changes in the larynx may cause the voice to become weaker and higher pitched. This situation can be alarming to the aged man who may fear that he is becoming demasculinized, and thus problems with sexuality may result.

ALTERATIONS OF HEALTH IN LATER ADULTHOOD

It has already been mentioned that as one ages, the possibility of becoming ill increases. However, numerous physical problems can be controlled and sometimes prevented if identified early by routine health examinations and screening programs and treated appropriately. The aged should seek dental, visual, and general medical supervision at least once each year. Health problems may be complicated by fear of death or disability; the elderly person may hide his or her head in the sand like an ostrich and pretend that health is optimal or symptoms of illness are inconsequential. Consequently, the avoidance of health care may allow the fulmination of an otherwise simple disease process or low level wellness.

Skeletal and Joint Problems

Osteoporosis is the most common metabolic bone disorder affecting older females. The affected bone loses the calcium and phosphate salts that are responsible for bone density. As a result, weight-bearing bones break easily, and these fractures are difficult to repair. Most osteoporosis is caused by a decrease in estrogen levels and by immobilization [53]. Adequate calcium intake and hormone therapy can help to slow this process in women [42]; however, women should be cautioned regarding the dangers of estrogen therapy, such as increased incidence of breast cancer and hypertension [41] (see also Chap. 36).

Falls by the elderly will commonly lead to fractures of the hip. Modern surgical techniques with the use of pins, nails, and prostheses have greatly shortened the hospitalization period and have done much to lessen the debilitating effect of long-term traction and immobilization. However, prevention is the best treatment for hip fracture [51].

Two forms of joint dysfunction in the aged are rheumatoid arthritis and osteoarthritis. The degree of deformity as well as how one reacts to the disability determine the degree of independence the individual maintains. Rheumatoid arthritis usually does not have an acute onset. There is a gradual increase in the joint symptoms, such as aching, stiffness on arising, swelling, pain on motion, tenderness, limitation of motion, malaise, and muscle weakness, which may be out of proportion to the degree of muscle atrophy. Large joints, such as the shoulder and the hip, may also be involved. Osteoarthritis is a widespread degenerative joint disease with softening and roughening of cartilage. The elderly person may experience aching pain on movement and relief of pain with rest [15].

The treatment of both joint diseases has four major objectives: to relieve pain, to reduce inflammation, to prevent deformity, and to maintain function. Active and passive exercises to maintain muscle tone and to prevent atrophy are helpful, provided the pain does not persist after the exercise.

Cardiopulmonary Problems

A variety of cardiopulmonary problems occur in the older adult. Hypertension (elevated blood pressure) can cause impairment of circulation to vital body organs. Hypertension may be caused by deposits of lipids (fats) in major arteries, the loss of elasticity of the aorta and large arteries, and reduced vascular compliance [14]. If blood flow to the brain is altered, the aged person can experience memory lapse, fainting, or light-headedness. Persons over age 60 with a blood pressure higher than 160/95 mmHg should receive therapy [14].

CORONARY ARTERY DISEASE

Some coronary atherosclerosis occurs as a normal part of the aging process, but it is also a major cause of heart disease in the elderly. Angina pectoris, myocardial infarction, and congestive heart failure can result from inadequate coronary circulation. Regular exercise and a well-balanced diet are thought to be preventive measures for this disease. Regular health checkups can detect early warning signs so that steps can be taken to reduce the possibility of coronary thrombosis.

BRONCHITIS

Bronchitis is a chronic pulmonary infection that is frequently found in the elderly. The mucous membrane of the lung may atrophy, and the bronchial walls fibrose and become thick and inelastic. A persistent cough and excessive sputum production also occur. Some aged persons can become dyspneic, or short of breath, as a result of coughing episodes.

EMPHYSEMA

Emphysema reduces lung flexibility to such an extent that pulmonary vital capacity is impaired. The elasticity of the lung decreases, and the bronchiole walls lose their support and enlarge. Emphysema is more common in males. As the disease progresses, air becomes trapped in the alveoli and the chest assumes a barrel-shaped appearance. Smoking appears to accelerate and aggravate the symptoms. Careful medical management is imperative.

Visual Problems

Both glaucoma and cataracts are conditions that can cause loss of vision. The result may be a reduction in one's independence. The occurrence of cataracts, or clouding of the lens, is frequently a part of the normal aging process and is the most prevalent ocular disease [35]. The loss of vision is gradual, decreasing with increased opacity, or blocking of the passage of light into the eye. Double images, color blindness, and dimness of vision are also symptoms of cataracts. Blindness is no longer a necessary outcome, since cataracts can be removed by surgery.

Glaucoma, or increased intraocular pressure of the eye, is manifested by an inability to adjust the eye to darkened areas, loss of side vision, blurred or foggy vision, rainbow-colored halos around lights, and difficulty in focusing on close work. Periodic examinations with tonometry can detect this problem. Glaucoma is treated with medication that must be continued for the rest of one's life.

Renal Problems

URINARY INCONTINENCE

The elderly may have bouts of incontinence when they cough, sneeze, or laugh. Incontinence can occur as a result of neurogenic disease, stress, overdistention of

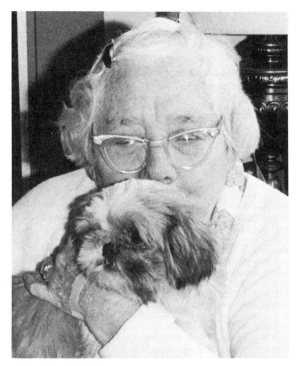

Figure 39–6. Animals offer social and sensory stimuli and are a source of companionship and reinforcement for the elderly.

the bladder, obstructive lesions, or urinary tract infection. With age, there is a change in supportive muscles and tissues, and the bladder tends to become funnel-shaped. Since the bladder capacity is also frequently diminished, the desire to empty the bladder may be urgent [41]. The older adult may be embarrassed because clothing becomes damp or soiled or because of unpleasant odor. A person who is unable to control the process of urination may begin to think that he or she has little ability to control other aspects of life. A regimen of urinary training can be initiated to help the person to empty the bladder every 2 hours by exerting gentle pressure over the bladder. Elderly persons should be encouraged to give themselves ample time to get to the lavatory and remove necessary clothing.

PROSTATIC HYPERTROPHY

The older male adult may discover that he has an enlarged prostate gland when he experiences a decrease in the urinary stream, a difficulty in urinating, or the inability to void at all. Surgery can successfully treat this problem. Four types of operations are performed to correct the enlarged prostate. Three of these oper-

ations will leave the individual sterile but not impotent; the fourth will leave him both impotent and sterile. Sexual function should be discussed with the man and his family before and after surgery.

MAINTAINING HEALTH IN LATER ADULTHOOD

Although numerous body changes occur as one ages, many older persons maintain an active, productive life. The focus of health today is on preventing disease and maintaining health. An awareness of the expected structural and functional changes that will occur over the life span encourages positive health behaviors, but allows the aging individual to adjust with less anxiety to necessary changes in activities and life style. The energies of the service-oriented professions should be focused toward assisting the elderly to adapt to changes and to function independently within their individual potentialities rather than the assumption of almost total responsibility for the elderly and their functioning.

Rest and Sleep Needs

The process of aging affects sleep in three major areas: length of sleep, distribution of sleep during a 24-hour day, and the sleep stage patterns [31]. Spontaneous interruption of sleep increases with age; as a result, the time spent in bed appears to increase after the fourth decade. The deepest sleep, stage IV, appears to be absent, and the amount of random eye movement (REM) sleep declines in old age [29]. The aged are aroused fairly easily from sleep and can gain rest in short naps throughout the day. Total sleep time is difficult to measure because of frequent and prolonged waking periods. Insomnia is common in the aged person. Pain, fear, anxiety, lack of exercise and depression contribute to difficulty in sleeping; other factors that may interfere with a restful sleep include grief over the realization of declining functions and awareness of the inevitability of death [29]. Sleep histories can be important in learning how well the older adult is sleeping and what personal rituals might add to, or detract from, the ability to sleep. In addition, the amount and type of daily activity as well as environmental conditions may help the health care worker to initiate a plan to improve the quality of sleep an older adult receives.

Rest is very important to the aged person even though the individual does not get the same number of hours of deep, restful sleep as in earlier years. Those who do not recognize the decreased need for sleep may resort to taking sleeping pills. Various measures may be tried to facilitate relaxation, such as listening to soft music, reading, or thinking of happy experiences. The practice of napping or "just resting one's eyes" provides needed rest that can replace the sleep lost at night. An involvement in constructive activities can relieve boredom and the need to escape life through sleeping. Little is known about the effect that aging has on biorhythms. Those persons who work with older adults should be aware of the twenty-four-hour life patterns of an individual, so that the normal sleep-wake cycle is not disrupted and the best times for introducing activity or therapy are identified.

Activity and Exercise Needs

EXERCISE

Older adults should view exercise and activity as a means of promoting and maintaining their health. Activity and exercise can help to keep an individual in shape and to maintain an optimal functioning level. Unfortunately, culturally imposed ageisms tend to dis-courage the elderly person from any type of daily exercise or exertion. Phrases such as "Don't exert yourself," "Sit back and enjoy life," "Don't lift a finger," and "You deserve a rest" convey the mistaken idea that the older adult should not engage in normal physical activity. Newspapers tell of persons who die suddenly after shoveling a driveway full of snow. The healthy older adult probably can and should shovel the driveway; it will take longer, however, and the individual should have ample rest periods. Since there is a decline in exercise tolerance and work capacity as one ages, exercise does place greater demands on all body systems. Physiological changes require that the aged person take up new activities gradually in order to give the body time to adjust to new situations.

A regular program of daily exercise helps to slow the aging process and to give the individual a greater feeling of well-being. Two concepts are central to outlining an exercise program for the older adult: (1) physical activity, if sensibly paced and gradually increased, is helpful in maintaining optimal functioning as one ages;

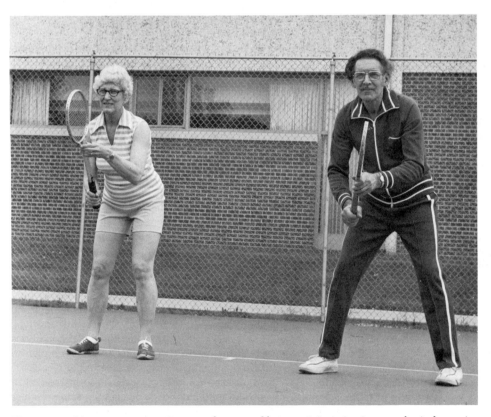

Figure 39–7. Many persons over 65 years of age are able to participate in vigorous physical exercise. Exercise may actually slow the aging process.

and (2) the elderly are capable of achieving higher levels of physical fitness and better performance with training [21]. If one does not exercise a part of the body, its use declines.

The forms of exercise that are appropriate to the older adult include dancing; swimming; bowling; golf; games, such as horseshoes or shuffleboard; walking; and jogging alternated with walking. Senior-citizen groups have instituted daily exercise programs under the direction of a physical education specialist, physical therapist, or other professional, in which seniors participate in group exercises geared to their capabilities [17]. Some communities have organized baseball teams for older persons. Other forms of daily exercise involve home and garden chores, travel, hobbies, and various activities and projects. Physical competition with another individual should be limited to one's own age group; for example, engaging in arm wrestling with a 22-year-old football player may be disastrous.

Exercise should be considered a natural physiological source of stimulation that is necessary for the proper and harmonious functioning of the human organism at all ages, including older adults. Very few people reach 80 years of age without establishing a viable routine for work or physical activity [57]. The benefits and purposes of exercise are to improve circulation, improve blood pressure readings, improve respiratory function, maintain muscle tone throughout the body, reduce muscle tension, reduce muscle pain, and promote relaxation. The lack of this stimulation causes dysfunction and atrophy. To be fit is not just to have strong muscles and good coordination; exercise improves the individual's resistance to other stressors besides improving stamina and self-reliance [21].

MOBILITY

Mobility is the ability of a person to move within his or her environment and thus to facilitate interaction with the environment. Mobility may be restricted by a variety of physical problems of the bones, muscles, or cardiovascular system or simply by the feebleness and weakness of being very old. For the older adult, mobility promotes independence, enhances self-esteem, helps to maintain relationships with family and friends, and facilitates the maintenance of interests and activities.

If physical disabilities limit any person's ability to move about independently, special attention should be given to obtaining canes, walkers, wheelchairs, or other devices to help the individual to achieve and to retain mobility. Wheelchairs are easily manageable and can promote self-mobility. A walker can be a valuable asset to the older adult who has problems with balance and walking strength. To many elderly persons, canes are a bother because they are seen as a reminder of decreasing body function. Encouragement and the proper teaching of cane use are necessary in assisting older adults to use this aid safely for negotiating the environment. When one is unable to achieve independent mobility, another alternative is to provide transportation for the immobile individual within his or her environment, thus allowing the enjoyment of a broader radius of interaction. In many communities, senior citizen buses or "Dial-A-Ride" will provide transportation to and from recreation centers, clinics, and shopping areas.

TERRITORIALITY

Territoriality is a concept that indicates the space perceived by the individual as belonging to him or her. Each of us needs this personal space and privacy, a place to call our own and to house our personal belongings. The older adult also needs to have a niche that is identified as his or her own. Having an identified life space allows for more independence and self-confidence on the part of the elderly in providing self-care.

The concept of territoriality may give clues as to how a person communicates with the environment and other people. The older adult will place objects in certain places and may get very upset if they are moved. A sense of possessiveness is illustrated by this maneuver. At one center for the aged, one of the authors made the mistake of sitting in an empty chair at a table; she was told immediately that the chair belonged to Mrs. S. Mrs. S. had "squatter's rights" to that position, although the dining area was nearly empty. The author had invaded the territory of Mrs. S., which was being protected by her peers.

Some older persons are shifted from household to household by their families. They may spend a few weeks or months with one person and then move on without ever having an identified space at any of these residences. Many older adults are staying in their own homes because private and governmental agencies provide programs that offer personal and health care services to older persons. This encourages autonomy and promotes a sense of belonging.

Safety Needs

ENVIRONMENTAL FACTORS

Older adults need to be aware of safety precautions that should be taken in their immediate environment.

Since much time is spent in the home, this is where many accidents occur. The elderly need to adhere more closely to safety rules because they are unable to respond quickly to potentially harmful stimuli.

Falling is the most prevalent home accident. Hand rails should be placed on all stairs and in the bathroom. Light switches should be conveniently located with adequate lighting in areas of activity. Furniture should not be moved unless thoughtful consideration is given to the movement patterns of the older person. Throw rugs and a highly polished floor should be exchanged for nonskid wax and tacked-down rugs. Electric cords or other hazards to unimpeded walking should be removed from the environment. Outside walkways should be in good repair; a minor crack or unevenness can catch a heel and precipitate a fall. A good pair of supporting shoes can help the older person maintain balance in walking. Numerous accidents occur at night when elderly persons wake to use the bathroom. They may rise too quickly, become confused, and move around aimlessly in the dark. Supplying a flashlight or night light and suggesting that they move slowly can help to reduce accidents at night.

Fires are caused by the elderly in many ways. Burners may be left on, or frayed electrical cords may be left unrepaired. The elderly may not smell or notice smoke until the fire is out of control. Friends and relatives should encourage older persons to cook carefully, to turn off burners, to remove pots from the burners, and to keep electrical cords and appliances in good repair. The careless use of matches and cigarettes when smoking in bed or napping in a chair while watching television can result in a fire being started. When home fires do break out, the elderly may be unable to get themselves out of the house in time. A smoke detector or some other early warning system may be a good investment.

Driving a car can be a hazard for the aged person as well as for riders in the car, pedestrians, and other drivers. Signs may confuse the elderly because they may be unable to read or to understand them. Their reaction time is decreased, and they are unable to respond to abrupt changes. The aged person tends to drive slowly, to change lanes less quickly, and to misjudge distances. Night driving can be particularly hazardous because of the decreased visual acuity that accompanies the changes that occur in the eye. Some elderly persons must be helped to accept the fact that they are no longer capable of driving safely. One should encourage older drivers to drive during less crowded times, to select routes that are less congested, and to

allow adequate time for trips. The elderly person should avoid fatigue, make frequent rest stops, and keep the automobile in good running order.

DRUG USE AND ABUSE

Persons over age 65 constitute only 10 percent of the population, but they use 22 percent of the total prescribed and over-the-counter drugs [27]. They may be taking one or sometimes many prescribed drugs. A study of drug administration errors showed that the elderly omit doses, choose their own medications, take incorrect doses, take drugs at the wrong times, and have incorrect knowledge about drugs [49]. There are proportionally more drug-induced illnesses leading to hospitalization for persons who are more than 61 years of age than for those less than age 61 [13]. The elderly may have difficulty in understanding the directions for taking the medication, or they may forget or misplace the directions. Older persons may also exchange drugs with one another or use an outdated drug for a recurring malady.

Correct drug usage is extremely important in this age group because the elderly have a reduced tolerance to drugs, an altered response to some drugs, and they are unusually susceptible to adverse drug effects. Absorption of drugs is diminished by the rise in gastric pH, the decreased intestinal motility, and the decrease in renal function [27]. Drugs should be prescribed with great caution and in the minimum effective dosages. Delayed drug reactions can occur because of the reduction in the rate at which drugs are metabolized or eliminated [43]. The principles to follow when helping an older adult with drugs are as follows: (1) determine if the drug is necessary, (2) assess the knowledge the person has about the drug (or drugs), (3) check the person's ability to take the drug (i.e., can he or she read, follow directions, and remember when the drug was taken?), (4) label bottles clearly, and (5) write out a medication schedule to facilitate remembering and to reduce confusion.

Elderly persons use many over-the-counter drugs to ease their complaints instead of seeking the advice of health personnel. Laxatives are used extensively, some of which can cause liver damage. Overuse of aspirin can produce vitamin K deficiency. Cough remedies have sugar, a narcotic, or alcohol as their principal ingredients, which might make the person taking them feel good, but they can be addicting. Other readily available popular self-remedies are cold remedies, sleep aids, antidiarrheals, and antacids. Older adults should be cautioned against using unprescribed drugs or overusing drugs because of their extreme vulnerability to drug reactions.

PROTECTIVE SERVICES

Protective services are defined as those psychosocial, physical, and legal services that provide assistance to older people who are unable to cope independently with activities of everyday living. The purposes of protective services for older individuals are (1) to prevent deterioration of those individuals who cannot care for themselves or manage their financial affairs; (2) to protect them from unfavorable conditions, physical abuse, financial mismanagement, or exploitation; (3) to support them in their attempts to live independently, if feasible, in their chosen life-styles; and (4) to rehabilitate those who are temporarily unable to manage their care, environment, or finances [33].

Some communities provide day care centers that offer the elderly service, care, and recreation during the daytime hours if they are unable to meet their own needs while family or friends are working. Many housing projects and apartments where large numbers of older adults live will hire security guards to monitor the grounds and buildings. Legal aid societies give counsel regarding finances and property: The elderly are frequently easy prey to unscrupulous swindlers who attempt to cheat them out of their life savings or property. Homemakers' services provide personal and household assistance for those who are unable to do their own housekeeping chores. This service often helps couples to remain together or helps the single elderly person to continue living in his or her own home.

Immunization Needs

Both healthy and ill older adults should avail themselves of recommended immunizations against communicable diseases because of their greater susceptibility to the morbidity and mortality that is associated with acute illness. Since older adults may engage in gardening and other outdoor activities, any wound should receive immediate attention, and the individual should receive a tetanus immunization when it is indicated. Those who live in rural areas should also receive tetanus toxoid periodically. More physicians are recommending that the older adult receive immunization for influenza and pneumococcal pneumonia as a preventive for respiratory problems to which the older adult is more vulnerable. Tuberculosis screening is being initiated in some areas that are at risk for this health problem.

Nutritional Needs

NORMAL NUTRITION

Adequate nutrition for elderly persons can help to prevent disease and disability by increasing the body's ability to cope with stress, illness, and injury. Mealtimes offer opportunities for social exchange and serve to stimulate all the senses of the older adult. A large percentage of older adults have health problems that are related to nutrition. Females generally tend to eat better than males, although elderly males will eat a more balanced diet if they are living with a family or relatives [22]. If a person has practiced good nutrition during the younger years, he or she is more likely to continue to eat a balanced diet. At times, however, the individual may lose the motivation to apply known principles when preparing food. Many communities have recognized the problem of nutrition for the aged and have set up programs that serve well-balanced noon-time meals in a community setting that offer respite from home cooking. A service called "Meals on Wheels" will deliver nutritious meals for a small fee.

The nutritional requirements of older people are similar to those of the younger adult. However, fewer calories are needed by the elderly person because of the lower basal metabolic rate and decreased physical activity. Caloric intake can be decreased by reducing the consumption of sugar. Reduced free sugar in the diet can also cut down on dental caries. Fat provides a source of energy, essential fatty acids, as well as fat-soluble vitamins. A reduced intake of saturated fat and cholesterol is thought to slow down the development of arteriosclerosis. Eating less fried food, trimming excess fat, and using low-fat milk help to reduce fat intake. Protein intake should provide 15 to 20 percent of total daily calories [22]. The complete proteins found in meat, fish, poultry, eggs, and milk or milk products are essential in the diet for maintaining and repairing tissue.

Advertisements suggest to the aged that they need "geriatric vitamins," which implies that the requirement for vitamins increases with age. Most studies, however, show no increase in the requirement for vitamins as one ages. A well-planned, balanced diet offers an adequate quantity of essential vitamins, although many physicians still recommend daily vitamins as a precautionary practice.

Sufficient roughage and water should be ingested to maintain bowel regulation. Stewed fruits, prune juice, cereals, bran, and vegetables provide good roughage. The elderly, like other people, need to be reminded to

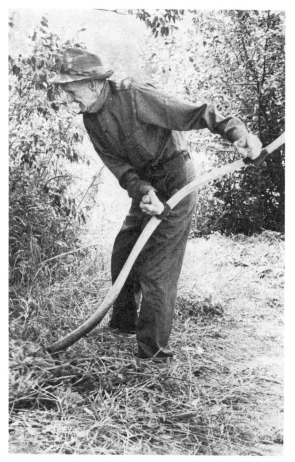

Figure 39–8. Each individual must adapt to the aging process in some way. Most tasks can still be accomplished by spreading the work over a longer period of time or using alternative tools.

drink water. A decrease in salt (sodium) consumption is recommended to aid in preventing fluid retention and elevated blood pressure.

The longevity of the inhabitants of Abkhasia (a region of the Soviet Union) is attributed to their diet. The diet, which relies mainly on fresh vegetables and fruits, consists of foods that are high in vitamins, especially vitamin C. Beef, goat, and fowl are eaten only twice each week. Honey replaces sugar, and these persons never drink tea or coffee. They do drink a dry red wine and large amounts of buttermilk as well as a type of yogurt called "matsoni." The inhabitants of Abkhasia remain active and productive in later life and live well over 100 years [11]. The longevity of these people may also be attributed to a genetic potential for longer life

and their relative isolation from potentially life-shortening diseases.

UNDERNUTRITION

Vitamin and mineral deficiencies in the aged, especially vitamin C and iron levels, are fairly prevalent and add to existing health problems. In the United States 40 percent of people who are more than 60 years of age suffer from iron-deficiency anemia, resulting from an insufficient iron intake and the poor absorption and utilization of iron [4]. The signs of anemia include pallor, weakness, tiredness, and nervousness. The iron needs of women may decrease when menstruation ceases. There is much controversy over the use of vitamin E, which is thought to protect the lipids that construct the cell wall and thus maintain its strength and integrity, which otherwise may diminish with age [22]. Some physicians and nutritionists recommend supplements of this vitamin for the aging person. Deficiencies in vitamin B cause mental confusion, while deficiencies in vitamin A affect vision and reduce the integrity of epithelium. The diet of elderly persons may be low in calcium, since milk, the best source, may be avoided because it is constipating for some individuals.

Although budget constraints are frequently cited as one cause of poor nutrition, the Ten State Nutrition survey [56] revealed that undernutrition in individuals more than 60 years of age is not limited to any one socioeconomic or ethnic group. This study found that the elderly make poor food choices, which result in diets that are inadequate. In addition, they do not budget money well when purchasing food.

Other factors that contribute to the undernutrition of the elderly are tooth and gum problems and difficulty in chewing and swallowing. Poor eating habits of an entire lifetime show up in the aged. Some persons are unable to prepare an adequate meal because of poor finances, inadequate cooking facilities, or the purchase of nonnutritive expensive foods that require little fussing. Loneliness and depression may prevent the elderly from enjoying the experience of eating.

OVERNUTRITION

There are many causes of overnutrition in the elderly. A person may increase food intake in response to frustration or anxiety that is related to loss of job; loss of independence; loss of identity; or loss of home, friends, or relatives. Inactivity without reduction of caloric intake may lead to weight gain. Any excess weight can be particularly hazardous to the older adult. Some of the problems associated with obesity are cardiovascular complaints, hypertension, atherosclerosis, and diabetes.

The elderly find it very difficult to change a lifetime of eating patterns. Much thoughtfulness, patience, and understanding are necessary on the part of the practitioner who is assisting an older adult to adjust a diet. A point to keep in mind when restricting an elderly person's diet is that radical changes in one's environment can reduce the body's resilience to stressors [4]. A large or sudden decrease in calories or an excessively rapid weight loss can throw the aged person into physiological disequilibrium.

Sexual Needs

Sexual interest shows some decline with increasing age, but the older adult certainly does not have to lead a life of celibacy. There is much variation in the individual sexual needs and desires of the aged. A study at Duke University of 254 males and females between 60 and 94 years of age found that (1) in general, elderly males are sexually more active than females; (2) continued sexual activity among 80- and 90-year-old males is not a rarity; (3) although sexual interest declines with age, one-half of subjects in their eighties and nineties report that they continue to have mild sexual interest; (4) unmarried males have approximately the same level of sexual interest and activity as married males; and (5) approximately one-fourth of the males report an increase in the degree of sexual activity or interest [58].

The authors have found that when given the opportunity to share their feelings, 60- to 80-year-old females frequently express unmet sexual longings. Some of the concerns voiced by women in a senior health assessment clinic included: "I'd love to make love to a man once more before I die"; "I want to be kissed"; "No one has hugged me since my husband died three years ago"; "Do mechanical stimulators help someone my age?" and "How can I get a date at 82?" This brief listing seems to indicate that elderly females and males think about sex and try to find ways to satisfy their sexual needs.

Families and friends must realize that the desire for gratification of sexual needs is as normal for the aged as it is for any other age group. Myths indicate that the aged are too old to participate actively in intercourse, that they do not have sexual desires, that they are too fragile and physically unattractive to engage in sexual activities, and that the elderly who do engage in sex are shameful and perverse (the concept of the "dirty old man"—or woman) [55]. Sex may no longer have a

reproductive function for the aged, but it is recreational. A variety of stimulating techniques may be used in place of traditional sexual intercourse. Sexual activity for the elderly may include stroking, kissing, or using vibrators on various erogenous areas. One aim of the sexual activity of older persons is to develop and maintain excitation. Whereas in younger years orgasm was an objective of sexual activity, in later years the joy of close contact and the enjoyment of mutual intimacy appear to be of prime importance.

The need for the expression of sexuality as one ages should receive as much attention by the practitioner as any other biological need. The older adult is physiologically capable of expressing sexual needs and should be encouraged to do so. There is no biological limitation to the sexual capacity of the aging female, and she can be an active and enthusiastic sexual participant. The elderly man is capable of a sustained erection for longer periods without the urge for ejaculation that he experienced as a youth. Biological changes do not necessarily decrease the mutual satisfaction enjoyed by elderly sexual partners. Homes for the aged should provide opportunities for elderly persons to enjoy sexual intimacy in privacy and without fear of ridicule or censorship from others.

If no sexual contact is possible or available, other forms of sexual release are possible and can be suggested to the elderly. For some, fantasizing can be a form of expressing their sexual needs. Daydreaming about sex can be healthy as long as it does not preclude all other activity. Some elderly persons may need to be told that fantasizing is a normal way to release sexual tensions.

Some nursing homes have reawakened the sexual responses of the elderly by hanging artwork depicting nudes in strategic spots. One nursing home reported that a previously immobile male eventually moved out of his room to view a picture of a nude. Magazines, movies, and stories can also stimulate the elderly to think about their sexuality.

One should remember that sexuality and sex are a very personal matter and have a recreational as well as a relational component. The aged may find it difficult to find a socially acceptable sex partner, or the standards and values of the aged may prevent them from having sexual activity with anyone except a spouse. Each aged individual has personal preferences in regard to sexual expression, needs, interests, and desires. Some older persons no longer desire any sexual contact or express any sexual needs, while on the other end of the continuum, some may be experiencing a very active sex life.

Perceptual Needs

Sensory deprivation may occur when an individual resides in environments where there is little color, sound, or activity. Sensory input is a necessary part of the life of an individual in order to avoid stimulus hunger. A person who lives alone or is isolated in a room in a nursing home usually does not receive enough stimulation from either the external or the internal environment. The lack of an adequate sensory input can contribute to the phenomenon of senility; the individual becomes disoriented in regard to time, person, and place. Restructuring the environment to increase meaningful stimuli can frequently help the individual to achieve higher levels of independent functioning in all domains.

Multisensory stimuli should be provided through smell, touch, vision, hearing, and taste. The environment of the elderly person should include a judicious use of color and various fabric textures. Hearing can be improved by screening out environmental noises and speaking directly to the older person. Extra food seasoning can be used to stimulate taste. Encouraging the aged to use perfume, shaving lotions, and makeup can help to maintain self-esteem and attractiveness. Interesting activities can take the person out of a room or a neighborhood and into the larger community. Visitors, field trips, and planned outings can help to keep the aged person oriented to the reality of his or her place in the world.

TACTILE STIMULATION

Touch is a valuable means of nonverbal communication; it conveys to the elderly person that someone is trying to communicate with him or her. The aged appear to have a great need to reach out and touch others. They need to touch surfaces, fabrics, and people in order to concretize the world that exists around them. An embrace, a hug, or a gentle pat on the arm or back can give an emotional boost to the older adult. The need for contact stimuli in the aged appears to be similar to the contact needs of the infant in the sensorimotor period of development.

Some older persons may get enjoyment from stroking the arms and feeling the skin of younger individuals. The "grabbing," "stroking," and touching done by the elderly is an attempt to satisfy both sensory and essential social needs. Visits from children can be very satisfying to both. Some facilities, recognizing the importance of these interactions between young children and the elderly, have combined nursing homes and child day care centers under the same roof [60].

COGNITIVE STIMULATION

Challenging the minds of the elderly to keep their minds active helps them to remain oriented to reality (the best way to prevent senility). Those who experience some loss of neurosensory function can become confused when too much information is given in a short time. They may not be able to interpret a mes-

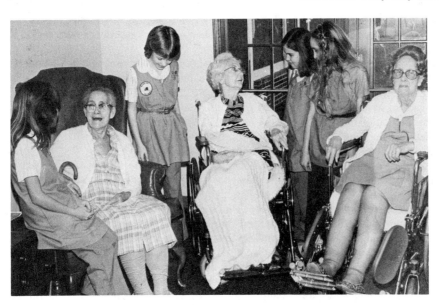

Figure 39–9. Persons in nursing homes frequently mention that they miss contact with children. Contacts can be mutually beneficial and highly enjoyable.

sage and provide a coherent answer, which results in language confusion. People should be aware that they must talk directly to an elderly adult in a slow manner, giving the person ample time to respond. Talking precisely and slowly does not mean that the caregiver thinks the person is infantile, slow-witted, or deaf, rather, the caregiver is showing awareness that the aged person's response time is lengthened. The "computer" of the elderly person has such vast information that retrieval time takes longer.

Learning in the elderly person is influenced by how he or she feels about the self. Ethnicity can influence this self-concept. Society should be aware that each person has an ethnicity (values and expectations that have been influenced by previous cultural and social groups) [37], which makes the individual a unique being. Support systems should be identified and utilized to help the elderly adult maintain continuity with earlier years and significant others.

Brearley presents two hypotheses about the needs of people who are growing old. He states that (1) the loss of significant relationships is likely to distress older people, and (2) the lack of adequate opportunities for mixing with others hinders adaptation to aging [7]. Attempts should be made by family, friends, or interested others to make alternative relationships available when significant others are absent. Maintaining interaction with others is one way to enhance the cognitive process of the elderly person. (Chaps. 40 and 41 will cover these concepts in more depth.)

Reminiscences can be an enjoyable experience for the older adult. It is a valuable therapeutic tool through which older adults can review life happenings, recall events of importance, and work through personal conflicts. Allowing a person to reminisce reinforces a sense of identity and helps maintain self-esteem. Listening to the life review provides the family members with clues to the older person's needs and how to meet them. Children and adolescents may be fascinated by the older person's stories of bygone days. The opportunities for sharing facilitate intergenerational bonding and provide a sense of cultural continuity and heritage.

Support systems are an important interactive segment for the elderly because they assist the older individual to maintain mastery of the environment by using his or her unique skills and potentials. Support systems are those people or agencies in the environment who interact with an individual to provide emotional and task-oriented assistance. An elderly person's family is a natural support system that can help the individual to achieve developmental tasks related to independence by providing transportation, food, shelter, or communication or by encouraging the elderly individual to take advantage of screening and other health-related services. Because of the differing ethnicity of the elderly, support systems vary greatly. Some elderly persons are too proud to utilize Medicare or Medicaid and choose to pay their own medical bills. Other older persons will not seek health care unless they are ill, while some will take full advantage of the many health-related services offered to the aged.

The older-aged population of the future will continue to be extremely heterogeneous and a valuable national resource. The older adult at the beginning of the twenty-first century will be even more educated, politically active, community-oriented, and productively engaged in a variety of pursuits. The older adult will need safe, secure housing; mass transit systems that are accessible, safe, and efficient; recreational facilities adapted for their abilities and capabilities; low-cost nutritious meals; and a health-delivery system designed for the special needs of the older adult. Educational programs designed to promote the concept of life-long learning should be encouraged and made available. The potential for future generations of older adults who are biologically and psychosocially healthier individuals lies in the emphasis on learning about life-span developments in the early school years.

The ultimate goal of health care should be to improve the quality of life for the aging. The elderly, with help, should be able to reach and to maintain their optimum level of functioning throughout the process of aging, which will allow them to have the independence, the mobility, and the energy required to enjoy life to its fullest.

SUMMARY

The health of the elderly can be improved by finding ways to make growing old more enjoyable and by developing more knowledge and understanding of the normal processes of aging. Both the young and the old need to develop a respect for the abilities, capabilities, and potentialities of the elderly.

REFERENCES

1. Alwell, N. Aging kidney. *Lancet* 2:635, 1978.
2. Baldwin, P. Nursing care of the elderly person with acute cardiovascular problem. *Nurs. Clin. North Am.* 18:2, 1983.
3. Benson, E. R., and McDevitt, J. Q. Health promotion by nursing in care of the elderly. *Nursing and Health Care* (January 1982):39.

4. Berger, R. Nutritional Needs of the Aged. In I. M. Burnside (Ed.), *Nursing and the Aged*. New York: McGraw-Hill, 1976.

5. Birren, J., and Renner, J. Research on the Psychology of Aging. In J. E. Birren and J. W. Schaie (Eds.), *The Psychology of Aging*. New York: Van Nostrand Reinhold, 1977.

6. Blazer, D., and Siegler, I. C. *A Family Approach to Health Care of the Elderly*. Menlo Park, CA: Addison-Wesley, 1983.

7. Brearley, P. Deprivation syndrome. *Nurs. Times* 71:1914, 1975.

8. Brocklehurst, J. How to define and treat constipation. *Geriatrics* 32:85, 1977.

9. Brody, H. Aging of the Vertebrate Brain. In M. Rockstein (Ed.), *Development and Aging in the Central Nervous System*. New York: Academic, 1973.

10. Burnside, I. M. (Ed.). *Nursing and the Aged* (2nd ed.). New York: McGraw-Hill, 1981.

11. Butler, R. N., and Lewis, M. I. *Aging and Mental Health: Positive Psychological Approaches* (3rd ed.). St. Louis: Mosby, 1982.

12. Calin, A. Immunology: A facet of aging. *Geriatrics* 32:54, 1977.

13. Camanasos, G., Stewart, R., and Cluff, L. Drug-induced illnesses leading to hospitalization. *J.A.M.A.* 228:713, 1974.

14. Chrysant, S., Frohlich, E., and Papper, S. Why hypertension is so prevalent in the elderly and how to treat it. *Geriatrics* 31:101, 1976.

15. Clark, H. Osteoarthritis: An interesting case? *Nurs. Clin. North Am.* 11:199, 1976.

16. Davison, A. Biochemical aspects of the aging brain. *Age Ageing Supplement* 4, 1978.

17. Diekelmann, N. *Primary Health Care of the Well Adult*. New York: McGraw-Hill, 1977.

18. Eisdorfer, C., and Wilkie, F. Auditory Changes. In E. Palmore (Ed.), *Normal Aging II*. Durham, NC: Duke University Press, 1974.

19. *Facts About Older Adults*. U.S. Department of Health and Human Services Publication No. 80–20006 1979.

20. Garn, S. Bone Loss and Aging. In R. Goldman and M. Rockstein (Eds.), *The Physiology and Pathology of Human Aging*. New York: Academic, 1975.

21. Gore, I. Physical activity in old age. *Nurs. Mirror* 142:49, 1975.

22. Grenby, M. Living to eat: Nutrition for senior citizens. *Can. Nurs* 73:42, 1977.

23. Gress, L. D., and Bahr, R. T. *The Aging Person: A Holistic Perspective*. St. Louis: Mosby, 1984.

24. Harris, R. Cardiac Changes with Age. In R. Goldman and M. Rockstein (Eds.), *The Physiology and Pathology of Human Aging*. New York: Academic, 1975.

25. Hess, B. B., and Markson, E. W. *Aging and Old Age*. New York: Macmillan, 1980.

26. Hess, P. A., and Day, C. *Understanding the Aging Patient*. Bowie, MD: Brady, 1977.

27. Hollister, L. Prescribing Drugs for the Elderly. *Geriatrics* 32:71, 1977.

28. Jaffe, J. Common Lower Urinary Tract Problems in Older People. In A. B. Chinn (Ed.), *Working with Older People: A Guide to Practice*. Volume 4. Rockville, MD: U.S. Department of Health, Education and Welfare, Public Health Services and Mental Health Administration, Community Health Services, 1972.

29. Kales, J. Aging and Sleep. In R. Goldman and M. Rockstein (Eds.), *The Physiology and Pathology of Human Aging*. New York: Academic, 1975.

30. Katch, M. P. A negative view of the aged. *J. Gerontological Nurs.* 9(12):656, 1983.

31. Kimmel, D. C. *Adulthood and Aging: An Interdisciplinary Developmental View* (2nd ed.). New York: Wiley, 1980.

32. Lindemann, R. Age Changes in Renal Functions. In R. Goldman and M. Rockstein (Eds.), *The Physiology and Pathology of Human Aging*. New York: Academic, 1975.

33. Long, J. M. (Ed.). *Caring for and Caring About Elderly People*. Rochester, NY: Rochester Regional Medical Program and the University of Rochester School of Nursing, 1972.

34. Maddox, C. L. The Social and Cultural Context of Aging. In G. Usdine and C. Hoflin (Eds.), *Aging: The Process and the People*. New York: Brunner/Mazel, 1978.

35. Marmor, M. The eye and vision in the elderly. *Geriatrics* 32:63, 1977.

36. McFarland, R., Tune, G., and Wolford, A. On driving of automobiles by older people. *J. Gerontol.* 19:190, 1964.

37. Moriwaki, S. Ethnicity. In I. M. Burnside (Ed.), *Nursing and the Aged*. New York: McGraw-Hill, 1976.

38. Morris, W. W., and Bader, I. M. (Eds.). *Hoffman's Daily Needs and Interests of Older People* (2nd ed.). Springfield, IL: Thomas, 1983.

39. Murray, R. B., and Zentner, J. P. *Nursing Assessment and Health Promotion Through the Life Span* (2nd ed.). Englewood Cliffs, NJ: Prentice-Hall, 1979.

40. Palmore, E., and Tindall, J. Skin Conditions and Lesions in the Aged. In E. Palmore (Ed.), *Normal Aging II*. Durham, NC: Duke University Press, 1974.

41. Pinel, C. Disorders of micturition in the elderly. *Nurs. Times* 71:2019, 1975.

42. Pinel, C. Metabolic bone disease in the elderly. *Nurs. Times* 72:1046, 1976.

43. Richey, D. Effects of Human Aging on Drug Absorption. In. R. Goldman and M. Rockstein (Eds.), *Physiology and Pathology of Human Aging*. New York: Academic, 1975.

44. Roberts, S. Cardiopulmonary Abnormalities in Aging. In I. M. Burnside (Ed.), *Nursing and the Aged*. New York: McGraw-Hill, 1976.

45. Rockstein, M. Aging in Humans—An Overview. In R. Goldman and M. Rockstein (Eds.), *Physiology and Pathology of Human Aging*. New York: Academic, 1975.

46. Rodstein, M. Heart Disease in the Aged. In I. Rossman (Ed.), *Clinical Geriatrics* (2nd ed.). Philadelphia: Lippincott, 1979.

47. Rossman, I. Human Aging Changes. In I. M. Burnside (Ed.), *Nursing and the Aged*. New York: McGraw-Hill, 1976.

48. Rowe, J. W., and Besdine, R. W. *Heart and Disease in Old Age*. Boston: Little, Brown, 1982.

49. Schwartz, D.   Safe self-medication for elderly outpatients. *Am. J. Nurs.* 75:1808, 1975.

50. Shafer, J.   Dysageusia in elderly. *Lancet* 1:83, 1965.

51. Shanck, A.   Musculoskeletal Problems in Aging. In I. M. Burnside (Ed.), *Nursing and the Aged.* New York: McGraw-Hill, 1976.

52. Shock, N.   System Integration. In C. E. Finch and L. Hayflick (Eds.), *Handbook of the Biology of Aging.* New York: Van Nostrand Reinhold, 1977.

53. Soika, C.   Combating osteoporosis. *Am. J. Nurs.* 73:1193, 1973.

54. Solomon, N., Shock, N., and Aughenbaugh, P.   The Biology of Aging. In A. M. Hoffman (Ed.), *The Daily Needs and Interests of Older People.* Springfield, IL: Thomas, 1970.

55. Stanford, D.   All about sex—after middle age. *Am. J. Nurs.* 77:608, 1977.

56. *Ten State Nutrition 1968-70. Highlights.* U.S. Department of Health, Education, and Welfare Publication No. (HSM) 72 8134. Atlanta: 1972.

57. Thacker, J.   Why do some live longer? Activity helps. *Perspectives Aging* 6(3):7, 1977.

58. Verwoerdt, A., Pfeiffer, E., and Wang, H.   Sexual behavior in senescence: I. *J. Geriatr. Psychiatry* 2:163, 1969.

59. Voors, A. W., et al.   Racial differences in blood pressure control. *Science,* 204:1091, 1979.

60. Vujovich, J.   Child day care livens a nursing home. *Geriatric Nursing* (January-February 1984):31.

61. Weg. R.   Changing Physiology of Aging: Normal and Pathological. In D. S. Woodruff and J. E. Birren (Eds.), *Aging: Scientific Perspectives and Social Issues.* New York: Van Nostrand Reinhold, 1975.

62. Weg, R.   Sexual Inadequacy in the Elderly. In R. Goldman and M. Rockstein (Eds.), *Physiology and Pathology of Human Aging.* New York: Academic, 1975.

63. Weg, R.   *Nutrition and the Later Years.* University Park, CA: University of Southern California Press, 1978.

64. Weiss, N., et al.   Decreased risk of fractures of the hip and lower forearm with post-menopausal use of estrogen. *N. Engl. J. Med.* 303:1195, 1980.

65. Williams, S. R.   *Essentials of Nutrition and Diet Therapy* (3rd ed.). St. Louis: Mosby, 1982.

66. *World Almanac and Book of Facts, 1984.* New York: Newspaper Enterprise Association, Inc., 1984.

Cognitive and Psychosocial Development of Older Adults

Robert Bornstein

Cato: "The great affairs of life are not performed by physical strength, or activity, or nimbleness of body, but by deliberation, character, expression of opinion. Of these old age is not only not deprived, but, as a rule, has them in a greater degree."

—Cicero, Old Age, VI

Clearly delineated life-span stages or age segments do not appear to be an inherent characteristic of human existence; they are simply "invented" whenever it is deemed useful from a biological, psychological, and/or sociocultural point of view to create classification systems for the purpose of clarification and organization [55]. The psychological study of old age and aging (gerontology) began in the late 1930s; however, the advent of World War II arrested its further development. Study was resumed after World War II with the founding of the Gerontology Society and the Division of Maturity and Aging of the APA (American Psychological Association) in 1945; the International Association of Gerontology in 1948; three White House conferences on aging in 1961, 1971, and 1981; and numerous research and training centers that have been sponsored by the government and universities [11].

At its inception, the field of gerontology (and the subspecialty of psychological gerontology) used the age of 65 years for the beginning of old age; everyone who attained or exceeded this age was considered old or elderly. It has now been suggested that a distinction be made between the young-old (those between 65 and 74 years of age) and the old-old (age 75 years and beyond). While limitations of space preclude the separate treatment of these two groups in this chapter, gerontological researchers and practitioners are well aware of the fact that these two groups of individuals differ from one another in several important quantitative and qualitative ways. In precisely the same manner that a seasoned practitioner would anticipate developmental differences between an infant and a child or a child and an adolescent, so must he or she expect and be sensitive to the individual differences that exist between the young-old and the old-old.

The relatively recent emergence of interest in psychological gerontology is, itself, a reflection of the confluence of three interrelated forces. One is the desire to extend or to expand upon previous knowledge about human development. In this case, the expansion has been sought within a formerly slighted and overlooked age-segment of the life span. A second force is more practical-minded in orientation. The general aging of human populations in large segments of the world, and the so-called "graying of America," in particular, have begun to create a number of very real and pressing problems for society. The plight of this nation's social security system, which has been well documented in governmental committee meetings and the mass media, is only one example of this phenomenon. Effective solutions to problems such as these will be found only after a far more expansive, accurate, and reliable knowledge base has been established. The third force is a partial derivative of the first two: The conventional wisdom about aging is often so inaccurate as to actually hinder any attempts to establish a sound base of knowledge.

This chapter will discuss the current state of theoretical and empirical knowledge about cognitive and psychosocial development in older adults. Unfortunately, to date, there are no well-delineated, fully encompassing theories of aging, only crude outlines that can serve as guides for the exploration of this relatively unstudied portion of the life-span. The status of the empirically derived knowledge base on aging also reflects the fact that our explorations are in their infancy. Remember, the discipline called psychological gerontology is, relatively speaking, only a few years old. Hence, this discussion will of necessity reflect the rather tentative and sometimes contradictory nature of what is presently known about old age and aging.

One very central concern for both the theoretical and empirical realms of gerontological study is the issue of successful versus unsuccessful aging, and this concern is reflected in the consistency and frequency with which this issue appears throughout the chapter. The reader is cautioned that the concepts of successful and nonsuccessful aging are complex ones that often have different meanings for different theorists and researchers. In most discussions, the concern is to spec-

ify a way of measuring the content or the quality of life of the older adult.

THEORIES OF RELEVANCE TO THE STUDY OF OLDER ADULTS

Biological Theories

We have not yet achieved a complete understanding of the degree and the nature of the relationship(s) between aging biological functions and their psychological and social reflections. Biological functioning across the life span does not necessarily parallel the life course of psychological and social developments. We know that biophysical defects and declines may sometimes limit an individual's ability to fully express his or her capacities even though the inner self (feelings, thought processes) remains basically intact and fully functioning (e.g., some forms of cerebral palsy and victims of stroke). Conversely, individuals who are apparently biologically normal or healthy are sometimes victimized by a variety of social and psychological disturbances. In general, the major discrepancy between the biological and psychological graphs is most likely to occur in old age where the curve representing biological status shows a well-documented and clearly downward trend that reflects declining function, while the trends for psychological and social development are less uniform and more difficult to trace. We therefore begin the discussion of theory with an examination of Roy Hamlin's utility theory, which proposes a bridge between the biological and psychosocial natures of human beings.

HAMLIN'S UTILITY THEORY

Roy Hamlin's utility theory is relatively simple and straightforward and is based on the following assumptions [19]:

1. Humans are capable of living to 140 years of age (the maximum life span).
2. Early development reflects the expansion of biological programs, which reach a steady state at approximately 30 years of age and then begin to deteriorate or break down at about age 65.
3. During the last half of life, behavioral programs, which are culturally determined and need not break down at any age, may be substituted for biological ones.
4. Whenever the individual ceases to utilize and expend energy, decline and then death result.

5. Energy is utilized and expended as long as the individual remains both active and useful.
6. As societies become more complex, the individual span of utility increases.

To obtain a better understanding of the concept of a behavioral program, we can consider the way in which our society has traditionally defined and structured "motherhood." Good mothers were expected to provide almost total, or around-the-clock, nurturance and care for their children; to serve as the facilitator of family harmony, especially in the realm of reducing frictions between the children and their father; and if necessary, to sacrifice their own personal welfare for the sake of other family members. While the successes of many dual-career women (homemaking plus outside employment) are causing us to take a second look at this traditional view of the good mother, the point to be made here is that any working woman who has accepted the more traditional view and then becomes a mother will either behave and act according to her traditional value system or experience some guilt. In essence, she has been behaviorally programmed. Any kind of cultural expectation or stereotype can serve as a behavioral program for the members of that culture. Thus, the stereotypic view of old people as debilitated and disengaged may program them to behave in precisely this way.

Hamlin is most concerned with those behavioral programs that would function to keep the individual active and useful during the later years of life and, by so doing, would function to increase life expectancy (see the fourth and fifth assumptions, above). His assumption that an individual's span of utility increases as the society becomes more complex appears to contradict the more commonly held assertion that the elderly are both more valued and more esteemed in so-called primitive societies. This apparent contradiction can be solved in two ways. First, there is no real evidence to support the assertion that primitive societies per se value their aged members more than do modern societies. When older persons control economic resources, they are esteemed and respected regardless of the state of development of their societies. Second, complexity means more than "industrialized" or "modernized" in this context; it refers to the number and the kinds of psychosocial roles that are available to individuals within a given society.

An important point to keep in mind is that Hamlin's theory deals with the relationship between energy utilization and expenditure on the one hand and life expectancy on the other. The activity and identity continuity theories, presented later in this chapter, will relate activity and energy levels to the degree of happiness or life satisfaction experienced by the older adult.

Some support for Hamlin's theory is derived from several fairly recent studies of societies that are characterized by unusual longevity. Each of these societies, although scattered throughout the world, seems to have evolved behavioral programs that maintain the individual's utility well into old age (often beyond the century mark). Individuals are expected to engage in meaningful and productive labor regardless of age. At the end of the day's work, the elders are called on to serve as consultants, counselors, and mediators for issues of importance both to other individuals and to the community as a whole. Other, more subtle aspects of behavioral programming may also exist; there appears to be provision for, and communal expectation of, a full and vigorous experiencing of life. Smoking and drinking may be quite heavy, dancing and other forms of social interaction are common, and the level of social and sexual attraction between older males and females appears to be quite high in these societies.

It can be argued, therefore, that behavioral programming (a psychosocial variable) can have a profound effect on one's life expectancy. However, it can also be argued that basic biological factors may account for both the unusual longevity and the behavioral manifestations of these societies. It seems likely that the unusual longevity is itself a result of a relatively homogeneous genotype that confers long lives on the members of these communities. It might also be argued that the stressors commonly associated with living in modern industrialized societies are absent in these communities, as are various forms of pollutants. Moreover, in spite of variations in diet from one of these societies to the next, food intake in general is much lower than that found in western societies. Findings from animal research, indicate that the food intake during the earliest period of life is a prominent determinant of the rate of development of the immunity system. Therefore, it remains a possibility that the individuals in these societies exhibit less decline in psychological and sociological functioning during their old age because of their eating habits and healthier biological states.

This particular bit of information is especially interesting to proponents of the autoimmune theory, a biological theory that is described in Chapter 36. According to one version of this theory, if the immune system develops early in life, it provides the individual with protection during infancy and early childhood, but places that same individual at relatively greater risk in later life when the system's functions are beginning to breakdown. However, if there is a delay in the development of the immune system, it places the infant or child at relatively greater risk, but confers a greater degree of protection against disease processes in later life because of the system's continued functioning. This latter pattern is commonly observed in populations of unusual longevity where infant mortality rates tend to be higher than average while mortality rates at older ages are somewhat lower than expected.

Psychological Theories

ERIKSON

With the introduction of Erikson's theory [16], this discussion will begin to focus on the developmental tasks that confront the older adult. Some of these tasks are overtly cognitive or psychosocial in nature; others are so only by inference. The term **ego integrity** denotes acceptance of the way one has lived and is still living one's life; it is the subjective realization that the life cycle had to be as it was, that it did not permit substitutions, and that the choices and the decisions made at various points were the best that could be made at those times. As the infant learned to trust life for the successful resolution of Erikson's first task, so the adult must learn to trust death for the successful resolution of Erikson's final task. It is also the subjective evaluation that one was, and still is, in control of one's life; and that it has been a life of dignity. In contrast, the term **despair** refers to a conflict about the way one has lived and is still living; it is the subjective experience of dissatisfaction, disappointment, or disgust with the course of one's life and the conviction that it would be lived differently if another chance were given to do so. Despair also denotes concern over future events and a sense of helplessness in facing them—a lack of control.

The healthy resolution of this developmental task consists of an abundance of ego-integrity and just enough despair to guarantee the possibility of life changes up until the moment of death. Resolutions of the task that deviate from this ideal ratio are said by Erikson to be associated with maladjustment. Of importance to Erikson's theory is the notion that the successful resolution of this eighth and final developmental task is contingent upon, but not guaranteed by, the degree to which adequate resolutions have occurred for the preceding seven developmental tasks. Thus the task of generativity versus stagnation is not only important to functioning during the middle years (see Chap. 37) but is also crucial to the quality of life in the later years.

We will return to Erikson's concept of ego-integrity versus despair when we begin to examine the course of psychosocial development in the older adult, especially the phenomenon of "the life review."

PECK

While Erikson theorizes that there is only one major developmental task of old age, Peck [42] hypothesizes that there are three. One of these tasks is **ego differentiation versus work-role preoccupation.** During the middle adult years, identity and feelings of worth are strongly dependent on one's work role or occupation. Therefore, the onset of retirement may signal a dramatic reduction in feelings of worthiness for some individuals. Individuals with well-differentiated egos possess a sense of worth that is defined along several different dimensions, any one of which can then be utilized to replace the work role or occupation, as the central defining characteristic for self-esteem. Thus there is a bipotentiality in the retirement situation; retirement can result in a weakened or lost sense of worth, or it can result in a reassignment of self-esteem that is healthier and more growth-oriented than the former one. Chapter 41 is devoted to this special topic.

A second developmental task, **body transcendence versus body preoccupation,** meshes well with Hamlin's third assumption. It is apparent that most biophysical changes in old age are in the general direction of declining function. The task then is to adjust to, and transcend, these bodily declines in order to maintain feelings of well being. A resolution in the opposite direction implies a dwelling on, or preoccupation with, these bodily declines to the extent that life satisfaction and happiness are reduced and psychosocial functioning is impaired.

Peck's third and final developmental task of old age is **ego transcendence versus ego preoccupation.** Ego transcendence denotes the acceptance of death, without undue fear or anxiety, as the inevitable conclusion of one's life. It is not a passive acceptance of death, but, rather, an active involvement with a future that extends beyond the boundaries of one's own mortality. Ego preoccupation denotes a refusal to let go of life, an immersion in a system of immediate self-gratification. Presumably, those individuals who resolve Erikson's task in favor of ego integrity over despair will be the same individuals who resolve Peck's task in favor of ego transcendence over ego preoccupation.

HAVIGHURST

The developmental tasks that Havighurst says characterize the older adult years in western society are listed in Appendix C.

The particular order in which these developmental tasks are listed does not imply a predetermined hierarchy; the tasks are to be mastered as they are presented by society to the older adult—one at a time, in various combinations, or all at once. According to Havighurst, failure to master these developmental tasks will result in high anxiety, maladjustment, and exposure to social disapproval. The likelihood of successful mastery is contingent upon the degree of mastery of the developmental tasks of previous life stages.

It is instructive to examine Havighurst's developmental tasks in light of the assumptions of the disengagement and activity theories. Since these two theories are to a large degree antithetical to one another, the proper resolutions of Havighurst's tasks take on a very different meaning from the perspective of the disengagement and activity theories.

Sociological Theories

DISENGAGEMENT THEORY

A major premise of disengagement theory [14] is derived from functional sociology: Given that individuals inevitably die but that the society to which they belong is continuous, it is therefore necessary for society to find ways of minimizing the social disruption or impact that results from the death of its members. In this way, the effective functioning of the system is minimally disrupted by the loss of the essential services provided by a specific subsystem. For example, the constitution of the United States provides for a line of succession to the presidency that guarantees that societal disruption will be kept to a minimum should the nation's leader die during tenure in office. On a larger scale, societal disruption is minimized by removing large numbers of older adults (who are more likely to die than their younger counterparts) from the mainstream of society prior to their deaths. Compulsory retirement is one mechanism for achieving this type of disengagement; another is age constraint norms (see the section, Psychosocial Functioning in the Older Adult, following). One can, in all likelihood, think of additional societal mechanisms for disengaging the older adult; many of these mechanisms would have a differential effect on males and females, since their roles have traditionally been structured differently in our society.

A second major premise of disengagement theory is that individuals undergo a self-disengagement process during the middle and later years of life. This process is characterized by a reduction in general energy levels, a reduction in societal involvement in the form of both fewer relationships and changes in the quality of those relationships that are maintained, an increased preoccupation with one's own needs and desires, and a reorientation from counting the years already lived to a consideration of the number of years of life that remain. There are obvious possibilities for relating the self-disengagement process to Erikson's concept of ego integrity versus despair as well as to Peck's developmental task of ego transcendence versus ego preoccupation.

Disengagement theory also generates a set of predictions about life satisfaction and morale during the late adult years. Given the fact that an individual may or may not want to disengage, and that society may or may not want that same individual to disengage, life satisfaction and morale should be highest in those individuals for whom there is a match-up with society's expectations. Satisfaction and morale should also remain relatively high for those individuals who wish to disengage even though society wishes them to remain within the mainstream. However, life satisfaction and morale may be quite low for those individuals who want to remain in the mainstream while society wishes them to disengage.

ACTIVITY THEORY

While disengagement theory predicts that for the majority of older adults, satisfaction and high morale will be associated with the general decline in activity that accompanies dropping out of the mainstream of society, the activity point of view assumes that successful aging involves the maintenance of high activity levels during old age. The term **activity level** refers to more than just physical exertion; it includes psychological as well as social activities and functions. Since this point of view recognizes the fact that some areas of activity and functioning may be lost or curtailed as a result of the normal vicissitudes of old age, it assumes that successful aging can still occur through the substitution of new activities for lost ones. For example, the reduction in physical strength and health that occurs in old age can be compensated for by an increase in psychological or social activities. Again, note the congruence with Hamlin's theory that higher activity levels function to extend one's life expectancy.

Activity level is now being used to explain successful

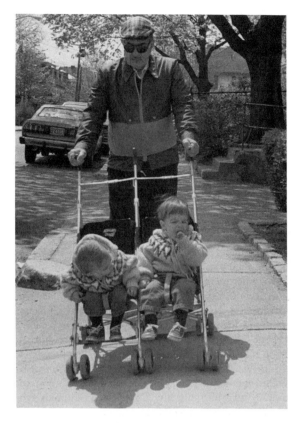

Figure 40–1. Many elderly persons thoroughly enjoy the time spent with their grandchildren and great-grandchildren. Generativity tasks can be continued through guidance of the younger generation. (Photo by Ed Slaman.)

aging; that is, why it is that some older individuals experience higher life satisfaction and morale than do others. For this reason, the activity point of view probably serves as the most prevalent theoretical basis for the creation of activity programming for older adults. Interestingly enough, this theory receives only partial support in empirical research, perhaps because research has not adequately differentiated between internally mediated activity and externally imposed activity (which to the observer may appear the same!). Although a relatively high degree of life satisfaction and morale is typically associated with moderate to high levels of activity, differences in the degree of activity within this range are no longer predictive of increasing levels of life satisfaction and morale.

IDENTITY CONTINUITY THEORY

The identity continuity theory [3] assumes neither a necessary reduction in activity levels (disengagement

theory) nor the necessity of maintaining high activity levels (the activity point of view). It does assume, however, that successful aging is associated with the ability of the individual to maintain those patterns of behavior that existed prior to old age. Therefore, it is the degree of continuity over time that is predictive of life satisfaction and morale—a continuity in one's behavioral patterns and one's life-style, regardless of the actual level of activity present in those patterns and styles.

Two psychological mechanisms, selective perception and situational reinforcement, have been utilized to explain how and why continuity over time occurs. **Selective perception** is the name given to the psychological process whereby experiences are reacted to on the basis of their relative congruence with currently held values, beliefs, and attitudes. Rather than being rejected per se, noncongruent events are simply screened out of awareness, ignored, or reinterpreted. Because we tend to pay attention only to the information that will serve to confirm our current values, beliefs, and attitudes, the existence of selective perception clearly serves to maintain previously established behavioral patterns. **Situational reinforcement** works in much the same way. The behaviors we tend to utilize are those that are rewarded; conversely, nonrewarded or punished behaviors tend to be reduced in usage. Since previously established behavioral patterns tend to be the ones that are still open to the reinforcement process that serves to strengthen them further, these behavioral patterns tend to be maintained to the exclusion of other behavioral possibilities.

It might be argued, however, that it becomes increasingly more difficult to maintain a specific behavioral pattern, or a certain style of life, when one is confronted by the developmental tasks of older adulthood in our society. There are also changes of fortune that are less clearly defined that by their very nature may be more insidious in their effects on the degree of satisfaction and morale experienced by the older adult. The minority group theory provides some insight into this aspect of aging.

MINORITY GROUP THEORY

Since individuals who are 65 years of age and older represent only slightly more than 11 percent of the current U.S. population, they constitute a minority group. Consequently, it becomes possible to apply to the elderly some of the principles that have been used by social scientists to understand the behavior of individuals belonging to other minority groups. The following statements represent, in simplified form, some of the major assumptions of minority group theory:

1. The majority discriminates against the members of the minority group, and it also evolves or develops a set of stereotyped concepts about them.
2. These stereotypes are typically worded in such a way that negative inferences can be drawn from the characteristics attributed to the members of the minority group.
3. As a result of having experienced discrimination and having come to accept these stereotypes as being accurate, the members of the minority group acquire feelings of inadequacy, self-pity, self-hatred, and low self-esteem.

Although the elderly do constitute a minority group in a numerical sense, they apparently do not do so in either a psychological or a sociological sense. For example, while older adults do experience job discrimination because of age, they are not automatically subjected to less respect and consideration in their day-to-day interactions with others. In addition, old people do not appear to feel the sense of group solidarity, group spirit, or consciousness of the kind that tends to characterize other minority groups [52]. Indeed, one cannot get many 80-year-olds to agree that they are old!

Aging is viewed negatively in our relatively youth-oriented society, and most stereotypes directed toward older adults reflect this orientation. Thus the potential for harm to the self-concept of the older adult does exist. However, the range of psychological and sociological differences among older adults is at least as great as that for any other adult group, which is why both the potential harm and the actual harm that is experienced tend to vary greatly from one aging individual to another. Many of these stereotypes, with their general lack of validity and their effects on older adults, will be explored in the section to which we now turn—the research data on the cognitive and psychosocial development of the older adult.

FUNCTIONAL CAPACITIES OF OLDER ADULTS

Cognitive Functioning in Older Adults

The existence of negative stereotyping is nowhere as evident as it is in the particular area of the intellectual functioning of older adults. These stereotypes would have us believe that thinking and problem solving become increasingly rigid with age, that the judgmental ability of the elderly is dramatically impaired, and that learning capacity is greatly reduced. The stereotypes also suggest that frequent lapses of memory, slower thinking processes, and periods of severe mental confusion are characteristic of the aging intellect [40]. These extreme stereotypes may represent an accurate portrayal of the mental functioning of that segment of the elderly population (10 to 15 percent) that suffers from some form of organic or functional pathology [6, 40]. However, the stereotypes are inaccurate for the vast majority. Some of our misperception arises out of the common usage of the term **senility** and its confusion with **senescence,** which literally means "growing old or aging." Since the terms are so similar in form and because the term senility has acquired the rather negative connotations of general mental and physical degeneration, it is rather natural to assume that senescent (aging or old) individuals are also senile (suffering from general mental and physical degeneration). In actuality, only a small minority of senescent individuals are also senile in the everyday sense of that word.

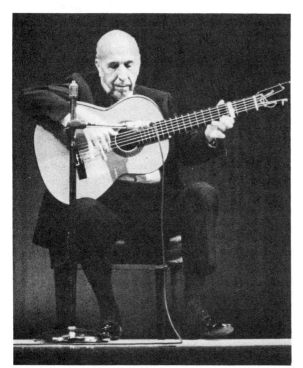

Figure 40–2. The skills of elderly persons can be highly valued by the culture.

THE COURSE OF INTELLECTUAL DEVELOPMENT

It has already been stated (in Chap. 37) that intellectual performance seems to peak during the middlescent period at approximately 50 years of age. The current controversy about the course of intellectual development revolves around the issue of whether or not this peak in middlescence is followed by a significant decline in intelligence during the "twilight years" of life.

The inability of researchers to arrive at a consensus on this issue, and hence the continuing controversy, is due in part to the ambiguity involved in interpreting the developmental data that have been collected via different research strategies. Thus for example, cross-sectional studies tend to demonstrate a general decline in intelligence beyond age 50, while longitudinal studies reveal little or no such general decline until the seventies [23, 46, 47]. Such differences in interpretation are exaggerated by the fact that each of these research strategies is subject to somewhat different sources of methodological bias. Also contributing to the controversy is the possibility that intelligence tests may be age-biased in favor of younger adults, thus artificially presenting a somewhat negative picture of intellectual development in later life.

Intelligence tests were originally designed to predict scholastic achievement in children, and the currently used standardized intelligence tests have tended to measure similar types of skills and abilities. Another pertinent problem resides in the relationship between intellectual competence or capacity on the one hand and intellectual performance on the other. One's performance is not always a clear indication of competence, since a number of factors or variables often intervene between the two. Unless these intervening variables are controlled for, or otherwise excluded from, consideration, any comparatively poor intellectual performance by the elderly can be dismissed by arguing that their intellectual competence or capacity could have been undiminished and the reduced performance attributable to intervening variables.

One additional point about this controversy merits our careful consideration. The debate has historically been couched in terms of a general intelligence decline, while the answer appears to require specificity in terms of both different types or forms of intelligence and different patterns of development for different people.

The distinction between the fluid and crystallized forms of intellectual skills was introduced in Chapters 27 and 37. The former type is basically determined by the status of the individual's neurological and physiological functionings. Since one's biological status begins to decline around age 30 with a rapid decline beginning about age 65 to 70, the skills that involve fluid intelligence can also be expected to decrease during the later years of life. Crystallized intelligence, on the other hand, is believed to arise out of any or all of those life experiences that affect an individual's general adjustment, motivational status, and overall level of knowledge. Hence, remaining in a reasonably stimulating environment should result in the maintenance or even the enhancement of these skills [24]. Total intelligence quotient (IQ) scores, which are based on the combination of both sets of skills, may decline somewhat in later life; but since certain specific intellectual skills (the crystallized ones) appear to hold relatively constant or improve throughout adulthood [22], how can one argue for a general intellectual decline?

It is also difficult to argue for a general intellectual decline in old age when one finds evidence that while many elderly individuals fit the expected pattern, a significant number also deviate from that pattern. Longitudinal studies of individuals indicate some remarkable gains in the level of performance from age 70 to age 84; others decline from age 20 to age 30. [45] What can account for these individual differences?

Those individuals whose intellectual performance is maintained or even enhanced into the later years of life seem to have the following common characteristics that distinguish them from those individuals whose intellectual performance declines earlier: They gained early experience in a rich and stimulating environment; they were more intelligent to begin with, as determined by early life assessments [51]; they obtained more years of formal education; and as adults, they tended to be in professional, executive, or managerial vocations. Schaie [45] concludes that "the maintenance and growth of intelligence of an adult may also have much to do with the complexity of his environment . . . we suggest that it will be possible to show that people who live in a varied environment are often the ones who show continued growth throughout life, while those who live in a static environment may be the ones who most likely show some decrement." This conclusion is strikingly similar to a proposal discussed in the theoretical section of this chapter; it would appear that some individuals have adopted behavioral programs that call for the continued use of intellectual functions, and that this practice results in the maintenance or even the strengthening of these skills and abilities.

It is too early to predict the final outcome of the debate about the course of intellectual development in later life. For now, it can be said that at a minimum, the continuing controversy has created an awareness of the possibility that the declines that do take place start later in life and are smaller in magnitude than previously thought and that these declines include fewer intellectual skills [10a].

LEARNING AND PROBLEM SOLVING

As is the case for intellectual development, cross-sectional studies of problem solving and learning indicate a decline in both of these skill areas throughout middle and old age. Although longitudinal studies indicate a delay in the onset of decline perhaps until the individuals' late sixties or early seventies, a slower rate of decline, and less overall decline, the decline nevertheless persists.

Thus, researchers have sought to discover whether the cause of the poorer performance stems from changes within the older adult's competence or capacity, or the poorer performance might be the result of other factors (intervening variables) that come into play when problem solving and learning are measured in subjects of different ages. In this regard, several situational determinants and personal variables have been identified that might place the elderly subject at a disadvantage relative to the younger one.

One case in point is the method of using timed tests to assess problem solving and learning ability. It is a well-established fact of biological functioning that reaction time, the interval between the onset of the stimulus and the subject's response to it, increases from about 20 years of age. The rate of increase becomes greater when the individual is more than 60 years of age, and this phenomenon is further exaggerated with the performance of complex tasks [5]. Thus older subjects whose reactions are slowed down are at a disadvantage when forced to perform under imposed time constraints. Indeed, in those studies in which the time constraints have been removed, the performance of older and younger subjects has tended to become more congruent [1, 15].

Another determinant is reflected in the motivational status of the older adult relative to the younger one. It has been suggested that as individuals grow older, they become increasingly cautious and resistant to taking risks. Consequently, older individuals are less likely to attempt a response unless they are relatively certain that it will be correct. As a result of this tendency, older subjects will respond less often thus earning poorer scores (a "no response" is typically scored as an error). This also creates a further hindrance to their problem-solving and learning abilities by diminishing the possibility of learning from their own mistakes [4, 9].

It has also been suggested that the tendency toward increasing cautiousness with age is, in and of itself, a reflection of a deeper motivational restructuring of the personality. Some theorists believe that the earlier portion of the life span can be characterized as expansion-oriented; that is, the individual tends to be externally oriented and driven by motivational forces that are achievement-, growth-, and acquisition-oriented. In contrast, the latter half of the life span is constriction-oriented; that is, the individual becomes increasingly internally oriented, concerned with self-serving needs, and preoccupied with holding on to what has already been gained [30]. One clear implication of this hypothesized personality restructuring is that the achievement-oriented younger adult will be more highly motivated to perform well on problem-solving and learning tasks, whereas older adults may find such tasks to be totally irrelevant to their personal concerns.

Another large body of literature indicates that the reduced performance of older adults is at least partially due to the existence of aging-related memory deficits. Two points of particular interest are generated from this research. The first is that the amount and type of memory loss is significantly less than the loss that appears in popularized and stereotyped accounts. For example, the evidence indicates that there is little or no decrement in long-term memory with age, and that significant short-term memory loss occurs only at significantly later ages than previously thought [23]. The second, and still highly tentative, point is that the major source of such memory deficits probably resides within the original encoding or registration of the material to be remembered rather than in its storage per se.

Thus, one explanation of the poorer short-term memory performance of older adults is that they tend to process information at a shallower level than do younger adults; that is, they tend to do so phonetically (by sound) rather than semantically (by meaning). It is further asserted that they rehearse less during memorization, and/or that they utilize less elaborate rehearsal strategies. Since one tends to retrieve information from memory storage by utilizing cues that are derived from the original encoding and rehearsal strategies, it is not surprising that retrieval from short-term memory is also somewhat adversely affected in the elderly.

This failure of older adults to process information at deeper levels could reflect a basic inability or incapacity to do so, or it could reflect a tendency of simply not doing so when formulating problem-solving strategies—a so-called spontaneous performance deficit.

According to the evidence available to date, the latter interpretation seems the more justifiable.

The likelihood of spontaneously processing information at deeper levels appears to be at least a partial function of the nature of the material to be memorized. Information that is familiar, meaningful, and/or relevant to the learner tends to be processed more deeply by both young and old alike [10]. This is probably the reason the memory performances of younger and older adult subjects on meaningful materials are more congruent (but still not equivalent) than those with unfamiliar, meaningless, and/or irrelevant information. Further support for the assertion of a spontaneous performance deficit rather than a basic inability or incapacity comes from studies in which older people have been coached or instructed on how, when, and why to process information more deeply. Generally speaking, these manipulations have had a substantially positive effect upon the memory performances of the elderly.

Mediational techniques, whose role in efficient

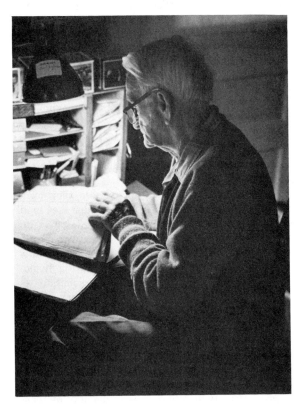

Figure 40-3. Some elderly persons pursue cognitive tasks (for which they had inadequate time during earlier years) with enthusiasm tempered by experience.

learning and problem solving has been well documented, provide an example of the encoding processes we have been talking about. **Mediators** can take the form of mental pictures or images. When an individual is asked to describe his or her bedroom, for example, the response is dictated by what is "seen" as the individual visualizes the bedroom. On the other hand, if a person is given the task of categorizing blocks of different sizes, shapes, and colors, the categories may be made on the basis of color (red or green), size (big or little), or shape (square or rectangle). Each of the terms appearing in parentheses can serve as a verbal mediator, since it represents a verbal abstraction of the stimulus property. Making categorizations on this basis is far more efficient than using a trial-and-error procedure that would require learning the correct response for each individual stimulus. According to the literature, older adults appear to be less likely to spontaneously generate verbal mediators while engaged in problem solving, and when they do, they tend to generate a different type of verbal mediator than do younger adults [13, 25].

One can find references to other variables scattered throughout the literature that have been identified as possible hindrances to the problem-solving and learning performance of older adults. Among these variables are sets and expectancies, functional fixedness, and nondirected thinking.

Sets and expectancies refer to the tendency of an individual to behave or to respond in a manner congruent with, and determined by, prior learning and problem-solving experiences. Such sets and expectancies are nominally neutral with regard to problem solving. Performance, therefore, should be facilitated when the individual's predetermined responses coincide with the proper solution to the current problem (positive transfer): performance should be hindered when the individual's predetermined responses are antagonistic to a proper solution to a current problem (negative transfer). According to the literature, it may be more difficult to arouse or to maintain task-appropriate sets and expectancies in older adults [8, 31], and therefore there may be differential positive and negative transfer effects for younger and older adults [17].

Functional fixedness refers to a specific form of learning set or expectancy—one in which the individual is unable to use a particular object for anything other than its traditional use or function. Such fixedness should increase with age, since more time will have been spent using a particular object in its customary or usual fashion. Therefore, when problems call for the creative use of objects in terms of their abstract rather than their functional properties, older adults should be affected more negatively than younger ones. However, one could argue just as well that older adults should have less fixedness over time because they have had more opportunities to see objects used in other than customary fashion over the years. Environment and motivation play significant roles.

Directed thinking is defined as thinking that is brought into focus when there is a problem to be thought through and solved; it is both voluntary and goal-oriented. **Nondirected thinking,** in contrast, is involuntary, unselected, purposeless, and is said to characterize fantasizing, reverie, and dreaming. Researchers who study fantasy and dreaming, however, argue that the nondirective thought processes involved are oriented toward problem solving, the problems usually being of a personal and conflictual nature. Regardless of the specific definitions involved, the argument being tendered is that older adults spend more time in nondirected thinking, and that this tendency is detrimental to their problem-solving performances. Perhaps the real distinction is the one made previously, that older adults are geared toward the solution of more personal types of problems, whereas younger adults are willing to spend more time working on the kinds of problems being presented in a laboratory setting.

Note how natural it is for several of these variables to interact with one another, and with yet other variables, to produce the problem-solving deficits that characterize old age. As but one example, processing information at deeper levels should facilitate memorization, which in turn is known to have a facilatory effect on problem solving. The depth of processing (including the use of mediators) at least partially depends, however, on the degree to which the material to be remembered is familiar, meaningful, and/or relevant to the learner. These factors are in turn dependent on both the learner's past experiences and current motivational status. Hence, it is not surprising to find that one's level of problem-solving skills is highly correlated with his or her years of formal schooling—the more years, the better the skills.

It is also well known that the years of schooling are positively related to early adulthood intelligence as well as to the pattern of intellectual change found in later life.

Simply stated, when older persons have had fewer years of formal schooling, they are likely to have missed some of those educational experiences that enable younger adults to outscore them. It must also be noted that even where years of education are matched, the nature of the curricula are likely to be quite different.

Furthermore, the time elapsed since formal schooling is much greater for older than for younger adults, another factor that may produce adverse effects when scores are based on formal testing procedures. Lastly, several of the motivational shifts mentioned previously could easily interact with missed educational experiences to reduce the overall meaningfulness or relevancy of these tasks for older adults.

The younger adult will outperform his or her aging counterpart when presented with identical formal lab problems to be learned or solved under identical situational constraints. It is one thing to say that an older learner or problem-solver is not as efficient as a younger one; it is an entirely different matter to say that the older adult is incapable of either learning or problem solving. Although learning and problem solving may not be as efficient in old age as in youth or middle age, both processes still occur, and they do so to a greater extent than is usually portrayed in stereotypes about the cognitive functioning of older adults. Furthermore, to the degree that we believe that optimization of one's functioning is the right of individuals of all ages, it behooves us to consider the various manipulations necessary for the creation of an optimal learning and problem-solving environment for the older adult.

An even more important point is that we have been talking about cognitive processes and change as measured by formalized, laboratory-type tasks and procedures. What about cognitive process and change in relation to the realm of day-to-day living? Some early findings derived from "naturalistic" studies of this type suggest that the elderly do define their problems differently than do the young: They utilize the realization that goals can and have already been changed to help them decide how to live their lives; and they recognize the necessity for taking advice, conserving time and resources, and distinguishing between critical and extraneous tasks and demands [6]. Their functioning is influenced by a different set of life experiences, and consequently, a different set of values and priorities.

In considering the real-life performance of older people, it is naive to regard them as passive victims of a cognitive degeneration of which they are helplessly unaware. On the contrary, older people may be said both to conserve and to exploit their intellectual resources more fully than do the young, to have a more subtle perception of the points where the complexity of decisions exceeds their capacities, and to avoid thereby unnecessary blunders. It is fitting to conclude with this reminder that the study of performance with age is not merely the study of " 'decrements in performance.' Unless we recognize that it is also the study of 'adaptation' to decrements of performance, we shall entirely miss the point" [43]. From the perspective of day-to-day living then, intellectual and cognitive functioning represents more than the accretion of formal knowledge and/or problem-solving techniques. It also includes the acquisition and utilization of what we commonly refer to as wisdom, and according to the previous comments, older adults score quite high in this regard.

Psychosocial Functioning in Older Adults

As was the case with cognitive development, the conventional wisdom with regard to the psychosocial development of older adults is overrun with myths and inaccurate stereotypes. One such myth is reflected in the assumption that little or no psychosocial change takes place during the middle and late adult years.

Although personality theories often differ from one another with regard to the specifics of the theory, they seem to share a single common core assumption—that the adult personality consists of a relatively set, stable, and enduring organization of behavioral traits and/or dispositions. Since behavior is the reflection of the action of one's personality on the environment, it is further assumed that adult behavior will also be relatively set, stable, and enduring. In contrast to personality theorists, social psychologists and sociologists have taken the position that behavior is determined less by what an individual brings to a situation, his or her personality, than it is by the situation per se. They argue, therefore, that adult behavior need not be either set or stable; when and if the individual's situations change, so should his or her behavior. In those studies that have pitted personality determinants against situational determinants, it has been the situational determinants that have proven to be the more influential in determining an individual's behavior [35]. Therefore, the behavioral patterns of adults may be neither as stable nor as enduring as personality theorists would lead us to believe and as the stereotypes portray.

STABILITY AND CONTINUITY IN BEHAVIOR

The data in support of the notion of stability and continuity in behavior over time take two basic forms: Behavioral patterns and styles (personality types) in old age seem to be extensions of those that existed earlier in life; and an individual's ability to adjust, and his or her style of adjustment, appears to remain relatively constant across the life span.

It is obvious to each of us that specific behaviors do indeed change as we grow older. However, it is not

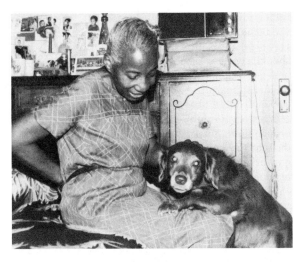

Figure 40–4. Pictures, pets, a familiar environment, friends, and family members can help the older adult to accept the changes in body functioning and energy levels as well as the loss of close family members.

specific behaviors that we are concerned with here but rather the patterns and styles of behavior. Thus one can examine an individual's behavior at a particular age and clearly recognize it as being a different but analogous form of the same behavior exhibited at an earlier or later age. The dependency of a 4-year-old and a 20-year-old are expressed differently, but it is still dependency being expressed. This notion of the "psychological equivalence" (sameness of meaning) of different behavioral expressions has helped researchers to demonstrate a marked degree of stability across adulthood for diverse behavioral patterns, such as those relating to activity levels, vocational interests, gender-expression, and life-style themes or values [18, 33].

On the basis of their own research, Neugarten, Havighurst, and Tobin [38] have concluded that behavioral patterns tend to remain stable throughout adulthood. They state that "[the individual] continues to exercise choice and to select from the environment in accordance with his own long-established needs. He ages according to a pattern that has a long history and that maintains itself, with adaptation, to the end of life."

This conclusion is all the more remarkable in that these researchers had identified a minimum of eight different personality types or patterns in 70- to 79-year-old men and women. The **reorganized, focused,** and **disengaged** personality types were represented by well-functioning individuals who had intact cognitive and psychosocial skills and a high degree of life satisfaction. These three types differed from one another in terms of their respectively decreasing commitments to various activities and roles. The **holding on** and **constricted** types were represented by striving, ambitious, and achievement-oriented individuals who tended to defend themselves against the anxiety generated by the realization of their aging. The former type did so by holding on to the patterns of their younger years, whereas the latter type tended to close themselves off from any and all experiences that would verify their growing older. Life satisfaction and morale remain high as long as these defenses work; if and when they fail, life satisfaction and morale are reduced. The **succor-seeking** and **apathetic** types were represented by passive-dependent individuals, the former being able to maintain themselves moderately well as long as someone responded to their emotional needs and the latter being characterized by extreme passivity. Note that the life satisfaction and morale of those individuals will be low unless they are cared for in a stable and nurturant environment. The eighth personality type was labeled the **disorganized** type and represented those individuals who had gross losses or deficits in psychological functions.

It thus appears that differences in personality types among the elderly are to some degree a reflection of the differences in personality that existed earlier in life. This point is further emphasized when the same researchers state that "There is considerable evidence that, in normal men and women, there is no sharp discontinuity of personality with age, but instead an increasing consistency. Those characteristics that have been central to the personality seem to become even more clearly delineated, and those values the individual has been cherishing become even more salient" [38]. It should be noted that these eight personality types do not represent an exhaustive listing of possibilities. Other researchers have identified additional variations in the aging personality.

Similar conclusions of persistence, stability, and continuity of psychosocial development are reached with regard to the evidence on adjustment and styles of adjustment. In two somewhat similar studies [44], researchers found evidence that an individual's style of adapting in old age is a direct extension of that individual's lifelong patterns of adjustment. In addition, Neugarten [37] has reached the conclusion, based on all previously accumulated evidence, that an individual's ability to adjust to the normal vicissitudes of life (to roll with the punches) remains relatively constant across the life span. Troll [54] concludes that "People

who are comfortable with themselves and their world continue to be able to cope in the face of life's transitions. Those who fall apart at critical points like menopause, retirement, or death of spouse are those who have been fragile or have fallen apart before. There is no point in the life cycle that can be called a 'falling to pieces' time." It appears that theorists, such as Erikson and Havighurst, are expressing a truism when they state that the resolution of previous conflicts, or the mastery of previous developmental tasks, is predictive of future resolutions and future mastery. Seligman (learned helplessness theory) [49] hypothesized that each time an individual effectively copes with a stressful situation, he or she actually enhances coping abilities and becomes less likely to feel and act helpless.

INSTABILITY AND NONCONTINUITY IN BEHAVIOR

The evidence that supports the notion of instability and noncontinuity in behavior over time also takes two basic forms: resocialization phenomena and reorientation of personality.

In the argument for stability and continuity, it was stated that researchers have been able to establish high correlations between some behavioral patterns exhibited by individuals at different periods of the life span. For example, Kagan and Moss [27] found that aggressiveness in childhood was moderately to highly predictive of aggressiveness in young adulthood for males, but not for females, and that dependency in childhood was equally predictive for young adult females, but not for males. The consistencies support the contention of stability over time; the inconsistencies in these data can be easily explained in terms of movement toward age-gender norms or socially mediated behavioral programs, and thus argue for instability. During adolescence, females are resocialized in such a way as to inhibit expressions of dependency. Therefore, some shifts in behavioral patterns do occur over time, and these shifts often seem to be in the direction of congruence with age-gender norms.

A more impressive finding is that resocialization is not restricted to the periods of childhood and adolescence. Neugarten, Moore, and Lowe [39] have demonstrated that as individuals grow older, they ascribe increasing importance to age norms and correspondingly place greater constraints upon adult behavior. Interestingly enough, at all ages tested, these same individuals assumed that others were more concerned with age norms than they were. These authors state that "although the actual occurrence of major life events for both men and women are influenced by a variety of life contingencies, and although the norms themselves vary somewhat from one group of persons to another, it can easily be demonstrated that norms and actual occurrences are closely related. Age norms and age expectations operate as prods and brakes on behavior, in some instances hastening an event, in others, delaying it. Men and women are aware not only of the social clocks that operate in various areas of their lives, but they are aware also of their own timing and readily describe themselves as 'early,' 'late,' or 'on time' with regard to family and occupational events" [39].

With regard to the possibility of a reorientation of personality, Neugarten [36] speaks of the age span of 50 to 59 years as one of increased "interiority," during which introspection, contemplation, reflection, and self-evaluation become increasingly salient components of mental life. Other researchers have reported that men and women enter a period of ambivalence and reassessment from as early as age 40 (to age 60) in which they desire some type of life change, although actual change may sometimes be feared [53]. This last statement raises an interesting point. The personality reorientation that is being described consists of an internal set of shifts. Whether or not these shifts are accompanied by changes in external behavior is problematical: A reassessment and self-evaluation may lead to the conclusion that no change in life-style or pattern is necessary; the individual may be unable to decide which changes to make; or the fear of unknown consequences may be too great to allow change. In any case, there is a general consensus that this internal reorientation of personality appears earlier and more consistently than does a reorientation in the external manifestations of personality.

It is a matter of conjecture as to whether or not this midlife reorientation is a precursor to the "life review," a phenomenon that occurs in older adults that is often associated with dramatic shifts in personality. According to Butler [12], the life review is a universal process that can occur at any age that an individual confronts his or her mortality. Its occurrence in older adults, however, is accompanied by a heightened intensity and vividness and an emphasis on putting one's life in order. The process itself consists of a progressive return to consciousness of one's life-history experiences, especially previously unresolved conflicts, which can once again be examined in a last attempt at resolution.

To the degree that one is successful in the life review process, fear and anxiety about death will be alleviated, a sense of serenity will exist, old wrongs will have been righted, and the individual will take pride in the accomplishments of his or her life. This outcome appears to be synonymous with Erikson's concept of ego integrity and Peck's notion of ego transcendence. An unsuccessful life review can result in severe depression, terror, anxiety, panic, or feelings of guilt—an outcome strikingly similar to the concepts of despair and ego preoccupation. Regardless of the outcome, it is obvious that in passing through the life review, each individual experiences an opportunity for a final integration of his or her past life with the present personality. When this happens, dramatic shifts in personality can and sometimes do take place.

SUCCESSFUL AND UNSUCCESSFUL AGING

Another set of myths and inaccurate stereotypes is that which portrays the elderly as debilitated, lonely, forgotten, unhappy, and dissatisfied individuals with poor self-concepts and low levels of self-esteem. Such outcomes, if true, would clearly constitute evidence of unsuccessful aging. Studies of self-esteem and self-concept in the older adult have yielded somewhat contradictory results. Some have found increases in self-esteem with age; others indicate little or no change over time; still others report slight declines. It therefore appears safe to conclude only that the self-esteem and the self-concept of older adults are about as positive as those of their younger counterparts [5].

A conclusion similar to that for self-esteem and self-concept has been reached for self-reported ratings of morale, happiness and life-satisfaction in older adults: They appear to score about as high as do younger adults on these three self-reported measures of psychological well-being.

MENTAL HEALTH STATUS

The data on the mental health status of older adults is somewhat equivocal; its interpretation often depends on the particular data sets being utilized and the mitigating circumstances that are considered. On the negative side are those statistics that show that suicide rates increase rapidly after 60 years of age, especially in the white male segment of the population. On the other hand, it is often argued that attempted suicide rates (another presumed measure of psychological nonwell-being) do not significantly differ across the adult years. The greater rate of suicide among the elderly may therefore be attributed to their greater resolve and efficiency rather than lowered levels of well-being.

Again on the negative side, although older adults (those 65 years of age and older) comprise slightly more than 11 percent of the United States population, they also account for 15 to 20 percent of first admissions to mental hospitals, and 30 percent of the chronic patient population. The vast majority of these individuals are admitted with a diagnosis of organic brain syndrome (OBS). On the other hand, the reported incidence of OBS, while certainly higher among the elderly, is probably grossly overstated, since this diagnostic label tends to be applied to a "catch-all" group of disorders that present somewhat similar clinical features. Many professionals feel that true OBS exists in only a very small percentage of individuals and that many persons diagnosed as having OBS are actually suffering from poor nutritional status, sensory-perceptual declines, or a lack of general environmental stimulation. The diagnosis itself is often made in light of the existence of "soft neurological signs or symptoms" rather than direct evidence of organic damage. (The reader is referred to Chap. 39 for a more detailed discussion of this general topic.)

Several prominent professionals adhere to the view that old age is, in and of itself, no more a period of mental health risk than is any other period. We know, for example, that poor mental health often results from a progressive accumulation of poor adjustments; it is therefore to be expected that mental illness rates will increase with age as some individuals continue to experience the kinds of stressors that result in progressively poorer and poorer adjustments. Furthermore, there is evidence to indicate that older adults are proportionately underrepresented in the use of mental health facilities, such as outpatient clinics, day-care programs, and community mental health center care programs [29]. Thus, with the exception of OBS, which does increase in frequency as individuals grow older, the frequencies of other forms of mental illness (e.g., psychoneuroses, functional psychoses, personality disorders, alcoholism) probably remain relatively static throughout middle and old age. Older adults are more likely, however, to receive treatments in mental hospitals, whereas their younger counterparts more often receive treatment in local community or outpatient facilities.

Although variables, such as self-esteem, happiness, self-concept, life satisfaction, and mental health status, are intuitively related to one another, a point of particular interest is that the variables that are highly predictive of any one of them are not necessarily predictive of the others or may be so to a much lesser degree.

LIFE CIRCUMSTANCES

It has been demonstrated experimentally that a rather large number of life-circumstance variables are related to psychological well-being in old age. Health status, income, educational level, socioeconomic class, activity level, marital and family statuses, and work status are several of the most frequently studied variables. In almost every case, the relationships between these variables and the outcome measures of well-being tend to be relatively slight but statistically significant. This means that while the variables are generally predictive

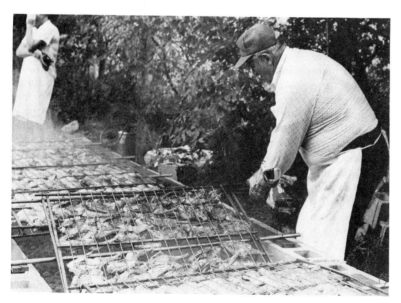

Figure 40–5. Individuals with the highest sense of ego integrity appear to be those who continue to be active in the community.

of well-being in the population as a whole, they do not account for much of the variability in the level of well-being experienced by individual members of that population [34].

In order to improve on these results, gerontologists have come up with a psychological refinement of these predictor variables. Rather than studying objectively defined life-circumstances, they have begun to examine the elderly individual's subjective reaction to, or perception/experience of, these circumstances. For example, instead of objectively studying the amount of time devoted to each of several spheres of activity, one researcher studied the effect on well-being of the discrepancies between individuals' reports of the amount of time they expected or desired to spend in each sphere versus the actual amount of time they devoted to those activities [48]. In general, studies that have utilized this more subjective approach have demonstrated a much higher degree of relationship between circumstantial variables and measures of well-being. The meaning given to an event is the significant factor in determining the effect of the event on the individual's satisfaction with life.

INTERPERSONAL SUPPORT SYSTEMS

An individual's capacity for dealing with potentially disruptive situations is to a large degree a function of the supportive resources available to that individual [41]. If the stereotypes of the elderly as isolated and forgotten are correct, then the elderly are obviously more susceptible to the apparent ravages of stress than are the young. Fortunately, however, these stereotypes also prove to be inaccurate [50].

In the United States, fully 80 percent of older males and 60 percent of older females live in a family unit; 49 percent of the elderly live within a 30-minute drive of at least one child; and 65 percent of those older adults who have children reported seeing at least one of their children during the previous 24-hour period. Moreover, adult children provide economic help, emotional gratification, personal health care, and assistance with household management for their elderly parents when it is necessary [21, 53]. Spouses, when still living, still represent the primary source of support. Spouseless and childless elderly adults tend to turn to siblings, close friends, and then neighbors for needed support and do so in the order given [26]. Even pets may serve as sources of comfort and solace in times of need.

Thus the typical or average older adult has access to many people and relationships, any of which may afford the support necessary for effectively coping with disruption. Sometimes, the necessary support is not available, in spite of the existence of such relationships. It is neither the number of relationships per se nor the frequency or duration of interpersonal contacts that is important; the crucial variable seems to be the quality of the interpersonal relationships. The availability of at least one close friend or confidant appears to be the single most important variable in distinguishing those older adults who cope effectively with disruption and those who do not [32].

GENERALIZATIONS ABOUT DEVELOPMENT IN OLDER ADULTS

Interindividual Differences in Development

The first generalization about development in older adults is somewhat paradoxical because it states that no generalization about older adults can be completely accurate or valid. In dealing with inaccurate stereotypes, it is important to point out their inaccuracies without creating opposite but equally inaccurate ones. Many older adults have intact intellectual abilities and problem-solving and learning skills; other older adults do not. Most older adults experience successful aging, possessing a high degree of self-esteem and positive self-concepts, having reasonable good mental health, and reporting relatively high degrees of life satisfaction; other older adults do not. Indeed, aging individuals are even more different from one another than are younger adults; as a result, stereotypes have no more general validity for the elderly than they do for the young. Differences in experiential background tend to create interindividual variability with age.

Intraindividual Differences in Development

While it is true that effectiveness in cognitive functioning and effectiveness in psychosocial functioning are generally predictive of one another, these processes and their subcomponents follow somewhat different developmental courses in any given individual. The data are quite clear on this point: Each psychological function ages in a different way and rate. The earliest decline is generally observed in the ability to perform vigorous physical activities; then there will be a decline in fine neuromuscular activities; next there will be a decline in general intellectual skills, some of which, like fluid intelligence, will decline earlier and others, like crystallized intelligence, will decline much later. It is hard to determine where psychosocial development fits into this overall scheme, since some theorists hold to the possibility of a final integration and optimization of self just prior to death.

SUMMARY

Throughout this chapter an attempt has been made to point out the key factors or variables that seem to make a difference in the course of cognitive and psychosocial development in older adults. The data in this regard seem to be straightforward. Those individuals who continue to live in intellectually stimulating environments that challenge them to use their learning and problem-solving skills tend to be those who maintain effective cognitive functioning well into old age. Those individuals who are able to maintain lifelong patterns and styles of psychosocial behavior, because of either a lack of disruption in their lives or the development of effective coping skills and personal support systems, are those who experience successful aging during the older adult years. The lesson in all of this is quite clear; One's general status as an older adult, although affected by the events and occurrences of old age, is also determined by the previous life history. Those persons who wish to experience the unique and special kinds of joy and happiness that are the mark of a long, productive, and successful life can, and must, begin to prepare for it during childhood and the young adult years.

ACKNOWLEDGEMENTS

The author wishes to express his sincerest appreciation to Dr. Robert C. Atchley, Dr. Mildred M. Seltzer, and Ms. Patricia L. Gump of the Scripps Foundation Gerontology Center, Miami University, for their encouragement, suggestions, and helpful criticism during the writing of this chapter.

REFERENCES

1. Arenberg, D. Age differences in retroaction. *J. Gerontol.* 22:88, 1967.
2. Ariès, P. *Centuries of Childhood: A Social History of Family Life.* Translated by R. Baldick. New York: Vintage Books, 1965.
3. Atchley, R. C. *The Social Forces in Later Life* (3rd ed.). Belmont, CA: Wadsworth, 1980.
4. Birkhill, W. R., and Schaie, K. W. The effect of differential reinforcement of cautiousness in intellectual performance among the elderly. *J. Gerontol.* 30:578, 1975.
5. Birren, J. E. *The Psychology of Aging.* Englewood Cliffs, NJ: Prentice-Hall, 1964.
6. Birren, J. E. Age and Decision Strategies. In A. T. Welford and J. E. Birren (Eds.), *Interdisciplinary Topics in Gerontology.* Basel: Karger, 1969.
7. Bischof, L. J. *Adult Psychology* (2nd ed.). New York: Harper & Row, 1976.
8. Botwinick, J. Drives, Expectancies, and Emotions. In J. E. Birren (Ed.), *Handbook of Aging and the Individual.* Chicago: University of Chicago Press, 1959.
9. Botwinick, J. Disinclination to venture response versus cautiousness in responding: Age differences. *J. Genet. Psychol.* 115:55, 1969.
10. Botwinick, J., and Storandt, M. *Memory, Related Function, and Age.* Springfield, IL: Thomas, 1974.
10a. Botwinick, J. Intellectual Abilities. In J. E. Birren and K. W. Schaie (Eds.), *Handbook of the Psychology of Aging.* New York: Van Nostrand Reinhold, 1977.
11. Brumer, S. as reported in K. F. Riegel's, History of Psychological Gerontology, in J. E. Birren et al. (Eds.), *Handbook of the Psychology of Aging.* New York: Van Nostrand, Reinhold, 1977.
12. Butler, R. N. The life review: An interpretation of reminiscence in the aged. *Psychiatry,* 26:65, 1963.
13. Canestrari, R. E. Age Changes in Acquisition. In G. A. Talland (Ed.), *Human Aging and Behavior.* New York: Academic Press, 1968.
14. Cumming, E., and Henry, W. E. *Growing Old: The Process of Disengagement.* New York: Arno Press, 1979.
15. Eisdorfer, C., Axelrod, S., and Wilkie, F. L. Stimulus exposure times as a factor in serial learning in an aged sample. *J. Abnorm. Soc. Psychol.* 67:594, 1963.
16. Erikson, E. H. *Childhood and Society* (Rev. ed.). New York: Norton, 1978.
17. Gladis, M., and Braun, H. W. Age differences in transfer and retroaction as a function of intertask response similarity. *J. Exp. Psychol.* 55:25, 1958.
18. Haan, N., and Day, D. A longitudinal study of change and sameness in personality development, adolescence to later adulthood. *Aging Hum. Dev.* 5:11, 1974.
19. Hamlin, R. M. Utility theory of old age. *Proceedings of the 74th Annual Convention of the APA.* 1:213, 1966.
20. Havighurst, R. J. *Developmental Tasks and Education* (3rd ed.). New York: McKay, 1972.
21. Hill, R. Decision Making and the Family Life Cycle. In E. Shanas and G. F. Streib (Eds.), *Social Structure and the Family: Generational Relations.* Englewood Cliffs, NJ: Prentice-Hall, 1965.
22. Hooper, F. H., and Storck, P. A. "A Life Span Analysis of Fluid vs. Crystallized Intelligence." Paper presented at the 25th Annual Meeting of the Gerontology Society, San Juan, Puerto Rico, 1972.
23. Horn, J. L. Organization of Data on Life-Span Development of Human Abilities. In L. R. Goulet and P. Baltes (Eds.), *Life-Span Developmental Psychology.* New York: Academic Press, 1970.
24. Horn, J. L. Intelligence: Why it grows, why it declines. *Transaction* 4:23, 1967.
25. Hulicka, I. M., and Grossman, J. L. Age-group compar-

isons for the use of mediators in paired-associate learning. *J. Gerontol.* 22:46, 1967.

26. Johnson, C. L., and Catalano, D. J. Childless elderly and their family supports. *Gerontologist* 21:610, 1981.

27. Kagan, J., and Moss, H. A. *Birth to Maturity: A Study in Psychological Development* (2nd ed.). New Haven: Yale University Press, 1983.

28. Kay, D. W. K., and Bergmann, K. Epidemiology of Mental Disorders Amongst the Aged in the Community. In J. E. Birren and R. B. Sloane (Eds.), *Handbook of Mental Health and Aging.* Englewood Cliffs, NJ: Prentice-Hall, 1980.

29. Kramer, M., Taube, C. A., and Redick, R. W. Patterns of Use of Psychiatric Facilities by the Aged: Past, Present, and Future. In C. Eisdorfer and M. P. Lawton (Eds.), *The Psychology of Adult Development and Aging.* Washington, D.C.: American Psychological Association, 1973.

30. Kuhlen, R. G. Personality Change with Age. In P. Worchel and D. E. Byrne (Eds.), *Personality Change.* New York: Wiley, 1964.

31. Levinson, B., and Reese, H. W. Patterns of discrimination learning set in preschool children, fifth-graders, college freshmen, and the aged. *Monogr. Soc. Res. Child Dev.* 32, No. 7, 1967.

32. Lowenthal, M. F., and Haven, G. Interaction and adaptation: Intimacy as a critical variable. *Am. Sociol. Rev.* 33:20, 1968.

33. Maddox, G. L. Persistence of life style among the elderly: A longitudinal study of patterns of social activity in relation to life satisfaction. *Proceedings of the 7th International Congress of Gerontology* 6:309, 1966.

34. Markides, K. S., and Martin, H. W. A causal model of life satisfaction among the elderly. *J. Gerontol.* 34:86, 1979.

35. Mischel, W. *Personality and Assessment.* New York: Wiley, 1968.

36. Neugarten, B. L. *Middle Age and Aging.* Chicago: University of Chicago Press, 1968.

37. Neugarten, B. L. Personality Change in Late Life: A Developmental Perspective. In C. Eisdorfer and M. P. Lawton (Eds.), *The Psychology of Adult Development and Aging.* Washington, D.C.: American Psychological Association, 1973.

38. Neugarten, B. L., Havighurst, R. J., and Tobin, S. S. Personality and Patterns of Aging. In B. L. Neugarten (Ed.), *Middle Age and Aging.* Chicago: University of Chicago Press, 1968.

39. Neugarten, B. L., Moore, J. W., and Lowe, J. C. Age norms, age constraints, and adult socialization. *Am. J. Sociol.* 70:710, 1965.

40. Palmore, E. Facts on aging: A short quiz. *Gerontologist* 17:315, 1977.

41. Palmore, E., et al. Stress and adaptation in later life. *J. Gerontol.* 34:841, 1979.

42. Peck, R. F. Psychological Developments in the Second Half of Life. In B. L. Neugarten (Ed.), *Middle Age and Aging.* Chicago: University of Chicago Press, 1968.

43. Rabbitt, P. Changes in Problem-solving Ability in Old Age. In J. E. Birren et al. (Eds.), *Handbook of the Psychology of Aging.* New York: Van Nostrand, Reinhold, 1977.

44. Reichard, S. K., Livson, F., and Petersen, P. G. *Aging and Personality: A Study of 87 Older Men.* New York: Arno Press, 1962.

45. Schaie, K. W. Age Changes in Adult Intelligence. In D. S. Woodruff and J. E. Birren (Eds.), *Aging: Scientific Perspectives and Social Issues.* Monterey, CA: Brooks/Cole, 1983.

46. Schaie, K. W., and Labouvie-Viel, G. Generational versus ontogenetic components of change in adult cognitive functioning: A fourteen-year cross-sequential study. *Dev. Psychol.* 10:305, 1974.

47. Schaie, K. W., and Strother, C. R. A cross-sequential study of age changes in cognitive behavior. *Psychol. Bull.* 70:671, 1968.

48. Seleen, D. R. The congruence between actual and desired use of time by older adults: A predictor of life satisfaction. *Gerontologist* 22:95, 1982.

49. Seligman, M. E. P. *Helplessness: On Depression, Development, and Death.* San Francisco: Freeman, 1975.

50. Shanas, E., et al. *Old People in Three Industrial Societies.* New York: Atherton, 1980.

51. Siegler, I. C., and Botwinick, J. A long-term longitudinal study of intellectual ability of older adults: The matter of selective subject attrition. *J. Gerontol.* 34:242, 1979.

52. Streib, G. F. Are the Aged a Minority Group? In B. L. Neugarten (Ed.), *Middle Age and Aging.* Chicago: University of Chicago Press, 1968.

53. Sussman, M. B. Relationships of Adult Children with Their Parents in the United States. In E. Shanas and G. F. Streib (Eds.), *Social Structure and the Family: Generational Relations.* Englewood Cliffs, NJ: Prentice-Hall, 1965.

54. Troll, L. E. *Early and Middle Adulthood: The Best is Yet to Be—Maybe.* Monterey, CA: Brooks/Cole, 1975.

55. Turner, J. S., and Helms, D. B. *Contemporary Adulthood* (2nd ed.). New York: Holt, Rinehart, & Winston, 1982.

41
Retirement

Judith Robinson

Everything can be taken away but one thing . . .
to choose one's attitude in any given set of
circumstances.

—Victor Frankl, *Man's Search for Meaning*

Retirement heralds anticipated and unanticipated changes in the life-styles of both men and women. Once a sign that the individual was "too old" to participate in the work force, retirement has increasingly become a phenomenon of the middle years. Although in 1978 the mandatory retirement age was elevated from 65 to 70 years of age, many workers choose to retire early, before poor health or arbitrary employment policies push them out. In 1975 only 22 percent of males and 8 percent of females over 65 years of age remained in the labor force compared to 60 percent in 1920 and 40 percent in 1950 [11, 21]. The decreasing number of older workers in the labor force coupled with the increasing life expectancies of current generations makes it clear that larger numbers of individuals will spend more years in retirement. This makes the transition to retirement a significant force in the structure and function of society as a whole as well as a significant fact of life for its members.

Viewed simplistically, retirement is the separation of the individual from a position of employment. Just as employment means different things to different people, the meaning of retirement varies for each individual. It may signify the end of a successful career or relief from a tedious, boring job; it may bring unlimited time to pursue more pleasurable endeavors, or it may signal the loss of social and economic livelihood. Whatever the meaning of retirement for the individual, it involves separation from a sphere of activity that has provided social order, economic remuneration, and some degree of personal identity and prestige for the greater part of the adult years. For many people, employment is the signifier of adult status and autonomy. Thus, retirement may require some major adjustments—both positive and negative—for the individual.

Traditionally, the emphasis has been placed on the negative aspects of this transition. Retirement frequently has been considered "a crisis situation precipitating personal and social disorganization, familial disruption, organic illness, physical deterioration, mental illness and even death" [23]. The underlying assumption of the degenerative-crisis view is that the work role is of central importance to the individual's self-concept and identity [46, 47]; thus the loss of that role by retirement is seen to cause an identity crisis and a disruption of social relationships. The disorganization created by retirement requires the difficult process of creating new meaning to life and finding a new source of identity.

Despite the prevalence of this point of view, the research conducted over the last two decades has generally failed to confirm that retirement is as disruptive as it has been depicted. Self-esteem has been found to be high in retirement [16], and self-concept differs little between workers and retirees [9]. Moreover, available evidence clearly indicates that most retirees are well-adjusted. Both cross-sectional data, comparing the well-being of older workers and retirees [2, 42, 65], and data from longitudinal studies [24, 48, 66] suggest that most persons make a very adequate adjustment to retirement.

The prevalence of this negative view of retirement, despite the existence of disconfirming data, may be understood better if retirement is viewed from a historical perspective. Prior to the creation of Social Security in 1930, retirement was often forced on older workers as a means of ridding the labor force of older employees to make way for younger persons with better training. Pensions were the exception rather than the rule, and most pensions were inadequate to meet the needs of the retiree [33]. In addition, the strong influence of the work ethic [70] placed a high value on the ability to work and degraded the receipt of a pension for any reason other than disability. In the 1950s, despite changes in retirement policy and provisions for retirement benefits, retirement was still deemed acceptable only in cases of physical impairment [1, 30]. Given these prevalent attitudes and the financial insecurities surrounding retirement in the 1930s (the depression years) and earlier, it is not surprising that retirement had a negative image that persisted for later generations of workers. In this historical context, the crisis view seemed an appropriate model by which to study retirement because it mirrored popular conceptions.

The biases of the people who studied retirement may also account in part for the persistence of the degenerative crisis view. It has been shown that people in professions that require long periods of occupational preparation tend to organize their identity around work and to have less favorable attitudes toward retirement than members of other occupational groups [26]. Based on such findings, it has been suggested that the degenerative crisis view of retirement is to some extent a projection of the researchers' own fears about separation from employment. Again, even though a crisis view may characterize preretirement fears, the current data clearly indicate that these fears do not realistically reflect the positive outcome of the postretirement experience [34, 66].

Over the past decade, the focus of retirement research has shifted away from the degenerative crisis

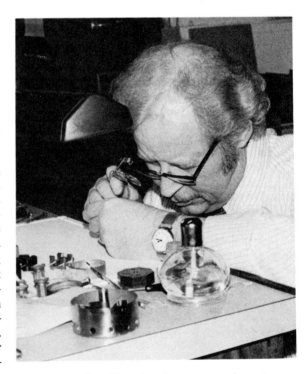

Figure 41–1. The self-employed person may choose to continue a career at his or her own pace as long as health and interest permit and the need for his or her skills exists in the community.

view and toward the factors that facilitate successful adjustment to retirement. The following sections of this chapter focus on the social and psychological aspects of retirement, especially those factors that account for the variability in adjustment to retirement and facilitate a successful transition to later life.

PERSPECTIVES ON RETIREMENT

Despite the common usage of the term, retirement is a complicated concept to define. In general, retirement is considered to be the separation from employment. But there are numerous ways to achieve this separation. Separation from employment may mean changing from a full-time position to a part-time one, or it may mean leaving a career to pursue an avocation. It may occur as the result of ill-health or the inability to acquire another job or suddenly or gradually over an extended period of time. To distinguish retirement from all the other ways in which a person can withdraw from employment, an individual must meet two criteria [5]. First, he or she is no longer employed at a full-time, year-round paying job. Second, his or her income comes at least in part from a retirement pension earned through previous years of employment. These criteria insure that retirement does not apply to persons who draw pensions yet remain fully employed (such as former military personnel) nor to persons who are not employed and do not receive a retirement pension (such as homemakers or those drawing a disability pension). Thus, these defining criteria generally restrict retirement to people at the end of an occupational career.

It is also necessary to understand the differing ways in which the term "retirement" may be used. Retirement has been used concurrently to describe an event, a role, and a process. In actuality, each of these usages is valid; however, the differences in the meaning of retirement lie in the functional aspects of the term.

As an **event**, retirement is the outward sign that the separation from employment has taken place. The retirement event conveniently provides a point for the individual to mark the assumption of the retirement role. Quite neatly, it signifies that the time preceding the event is preretirement and the time after the event is retirement. It is like a rite of passage into later life, much as acquiring employment may be viewed as a rite of passage into adulthood. But unlike rites of passage, retirement is not clearly marked by institutionalized ceremonies. The event may be celebrated with a party, the receipt of special cards and best wishes for

the occasion, or the bestowal of the customary gold watch as a token honor for years of service. The event can just as easily pass without notice as simply the last day of work or the first day of drawing retirement benefits. Little is known about the significance of the retirement event to the individual, but its importance is generally thought to be a part of the larger significance attached to the retirement transition.

Retirement as a **role** refers to the behavioral expectations applied to persons who are defined as "retired." Retirement has been described as a "roleless role," without expectations, rights, or responsibilities to guide behavior. However, Atchley [5] postulates that there are both norms and relationships associated with the retirement role, although more flexible and qualitative than the concrete, instrumental guidelines of the work role. The rights of retired persons include the right to economic support from an earned pension without a negative social stigma, and the right to autonomy in the management of time and other resources. At the same time, retired persons are expected to avoid full-time employment, to carry over skills from previous jobs, and to manage their own lives without becoming dependent on others. Previous relationships also continue into retirement through professional organizations and informal contacts. Overall, the retirement role is more flexible than the strictly defined work role, thereby creating some ambiguities. However, the flexibility allows the individual to continue some relationships while adopting new ones to meet the changing capacities and demands of physical and psychological aging.

Finally, retirement can be described as a **process,** involving the transition from full-time employment to some degree of unemployment. It is difficult to pinpoint the exact beginning of the retirement process. There is always a vague notion of the prospect of retirement and some set of beliefs about leaving the work force; however, the notions and concerns vary over the course of becoming retired. Atchley [5] outlines several phases in the process of retirement that are helpful in conceptualizing the different concerns of the transition. In **preretirement** the consequences of retirement are considered. The consideration is vague at first in the **remote** phase; but in the **near** phase a new attitude toward the work role is assumed in preparation for retirement, and fantasies about life in retirement are entertained. After the retirement event, the retiree enters the **honeymoon** phase in which the preretirement fantasies are lived out, fantasies that range from taking a lavish dream vacation to taking the time to clean all of the closets. The length of this phase depends largely on the resources and imagination of the retiree. Many retirees experience a period of **disenchantment** when resources and imagination are spent and with the realization that the retirement fantasy is finite and the honeymoon is over. Out of this realization, retirees enter a phase of **reorientation** in which a more realistic routine for daily living is established. A **stability** phase follows this reorientation, in which the retiree has well-developed sets of criteria for making decisions and has established a satisfying routine. When illness and disability change the routine established after retiring, retirement ceases to be relevant. At **termination,** it becomes impossible to carry out the retirement role as loss of health and independence curtail activities.

Despite the problems with this particular model [8], it does illustrate that retirement is a transition that requires some forethought about the event and the reorganization of economic, social, and psychological resources. It also emphasizes that retirement is a gradual process that may be accomplished at various rates with varying degrees of success. Later in the chapter, the factors that affect this process will be discussed.

THE DECISION TO RETIRE

The transition from the world of work to life in retirement is a process that requires some preparation. The individual must decide when to retire and, in some cases, whether or not to retire. This process often involves taking stock of the resources available in retirement and coming to terms with subjective feelings about assuming the retirement role. A variety of factors are involved in the formal and informal preparation for retirement. The following sections will address how they shape the process of retiring.

Attitudes toward Retirement

In social psychology, an attitude is defined as an affective evaluation that is determined by a set of beliefs or cognitions about the target object or event [18]. When looking at attitudes toward retirement, the focus is on the individual's subjective evaluation of retirement: whether it is perceived as a positive or a negative transition, freedom from mandatory daily toil, or assignment to "pasture." Although some variation in attitude is noted among occupational groups [32, 42, 66], only a few people actually express dread of retirement [41]. Most workers look forward to the event and increasingly see it as an earned reward for years of service that is taken up with joy. Although retirement is anticipated as a positive transition by most, there are

still some beliefs and situational considerations that may lead the individual to view retirement less favorably.

It is often hypothesized that distance from the retirement event influences the evaluation of separation from employment [5, 41]. The basis for this assertion is the belief that the closer one comes to the event, the less favorably the event is perceived. Presumably, proximity to retirement heightens the awareness of the negative aspects of the transition, such as the reduction in income and the lack of a set routine. Although some persons presume that such a relationship exists [32, 64], there is little longitudinal evidence to suggest that distance from retirement has anything to do with preretirement attitudes [8]. Although the attitude toward retirement may vary over the life course, retirement is not systematically viewed any more or less favorably as the event approaches.

The way one feels about work is also widely assumed to influence feelings about retirement. The orientation toward work may mean several things: It can refer to a sense of commitment to a vocation; to satisfactions received from work, such as a sense of purposeful activity, identity or status; or to general job satisfaction. While it seems logical to assume that a favorable orientation toward work would make it difficult to look forward to separation from that work, the nature of this relationship is unclear. Generally, research in this area has indicated that work orientation alone is unrelated to the evaluation of retirement [31, 52, 65]. Neither commitment to work nor deriving a sense of identity or status from work predicts how the individual feels about retiring. It appears that it is possible to value one's work as well as look forward to separation from that work in retirement. Although this relationship remains difficult to explain, it is possible that the carry-over of preretirement identity and status from work and the increasing preference for leisure time account for the lack of an effect.

The only instance in which work orientation appears to influence preretirement attitudes is when occupational status is taken into consideration. While retirement attitudes are generally favorable, workers in upper-status occupations, especially professionals, executives, and government officials, tend to express more apprehension about retirement [65, 68]. Clearly, a work-centered orientation is associated with upper-occupational strata, where the period of entry is long and job satisfaction and salaries are high. Such upper-level jobs offer not only more economic benefits but also more opportunities for intrinsic satisfactions. It is only for workers at this level that work attitudes have been related to the evaluation of retirement [17, 31].

The relationship between socioeconomic factors and retirement attitudes is obviously complex. While those in upper-status occupations may dread relinquishing the intrinsic rewards of a satisfying job, they are in the best position to enjoy the increased leisure time in retirement because of high levels of income and education. At the other end of the spectrum, the worker in a lower status occupation is more likely to welcome retirement as relief from a dissatisfying job but dread the economic insecurity of living on an inadequate pension. Certainly, the economic problems that plague lower-status workers can tarnish the retirement dream by reducing the number of resources available to make retirement pleasant, let alone to meet daily needs.

Health is also a major influence in retirement attitudes. Although retirement may mean relief from the physical demands of a job, older workers often realize that they may be forced to retire early by physical disability and thereby receive reduced benefits. This prospect of living in retirement produces a sense of despondency and less than favorable evaluations [36, 61].

Even though preretirement attitudes are postulated as playing a big part in the retirement decision, there is little substantive data to support a relationship between attitudes and actual behavior. However, hypothesizing about the influence of attitudes on the retirement decision continues. The subjective evaluation of retirement may not directly affect the decision to exit from the work force, but it can influence the amount of planning for the event and the attention given to information regarding the retirement process. Presently, little is known about the indirect effect of attitudes on the retirement decision.

Preretirement Preparation

Although retirement is nearly a universal phenomenon in our society, there is little in the way of formal preparation for this transition. Most people manage to adjust without formal preparation, even though retirement preparation programs can facilitate positive orientations toward, and coping with, retirement [7]. The actual number of existing preretirement programs is unknown, but they are on the increase. Almost all such programs are offered by government agencies or by companies whose employees have private pensions [5].

Retirement preparation programs can be categorized as either **limited** or **comprehensive.** A limited program provides information about the pension plan,

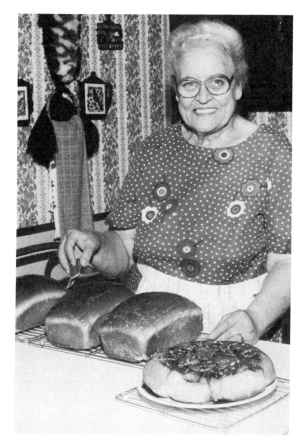

Figure 41–2. Housewives generally experience less change in life-style than persons who work out of the home, since they are able to capitalize on skills gained during earlier years.

Social Security benefits, retirement-timing options, and the level of benefits under the options. The comprehensive program provides financial information as well as discussion of health care planning, leisure-time activities, legal concerns, and housing options. Typically, the limited program involves one or more meetings between the company personnel manager and the prospective retiree. The comprehensive program consists of group meetings in which a variety of techniques are used to provide general information about retirement as well as to teach planning skills. Currently, limited programs outnumber comprehensive programs by two to one [6]. However, it is estimated that newer programs are more comprehensive in the presentation of information [50].

Despite the increased interest and presumed need for retirement preparation programs, only two studies have attempted to assess the information most needed in preretirement [19, 38]. A study of retirees found that preretirement planning for financial and health-related issues was considered to have potential benefits [38]. Similarly, the majority of older employees (70%) identified income inadequacy as a potential concern when asked what type of problems they anticipated at retirement [19]. Other problems that were frequently mentioned included health, lack of meaningful activities, and crime. Although most older employees identified potential problems, more than half (60%) reported having made no plans to deal with such problems: Only 10 percent had definite plans for coping with the difficulties they anticipated during retirement. Seventy percent indicated they would participate in a retirement planning program if one were available.

While it is assumed that preretirement planning in potentially problematic areas, such as health care and income, will decrease the disruptive effects of retirement, there has been little data to confirm the beneficial effects of such programs. In a study comparing the effectiveness of preretirement preparation programs, it was found that only those workers who participated in the comprehensive program had a significant increase in familiarity with retirement issues and reported feelings of preparedness for retirement [25]. Unlike the participants in the limited program and the controls who received no such preparation, these potential retirees made significantly more plans for retirement after their training. This finding was supported by the results of a "before and after" study of a comprehensive program, in which preretirement financial planning was increased by exposure to the training [20].

Although the data are sparse, it appears that preretirement preparation programs have the potential to facilitate planning areas that cause the greatest concern. However, the long-term effects of the training are unknown. In a 6-year follow-up of an earlier study [25], Glamser [27] found no systematic differences in length of adjustment, level of preparation, and adjustment in retirement. However, those retirees who participated in the training reported that it was a useful tool in the preparation for their retirement [20, 25]. Thus the real value of these programs is their positive impact on the informational and emotional support provided during the preretirement phase when anxiety over retirement-related issues is highest.

Unfortunately, those who could benefit most from preretirement planning are the least likely to participate. Atchley [5] points out that most participants have a high level of education, adequate retirement income, and good health. Conversely, the need for retirement planning is greatest among those workers from lower socioeconomic levels; yet these people are least likely to be exposed to preparation programs. The failure of preretirement programs to reach the potential retirees with the greatest need for assistance may in part account for the lack of demonstrated long-term effectiveness.

The Timing of Retirement

There are a variety of ways in which the individual can come to the decision to retire. Although the course to retirement is highly individualistic and is mediated by a combination of factors, there are three basic categories of retirement decisions [53]. First, retirement may occur as the result of a mandatory retirement policy that forces individuals to leave employment at an arbitrary age despite their willingness and ability to work. Second, retirement may be the consequence of ill-health or disability. And finally, retirement may occur as a willing act by those who do not desire to continue to work past the mandatory retirement age or by those who opt to retire even though they were not subject to a mandatory retirement policy. The characteristics of each of these types of retirement decisions will be examined in the following sections.

MANDATORY RETIREMENT

It is widely assumed that large numbers of workers are forced to retire, but mandatory retirement actually affects few older workers. In 1970 only 35 percent of older male workers and 23 percent of older female workers reported a compulsory retirement policy on their most recent job [57]. A longitudinal study of the retirement decision found that even though a mandatory retirement-age policy existed, only 3 percent of workers were forced to retire [53], leading to the speculation that more persons opt for voluntary retirement regardless of an employer's mandatory retirement age [5]. A 1978 congressional amendment to the Age Discrimination in Employment Act abolished mandatory retirement in federal civil service and raised the mandatory age from 65 to 70 for other employees, further reducing the number of people who are affected by induced retirement.

Mandatory retirement applies to a minority of individuals but has never been a popular policy, and the rationale for its existence has been sharply questioned. The rationale for mandatory retirement policy generally focuses on benefits to the employer and includes the following advantages:

1. It is an orderly method of managing employees that is simple and easy to administer.
2. It provides for equitable treatment free of discrimination, bias, or favoritism.
3. It opens channels of promotion for younger workers.
4. It sets an end to the work period that employees can anticipate and plan for [25, 51].

Yet there are numerous sound arguments against mandatory retirement. Foremost is the criticism of the inflexibility of the policy, resulting in the expulsion of valuable labor at an arbitrary age. In addition to the waste of talents and skills, such a policy has been criticized as discriminating against persons in a given age category by depriving them of the ability to generate income.

Within the last decade, attention has begun to shift away from the impact of mandatory retirement toward the factors that contribute to the decision to retire early. It has been suggested that the debate over the mandatory retirement policy has obscured the more significant decline in the minimum age at retirement: Rather than being forced from employment by retirement policy, the majority of retirees are leaving as soon as it is feasible. In fact, as soon as Social Security retirement benefits became available at age 62 rather than age 65, the mean age of retirement quickly went from 65 to 63 years of age [5]. Many individuals opt for early retirement even if it means a reduction in their benefits.

HEALTH-RELATED RETIREMENT

A major factor in the decision to retire early is health. Since physical health is necessary to continue in full-time employment, the loss of health or the onset of disability forces the individual to retire even if the individual desires to stay on the job. Of those persons retiring early under Social Security, most cited health as the reason for their decision [11, 56]. However, the prevalence of health-related retirement declined among those who retired closer to the traditional retirement age [11, 54]. It has been suggested that the prevalence of ill-health as a reason for early retirement may reflect the fact that it is seen as more socially acceptable than simply a desire for retirement [59].

VOLUNTARY EARLY RETIREMENT

While ill-health remains the most frequently cited rationale for early retirement, more and more older workers are selecting retirement for reasons other than health. The second most frequently reported reason for the decision to leave employment before the mandatory age is the availability of an adequate retirement income [11]. Although early retirement may mean some reduction in benefits, most workers retire as soon as it is financially possible. The previously cited decrease in the retirement age with the lowering of the criterion age for receipt of Social Security benefits attests to this trend. The availability of private pensions to supplement the retirement income prior to the receipt of full benefits makes it possible for many workers to retire earlier than is possible under Social Security alone. Even among college professors—an occupational group described as highly work-oriented—early retirement was viewed as acceptable and highly attractive with sufficient incentives and adequate financial arrangements [42]. Conversely, the lack of an adequate pension influences the older worker to remain in the work force despite a desire for retirement. Thus the retirement decision, free from health and policy considerations, is primarily an economic decision for many.

The characteristics of the job itself play some part in the decision to retire. Physically demanding jobs are associated with the accumulation of work-related injuries, and they often place undue stress on the physical energies of older persons. In addition, jobs with lower levels of task quality, such as rigidly mechanized routine work, are tedious and contribute to low job satisfaction. Overall, workers in jobs requiring heavy physical labor and lower skill levels prefer earlier retirement ages [39, 63] as a relief from the demands of their work.

Speculation continues about the role of attitudinal factors in the retirement decision. Several studies have found that retirement attitudes in conjunction with health and income are highly predictive of the timing of retirement [11]. Attitudes of friends and family can also indirectly influence the decision by influencing the worker's beliefs about retirement. Because of their own unfavorable attitudes about retirement, friends and family can point out the negative consequences of leaving employment, or their favorable attitudes may lead them to accentuate the positive aspects. The retirement experiences of friends may also serve as role models for prospective retirees. Some better measurements of retirement attitudes and an enhanced understanding of the relationship between attitudes and behavior may shed new light on the actual nature of the relationship between the subjective evaluation of retirement and the retirement decision.

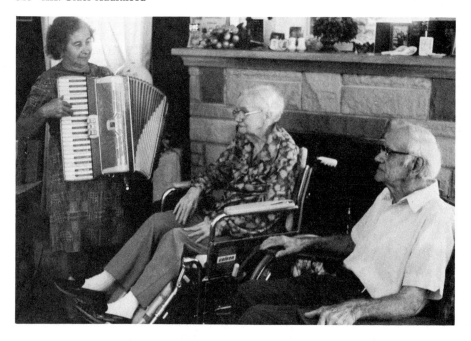

Figure 41–3. This couple, who have maintained their own home, appreciate the visit of other persons. The younger elderly often contribute to the welfare of the older elderly in these non-material ways.

ADJUSTMENT TO RETIREMENT

Despite the fact that retirement does not have negative consequences for the majority of individuals, it is a life change that requires some adjustments. These adjustments include changes in the daily routine, the handling of financial decisions, and often the location of residence. In addition to the adjustments that must be made to the living situation, the retiree faces adjustments in his or her intrapersonal evaluation of retirement life as well as changes in the nature of interpersonal relationships. The following sections will examine how the retiree copes with the transitions that accompany retirement.

Situational Adjustments

FINANCIAL CONSIDERATIONS
It is estimated that the number of older persons living on incomes below the poverty line reached 3.3 million in 1975; that was 15.3 percent of the aged population [12]. The poverty level is an estimate of the amount of income required for mere survival. Near poverty is considered 125 percent of the poverty level. The estimate takes into account the cost of food in different geographical locations, farming versus nonfarming

families, size of family and whether the age of the head of household is under or over age 65. The estimate of poverty levels for those over 65 years of age is based on the assumption that older people need less income because their families have fewer members, and they make fewer expenditures because they have accumulated assets. However, such an estimate does not take into consideration the additional expenses of health care and hospitalization that increase with age.

The income status of older members of racial and ethnic minorities and of older single females tends to be lower than the general population of older persons. Primarily because of previous employment discrimination, minority and female workers tend to have irregular work histories and poor pension coverage that result in lower retirement incomes. Minority females are likely to experience "double jeopardy," that is, having a higher risk of living in poverty than both white females and minority males.

An inadequate income precipitates a number of problems for the elderly. Without money, preventive health maintenance becomes a luxury rather than a necessity. Health care is postponed until problems are critical or necessitate hospitalization. Adequate nutrition suffers as cheaper foods are substituted for the more costly items containing protein, such as meats and dairy products. The necessary repairs on a home are postponed because of the cost involved in labor and materials. Where leisure activities exist, the poor elderly often cannot afford the cost of the activity or the transportation to the event. These problems illustrate just a few of the complications created for the older individual by the lack of sufficient income.

There are several direct and some indirect forms of assistance available in retirement. The primary source of income for most retirees are pensions of which there are several types that provide direct income in retirement. Social Security is a general, public retirement pension administered by the federal government. The program was created in 1935 to provide an old-age pension, and has since seen the addition of survivors' benefits, disability insurance, and Medicare. The program is set up so that employee and employer contributions are paid into the fund and benefits are paid out to the eligible individual during his or her retirement. Retirement benefits are computed on the basis of the average annual income of the 10 years of highest earnings. The recipient of the retirement benefit must have worked at a covered job for a specified minimum period of time and be at least 65 years of age to receive full benefits; those retiring earlier receive reduced benefits. Retirees may earn money in addition to their benefits, but there are restrictions on the amount of money that can be earned without being penalized with a reduction. However, persons 72 years of age or older may earn an unlimited amount without being penalized.

Social Security benefits provide a retired couple with 150 percent of the same pension that would be entitled to the covered single individual. Thus a working woman can draw retirement benefits on the basis of her own eligibility or as a spouse, whichever is greater. If a man is 62 years of age or older and dependent on his wife's income for at least one-half of his support, he can draw benefits on her claim. Survivor benefits are also available to widows, dependent widowers, unmarried children under 18 years of age, and dependent parents over 62 years of age.

Most recent figures indicate that Social Security is the sole source of income for 80 percent of retired Americans [5]. As the sole source of income, Social Security provides for a relatively low-level budget: the average annual Social Security pension in 1985 was $9,312 for married couples and $5,388 for single retirees. Although benefits have increased to meet the cost of living, many individuals receive the minimum benefit. The largest group receiving the minimum is single females; black retirees were also more likely than their white counterparts to receive the minimum benefit.

The factors that contribute to lower benefits for these groups include low earnings, irregular employment, and short periods of employment—the effects of past job discrimination. Unfortunately, these factors also make it unlikely that these retirees will have accumulated other sources of income for retirement.

PRIVATE PENSIONS

A private pension refers to a job-specific pension available only to those in a particular position of employment. Most private pension programs were created after the Social Security program was enacted and were intended to supplement Social Security benefits. Although benefits from private pensions are low and would provide little financial support alone, as an addition to Social Security benefits they can substantially raise the level of retirement income. However, a private-pension program was available to only 31 percent of workers in private industry in 1975 [5].

As with Social Security, eligibility for private pension benefits depends on the years of service. Employees pay into the pension fund and employers regulate the payment of benefits to eligible workers in retirement. In 1974, Congress passed the Employee Retirement Income Security Act (ERISA) in order to protect employees from losing benefits as a result of company closings or bankrupt funds and from being subjected to unreasonable terms of eligibility. This law protects workers from losing their pension rights by federally controlling the vesting and financing of private pension funds. Vesting insures that an employee is guaranteed a share of the fund that he or she has paid into, even if he or she leaves the employer before retiring. The law also creates a Pension Benefit Guarantee Corporation to protect workers when their pension plan folds, and establishes standards for the financing and administration of these plans.

PUBLIC PENSIONS

Another form of job-specific pensions are the public pensions paid to employees of federal, state, and local governments. Unlike private pensions, public pensions may or may not be intended to serve as supplements to Social Security benefits. They often comprise the major portion of retirement income in place of Social Security. In fact, public pensions tend to pay higher benefits than Social Security [5]. About 80 percent of civil servants are covered by public pensions.

OTHER SOURCES OF DIRECT INCOME

Sources of direct income other than pensions include earnings, assets, and cash gifts. Under Social Security,

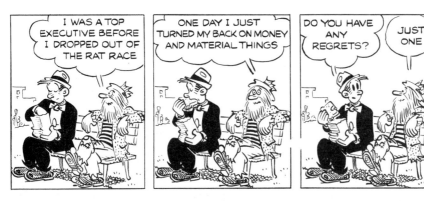

Figure 41–4. *Blondie,* Copyright © 1980. King Features Syndicate, Inc. With permission.

it is possible for a retired individual to earn money up to a certain amount. It is estimated that one-half of those persons employed in old age need the earnings to supplement inadequate pensions [5]. However, it is difficult to estimate how many more would supplement their pension with earnings if they could find employment. Financial assets, such as houses, cars, stocks, bonds, and savings, are also considered a source of income in retirement that provide housing, interest, dividends, and rents. Although one-half of the retired population reports income from assets, the level of income is generally low. Moreover, income from assets tends to be correlated with higher socioeconomic status and adequate pensions. Only a small percent (3%) report income from gifts.

For those older persons with little or no income from pensions, earnings, or assets, the Supplemental Secu-

rity Income Program (SSI) was created in January of 1974. The purpose of this program was to replace Aid for the Aged and two other public assistance programs administered by local welfare departments in order to guarantee a monthly income of a baseline amount to every older American. SSI is federally funded through the Social Security Administration, but is not part of the Social Security Act. The payments are made regardless of work history, so that they cannot be regarded as a pension. The eligibility for the program depends on the amount of assets, which may not exceed a given amount. The payments are made to provide income for those without Social Security and to supplement inadequate benefits. SSI has had a major role in reducing poverty among elderly Americans as well as relieving the stigma associated with receiving welfare.

INDIRECT SOURCES OF INCOME

Aside from the direct sources of income just discussed, retired persons receive economic benefits from indirect sources, such as public housing, food stamps, and Medicare. Such programs are methods for improving the economic status of the elderly without directly providing income. Through nutrition and transportation programs, rent subsidies, and tax exemptions, to name a few, many retirees are able to make their limited incomes go farther.

Perhaps the best example of a source of indirect income for the elderly is the national health insurance amendment to the Social Security Act. This 1965 amendment created two health insurance plans—Medicaid and Medicare—to reduce the staggering cost of health care for older Americans. Medicaid is a comprehensive health care program administered by local welfare departments, using federal funds, that is de-

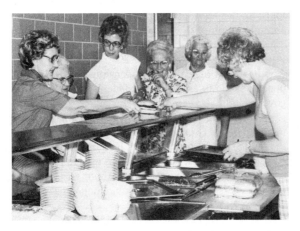

Figure 41–5. Most senior-citizen centers offer a well-balanced hot meal program at minimal cost.

signed to provide medical care to indigent persons of all ages. Medicare is administered by the Social Security Administration and consists of two parts. The hospital insurance is available to Social Security recipients to cover the major portion of hospitalization and extended care. The supplementary medical insurance is available to eligible persons for a small monthly premium: It covers the major portion of doctors' services and outpatient therapy. These programs contribute a significant amount to the income of infirm older Americans.

RESIDENTIAL ADJUSTMENTS

Once an individual fully retires, the workplace no longer ties him or her to a specific locality. Without having to report to work or to meet residential requirements, the retiree is free to live wherever he or she desires and can afford. Despite the fact it is widely believed that retirement spurs significant numbers of people to relocate, only slightly more people over 65 years of age move than those under age 65 [5]. Between 1965 and 1970, only 3.8 percent of the older population moved across state lines: one-half of these were from only five states—New York, Pennsylvania, Ohio, Illinois, and Michigan—and most moved to one state—Florida. Movers were more likely to be widowed, disabled, well-educated, or not living in their own households, but being retired, in and of itself, had little impact on relocation. The most significant effect of retirement is on movement across county lines, and it has the least effect on movement within counties [58]. However, the rate of relocation should not be confused with residential satisfaction [14]. Although older people may wish to change their residence, they are much less likely to realize this wish than younger people [15] primarily because of economic and physical limitations.

Most older Americans continue to live in single-family homes that they own. The preference for independent living in some part reflects the desire to remain self-sufficient and autonomous; however, it is also indicative of the lack of alternatives available to the older person. Many of the homes inhabited by the elderly are older and in need of repair. Seventy percent of these homes were built prior to 1950, and one-half of these were built earlier than 1940 [67]. Although considered an asset, these houses may also become burdens because of their low value relative to newer housing, the rising cost of maintenance necessitated by the age of the structure, and the increments in property taxes. While many older persons may desire to change their living situation, it is not known how many are limited

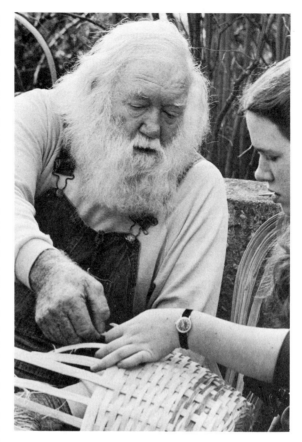

Figure 41–6. The ''new'' and the ''old'' generations frequently find a very special bond when they share a common interest. This gentleman maintains his generative orientation well into his eighties.

to their present arrangements by their inability to financially secure an alternative.

The consequences for the individual's social functioning of remaining in a single-family home are mixed. On the one hand, remaining in one's own home may facilitate a sense of continuity between preretirement and retirement life. Acquaintances in the neighborhood are maintained, and familiarity with the community and the pace of life make it easier to become involved in local affairs. In addition, the individual does not have to seek new physicians, new barbers, new pharmacists, or new stores. On the other hand, staying in a single-family community may have deleterious effects. Without adequate funds or transportation, the older individual can easily become isolated in his or her home. The activities and services provided, especially for senior citizens, may be too far away or may be too troublesome to reach. Even the familiar neighborhood can change around the older homeowner as many urban centers have, leaving the aging person with lower property values and higher crime rates. Other retirees find that residence in a private home area provides continuing contact with persons of all age groups—a factor that helps to keep them in the mainstream of life.

An alternative form of housing that is appealing and affordable for many older people is age-segregated multifamily housing. Multifamily housing refers to apartments, townhouses, or condominiums that are designed for older residents. This form of housing allows independent living while bringing the individual closer to group activities and services and enhances the sense of security that comes from group living. This type of housing has increased considerably over the past decade both under the federally assisted housing programs and in relatively affluent retirement communities that are privately owned. While moving to this new setting does mean leaving behind a familiar home and neighborhood, most movers report the favorable effects of improved housing on their social and psychological well-being [13], especially those moving from substandard housing. Some persons regret the lack of contact with other age groups, especially children.

A small percent of those over 65 years of age (4 to 6 percent) live in group housing. Group housing can be classified as either institutional or noninstitutional, depending on the degree of independence afforded the resident. In congregate housing, such as retirement hotels, the individual has a self-contained residence; thus he or she may remain independent from the rest of the community. Household help and nursing care are usually available but not as regular services. In personal care homes, such as retirement homes, the living unit is not self-contained nor self-sufficient. Partial care is available in terms of help with grooming, housekeeping, and meals; nursing care is provided when needed. These forms of group housing are considered noninstitutional. Institutionalized housing generally refers to nursing homes in which the resident is fully dependent on the staff for grooming, meals, and total health care.

In recent years, a new form of housing has evolved that provides several levels of living in one group setting. These retirement communities offer a continuum of care, from independent living in a single family unit to full nursing care. The aim of these facilities is to provide one location in which the retired person can settle, and as physical abilities decline and more ser-vices are needed, the individual can receive a higher level of care. The emphasis is on encouraging independence as long as possible and changing arrangements only as needed, thereby minimizing the traumatic effects of being transferred to another facility [28].

Changes in Health

Retirement is widely assumed to have an adverse effect on health. However, such assumptions neglect to consider that failing health and disability are often the impetus to retire rather than the consequences. When the health of willing retirers is compared to that of workers of the same age, no differences are found [61, 66]. In fact, retirement has been associated with improvements in health [66]. Although the incidence of health problems and disability increases with age, retirement does not directly affect physical well-being.

Conversely, health does have a significant impact on retirement. Poor health restricts the range of activities in which the retiree can participate and places a burden on finances. Health plays an important part in determining the resources available to the retiree in coping with the retirement transition. A lack of physical well-being can substantially drain the energies that could be devoted to pleasurable activities, and it often isolates the individual by making it difficult to fulfill the retirement role. In addition to the social and economic ramifications, poor health can have deleterious effects on psychological well-being in retirement by increasing feelings of dependency and uselessness and clouding the prospect of living a full life.

Affective Adjustment

The emotional reaction to retirement has most often been assessed by looking at morale and life satisfaction. Overall, studies of the affective response to retirement have found no relationship between separation from employment and morale [24, 65], life satisfaction [66], self-esteem [16], or identity [48]. Perhaps one-third of those who retire have difficulty in adjusting to retirement [3, 34, 62], but research shows rather convincingly that other factors, such as health, income, and activity level, have much more influence on well-being than does leaving the workforce per se [65].

Although the level of adjustment remains high in retirement, there is a slight decline in self-ratings of involvement. One research study [9] examined three dimensions of self-concept: involvement, optimism, and autonomy. While self-ratings of optimism and autonomy remained high, retirees scored lower than

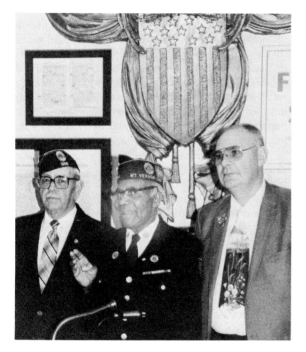

Figure 41-7. Elderly persons are frequently recognized publicly for their life-long contributions to the welfare of the community.

older workers on the measure of involvement. Other studies [66] also report a small decline in feelings of usefulness. Apparently, self-ratings of instrumentality are related to retirement; however, more global ratings of identity indicate continuity with preretirement ratings.

Several social-status and situational variables account for individual differences in the response to retirement. In addition to health, economic status is a major influence in the affective response to retirement. Much of the reported lower levels of satisfaction in retirement are attributable to lower levels of income [22]. Just as poor health restricts mobility, inadequate income limits the type of activities available to make retirement enjoyable; but more significantly, a limited income jeopardizes the ability to meet the needs of daily living and increases the worry associated with insufficient resources.

Not only does the adequacy of income influence the ability to cope with the retirement transition but, generally, socioeconomic status affects the way in which the individual responds to retirement. Socioeconomic status includes income level as well as educational and occupational statuses. Retirees in upper statuses are

less likely to experience difficulty in adjusting to retirement [36, 66], owing largely to better levels of health and income. Upper-status workers may experience less difficulty and are more satisfied because they have greater role flexibility [45]. However, it must also be noted that upper-status workers have more orderly work histories, more satisfying jobs, more opportunities to express themselves through work and leisure, and higher levels of involvement in society than lower-status workers.

While health and socioeconomic status are critical variables in retirement adjustment, part of their impact occurs indirectly through their influence on the level of activity in retirement. The relationship between activity level, health, age, and income adequacy is complex. Most research indicates that higher levels of activity are associated with better adjustment in later life [2, 48]. Maintaining a satisfying level of activity lessens feelings of social isolation and uselessness while providing a routine for living. There is no certain level of activity that insures adjustment: what matters is that the retiree is satisfied with the amount of activity.

Very little detailed information is available concerning the effect of social support systems on retirement adjustment. One study [24] reports a significant relationship between marital status and retirement adjustment for males. A satisfying marital relationship can improve the response to retirement in that a spouse can provide emotional support and serve as a resource for ideas about the use of time. Little is known about the support provided by other family members and peers. However, it is speculated that the activities involved in maintaining family ties can provide a sense of involvement and satisfy expressive needs for the retiree. The grandparent role, because it is contiguous with retirement, is considered an especially pleasurable substitute for the activities associated with work.

Most of the research on retirement adjustment has focused exclusively on male retirees. However, (despite prior assumptions about women's lack of commitment to employment outside the home), the available evidence suggests that women are just as work-oriented as men [60], have less positive attitudes toward retirement, and exhibit poorer adjustment and longer adjustment periods [2, 16, 66], particularly if divorced or widowed [22, 40]. The effect of gender on retirement may primarily be a function of its interaction with other variables, such as marital status and income. For example, women are more likely to have irregular work histories, and substantially lower incomes, and they often enter and leave the work force for different reasons than do men. In addition, women are more likely to experience widowhood and economic hardship in conjunction with retirement. Further research in this area will shed more light on gender differences in work experience and the process of retiring.

Social Adjustment

CHANGES IN THE MARITAL RELATIONSHIP
The social adjustments to retirement involve negotiations in relationships with other people and changes in the way the individual relates to the world. Perhaps the most important adjustment occurs within the marital dyad. Most retired people are married and living with their spouse.

Since women have generally carried the role of homemaker in addition to volunteer work or employment responsibilities, on retirement they simply spend more time on household chores. They slow down the work pace and "catch up" on all those little jobs they never had time to get around to. For husbands, the increased leisure time of retirement can create problems. Some wives dread the intrusion and complain about their spouse's interference in their daily household routine [43]. With increased numbers of working wives and more equalization of household duties between spouses, this problem may occur less often in the future. Many couples experience a new level of companionship in the sharing of household activities. Renegotiation and reallocation of household and home responsibilities require reassessment of past gender-roles coupled with patience and humor while each assumes and learns new skills.

The couple's adjustment to retirement is largely influenced by their socioeconomic status. A widely cited study [43] found that the increased involvement of the husband in household activities was viewed differently by couples of differing socioeconomic levels. In upper- and middle-level couples, where activities are often shared by husband and wife, the increase was seen as desirable by both spouses. In lower economic levels, where activities are more often relegated to separate spheres for men and women, the wife is more likely to resent the invasion of the husband into her exclusive domain.

In addition, the couple's focus on expressive, nurturant roles versus instrumental, functional roles is important. The middle- and upper-class couple is more likely to have a relationship based on expressivity and understanding, so that the loss of the instrumental role with retirement is not a major destructive force to the marital relationship. But the lower-class couple who generally base the relationship on a traditional gender division of instrumental/expressive roles, may find it difficult to adjust to the loss of the instrumental role [44, 69]. Generally, retirement can provide the time to relish and revitalize a mutually satisfying relationship, but it can also place strain on marriages that were unhappy prior to the event [37]. Flexibility is a cardinal feature of a successful adjustment.

CHANGES IN PEER RELATIONSHIPS
Little is known about the changes that retirement brings to peer relationships. Obviously, retirement necessitates some alteration of the formal relationships associated with the work place. Yet it is the informal relationships that provide the most support for the individual, and these need not be renegotiated with retirement because they are often unrelated to the workplace. In fact, retirement allows more time to spend with friends [16]. The positive experiences of retired friends may even influence the retirement decision and aid in the planning for life as a retiree.

USE OF LEISURE TIME
Perhaps the most dramatic impact of retirement is the sudden increase in leisure time. Because people are retiring earlier and living longer, the problem facing many individuals is how to make leisure time meaningful and satisfying. There are three basic functions of leisure activities in retirement [29]. First, leisure-time activities tend to replace the focus on work-related instrumental activities with more informal forms of expressiveness, such as acceptance and empathy (e.g., the process, or the relationship tends to take precedence over the product). Second, leisure-time activities provide the opportunity to develop one's creative potentials (a factor that can combat depression). And finally, leisure activities structure the abundance of free time by setting a routine. If the individual has the physical and economic resources to pursue desired activities, retirement can be a very rewarding and integrated phase of life.

Leisure activities in retirement range from those engaged in for pure diversion or self-expression to those that are educational or lend a helping hand. Despite the physical limitations of aging, the pattern of activities an individual pursues remains rather constant over the course of a life [49, 71], with socioeconomic status determining the type of preferred activities [35]. Those of the upper and middle socioeconomic levels tend to prefer volunteer work, travel, reading, and gardening; those of the lower socioeconomic levels tend to prefer visiting with family and relatives. These patterns are established early in life and continue to be prevalent in retirement.

Cross-sectional studies have found a few differences in the leisure pursuits of older and younger people. These studies suggest that older individuals are more interested in current events [58] but unlike younger persons are less likely to participate in outdoor activities, or to attend sporting events, movies, plays, concerts, or dances [29, 34]. Travel is a more frequent activity of the aged than might be expected given the economic strain of retirement; but older people still travel less often than other age groups [29]. It is not clear exactly which factors contribute to the differences in activities. Of course, the physical and economic limitations of many retirees prohibit participation in a number of activities, such as vigorous sports, travel, or dining out regularly. Restricted mobility from either a physical disability or simply a lack of transportation also makes it difficult to pursue activities outside the home, such as attending social gatherings, shopping, or visiting. In addition, the increasing introspection noted with age may result in a preference for activities that can be enjoyed in solitude.

While the type of activities remains somewhat the same in retirement, the time spent in these activities does increase. The nature of this change appears to be highly individualistic. Some people welcome retirement as the chance to reduce the level of activity just as the disengagement theory predicts (see Chap. 40); others try to fill the void of retirement with new activities, following the pattern predicted by the activity theory. However, the majority of retirees appears to continue its preretirement levels of activity, increasing slightly its participation in usual activities. Atchley [4, 5] suggests that the time formerly occupied by full-time employment often becomes filled with meeting the obligations of daily living more fully than before. Thus, balancing the checkbook, shopping, puttering around the house, and corresponding with friends are more thoroughly attended to than they were prior to retirement.

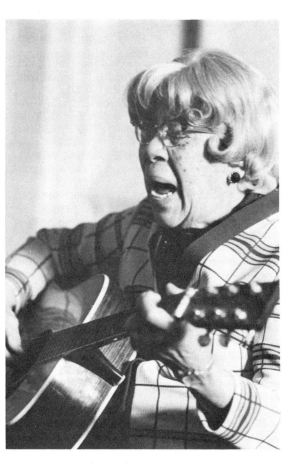

Figure 41–8. Elderly persons can be treasured resources of cultural tradition and healthy models for graceful aging.

CONCLUSION

The ultimate goal of the study of the retirement transition is an understanding of the process, so that the experience of retirement can be made as effective, functional, or rewarding as possible. As more and more people reach the age of retirement and the older population swells, this goal becomes particularly important. While steps are presently being taken to reduce the most problematic aspects of life in retirement and to enhance the advantages, continuous consideration must be given to the implications of retirement for the individual and society: As the aging population changes in size and character, we must come up with new ways to enhance the retirement experience.

In general, retirement is, and should continue to be, a pleasurable experience. Most people accommodate to changes in finances and in use of time; they relish the time to pursue nonwork activities, to take on more expressive roles within the family, to be introspective, and to integrate past experiences. For the most part, this is a transitional crisis from which a new identity and new roles emerge. While poor health and inadequate income are real problems for some persons, the majority of retirees have sufficient resources to enjoy their retirement.

The question is how the retirement experience can be made better. Although it is a pleasant time of life for most, there is some anxiety associated with the preparation for retirement that could be alleviated by preretirement planning. While the number of preretirement preparation programs is on the rise, education about retirement remains sadly lacking for the majority of prospective retirees. These programs reach only a small and elite percentage of workers, and they provide information only shortly preceding the retirement event. To dramatically enhance the long-term effectiveness of such programs, their exposure must increase among lower and lower-middle level workers who are in the greatest need of financial planning. Only then can the effect of preparation be seen on the use of fixed resources. In addition, the extension of preparation across the work-life via a continuous program of education would optimize the effect. By providing information programs about retirement for workers during their years of employment, misinformation and stereotypes about retirement could be dispelled and workers would be encouraged to make long-range financial plans and to establish enjoyable patterns of leisure that would facilitate the adjustment to retirement.

Retirement can also be optimized for the benefit of the individual and of society by a better utilization of the skills of the retired population. Programs exist already that use the know-how and experience of retirees to train and encourage younger people. Such programs not only provide purposeful activity for the older individual but insure that their skills are not wasted. With the increasing size of the population of those more than 60 years of age and the decrease in the number of younger workers, older adults may become a resource that society cannot afford to ignore.

As for the future of retirement, it is difficult to make predictions. Although it is a certainty that larger numbers of people are approaching and living well beyond retirement age, it is not clear how economic changes will influence the average age of retirement; it is currently decreasing, but economic hardship and lack of resources may entice more people to opt for later retirement. The declining number of younger workers may also result in employers encouraging a later retirement. In addition, as the period of technical training lengthens and entry into the job market is postponed, future generations of workers may have to remain in the labor force in order to accumulate the required number of years of service to be eligible for an adequate pension. The increasing levels of educa-tion and physical health will also change the character of the retirement population in that future retirees will have an interest in, and the aptitude for, different leisure pursuits and a different attitude toward work and retirement. While the future may bring unforeseen difficulties for retirement living, the prospect of larger numbers of healthier and better educated retired individuals suggests that retirement may be seen as a more desirable and purposeful phase of adulthood by generations to come.

REFERENCES

1. Ash, P. Preretirement counseling. *Geront.* 6:97, 1966.
2. Atchley, R. C. Retirement and work orientation. *Geront.* 11:29, 1971.
3. Atchley, R. C. Adjustment to loss of job at retirement. *Intl. J. Aging and Hum. Dev.* 6:97, 1975.
4. Atchley, R. C. *The Sociology of Retirement.* Cambridge, MA: Schenkman, 1976.
5. Atchley, R. C. *The Social Forces in Later Life* (3rd ed.). Belmont, CA: Wadsworth, 1980.
6. Atchley, R. C. What Happened to Retirement Planning in the 1970s? In N. McCluskey and E. F. Borgatta (Eds.), *Aging and Retirement.* Beverly Hills, CA: Sage, 1981.
7. Atchley, R. C., Kunkel, S. R., and Adlon, C. *An Evaluation of Preretirement Programs: Results from an Experimental Study.* Oxford, OH: Scripps Foundation Gerontology Center, 1978.
8. Atchley, R. C., and Robinson, J. L. Attitudes toward retirement and distance from the event. *Res. on Aging* 4:299, 1982.
9. Back, K. W., and Guptill, C. S. Retirement and Self-ratings. In I. H. Simpson and J. C. McKinney (Eds.), *Social Aspects of Aging.* Durham, NC: Duke University Press, 1966.
10. Bixby, L. Income of people aged 65 and over: An overview from the 1968 survey of the aged. *Social Security Bull.* 33:3, 1970.
11. Bixby, L. Retirement patterns in the United States: Research and policy interaction. *Social Security Bull.* 39:3, 1976.
12. Brotman, H. Income and poverty in the older population in 1975. *Geront.* 17:22, 1977.
13. Carp, F. M. Short-term and long-term prediction of adjustment to a new environment. *J. Geront.* 29:444, 1974.
14. Carp, F. M. Housing and Living Environments of Older People. In R. H. Binstock and E. Shanas (Eds.), *Handbook of Aging and the Social Sciences.* New York: Van Nostrand, Reinhold, 1976.
15. Clark, M. Patterns of aging among the elderly poor of the inner city. *Geront.* 11:58, 1971.
16. Cottrell, W. F., and Atchley, R. C. *Women in Retirement.* Oxford, OH: Scripps Foundation Gerontology Center, 1969.

17. Fillenbaum, G. G.   On the relationship between attitude to work and attitude to retirement. *J. Geront.* 32:196, 1977.

18. Fishbein, M.   Attitude and the Prediction of Behavior. In M. Fishbein (Ed.), *Readings in Attitude Theory and Measurement*. New York: Wiley, 1967.

19. Fitzpatrick, E. W.   An industry consortium approach to retirement planning—A new program. *Aging and Work* 1:181, 1978.

20. Fitzpatrick, E. W.   Evaluating a new retirement planning program: Results with hourly workers. *Aging and Work* 2:87, 1979.

21. Foner, A., and Schwab, S.   *Aging and Retirement*. Monterey, CA: Brooks/Cole, 1981.

22. Fox, J. H.   Effects of retirement and former work life on women's adaptation in old age. *J. Geront.* 32:196, 1977.

23. Friedmann, E. A., and Orbach, H. L.   Adjustment to Retirement. In S. Arieti (Ed.), *American Handbook of Psychiatry*, Vol. I: *The Foundation of Psychiatry*. New York: Basic Books, 1974.

24. George, L. K., and Maddox, G. L.   Subjective adaptation to loss of the work role: A longitudinal study. *J. Geront.* 32:456, 1977.

25. Glamser, F., and DeJong, G.   The efficacy of preretirement preparation programs for industrial workers. *J. Geront.* 30:595, 1975.

26. Glamser, F.   Determinants of a positive attitude toward retirement. *J. Geront.* 31:104, 1976.

27. Glamser, F.   The impact of preretirement programs on the retirement experience. *J. Geront.* 36:244, 1981.

28. Golant, S.   Residential concentrates of future elderly. *Geront.* 15:16, 1975.

29. Gordon, C., Gaitz, C. M., and Scott, J.   Leisure and Lives: Personal Expressivity Across the Life Span. In R. H. Binstock and E. Shanas (Eds.), *Handbook of Aging and the Social Sciences*. New York: Van Nostrand Reinhold, 1976.

30. Gordon, M. S.   Work and Patterns of Retirement. In R. W. Kleemeier (Ed.), *Aging and Leisure*. New York: Oxford University Press, 1961.

31. Goudy, W. J., Powers, E. A., and Keith, P.   Work and retirement: A test of attitudinal relationships. *J. Geront.* 30:193, 1975.

32. Goudy, W. J., et al.   Changes in attitudes toward retirement: Evidence from a panel study of older males. *J. Geront.* 35:942, 1980.

33. Graebner, W.   *A History of Retirement*. New Haven, CT: Yale University Press, 1980.

34. Harris, L.   *The Myth and Reality of Aging in America*. Washingon, DC: National Council on Aging, 1975.

35. Havighurst, R. J.   Social Roles, Work, Leisure, and Education. In C. Eisdorfer and M. P. Lawton (Eds.), *The Psychology of Adult Development and Aging*. Washington, DC: American Psychological Association, 1973.

36. Heidbreder, E. M.   Factors in retirement adjustment: White collar/blue collar experience. *Indust. Geront.* 12:69, 1972.

37. Heyman, D. K., and Jeffers, F. C.   Wives and retirement: A pilot study. *J. Geront.* 23:488, 1968.

38. Holley, H. A., and Field, J. H.   Design of a retirement preparation program: A case history. *Personnel J.* 53:527, 1974. *Geront.* 1:49, 1974.

39. Jacobsohn, D.   Willingness to retire in relation to job strain and type of work. *J. Indust. Geront.* 13:65, 1972.

40. Jaslow, P.   Employment, retirement, and morale among elderly women. *J. Geront.* 31:212, 1976.

41. Keatona, G.   *Private Pension and Individual Savings*, Monogram No. 40. Ann Arbor, MI: University of Michigan, Institute for Social Research, 1965.

42. Kell, D., and Patton, C. V.   Reaction to induced early retirement. *Geront.* 18:173, 1978.

43. Kerckhoff, A. C.   Husband–wife Expectations and Reactions to Retirement. In I. H. Simpson and J. C. McKinney (Eds.), *Social Aspects of Aging*. Durham, NC: Duke University Press, 1966.

44. Lipman, A.   Role Conceptions of Couples in Retirement. In C. Tibbitts and W. Donahue (Eds.), *Social and Psychological Aspects of Aging*. New York: Columbia University Press, 1962.

45. Loether, H. J.   The Meaning of Work and Adjustment to Retirement. In A. B. Shostak and W. Gomberg (Eds.), *Blue Collar World*. Englewood Cliffs, NJ: Prentice-Hall, 1964.

46. Maddox, G. L.   Retirement as a Social Event. In J. S. McKinney and F. T. de VyVer (Eds.), *Aging and Social Policy*. New York: Appleton-Century-Croft, 1966.

47. Miller, S. J.   The Social Dilemma of the Aging Leisure Participant. In A. M. Rose and W. A. Peterson (Eds.), *Older People and Their Social World*. Philadelphia: Davis, 1966.

48. Mutran, E., and Reitzes, D. C.   Retirement, identity and well-being: Realignment of role relationships. *J. Geront.* 36:733, 1981.

49. Oliver, D. B.   Career and leisure patterns of middle-age metropolitan out-migrants. *Geront.* 11:13, 1971.

50. Olson, S. K.   Current status of corporate retirement preparation programs. *Aging and Work* 4:175, 1981.

51. Palmore, E.   Compulsory versus flexible retirement: Issues and facts. *Geront.* 12:343, 1972.

52. Parnes, H. S., et al.   *Manpower Administration*. Manpower Research Monogram No. 15, U.S. Department of Labor, Washington, DC: 1970.

53. Parnes, H. S., and Nestel, G.   The Retirement Experience. In H. S. Parnes (Ed.), *Work and Retirement: A Longitudinal Study of Men*. Cambridge, MA: MIT Press, 1981.

54. Pollman, A. W.   Early retirement: A comparison of poor health to other retirement factors. *J. Geront.* 26:41, 1971.

55. Reibel, E.   Retirement. In C. S. Schuster and S. S. Ashburn (Eds.), *The Process of Human Development: A Holistic Approach*. Boston: Little, Brown, 1980.

56. Reno, V. P.   Why men stop working at or before age 65. *Social Security Bull.* 34:3, 1971.

57. Reno, V. P.   Compulsory retirement among newly entitled workers: Survey of new beneficiaries. *Social Security Bull.* 35:3, 1972.

58. Riley, M. W., and Foner, A. *Aging and Society,* Vol. I: *An Inventory of Research Findings.* New York: Russell Sage Foundation, 1968.

59. Schulz, J. H. The economic impact of an aging population. *Geront.* 13:111, 1973.

60. Seltzer, M. M., and Atchley, R. C. The impact of structural integration into the profession on work commitment, potential for disengagement, and leisure preferences among social workers. *Sociolog. Focus* 5:9, 1971.

61. Shanas, E. Health and adjustment in retirement. *Geront.* 10:19, 1970.

62. Shanas, E., et al. *Older People in Three Industrial Societies.* New York: Atherton Press, 1968.

63. Sheppard, H. L. *Where Have All the Robots Gone?—Work Dissatisfaction in the 1970s.* New York: Free Press-Macmillan, 1972.

64. Sheppard, H. L. Work and Retirement. In R. H. Binstock and E. Shanas (Eds.), *Handbook of Aging and the Social Sciences.* New York: Van Nostrand Reinhold, 1976.

65. Simpson, I. H., Back, K. W., and McKinney, J. C. Orientation Toward Work and Retirement, and Self-evaluation in Retirement. In I. H. Simpson and J. C. McKinney (Eds.), *Social Aspects of Aging.* Durham, NC: Duke University Press, 1966.

66. Streib, G. F., and Schneider, C. J. *Retirement in American Society.* Ithaca, NY: Cornell University Press, 1971.

67. Struyk, R. The housing situation of elderly Americans. *Geront.* 17:130, 1977.

68. Thompson, W. E. Preretirement anticipation and adjustment in retirement. *J. Social Issues,* 14:34, 1958.

69. Troll, L. E. The family of later life: A decade review. *J. Mar. Fam.* 33:263, 1971.

70. Weber, M. *The Protestant Ethic and the Spirit of Capitalism.* New York: Scribner's, 1958.

71. Zborowski, M. Aging recreation. *J. Geront.* 17:302, 1962.

XIII
Epilogue

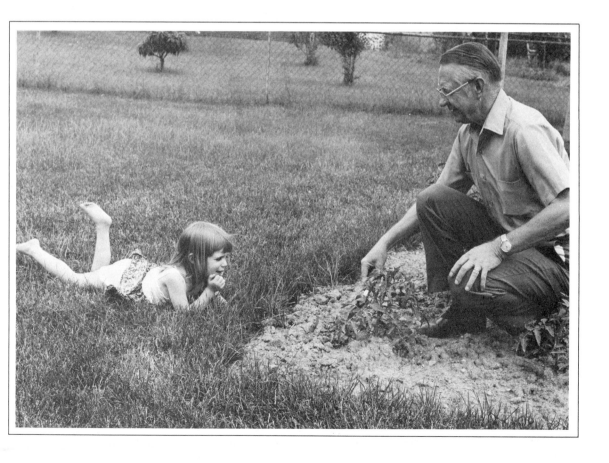

42

To Live—Not Somehow, but Triumphantly!*

Clara S. Schuster

It was the best of times, it was the worst of times, it was the age of wisdom, it was the age of foolishness, it was the epoch of belief, it was the epoch of incredulity, it was the season of Light, it was the season of Darkness, it was the spring of hope, it was the winter of despair, we had everything before us, we had nothing before us.

. . .

—Charles Dickens, *A Tale of Two Cities*

In 1970 Alvin Toffler startled the world with his provocative treatise on the relationship between technology and the quality of life. In his book, *Future Shock* [43], he observed that as technological knowledge increases, the entire pace of life is accelerated. Individuals experience changes in employment and thus in their places of residence and have to learn to adapt to new places, people, and things. Relationships become more transient, and the individual is forced to cope with an increasing number of novel experiences in a shorter period of time. Toffler expressed concern that

As change accelerates in society, it forces a parallel acceleration within us. New information reaches us and we are forced to revise our image-file continuously at a faster and faster rate. Older images based on past reality must be replaced, for, unless we update them, our actions become divorced from reality and we become progressively less competent. We find it impossible to cope [44].

In order to cope successfully with this rapid change, commitments to others and involvement in the life of the community may be decreased, which threatens the very core of interpersonal and intrapersonal relationships. The patterns of response and the skills learned in earlier years may become outdated; they may no

*Bertha Munro

longer be adequate to meet the demands of daily living. Our very survival may be threatened!

In primitive, nomadic, and agrarian cultures, cultural change was slow. Children were able to use their parents as models for desirable and adaptive behaviors. Entire cultures and their mores were transmitted intact to generation after generation [44]. The family was the core unit of society, and cooperation was essential to survival. With the industrial revolution, changes in technology created radical changes in types of employment, community size, educational needs, and family structure. The large, extended family, which thrived in a permanent location with all of its members involved in some way in family concerns, gave way to the smaller, mobile nuclear family that was free to move easily to various places of employment [44].

Today western cultures are immersed in another cultural revolution [50]. Practitioners and lay persons alike face the startling reality that the present world is vastly different from the world in which they were reared, and it promises even more changes in the future. We are on the crest of what Toffler terms "the third wave" of major cultural change [44]. Computers have not only reduced our work load, but in some situations, have made human efforts obsolete. Our culture and the in-

dividuals within it are threatened by the very technology we have created [1]. To question our ability to survive might seem to the reader to disregard the obvious lessons of history. We seem not only to have survived, but to have transcended what were earlier regarded as the fixed limits of our world. It would appear then that our adaptive capabilities are infinite. However, we are concerned with more than just physical survival, more than the provision of safety, more than the protection of the physical self. Professional persons and political leaders must also address psychological and spiritual survival—in short, the **quality** of life. Can we continue to cope with the rapid pace of change and to maintain high level wellness as societies, as families, and as individuals?

Although it is recognized that not everyone is caught up in the technological revolution, we are all, nevertheless, influenced by various technological advances, such as new modes of travel, new forms of entertainment, new banking systems, and new communication systems. The educational programs implemented in our schools and the health care services provided for our citizens influence the quality and philosophy of daily life as well as our future. These social changes precipitate concurrent changes in personal areas, such

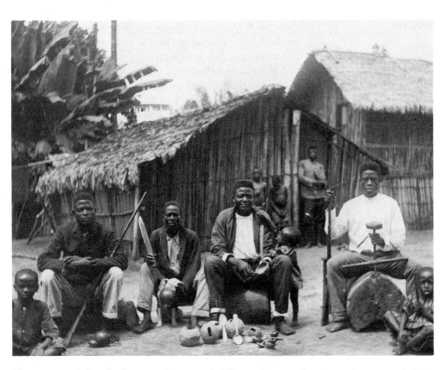

Figure 42–1. Cultural values, traditions, and skills can be passed on intact in more primitive cultures.

as hair and clothing styles, language usage, interpersonal relationships, leisure-time activities, and moral codes.

Change is especially stressful when certain conditions exist: (1) when the pace of change is accelerating so rapidly that an individual is exposed to two or even more major cultures, or critical suprasystems, within a life span; (2) when there is inadequate preparation in the skills needed to adapt to the new requirements; (3) when there are inadequate or insufficient models with whom to identify who exhibit the critical personal skills necessary for adapting to change; or (4) when change results in conflict with, or widespread questioning or rejection of, commonly accepted beliefs and values.

From the first days of life, we attempt to organize incoming information into meaningful units or schemata that can be retrieved and used to predict or to control the outcome of events. This organizational skill becomes even more critical as more information comes to us and as events require rational decisions on our part. Information overload, in the form of too many novel experiences, taxes our ability to process the information, to organize it, and to make effective, rational decisions [43]. The existence of only one or two of the above conditions is sufficient to jeopardize effective coping; the presence of all of them creates an overwhelming sense of overload and may threaten one's ability to survive—socially, affectively, cognitively, and even in some few cases, physically.

A number of eloquent voices from within the social and life sciences have expressed uneasiness about the individual's ability to live holistically in today's world [29, 31, 35, 44]. People obviously do not possess an endless plastic ability to adapt to life change [40]. It is important, therefore, that we have a better understanding of the specific nature of these threats to our survival in order to learn how to work with the environment [31, 32] and with the new technologies [44] to create new, more vibrant and meaningful life-styles. The question becomes: What have we learned from the past that can help us in the present to prepare for the future?

THREATS TO SURVIVAL: A PERSPECTIVE ON CONTEMPORARY STRESSORS

The very nature of a technological society breeds a threat to well-established coping responses. Technology requires change as a condition for improvement. It follows then that if society is becoming increasingly

dependent on technological improvement, significant and frequent change will be the inevitable result. With the current rate of technological advance and its impact on life-style, we are forced to consider and to develop strategies for maintaining psychosocial and cognitive equilibrium. We must balance our responsibilities and needs against our skills and assets in order to cope with what appears to be the advent of perpetual change.

Increased system stress is an inevitable response to perpetual change. Stress arises from three sources: pressure, frustration, and conflict. Pressure stems from both internal feelings and external circumstances when there is a demand to speed up or intensify efforts. Frustration occurs when the ability to achieve a desired goal is impeded or blocked. Conflict occurs not from a single obstacle, but when a choice must be made between two or more goals. All three types of stress are closely interrelated and are usually combined to form the total stress pattern of a person's life.

Stress can occur on physiological or psychological levels. It is often difficult, however, to make a clear-cut distinction between the two, since they interact and the human organism generally responds as a total unit. The severity of stress refers to the degree of disruption to the person-as-a-system and is determined primarily by the importance, duration, frequency, multiplicity, and complexity of the demands on the individual. The longer a stressor operates, the more severe it is likely to become. This is not to indicate that the stressor per

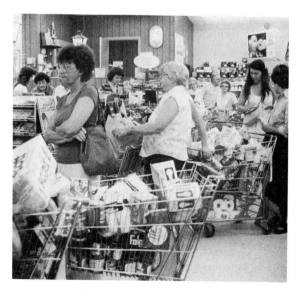

Figure 42-2. A hallmark of today's society: Hurry up and wait.

se intensifies but, rather, the person's ability to cope with the stressor often begins to weaken, causing an increase in the amount of stress felt by the individual. Similarly, a number of stressors that are operating at the same time or in a rapid sequence are cumulatively more decompensating than if these events had occurred separately or over a longer period of time. Severe or multiple stressors lead to overloading, a situation that dramatically interferes with the ability of the human organism to adapt to change. The four characteristics of technological societies that are most likely to produce feelings of stress are discussed below.

Too Much Change Too Soon

The hypothesis that severe and frequent changes threaten our coping abilities has resulted in a new surge of research. Among the most prominent researchers who are evaluating the effect of rapidly changing life-styles and environments on humans are Thomas Holmes and Richard Rahe [19]. After extensive clinical observations and research, they devised a social readjustment rating scale (SRRS), which assigns a life change unit (LCU) to events that normally disrupt "everyday stability." The SRRS for persons living in the United States is shown in Table 42–1.

An analysis of the list indicates that most of the items concern concrete social events, many of which are desirable, such as going on vacation, achieving an outstanding personal goal, or completing one's education. Nevertheless, because of the disruption in daily patterns of living brought about by such events, the potential for confrontation with novel experiences and the need for making conscious decisions is increased, which in turn increases the stressors. Any stressor, whether real or perceived, external or internal, will elicit physiological responses. Once adaptation occurs, homeostasis will return. But prolonged or repeated stressors can lead to permanent alterations in body functioning, especially if a major body system is involved [28]. Therefore, the individual who is exposed to too many social changes in too short a time will experience an erosion of the system's recuperative powers, which may result in physiological illness [27].

Holmes and Rahe define a "life crisis" as any clustering of life changes whose individual values add up to 150 or more LCU in 1 year. In their studies, they found that 37 percent of individuals with 150 to 199 LCU, 51 percent of individuals with 200 to 299 LCU, and 79 percent of individuals with 300 or more LCU became ill within 6 months [18]. Both the severity and the frequency of illness correlate with higher LCU ratings. Although the research of Holmes and Rahe was

Table 42-1. Social Readjustment Rating Scale

Life Event	Life Change Unit (LCU) Value
Death of spouse	100
Divorce	73
Marital separation	65
Jail term	63
Death of close family member	63
Personal injury or illness	53
Marriage	50
Fired at work	47
Marital reconciliation	45
Retirement	45
Change in health of family member	44
Pregnancy	40
Sex difficulties	39
Gain of new family member	39
Change in financial state	38
Death of close friend	37
Change to different line of work	36
Change in number of arguments with spouse	35
Mortgage over $10,000	31
Foreclosure of mortgage or loan	30
Change in responsibilities at work	29
Son or daughter leaving home	29
Trouble with in-laws	29
Outstanding personal achievement	28
Wife beginning or stopping work	26
Beginning or ending school	26
Revision of personal habits	24
Trouble with boss	23
Change in work hours or conditions	20
Change in residence	20
Change in schools	19
Change in social activities	18
Mortgage or loan less than $10,000	17
Change in sleeping habits	16
Change in number of family get-togethers	15
Change in eating habits	15
Vacation	13
Minor violations of the law	11

Source: From T. H. Holmes and R. R. Rahe, The social readjustment rating scale *J. Psychosom. Res.* 11:216, 1967. Copyright 1967, Pergamon Press, Ltd. Used with permission.

geared more toward the relationship between life change and susceptibility to physical illness, their conclusions have significance for any kind of massive or frequent changes within the individual's external or internal environment.

The effect of an event may be contingent on context and may also be closely related to what the individual expects the stress level to be. In other words, perception of stress may be culturally mediated [8]. Stress is aggravated when the person feels out of control of changes or choices or feels subject to the whims of the environment; helplessness syndrome will then ensue.

Erosion of Values without Adequate Replacement

One of the more profound consequences of the technological age with its radical and repeated change has been the relativizing of once securely grounded values. With biological knowledge doubling every 5 years and genetic knowledge doubling every 2 years [32], we face moral and ethical issues undreamed of even 10 years ago. With rapid total world communication a reality, one begins to realize that a personal point of view might be conditioned and culture-specific. People appear to be stripped of any claim to ultimate truth. Traditional values frequently appear to lose validity in the pressure of contemporary problems and situations and may instead represent what a person at a particular time and place might hold to be desirable. The acquisition of a healthy sense of identity involves a cohesive blending and acceptance of a wide range of internalized ideals and role images as well as a sense of affirmation by one's environment. This internal and external acceptance leads to a sense of security about one's place in the world and a confidence about the future [49].

When the work ethic is no longer essential to one's survival or even to one's self-esteem, then new role expectancies must replace this value. Each of us must have a *raison d'être*. Life without a goal or a purpose gives rise to severe psychosocial disequilibrium [49]. Having a purpose to one's life is one of the main reasons why individuals who have the finances to remain unemployed (e.g., members of wealthy families, retirees, and many homemakers) may still seek gainful employment or may become deeply involved in the arts, community projects, politics, or volunteer services.

It has become blatantly obvious that a cultural revolution is transforming the rules that once guided everyday life and personal decisions [50]. As traditional values are relinquished, they are replaced by the pursuit of self-fulfillment and affluence [35, 50]. Consequently, work may lose its meaning for the individual unless it contributes to personal goals. A hedonistic mentality encourages some individuals to "do their own thing"—a factor that can precipitate social chaos [50]. Respect for individuality actually begins to diminish, and conflict and confusion can ensue. Yankelovich observes that a concentration on one's own perceived needs serves as a barrier to the achievement of meaningful interpersonal relationships or employment

positions of responsibility, because these require one to balance self-needs with those of others to achieve mutuality and compatability [50].

Today we have the technology to set up the conditions for the creation of life (e.g., cloning of animals, gene construction, and extrauterine conception), to sustain life after clinical death, to transplant body organs, to maintain life with artificial blood, and to implant an artificial heart. Such technological advances present problems and ethical questions undreamed of in earlier generations. Arnold Toynbee warns that we need to "redirect our attention and energy from mastery of the biosphere . . . to the mastery of ourselves and of our relations with each other. This is what all the historical religions and philosophies have been telling us with one voice for a long time. . . . We must somehow master ourselves—master ourselves in the sense in which the historic religions and philosophies all beseech us to master ourselves, and until we can do that and unless we can do that, we shall be under threat from the technosphere which is our own . . . creation" [46]. Toffler [44] agrees, stating that technology offers us the potential for improved personal and family life.

Toynbee contends that we are social creatures—we would perish otherwise—but he expresses concern that we may not be social enough to hold our power in check. "Ethics and values maintain the checks and balances between science and politics" [6]. However, "today, too many decisions appear to be made on the basis of expediency rather than integrity" [2]. Watergate is a case in point. Most people realize that a life without values, order, and goals is a meaningless one and attempt to find some structure and values to guide their behaviors [7, 44].

Rifkin [32] challenges us to find enduring values to guide our ethical decisions. We define a **value** as any philosophy, event, person, place, or object which, when freely chosen and acted upon, contributes to the meaning of an individual's life and enhances growth. By definition, then, a value assists one in finding meaning; this distinguishes a value from other objects or events that may motivate behavior. The act of valuing is to choose voluntarily to be deeply influenced by certain philosophies, theologies, objects, persons, or events in the environment. Values give strong meaning, direction, goals, order, and even roles to one's life.

One of the most interesting conclusions about the impact of environmental challenge on value systems is suggested by the studies of Milton Rokeach [34]. Since thousands of beliefs cannot be equally important to an individual, a hierarchy or priority value tends to be assigned to each belief held by a person. Rokeach's research indicates that there are five levels of belief systems, arranged here in descending order according to their significance to the individual:

1. **Primitive** beliefs, the most important, are comprised of a core of values that a person holds because they are derived from cultural consensus. Consequently, they are the most resistant to any change, but when they do change, they greatly influence personal functioning.
2. **Deep personal experience** beliefs, which are based on subjective experiences, have inordinate value to the believer whether or not anyone else accepts them.
3. **Authority** beliefs are values that we hold because an authority figure whom we trust also holds them. They do not necessarily have to be grounded in reality to be viable to a person; they are based on the confidence one has in the authority figure.
4. **Peripheral** beliefs come from a variety of sources, and represent many opinions that can easily change as new data or experiences come into one's consciousness.
5. **Inconsequential** beliefs are superficial and largely untested ideas that do not necessarily influence the functioning of the total system.

Rokeach concludes that when a higher priority belief is challenged and rendered less viable, the individual will experience a higher degree of disequilibrium and decreased adaptive functioning. This disequilibrium points to a major adjustment problem in periods of rapid change. When deeply held values are challenged and rejected with an inadequate lead time to reformulate them, one's sense of identity and integrity is gravely threatened. The vacuum may be filled with a "pragmatic" code of conduct, by which individuals take over the ultimate judgment for themselves or others as to what is right or wrong. A situational ethic based on one's response to certain events rather than on adherence to an abiding principle creates its own stress, since a new decision must be created each time.

Maslow observes that "We need something 'bigger than we are' to be awed by and to commit ourselves to in a new, naturistic, empirical, non-churchly sense" [23]. There are so many different systems of values wrapped up in the life of a society, challenging traditional belief systems, that people are profoundly affected, often becoming indecisive about which values or goals make sense to them. Consequently, some people will fill the vacuum by accepting the ready-made values of another person, usually a strong leader. This choice offers structure, safety, and security, since one does not have to extend efforts to "recreate the wheel," or find values to live by. Bugental warns, however, that values must be tempered with realism. To accept another's values without question or to strive for perfection as a value in itself, may be counterproductive or even destructive, leading to a "loss of humanness in experience" [7]. One of the privileges of being human is the ability to choose among alternatives. When one abdicates this choice to another, does it free the individual to pursue other interests, or does it restrict him or her? The Jonestown, Guyana, tragedy of 1978, in which more than 900 people committed suicide in obedience to their "leader," offers an extreme case in point. "The cult sells community, structure, and meaning at an extremely high price: The mindless surrender of self" [44].

In the face of a changing culture, individuals must address the question of meaning if they are to survive holistically. They must "rediscover and scrutinize the immutable and the permanent which constitute the dynamic, unifying aspect of life" [1]. Perhaps a starting point for discovering these values is to explore religious traditions. Heath observes that "religious traditions agree in most of their basic assumptions about healthy adult growth. . . . maturing involves persistent, disciplined commitment [stable values] that brings inner certitude, serenity, calm, repose, and self-confidence [stability of the self]; as a person matures, he becomes more alive, joyful, and spontaneous, and transcends [or becomes more autonomous of] the reality of his body and surrounding world" [17]. Heath's definition is very supportive of Maslow's theory of human development. It should be noted that in this context, religion—"the feelings, aspirations and acts of man, as they relate to total reality" [1]—is not synonymous with a particular theory or doctrine.

Margaret Mead observed that "Most Americans—even though they acknowledge some slight connection with religion, accept the label of some denomination, and obey a certain set of ritualistic requirements—do not admit the existence of a significant connection between the lives they lead, the careers they pursue, the thoughts they think, and their relationship to God or their spiritual existence" [26]. Most religions emphasize that "to **be** is more important than to **have** since **being** leads to transcendence and joy, while **having** only leads to apathy and despair" [1]. One's values, then, facilitate the integration of an inner life with outer behaviors. Stable core values can decrease the energy expended in decision-making processes, since the answer is often an integral part of the values held. An adherence to values can reduce conflicting decisions and enhance integration of one's identities.

Values can offer continuity from the past, through the present, and into the future. When one's value system no longer appears to offer an adequate frame for decision making, stress is increased unless a solid replacement is identifiable. Whatever the approach taken, the search for abiding values is essential to survival in a technological age.

The Inability to Meet Changing Demands with Existing Skills

Chapter 19 contained a discussion of the problems encountered when skill development is inadequate to meet the demands of the environment. Skill building is an integral part of personality development. Mastery of specific skills, whether culturally, developmentally, or personally imposed, is critical to the development of self-confidence and self-esteem. It is essential that a number of skills develop simultaneously in a holistic fashion in order for the individual to meet the demands of the environment. These skills fall into four general areas [15]:

1. Systemic skills. The skills essential for coping with the basic systems (e.g., the use of one's body, communication skills for interacting with family and social institutions, self-care)
2. Instrumental skills. The task-oriented skills that one can rely on to complete jobs adequately, such as general skills (reading and writing), functional skills (the use of tools), and professional skills (practicing medicine or law)
3. Interpersonal skills. The ability to enter into deeply satisfying, reciprocal human relationships
4. Imaginal skills. The ability to bring fantasy, emotions, and the reflective intellect into creative and productive thought

The onset of rapidly changing social and technological demands for one category of skills can have implications for other areas. The individual may find that the interpersonal skills that facilitated rich relationships in a rural environment are inadequate in a fast-paced urban area where truncated relationships are common. When existing instrumental skills are inadequate to cope with changing demands, the individual who fails to update skills or is unable to do so may become unemployable. The stress generated by the change of life-style or a perceived personal inadequacy generally further jeopardizes systemic, interpersonal,

and imaginative skills. Thus once efficient adaptation in one area is lowered, it becomes increasingly difficult for the individual to function effectively in other aspects of life.

The commonly held understandings, meanings, and rules of a culture increase internal and external predictability as well as control. Ethnic groups, which are comprised of individuals who are kept together by their regard for common symbols and skills, establish their own rules and rituals as cultural norms. This is as true for life in a New York ghetto or a wealthy Chicago suburb as it is for life on a Navajo reservation or in a mining town in Kentucky. Enmity between groups seems to be strongest when the groups feel a need to protect their identity or individuality. Parents and adolescents sometimes find themselves belonging to two different cultures or ethnic groups. The parents' traditional, instrumental, skill-oriented culture may be rejected by the teenage culture, which is centered around interpersonal and imaginal skills [22]. When adolescents see the parents' culture fixated on an adherence to roles imposed by external sources, they fight the artificiality of such structured relationships and struggle to increase the interpersonal skills they feel their parents were unable to model for them. They sense that in an impersonal technological environment, their psychological survival may depend on achieving psychological intimacy [29], and therefore strip away the roles and social games that interfere with knowing and being known.

The family system as well as the individual may be affected by changing demands. The interpersonal skills of chronically unemployed families are considerably retarded. However, it is not just the lack of adequate finances that precipitates depressed behaviors. Martin Seligman's research on the helplessness syndrome has relevance here as well as to childhood development (see Chap. 14). Learned helplessness is accompanied by a general sense of inadequacy caused by events that the individual or family members perceive are beyond their control. The adult discovers that his or her behavior no longer produces the desired responses from the environment (i.e., gainful employment). In order for an individual to maintain self-confidence and self-esteem, each new challenge of the environment requires that the individual develop skills to control the outcome adequately. When it becomes apparent that one cannot produce responses that will have a predictable effect on the environment, the feeling of helplessness can then become a self-perpetuating phenomenon. It sabotages the desire to respond to environmental demands, retards the ability to perceive success, and results in a greatly heightened sense of hopelessness and helplessness [38]. Seligman's theory may be as relevant to family system functioning as it is to individual system functioning.

The Feeling of Depersonalization in a Technological Age

One of the by-products of the technological age is the loss of true community and the resultant loss of personal identity. Whatever the cause (e.g., mobility, computerized accountability to the environment), it contributes to a feeling that one's individuality is insignificant or undervalued. Rapidly changing events tend to encourage people to relate and disengage quickly. Under such conditions, one may avoid intimacy with another individual or an idea because the nature of the relationship or the truth of the concept could change, and one may have invested too heavily to change these relationships or concepts effectively. The result is depersonalization, a sense of loneliness or isolation, the consciousness of being out of meaningful contact with one's environment.

Abraham Maslow's theory of hierarchical needs has relevance here. Maslow believes that each person has a biologically based inner nature which is pushing towards self-actualization, but which is nevertheless weak and easily overcome by a rapidly changing and incorrectly perceived environment. He believes that in an environment in which proper stimulation, justice, freedom, and orderliness exist, the basic hierarchy of survival and deficiency needs will be met. The individual will be allowed to expand horizons, to become more fully integrated; as a result, one is more likely to recognize and actualize potentials [23]. Maslow's hierarchy of motivating concepts is illustrated in Figure 42–3.

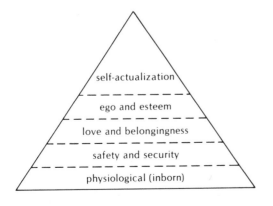

Figure 42–3. Maslow's hierarchy of human needs.

While Maslow's theory explains some of the environmental conditions that are essential in allowing people to actualize their potentials, it also indicates why some people never develop or meet the higher-order needs. Maslow indicates that only about 1 percent of individuals are able to actualize their potentials fully [23]. A rapidly changing, inadequately supportive, stressful environment forces many people to deal continually with threats of deprivation of lower-level needs. As a result, life is dominated by an overriding urgency to survive—if not physically, then psychologically. Brennecke contends that in this technological age, the dissolution of predictability threatens the need structure of the personality so massively that many people are still preoccupied with the basic survival needs of bodily comfort, security, and love and are doing little or nothing to fulfill their potentials. Under such stress, it is all they can do to maintain an appearance of self-confidence and a semblance of balance in their lives [4].

Maslow observes that "Striving, the usual organizer of most activity, when lost, leaves the person unorganized and unintegrated" [23]. Consequently, increased leisure time (whether resulting from unemployment or shorter working hours) can precipitate stress in the individual. For many people the goal of work is leisure, but when too much unoccupied free time is available, it becomes a greater burden than too little free time [33]. Hans Selye, the leading authority on the study of stress, contends that too much leisure leads to boredom—a significant stressor [39]. Persons from widely varying backgrounds recommend that individuals develop specific, meaningful activities to occupy leisure time. Benjamin Spock recommends developing one's creative skills or engaging in activities that will enhance the community welfare [41]. Arnold Toynbee feels that if individuals are educated in the proper use of leisure time, our culture has the capability of becoming a second Renaissance instead of a parasitic society [45].

The very advances, therefore, that absorb our jobs and seem to make our humanness obsolete can actually allow us to become more human and can give us the freedom to spend more time in service to others—to actualize our own and the community's potentials. This will be accomplished, however, only by a reevaluation of values, goals, and roles.

COPING WITH EXTERNAL STRESS

When an external stimulus evokes stress, the individual usually attempts to eliminate either the stimulus or the unpleasant emotional state aroused by it. Some persons, however, like Theseus in Greek mythology, will attempt to control the stressor or to "harness" the energy it elicits in order to capitalize on an otherwise difficult situation (for example, channeling stage fright into a brilliant piece of acting). Gail Sheehy observes that this skill is a trademark of persons of high well-being [36]. The route chosen will depend on past experience, the circumstances, and one's philosophical approach to life. We will explore four major theoretical positions explaining how individuals adapt to specific stressors (as opposed to the cumulative stressors discussed in the previous section) or the emotional state aroused by them.

Social Learning Theory

The principles of learning have emerged from the observation that individuals tend to repeat those behaviors that result in desirable effects: (A) The individual who becomes aware that the **antecedent** (stimulus or appropriate conditions) is present, (B) **behaves** (gives a response or performs a skill) in a way that (C) has elicited a desirable **consequence** in previous situations. Consequently, behaviors learned through personal experience are very tenacious. After several experiences, the behavior can be labeled a habit—behavior that is repeated without much forethought. This basic paradigm is as valid for learning how to remain upright on a bicycle as it is for obtaining a desired object from the parent. Habits help to avoid stress by reducing the amount of energy one must expend in deciding how much to move a muscle to get the desired result or how to approach a social relationship.

Superstitious fears can result when an innocent stimulus is accidently paired with a noxious stimulus. The child or individual may blame the wrong stimulus for the unpleasant experience and feel increased stress in the presence of the innocent party (e.g., being scratched by a berry bush when a dog is present may lead to fear of all dogs). If one's behavior appears to prevent recurrence of the stressful stimuli, then a continuing link between the stimulus and one's response is formed.

Behaviors, once learned, can be either adaptive or maladaptive. Some behaviors may be highly useful in alleviating anxiety and dealing with life's stressors when, for example, a special sensitivity to an environmental threat creates a healthy vigilance, caution, and openness that leads to more effective coping behaviors. In fact, a moderate amount of anticipatory fear about realistic threats is necessary for the development of effective inner defenses for coping with the threat

(avoidance). However, too many previously negative responses from the environment following efforts to cope with a situation may effectively extinguish the individual's attempts to take positive action to meet a problem situation.

Novel experiences generally produce stress because the individual (1) has not had sufficient experience to discriminate the relevant cues in the situation (and thus must depend on trial and error or overgeneralization), and (2) is not sure of the environmental response to the behavior (i.e., whether it will be reinforced or punished). Individuals need models to imitate, assistance in discriminating cues, and information about the response system to allay anxiety in novel situations, especially during the earlier years. Conditioned responses can exact a high price if they are too defensive in nature, prevent meaningful interaction, or are inadequate to cope successfully with a changing environment.

Psychodynamic Theories

Like learning theories, psychodynamic approaches are difficult to summarize adequately in a few paragraphs. Whereas learning theory approaches stress from a conditioning standpoint, psychodynamic theories approach it from the perspective of developmental inadequacies. Defensive behaviors are employed to protect the ego from disintegrating trauma. The sense of "I" is protected at all costs.

It should be pointed out that the use of defense mechanisms is not necessarily maladaptive; everyone uses one or more of them regularly because they serve to reduce stress levels and the accompanying biophysical and psychic anxiety. However, when an individual uses defense mechanisms extensively, to the point where he or she is no longer assessing and dealing effectively with reality (reality distorting), then the integrity of the affective or cognitive domain (or both) is gravely threatened. Many therapists believe that the excessive use of defense mechanisms is the basic pathology of mental illness. Defensive behaviors can seriously interfere with reality functioning and essentially prevent adaptive functioning, thus leading to failure and tremendous frustration. Effective intervention can reverse the process and help the person to develop more effective strategies for dealing with stress.

The basic ingredients for evoking stress, from the psychodynamic viewpoint, are the instincts and their insatiable need for gratification. The founding father of the movement, Sigmund Freud, believed that biological instincts are an inherent part of human nature. A certain amount of internal tension or stress always exists simply because the organism experiences deprivation or inadequate satiation of these impulses as a normal process of biological functioning [14].

Psychodynamic theorists believe that there are three basic types of instincts: self-preservation, sexual, and actualization instincts. (Later in his life, Freud postulated the existence of the death instinct, but this is of little concern to our presentation.) Most theorists say that gratification of instincts per se is ineffective in reducing stress; one must act intelligently. The ego, the part of the mind that comprises the thought and perceptual processes, aids the individual in finding satisfaction for instinctual needs in the external world. The superego, which becomes differentiated to represent the rules and regulations of society to the self, uses an experience of guilt to raise tension and thus to direct the meeting of instinctual needs (or the reduction of stress induced by need deficit) by more appropriate means, through the ego. Freud calls this function "reality principle functioning" [14].

Anxiety arises whenever an externally or internally motivated instinct becomes strong enough to arouse conflict. This anxiety recalls the anticipation of punishment and guilt and triggers the defensive process. According to psychodynamic thought, defense mechanisms are used to maintain homeostasis by balancing the two stress sources. A defense mechanism eases the conflict between the demands of the instincts and those of the environment by forging out a compromise between them. The defense behavior channels that energy into action that may or may not be acceptable to others and to one's own superego.

Psychodynamic thought tends to see most coping behavior as defensive—that is, reactive rather than proactive. Most defenses function outside of our conscious awareness. Some of the commonly found defense mechanisms are given in the following list:

Denial. Suppressing awareness of other things, people, events, or consequences that could arouse anxiety or threaten one's psychic integrity

Repression. Involuntary denial of instinctual wishes, feelings, and experiences, so that associated anxiety will not be experienced

Suppression. Conscious exclusion of events from memory or refusal to acknowledge instinctual needs

Sublimation. Focusing attention and interest on a substitute for an unacceptable feeling; usually, consciously diverting energies into creative, constructive, socially acceptable activities

Displacement. Shifting emotional energies from one object, idea, person, or situation to another that is less threatening

Compensation. Overemphasizing a desirable attribute or skill to make up for a perceived or real disability

Projection. Attributing negative wishes, feelings, and impulses to other persons while denying that they originate in oneself

Introjection. Crediting oneself with another's values, attributes, and behaviors in order to avoid conflicts, to enhance acceptance, or to avoid the threatening nature of one's own instincts

Rationalization or intellectualization. Losing awareness of the significance of one's own wishes and impulses while offering a socially acceptable, fairly logical explanation for one's behaviors, feelings, or decisions

Regression. Retreating to more primitive patterns of coping (associated with earlier developmental stages) to avoid the challenges of the higher forms of behavior

Undoing. Emitting behaviors that seek to cancel out or atone for what are considered unacceptable thoughts of previous behaviors

Ego restriction. Abandoning an activity because of inferiority feelings and thus restricting one's range of adaptability or the horizons of one's life

Reaction formation. Going to the opposite extreme in order to avoid behaviors that would allow expression of one's impulses

Systems Viewpoint

Herman Witkin [48] was greatly interested in the relationship of defensive behavior to the individual's level of maturity and stress. However, he saw the relationship in terms of psychological differentiation rather than psychosexual development. Like Werner, Witkin hypothesized that the individual begins life in a highly undifferentiated state. As the individual matures, the subsystems of psychological operations within the individual (e.g., feeling, perceiving, and thinking) become more heterogeneous and specialized. The more highly differentiated psychological functioning enables the individual to differentiate between the self-system and others, and to make more specific responses to a specific stimulus instead of a diffuse response to many stimuli. Poorly differentiated persons tend to rely on, or are more likely to be influenced by, the behaviors, values, and decisions of others, whereas highly differentiated persons are able to identify their own ideas, feelings, and values.

Witkin's studies [48] indicate that poorly differentiated or **field-dependent** individuals tend to be characterized by low self-esteem, difficulty with organization and priority setting, a tendency to deny or to repress their emotional responses, passivity, and an inability to function independently. His research indicates that field-dependent individuals use more rudimentary forms of defense mechanisms in the turning away from their own perceptions through the use of repression and denial. Because of their inability to differentiate clearly between their ideas and the ideas of others or between their emotional and intellectual domains, field-dependent persons exhibit more stress responses because they are unable to channel energies to pursue a specific goal.

Field-independent persons, on the other hand, because of their more highly developed or differentiated affective skills, perceive events differently and are able to respond to specific elements or factors within a situation without undue influence from other events or other persons [48]. Field-independent individuals are more likely to use intellectualization or sublimation to cope with adverse, stress-producing stimuli, since they generally possess richer and more diversified resources for coping than does the less differentiated person. As a result, according to Witkin, the former individuals think more clearly, respond more specifically, initiate actions, exhibit more control over external events as well as their own responses and behaviors, are highly organized, and exhibit high self-esteem [48].

The internalization of one's own values, standards, and goals guides perception and self-control. Therefore, according to Witkin, the ability to identify and to internalize goals becomes a critical factor in determining one's level of maturity (the degree of differentiation and effectiveness of integration of the various subsystems of the psychological domain) [48]. Classic psychodynamic thought, coupled with more contemporary research, such as that of Witkin, shows clearly the importance of stress management and of developing the essential skills for responding properly to the crescendo of environmental stressors. The importance of reducing stress through accurate, realistic insight, mature, internalized values, and creative coping responses cannot be overestimated.

Cognitive Viewpoints

Despite the striking differences between social learning, psychodynamic, and systems theories, they share a basic assumption: The emotionally stressed person is victimized by forces over which he or she has no control. Learning theory regards the disturbance in terms of involuntary reflexes based on accidental conditionings that occurred previously in one's life. Since the individual cannot modify these conditioned reflexes merely by knowing about them and trying to will them away, the application of counter-conditioning by a competent therapist is required. Psychodynamic thought attributes the individual's reaction to stress to unconscious psychological factors that are sealed off by defensive behavior. The systems view stresses system immaturity that affects the processing of input and, consequently, the output behaviors. The inability to adequately separate the affective and cognitive domains prevents the effective functioning of either. While later psychodynamic theorists emphasized the role of an autonomous ego and the conscious mind [16], it is the cognitivists who highlight proactive responses.

Cognitive theory assumes that each person has the potential for various rational techniques to deal with disturbing elements in the consciousness. It suggests that stress reduction can be better understood by assuming that a person has the key to understanding and solving a disturbance within the scope of his or her own awareness. Cognitive theorists hold that most stress problems stem directly from a person's magical, superstitious, empirically unvalidated thinking, and that "if disturbance-creating ideas are vigorously and persistently disputed by the rigorous application of logico-empirical thinking, they can almost invariably be eliminated" [10]. Misconceptions that produce stress can be corrected with the same problem-solving apparatus that one has achieved through the various stages of development. In this approach, a person regards a disturbance as a misunderstanding or misinterpretation that can be resolved either through acquiring more adequate information or by recognizing the logical fallacy of these misunderstandings.

Cognitive theorists are optimistic about the individual's ability to filter large amounts of information; they believe that one can label all external stimuli efficiently, monitor imagination, and distinguish between the real and imaginary elements of a situation. They believe that individuals are able to hypothesize and test accumulated inventories of formulas, equations, and axioms that enable them to make deductions when confronted with problems similar to those previously resolved [3].

Cognitive psychologists feel that in the course of development, individuals acquire many techniques and generalizations that enable them to judge whether or not they are reacting realistically to situations. The individual processes, decodes, and interprets incoming messages by a self-regulating system that issues instructions and prohibitions, self-praise, or self-reproaches. According to the cognitive theorist, a person can respond effectively to the environment to the extent that the input of the environment is meshed with the individual's internal psychological system. If this system shuts out or twists around the signals from the outside, the individual will be completely out of phase with what is going on around him or her [3].

Human events are often controlled by causal factors beyond one's will. Nevertheless, individuals have a uniquely rational dimension to their functionings and the possibility, difficult though it may be, of taking action that will change and control their futures. Since reaction to stress is often the result of irrational and illogical thinking and is thus determined not so much by external circumstances but by perceptions and attitudes toward those circumstances, a reorganization of these perceptions and thinking can help one to develop adequate coping behaviors to deal effectively with stressors [11]. Thus one can become proactive instead of reactive to life.

The belief in the ability of the individual to determine personal behavior and emotional experience is expressed in Ellis's "A-B-C" theory of personality. "A" is the existence of the fact, event, behavior, or attitude of another person; "C" is the reaction of the individual (e.g., emotional disturbance or unhappiness) that follows from "A." However, it is not "A" that is the cause of "C," but "B," which is the self-verbalization by the individual about the meaning of "A"—the definition or interpretation of "A" as being awful, terrible, good, or solvable. It is, therefore, not so much the environmental cues as one's definition and interpretation of these cues that becomes the cause of maladaptive thinking and behavior. Thus the mind plays a unique role in coping successfully or unsuccessfully with a stressful environment.

Each of the major theoretical schools has touched on important ingredients of stress situations. The learning theorists have shown us the power of environmental cues in disrupting and in shaping our lives. Psychodynamic theorists reveal to us how the needs and drives of the human personality can retard reality functioning and response to stress from within. The systems viewpoint stresses the intrapersonal and interpersonal differentiation of the individual as a critical factor in stress perception and management. The cognitive theorists have stressed the inhibiting or liberating effect of one's own information processing system. While all four views clarify the ways in which individuals react adversely to stress, it remains for us to suggest ways in which individuals can better cope with the rapid and profound changes that all people are experiencing. In these next sections we will discuss how one can build on this large theoretical base to provide concrete suggestions for coping with the stressors inherent in a technological society.

IMPLICATIONS FOR FOSTERING OPTIMAL DEVELOPMENT OF HUMAN POTENTIALS

Douglas Heath [17], in his cross-cultural research on maturity and competence, discovered that persons who were considered mature within their culture by their peers consistently differed from immature persons in similar ways. He found that "mature persons are able to symbolize their experiences; they are also more allocentric [opposite of egocentric], integrated, stable, and autonomous in their cognitive skills, concepts of themselves, values, and personal relationships" [17]. He hypothesized that a successful adaptation or achievement of a new level of maturity releases affective energy that results in increased enthusiasm, joy, humor, and a sense of power, since such experiences foster identity integration that in turn encourages integrity and results in spontaneity [17]. After research in cultures as diverse as rural Turkey and urban America, Heath was able to identify a core set of traits possessed by mature persons: (1) ability to anticipate consequences; (2) calm and clear thinking; (3) potential fulfillment; (4) orderly, organized approaches to life's problems; (5) predictability; (6) purposefulness; (7) realisticness; (8) reflectiveness; (9) strong convictions; (10) implacability.

Heath's research blends well with the theories of Seligman, Maslow, Witkin, Sheehy, and many others in the concept that previous successes foster sufficient self-confidence to risk initiating active efforts to cope when novel situations arise that force one to generalize from previous experiences or to create new solutions to problems. Heath observes, however, that a sense of competence does not mature in a vacuum. "Effectiveness is associated not only with a private sense of competence or self-esteem, but also with a belief that others also judge one's self to be able to cope successfully" [17]. Thus we are affected by the suprasystems, the family, and the culture in which we are reared—their support, the opportunities offered, and the competencies valued.

In 1970 the White House Conference on Children and Youth observed that "We are experiencing a breakdown in the process of making human beings human" [5]. Talbot observes that "Millions of children grow up in conditions that stunt their intellectual and emotional growth as well as their physical growth" [42]. "To be fully human, one must be attached to, care for, and be interdependent with other human beings. To be totally self-absorbed, as we learn from the writings of the new narcissists, is finally to feel lonely, bored, and despairing in the face of the meaninglessness of life" [9].

With these remarks in mind, we shall review what research and child development experts indicate assists the child to develop a sense of competence and to foster high self-esteem during the developmental years. However, "being a person is not something we get set or that we construct, once and for all. It is a constant, evolving, changing thing. This focus on process, on the evolution of experience, is something that changes our expectancies of ourselves" [7].

Infancy

Selma Fraiberg notes that "our survival as a human community may depend as much upon our nurture of love in infancy and childhood as upon the protection of our society from external threats" [12]. Such love, security, and the opportunity for healthy attachment are best realized in a family who plans for and eagerly anticipates the child's arrival. In such an environment, the potential for parental commitment and devotion and their ability and willingness to sacrifice personal goals temporarily for the needs of the infant are increased. The presence of caring adults is the most critical component for healthy development during infancy.

Erikson speaks about the need to develop trust. Mahler emphasizes that primary narcissism, or autistic behavior, is characteristic of the early months. Thus regularity is required in meeting the child's basic physiological needs. This regularity of experiences helps the child to organize information into meaningful, useful schemata. A regular but flexible schedule helps the child to begin to predict events, yet allows both the parents and the child to meet their individual needs.

The parents must be able to invest themselves in the child so fully that synchrony of interaction is established early. This means that the parent and young child take turns during periods of communication or play. Each plays an equal role in maintaining the interaction. Each responds specifically to the behaviors of the other and initiates new directions. Communication is not unidirectional with the adult initiating all contacts, toy uses, or communication topics. This early respect as communication partners facilitates attending and engenders trust. Through brief interactions,

the child begins to associate specific behaviors with predictable, pleasant events. This association is the beginning of competence—learning to control the outcome. Seligman's theory on learned helplessness is very significant at this stage of development.

Even the infant needs a change of pace and exposure to new experiences to prevent boredom and further withdrawal into his or her own world. However, new experiences or stimuli must be modified or presented gradually if they are to capture and maintain the infant's interest; otherwise they may cause withdrawal because of "flooding" or sensory overload [47]. Mobiles can be used to capture visual interest; their slow movement allows practice in visual following. Parental conversation should generally be slower, restricted in word usage, and repeated often. Gentle tactile and kinesthetic stimulation, such as holding, patting, caressing, and changing position, is essential for neurophysical maturation as well as emotional well-being [12]. Repetitive body games, such as "creepy spider" and "peek-a-boo," provide variation, yet allow the infant to anticipate the end result. A gradual change of stimulus and the provision of a variety of social, sensorimotor, language, and kinesthetic experiences help to prepare the infant for more active involvement with the environment during the toddler years.

The infant needs a stable person to cathect to or to "fall in love with." This factor more than any other is essential to the development of those most human qualities of sensitivity, caring, and giving. Inadequate physical as well as emotional contact during infancy hinders identification with a significant adult [23]. Lap games become an essential vehicle for early sharing of the culture (e.g., pat-a-cake) as well as exchanges of tenderness.

Selma Fraiberg, from her studies of child development, infants with failure-to-thrive, and family relationships, feels that there is a very close link between the love-respect relationships of adulthood and the love-acceptance relationship experienced during infancy. "In every act of love in mature life there is a prologue which originated in the first year of life. There are two people who arouse in each other sensual joy, feelings of longing, and the conviction that they are absolutely indispensable to each other—that life without the other is meaningless. Separation from the other is intolerable. . . . To a very large extent the disease of non-attachment can be eradicated at the source, by ensuring stable human partnerships for each baby" [12].

The infant also needs opportunities to practice the skills already possessed—whether they are looking behaviors, manipulating an object, eating solid foods, or communicating. Since initial efforts are generally fleeting and weak, reinforcement of early skills is essential as a stepping-stone to the development of stronger or more complex skills. The provision of toys that respond easily with only minimal effort on the infant's behalf is critical during the early months and years. Thus reinforcement for one's efforts at control is "cost-effective." The behaviorists' concept of successive approximations, which emphasizes the reinforcement of rudimentary skills, is very appropriate for the development of competency that leads to initiative in later childhood.

Toddlers and Preschoolers

According to Erikson, the toddler and preschooler are developing autonomy and initiative. Once they learn that their actions can affect the environment, they become "drunk with their own power" and try to control the whole world. It is important, therefore, that parents help the child to develop appreciation for the limits of his or her power in order to maintain both physical and psychological safety. This need is often difficult to balance with the child's continuing need to practice emerging skills. However, the child who has parents who set consistent, reasonable limits, and who follow through with the guidance and limits they offer, gradually begins to internalize limits, learns to control impulses, and thus develops self-discipline. The child recognizes his or her own ability to tell the self "no." This recognition enhances the child's self-esteem and self-confidence (since the child can begin to trust the self), especially if the parents notice and reinforce efforts at self-control.

The child's needs for physical affection, love, and acceptance do not diminish during the preschool years. Although the child may want the attention less frequently or in a different form (parents need to respect the child's pace and preferences), the toddler or preschooler still needs tangible and frequent evidence of the parent's love, which affirms his or her value to them. One of the best ways to offer this reassurance is to spend time with the child. Toys and other material possessions are secondary to the child when compared to social play time with the parents. Social play time offers an opportunity for synchronized, cooperative use of language, which is essential to the development of language and cognitive skills as well as social skills. The turn-taking play and communication patterns established during infancy must continue during this period of life. The typical adult directed conversation consists of a series of questions to help the child remember past events or show off knowledge to another

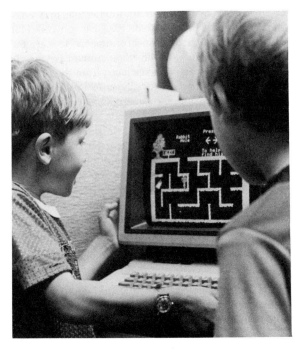

Figure 42–4. Computer games familiarize preschoolers with the type of equipment they will be using in school and in later careers.

adult. This is not turn-taking since the adult is initiating all the topics of interaction. The young child's tension level rises with increased behavior problems and decreased cooperativeness. The child may feel as if he or she is taking an examination! Many of the typical resistive behaviors of young children can be avoided through sensitive listening and responding.

The child's exposure to adult language is just as important as the parent's ability to understand and respond specifically and sensitively to the child's attempts to communicate. From infancy and throughout life, "the more empathetically and accurately parents read their children's signals, and the more sensitively they respond to them from the heart, the more likely the child will be protected from erosions in mental health. Children who know they are operating from a firm base do not 'spoil'; instead they are able to draw on a well of security lasting a lifetime. Don't hold back on the instincts of love and caring" [37]. The social play time offers an opportunity to develop this sensitivity on the part of the parent, while fostering the child's optimal development.

The toddler and especially the preschooler need exposure to models who possess both similar and valued characteristics with whom they can identify. Models serve to stimulate the desire to develop similar skills and provide the child with a feeling of power and virtue. The opportunity to play with peers helps the child to develop cooperative social skills, to practice language, and to compare self-competencies with more realistic performance levels.

Stability of experiences is critical during these early years when children are learning roles and relationships, and when cognitive organizational skills are still limited. Their ability to be flexible or to adapt to entirely new circumstances is limited. When a move to a new neighborhood, a hospitalization, or a separation from family members is unavoidable, every effort needs to be extended to continue as much stability in relationships and routines as possible. The practices of parents do affect and shape a child, but it is a dynamic relationship that is constantly changing; therefore, no **one** experience will ensure success or failure in later life. However, parents do need to attempt to ensure as much stability as possible [37] in order to provide information that facilitates the child's ability to organize and to predict events and thus control outcomes. It is the continuity between the internal prediction and the external outcome that fosters the child's sense of competence and high self-esteem.

Young children need challenges to help stretch their burgeoning skills. Many parents try to spare their children "the necessity of overcoming any kind of obstacle, including, of course, any kind of contradiction from their parents. The result is intolerably aggressive and, at the same time, neurotic children. Quite apart from the fact that trying to raise unfrustrated human beings is one of the most cruel deprivation experiments possible, it puts its unfortunate victim in a position of tormenting insecurity. . . . Small wonder their world breaks down and they become openly neurotic when they are suddenly exposed to the stress of public opinion" [22]. Environmental and social challenges are essential for learning how to solve a problem, how to work, how to assess one's self against a standard. Rules and developmentally appropriate challenges give a child structure, security, motivation, and a valid source of self-esteem.

School-Age Children

Erikson feels that the development of industry—the ability to work—is critical during the school-age years. Children continue to need opportunities to master skills during the school years [21]. In fact, individuals at each age need opportunities not only for exposure to new, meaningful skills, but to practice them as an end in themselves until they are mastered to the extent that they can be used as a tool to accomplish other, more complex skills. Both the school and the home can help children to discover and to develop their unique potentials while they also offer them the opportunity to gain those skills that are deemed critical to successful adaptation in the culture (e.g., reading, computational skills, self-care skills).

The White House Conference of 1970 recognized that both the home and the school need to involve children in genuine responsibilities—not duties or busy work—so that they learn to "deal constructively with personal and social problems . . . to acquire the capacity to cope with difficult situations" [5]. Such genuine involvement enhances self-esteem in that it offers respect for and confidence in the child's capabilities; it makes the child a genuine part of the team, an integral part of the system's functioning. At the same time, it helps to develop the skills of perseverance and cooperation, brings the pride of accomplishment, and leads to a feeling of competence—all integral parts of the task of industry. When a number of responsibilities are assigned, children can learn how to organize their time and to establish priorities. Some parents try to absorb all responsibilities from children—a task that becomes increasingly easy in a technological society—because they feel that childhood is a time for fun, not for responsibility. They overlook the fact that childhood is also a time of preparation for adult responsibilities, and it is much easier to learn those responsibilities through successive approximations. The assumption of responsibilities involves the development of the affective domain, or attitudes, as well as the acquisition of appropriate psychomotor skills. As an anonymous sage has observed, "One's greatest opportunities frequently come cleverly disguised as unsolvable problems." Affective growth can occur when problems are faced and mastered; one learns how to establish priorities and weigh outcomes. Such skills are learned gradually. Each choice or decision involves not only the attainment of one goal, but the relinquishing of an alternative [7]. Living with the results of one's decisions in childhood can help to prepare one to make more astute decisions during the adult years, when a single decision may in fact change the entire course of one's life.

Peers, an essential ingredient to the psychosocial development of children of all ages, become increasingly important to school-agers. Parents may help children to select their friends through the modeling of what they deem to be desirable behaviors, attitudes, and values. However, "Mothers and fathers will serve children best if they accept the power of their children's friends, recognize their presence, and work with rather than against them. . . . the child's indiscriminate choice of friends is most likely when family ties are weak and when the child's sense of belonging is fragmented" [37]. Bronfenbrenner and many others observe that negative or unhealthy "attachment to age-mates appears to be influenced more by a lack of attention and concern at home than by any positive attraction of the peer group itself. In fact, these children have a rather negative view of their friends and of themselves as well. They are pessimistic about the future, rate lower in responsibility and leadership, and are more likely to engage in anti-social behavior, such as lying, teasing other children, 'playing hooky,' or 'doing something illegal' " [5]. Warm, readily available models in the form of parents, teachers, and peers who possess skills and characteristics that the child regards as culturally or personally desirable offer the child stable relationships and goals toward which to focus energies while striving for mastery of tasks that lead to higher levels of competence and self-esteem.

Although technology may be calling for different instrumental skills, various alternative interpersonal skills, and the reassessment of priorities, some intrapersonal values remain stable and may indeed assume even greater salience in the new culture. These values are best taught in the home by the example of the parents as they deal with the exigencies of daily life. Five enduring values include [47]: **joy,** the habit of being

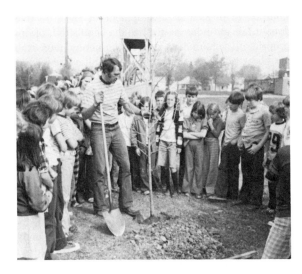

Figure 42–5. Planting a tree often helps to give a child a sense of belonging to the community and a link to the future. (Photograph by Candy Shultz.)

pleased; **love,** the sense of identification with another person; **honesty,** the quality of being able to be trusted; **courage,** the ability to face crisis with optimism; **faith,** something to believe in. Such values transcend cultural change.

Adolescence

The basic needs of adolescents are really not very different from those of younger chlidren; they still need warm, caring parents who continue to serve as role models and continue to respect the need for turn-taking and mutual responsibility in initiating ideas during conversations. However, they also need expanded opportunities to have contact with other adults who model characteristics of career skills that the young person regards as desirable and compatible with his or her unique abilities and interests. They need opportunities to develop skills in preparation for assuming adult roles and responsibilities; this may involve part-time or volunteer work.

Probably one of the most critical tasks of adolescence is the opportunity to develop one's own ideology, values, and roles. Benjamin Spock observes that children who are reared by parents who are sure of their own convictions and ethical standards and who share these values constructively with their children have children who are more considerate, easier to live with, and happier in themselves [41]. There comes a point, however, when individuals must identify their own values as being separate from those of their parents (even though they may end up with an identical value system) if they are to become field-independent. What one believes is central to personal integrity. One must learn to acknowledge and to accept inner feelings as a natural, normal part of life experiences without denial or suppression. These feelings can be important signals to the individual's level of functioning and areas that need attention [7]. It is through attending to one's real feelings and assessing priorities and goals that one's true values begin to be identified. Adolescents often experience conflict with the family as they attempt to prove to themselves and the world that what they believe is not a "warmed-over version borrowed from [the] family" [21].

Eisenberg observes that "At their best, the adolescent years are characterized by the development of idealism and concern for the general welfare. No educational task is more critical than the cultivation of these most human of all qualities by providing experiences to permit their fullest flowering" [10]. Such opportunities can be offered through the Red Cross, scouting, and other organizations. Adolescents thrive

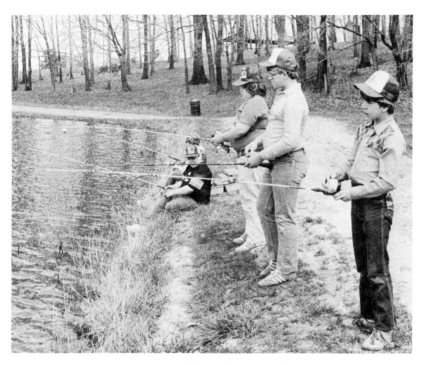

Figure 42–6. Leisure-time activities and attitudes learned during school years are likely to continue into the adult years.

on activities, such as helping younger children to learn to read or play a game; helping disabled children or adults to learn a new skill; beautifying or improving the community; or assisting older persons with letter writing, transportation, or self-help needs. Such activities reduce feelings of alienation, increase feelings of competence and involvement, and provide a constructive outlet for leisure time—all excellent preparations for living in a technologically advanced society [9]. Talbot observes that "One of the basic issues today is the survival of a society in which people are useful to each other, glad to be alive, and of value to themselves" [42].

Young and Middle Adult Years

Happiness, personal peace, or lack of anxiety are often identified as goals during the adult years. But one does not find happiness as an end in itself. True happiness is not the absence of stress but a by-product of a conquered challenge. The experience of some stress is an essential prerequisite. As a person identifies a need and overcomes it through personal efforts, a deep sense of confidence, contentment, and competence ensues—all components of personal peace. Happiness appears to

be the antithesis of helplessness. Happiness (or helplessness and overpowering stress) is most likely to evolve from four situations during the adult years: (1) general personal relationships, (2) employment, (3) personal time, or (4) specific personal relationships.

The potential for conflict is an integral part of any relationship. Differences, however, can be a "positive source of nourishment for the relationship" [7], which can be used for the growth of the individuals involved when both partners of the interaction recognize that they are equally responsible for the outcome of the relationship. Planned or controlled encounters can be painful but can lead to greater authenticity and genuine mutuality, which helps us to appreciate the humanity of each person with whom we have contact [7]. "Game playing" has no place in this type of relationship.

Reich notes that "As the individual is drawn into the meritocracy, his working life is split from his home life, and both suffer from a lack of wholeness" [29]. Many individuals today are rejecting occupations with high financial remuneration and seeking those that provide dignity [31] and allow them to be more fully human [50]. "Money, important as it is to comfortable survival

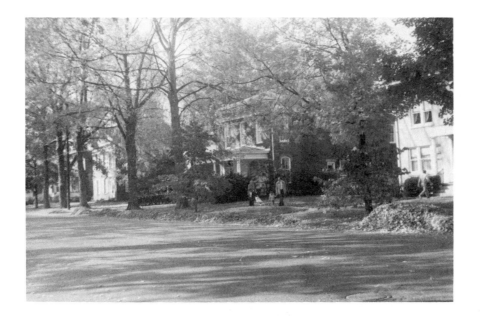

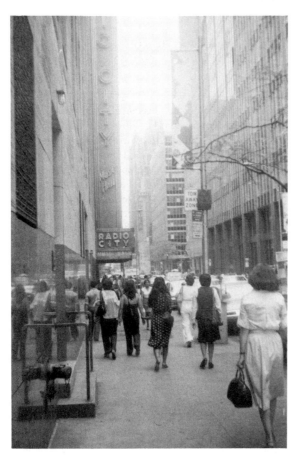

Figure 42–7. The individual's attitudes and pace of life are strongly affected by the community in which he or she resides. The community of origin may differ greatly from the community of residence.

in the modern world, is not an end in itself but a means to an end, and . . . vocational choices should be made on broader bases than just how much a job pays. Life satisfaction derives from doing something constructive that one likes to do and does well" [42]. Stress evolves when employment conflicts with one's values, goals, or priorities. It is easy to get caught up in a "role" imposed by employment, status, or social conventions. A person can literally become a stranger to one's self because so much attention is focused on external constraints rather than internal guidelines.

In a harried world, one may sometimes feel like crying, "Stop the world—I want to get off." This attitude reveals a critical component of reducing stresses. Every individual needs some private time each day in which to reflect, to pursue a hobby, or to unwind in a personal way. Since we can predict the results of "flooding" by sensory or experiential overload, we can also prevent it [26]. Thirty minutes of watching a sunset or a sunrise; praying silently; watching a flight of birds or a snowfall; or listening to quiet music, rain, the muffled sounds of children playing, or the rustle of leaves can allow a person to slow down, to "regroup"—to restore adequate equilibrium to face life's responsibilities once again. Many religions stress the necessity of setting aside a Sabbath day for rest. "Quiet time" allows one to release instrumental values for sacred or expressive ones and to find a deeper meaning and purpose to life [50].

Commitment to a specific personal relationship—to belong to someone—appears to be another critical component in reducing stress. The ability to love appears to be the most critical and fundamental characteristic of happy individuals. Spock observes that an individual who genuinely loves at least one other person is more likely to have a stable, gratifying career, comfortable relationships with other persons, and a good marriage [41]. Maslow defines love based on mutuality as follows: "Two separate sets of needs become fused into a single set of needs for the new unit. Or love exists when the happiness of the other makes me happy, or when I enjoy the self-actualization of the other as much as I do my own, or when the differentiation between the word **other** and the words **my own** has disappeared" [24]. This degree of commitment must not be confused with a fused ego identity. Quite the opposite is true. Each recognizes and values the individuality of the self and the other, but each is so committed to the well-being of the other as well as the self that the concentration of selfish interests is obliterated by genuine concern and caring for the other with the same sensitivity and respect offered to the self.

Family Relationships

In the technological society of today, schools are consolidating, both parents are frequently working and thus are spending less time with their children, and surrogate caretakers are becoming essential to provide child care during parental absence. Families are changing residences, neighborhoods, schools, and friends at alarming rates [5]. This mobility attenuates ties to extended family members and friends, as well as neighborhood commitments. As a result, "the nuclear family has become almost the sole source of affective sustenance. . . . With all our emotional eggs in the nuclear family basket, breakage is both more inevitable and more devastating when it does occur" [10]. The family becomes even more important in a technological age as a refuge from the stressors of life, as a source of stability, and the central focus of fulfillment [20].

Urie Bronfenbrenner suggests that as a society, therefore, we need to support the integrity of the family and to provide opportunities for more and more meaningful relationships between parents and their children [20]. Some suggestions include more flexible work hours (those who have tried it report reduced stress, increased work productivity, and improved family relationships); community family activity centers; easily accessible day care programs that allow parents to visit during the day; opportunities for children to visit the parents' place of employment; and more part-time employment options for parents who wish to spend more time with the family [5].

Alvin Toffler [44] observes that the technological society offers opportunities to improve the quality of family life. With increased use of computers, many people will be able to have a terminal in their own home instead of going to a central office to work. This option translates into financial savings for the business (less office and parking space), and to the individual (transportation and clothing). Reduced transportation also means reduced air pollution. Terminals in the home will allow the adults to set their own working hours and to share the job with each other or even with the children. This can translate into reduced personal stress, increased family cooperation, better role modeling for the children, earlier development of positive work attitudes, and more leisure time [44].

The community can also benefit from an increased community stability. An individual no longer needs to move to the locale of a new job. The computer can hook up with any central location. With increased stability of residence, community commitment and participation will be increased. So while many decry the destructive impact of technology and the development of modular relationships that are frequently and easily fractured (increasing stress and the use of coping skills), Toffler heralds the generative potentials of technological advances.

Studies by Fraiberg and many others support the importance of the family to the developing child—the adult of tomorrow. However, the family is also important to the continued development of its adult members. Chapter 30 emphasized the necessity of choosing one's partner wisely. A good marriage does not just happen; the partners must work hard to maintain the spontaneity, joy, and love of the early months. Mutual respect must be maintained. All of this requires commitment to the conjugal bond and to the other members—commitment that can be eroded by rapid changes in other areas of one's life. One's values, priorities, and goals, then, again become critical in influencing commitments and focusing one's energies. True interdependence and sharing become critical elements in developing this "commitment and the sense of community which underpin love, generosity, and caring" [9]. The family allows for mastery of Erikson's tasks of intimacy and generativity as well as satisfying Maslow's need to love and to belong.

Late Adult Years

Because of the separation of extended family members and the need for small, transportable families in a highly technological era, elderly persons may be widely separated from their own siblings or their children, or both. Consequently, many older adults may feel that they no longer belong; they no longer have anywhere to offer their assistance; they are not needed; and they will have no one to care for them should they need assistance. Some may even die for lack of someone who cares. In short, feelings of alienation may be very acute. When problems do arise, they may be forced to turn to government agencies for aid; this may increase their stress if they value self-reliance and independence and feel that such agencies are only for indigent, disabled, or incompetent persons.

Many communities are resolving this problem by establishing community centers for senior citizens where they can share skills with each other, or more important, actively involve themselves in the welfare of the community through part-time employment services and volunteer programs. Older citizens offer a large untapped source of stability and involvement for communities. Many elderly persons are beginning to assist with tutoring services in the schools or to offer foster grandparent services for children in institutional settings or even to neighbors whose natural grandparents

live too far away to maintain close contact. Others offer their expertise in constructing equipment for Head Start programs, recreational centers, church schools, or neighborhood child care centers.

Many older persons are merely waiting for someone to tell them that they are wanted and needed. **At each age, individuals need to feel wanted, needed, appreciated, and an integral part of the significant suprasystems to which they belong.** The elderly are a national treasure. In recognition of this, Presidential greeting cards are sent (if requested by friend or relative) to persons 80 years of age or more and to couples marking their fiftieth wedding anniversary. Those celebrating their one hundredth birthday are sent a personal presidential letter. (Greeting Office, Room 39, The White House, Washington, DC, 20050)

CONCLUSIONS

We have been discussing fostering individual high level wellness in light of rapidly changing technological advances. Yet the survival of the individual is affected not only by the immediate system of which he or she is a part (the family), but also by the suprasystem in which the family is embedded (the society). It should be clear by now that if change is too severe and too frequent, one's adaptive efficiency is lowered, resulting in both psychological and physiological deterioration. The appropriate experiences during earlier developmental years can help an individual to develop skills in problem solving and value clarification that will lead to greater stability and flexibility. Appropriate challenges and experiences offered during developmental years can increase the coping resources of the individual and result in a firm self-confidence, which immunizes the individual against the helplessness syndrome.

Those who are preparing children to cope with a technological society should be aware that, throughout childhood, children need:

1. To be wanted and loved by warm, caring adults who provide a stable family system
2. To be valued, accepted, and offered respect for personal interests, ideas, needs and talents
3. Stable models with whom to identify
4. Challenges to stimulate the desire to use higher level skills
5. Assistance in mastering age-appropriate skills that foster the development of competence and responsibility.

6. Opportunities to identify and to explore all their feelings—both positive and negative

7. Opportunities to participate in a variety of experiences in order to develop flexibility and a wide continuum of skills

8. Opportunities to organize responsibilities, to establish priorities, and to solve problems and then to live with the consequences

9. Opportunity to belong and to become involved in helping others in order to strengthen their own skills while developing a sense of commitment to others

10. Encouragement to think for themselves—to develop their own standards, values, and goals

Individuals who are offered these experiences during the early developmental years are more likely to develop the characteristics of competence and maturity, as identified by Heath, and the characteristics of

Dennis the Menace

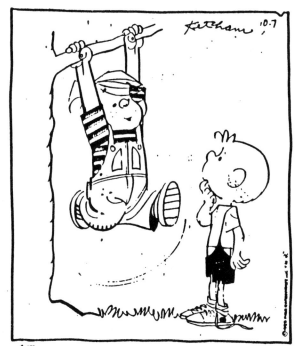

" THE BEST THING YOU CAN DO IS TO GET VERY GOOD AT BEING YOU."

Figure 42–8. *Dennis the Menace.* Copyright used by permission of Hank Ketcham and © by News Group Chicago, Inc.

field-independent individuals as described by Witkin. They are also more likely to be able to integrate their various identities into a stable view of self, as proposed by Erikson. Since they have met lower-level needs, they are freed to expend energies in actualizing their unique potentials, as described by Maslow. They will be prepared to function with relatively little guidance from others and to maintain their own direction in spite of the contradicting attitudes, judgments, and values of others—all of which is excellent preparation for the adult years in a rapidly changing society.

Every person faces challenges and even disasters at some point in life. It is not the situation that creates a tragic life, but the individual's response to the circumstances. Gail Sheehy, in her book *Pathfinders*, documents life stories of persons both famous and unknown who have faced impossible situations, yet have survived not somehow, but triumphantly, to become family, community, and even national leaders. One major key was attitude—the ability, the desire, the commitment to find growth and challenge instead of failure in the most trying circumstances. Through a creative handling of past transitions, an identification of a specific meaning and direction in life, a working toward achievement of long-term goals, and a satisfaction with one's own growth and development, these individuals develop a sense of happiness and well-being that undergirds their lives through transitions as well as life's most tragic accidents [36]. These persons have found the balance between their personal development and the development of others, and it frees them to be more fully themselves. They found a way to "bloom" where they were "planted" in spite of rocky soil or inadequate rain.

Arnold Toynbee observes that: "The material side of life is not an end in itself. It is only a means to an end. I have already shown that I believe that the true purposes of human life are spiritual; surely we ought to try to make machinery our servant for helping us to carry out these spiritual purposes. It will be our master, perhaps, in the sense that we shall have to live in the uncongenial environment of factories and offices in great cities; but, in any environment, we can lead the spiritual life; and this is what man is for" [45]. Victor Frankl [13] made the same observation at the close of World War II: It is not the circumstances, but one's attitude toward them, that give meaning and value to one's life. Humans possess remarkable resiliency. Even the most difficult of circumstances can have a positive outcome [30]. "Man's religion and ethics will once again express the true realities of his way of life: Solidarity with his fellow man, a genuine community representing a balanced moral-aesthetic order, and a continuing expansion of man's inner capacities" [29].

This is the purpose and the challenge of life: To help each person to maximize his or her potentials—to live life not somehow, but triumphantly. Such a goal, however, will be achieved only through self-respect and mutual respect. This means recognition of ourselves as a part of the universe [31] rather than as an autonomous unit: It means creating a niche for ourselves in the social environment, identifying a core value system by which to live, and finding a meaning to life through commitment to values higher than ourselves. Each of us must do our part to create a high-quality life for ourselves and for others, a life which is found by respecting the balance between the rights and the responsibilities of ourselves and others within our various suprasystems.

May you live all the days of your life.
—Jonathan Swift

REFERENCES

1. Anshen, R. N. Introduction. In M. Mead, *Twentieth Century Faith: Hope and Survival.* New York: Harper & Row, 1972.
2. Archer, J. Personal communication, 1977.
3. Beck, A. T. *Cognitive Therapy and The Emotional Disorders.* New York: New American Library, 1979.
4. Brennecke, J. H., and Amick, R. G. *The Struggle for Significance* (3rd ed.). Encino, CA: Glencoe, 1980.
5. Bronfenbrenner, U. The Roots of Alienation. In N. B. Talbot (Ed.), *Raising Children in Modern America: What Parents and Society Should Be Doing for Their Children.* Boston: Little, Brown, 1976.
6. Brown, B. S. Mental health in the future: Politics, science, ethics and values. *Annals of the American Academy of Political and Social Science,* Vol. 408, July 1973.
7. Bugental, J. F. T. Changes in Inner Human Experience and the Future. In S. C. Wallia (Ed.), *Toward Century 21: Technology, Society, and Human Values.* New York: Basic Books, 1970.
8. Dohrenwend, B. S., and Dohrenwend, B. P. Life Stress and Illness: Formulation of the Issue. In B. S. Dohrenwend and B. P. Dohrenwend (Eds.), *Stressful Life Events and Their Contexts.* New Brunswick, NJ: Rutgers University Press, 1984.
9. Douvan, E. The caring society. *Educational Horizons* 57(1):3, 1978.
10. Eisenberg, L. Youth in a changing society. In V. C. Vaughan and T. B. Brazelton (Eds.), *The Family—Can It Be Saved?* Chicago: Year Book, 1976.
11. Ellis, A., and Harper, R. A. *A New Guide to Rational Living.* N. Hollywood, CA: Wilshire, 1979.
12. Fraiberg, S. H. *Every Child's Birthright: In Defense of Mothering.* New York: Bantam Books, 1978.
13. Frankl, V. E. *Man's Search for Meaning: An Introduction to Logotherapy.* Translated by I. Lasch. Boston: Beacon Press, 1962.
14. Freud, S. *New Introductory Lectures on Psycho-analysis.* In Standard Edition, Vol. 22. London: Hogarth Press, 1964.
15. Hall, B. P., and Smith, P. *Development of Conscience: A Confluent Theory of Values.* New York: Paulist Press, 1976.
16. Hartmann, H. *Ego Psychology and the Problem of Adaptation.* Translated by D. Rappaport. New York: International Universities Press, 1958.
17. Heath, D. H. *Maturity and Competence: A Transcultural View.* New York: Gardner Press, 1977.
18. Holmes, T. H., and Masuda, M. "Life Change and Illness Susceptibility." From Symposium on Separation and Depression: Clinical Research Aspects. Chicago: American Association for the Advancement of Science, Annual Meeting, Dec. 26–30, 1970.
19. Holmes, T. H., and Rahe, R. R. The social readjustment rating scale. *J. Psychom. Res.* 11:213, 1967.
20. How will we raise our children in the year 2000? *Saturday Review of Education* 1(2):29, 1973.
21. Kagan, J. The Psychological Requirements for Human Development. In N. B. Talbot (Ed.), *Raising Children in Modern America: What Parents and Society Should be Doing for Their Children.* Boston: Little, Brown, 1976.
22. Lorenz, K. The Enmity Between Generations and its Probable Ethological Cause. In M. W. Piers (Ed.), *Play and Development.* New York: Norton, 1972.
23. Maslow, A. H. *Toward a Psychology of Being* (2nd ed.). Princeton, NJ: Van Nostrand, 1968.
24. Maslow, A. H. A Theory of Human Motivation: The Goals of Work. In F. Best (Compiler), *The Future of Work.* Englewood Cliffs, NJ: Prentice-Hall, 1973.
25. McCamy, J. C., and Presley, J. *Human Life Styling: Keeping Whole in the Twentieth Century.* New York: Harper & Row, 1978.
26. Mead, M. *Twentieth Century Faith: Hope and Survival.* New York: Harper & Row, 1972.
27. Rahe, R., and Arthur, R. Life change patterns surrounding illness experience. *J. Psychosom. Res.* 11:341, 1968.
28. Rahe, R. H. Developments in Life Change Measurement: Subjective Life Change Unit Scaling. In B. S. Dohrenwend and B. P. Dohrenwend (Eds.), *Stressful Life Events and Their Contexts.* New Brunswick, NJ: Rutgers University Press, 1984.
29. Reich, C. A. *The Greening of America.* New York: Random House, 1970.
30. Richardson, G. A., and Kwiatkowski, B. M. Life-span developmental psychology: Non-normative life events. *Hum. Dev.* 24:425, 1981.
31. Rifkin, J. *Entropy.* New York: Viking Press, 1980.
32. Rifkin, J. *Algeny.* New York: Viking Press, 1983.
33. Robinson, J. P. *How Americans Use Time: A Social-Psychological Analysis of Everyday Behavior.* New York: Praeger, 1977.

34. Rokeach, M. *Beliefs, Attitudes, and Values: A Theory of Organization and Change.* San Francisco: Jossey-Bass, 1976.

35. Schaeffer, F. A. *How Then Should We Live? The Rise and Decline of Western Thought and Culture.* Westchester, IL: Crossway Books, 1983.

36. Sheehy, G. *Pathfinders.* New York: Morrow, 1981.

37. Segal, J., and Yahraes, H. Protecting children's mental health. *Child. Today* 7(5):23, 1978.

38. Seligman, M. E. P. *Helplessness: On Depression, Development, and Death.* San Francisco: Freeman, 1975.

39. Selye, H. *Stress Without Distress.* Philadelphia: Lippincott, 1974.

40. Skinner, B. F. *Beyond Freedom and Dignity.* New York: Knopf, 1980.

41. Spock, B. M. *Raising Children in a Difficult Time.* New York: Norton, 1974.

42. Talbot, N. B., and Wells, L. Implications for Action. In N. B. Talbot (Ed.), *Raising Children in Modern America: Problems and Prospective Solutions.* Boston: Little, Brown, 1976.

43. Toffler, A. *Future Shock.* New York: Random House, 1970.

44. Toffler, A. *The Third Wave.* New York: William Morrow, 1980.

45. Toynbee, A. J. *Surviving the Future.* New York: Oxford University Press, 1971.

46. Toynbee, A. J. Technical Advance and the Morality of Power. In G. R. Urban (Ed.), *Can We Survive Our Future? A Symposium.* New York: St. Martin's Press, 1971.

47. Whitman. A. Five enduring values for your child. *Reader's Digest* 118(710):163, 1981.

48. Witkin, H. A., et al. *Psychological Differentiation: Studies of Development.* New York: Wiley, 1974.

49. Wixen, B. N. *Children of the Rich.* New York: Crown, 1973.

50. Yankelovich, D. New rules in American life: Searching for self-fulfillment in a world turned upside down. *Psychology Today* 15(4):35, 1981.

Appendixes

A
Glossary

accommodation: according to Piaget, the creation of a new schema or the modification of an old one in order to differentiate more accurately a behavior or stimulus from already categorized schemata.

adaptation: process of adjusting successfully to new and different conditions.

adolescence: the period of physical, social, and emotional transition between childhood and adulthood (with emphasis on the social and emotional components). Adolescent thought and behavior patterns may continue on into the twenties and thirties or later.

affective domain: encompasses all of one's emotional aspects: feelings, longings, values, motivations, aspirations, frustrations, and identifications; includes one's internal responses to external events.

allocentric: other-centered; concerned about the well-being of other persons (the opposite of egocentric).

alveolus (pl. alveoli): a small, saclike dilation. Pulmonary alveoli are structures in the respiratory system through which gas exchange occurs between inspired air and pulmonary capillary blood. Mammary alveoli are the structures of the female breast that secrete milk.

anomaly: malformation; marked deviation from the expected standard.

aspirate: to inhale, to take a foreign substance into the lungs.

assimilation: according to Piaget, the process whereby stimuli are recognized and integrated into an already existing schema.

attachment: the primary social bond that evolves between an infant and the principal caretaker.

BMR (basal metabolic rate): the rate at which the body uses oxygen and sugar (energy expenditure) under conditions of absolute rest.

behavior: any act that can be observed, described, and measured.

biophysical domain: includes all aspects of the active, interactive physical self, from the genetic, cellular, and chemical levels to the organ and body system levels of functioning.

bonding: emotional reciprocity between two individuals. Particularly used to identify the attachment of the parent to his or her infant.

client: a person who engages the professional services of another; in specific settings is synonymous with patient, student, recipient, etc.

cognition: the process of obtaining knowledge about one's world; the internal manipulation of external or hypothetical events through the use of symbols.

cognitive domain: encompasses all those aspects involved in perceiving, interpreting, organizing, storing, retrieving, coordinating, and using stimuli received from one's internal and external environments.

concept: a thought or abstract idea about a given phenomenon extracted from an individual's experiences and mediated by mental operations; one's comprehension of essential attributes or relationships.

congenital: born with; a condition existing at birth.

contingency: a prerequisite for an event to occur.

crisis: any internal or external event that taxes the coping skills of the individual, or requires a major adjustment in patterns of daily living, or both.

dependency: the extent to which one individual relies on another for his or her existence or level of functioning.

deprivation: the withholding of a need-satisfying stimulation or object.

development: the refinement, improvement, or expansion of a component or skill. The increased differentiation of subsystems with concomitant hierarchical integration.

developmental task: a growth responsibility that arises at a certain time in the life cycle of an individual; the successful accomplishment of a developmental task builds a foundation for potential success in subsequent tasks.

deviation: an alteration in behavior, value, or characteristics that goes beyond predictable and expected normal parameters.

disability: an inability to execute some skill or to perform some function, usually arising from an impairment.

discipline: the process and methods used by adults to guide children toward desired behavior.

drives: energy structures which, by responding to needs, activate physiological processes in appropriate organ systems to eliminate the need and thus secure survival.*

egocentrism: cognitively, the tendency of an individual to think that others see things from the same point of view and experience the same feelings as her- or himself.

electrolyte: a substance dissolved in water that possesses an electric charge.

ethnocentrism: the viewing of life and life-styles through the eyes of one's own social, cultural, and national milieu.

family: a social system comprised of two or more interdependent persons, which remains united over time and serves as a mediator between the needs of its members and the forces, demands, and obligations of society.

fractionalization: refers to the disunity of a family that is brought about by stressors. The stressors may be initially induced by an individual family member, several family members, or the socioaffective or biophysical environment.

gamete: a haploid or "half" cell produced by the male and female reproductive systems for the purpose of procreation of the species (i.e., ovum, sperm).

genotype: the genetic makeup of an individual.

grief: feelings associated with the loss of an object relationship.

growth: the addition of new components or skills.

health: the state of adaptation of a system to its suprasystems and subsystems.

helplessness syndrome: according to Seligman, a psychological state that results when an individual be-

*E. J. Anthony and T. Benedek (Eds.), *Parenthood: Its Psychology and Psychopathology* (Boston: Little, Brown, 1970), p. 168.

lieves or learns that he or she cannot control events; therefore, either no effort or ineffective effort is made to affect one's life events.

high level wellness (high level health): the optimal level of functioning of which a person is capable when total assets and liabilities (powers and loads, strengths and weaknesses) are considered.

holistic: recognizing the individual as a total entity; considering the interdependent functioning of the affective, biophysical, cognitive, and social domains.

hyperplastic cell growth: an increase in the number of tissue cells; increased number of nuclei.

hypertrophic cell growth: an increase in the size of an individual cell; increased amount of cytoplasm.

identification: the process that leads a child to think, feel, and behave as though the characteristics of another person belong to him or her.*

ideology: a systematic body of concepts that includes one's moral principles.

individuation: according to Mahler, the recognition of one's separate identity from that of one's primary caretaker, with the assumption of one's unique affective and social behaviors.

learning: the dynamic process by which systematic changes occur in behavior in response to environmental input.

loss: an acute awareness of being deprived of a desired relationship to a person, object, goal, state, or self.

lunar month: 28 days, or 4 weeks.

maturation: the process of achieving full or optimal development of a component or skill.

maturational crisis: the confrontation of an individual with a developmental task. This process usually evolves gradually over a period of time, but may be resolved during a situational crisis (e.g., learning to walk, transition to adolescence, climacteric).

maximization of potentials: optimal utilization of one's powers or assets in order to keep energy expenditures at a minimum while focusing toward achievement of a goal.

need: a necessity or requirement for an individual's continued growth and development; deprivation thereof leads to signs of disequilibrium.

object relationship: the emotional investment in, or the

significance ascribed to, the things in one's environment—people or objects.

ordinal position: the hierarchical status held by a child within the family system.

parameter: a particular value characterizing the limits of a specific function or population.

peers: one's equals; one's companions or counterparts.

perception: interpretation of a sensory stimulus.

perineal: pertaining to the pelvic floor and the associated structures occupying the pelvic outlet.

personality: the integrated totality of the characteristic habits, attitudes, and ideas of an individual and the distinctive organization of his or her responses to social stimuli.*

phenotype: the characteristics an individual displays for a particular trait based on genetic makeup.

practitioner: any professional person engaged to offer specific services directed toward helping another person to prevent illness, alleviate stress, or maximize potentials in one or more domains. Includes occupations such as minister, lawyer, social worker, nurse, dietitian, teacher, physical therapist, physician, psychologist, etc.

preadolescence (pubescence): the period between childhood and adolescence, marked by physical and emotional transition to adolescence.

proactive: growth producing, adaptive behaviors. Behaviors guided by one's values and goals, which allow the individual to maintain control of personal response systems or environmental events. Opposite of reactive, when the individual exhibits little or no control over personal responses to environmental stimuli or events.

psychosocial: the intrapersonal and interpersonal responses of an individual to external events.

pubertal period: the span of time surrounding puberty when the body undergoes primary and secondary sexual changes that prepare the individual for reproduction.

puberty: that point in time when the individual is first capable of reproduction; the initial production of gametes.

pubescence: see **preadolescence.**

RBC: red blood cells.

reciprocity: interdependence; a complementary inter-

---

*From P. H. Mussen, J. J. Conger, and J. Kagan, *Child Development and Personality* (4th ed.) (New York: Harper & Row, 1974), p. 395.

*From W. C. Smith, *The Stepchild* (Chicago: University of Chicago Press, 1953), p. 202.

change or turn taking; a state of mutual dependence, requiring cooperation and respect.

reflex: a naturally occurring, involuntary, unlearned neuromuscular response to a stimulus.

refueling: a term coined by Furer that describes the young child's attempts to reestablish bodily contact with the primary caretaker in order to restore sufficient affective energy to allow for independent exploration and interaction with the environment.

schema (pl. schemata): according to Piaget, a unit or category of thought; a classification for a phenomenon, behavior, or event.

sensorimotor: those behaviors that involve the combined use of perceptual senses and body movements to bring about interaction with the environment.

sibling: an individual sharing the same parents as the target person.

situational crisis: any event arising from the individual's interaction with the environment that constitutes a stressor. These events usually occur suddenly (e.g., confrontation with authority, illness, natural disaster, separation from significant others).

social domain: includes one's external response to internal and external events; encompasses roles, affiliations, communication styles, adaptive behaviors, and interpersonal relationships.

somatic: pertaining to the body.

sphincter: a ringlike band of muscle fibers that constricts a passage or closes a natural opening.

state 4: the quiet alert, awake state of consciousness found in the neonate and young infant. The child is most attentive to environmental stimuli in this state.

stimulus (pl. stimuli): an event, agent, or action that is perceived through the senses and causes or elicits a response.

stressor: any consciously or unconsciously perceived threat to the integrity of an individual that requires an adaptive response to maintain effective functioning.

subsystem: the components of the target unit of study.

successive approximations: the gradual changing of behaviors toward a desired end behavior. At each step, a higher level of performance (incorporating more aspects of the terminal skill) is acquired until the end behavior is achieved.

suprasystem: any selected unit or group to which the target unit of study belongs.

synthesize: to combine components to form a whole or a total integrated entity.

system: the target unit of study.

trimester: a 3-month period of time, usually connected with the pregnancy process.

variable: a characteristic or value that is subject to change; an arbitrary factor that may or may not affect the functioning of the unit under study.

variation: an alternative behavior, value, or characteristic that is predictable and within normal parameters.

B
Selected Theories of Development

Shirley S. Ashburn

Nothing is so firmly believed as what we least know.

—Michel de Montaigne

Sigmund Freud

Alfred Adler

Erich Fromm

Harry Stack Sullivan

Erik H. Erikson

Carl Rogers

Abraham Maslow

B. F. Skinner

Robert J. Havighurst

Jean Piaget

Human behavior is complex, and the theories proposed to explain it are diverse and, at times, in conflict. It becomes evident in reading selected theorists that there is no ultimate answer that consistently or comprehensively describes human behavior. At best, the available theories give only a partial view of development—explaining a limited domain or only a brief period of the life cycle. However, the authors believe that each of the theorists selected has, in part, something unique and valuable to say about people.

SIGMUND FREUD [1856–1939]

Sigmund Freud offered the first formal theory of personality. His ideas have probably influenced contemporary personality theory more than the thoughts of any other single individual. It is therefore logical to introduce Sigmund Freud and his subject matter first in this brief discussion of theorists and theories.

Freud's concept of personality development, like those of others to be studied, was heavily influenced by his own early childhood experiences. The confidence and pride expressed by Freud's mother is reflected in his lifelong characteristic of an extremely high degree of self-confidence [23]. Freud loved his mother dearly and worked hard to retain her favor. He originally chose medicine as a career because he thought that medical study would help him to attain the personal goal of scientific research. However, after receiving his medical degree at the University of Vienna, Freud lacked the independent income needed to expedite this goal. He therefore established a practice as a clinical neurologist and began to study the personalities of those experiencing emotional disturbances. It was during these years that Freud was greatly influenced by the process of hypnosis, as well as by Dr. Josef Breuer's "talking-cure" method. Using these methods, Freud worked very intensely with his patients and listened carefully as his patients described their childhood experiences. From these situations, he gradually developed a theory about the processes and functions of the individual personality.

As Freud's popularity grew, he attracted many followers (most of whom were physicians), who often met with him weekly. The Nazis considered Freud an "enemy of the state," but it was not until after the arrest of his daughter, Anna, that he fled from Vienna to London. He died in London in 1939, having continued his work almost until his death.

Freud's Major Concepts and Terms

Freud defined "instinct" as the representation in the mind of energy that originates within the body. He viewed this stimulus as being basic to the personality and as the force that drives and gives direction to behavior. Freud's notion of psychic structure organizes the personality into the id, the ego, and the superego (see Chap. 18).

Freud viewed anxiety as the source of neurotic and psychotic behavior. He conceived of three types of anxiety, all differing in their potential threat to the individual. It was his daughter, Anna Freud, who described defense mechanisms, which are viewed as the responses that an individual makes in an attempt to cope with and reduce anxiety (see Chap. 42).

Freud's Concept of Human Growth and Development

Freud believed that a person's unique character develops from the quality of the mother-child interaction. He explained behavior by analyzing the conflicts among instincts, reality, and society. He grouped instincts into two categories: the life instincts and the death instincts. Life instincts are oriented toward growth and development, trying to satisfy the individual's needs for food, water, air, and sex. Freud termed the form of psychic energy manifested by the life instincts as the "libido." He postulated the "aggressive drive" as an important component of the death instinct—the wish to die turned against objects other than the self.

Freud theorized that the development of these life forces follows certain stages, during which the foci or body sites of energy change as the concomitant tasks related to them are mastered. He concentrated on the mouth, anus, and sex organs as these foci. Freud stated that in each stage a conflict exists that must be resolved satisfactorily before the individual can progress to the next stage. He believed that people could become fixated at any stage or any part of these stages and that this fixation would be demonstrated in their adult behavior. Freud's concepts of the life forces' interaction in relation to the id, ego, and superego are referred to throughout this text, and with special emphasis in Chapter 18.

Freud's Technique of Inquiry

Since Freud considered the major motivation force in human life to be the unconscious, he devised free association and dream analysis as his two basic methods of acquiring data. He felt that, in his presence as therapist, relaxed individuals who truly said out loud everything that came to their minds might eventually purify problems from repressed experiences. Freud also believed that the analysis of dreams could unravel unpleasant memories that had long been repressed.

Freud allowed no one else to observe or interpret the data his patients gave him, and this behavior led to much criticism of his theory. Many of his followers modified his theory and thus gave birth to new concepts—their theories follow in the next few pages.

Applicability of Freud's Theory

Experimental psychologists often complain that psychoanalysis is not based on systematic, controlled research. It should be pointed out, however, that most experimental psychologists also disagree with most personality theorists and their various approaches to interpreting human behavior.

Some of Freud's critics feel that people are more strongly shaped by social experiences, with less emphasis on sexual experiences. Others believe that people have more control over their behavior than Freud credits to them. The fact that Freud based his theory on observations of many emotionally crippled individuals is another reason his concepts are not always fully accepted. Another argument is based on the fact that Freud's basic assumptions (e.g., the Oedipal complex) do not appear to have cross-cultural applicability.

Despite all these criticisms, Freud presented a foundation for personality theory that has not been equaled.

His theory can be used in implementing psychotherapy, guiding parent-child relations, and interpreting abnormal behavior.

ALFRED ADLER [1870–1937]

Alfred Adler's concepts of the uniqueness of man represented the first major departure from Freud's theory. Adler emphasized the conscious as being the core of personality. Believing that personality is shaped by one's individual social environments and interactions, he proposed that individuals can actively guide and fashion their own growth and development.

Adler was the second-born of six children of a Viennese merchant. It is easy to assume that Adler drew experiences from his unhappy childhood when he proposed in his theory that a person can compensate for feelings of inferiority. (Adler was unable to run and play with other children because he had rickets. When he was 3 years old, he saw his younger brother die in the bed next to him.) Initially viewed as awkward and unattractive, Adler expended much energy to gain acceptance from his peers. He wanted to increase his sense of worth—a positive feeling he had not attained within his home and family. Adler rose from being considered a mediocre student who should not pursue an academic career to become the best student in the class [23].

After studying medicine at the University of Vienna and after several attempts at various fields of medicine, he entered neurology and psychiatry. Adler worked closely with Sigmund Freud for 9 years; however, their relationship was not a particularly friendly one. After World War I, Adler organized many government-sponsored child counseling clinics in Vienna. He was very busy in the following years, frequently visiting the United States to lecture. It was on a lecture tour that he succumbed to a heart attack in 1937 [23].

Adler's Concepts and Terms

Adler believed that inferiority feelings are ever-present in humans and are the stimulus for growth. He felt that a person could compensate for either imagined or real inferiorities. Adler proposed that a person could develop an "inferiority complex" or "an inability to solve life's problems" (1) by being organically inferior, (2) by being spoiled and then having to meet rejection, or (3) by being neglected. He believed that people strive for "superiority" or "perfection" and are always seeking improvement. This quest for superiority increases tension and thus calls forth more efforts. Adler also believed that the best situation for making these efforts was that of a self-reliant individual working cooperatively with others within his culture [2].

Adler's Emphasis on Human Growth and Development

Adler believed that each individual cultivates a unique pattern of striving for superiority; that is, every person formulates a life-style or character. This life-style is learned from early parent-child interactions. Adler postulated that one's life-style is firmly set by early childhood [1]. Even the very young, he said, are free to interpret their experiences. An individual may choose to change in later years only if it is realized that inappropriate and disturbing responses are inadequate "holdovers" from childhood [2]. Adler believed that getting along with others is the first task one encounters in life; this way of coping becomes a basis for later behavior. He also proposed birth order as one of the major social factors in one's childhood that affects the type of life-style one chooses.

According to Adler, all individuals must solve three categories of problems during their lifetime—problems involving behavior toward others, problems of occupation, and problems of love. He spoke of four basic styles that people use in working through these problems—avoidance, expecting to get everything from others, dominating others, and cooperating with others by acting in accordance with their needs [23].

Adler's Techniques of Inquiry

Adler developed this theory from information he gained in informal conversations with his patients. He paid particular attention to body language (the expression of feelings or thoughts by means of bodily movements). Adler also gained information from his patients, and thus for his theory, by assessing their order of birth and their dreams, and by asking them to recall their first memories of childhood [17].

Some criticize Adler's theory for its simplicity; others state that he was not always systematic and that he left many questions unanswered. There are also those who question how a child less than 5 years of age can choose his or her own life-style.

Alfred Adler's theory has become most applicable to school guidance counseling, penal reform, psychosomatic medicine, and individual psychology.

ERICH FROMM [1900–1980]

Like Adler, Erich Fromm is often referred to as a social-psychological theorist. He viewed an individual's personality as influenced more by culture than by biological forces. Fromm maintained the optimistic view that human beings possess the ability to solve the very problems they have created.

It has been written that Fromm's father was prone to being moody and anxious and that his mother was often afflicted by depression [23]. When Fromm was 12 years of age, a family friend committed suicide; Fromm could not understand why such a lovely and talented person would do such a thing. Several other tragedies (both cultural and individual) also had a profound effect on Fromm—especially the hate, human slaughter, and arrogance of World War I.

Although he never became a Party member, Fromm subscribed to socialist ideas. His quest for righting social conditions led him to become most familiar with the works of Karl Marx, Max Weber, and other political leaders. Although he underwent psychoanalytic training, Fromm later criticized Freud's theory because it did not recognize the effect of socioeconomic forces on personality. Many of Fromm's books are so popular that they have reached best-seller status.

Fromm's Major Concepts and Terms

Fromm asserted that people are free of the "instinctive biological mechanisms" that dictate the behaviors of lower animals on the phylogenetic scale. He believed that humans are gifted with reason and that an individual has an awareness of self, fellow human beings, the past, and the possibilities of the future [9].

Fromm also contended that people today have more freedom than mankind has ever had. This powerful freedom, he said, causes them to experience feelings of loneliness, insignificance, and alienation. The basic needs of humans, therefore, are to discover meaning in life, to develop a sense of belonging, and to avoid feelings of isolation.

Fromm postulated mechanisms of escape that people use to regain lost security, ranging from destroying others in order to obtain power to losing one's self-identity by surrendering to total conformity. He also proposed the existence of "character traits," the forces that underlie all behavior, by which a person relates the self to the world.

Fromm's Concept of Human Growth and Development

Fromm believed that all human beings are born with an inherent set of psychological qualities by which they can shape their personalities. He concluded that the person who fails to realize his or her positive potentialities toward justice and truth will have unhappiness and mental illness as an outcome [9].

Fromm also contended that as a child grows and develops, he will gain increasing freedom and independence. Loss of security is experienced as this freedom grows, and the child then attempts to regain this security, using one of the escape mechanisms conceived by Fromm. The nature of the parent-child relationship determines which mechanism the child employs.

The child who uses "symbiotic relatedness" never becomes an independent person. Instead, the child "becomes a part of someone else" and either remains totally dependent on the parents by submitting to their every wish (resulting in masochism) or is allowed to manipulate the parents to the point of exploitation (resulting in sadism). The child who chooses Fromm's "withdrawal-destructiveness" mechanism will be a person who maintains distance from others. To do this, Fromm said, the child will either passively withdraw or aggressively destroy, depending on the parental behavior with which the child identifies [9].

"Love" is the third, and most desirable, form of parent-child interaction. The individual who as a child experiences opportunities to develop in an environment that promotes respect and a balanced ratio of security and responsibility will become a person who can love the self as well as others. Fromm stressed that the significant person (or persons) in a child's life must have faith in the child's potentials [9].

Fromm agreed with Freud in identifying the first 5 years of life as crucial to personality development, but he did not hold that the personality is firmly fixed by that time. He believed that later events can be just as effective in influencing an individual's personality. Reaction to these later events is, in part, prescribed by the culture in which one lives.

Fromm's Techniques of Inquiry

Compared to the other psychoanalysts discussed thus far, Fromm wrote little about how or from where he received his data. He did use free association and strongly believed in the importance of dream analysis.

Applicability of Fromm's Theory

Fromm obviously pulled knowledge from several disciplines to compose his theory; this is perhaps why critics with expertise in only one discipline attack only a part of his theory and do not criticize it in totality. As mentioned previously, Fromm did not reveal any specific supportive data, which left him open to criticism. Many theorists and some readers felt that Fromm should have recognized the current developments of the humanistic psychologists (those who assume that people are motivated toward autonomy and self-reliance) in his publications. Fromm's books, however, have attained worldwide popularity. He purposely wrote his books for the lay audience, because he believed they are the target population to reach if we are to learn about ourselves and how we must cope in today's world.

Fromm has certainly conveyed the idea that mankind is a capable entity composed of individuals who have great potential for conquering social problems.

HARRY STACK SULLIVAN [1892–1949]

Harry Stack Sullivan's conception of personality is a unique blend of biology, sociology, psychiatry, and social psychology. He believed that an individual should be studied only in terms of interactions with others. He did not feel that one's personality is firmly fixed during the preschool years; he conceived that personality could change greatly until and during the adolescent years.

After Sullivan's family moved to a New York farm when he was 3 years old, his closest "friends" were the farm animals. The Sullivans were the only Roman Catholic family in a Yankee Protestant community, and he was the only surviving child in his immediate family—he apparently knew loneliness from early childhood. One of Sullivan's close friends claims that Sullivan was finally able to establish a comfortable relationship with his father in Sullivan's adult years only after his mother died [16].

Sullivan is reported to have felt very "out of place" during his school years and to have had a traumatic adolescence. During his early twenties, when he was in medical school, he studied psychoanalysis and entered into it as a patient. Later, as an executive medical officer in a rehabilitation division of the Federal Board for Vocational Education, he became interested in working with individuals with neuropsychiatric conditions; he especially wanted to know what kept the neurotic from becoming schizophrenic. Sullivan believed that the cultural environment greatly shapes a person's personality. Studying patients' behavior as a psychiatrist both in hospital settings and in his private office, he focused on their interpersonal relations.

Sullivan's Major Concepts and Terms

Personification was Sullivan's term for a group of related attitudes, feelings, and concepts about oneself or another that have been acquired from extensive experience. He referred to "experience" as events that the individual participates in and that become more distinct and ordered during development [22].

Sullivan identified three ways of experiencing the world around us—three levels of thinking by which a person relates to others, called the **prototaxic, parataxic,** and **syntaxic** experiences. These various perceptions range from simply perceiving sensations immediately as they occur to learning logical relationships and being able to test one's perceptions against those possessed by others (refer to Chaps. 9 and 12).

Sullivan's Concept of Human Growth and Development

Sullivan focused on the individual as a product of the interpersonal environment. Like many other theorists, he believed that development of the self is sequential with the individual's accumulating significant experiences [25]. Sullivan thought that the juvenile era (see the list below) was the first developmental stage in which the limitations and peculiarities of the home as a socializing agent began to be open for remedy. If the limitations of the home were not remedied during this time, he thought, subsequent development might be warped [16]. He stressed that tension and anxiety arise from a person's interaction with the environment. He also believed that the individual consists relatively equally of rational cognitive processes and irrational emotional processes.

Sullivan divided the life cycle as follows:

1. Infancy lasts to the maturation of the capacity for language behavior.
2. Childhood lasts to the maturation of the capacity for getting along with peers (until about 5 or 6 years of age).
3. The juvenile era lasts to the maturation of the capacity for "isophilic intimacy" (Sullivan's term for affection or liking for others of the same sex, such affection lacking the genital element characteristic of homosexuality), until about 9 or 10 years of age.
4. Preadolescence lasts to the maturation of the "genital lust dynamisms," i.e., "chumships" or the "first reciprocal love relationship" (from about 10 or 11 to 13 years of age).
5. Early adolescence lasts to the maturation of the patterning of lustful behavior (until the age of about 17 years).
6. Late adolescence lasts to maturity (until the early twenties) [25].

During a person's early twenties, Sullivan says, if all positive components of his theory have been met by the individual, then the individual is ready to take a place as a full-fledged member of society [23].

Sullivan's Techniques of Inquiry

Although he used some dream analysis, Sullivan gained most of his data from his patients through interviews. His interviewing approach was unique in that he believed that as the therapist he should be both a participant and an observer. This approach led to a lengthy series of interviews involving significant interpersonal interactions.

Applicability of Sullivan's Theory

Very little criticism of Sullivan's theory exists. Perhaps part of the reason for this is that most of his works were lectures and papers published posthumously; these unsystematic works have not led to much research or critique of his theory. Nevertheless, his emphasis on working with an individual's potentials and his methods of treatment of individuals experiencing schizophrenia are becoming widely admired. Areas in which Sullivan's theory can be of great value are psychotherapy, interpersonal communication, parent-child relations, and education.

Sullivan collaborated with many scientists and devoted much of his time and energy to international affairs in the pursuit of world peace. Dr. Charles S. Johnson, then President of Fisk University, made the following remark at memorial services for Sullivan: "[Sullivan was the] hope of understanding and controlling the group tensions and international conflicts by which our civilization is now so darkly endangered" [25]. Patrick Mullahy, a noted author and psychiatrist, has stated his belief that "in the history of modern psychiatry, Sullivan will be ranked second only to Freud" [16].

ERIK H. ERIKSON [1902–   ]

Erik Erikson was trained by Sigmund Freud's daughter, Anna Freud. He augmented Freud's theory by adding culture and society (in addition to biological forces) as factors that influence personality development. Erikson also believes, unlike Freud, that personality continues to develop through the life cycle. Unlike most other psychoanalysts, Erikson has made special efforts to have experiences with children who were not emotionally disturbed as well as with those who were.

Erikson's career has been most diverse. He was born of Danish parents in Frankfurt, Germany. His father died soon after his birth, and his mother later married a pediatrician who had cured young Erikson of a childhood illness. Because his stepfather adopted him, some of Erikson's early papers are written under the name Homberger. Later, when he became an American citizen in 1939, he chose to be known by his original name [13].

Erikson, who coined the term **identity crisis,** apparently experienced several such crises during his younger years. For example, he was not told for several years that Homberger was not his biological father. Erikson later labeled this situation as one of "loving deceit." Erikson was rejected by his peers both at school and at synagogue; his German classmates rejected him because he was Jewish, and his Jewish friends rejected him because his appearance, that of a tall, blond Dane, caused him to look very unlike the rest of them [23].

After achieving only mediocre grades in school, Erikson "dropped out" of society. He made two attempts at attending art school during that period, but each time he chose to leave and resume his wandering throughout Germany and Italy (he says that he spent his time "neurotically" reading, recording his thoughts in a notebook, and observing the life around him) [23].

At the age of 25, Erikson began his professional career. He accepted an invitation to teach at a small school in Vienna that had been established for the children of Sigmund Freud's patients and friends. At this time he received training in psychoanalysis that was conducted by Anna Freud, and her special interest in the psychoanalysis of children became his as well.

Erikson later settled in Boston and set up a private practice specializing in the treatment of children [23]. In 1936 Erikson accepted an invitation from the Institute of Human Relations at Yale University to teach. It was at Yale that he and an anthropologist focused their studies on the ways children were reared among the Sioux Indians of South Dakota. This study affected Erikson's thoughts on the influence of culture on childhood events. He noticed symptoms related to a feeling of being alienated from one's cultural customs that resulted in an unclear, confused self-image or identity; he noted similar symptoms when he observed emotionally disturbed World War II veterans who had experienced crisis-filled war situations. Erikson called this phenomenon "identity confusion," a concept that could not be described or applied while using only Freudian theory.

Erikson taught both at the Institute of Child Welfare at the University of California at Berkeley and at Harvard University before he retired in 1970. At this writing, Erikson continues to be involved in psychohistorical analyses that explain the role of identity confusion in the lives of influential persons.

Erikson's Major Concepts and Terms

Erikson is concerned with psychosocial development, or human development viewed in terms of its dependence on interaction with others. He views experience as feeding into ego-identity, the synthesis of accumulated experiences of the individual's view of self. He defines eight stages of growth for humans, each stage being a crucial period of development. Simultaneously, within each developmental phase, two opposing forces cause a crisis and demand a solution. Erikson defines successful resolution as giving one the opportunity to advance to the next of his "eight stages of man." He sees failure or delay as an obstacle to the optimal development of the individual. However, an unsuccessful resolution may be resolved later in life under positive circumstances.

Erikson's Concept of Human Growth and Development

Unlike Freud, Erikson believes that an individual's social view of self is more important than libidinal urges. Erikson's relatively more optimistic outlook on human growth and development also speaks to new opportunities for particular strengths to develop at each stage. These "basic virtues" emerge only when each crisis is met and must be continuously upheld throughout a person's lifetime to be useful. The reader should refer to Appendix C to review Erikson's stages of the life cycle; they are discussed throughout the chapters in this text.

Erikson's Techniques of Inquiry

Erikson holds that no one technique of data collection can be applied in the same way to every subject. Instead, he believes the technique should be highly individualized. His techniques varied from watching children play with toys to being a participant-observer among Indian tribes. He is well known for his psychohistorical approach to prominent people. Using what he calls "disciplined subjectivity," he attempts to incorporate other people's perceptions of their own lives as his own so that he can better explain how they dealt with various crises in their lives.

Erikson's works are sometimes criticized because he has not defined some of his concepts (e.g., fidelity, hope) well enough for further research. There are also those who disagree with Erikson's concept of "identity" as applied to women; these critics, in contrast to Erikson, suggest that women do not attain identity until after marriage. (On the other end of the continuum, it is interesting that today many married women wish to maintain their maiden names so they will not lose their identity!)

Applicability of Erikson's Theory

Erikson is a very influential theorist. His developmental framework offers a guide to rearing and understanding children. His theory is also applied in psychotherapy, psychiatry, education, and the psychoanalytic meaning of moral responsibility.

CARL ROGERS [1902–   ]

Carl Rogers is known to many as the creator of client-centered psychotherapy. He prefers to refer to his patients as "clients" and believes that each of them possesses both the ability and the responsibility to improve his or her personality. He views his role as therapist as being one of facilitator, not director, of such change.

Rogers' theory reflects his ideas about how the therapy is implemented: He sees humans as rational beings who are guided by their conscious world. Although he accepts the hypothesis that past experiences of childhood can affect adult perception, he recognizes a person's present feelings and emotions as being more significant in influencing the growth of personality. A basic tenet of his theory is that an individual's perception of experience must be understood, whether or not it is in concert with reality. He promotes the concept of actualization of the self as being an individual's ultimate goal.

Rogers discloses that he spent much of his time as a boy in the world of fantasy and solitude. He loved to read any book he could find, including the dictionary and the encyclopedia. When he was 12 years of age, Rogers' family moved to a farm, providing him with new and rich experiences in nature and science. He later chose to study agriculture at the University of Wisconsin. It is also understandable, in view of his religious family background, that at a later time he transferred the focus of his studies from scientific agriculture to the ministry.

It was at this time that he was selected to attend a World Student Christian Federation Conference in China. As a result of these travels, he departed from the beliefs of his early family teachings and became very liberal. This action on his part also remained in his mind and became the foundation of his theory of personality—that an individual must depend on his experiences as the best guide.

In the years to follow, Rogers became interested in

clinical and educational psychology. He made many worthwhile contributions to the care of emotionally disturbed, underprivileged, and delinquent children. Having received several awards and honors, he is currently a Fellow at the Center for Studies of the Person in La Jolla, California.

Rogers' Major Concepts and Terms

Rogers maintains that people are born with a major motivation: a tendency to "actualize," that is, to develop all abilities and potentialities, from the strictly biological to the most sophisticated psychological aspects. Rogers believes that all living things (including plants and animals) possess this actualizing tendency. He asserts very positively that even under the most threatening and hostile conditions an organism can not only survive, but adapt to grow and develop. This actualization trait does more than just keep the individual alive; it also encourages improvement of the whole organism.

Experience, Rogers believes, is the best stimulus to growth. He sees the end product of psychological development and social evolution as evidenced by a person's "awareness of all experiences"—whether they are regarded as positive or negative by the beholder. He labels such an individual "the fully functioning person."

Rogers' Concept of Human Growth and Development

Rogers asserts that although a person's biological changes (and some psychological changes) are genetically determined, the individual's progress is often one of struggle. The tendency to grow, he adds, is much stronger than any urge to regress. Rogers writes that higher levels of development increase the meaning of one's experiential world and, in doing so, lead to the formation of the "self."

Rogers states that as an infant develops an experiential field, a self-concept emerges that consistently searches for congruence among the person's images of what he or she is, what he or she should be, and what he or she might like to be. At this time, the infant develops a need for "positive regard." Found in all human beings, it is a need for acceptance, love, and approval.

Next, the infant develops a concept of "conditions of worth," viewing the self as worthy only under certain conditions. From this experience, the individual learns to reward or punish the self.

Rogers conceives of the fully functioning person as one who can live fully and richly each and every moment. He goes on to say that such an individual trusts the judgment of the self. Rogers states that the self-actualizing person is continually growing and changing, which obviously involves much trial and challenge.

Rogers' Techniques of Inquiry

The only way to study and to understand personality, Rogers firmly believes, is through studying the individual's experiential field. He says that this means acceptance of clients "as they are for what they are." He is most opposed to free association, psychological testing, and case histories; all these, he says, make the therapist too threatening to the client. He did, however, introduce tape recording and video filming of sessions. The data for his theory come from his therapy sessions as well as from research on the therapy process itself.

Applicability of Rogers' Theory

Rogers' concepts promote the importance of one's self-concept. Criticisms of his theory are directed at (1) his failure to offer an exact definition of a person's innate, predetermined abilities, and (2) his principle that the only way to study personality is through understanding what are supposed to be an individual's subjective perceptions.

His approach to therapy and his theory have been met with much enthusiasm by those who favor an optimistic view of humanity. His works have wide relevance to sensitivity training, encounter groups, psychology, education, and family life research.

ABRAHAM MASLOW [1908–1970]

Abraham Maslow is renowned for his contributions to humanistic psychology. Maslow believed that in order to determine the apex of human potential, he had to study what he considered to be the very best representatives of the species. He diligently studied a large group of personalities, some of whom were no longer living (e.g., case histories of Abraham Lincoln and Thomas Jefferson) in order to extract what he believed to be the salient factors for successful development.

Born of Russian Jewish immigrant parents who wanted their son to rise above their lot in life, Maslow unhappily maintained his minority group status throughout his childhood. Out of loneliness he began to read, and he perceived that learning would pave the way out of the Brooklyn ghetto into which he had been born. He said that he wanted to study "everything"! At the University of Wisconsin, he received training from Harry Harlow (working with behaviorism and experiments with monkeys). It was also during this time that he married his fiancée of 4 years. (He proclaimed that it was only with his marriage and entry to the University of Wisconsin that his life began.) He attributed the birth of his first child as the culminating force that pulled him away from behaviorism ("I was stunned by the mystery and by the sense of not really being in control") and thrust him toward the development of his humanistic theory. A deeply sensitive man, Maslow was so disturbed by World War II that he dedicated himself to improving the human condition. In addition to engaging in research at several institutions of higher learning, he also formulated a political, economic, and ethical philosophy (with an obvious humanistic psychology base) while working under a foundation grant at Brandeis.

Maslow's Major Concepts and Terms

Maslow proposed a hierarchy of needs that must be met by each individual in order to reach his or her potentials. Those forces motivating development in the first stages must be satisfied before the forces of the next stage can become the focus. However, one stage (or need) does not have to be fully conquered before the next sequential one is undertaken. Partial satisfaction of needs will allow the person to work on the next stage, but with a decreasing percentage of satisfaction in each need as a person climbs the hierarchy. However, only one of these needs can be dominant at a time.

At the bottom of Maslow's hierarchy, the physiological needs assume priority. Once these needs have been satisfied, safety needs become the focus. Next in importance are the needs for "belongingness" and love, followed by the need for esteem. Potentials are realized when the final stage of self-actualization is reached. After reaching this stage, the individual must continue to "be" or to be actively engaged in "doing one's thing"; otherwise, that person's potentials will cease to be fully utilized. Obviously, several prerequisites exist that enable a person to attain or to maintain a state of self-actualization; among these are freedom from either self-restraints or cultural restraints and the individual's realistic assessment of self.

Maslow estimated that only 1 percent or less of the population ever become self-actualizing individuals. He postulated that self-actualization, although an innate need, cannot be universal, because the other four needs in his hierarchy are hard to meet in a poverty-stricken,

emotionally deprived environment. He also believed that the hierarchy does not apply to all individuals, because some people may become satisfied with meeting lower-level needs.

Maslow's Concept of Human Growth and Development

Maslow stated that because any individual's "inner nature is good or neutral rather than bad, it is best to bring it out and to encourage it rather than to suppress it" [15]. Although he emphasized the important influence of early childhood on later development, he did not believe that a person was a slave to his past. He felt, for example, that excessive freedom in childhood could lead to an insecure adulthood. What Maslow termed "freedom within limits" was the correct equation for laying the foundation for a potentially self-actualizing person. He also stressed that satisfaction of basic needs was crucial within the first 2 years of life if a child was to become a secure adult (the need for safety being strongest, he said, during the infant years). Maslow pointed out that most normal adults still require some degree of security.

Maslow also believed that the need to know and to understand begins in late infancy and in childhood. Inhibiting a child's curiosity could, he said, retard the child's development of a fully functioning personality. He made many statements about the tasks a healthy child must accomplish (although he did not arbitrarily attach these tasks to any age groups)—he said that a child "must give up being good out of fear" and rather should be good because he wants to be. He also said that the child "must become responsible rather than dependent, and hopefully must become able to enjoy this responsibility" [15].

Maslow's Techniques of Inquiry

Maslow concluded that self-actualizing people possess a common pattern of personal characteristics. In his search for these characteristics in others, he soon decided that college students in Western culture had not yet developed traits that could be labeled as self-actualizing. After studying middle-aged and older individuals, he concluded that very few people attain that stage of his hierarchy. To study the subjects whom he thought self-actualized, Maslow explained that he used any available technique that appeared to be appropriate; the techniques ranged from analyzing biographical sketches of deceased individuals to administering the Rorschach ink blot test to those persons still living.

Applicability of Maslow's Theory

Maslow's concern for humanity was evident from his writings and from the dedication of his life. Maslow realized that critics would be skeptical of his lack of systematic research in forming his theory. (His reply was that since the problem could not have been studied by rigorous scientific procedures, the only alternative would have been not to study it at all [23].) The fact that Maslow claimed that self-actualization is an innate need has also been questioned.

It goes without saying that Maslow's theory has prompted more research on the problems of realizing human potential. His theory has become immensely popular among the young, among psychologists, and among the educated public. Sensitivity training group sessions make use of his ideas. There are even heads of business who incorporate Maslow's concepts as a way of increasing employee drive.

B. F. SKINNER [1904–   ]

The reader might wonder why B. F. Skinner, a controversial theorist who does not speculate on (or consider very important) the topic of personality, is included in this section of the text. The answer is that not only has his viewpoint been extremely productive of research, but his attempt to account for all human behavior strictly in terms of what can be observed remains a strong force in psychology today. Skinner does not believe that a person is controlled by any innate or inner conscious drive; he says that the only way to predict and control behavior is by correlating the person's behavior with what is occurring in the person's environment.

It would appear that many events in Skinner's adult life (as well as basic concepts in his theory) were founded in his childhood experiences. He was born in Susquehanna, Pennsylvania, to a family that administered continuous admonitions about what God, other people, and the police might think about his actions. As a child he loved animals and the study of animal behavior. He later even taught pigeons to play Ping-Pong [23].

Skinner enjoyed school so much that he was usually the first to arrive each day. Later, while majoring in English at Hamilton College in New York, he became disenchanted with many different facets of the collegiate scene—sports (in which he did not excel), curriculum requirements (he did not feel that any were necessary), and his fellow students (he thought they

lacked academic motivation). His discontent grew, as did his mischievous pranks. At one point he was cautioned that he would have to behave during his commencement exercises if he wished to graduate (it would appear that he had already established his pattern of not really caring if he was considered different by others). After graduation, his intention and desire were to become a writer. Although he constructed a study in his parents' attic, he soon found that he used his time in that room for everything, it seemed, except writing—listening to the radio, building ship models, and, eventually, wondering if he needed to see a psychiatrist. He moved to Greenwich Village in New York City and later toured Europe. During this time he decided that he himself had "nothing to write" but that he still wanted to understand human behavior. Inspired by the writings of Pavlov and Watson, he entered Harvard graduate school to study psychology. By adhering to an extremely rigid schedule, he completed his doctoral studies in three years.

Skinner's Major Concepts and Terms

Skinner displayed little interest in the individual person; he was searching for general laws of human behavior in terms of stimulus and response. He accounted for differences in human behavior by saying that experiences evoke varying responses, or reinforcement value. He views the human being as a machine that always operates according to fixed laws. Very simply, he states that all behavior can be controlled. It is the kind and the extent of reinforcement that follows a behavior that determines if that behavior will be repeated.

Skinner identifies two kinds of behavior—"respondent" and "operant." Respondent behavior occurs when a response is elicited by a known and specific stimulus. Respondent behaviors can be simple, as in the initiation of a reflex action, or learned, such as those behaviors involved in conditioning. Operant behaviors are those that are emitted in order to obtain a response or reinforcement from the environment or from other persons.

Skinner's Concept of Human Growth and Development

Skinner believes that beginning in infancy, selected human behaviors become reinforced in such a way that they form patterns. These patterns of behavior are referred to as "personality" by Skinner (it must be noted that he discusses this concept infrequently, because he believes it is of no relative significance [3]).

Since Skinner believes that all aspects of behavior are controlled from without and that a person is a product of past reinforcements, it follows that his thoughts on child-rearing deal with manipulating a child's environment so that certain behaviors will be reinforced at certain intervals over a period of time. He does believe that, later in life, people can control their futures by controlling their environments.

Skinner's Techniques of Inquiry

Skinner's methods of research are extremely different from those of the other theorists mentioned in this section: First, he derived his theories from studies of animals. Rationalizing that all behavior follows the same laws, he reasoned that animals and humans are alike (the only difference being that humans can learn to control not only themselves but the environment as well). In addition, Skinner chose to study one subject at a time. He believes that since all behavior is guided by the same rules, any information gained can be applied to all animals (including humans). He made use of an operant conditioning apparatus that has come to be known as a "Skinner box." Using this apparatus, the experimenter can control subject behavior by limiting stimuli and controlling the reinforcement schedule.

Applicability of Skinner's Theory

Although application of Skinner's theory is readily apparent in many areas, his approach has been censured, especially by humanistic critics. He is criticized especially for his generalization of animal research to human beings. However, one must note that his theory has been effectively used with members of every phylogenetic level, including humans (even gifted adults). Many find the concept of human behavior being totally controlled by external forces as dehumanizing and threatening. Others claim that Skinner's theory is derived from unscientific, broad generalizations. Nevertheless, he remains an influential force in psychology. His principle of operant conditioning has led the way to effective use of behavior modification in classrooms, prisons, and residential and mental institutions, and even in the home by parents.

Skinner maintains that he cannot be bothered by his critics (who, he says, do not understand him) and that his research proves that humans can make the world a better place in which to live through systematic alteration of the environment. After having taught in several universities, Skinner is now Professor Emeritus of Psychology at Harvard University.

ROBERT J. HAVIGHURST [1900–   ]

No text that discusses human growth and development would be complete without mention of Robert Havighurst's concept of developmental tasks. He did not originate the concept of developmental tasks, but rather identified those tasks he felt are critical to healthy development. Havighurst believes that "living in a modern society is a long series of tasks to learn, where effective learning will bring satisfaction and reward; while learning poorly brings unhappiness and social disapproval" [11]. Havighurst says that he was greatly influenced by Erikson's theory of psychosocial development, and especially by his publications on adolescence and identity [11].

Havighurst's Major Concepts and Terms

Havighurst defines a developmental task as "the task which arises at or about a certain period in the life of the individual, successful achievement of which leads to his happiness and to success with later tasks, while failure leads to unhappiness in the individual, disapproval by the society, and difficulty with later tasks" [11]. He adds that such a task is midway between an individual need and a social demand.

Some developmental tasks arise primarily because of physical maturation (e.g., learning to walk). Others arise mainly from the cultural pressure of society (e.g., learning to read). Still another source of developmental tasks, according to Havighurst, is the personal values and goals of the individual. He believes that by 3 or 4 years of age, the individual's personality is active in identifying and mastering developmental tasks.

Havighurst states that there may be critical periods in the development of an individual when the organism is maximally receptive to specific stimuli. He therefore places many of his tasks at what he deems critical points, or "teachable moments." He does point out that some tasks are recurrent through life (e.g., "learning to get along with age-mates").

Havighurst's Concept of Human Growth and Development

Havighurst summarized and discussed the principal developmental tasks of six age periods, each period, in turn, containing six to ten developmental tasks. The reader will find his developmental tasks listed in Appendix C.

Havighurst's Techniques of Inquiry

Havighurst gained much of his insight and formed many of his concepts while studying growth and development in the academic world and while working under the auspices of the General Education Board at the Rockefeller Foundation. He also profited from associations with other well-known theorists.

Applicability of Havighurst's Theory

Havighurst's developmental task concept "occupies middle ground between the two opposing theories of education: the theory of freedom—that the child will develop best if left as free as possible, and the theory of constraint—that the child must learn to become a worthy, reponsible adult through restraints imposed by his society" [11].

There are those who criticize the way Havighurst divides the life cycle (especially his inclusion of so many significant developmental milestones in just one period—infancy and early childhood). His tasks are limited to what he calls the American culture, and although at times he speaks to the different foci emphasized by various socioeconomic levels, he still adheres for the most part to middle-class norms. Some critics feel that his work is outdated in parts; for example, he describes early adulthood as a time to marry and rear children (not everyone today has a similar goal), and he speaks of middle-aged people as strengthening their occupational associations (many "occupationally mobile" people in this age group today leave one job for another, and the types of work may be completely unrelated and in different fields).

Regardless of these criticisms, Havighurst's ideas have proved useful to many people who seek a general understanding of development in American culture. Havighurst is currently a professor of education and human development and a member of the Committee on Human Development at the University of Chicago.

JEAN PIAGET [1896–1980]

Jean Piaget was one of the most influential contemporary psychologists. The works written by Piaget and his associates (originally in French) center on the cognitive development of childhood. Piaget's concepts have been adopted especially by those who respect humans as thinking organisms interacting with their environment. Piaget is especially interested in **how** the mind works, rather than in **what** it does [18].

Piaget was born in 1896 in Neuchatel, Switzerland. He said that his intelligent parents influenced him in several ways to study both psychology and genetic epistemology (study of how knowledge is acquired). Piaget recalled that his scholarly father stirred him to ask questions and to explore at an early age. The 10-year-

old Piaget published his first scholarly paper, which described a partially albino sparrow he had observed in a public park [26]. By the age of 15, he had decided to study knowledge as an entity in itself and to explain it biologically. Piaget said that his mother's neurosis initially encouarged him to question psychoanalysis and pathological psychology, but that he continued to prefer to study ranges of normalcy and not to focus on the "tricks of the unconscious" [13].

At the age of 18, Piaget received his baccalaureate from the University of Neuchatel. In 1918, three years later, he received his doctorate in the natural sciences from the same institution. During this time Piaget studied mollusks and their adjustment over time to a changing environment. It was from this long-term study that he became interested in the concept of interaction with the environment (which later became a cornerstone of his theory of mental development).

As soon as Piaget had completed his doctorate, he became intrigued with psychology. This interest took him to Paris to work with Alfred Binet in a grade school, where his task was to aid in standardizing tests. Piaget soon became occupied in analyzing the *incorrect* answers that the children gave as responses to questions. From that time on, he used clinical observation and structured questioning of children to provide data for analyzing and understanding how intelligence developed.

By 30 years of age, Piaget was famous for his work in psychology. Although he is often considered a child psychologist, he wished to be known as a person who was primarily concerned with describing and explaining in a very systematic way the growth and development of intellectual structures and knowledge [26].

In 1955 with the aid of a Rockefeller Foundation grant, the Centre International d'Epistémologie Génétique was established in Geneva. Under this program, three scholars were chosen every year to visit and to do research with Piaget and his associates.

Having published more than 80 books and hundreds of journal articles, Piaget remained a prolific author. Each year after the results of a year's research had been completed, Piaget traveled to an isolated farmhouse in the Alps to write for the summer.

Piaget held several honorary degrees from prominent universities around the world. His works have generated more interest and research than those of any other person in psychology during the last 50 years [26].

Piaget's Major Concepts and Terms

From his early work in biology, Piaget came to believe that biological acts (as well as intellectual acts) are the "adaptation" to and "organization" of the perceived environment. To understand these processes of intellectual organization and adaptation as they are viewed by Piaget, four basic concepts are required—the concepts of "schema," "assimilation," "accommodation," and "equilibration," which are used to explain how and why mental development occurs:

1. **Schema** (plural, **schemata**). The cognitive structures by which individuals intellectually adapt to and organize the environment. These structures are inferred to exist much in the same way as Freud's id and ego. Schemata can be simplistically thought of as categories or units of information—a set.
2. **Assimilation.** The cognitive process by which the person integrates new perceptual matter or stimulus events into existing schemata or patterns of behavior.
3. **Accommodation.** The establishment of a new schema or the modification of an old schema. This results in a change in, reorganization of, or development of cognitive structures (schemata).
4. **Equilibration.** The balance between assimilation and accommodation. When disequilibration occurs, it provides motivation for the individual to assimilate or to accommodate further.

Piaget believed that mental development is a process that begins the day the infant is born (and possibly sooner). He also theorized that the path of cognitive development is the same for all people, although they progress at different rates. His stages of development are discussed throughout this book.

At each new level of cognitive development, previous levels are incorporated and integrated. Schemata are continually being modified through the life cycle. Although qualitative changes in cognitive structure cease after the development of formal operations, quantitative changes in content and function of intelligence continue.

Piaget's Techniques of Inquiry

Piaget's investigations were primarily clinical. His usual procedure was to observe a child's behavior in natural surroundings, and to formulate a hypothesis concerning the structure that underlies the child's response to, or interaction with, the material and events in the environment. He tested the hypothesis by altering the child's surroundings. This alteration was accomplished by rearranging the materials, by posing the problems in a different way, or by overtly suggesting to the subject a response different from the one predicted by the theory. Piaget made many first-hand, longitudinal observations of his own three children. Although most of his early works were rather intuitive, some of his more recent endeavors employed rigid experimental strategies (using, for example, statistical findings and adequate sample sizes). Piaget said that the important thing is to "make contact with the child's thinking" [5].

Applicability of Piaget's Theory

The current interest in Piaget's efforts evolved as psychologists began to recognize the importance of what he had to say. His research has been criticized by some, however, because of the small sample size and its less rigid, "nonexperimental" mode. (Of course, if one accepts Piaget's assumption that the general course of development of intellectual structures is the same in all individuals, the small sample size poses no problem.)

In 1972 Piaget answered some of his critics who contested that his theory covered only the years from birth to about 15 years of age. As a result, Piaget performed additional research and hypothesized that individual differences in cognitive processes among adults are influenced more by aptitudes and experiences, such as career and education, than by the general characteristics determining the individual's type of formal thinking.

Piaget's works are frequently utilized by those who find themselves in daily contact with children. Teachers, counselors, school psychologists, and, lately, many parents are using the practical implications of Piaget's theory to aid in enhancing the individual cognitive potential of the children for whom they provide care.

REFERENCES

1. Ansbacher, H. L., and Ansbacher, R. R. (Eds.). *The Individual Psychology of Alfred Adler.* New York: Harper & Row, 1967.
2. Beecher, W., and Beecher, M. Memorial to Dr. Alfred Adler. In H. H. Mosak (Ed.), *Alfred Adler: His Influence on Psychology Today.* Park Ridge, NJ: Noyes Press, 1973.
3. Carpenter, F. *The Skinner Primer: Behind Freedom and Dignity.* New York: Free Press, 1974.
4. Crain, W. C. *Theories of Development: Concepts and Applications.* Englewood Cliffs, NJ: Prentice-Hall, 1980.
5. Duckworth, E. Language and Thought. In M. Schwebel and J. Ralph (Eds.), *Piaget in the Classroom.* New York: Basic Books, 1973.
6. Erikson, E. H. *Childhood and Society* (2nd ed.). New York: Norton, 1963.
7. Flavell, J. H. *The Developmental Psychology of Jean Piaget.* New York: Van Nostrand, 1963.

8. Freud, S. *A General Introduction to Psycho-analysis.* Authorized English translation of the revised edition by J. Rivière. New York: Liveright, 1935.

9. Fromm, E. *The Art of Loving.* New York: Harper & Row, 1974.

10. Hall, E. A conversation with Erik Erikson. *Psychology Today* 17(6):22, 1983.

11. Havighurst, R. J. *Developmental Tasks and Education* (3rd ed.). New York: McKay, 1972.

12. Jones, E. *The Life and Work of Sigmund Freud.* New York: Basic Books, 1981.

13. Maier, H. W. *Three Theories of Child Development* (3rd ed.). New York: Harper & Row, 1978.

14. Maslow, A. H. A theory of human motivation. *Psychol. Rev.* 50:370, 1943.

15. Maslow, A. H. *Toward a Psychology of Being* (2nd ed.). New York: Van Nostrand Reinhold, 1982.

16. Mullahy, P. *Psychoanalysis and Interpersonal Psychiatry; The Contributions of Harry Stack Sullivan.* New York: Science House, 1970.

17. Orgler, H. *Alfred Adler: The Man and His Work* (4th ed.). London: Sidgwick & Jackson, 1973.

18. Phillips, J. L. *The Origins of Intellect: Piaget's Theory.* San Francisco: Freeman, 1975.

19. Piaget, J. Piaget's Theory. In P. H. Mussen (Ed.), *Carmichael's Manual of Child Psychology* (3rd ed.). New York: Wiley, 1970.

20. Piaget, J. *Psychology and Epistemology.* Translated by A. Rosin. New York: Viking, 1972.

21. Rogers, C. R. *Freedom to Learn for the 80s.* Columbus, OH: Merrill, 1983.

22. Schell, R. E., and Hall, E. *Developmental Psychology Today* (4th ed.). New York: Random House, 1983.

23. Schultz, D. P. *Theories of Personality* (2nd ed.). Monterey, CA: Brooks/Cole, 1981.

24. Skinner, B. F. Origins of a behaviorist. *Psychology Today* 17(9):22, 1983.

25. Sullivan, H. S. *The Fusion of Psychiatry and Social Science.* New York: Norton, 1971.

26. Wadsworth, B. J. *Piaget's Theory of Cognitive and Affective Development.* New York: Longman, 1984.

27. Wall, W. D. Jean Piaget: 1896–1979. *J. Child Psychol. Psychiatry and Allied Disciplines* 23(2):97, 1982.

C

Developmental Frameworks of Selected Stage Theorists

Clara S. Schuster

Evelyn Millis Duvall
Development of the Family System

Jean Piaget
Levels of Cognitive Development

Erik H. Erikson
Psychosocial Developmental Levels

Robert J. Havighurst
Developmental Tasks of Life Phases

Abraham H. Maslow
Levels of Motivating Needs

Evelyn Millis Duvall

Development of the Family System*

A. Stages
1. Married couple
2. Childbearing family
3. Family with preschool children
4. Family with school-age children
5. Family with teenagers
6. Family as a launching center
7. The "empty nest" family
8. The aging family
B. Tasks of each stage
1. Physical maintenance
2. Allocation of resources
3. Division of labor
4. Socialization of family members
5. Reproduction, recruitment, and release
6. Maintenance of order
7. Placement of members into the larger society
8. Maintenance of motivation and morale

Each stage must successfully accomplish all eight tasks in order to function optimally. The tasks of the family support and complement the development of its individual members.

*From E. R. M. Duvall, *Family Development* (4th ed.) (Philadelphia: Lippincott, 1971), pp. 116–117, 149.

Jean Piaget

Levels of Cognitive Development*

Period	Age	Characteristics
Sensorimotor	0–2 years	Thought dominated by physical manipulation of objects and events
Substage 1	0–1 month	Pure reflex adaptations No differentiation between assimilation and accommodation
Substage 2	1–4 months	Primary circular reactions Slight differentiation between assimilation and accommodation Repetition of schemata and self-imitation, especially vocal and visual Reflex activities become modified with experience and coordinated with each other
Substage 3	4–8 months	Secondary circular reactions Differentiation between assimilation and accommodation, still overlap Repeat action on things to prolong an interesting spectacle Beginning to demonstrate intention or goal-directed activity
Substage 4	8–12 months	Coordination of secondary schemata Clear differentiation between assimilation and accommodation Application of known schemata to new situation Schemata follow each other without apparent aim Beginning of means-ends relationships
Substage 5	12–18 months	Tertiary circular reactions Ritualistic repetition of chance schema combinations Accentuation and elaboration of ritual Experimentation to see the result, find new ways to solve problems
Substage 6	18–24 months	Invention of new solutions through mental combinations Primitive symbolic representation Beginning of pretense by application of schema to inadequate object A symbol is mentally evoked and imitated in make-believe A symbolic schema is reproduced outside of context; thus, transition between practice play and symbolic play proper
Preoperational	2–7 years	Functions symbolically using language as major tool
Preconceptual	2–4 years	Uses representational thought to recall past, represent present, anticipate future Able to distinguish between signifier and signified Egocentric, uses self as standard for others Categorizes on basis of single characteristic
Intuitive	4–7 years	Increased symbolic functioning Subjective judgments still dominate perceptions Beginning ability to think in logical classes Able to see simple relationships Able to understand number concepts More exact imitations of reality
Concrete operations	7–11 years	Mental reasoning processes assume logical approaches to solving concrete problems Organizes objects, events into hierarchies of classes (classification) or along a continuum of increasing values (seriation) Reversibility, transitivity, and conservation skills attained
Formal operations	11–15 years	True logical thought and manipulation of abstract concepts emerge Hypothetical deductive thought Can plan and implement scientific approach to problem solving Handles all kinds of combinations in a systematic way

*From J. Piaget, *The Psychology of Intelligence*, Transl. by M. Piercy and D. E. Berlyne (Totowa, NJ: Littlefield, Adams, 1973), and *Play, Dreams and Imitation in Childhood*, transl. by C. Gattengo and F. M. Hodgson (New York: Norton, 1951). Also from J. H. Flavell, *The Developmental Psychology of Jean Piaget* (New York: Van Nostrand, 1963).

Each level incorporates and integrates processes from previous levels. Schemata are continually added and modified throughout life. Quantitative changes continue to occur throughout life, but qualitative changes cease after the development of formal operational thought.

Erik H. Erikson

Psychosocial Developmental Levels*

Developmental Level	Basic Task	Negative Counterpart	Basic Virtues
1. Infant	Basic trust	Basic mistrust	Drive and hope
2. Toddler	Autonomy	Shame and doubt	Self-control and willpower
3. Preschooler	Initiative	Guilt	Direction and purpose
4. School-ager	Industry	Inferiority	Method and competence
5. Adolescent	Identity	Role confusion	Devotion and fidelity
6. Young adult	Intimacy	Isolation	Affiliation and love
7. Middlescent	Generativity	Stagnation	Production and care
8. Older adult	Ego-integrity	Despair	Renunciation and wisdom

*From E. H. Erikson, *Childhood and Society* (2nd ed.) (New York: Norton, 1963).

A specific age should not be attached to developmental levels, since each person progresses at his own rate. A child may be in several developmental levels simultaneously, may advance in spurts, or may regress to an earlier level in adverse circumstances. Both genetic and environmental factors can influence the rapidity with which one progresses through the stages. Failure to achieve positive growth will lead to the development of the negative counterpart and, according to Erikson, mental illness.

Robert J. Havighurst

Developmental Tasks of Life Phases*

1. Infancy and early childhood
   a. Learn to walk
   b. Learn to take solid food
   c. Learn to talk
   d. Control elimination of body wastes
   e. Learn sex differences and sexual modesty
   f. Form concepts and learning language to describe social and physical reality
   g. Get ready to read
   h. Learn to distinguish right and wrong and begin to develop a conscience
2. Middle childhood
   a. Learn physical skills necessary for ordinary games
   b. Build wholesome attitudes toward oneself as a growing organism
   c. Learn to get along with age-mates
   d. Learn an appropriate masculine or feminine social role
   e. Develop fundamental skills in reading, writing, and calculating
   f. Develop concepts necessary for everyday living
   g. Develop conscience, morality, and a scale of values
   h. Achieve personal independence

   i. Develop attitudes toward social groups and institutions
3. Adolescence
   a. Achieve new and more mature relations with age-mates of both sexes
   b. Achieve a masculine or feminine social role
   c. Accept one's physique and use body effectively
   d. Achieve emotional independence of parents and other adults
   e. Prepare for marriage and family life
   f. Prepare for economic career
   g. Develop an ideology—a set of values and an ethical system as a guide to behavior
   h. Achieve socially responsible behavior
4. Early adulthood
   a. Select a mate
   b. Learn to live with a marriage partner
   c. Start a family
   d. Rear children
   e. Manage a home
   f. Start an occupation
   g. Assume civic responsibility
   h. Find a congenial social group
5. Middle age
   a. Assist children to become responsible and happy adults

*From R. J. Havighurst, *Developmental Tasks and Education* (3rd ed.) (New York: McKay, 1972).

(continued)

Robert J. Havighurst (cont.)

    b. Achieve adult social and civic responsibility
    c. Attain and maintain satisfactory performance in occupation
    d. Develop adult leisure-time activities
    e. Relate to spouse as a person
    f. Accept and adjust to physiological changes
    g. Adjust to aging parents
6. Later maturity
    a. Adjust to decreasing physical strength and health
    b. Adjust to retirement and reduced income
    c. Adjust to death of spouse
    d. Establish affiliation with one's age group

    e. Adopt and adapt to social roles in a flexible way
    f. Establish satisfactory physical living arrangements

Havighurst feels that development is a cognitive learning process. Tasks develop out of a combination of pressures arising from physical development, cultural expectations, and individual values and goals. He postulates the ocurrence of "teachable moments" when a special sensitivity or readiness to learn a task arises from the unique combination of physical, social, and psychic readiness.

Abraham H. Maslow

Levels of Motivating Needs*

A. Primary motives (basic needs): survival needs, vital for continuing existence
    1. Oxygen
    2. Water
    3. Nutrition
    4. Elimination
    5. Physiological homeostasis
    6. Rest and sleep
    7. Avoidance of pain
    8. Sex (basic motive, but not considered essential to survival)
B. Secondary motives: social needs, learned or acquired
    1. Security
    2. Social approval
    3. Affiliation
    4. Status
    5. Knowledge acquisition
    6. Achievement
C. Hierarchy of motives
    1. Physiological (inborn)
    2. Safety and security
    3. Belongingness and affection
    4. Esteem and self-respect

    5. Self-actualization
      a. Self-fulfillment
      b. Desire to know and understand
      c. Aesthetic need

As lower-level needs are met and found to be satisfying, the individual moves on to the next level. Levels are not fixed. Lower-level needs are always present, but as need tension is reduced, the person is free to concentrate on higher-level needs. Adverse environmental circumstances can require increased attention to lower-level needs. Those who remain at a given level after the needs have been satisfied become bored, fatigued, and resentful. Satisfaction of higher-level needs produces more genuine happiness, serenity, and richness of inner life; therefore, the needs of that level are more highly valued by persons who have experienced gratification at that level. Pursuit of higher-level needs indicates a trend toward psychological health. However, Maslow believes that only about 1 percent of the adult population is actually in the process of true self-actualization, even though the people in this group may be involved in many creative endeavors.

*From A. H. Maslow, *Motivation and Personality* (2nd ed.) (New York: Harper & Row, 1970), and *Toward a Psychology of Being* (2nd ed.) (Princeton, NJ: Van Nostrand, 1968).

D

Physical Growth:
NCHS Percentile Charts

BOYS: BIRTH TO 36 MONTHS
PHYSICAL GROWTH
NCHS PERCENTILES*

NAME _____ RECORD # _____

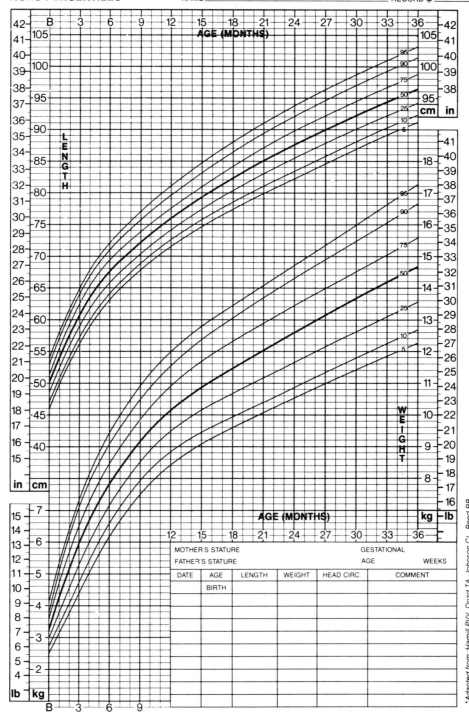

*Adapted from: Hamill PVV, Drizd TA, Johnson CL, Reed RB, Roche AF, Moore WM: Physical growth: National Center for Health Statistics percentiles. AM J CLIN NUTR 32:607-629, 1979. Data from the Fels Research Institute, Wright State University School of Medicine, Yellow Springs, Ohio.

© 1982 ROSS LABORATORIES

BOYS: BIRTH TO 36 MONTHS
PHYSICAL GROWTH
NCHS PERCENTILES*

NAME_____ RECORD #_____

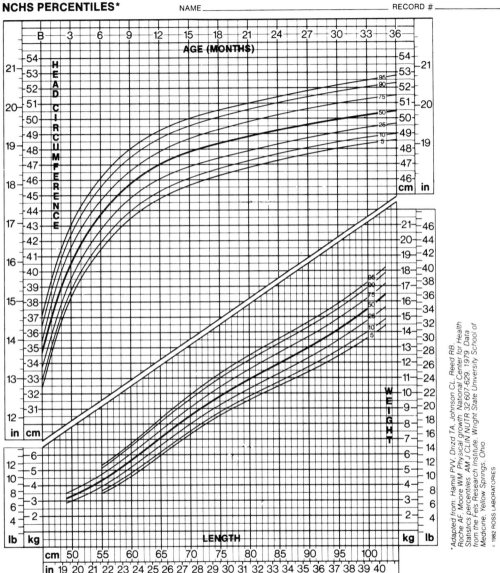

*Adapted from: Hamill PVV, Drizd TA, Johnson CL, Reed RB, Roche AF, Moore WM. Physical growth: National Center for Health Statistics percentiles. AM J CLIN NUTR 32:607-629, 1979. Data from the Fels Research Institute, Wright State University School of Medicine, Yellow Springs, Ohio

© 1982 ROSS LABORATORIES

BOYS: 2 TO 18 YEARS
PHYSICAL GROWTH
NCHS PERCENTILES*

NAME _____ RECORD # _____

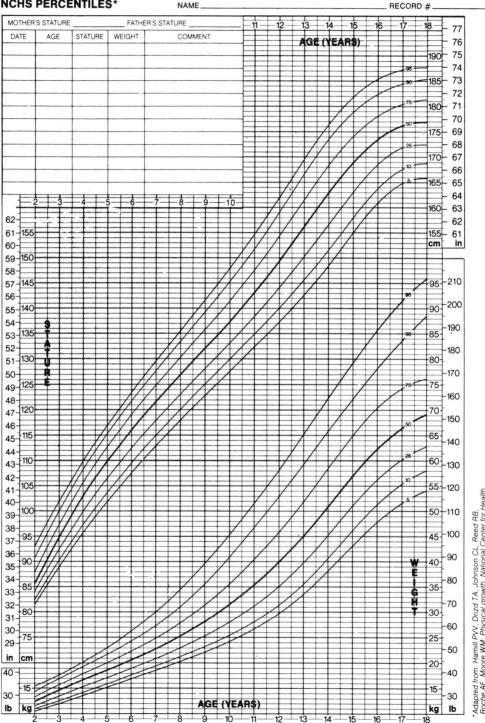

*Adapted from: Hamill PVV, Drizd TA, Johnson CL, Reed RB,
Roche AF, Moore WM. Physical growth: National Center for Health
Statistics percentiles. AM J CLIN NUTR 32:607-629, 1979. Data
from the National Center for Health Statistics (NCHS) Hyattsville,
Maryland.

© 1982 ROSS LABORATORIES

BOYS: PREPUBESCENT
PHYSICAL GROWTH
NCHS PERCENTILES*

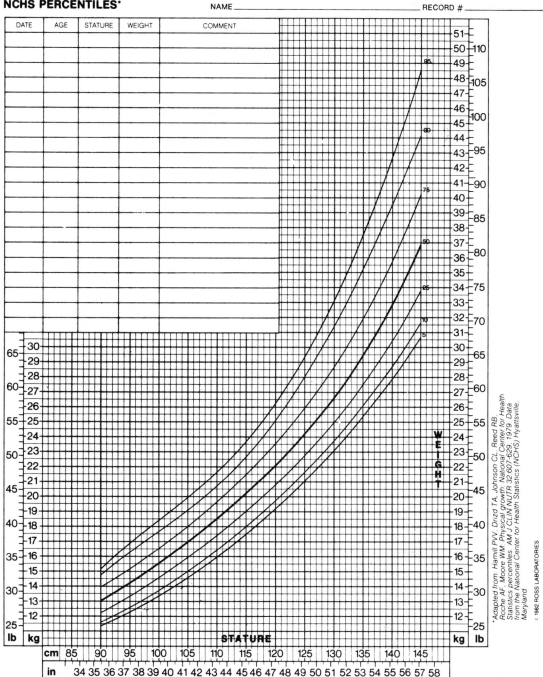

GIRLS: BIRTH TO 36 MONTHS
PHYSICAL GROWTH
NCHS PERCENTILES*

NAME _____ RECORD # _____

*Adapted from: Hamill PVV, Drizd TA, Johnson CL, Reed RB, Roche AF, Moore WM. Physical growth: National Center for Health Statistics percentiles. AM J CLIN NUTR 32:607-629, 1979. Data from the Fels Research Institute, Wright State University School of Medicine, Yellow Springs, Ohio.

© 1982 ROSS LABORATORIES

GIRLS: BIRTH TO 36 MONTHS
PHYSICAL GROWTH
NCHS PERCENTILES*

NAME _____ RECORD # _____

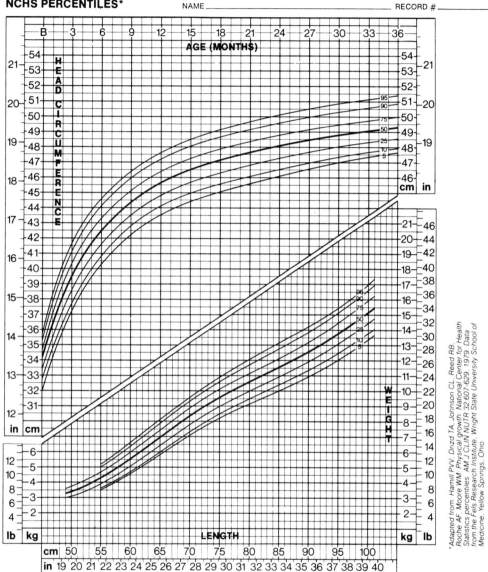

*Adapted from: Hamill PVV, Drizd TA, Johnson CL, Reed RB,
Roche AF, Moore WM. Physical growth. National Center for Health
Statistics percentiles. AM J CLIN NUTR 32:607-629, 1979. Data
from the Fels Research Institute, Wright State University School of
Medicine, Yellow Springs, Ohio
© 1982 ROSS LABORATORIES

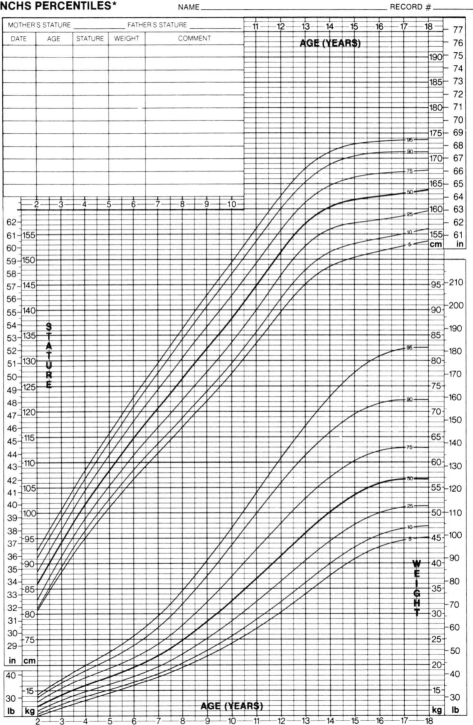

GIRLS: 2 TO 18 YEARS
PHYSICAL GROWTH
NCHS PERCENTILES*

NAME_____ RECORD #_____

*Adapted from: Hamill PVV, Drizd TA, Johnson CL, Reed RB, Roche AF, Moore WM: Physical growth: National Center for Health Statistics percentiles. AM J CLIN NUTR 32:607-629, 1979. Data from the National Center for Health Statistics (NCHS) Hyattsville, Maryland

© 1982 ROSS LABORATORIES

GIRLS: PREPUBESCENT
PHYSICAL GROWTH
NCHS PERCENTILES*

NAME _____   RECORD # _____

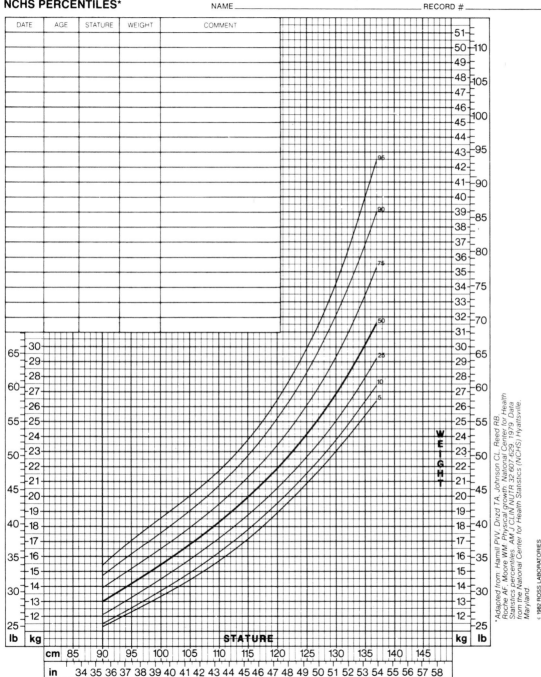

*Adapted from Hamill PVV, Drizd TA, Johnson CL, Reed RB, Roche AF, Moore WM. Physical growth: National Center for Health Statistics percentiles. AM J CLIN NUTR 32:607-629, 1979. Data from the National Center for Health Statistics (NCHS) Hyattsville, Maryland.

E

Normal Physiological Parameters Through the Life-Span

Table 1

Age	Vital Signs			Height		Weight		Blood Values		
	Pulse	Resp.	B/P	Cm	Inches	Kg	Pounds	Hgb (gm)	Hct	WBC/cu mm
Birth	140 ± 20	55 ± 25	80 ± 16 / 46 16	50 ± 2	20 ± 1	3.4 ± .6	7.5 ± 1	20 (14–24)	53 (44–64)	19,000 (9–30)
14 days	135 ± 15	40 ± 15						17 (15–20)	46 (42–60)	12,000 (5–21)
1 month	130 ± 20	35 ± 10	80 ± 20 / 50 10	53 ± 2.5	21 ± 1	4.4 ± .8	10 ± 1.5	15 (11–17)	43 (35–49)	10,800 (5–19.5)
3 months				60 ± 2	23.5 ± 1	5.7 ± .8	12.5 ± 2	11 (10–13)	37 (31–41)	11,000 (5.5–18)
6 months	120 ± 20	31 ± 9	90 ± 28 / 60 10	65.5 ± 3	26 ± 1	7.4 ± 1	16.5 ± 2.5	11.5 (10.5–14.5)	37 (30–40)	11,900 (6–17.5)
12 months	115 ± 20	30 ± 10	96 ± 30 / 66 24	74.5 ± 3	29 ± 1.5	10 ± 1.5	22 ± 3	12.5 (11–15)	37 (33–42)	11,400 (6–17.5)
2 years	110 ± 20	25 ± 5	98 ± 26 / 64 24	87 ± 4	34 ± 2	12.4 ± 2	27.5 ± 4	13 (12–15)	38 (33–42)	10,500 (6–17)
3 years	105 ± 15		100 ± 24 / 66 22	96 ± 5.5	38 ± 2	14.5 ± 2	32 ± 5			
4 years	100 ± 10	24 ± 4	100 ± 20 / 66 20	103 ± 6	40.5 ± 2.5	16.5 ± 3	36.5 ± 5	13.5 (12.5–15)		9,000 (5.5–15.5)
5 years	95 ± 15	22 ± 3	100 ± 14 / 60 10	109 ± 6	43 ± 2.5	18.4 ± 3	40.5 ± 6		40 (31–43)	
6 years	90 ± 15	21 ± 3	100 ± 16 / 60 10	117 ± 7	46 ± 2.5	21.5 ± 4	47.5 ± 8			8,500 (5–14.5)
8 years	85 ± 10	20 ± 3	102 ± 16 / 60 10	129 ± 7.5	50.5 ± 3	27 ± 5	59 ± 11	14 (13–15.5)		
10 years	80 ± 10	19 ± 3	106 ± 16 / 60 10	139.5 ± 8	55 ± 3	32.5 ± 7	71 ± 14		42 (33–44)	8,000 (4.5–13.5)

From C. S. Schuster, Normal physiological parameters through the life cycle, *The Nurse Practitioner: A Journal of Primary Nursing Care*, 2:25–28, Jan.–Feb. 1977.

Table 2

Age	Vital Signs			Height		Weight		Blood Values			Calories/24 hr		Protein
	Pulse	Resp.	B/P	Cm	Inches	Kg	Pounds	Hgb (gm)	Hct	WBC/cu mm	/Pound	Total	Gm/24 hr
Males													
12 years	69 ± 9	19 ± 2	$\frac{110 \pm 12}{64 \pm 16}$	150 ± 8	59 ± 3	39 ± 9	85 ± 12	13 (11–16)	38 (34–40)	8,000 (4.5–13.5)	30	2,400	48
14 years	65 ± 8	19 ± 3	$\frac{114 \pm 14}{68 \pm 14}$	163 ± 9	64 ± 4	49 ± 11	108 ± 20	14 (13–16)	41 (37–43)		31	2,800	54
16 years	63 ± 8	17 ± 3	$\frac{116 \pm 12}{70 \pm 14}$	172 ± 8	68 ± 4	59 ± 9	130 ± 20	15.5 (13–17)	45 (40–48)	7,800 (4.5–13)	31	3,000	58
18 years	61 ± 8	16 ± 3	$\frac{120 \pm 16}{72 \pm 14}$	174 ± 8	68.5 ± 4	63 ± 10	140 ± 20				25	3,200	62
18–22 years								16 (14–18)	47 (42–52)			3,000	60
23–50 years	70 ± 10	18 ± 2	$\frac{126 \pm 26}{74 \pm 16}$	175 ± 8	69 ± 4	68 ± 12	150 ± 25			7,500 (4.5–11.5)	18–25	2,700	
51+ years												2,400	56
Females													
12 years	71 ± 9		$\frac{110 \pm 10}{64 \pm 12}$	152 ± 8	60 ± 3	40 ± 10	88 ± 20	13 (11–16)	38 (34–40)	8,000 (4.5–13.5)	30	2,300	50
14 years	68 ± 8	19 ± 3	$\frac{112 \pm 10}{66 \pm 12}$	160 ± 7	63 ± 3	50 ± 10	110 ± 18	13 (12–16)	39 (35–42)	7,800 (4.5–13.0)	24	2,400	51
16 years	66 ± 8	18 ± 3	$\frac{114 \pm 14}{70 \pm 12}$	162 ± 7	63.5 ± 3	53 ± 11	117 ± 17				21		53
18 years	65 ± 8		$\frac{120 \pm 16}{70 \pm 12}$			54 ± 11	120 ± 20	13.5 (12–16)	40 (36–44)		19	2,300	55
18–22 years													50
23–50 years												2,000	
		17 ± 3	$\frac{126 \pm 26}{74 \pm 16}$	163 ± 7	64 ± 3		130 ± 25	14 (12–16)	42 (37–47)	7,500 (4.5–11.5)			46
51+ years	70 ± 10					60 ± 12					15–20	1,800	
Pregnant							+15–30	12 (11–15)	36 (34–40)			+300	+30
Lactating							+2–5					+800	+20

Table 3

Age	Calories /lb	Calories /kg	Calories total	Protein gm	Protein oz/lb	Water cc/kg	Water total	Output urine/24 hr	Sleep /24 hr	Head Circum. (cm)
Birth							45–90	15–60	22	
3 days	55	117	kg × 120		2¼	80–100	250–300	40–400	16–22	34 ± 2.5
14 days				kg × 2.2		125–150	400–500			
1 month	50	110	kg × 110			140–160	750–850	250–450	15–18	36.5 ± 2.5
3 months										40 ± 2.5
6 months		108		kg × 2.0		130–145	950–1,100	400–550	15–16	43 ± 3
12 months			1,100			120–135	1,100–1,300		13–15	46 ± 3
2 years	45	100	1,200	23	2	115–125	1,300–1,500	500–600	12–14	49 ± 3
3 years			1,300							50 ± 3
4 years	41	90	1,400	30	1½	100–110	1,600–1,800	600–750		50.5 ± 3
5 years			1,600			90–100	1,800–2,000		11–12	51 ± 2.5
6 years			1,800					650–1,000		51.5 ± 2.5
8 years	36	80	2,000	36		70–85	2,000–2,500			52.5 ± 2.5
10 years			2,200		1				9–11	53 ± 3
10–12 years						60–75				53.5 ± 3
12–14 years						50–60	2,200–2,700	700–1,500		54 ± 3
14–16 years						40–50			8–9	54.5 ± 3
16–18 years										55 ± 3
18–22 years			see Table 2		¾				7–9	
23–50 years						50	2,000–3,000			
51+ years								1,000–2,000	5–7	55.5 ± 3
Pregnant women										
Lactating women							3,000–4,500		9–10	

F
Desirable Weights for Adults

1983 Metropolitan Height and Weight Tables

Men					Women				
Height		Small	Medium	Large	Height		Small	Medium	Large
Feet	Inches	Frame	Frame	Frame	Feet	Inches	Frame	Frame	Frame
5	2	128–134	131–141	138–150	4	10	102–111	109–121	118–131
5	3	130–136	133–143	140–153	4	11	103–113	111–123	120–134
5	4	132–138	135–145	142–156	5	0	104–115	113–126	122–137
5	5	134–140	137–148	144–160	5	1	106–118	115–129	125–140
5	6	136–142	139–151	146–164	5	2	108–121	118–132	128–143
5	7	138–145	142–154	149–168	5	3	111–124	121–135	131–147
5	8	140–148	145–157	152–172	5	4	114–127	124–138	134–151
5	9	142–151	148–160	155–176	5	5	117–130	127–141	137–155
5	10	144–154	151–163	158–180	5	6	120–133	130–144	140–159
5	11	146–157	154–166	161–184	5	7	123–136	133–147	143–163
6	0	149–160	157–170	164–188	5	8	126–139	136–150	146–167
6	1	152–164	160–174	168–192	5	9	129–142	139–153	149–170
6	2	155–168	164–178	172–197	5	10	132–145	142–156	152–173
6	3	158–172	167–182	176–202	5	11	135–148	145–159	155–176
6	4	162–176	171–187	181–207	6	0	138–151	148–162	158–179

Note: Weights at ages 25–59 based on lowest mortality. Weight in pounds according to frame (in indoor clothing weighing 5 lb. for men and 3 lb. for women; shoes with 1 in. heels). Source of basic data: 1979 Build Study, Society of Actuaries and Association of Life Insurance Medical Directors of America, 1980. Copyright 1983 Metropolitan Life Insurance Company. Reprinted with permission.

G
Living Will

To Make the Best Use of Your Living Will*

1. Sign and date the Living Will before two witnesses. (This is to ensure that you signed of your own free will and not under any pressure.)
2. If you have a physician, give him a copy for your medical file and discuss it with him to make sure he is in agreement. Give copies to those most likely to be concerned "if the time comes when you can no longer take part in decisions for your own future." Enter their names on the bottom line of the Living Will. Keep the original nearby, easily and readily available.
3. Above all, discuss you intentions with those closest to you, **now.**
4. It is a good idea to look over your Living Will once a year and then to redate it and initial the new date to make it clear that your wishes are unchanged.

(continued)

*Reprinted with the permission of the Euthanasia Educational Council, 250 West Fifty-Seventh Street, New York, New York 10019. Copies available on request.

TO MY FAMILY, MY PHYSICIAN, MY LAWYER, MY CLERGYMAN
TO ANY MEDICAL FACILITY IN WHOSE CARE I HAPPEN TO BE
TO ANY INDIVIDUAL WHO MAY BECOME RESPONSIBLE FOR MY HEALTH, WELFARE OR
AFFAIRS

Death is as much a reality as birth, growth, maturity and old age—it is the one certainty of life. If the time comes when I, _____, can no longer take part in decisions for my own future, let this statement stand as an expression of my wishes, while I am still of sound mind.

If the situation should arise in which there is no reasonable expectation of my recovery from physical or mental disability, I request that I be allowed to die and not be kept alive by artificial means or "heroic measures." I do not fear death itself as much as the indignities of deterioration, dependence and hopeless pain. I, therefore, ask that medication be mercifully administered to me to alleviate suffering even though this may hasten the moment of death.

This request is made after careful consideration. I hope you who care for me will feel morally bound to follow its mandate. I recognize that this appears to place a heavy responsibility upon you, but it is with the intention of relieving you of such responsibility and of placing it upon myself in accordance with my strong convictions, that this statement is made.

Signed _____

Date _____

Witness _____

Witness _____

Copies of this request have been given to _____

_____

_____

_____

Index

Names of contributing authors and page number references to figures are italicized in this index.